ATLAS OF

Gastroenterology

Third Edition

ATLAS OF

Gastroenterology
Third Edition

EDITOR

TADATAKA YAMADA, M.D.

Adjunct Professor
Department of Internal Medicine
Division of Gastroenterology
University of Michigan Health System
Ann Arbor, Michigan

ASSOCIATE EDITORS

DAVID H. ALPERS, M.D.

William B. Kountz Professor of Medicine
Department of Internal Medicine
Division of Gastroenterology
Washington University School of Medicine
St. Louis, Missouri

NEIL KAPLOWITZ, M.D.

Brem Professor and Chief
Division of Gastrointestinal and Liver Diseases
Director, USC Liver Disease Research Center
Keck School of Medicine of the University
   of Southern California
Los Angeles, California

LOREN LAINE, M.D.

Professor
Department of Medicine
Keck School of Medicine of the University
   of Southern California
Chief, Gastroenterology Section
Los Angeles County and University of Southern
   California Medical Center
Los Angeles, California

CHUNG OWYANG, M.D.

Professor of Internal Medicine
H. Marvin Pollard Collegiate Professor and Chief
Division of Gastroenterology
University of Michigan Health System
Ann Arbor, Michigan

DON W. POWELL, M.D.

Associate Dean for Research
School of Medicine
Professor, Internal Medicine
Professor, Physiology and Biophysics
The University of Texas Medical Branch
Galveston, Texas

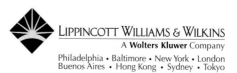

LIPPINCOTT WILLIAMS & WILKINS
A **Wolters Kluwer** Company
Philadelphia • Baltimore • New York • London
Buenos Aires • Hong Kong • Sydney • Tokyo

Acquisitions Editor: Beth Barry
Developmental Editor: Anne Snyder
Production Editor: Elaine Verriest McClusky
Manufacturing Manager: Colin Warnock
Cover Designer: QT Design
Compositor: Techbooks

© 2003 by LIPPINCOTT WILLIAMS & WILKINS
530 Walnut Street
Philadelphia, PA 19106 USA
LWW.com

Printed in the USA

Library of Congress Cataloging-in-Publication Data

Atlas of gastroenterology / editor, Tadataka Yamada; associate
editors, David H. Alpers . . . [et al.]. — 3rd ed.
    p.   cm.
    Includes index.
    ISBN 0-7817-3081-3
      1. Gastroenterology—Atlases. 2. Gastrointestinal system—
Diseases—Atlases. I. Yamada, Tadataka. II. Alpers, David H.
   RC801.T48 2003 Suppl.
   616.3'3—dc21   2002034137

CONTENTS

Paul C. Adams, M.D., F.R.C.P.(C.)
Professor, Department of Medicine, University of Western Ontario; and Chief, Department of Gastroenterology, London Health Sciences Centre, London, Ontario, Canada

David A. Ahlquist, M.D.
Professor of Medicine, Department of Internal Medicine/Gastroenterology and Hepatology, Mayo Clinic, Rochester, Minnesota

Aijaz Ahmed, M.D.
Assistant Professor of Medicine, Division of Gastroenterology and Hepatology, Department of Medicine, Stanford University School of Medicine, Palo Alto, California

David H. Alpers, M.D.
William B. Kountz Professor of Medicine, Department of Internal Medicine, Division of Gastroenterology, Washington University School of Medicine, St. Louis, Missouri

Dana K. Andersen, M.D.
Professor and Chairman, Department of Surgery, University of Massachusetts Medical School, UMASS Memorial Medical Center, Worchester, Massachusetts

Jeffrey L. Barnett, M.D.
Adjunct Professor, Department of Internal Medicine, Division of Gastroenterology, University of Michigan Health System, Ann Arbor; and Huron Gastroenterology Associates, Ypsilanti, Michigan

Nathan M. Bass, M.D., Ph.D.
Professor of Medicine, Division of Gastroenterology, University of California, San Francisco; and Medical Director, Liver Transplant Program, UCSF Medical Center, San Francisco, California

Michelle L. Bennett, M.D.
Assistant Professor, Department of Dermatology, Wake Forest University School of Medicine, Winston-Salem, North Carolina

Stephen J. Bickston, M.D.
Associate Professor, Department of Internal Medicine, University of Virginia; and Medical Director, Inpatient Digestive Health Center of Exellence, University of Virginia Health System, Charlottesville, Virginia

Elisa H. Birnbaum, M.D.
Associate Professor, Department of Surgery, Section of Colon and Rectal Sugery, Washington University School of Medicine at Barnes-Jewish Hospital, St. Louis, Missouri

David J. Bjorkman, M.D., M.S.P.H., S.M. (Epid.)
Senior Associate Dean, School of Medicine; and Professor, Division of Gastroenterology, University of Utah Health Sciences Center, Salt Lake City, Utah

Andres T. Blei, M.D.
Professor of Medicine, Department of Medicine, Division of Hepatology, Northwestern University, Feinberg School of Medicine, Chicago, Illinois

C. Richard Boland, M.D.
Professor, Department of Medicine, University of California San Diego School of Medicine; and Chief of Gastroenterology, Department of Medicine, University of California at San Diego, San Diego, California

Gregory A. Boyce, M.D.
Gastroenterology Clinic, St. Francis Medical Center, Monroe, Louisiana

H. Worth Boyce Jr., M.D.
Professor of Medicine, Department of Internal Medicine; and Director, Center for Swallowing Disorders, University of South Florida College of Medicine, Tampa, Florida

Robert S. Bresalier, M.D.
Professor of Medicine and Chairman, Department of Gastrointestinal Medicine and Nutrition, The University of Texas M. D. Anderson Cancer Center, Houston, Texas

Randall W. Burt, M.D.
Professor of Medicine, Department of Internal Medicine, University of Utah School of Medicine; and Senior Director for Prevention and Outreach, Huntsman Cancer Institute at the University of Utah, Salt Lake City, Utah

Michael Camilleri, M.D.
Professor of Medicine and Physiology, Mayo Medical School; and Consultant in Gastroenterology, Mayo Clinic, Rochester, Minnesota

Mitchell S. Cappell, M.D., Ph.D.
Associate Professor, Department of Medicine, State University of New York Downstate Medical Center; and Vice Chairman, Department of Medicine, and Chief, Division of Gastroenterology, Woodhull Medical and Mental Health Center, Brooklyn, New York

Kyung J. Cho, M.D., F.A.C.R.
Professor, Department of Radiology, University of Michigan Health System, Ann Arbor, Michigan

Poonputt Chotiprasidhi, M.D.
Clinical Assitant Professor II, Department of Internal Medicine, Division of Gastroenterology, University of Michigan Health System, Ann Arbor, Michigan

Paul J. Ciclitira, M.D., Ph.D., F.R.C.P.
The Rayne Institute, St. Thomas Hospital, Gastroenterology Unit, London, United Kingdom

Steven M. Cohn, M.D., Ph.D.
Paul Janssen Associate Professor, Digestive Health Center of Excellence, University of Virginia Health System; and Attending Physician, Digestive Health Center of Excellence, University of Virginia Hospital, Charlottesville, Virginia

David H.B. Cort, M.D.
Consultant, Department of Gastroenterology, St. Luke's Hospital; and Private Practice, St. Louis, Missouri

David Crabb, M.D.
John B. Hickam Professor and Chairman, Department of Medicine, Indiana University, Indianapolis, Indiana

Khaldoun A. Debian, M.D.
Division of Gastrointestinal and Liver Diseases, Keck School of Medicine of the University of Southern California, Los Angeles, California

Laurie D. DeLeve, M.D., Ph.D.
Division of Gastrointestinal and Liver Diseases, Keck School of Medicine of the University of Southern California, Los Angeles, California

Silvia Delgado-Aros, M.D., M.Sc.
Research Associate, Clinical Enteric Neuroscience Translational and Epidemiological Research (C.E.N.T.E.R.) Program, Mayo Clinic, Rochester, Minnesota

John Del Valle, M.D.
Professor and Senior Associate Chair of Internal Medicine, University of Michigan Health System, Ann Arbor, Michigan

John A. Donovan, M.D.
Assistant Professor of Clinical Medicine, Division of Gastrointestinal and Liver Diseases, Keck School of Medicine of the University of Southern California, Los Angeles, California

John P. Duffy, M.D.
Resident, Division of General Surgery, David Geffen School of Medicine at the University of California at Los Angeles, Los Angeles, California

Frederic E. Eckhauser, M.D.
Professor, Department of Surgery, Johns Hopkins Hospital; and Chairman of Surgical Sciences, Johns Hopkins Bayview Medical Center, Baltimore, Maryland

Grace H. Elta, M.D.
Professor, Department of Internal Medicine, Division of Gastroenterology, University of Michigan Health System, Ann Arbor, Michigan

B. Mark Evers, M.D.
Professor and Robertson-Poth Distinguished Chair in General Surgery, Department of Surgery, The University of Texas Medical Branch, Galveston, Texas

Douglas O. Faigel, M.D.
Associate Professor of Medicine, Department of Medicine, Division of Gastroenterology, Oregon Health and Science University, Portland Veteran Affairs Medical Center, Portland, Oregon

George T. Fantry, M.D.
Associate Professor, Department of Medicine, University of Maryland School of Medicine; and Director, Clinical Gastroenterology, Department of Medicine, University of Maryland Medical Center, Baltimore, Maryland

Lori E. Fantry, M.D., M.P.H.
Assistant Professor and Medical Director, Infectious Diseases Clinic, Department of Medicine, University of Maryland, Baltimore, Maryland

Richard N. Fedorak, M.D., F.R.C.P.C.
Professor, Department of Medicine, University of Alberta; and Director, Division of Gastroenterology, University of Alberta Hospital, Edmonton, Alberta, Canada

Robert S. Fisher, M.D.
Professor, Department of Medicine, Temple University School of Medicine; and Chief, Gastroenterology Section, Temple University Hospital, Philadelphia, Pennsylvania

Richard Garcia-Kennedy, M.D.
Department of Pathology, California Pacific Medical Center, San Francisco, California

Robert M. Genta, M.D.
Adjunct Professor of Pathology, Medicine, and Molecular Virology and Microbiology, Baylor College of Medicine, Houston, Texas; and Professor and Chairman, Division of Clinical Pathology, Hôpital Cantonal Universitaire, University of Geneva, Switzerland

Robert G. Gish, M.D.
Associate Clinical Professor, Department of Medicine, University of California San Francisco; and Medical Director Liver Transplant Program, California Pacific Medical Center, San Francisco, California

Fred S. Gorelick, M.D.
Professor, Department of Medicine and Cell Biology, Yale University School of Medicine, New Haven; and Staff Physician, Department of Medicine and Research, Veterans Affairs Healthcare Connecticut, West Haven, Connecticut

Gregory J. Gores, M.D.
Professor, Department of Medicine, Mayo Clinic, Rochester, Minnesota

Sugantha Govindarajan, M.D.
Professor, Department of Pathology, Keck School of Medicine of the University of Southern California, Los Angeles, California

David Y. Graham, M.D.
Professor, Department of Medicine; and Chief, Department of Gastroenterology, Veterans Affairs Medical Center, Houston, Texas

Leah M. Gramlich, M.D.
Associate Clinical Professor, Department of Medicine, University of Alberta; and Chief, Division of Gastroenterology, Department of Medicine, Royal Alexandra Hospital, Edmonton, Alberta, Canada

Richard J. Grand, M.D.
Professor, Department of Pediatrics, Harvard Medical School; and Director, Center for Inflammatory Bowel Disease, Children's Hospital, Boston, Massachusetts

Harry B. Greenberg, M.D.
Senior Associate Dean for Research and Professor of Medicine and Microbiology and Immunology, Department of Medicine, Stanford University, Stanford; and Staff Physician, Department of Medicine/Gastroenterology & Hepatology, Stanford Medical Center and Veterans Affairs Palo Alto Health Care System, Palo Alto, California

Rodger C. Haggitt, M.D. (deceased)
Professor, Department of Pathology, University of Washington; and Director of Hospital Pathology, Department of Pathology, University of Washington Medical Center, Seattle, Washington

Peter C. Hayes, M.D., Ph.D.
Professor of Hepatology, Department of Internal Medicine, University of Edinburgh; and Honorary Consultant Physician, Liver Unit, Royal Infirmary, Edinburgh, United Kingdom

E. Jenny Heathcote, M.B, B.S., M.D., F.R.C.P., F.R.C.P. (C.)
Professor, Department of Medicine, University of Toronto; and Staff Gastroenterologist, Department of Medicine, University Health Network, Toronto Western Hospital, Toronto, Ontario, Canada

Gail Hecht, M.D.
Professor, Department of Medicine, University of Illinois at Chicago; and Chief, Section of Digestive Diseases and Nutrition, University of Illinois Medical Center, Chicago, Illinois

Hans Herlinger, M.D., D.M.R.D., M.R.C.R., M.R.C.P.
Professor Emeritus, Department of Radiology, University of Pennsylvania; and Radiologist, University of Pennsylvania Hospital, Philadelphia, Pennsylvania

Ikuo Hirano, M.D.
Assistant Professor, Department of Medicine, Northwestern University, Feinberg School of Medicine; and Attending Physician, Department of Gastroenterology, Northwestern Memorial Hospital, Chicago, Illinois

Richard A. Hodin, M.D.
Associate Professor, Department of Surgery, Harvard Medical School; and Department of Surgery, Massachusetts General Hospital, Boston, Massachusetts

Mark Holodniy, M.D.
Associate Professor, Department of Medicine, Stanford University, Stanford; and Director, AIDS Research Center, Veterans Affairs Palo Alto Health Care System, Palo Alto, California

Arnold F. Jacobson, M.D., Ph.D.
Associate Director, Clinical Research, Amersham Health, Princeton, New Jersey

Russell F. Jacoby, M.D.
Associate Professor, Department of Medicine, University of Wisconsin; and Director, Colon Cancer Prevention Program, University of Wisconsin Comprehensive Cancer Center, Madison, Wisconsin

Oliver F.W. James, F.R.C.P., F.Med.Sci.
Professor and Head of School, School of Clinical Medical Sciences, University of Newcastle upon Tyne; and Physician, The Liver Unit, Freeman Hospital, Newcastle upon Tyne, United Kingdom

Stephen P. James, M.D.
Deputy Director, Division of Digestive Diseases and Nutrition, NIDDK/National Institutes of Health, Bethesda, Maryland

R. Brooke Jeffrey Jr., M.D.
Professor, Department of Radiology, Associate Dean for Academic Affairs, Stanford University School of Medicine, Stanford, California

Robert T. Jensen, M.D.
Chief, Digestive Diseases Branch, NIDDK/National Institutes of Health, Bethesda, Maryland

Joseph L. Jorizzo, M.D.
Professor and Former (Founding) Chair, Department of
Dermatology, Wake Forest University School of Medicine,
Winston-Salem, North Carolina

Peter J. Kahrilas, M.D.
Gilbert H. Marquardt Professor of Medicine and Chief,
Division of Gastroenterology, Northwestern University, Feinberg School of Medicine and Northwestern Memorial Hospital, Chicago, Illinois

Robert A. Kane, M.D.
Professor, Department of Radiology, Harvard Medical School;
and Director, Ultrasound Section, Radiology Department,
Beth Israel Deaconess Medical Center, Boston, Massachusetts

Gary C. Kanel, M.D.
Professor of Clinical Pathology, Department of Pathology,
Keck School of Medicine of the University of Southern
California, Los Angeles; and Associate Pathologist,
Department of Pathology and Laboratories, Rancho Los
Amigos National Rehabilitation Center, Downey, California

Umaprasanna S. Karnam, M.D.
Consultant, Department of Gastroenterology and Hepatology,
Central Utah Medical Clinic, American Fork, Utah

Emmet B. Keeffe, M.D.
Professor of Medicine, Division of Gastroenterology and
Hepatology, Department of Medicine, Stanford University
School of Medicine, Palo Alto; and Chief of Hepatology,
Co-Director, Liver Transplant Program, Stanford University
Medical Center, Stanford, California

Asif Khalid, M.D.
Assistant Professor, Department of Medicine, University
of Pittsburgh; and Chief of Endoscopy, Division of
Gastroenterology, V.A. Pittsburgh Health Care System,
Pittsburgh, Pennsylvania

Michael B. Kimmey, M.D.
Professor, Department of Medicine, Division of
Gastroenterology, University of Washington; and Chief of
Gastroenterology, University of Washington Medical Center,
Seattle, Washington

James A. Knol, M.D.
Associate Professor, Department of Surgery, and Attending
Surgeon, Section of General Surgery, University of Michigan
Health System, Ann Arbor, Michigan

Cynthia W. Ko, M.D., M.S.
Acting Assistant Professor, Department of Medicine,
University of Washington; and University of Washington
Medical Center, Seattle, Washington

Richard A. Kozarek, M.D.
Clinical Professor of Medicine, University of Washington;
and Chief of Gastroenterology, Virginia Mason Medical
Center, Seattle, Washington

M. Peter Lance, M.D.
Professor, Departments of Medicine and Molecular and
Cellular Biology; and Attending Physician, Section of
Gastroenterology, Arizona Health Sciences Center, Tucson,
Arizona

Jacob C. Langer, M.D.
Professor of Surgery, University of Toronto; and Chief,
Pediatric General Surgery, Hospital for Sick Children,
Toronto, Canada

James Y.W. Lau, M.D.
Consultant Surgeon, Department of Surgery, Prince of Wales
Hospital, Shatin, New Territories, Hong Kong

Igor Laufer, M.D.
Professor, Department of Radiology, University of
Pennsylvania School of Medicine, Philadelphia, Pennsylvania

Sum P. Lee, M.D., Ph.D.
Professor and Division Head, Department of Medicine,
Division of Gastroenterology, University of Washington; and
Section Chief, Gastroenterology Section Primary and
Specialty Medical Care, Veterans Affairs Puget Sound Health
Care System, Seattle, Washington

William M. Lee, M.D.
Professor, Department of Internal Medicine, University of
Texas Southwestern Medical School; and Attending
Physician, Department of Internal Medicine, Parkland
Memorial Hospital, Dallas, Texas

Glen A. Lehman, M.D.
Professor of Medicine and Radiology, Department of
Gastroenterology and Hepatology, Indiana University
Medical Center, Indianapolis, Indiana

Wai K. Leung, M.D.
Associate Professor, Department of Medicine and
Therapeutics, The Chinese University of Hong Kong; and
Honorary Senior Medical Officer, Department of Medicine
and Therapeutics, Prince of Wales Hospital, Shatin, New
Territories, Hong Kong

Marc S. Levin, M.D.
Associate Professor, Department of Medicine, Washington
University School of Medicine, St. Louis, Missouri

Joel S. Levine, M.D.
Professor, Department of Medicine, University of Colorado
Health Sciences Center, Denver, Colorado

Marc S. Levine, M.D.
Professor, Department of Radiology, University of Pennsylvania
School of Medicine; and Chief, Gastrointestinal Radiology
Section, Hospital of the University of Pennsylvania,
Philadelphia, Pennsylvania

Ellen Li, M.D., Ph.D.
Professor, Department of Internal Medicine, Washington
University; and Attending Physician, Barnes Hospital, St.
Louis, Missouri

T. Jake Liang, M.D.
Chief, Liver Diseases, NIDDK, National Institutes of
Health; and Chief Staff Physician, Hepatology Service,
National Institutes of Health Clinical Center, Bethesda,
Maryland

Mark L. Lloyd, M.D.
Private Practice, Meridian, Idaho

Mark A. Lovell, M.D.
Associate Professor, Department of Pathology, University
of Colorado Health Sciences Center; and Pathologist,
Department of Pathology, The Children's Hospital, Denver,
Colorado

Charles C. Lu, M.D.
Emeritus Professor, Department of Radiology, University of
Iowa Carver College of Medicine; and University of Iowa
Hospitals and Clinics, Iowa City, Iowa

Shelly C. Lu, M.D.
Professor of Medicine, Department of Internal Medicine,
Keck School of Medicine of the University of Southern
California, Los Angeles, California

Lawrence Lumeng, M.D.
Professor of Medicine and Biochemistry/Molecular Biology,
Indiana University School of Medicine; and Chief, Division
of Gastroenterology and Hepatology, Department of
Medicine, Indiana University School of Medicine and
Richard L. Roudebush Veterans Affairs Medical Center,
Indianapolis, Indiana

Finlay A. Macrae, M.D., F.R.A.C.P., F.R.C.P.
Professor, Department of Medicine, University of
Melbourne, Parkville; and Head, Colorectal Medicine
and Genetics, The Royal Melbourne Hospital, Victoria,
Australia

Ismael Maguilnik, M.D.
Head of Internal Medicine, Department of Internal
Medicine, Faculdade de Medicina UFRGS; and Head
Endoscopy Unit, Department of Gastroenterology, Hospital
de Clínicas de Porto Alegre, Porto Alegre, Brazil

Suzanne M. Matsui, M.D.
Assistant Professor, Department of Medicine, Division of
Gastroenterology and Hepatology, Stanford University
School of Medicine, Stanford; and Physician, Medical
Service, Veterans Affairs Palo Alto Health Care System, Palo
Alto, California

Marlyn J. Mayo, M.D.
Assistant Professor, Department of Internal Medicine,
University of Texas Southwestern Medical Center at Dallas,
Dallas, Texas

Alec J. Megibow, M.D., M.P.H., F.A.C.R.
Professor, Department of Radiology, New York University
School of Medicine, New York, New York

Michel H. Mendler, M.D.
Assistant Professor of Clinical Medicine, Division of
Gastrointestinal and Liver Diseases, Keck School of Medicine
of the University of Southern California, Los Angeles,
California

Raphael B. Merriman, M.D., M.R.C.P.I.
Clinical Instructor of Medicine, Department of Medicine,
University of California, San Francisco; and Attending
Hepatologist, University of San Francisco Medical Center,
San Francisco, California

Klaus E. Mönkemüller, M.D.
Assistant Professor, Department of Medicine, University of
Alabama at Birmingham; and Chief of Endoscopy, Department
of Gastroenterology, Veterans Affairs Medical Center,
Birmingham, Alabama

Richard H. Moseley, M.D.
Professor, Department of Internal Medicine, Division of Gas-
troenterology, University of Michigan Health System; and
Chief, Medical Service, Ann Arbor Veterans Affairs Medical
Center, Ann Arbor, Michigan

Michael W. Mulholland, M.D., Ph.D.
Professor and Chairman, Department of Surgery, University
of Michigan Health System, Ann Arbor, Michigan

V. Raman Muthusamy, M.D.
Assistant Clinical Professor, Department of Medicine,
University of California San Francisco; and Director,
Endoscopic Ultrasound, Department of Medicine, Division
of Gastroenterology, UCSF-Mt. Zion Medical Center, San
Francisco, California

Anil Nagar, M.D.
Department of Internal Medicine, Section of Digestive
Diseases, West Haven Veterans Affairs and Yale University,
West Haven, Connecticut

Garry A. Neil, M.D.
Senior Vice President, Drug Development, Johnson & John-
son Pharmaceutical Research & Development, Titusville,
New Jersey

H. Juergen Nord, M.D.
Professor, Department of Medicine, and Director, Division
of Digestive Diseases and Nutrition, University of South
Florida College of Medicine, Tampa, Florida

Jeffrey A. Norton, M.D.
Vice Chair and Professor, Department of Surgery,
University of California San Francisco; and Professor,
Department of Surgery, UCSF Medical Center, San
Francisco, California

Timothy T. Nostrant, M.D.
Professor, Department of Internal Medicine, Division of
Gastroenterology, University of Michigan Health System,
Ann Arbor, Michigan

Ward A. Olsen, M.D.
Professor, Department of Medicine, University of Wisconsin; Head, Gastroenterology Section, Department of Medicine, University of Wisconsin Hospitals and Clinics; and Chief, Gastroenterology Section, William S. Middleton Veterans Hospital, Madison, Wisconsin

Eric K. Outwater, M.D.
Professor, Department of Radiology, The University of Arizona; and Head, Cross-Sectional Imaging Section, Department of Radiology, Arizona Health Sciences Center, Tucson, Arizona

Chung Owyang, M.D.
Professor of Internal Medicine, H. Marvin Pollard Collegiate Professor and Chief, Division of Gastroenterology, University of Michigan Health System, Ann Arbor, Michigan

John E. Pandolfino, M.D.
Assistant Professor of Medicine, Division of Gastroenterology, Feinberg School of Medicine, Northwestern University, Chicago, Illinois

Julián Panés, M.D.
Assistant Professor, Department of Medicine, University of Barcelona; and Consultant, Department of Gastroenterology, Hospital Clinic, Barcelona, Spain

Sareh Parangi, M.D., F.A.C.S.
Attending Surgeon, Department of Surgery, Harvard Medical School; and Assistant Professor of Surgery, Department of General Surgery, Beth Israel Deaconess Medical Center, Boston, Massachusetts

Henry P. Parkman, M.D.
Associate Professor, Department of Medicine, Temple University School of Medicine; and Director, GI Motility Laboratory, Temple University Hospital, Philadelphia, Pennsylvania

Richard D. Pearson, M.D.
Professor, Departments of Medicine and Pathology, Division of Infectious Diseases and International Health, University of Virginia Health System, Charlottesville, Virginia

Marion G. Peters, M.D.
Professor of Medicine and Chief of Hepatology Research, Department of Medicine, Division of Gastroenterology, University of California at San Francisco, San Francisco, California

Josep M. Piqué, M.D.
Associate Professor, Department of Medicine, University of Barcelona; and Chief, Department of Gastroenterology, Hospital Clinic, Barcelona, Spain

Don W. Powell, M.D.
Associate Dean for Research, School of Medicine; Professor, Internal Medicine; and Professor, Physiology and Biophysics, The University of Texas Medical Branch, Galveston, Texas

Chandra Prakash, M.D., M.R.C.P.
Assistant Professor of Medicine, Division of Gastroenterology, Washington University School of Medicine, St. Louis, Missouri

John C. Rabine, M.D.
Adjunct Professor, Division of Gastroenterology, University of Michigan Health System, Ann Arbor, Michigan; and Chief of Gastroenterolgy, Department of Internal Medicine, David Grant Medical Center, Travis Air Force Base, California

Emad Y. Rahmani, M.D., F.A.C.P.
Associate Professor, Department of Medicine, Indiana University School of Medicine; and Director of Gastrointestinal Endoscopy, Department of Medicine, Wishard Memorial Hospital, Indianapolis, Indiana

David S. Raiford, M.D.
Associate Professor, Department of Medicine, Division of Gastroenterology, Hepatology, and Nutrition, Vanderbilt University School of Medicine; and Director, Liver Service, Vanderbilt University Medical Center, Nashville, Tennessee

Philip W. Ralls, M.D.
Professor and Vice Chair, Department of Radiology, Keck School of Medicine of the University of Southern California; and Department of Radiology, Los Angeles County and University of California Medical Center, Los Angeles, California

Jean-Pierre Raufman, M.D.
Moses and Helen Golden Paulson Professor of Medicine and Head, Division of Gastroenterology and Hepatology, University of Maryland School of Medicine, Baltimore, Maryland

Howard A. Reber, M.D.
Professor of Surgery, Division of General Surgery, Section of Gastrointestinal Surgery, David Geffen School of Medicine at the University of California Los Angeles, Los Angeles, California

K. Rajender Reddy, M.D.
Professor of Medicine and Surgery, Director of Hepatology, and Medical Director of Liver Transplantation, University of Pennsylvania, Philadelphia, Pennsylvania

Douglas K. Rex, M.D.
Professor of Medicine and Director of Endoscopy, Indiana University School of Medicine, Indianapolis, Indiana

Joel E. Richter, M.D.
Professor of Medicine, The Cleveland Clinic Lerner College of Medicine of Case Western Reserve University; and Chairman, Department of Gastroenterology and Hepatology, The Cleveland Clinic Foundation, Cleveland, Ohio

Michelle L. Robbin, M.D.
Associate Professor and Chief of Ultrasound, Department of Radiology, University of Alabama at Birmingham, Birmingham, Alabama

Lewis R. Roberts, M.D., Ph.D.
Assistant Professor, Department of Medicine, Mayo Medical School; and Senior Associate Consultant, Division of Gastroenterology and Hepatology, Mayo Clinic, Rochester, Minnesota

Stephen E. Rubesin, M.D.
Professor, Department of Radiology, University of Pennsylvania School of Medicine; and Radiologist, Department of Radiology, Hospital of the University of Pennsylvania, Philadelphia, Pennsylvania

Cyrus E. Rubin, M.D.
Professor Emeritus, Departments of Pathology and Medicine, University of Washington; and Gastrointestinal Pathologist, Department of Anatomic Pathology, University of Washington Medical Center, Seattle, Washington

Deborah C. Rubin, M.D.
Associate Professor of Medicine, Division of Gastroenterology, Department of Medicine, Washington University School of Medicine; and Attending Physician, Department of Internal Medicine, Barnes-Jewish Hospital, St. Louis, Missouri

Bruce A. Runyon, M.D.
Professor of Medicine, Division of Gastrointestinal and Liver Diseases, Keck School of Medicine of the University of Southern California, Los Angeles; and Chief, Liver Service, Department of Medicine, Rancho Los Amigos National Rehabilitation Center, Downey, California

Anil K. Rustgi, M.D.
T. Grier Miller Professor, Department of Medicine and Genetics; and Chief of Gastroenterology, Department of Medicine, University of Pennsylvania, Philadelphia, Pennsylvania

M. Hossein Saboorian, M.D.
Associate Professor, Department of Pathology, University of Texas Southwestern Medical Center, Dallas, Texas

Michael G. Sarr, M.D.
Professor, Department of Surgery, Mayo Medical School; Consultant, Division of Gastroenterology and General Surgery, Mayo Clinic, Rochester, Minnesota

James M. Scheiman, M.D.
Associate Professor, Department of Internal Medicine, Division of Gastroenterology; and Director, Endoscopic Ultrasound Program, University of Michigan Health System, Ann Arbor, Michigan

Frank V. Schiødt, M.D.
Assistant Professor, Department of Gastroenterology, University of Copenhagen; and Rigshospitalet, Copenhagen, Denmark

Neal E. Seymour, M.D.
Chief, Section of General Surgery, Vice Chairman of Surgery, Baystate Medical Center, Springfield, Massachusetts

Fergus Shanahan, M.D.
Professor and Chair, Department of Medicine, University College Cork, National University of Ireland; and Professor, Department of Medicine, Cork University Hospital, Cork, Ireland

Elizabeth F. Sherertz, M.D.
Skin Surgery Center, Winston-Salem, North Carolina

Stuart Sherman, M.D.
Professor, Departments of Medicine and Radiology, Indiana University Medical Center; and Director, ERCP Service, Indiana University Medical Center, Indianapolis, Indiana

Diane M. Simeone, M.D.
Assistant Professor, Department of Surgery, and Attending Surgeon, Section of General Surgery, University of Michigan Health System, Ann Arbor, Michigan

Kenneth J. Simpson, M.D., Ph.D.
Senior Lecturer, Department of Medicine, University of Edinburgh; and Consultant Physician, Scottish Liver Transplant Unit, Royal Infirmary, Edinburgh, United Kingdom

Phillip D. Smith, M.D.
Mary J. Bradford Professor in Gastroenterology, Professor of Medicine and Microbiology, Department of Medicine, University of Alabama at Birmingham; and Staff Physician, Veterans Affairs Medical Center, Birmingham, Alabama

Ronald J. Sokol, M.D.
Professor and Vice Chair, Department of Pediatrics, University of Colorado Health Sciences Center; and Director of Pediatric GCRC, Pediatric Liver Center, The Children's Hospital, Denver, Colorado

Nathaniel J. Soper, M.D.
Professor, Department of Surgery, Washington University School of Medicine; and Head, Minimally Invasive Surgery, Department of Surgery, Barnes-Jewish Hospital, St. Louis, Missouri

Samuel L. Stanley Jr., M.D.
Professor, Department of Medicine, Washington University School of Medicine; and Attending Physician, Department of Medicine, Barnes-Jewish Hospital, St. Louis, Missouri

William F. Stenson, M.D.
Professor, Department of Medicine, Division of Gastroenterology, Washington University School of Medicine, St. Louis, Missouri

Robert W. Summers, M.D.
Professor, Department of Internal Medicine, University of Iowa; and Director of Clinical Activities, James A. Clifton Center for Digestive Diseases, University of Iowa Health Care, Iowa City, Iowa

Joseph J.Y. Sung, M.D., Ph.D.
Professor of Medicine, Department of Medicine and Therapeutics, The Chinese University of Hong Kong; and Chief of Gastroenterology and Hepatology, Department of Medicine and Therapeutics, Prince of Wales Hospital, Shatin, New Territories, Hong Kong

Jayant A. Talwalkar, M.D., M.P.H.
Instructor of Medicine, Department of Internal Medicine, Mayo Medical School; and Senior Associate Consultant, Division of Gastroenterology and Hepatology, Mayo Clinic, Rochester, Minnesota

Stephan R. Targan
Director, Division of Gastroenterology, and Director, Inflammatory Disease Center, Cedars Sinai Medical Center; and Professor in Residence, University of California Los Angeles School of Medicine, Los Angeles, California

Alicia M. Terando, M.D.
Resident in Surgery, Department of Surgery, University of Michigan Health System, Ann Arbor, Michigan

Dwain L. Thiele, M.D.
Professor of Internal Medicine, Interim Chief, Digestive and Liver Diseases; Chief of Hepatology, Department of Internal Medicine, University of Texas Southwestern Medical Center at Dallas; and Chief, Liver Diseases, Department of Internal Medicine, Parkland Memorial Hospital, Dallas, Texas

Anthony C. Thomas, M.B., Ph.D., F.R.C.Path., F.R.C.P.A.
Associate Professor, Department of Anatomical Pathology, Flinders University of South Australia; and Senior Specialist, Department of Anatomical Pathology, Flinders Medical Centre, Bedford Park, South Australia, Australia

William J. Tremaine, M.D.
Professor of Medicine, Department of Gastroenterology and Hepatology, Mayo Medical School, Rochester, Minnesota

Jerrold R. Turner, M.D., Ph.D.
Assistant Professor, Department of Pathology, The University of Chicago; and The University of Chicago Hospitals, Chicago, Illinois

Guido N.J. Tytgat, M.D., Ph.D.
Professor, Department of Gastroenterology and Hepatology, Faculty of Medicine, University of Amsterdam; and Chief, Department of Gastroenterology and Hepatology, Academic Medical Center, Amsterdam, The Netherlands

Peter Vilmann, M.D.Sc.
Associate Professor, Copenhagen University; and Consultant Surgeon, Department of Surgical Gastroenterology, Gentofte University Hospital, Hellerup, Denmark

Arnold Wald, M.D.
Professor of Medicine, Division of Gastroenterology, Hepatology, and Nutrition; and Director, Fellowship Training in Gastroenterology, Hepatology, and Nutrition, Department of Medicine, University of Pittsburgh Medical Center, Pittsburgh, Pennsylvania

Jerome D. Waye, M.D.
Clinical Professor of Medicine, Department of Medicine, Division of Gastroenterology, Mount Sinai Medical Center; Director of Endoscopic Education, Mount Sinai Hospital; and Chief, Gastrointestinal Endoscopy Unit, Lenox Hill Hospital, New York, New York

Joel V. Weinstock, M.D.
Professor, Department of Internal Medicine, University of Iowa; and Director, Division of Gastroenterology and Hepatology, Department of Internal Medicine, University of Iowa Hospitals and Clinics, Iowa City, Iowa

David C. Whitcomb, M.D., Ph.D.
Professor of Medicine, Cell Biology and Physiology, and Human Genetics; Chief, Division of Gastroenterology, Hepatology and Nutrition; and Director, Center for Genomic Sciences, University of Pittsburgh, Pittsburgh, Pennsylvania

Russell H. Wiesner, M.D.
Professor of Medicine, Mayo Clinic Transplant Center, Mayo Medical School; and Director of Viral Hepatitis, Liver Transplant Center, Mayo Clinic, Rochester, Minnesota

C. Mel Wilcox, M.D.
Professor, Department of Medicine and Director, Division of Gastroenterology and Hepatology, University of Alabama at Birmingham, Birmingham, Alabama

John W. Wiley, M.D.
Associate Professor, Department of Internal Medicine, Division of Gastroenterology, University of Michigan Health System; and Program Director, General Clinical Research Center, University of Michigan, Ann Arbor, Michigan

Christopher B. Williams, B.M., F.R.C.P., F.R.C.S.
Consultant Physician, Wolfson Unit for Endoscopy, St. Mark's Hospital, London, United Kingdom

Francis Y. Yao, M.D.
Associate Clinical Professor, Department of Medicine; and Associate Medical Director, Liver Transplantation, University of California San Francisco, San Francisco, California

Graeme P. Young, M.B., B.S., M.D., F.R.A.C.P.
Professor of Gastroenterology, Department of Medicine, Flinders University of South Australia; and Director, Department of Gastroenterology, Flinders Medical Centre, Adelaide, Australia

Tonia M. Young-Fadok, M.D., M.S., F.A.C.S., F.A.S.C.R.S.
Associate Professor, Department of Surgery, Mayo Medical School; and Consultant, Division of Colon and Rectal Surgery, Mayo Clinic, Rochester, Minnesota

The practice of gastroenterology has undergone a dramatic metamorphosis in recent years. With the advent of endoscopic instruments it has become possible to directly visualize a large portion of the gastrointestinal tract and to obtain biopsy specimens from these sites. This has enabled clinicians to diagnose and treat many illnesses that otherwise might have gone unrecognized until a much later stage. In addition to these advances that have improved the direct visualization of gastrointestinal pathology, a number of advances in imaging techniques have also enhanced the ability to approach gastrointestinal problems indirectly. Double contrast radiography, computed tomography, isotopic scintigraphy, ultrasonography, magnetic resonance imaging, and even more experimental technologies such as positron emission tomography have facilitated the approach to diagnosing gastrointestinal disorders. The dramatic advances in these technologies and their impact on the practice of gastroenterology are chronicled in the Fourth Edition of our *Textbook of Gastroenterology*. Yet, the old adage that "a picture is worth a thousand words" could not be more applicable to anything other than to the teaching of gastroenterology—for ours is a visual science. With this in mind, we have endeavored to provide the Third Edition of the *Atlas of Gastroenterology* with additional graphic material that enhances the reader's understanding of the written material in the *Textbook*. The Third Edition of the *Atlas* expands on the material presented in the Second Edition by the addition of figures to existing chapters and by the addition of chapters covering new subject matter. Of particular note are the new chapters that cover the subject of liver diseases.

Although numerous excellent gastroenterology atlases are available, we have designed ours to be especially useful in conjunction with the *Textbook*. Accordingly, we have designed the *Atlas* in distinct chapter format to correspond to chapters in the *Textbook*. There is inevitably some duplication of material, but it is our intention to make it as convenient as possible for the *Atlas* reader to examine visual material according to various groupings (e.g., symptoms, diseases, and techniques). Not all of the *Textbook* chapters have a corresponding chapter in the *Atlas;* indeed, only those chapters that could be enhanced by additional graphic images were selected for expansion in the *Atlas*. The vast majority of the figures presented in the *Atlas* are new and original material provided by the authors, but in some instances isolated figures from other published sources were borrowed because of their unique appropriateness in depicting a particular problem. In this regard, we are particularly grateful to Dr. F.A. Mitros for material published in the *Atlas of Gastrointestinal Pathology* (J.B. Lippincott, Philadelphia, PA, 1988); Drs. J.J. Misiewicz, A. Forbes, A.B. Price, P.J. Shorvon, D.R. Triger, and G.N.J. Tytgat for material published in the *Atlas of Clinical Gastroenterology* (Wolfe, London, 1994); Drs. F.E. Silverstein and G.N.J. Tytgat for material published in *Gastrointestinal Endoscopy* (Mosby-Wolfe, London, 1997); and Dr. R.L. Eisenberg for material published in *Gastrointestinal Radiology: A Pattern Approach* (Lippincott Williams & Wilkins, Philadelphia, PA, 2003). For the sake of coherence and clarity, some figures from the *Textbook* also appear in the *Atlas*.

The written text in the *Atlas* provides only an abbreviated introduction to the graphic material, and the reader is referred to the *Textbook* for more detailed information. Although the *Atlas* is meant to be especially useful to the reader of the *Textbook*, the quality of many of the figures is unique and not to be found readily in existing publications. Thus, we hope that the *Atlas* will serve as a valuable educational resource for all readers, independent of their familiarity with the *Textbook*.

Tadataka Yamada, M.D.

ACKNOWLEDGMENTS

The work of the editors was greatly facilitated by the expert assistance of Lori Ennis and Barbara Boughen who collaborated as a team complementing editorial talents with interpersonal skills, maintaining the high quality of the text, and delivering the manuscripts in a timely fashion.

The editors are also indebted to the critical roles played by Carol Arnold, Robbie Loftin, Frances Powell, Terri Kirschner, Sue Sparrow, JoAnn Wilson, and Maria Vidrio. The editors wish to express their gratitude to their superlative colleagues at Lippincott Williams & Wilkins who demonstrated throughout the entire project their commitment to quality, integrity, and excellence. Of the many people at Lippincott Williams & Wilkins involved in the publication of this atlas, Beth Barry deserves special recognition. The book would not have been possible without her exceptional talents.

PART ONE

APPROACHES TO COMMON GASTROINTESTINAL PROBLEMS

1

APPROACH TO THE PATIENT WITH GROSS GASTROINTESTINAL BLEEDING

GRACE H. ELTA

Gastrointestinal (GI) bleeding is a common clinical problem that requires more than 300,000 hospitalizations annually in the United States. Most bleeding episodes resolve spontaneously; however, patients with severe and persistent bleeding have high mortality rates. Evaluation of a patient with bleeding begins with assessment of the urgency of the situation. Resuscitation with intravenous fluids and blood products is the first consideration. Once the patient's condition is stable, a brief history and physical examination will help determine the location of the bleeding. For probable or known upper GI bleeding, a nasogastric (NG) tube is placed to help determine the location of bleeding and to monitor the rapidity of the bleeding. The following algorithm is a general guideline for evaluation of nonvariceal upper GI bleeding. There is an important exception to this algorithm: endoscopy may be used urgently in *all* patients with upper GI bleeding irregardless of whether their bleeding has stopped spontaneously, allowing triage of patients to outpatient, inpatient, or intensive care. This practice has been shown to be safe and leads to significant cost saving because patients without risk factors such as coagulopathy, serious concomitant diseases, or bleeding stigmata do not require hospitalization.

Algorithm 1

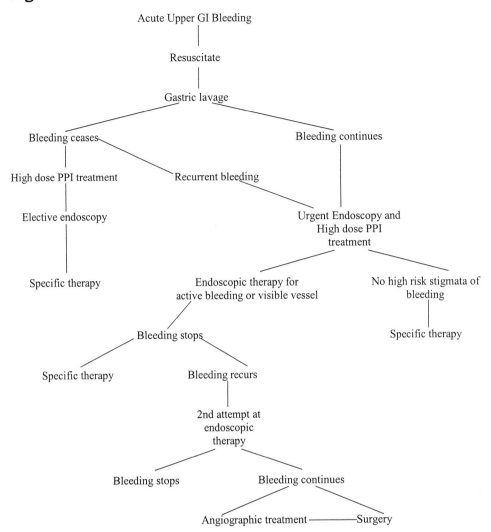

PPI, proton pump inhibitor.

Patients with liver disease or other causes of portal hypertension have a potential variceal source of hemorrhage. Urgent diagnostic endoscopy is indicated to confirm the bleeding source, because between one third and one half of these patients have bleeding from nonvariceal sites, and future management is different for bleeding varices. The following algorithm is for the evaluation and management of variceal hemorrhage. *TIPS* indicates transjugular intrahepatic portosystemic shunt.

Algorithm 2

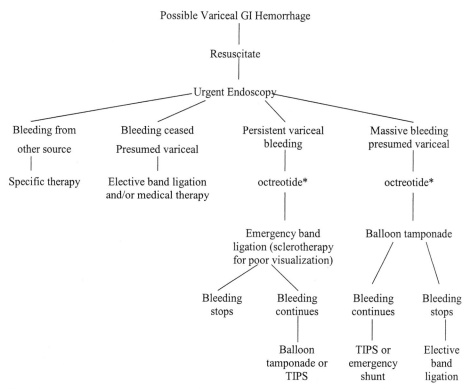

*If bleeding is persistent or massive, octreotide may be used prior to and concomitantly with endoscopy.

Lower GI bleeding is defined as bleeding from below the ligament of Treitz. When patients hospitalized for GI bleeding are identified, lower GI sources account for one quarter to one third of all bleeding events. When the location of bleeding is suspected to be the lower GI tract, an NG tube and even upper endoscopy may still be needed to rule out an upper GI source of hemorrhage. It is important to remember that as many as 10% of patients with hematochezia have an upper GI source, and that results of NG aspiration can be falsely negative when bleeding is duodenal and there is no duodenogastric reflux, or when the bleeding has ceased. The following algorithm is for evaluation of lower GI bleeding.

Algorithm 3

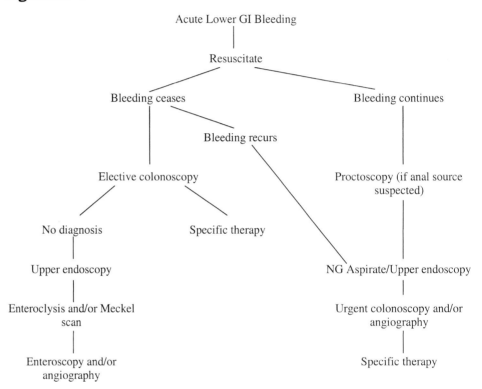

Unfortunately, some patients have both upper and lower GI bleeding sites that defy diagnosis despite the numerous diagnostic modalities available. They need repeated studies if bleeding recurs or becomes a management problem.

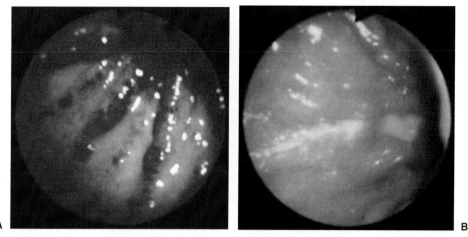

FIGURE 1-1. **A:** Endoscopic view of the antrum of a patient with watermelon stomach. Vascular ectasias are present on top of rugal folds giving the characteristic "striped" appearance to the mucosa. This patient presented with chronic gastrointestinal blood loss that necessitated transfusions. **B:** Antral view of the same patient 2 weeks after the second yttrium-aluminum-garnet (YAG) laser treatment of the vascular lesions. There was no further endoscopic evidence of the vascular lesions. A linear ulcer caused by the laser treatment is present. The patient needed no further transfusions in 10 months of follow-up care.

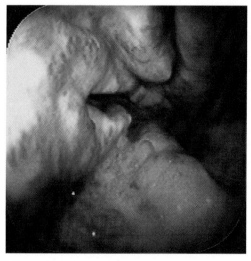

FIGURE 1-2. Endoscopic view of moderate-sized esophageal varices with multiple red marks.

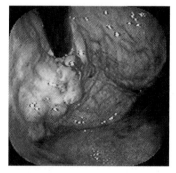

FIGURE 1-3. Retroflexed view of a cluster of gastric varices on the lesser curvature.

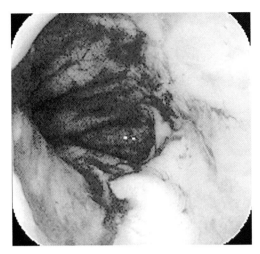

FIGURE 1-4. Endoscopic view of an oozing distal esophageal ulcer in a middle-aged man with chronic heartburn who cannot afford acid-reducing medicines and presented with a 6-unit upper gastrointestinal bleed.

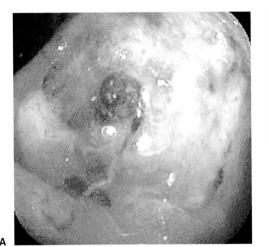

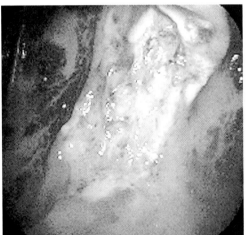

A   B

FIGURE 1-5. **A:** Sigmoid colon view of a polypectomy site with a visible vessel in a 65-year-old woman who presented with hematochezia 3 days after polypectomy of a sessile polyp with snare electrocautery. **B:** Same view of the postpolypectomy site after treatment with multipolar electrocoagulation.

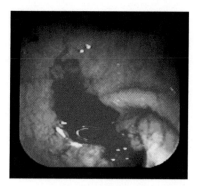

FIGURE 1-6. Duodenal bulb view of an actively bleeding Dieulafoy lesion in the distal bulb. After cleansing, there was no associated erosion or ulcer. This lesion was managed successfully with electrocautery. (Courtesy of W.D. Chey.)

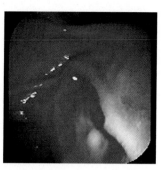

FIGURE 1-7. A 52-year-old man without a history of abdominal pain presented with his third episode of hematemesis in 5 months. Two previous upper endoscopic examinations did not show a bleeding source. At a third endoscopic examination, blood was found in the second portion of the duodenum, and examination with a side-viewing duodenoscope revealed hemobilia. Subsequent endoscopic retrograde cholangiopancreatography revealed a small stone in the distal common bile duct. The stone was removed after sphincterotomy.

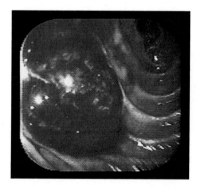

FIGURE 1-8. A 57-year-old woman with known metastatic carcinoma of the breast presented with melena and lightheadedness. This lesion in the second portion of the duodenum was found at biopsy to be metastatic adenocarcinoma. (Courtesy of W.D. Chey.)

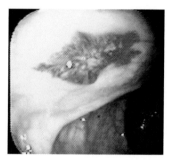

FIGURE 1-9. An 82-year-old man presented with a history of hematochezia for 24 hours and mild anemia. Colonoscopy after preparation revealed vascular ectasia in the right colon.

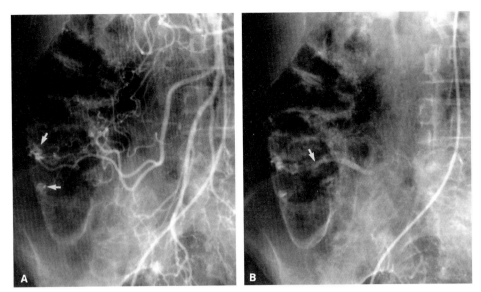

FIGURE 1-10. **A:** Angiographic demonstration of two vascular tufts (*arrows*) consistent with cecal angiodysplasia. **B:** Venous image from the same arteriogram demonstrated early venous filling (*arrow*), reflecting arteriovenous communication through a dilated vascular ectasia.

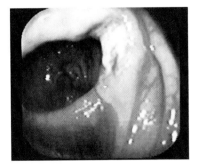

FIGURE 1-11. A 32-year-old man presented with maroon stools 4 days after running a marathon. Colonoscopy revealed two ulcers in the right colon. Biopsy findings were consistent with ischemia. The patient denied a history of use of non-steroidal antiinflammatory drugs. (Courtesy of W.D. Chey.)

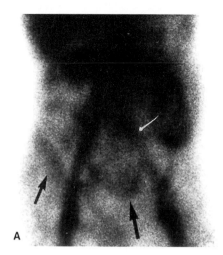

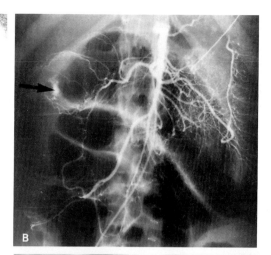

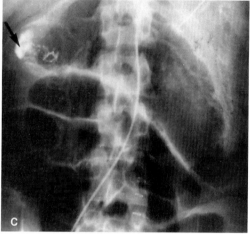

FIGURE 1-12. **A:** Five-minute image from a technetium-99m pertechnetate–labeled red cell scan of a 23-year-old woman postpartum with diffuse intravascular coagulation and gross hematochezia. The radioactivity appears to extend from the hepatic flexure to a location distal to the splenic flexure (*arrows*). **B:** Angiographic injection of the superior mesenteric artery of the same patient as in **A** immediately after the scintigraphic study demonstrated active bleeding in the hepatic flexure area of the colon (*arrow*). **C:** Later image during the angiographic study shows persistent extravasation of contrast medium in the lumen of the colon (*arrow*).

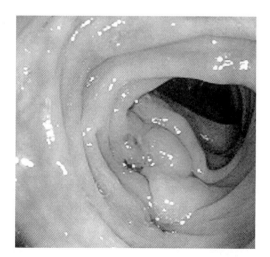

FIGURE 1-13. Sigmoid colon view of a bleeding diverticulum in a 68-year-old man taking one aspirin per day after the bleeding was controlled with injection of 8 mL of 1:10,000 epinephrine.

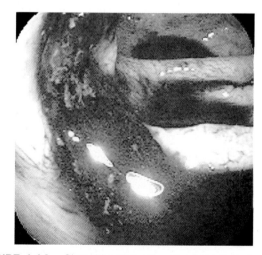

FIGURE 1-14. Sigmoid colon view of a bleeding diverticulum at 35 cm in a 58-year-old woman. The bleeding stopped after injection of diluted epinephrine and treatment with multipolar coagulation. The diverticula were limited to the sigmoid and descending colon. Four days later she had recurrent hematochezia and was taken to the operating room for a sigmoid colectomy.

APPROACH TO THE PATIENT WITH OCCULT GASTROINTESTINAL BLEEDING

DAVID A. AHLQUIST

Occult gastrointestinal (GI) bleeding is by definition not apparent on inspection of stools. Its presence is either suggested indirectly by the finding of iron deficiency with or without associated microcytic anemia or demonstrated directly by a fecal blood test. As with overt GI bleeding, occult bleeding may be acute or chronic, intermittent or continuous. Occult GI bleeding may arise at any level from the oropharynx to the distal rectum and there are many causes. As such, the clinician's judgment is challenged when faced with occult GI bleeding.

Iron deficiency anemia is the critical metabolic consequence of chronic occult GI bleeding. Occult GI bleeding may lead to iron deficiency in patients of any age, but is by far the most frequent etiology in men and postmenopausal women. Iron deficiency is exceedingly common, with a worldwide prevalence estimated at 15%; an appreciation of its causal association with occult GI bleeding is important.

Occult GI bleeding ranges from small physiological losses of 1 to 2 mL per day to marked pathological elevations. As much as 200 mL blood may be lost from the upper GI tract and remain occult. Generally, average blood losses of 5 to 10 mL per day or more are required to overcome compensatory mechanisms, deplete iron stores, and eventuate in anemia.

Occult GI bleeding involves a defect in the continuity of the epithelium and thus may be due to inflammatory, neoplastic, infectious, vascular, or traumatic mechanisms. Most clinically important occult bleeding arises from the upper GI tract. As a group, acid-peptic disorders are the most common cause of occult bleeding and anemia in industrialized countries. Malignant tumors of the GI tract represent another frequent cause; colorectal and gastric cancers are most common. On a global scale, however, hookworm infestation accounts for the largest number of persons with anemia from occult GI bleeding. Medications, especially aspirin and related nonsteroidal antiinflammatory drugs, commonly induce occult bleeding. Other causes of occult bleeding include the heterogeneous array of acquired and inherited vascular malformations, large hiatal hernias with associated Cameron erosions, inflammatory bowel disease, and certain endurance sports, especially long-distance running.

Because clinically significant lesions do not always bleed and not all occult bleeding results in iron deficiency, hematologic and fecal blood assessment are complementary diagnostic tests and can be interpreted only in the context of all clinical information about the patient. In patients with new onset iron deficiency and occult GI bleeding, a hemorrhagic GI lesion should be aggressively sought.

Several types of tests for detection of fecal occult blood are available. These tests assay different portions of the hemoglobin molecule. Because hemoglobin globin and heme are altered during digestive transit, immunochemical- and guaiac-type tests, which respectively target these analytes, often fail to detect proximal gut bleeding. In contrast, the heme-porphyrin test is unaffected by the anatomic level of bleeding. As such, each type of test has advantages and disadvantages according to the clinical indication. For colorectal cancer screening, guaiac- or immunochemical based tests may be preferable, because of their simplicity, qualitative nature, and insensitivity for upper GI bleeding. For the evaluation of iron deficiency, the heme-porphyrin–based test is most ideal because detection is quantitative and includes occult bleeding from all potential sites.

Effective treatment is dictated by the type of lesion found. The combination of extended upper endoscopy and colonoscopy will successfully identify the culprit lesions in more than 80% to 90% of instances. However, the diagnostic evaluation may be complex in the remaining small proportion. The extent of evaluation in cases of obscure occult bleeding must be weighted by the refractoriness of anemia, presence of co-morbidities, and other factors. Most obscure GI bleeding is due to vascular malformations occurring in the small intestine.

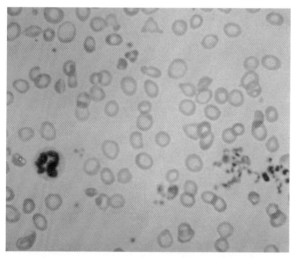

FIGURE 2-1. Peripheral blood smear from a patient with iron deficiency anemia. The red cells are small (microcytic), low in hemoglobin content (hypochromic), and variable in shape (anisocytic). However, these morphologic features may occur with other conditions, including anemia of chronic disease, thalassemia, sideroblastic anemia, the presence of hemoglobin E, and copper deficiency. Iron stores should be assessed when microcytic anemia is discovered. Because anemia is a late manifestation of iron deficiency, iron stores are always low when anemia is caused by iron deficiency.

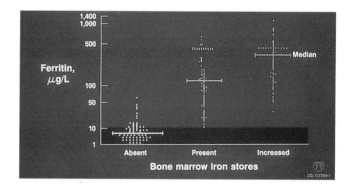

FIGURE 2-2. Relation between histologically assessed marrow iron stores and serum ferritin concentrations. All patients with ferritin values in the shaded region have absent storage iron. Thus, a low serum ferritin level is pathognomonic for iron deficiency. Causes of microcytic anemia other than iron deficiency are associated with normal or increased iron stores and ferritin levels.

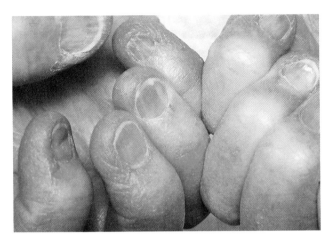

FIGURE 2-3. Koilonychia. These nail changes are characteristic of iron deficiency and consist of spooning concavity, longitudinal ridging, and brittleness. This patient had profound iron deficiency anemia caused by chronic occult bleeding from watermelon stomach.

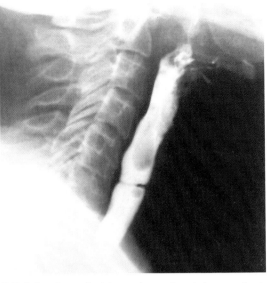

FIGURE 2-4. Postcricoid esophageal web in a patient with iron deficiency anemia (Plummer-Vinson or Paterson-Kelly syndrome). These webs are eccentric, sometimes multiple, proximally located, and more common among women. They may resolve with iron replacement.

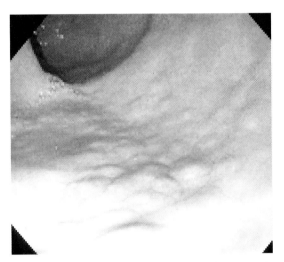

FIGURE 2-5. Antral mucosal nodularity with *Helicobacter pylori* gastritis. *H pylori* gastritis may be associated with iron deficiency even in the absence of endoscopically demonstrated erosions or ulcerations. Collectively, peptic diseases of the esophagus, stomach, and duodenum are the most common cause of occult gastrointestinal bleeding and iron deficiency in adults from industrialized countries.

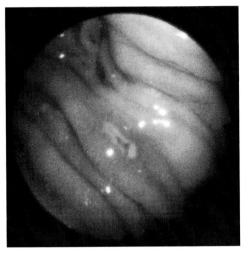

FIGURE 2-6. Endoscopic photograph of a Cameron erosion. This characteristic gastric mucosal lesion may accompany large hiatal hernias, which are found among as many as 10% of adults with iron deficiency anemia. Chronic occult bleeding results from these longitudinal erosions that straddle the diaphragmatic hiatus. Cameron erosions are probably caused by mechanical trauma from breathing.

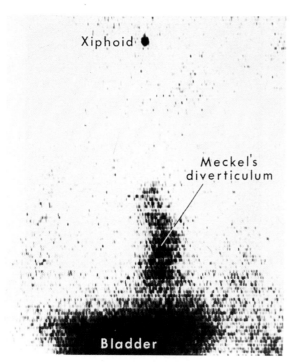

FIGURE 2-7. A pertechnetate scintigram shows abnormal tracer accumulation in Meckel diverticulum. Although commonly a cause of overt bleeding among children and young adults, Meckel diverticulum may produce chronic occult blood loss and anemia, as was the case for this 38-year-old woman.

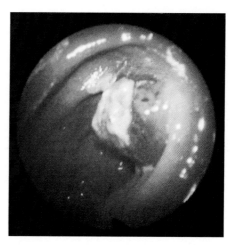

FIGURE 2-8. Endoscopic photograph of a rare cause of occult bleeding. This ulcerated lipoma in the descending colon caused occult bleeding in a patient taking long-term anticoagulant therapy. Elevated fecal blood levels for a patient taking anticoagulants usually reflect underlying gastrointestinal disease.

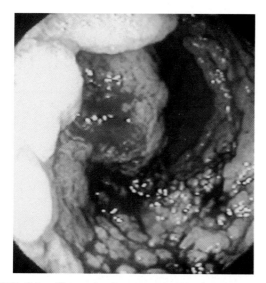

FIGURE 2-9. Hemorrhagic gastric adenocarcinoma in an elderly woman with profound iron deficiency anemia and negative immunochemical fecal blood test results. Because the globin portion of hemoglobin is digested by upper gastrointestinal peptidases, immunochemical tests may fail to detect occult bleeding from the proximal gut.

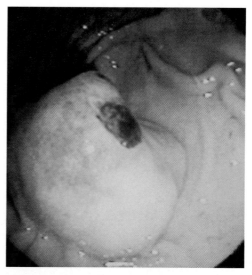

FIGURE 2-10. Large leiomyosarcoma in the gastric antrum that presented with occult gastrointestinal bleeding and iron deficiency anemia. Such lesions are characteristically smooth-walled with a central depressed ulceration.

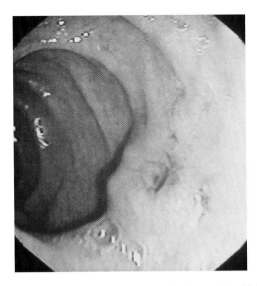

FIGURE 2-11. Ulcerated leiomyoma in the proximal jejunum found on extended upper endoscopy. The initial evaluation in this 40-year-old man with iron deficiency and occult gastrointestinal bleeding included a negative upper endoscopy, colonoscopy, and small bowel barium x-ray.

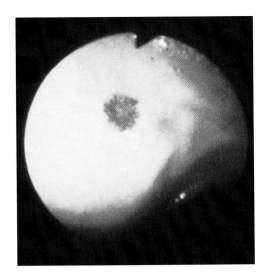

FIGURE 2-12. Endoscopic photograph of mulberry-type gastric vascular malformation. Vascular malformations of the gastrointestinal tract are heterogeneous in size, number, configuration, and location. Together they may explain 0.4% to 6.0% of all iron deficiency anemias among adults in the western world. Even when producing transfusion-dependent anemia, bleeding from vascular malformations remains occult in nearly half of cases.

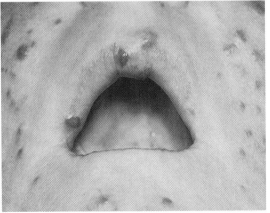

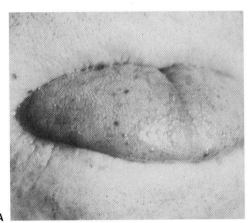

FIGURE 2-13. Hereditary hemorrhagic telangiectasia (Osler-Weber-Rendu) syndrome. Characteristic circumoral and lingual telangiectasia may be subtle (**A**), moderately dense (**B**), or florid (**C**). Similar-appearing lesions occur throughout the gastrointestinal (GI) tract, especially in the gastroduodenal region. GI bleeding, usually occult, often becomes problematic in middle age.

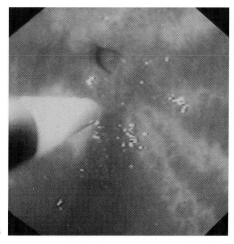

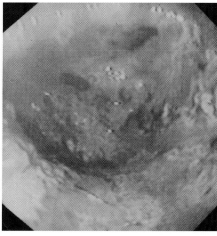

A, B

FIGURE 2-14. Watermelon stomach. Linearly arrayed vascular tissue radially distributed in the antrum looks like watermelon stripes (**A**). Painless occult gastrointestinal bleeding with anemia in an elderly woman is the most typical presentation. This lesion is amenable to endoscopic thermal ablation, and the lesion shown was treated by argon plasma coagulation (**B**).

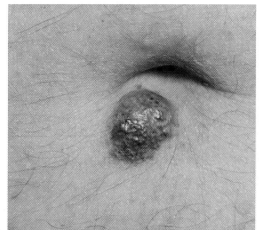

A

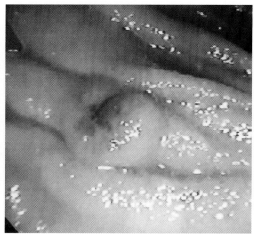

C

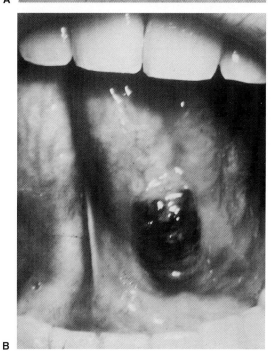

B

FIGURE 2-15. Blue rubber bleb nevus syndrome. This rare syndrome associated with occult gastrointestinal (GI) bleeding is characterized by congenitally acquired bluish hemangiomas that may occur on the skin (**A**) and mucus membranes of the mouth (**B**) or GI tract (**C**). The GI lesions are amenable to endoscopic thermal ablation if they can be reached.

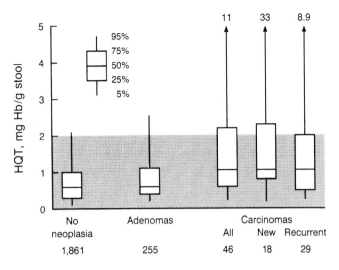

FIGURE 2-16.   Fecal blood distribution measured by means of the HemoQuant test (Mayo Medical Laboratories, Rochester, MN) among persons without symptoms undergoing routine postoperative surveillance. The presence or absence of colorectal neoplasia was established by means of imaging (normally colonoscopy but occasionally sigmoidoscopy plus barium enema). The *shaded zone* represents the normal range as defined by the HemoQuant assay at a reported specificity of 95%.

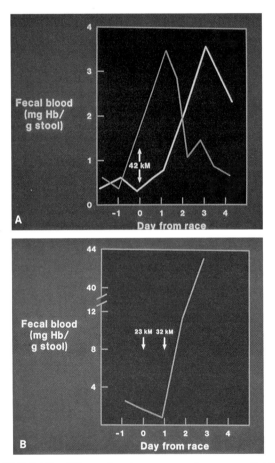

FIGURE 2-17.   Effect of endurance sports on occult bleeding. Fecal blood levels of two runners before and after a marathon (**A**) and one runner after consecutive days of long-distance races (**B**). Occult gastrointestinal bleeding may contribute to the relatively common finding of iron deficiency among endurance runners.

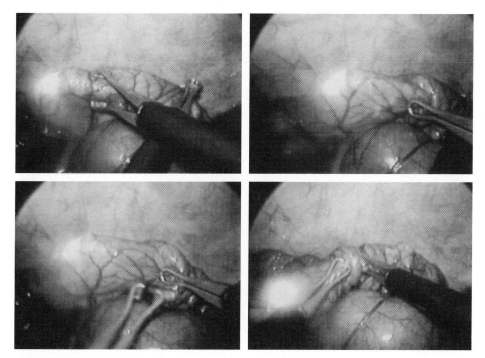

FIGURE 2-18. Laparoscopy-assisted panenteroscopy. This novel approach may provide a less invasive alternative to intraoperative endoscopy in the evaluation of obscure gastrointestinal bleeding.

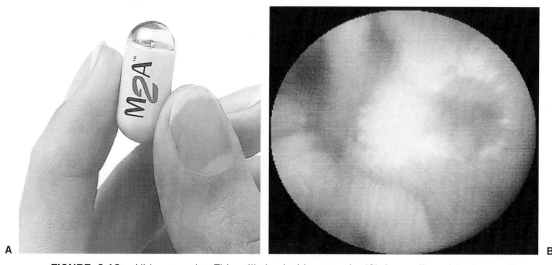

A   B

FIGURE 2-19. Videocapsule. This pill-sized videocapsule (**A**) is swallowed to transmit images of the gastrointestinal tract during its oro-anal passage. A videocapsule image of a small intestinal vascular malformation is shown (**B**). Early studies suggest that this may be an accurate and feasible minimally invasive approach to inspect the small intestine, which is unreachable by conventional endoscopy. (Photographs are courtesy of Given Images, Inc., Norcross, GA.)

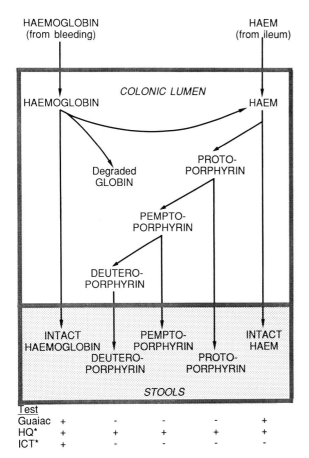

Test					
Guaiac	+	-	-	-	+
HQ*	+	+	+	+	+
ICT*	+	-	-	-	-

* HQ - HemoQuant; ICT - immunochemical test

FIGURE 2-20. The fate of hemoglobin and heme in the large bowel, the products found in feces, and the products detected by means of each of the three main occult blood test technologies. **Upper box:** Events occurring in the colonic lumen. **Bottom shaded box:** Derivatives found in stools. Dietary heme transiting through the ileum or hemoglobin arising from bleeding is composed of protoheme. Fecal bacteria act on the heme to remove the iron and modify the side chains, producing a range of heme-derived porphyrins. Hemoglobin itself in the feces is subject to degradative action by bacteria, which release the heme for further modification and degrade the globin. Degraded globin loses its immunoreactivity. **Bottom panel:** Derivatives found in stools that are detected with the various fecal occult blood tests. (Courtesy of Graeme Young, M.D.)

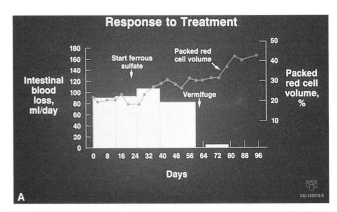

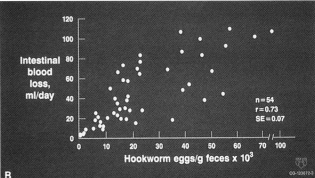

FIGURE 2-21. Hookworm infestation. **A:** Hookworm-induced occult bleeding and response to vermifuge therapy. **B:** Relation between fecal blood loss and hookworm burden. More than 600 million persons are host to this infestation, which is the most common reason for blood loss anemia worldwide.

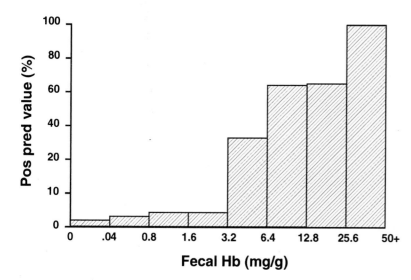

FIGURE 2-22. Positive predictive value of fecal hemoglobin (Hb) for presence of hemorrhagic gastrointestinal (GI) lesions. The positive predictive value increases in proportion to the fecal Hb level. Values are based on Mayo Clinic data from 1000 patients tested by the quantitative HemoQuant assay prior to GI investigation. Lesions included ulcers or erosions, vascular malformations, and malignancies.

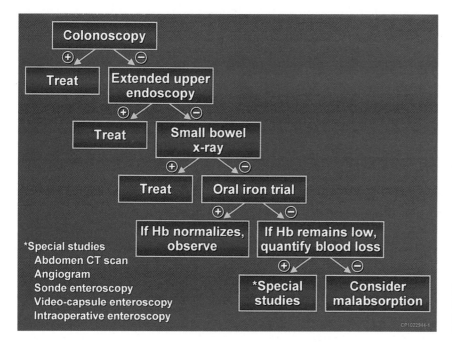

FIGURE 2-23. Suggested algorithm for evaluation of an asymptomatic adult patient with iron deficiency anemia and occult gastrointestinal bleeding.

APPROACH TO THE PATIENT WITH ACUTE ABDOMEN

MICHAEL W. MULHOLLAND

The term *acute abdomen* describes a syndrome of sudden abdominal pain with accompanying symptoms and signs that focus attention on the abdominal region. It is clinically useful to limit discussion to cases in which the pain has been present for less than 24 hours. Associated symptoms such as nausea, vomiting, constipation, diarrhea, anorexia, abdominal distention, and fever often are present and sometimes are confusing. Although operative therapy is not required for all cases of acute abdomen, unwarranted operative delay can have serious, potentially fatal consequences. Successful management is based on a careful initial assessment that incorporates history taking and physical examination; delineation of clinical priorities; and concurrent resuscitation, diagnosis, and therapy.

Treatment of patients with acute abdominal processes differs in a fundamental way from care delivered to patients with long-term problems. The potential for pathological processes to be rapidly progressive and for serious adverse consequences to result from therapeutic delay places a time constraint on diagnosis and treatment. An accurate diagnosis should lead promptly to specific therapy. A complete and accurate history and physical examination are the most important requirements for success.

The treating physician should first focus on the nature and timing of the abdominal pain. The pattern of onset and the progression of pain provide valuable clues to the cause. The pain associated with perforation of a duodenal ulcer or rupture of an abdominal aortic aneurysm is incapacitating, begins suddenly, and quickly reaches peak intensity. Because the onset of pain is so dramatic, patients may be able to provide detailed information about the time of onset or their activities at that moment. In contrast, pain associated with appendicitis increases over a period of one to several hours. Similarly, pain caused by acute cholecystitis increases over hours before reaching a steady intensity. The duration of painful symptoms is important. Biliary colic typically lasts for several hours before rapidly resolving, presumably as a result of dislodgment of the offending stone from the cystic duct. Pain caused by acute pancreatitis is unrelenting. Patients with mechanical obstruction of the small intestine initially may feel remarkably well between episodes of intense and debilitating colic.

The physical examination should be conducted in a systematic and unhurried manner. A complete abdominal examination requires unhindered visualization of the area between the nipples and the midthigh, anteriorly and posteriorly. The examination begins with observation of the patient's expression and behavior. A patient with serious intraperitoneal abnormalities usually has an anxious, pale face. Sweating, dilated pupils, and shallow breathing are common. In the presence of chemical or bacterial contamination of the peritoneum, the patient tends to lie immobile to minimize movement of inflamed viscera against the parietal peritoneum. Knees may be flexed, the abdomen scaphoid, breathing shallow. Inhaling deeply or coughing aggravates the pain. With ureteral colic or mesenteric ischemia, by contrast, the patient may appear restless with frequent changes in posture in an attempt to relieve discomfort. During inspection, the location of all surgical scars, masses, external hernias, and stomas is determined.

Auscultation precedes abdominal palpation. All four quadrants are auscultated for tone and quantity of bowel sounds and the presence of vascular bruits. Bowel sounds are considered to be absent only if no tones are heard over a 2-minute period of auscultation.

Next, the abdomen is palpated. To determine areas of tenderness and the vigor with which palpation may be pursued, it is useful first to ask the patient to demonstrate the point of maximal discomfort. Palpation begins in the abdominal quadrant farthest from the area of suspected pathological change. Gentle pressure to elicit tenderness and muscular resistance ensues. Progressively deeper palpation is attempted to delineate masses. Intentional efforts to reproduce abdominal pain by means of deep palpation and rapid release of pressure, termed *rebound tenderness,* are not helpful and *should not be attempted*. Production of rebound tenderness provides no information that is not available through gentle examination, causes the patient to guard voluntarily, and eliminates the possibility of meaningful serial abdominal examinations. The best evidence of a localized inflammatory process is demonstration of point tenderness, caused by movement of parietal peritoneum against the inflamed surface of a diseased viscus. Point tenderness is sought by means of palpation in the area of maximal discomfort, but also may be elicited by means of grasping the patient's hips and gently rocking the pelvis; the movement of inflamed peritoneum is presumed to cause pain. A stethoscope may be used to palpate the abdominal quadrants.

Every patient must undergo a digital rectal examination. If an inflamed appendix lies deep within the pelvis, point tenderness may sometimes be elicited only by means of palpation through the right rectal wall. Stool is tested for guaiac positivity. For female patients, manual and speculum vaginal examinations are required; vaginal secretions are obtained for Gram stain and culture. All external stomas, wounds, and fistulae are explored digitally.

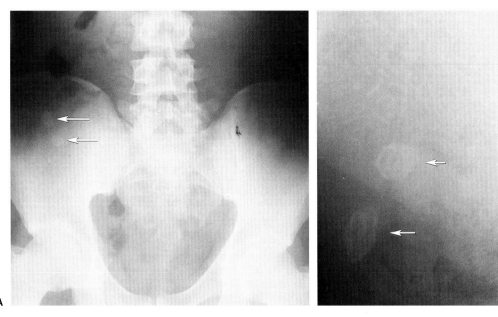

A   B

FIGURE 3-1.   Appendicitis. **A:** The plain abdominal radiograph of a young man with acute appendicitis. Two rounded areas of opacification are present in the right lower quadrant (*arrows*). These represent fecaliths, present in only 2% of the population. The presence of fecaliths correlates strongly with the presence of acute appendicitis in patients with acute abdominal pain. **B:** Magnified view of **A**.

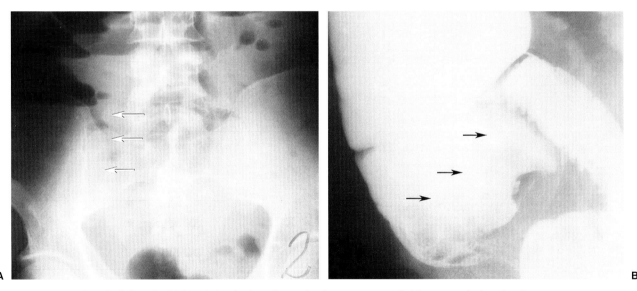

A   B

FIGURE 3-2.   **A:** Plain abdominal radiograph demonstrates fluid accumulation in the cecum (*arrows*) and colonic gaseous distention in perforated appendicitis. **B:** Barium enema radiograph of the same patient as in **A** demonstrates effacement of the cecum (*arrows*) by a periappendiceal abscess.

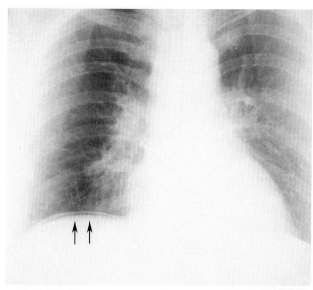

A

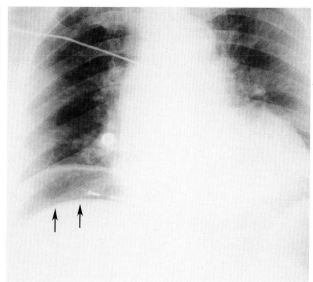

B

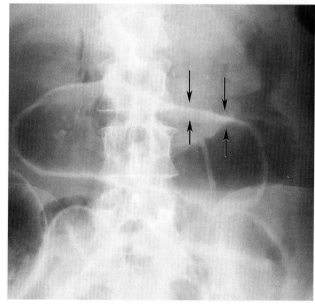

C

FIGURE 3-3. **A, B:** Upright chest radiographs of patients with pneumoperitoneum demonstrate minimal and large collections of air (*arrows*) under the right hemidiaphragms. **C:** Flat abdominal radiograph demonstrates the double-wall sign of pneumoperitoneum (*arrows*). Free intraperitoneal air outlines the serosal surface of the bowel, and intralumenal gas outlines the mucosal surface.

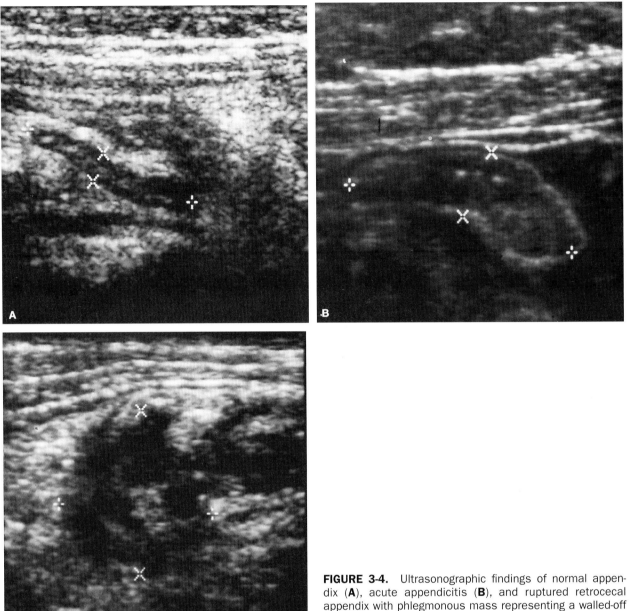

FIGURE 3-4. Ultrasonographic findings of normal appendix (**A**), acute appendicitis (**B**), and ruptured retrocecal appendix with phlegmonous mass representing a walled-off abscess (**C**). The retrocecal appendix (*middle two cursors*) is surrounded by echogenic amorphous material, representing the phlegmon.

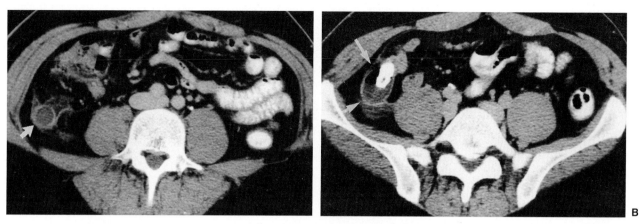

FIGURE 3-5. Computed tomographic findings of acute appendicitis. **A:** Dilated, fluid-filled appendix (*arrow*) lies posterior to the cecum and is surrounded by edematous fat. **B:** A periappendiceal abscess (*arrows*) is present 5 cm inferiorly. It contains gas, fluid, and a calcified appendicolith.

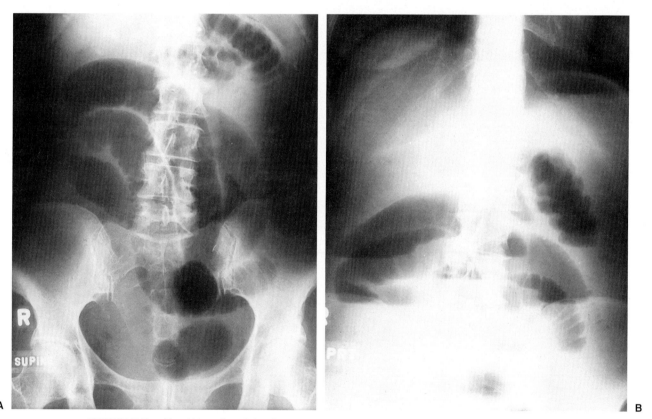

FIGURE 3-6. Flat (**A**) and upright (**B**) abdominal radiographs in the setting of obstruction of the small intestine. Distended, air-filled loops of small bowel and multiple air-fluid levels are present (**B**), and air is absent in the colon.

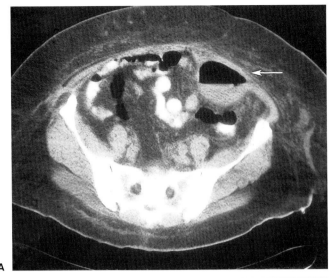

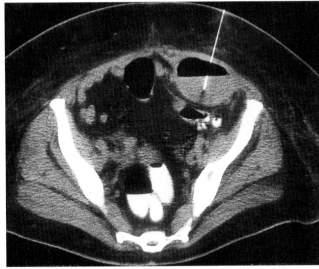

FIGURE 3-7. A, B: Computed tomogram of a patient with perforated sigmoid diverticulitis and associated pericolic abscess (*arrow*). The abscess was amenable to percutaneous drainage. **B:** Needle aspiration of the abscess preparatory to drain placement.

APPROACH TO THE PATIENT WITH ILEUS AND OBSTRUCTION

ROBERT W. SUMMERS ■ CHARLES C. LU

CLINICAL BACKGROUND

A wide spectrum of pathophysiological mechanisms may come into play when ileus or obstruction involves the small and large intestines. The most life-threatening abnormality is ischemic necrosis that occurs as a result of complicated obstruction. When blood flow is compromised, the most vulnerable bowel layer, the mucosa, becomes nonviable. This disrupts the normal functions of absorption and secretion, but more important, it destroys the protective barrier against intralumenal microorganisms. Lethal bacteria and toxins traverse the intestinal wall, causing peritonitis, abscesses, toxemia, and sepsis. The process is accelerated if transmural necrosis and perforation occur. Because of the high mortality rate associated with this complication, prevention is the best clinical plan. Early recognition is not sufficient, because it is often too late to intervene when clinical signs become apparent. Anticipation of this lethal complication and early surgical intervention should be adopted as the therapeutic strategy in many, if not most cases of obstruction of the small and large intestine.

Because of intestinal stasis in progressive obstruction, the normal gram-positive aerobic flora of the small intestine is replaced by anaerobic and gram-negative flora. If ileus or obstruction is incomplete, the result may be maldigestion because of bacterial overgrowth. If the stasis is complete, especially if accompanied by ischemia, severe infectious complications may occur. The same complications may occur as a result of surgical procedures involving enterotomy, making preoperative administration of antibiotics an important therapeutic intervention.

As a result of ileus or obstruction, the normal processes of fluid and electrolyte transport are altered. In the small bowel, secretory processes are enhanced, resulting in accumulation of fluid and electrolytes in the lumen. Normal gastric, biliary, and pancreatic secretions also accumulate, causing vomiting. Oral intake is frequently reduced or absent. Treatment involves correction of fluid and electrolyte losses, restoration of acid-base balance, and provision for maintenance fluid and electrolyte requirements through intravenous infusion.

In addition to fluid in the lumen, gas accumulates largely from swallowed air but also from bacterial metabolism of nutrients. This produces marked dilation of the bowel and abdominal distention, causing abdominal pain, respiratory embarrassment, and changes in intestinal and colonic motility. Initially in obstruction of the small intestine, the peristaltic reflex is activated, causing stimulation of motor activity and abnormal motor patterns proximal to the obstruction and inhibition of motor activity distal to the obstruction. As tension in the wall increases, inhibitory intestinointestinal reflexes are activated, causing progressive inhibition in the gut proximal to the obstruction. Decompression of the dilated bowel should be accomplished by means of intermittent nasogastric aspiration in essentially all cases of ileus and obstruction to relieve symptoms of pressure, vomiting, and pain, and to reduce the risk for perforation and many of the pathophysiological problems described previously.

For both ileus and obstruction, the differential diagnosis is varied and lengthy. Recognition and management of ileus involves recognition and management of the underlying cause of the problem. Surgical therapy must be avoided unless associated emergency disorders exist. However, in most instances of obstruction, the problem is anatomic and mechanical; definitive therapy necessitates surgical intervention in most instances. There are some important exceptions when surgical intervention should be avoided or alternative treatments are preferred. When obstruction is partial, recurrent, and due to prior multiple surgical procedural adhesions, it is usually wise to avoid another operation. Untwisting or decompression of volvulus, laser vaporization of tumors, and pneumatic dilation of strictures are a few of the treatments that can be accomplished with endoscopy. Radiologic and other nonsurgical approaches can provide other therapeutic alternatives.

The laboratory can play an important role in establishing the underlying problem in many cases of ileus, but radiologic techniques are the most useful tools in the differentiation of ileus from obstruction, and in identifying the level and the cause of obstruction.

PLAIN ABDOMINAL RADIOGRAPHS

When clinical suspicion of intestinal obstruction or ileus arises, plain abdominal radiographs (anteroposterior, upright, and supine) are the first radiologic modality to perform. In the normal, unobstructed condition, there is usually some gas in the stomach and colon; in the colon, the gas may or may not be mixed with feces. A small amount of gas may be present in the small intestine of children; however, in adults there is almost none.

In several situations, the radiographic gas patterns on plain radiographs are so characteristic of intestinal obstruction that no further contrast study or other radiologic modality is needed to make a diagnosis. Complete obstruction of the small intestine (Fig. 4-1), mesenteric vascular accident with compromised vascular flow resulting in functional obstruction (Figs. 4-2 and 4-3), volvulus of the sigmoid colon (Fig. 4-4) or the cecum (Fig. 4-5), and toxic megacolon (Fig. 4-6) are some conditions with characteristic radiographic findings. High-grade mechanical obstruction of the postbulb or proximal duodenum may show a double bubble sign, which also is diagnostic (Fig. 4-7).

Sometimes radiographic findings in addition to the intestinal gas pattern help the clinician make specific diagnoses on plain radiographs. Examples are air in the biliary tree in gallstone obstruction (Fig. 4-8), free intraperitoneal air or a calcified appendicolith associated with dilated ileum in perforated appendicitis (Fig. 4-9), presence of calcifications in the pancreas associated with dilation of the bowel from acute exacerbation of pancreatitis causing functional obstruction (Fig. 4-10), or presence of hernia containing a closed loop of intestine (Fig. 4-11).

TESTS AND TREATMENT BEYOND PLAIN ABDOMINAL RADIOGRAPHS

Patients with obstruction generally have episodes of severe cramping abdominal pain and abnormal hyperactive bowel sounds. Those with ileus usually complain of only mild discomfort and have reduced bowel sounds. However, radiographic studies are complementary to the clinical examination. The first study usually considered is the routine plain anteroposterior supine and upright abdominal radiograph. However, there are situations in which plain radiographs are inconclusive and additional studies are needed to establish the underlying diagnosis (Fig. 4-12). Barium contrast studies and abdominal imaging studies, including ultrasonography, computed tomography (CT), and magnetic resonance imaging (MRI), may be helpful to establish a preoperative diagnosis (Fig. 4-13). Abdominal CT and MRI are increasingly used because they can often elucidate the underlying etiology of obstruction (Fig 4-14).

Endoscopy is not ordinarily recommended in this setting because insufflating air into an already dilated bowel may worsen the situation. However, endoscopy can be therapeutic. It can be helpful to aspirate air from a massively dilated colon (acute colonic pseudoobstruction) or to decompress acute sigmoid volvulus. If insufflation is needed, CO_2 can be used instead of air. The use of self-expandable metallic stents, placed endoscopically or radiologically, permits decompression and establishes patency in acute malignant obstruction (Fig 4-15). It should be emphasized that in most situations, differentiating obstruction from ileus is the important decision that governs therapy. In these cases, it is neither useful nor desirable to perform multiple diagnostic tests that would delay appropriate surgical therapy.

DIFFERENTIATION OF ILEUS AND BOWEL OBSTRUCTION

If the loops of small intestine appear equal to or larger than the transverse colon, either right-sided colonic obstruction or small-intestinal obstruction should be considered. A barium enema examination that includes the ileocecal valve is necessary to search for a right hemicolonic lesion (see Fig. 4-5). A small-intestine series may be obtained (Figs. 4-16 through 4-18) for obstruction of the small intestine, but enteroclysis is the examination of choice, particularly for postoperative patients.

Radiologic signs of distal colonic obstruction on plain radiographs of abdomen are dilation of the colon with an empty rectum, marked retention of either solid or liquid stools (Fig. 4-19), and multiple air-fluid levels in the dilated proximal colon (Fig. 4-20). The small intestine may or may not be dilated, but the loops of small bowel proximal to the transverse colon retain a diameter smaller than that of the transverse colon (Fig. 4-21). This picture can be confused with that of paralytic ileus, but the issue can be resolved with performance of a barium enema examination or colonoscopy.

Differentiation of ileus from mechanical obstruction is usually but not always possible with plain abdominal radiographs (Fig. 4-22). In ileus, both the colon and small bowel are dilated, and the diameter of the colon is greater than that of the ileum. In such cases, administration of contrast medium is essential to determine the presence or absence of obstruction. Before administering barium into the upper gastrointestinal tract, it is critical to establish that the level of obstruction is not in the colon. If barium is given orally and reaches an obstruction in the colon, it stops at that point. Water is extracted, and the barium forms a cement-like concretion that is difficult and hazardous to remove surgically. If *there is any question* about colonic obstruction, a barium enema examination should be performed first.

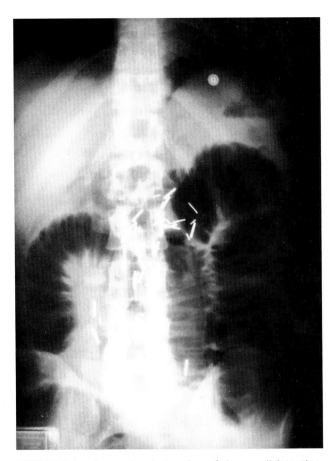

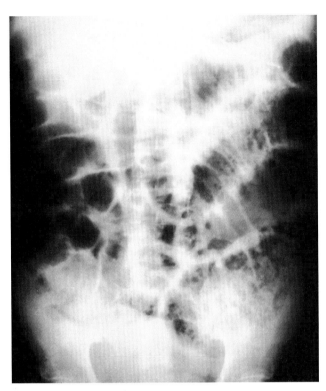

FIGURE 4-1. Complete obstruction of the small intestine. Multiple loops of the dilated small intestine are present on this upright abdominal radiograph without noticeable colonic gas in this acutely ill, middle-aged woman. The findings suggest mechanical obstruction of the small intestine. Numerous surgical clips testify to previous operations. Multiple adhesions causing obstruction were found in the distal jejunum at operation.

FIGURE 4-2. Mesenteric ischemia (ileus). Several loops of small intestine located on the left side of the abdomen appear irregular and distended with gas bubbles. A large amount of gas is present in the rest of the small intestine. A small amount of air is present in the colon. Ischemic enteritis was suspected because of these findings, and the patient underwent an operation. A loop of necrotic jejunum measuring 80 cm in length was resected.

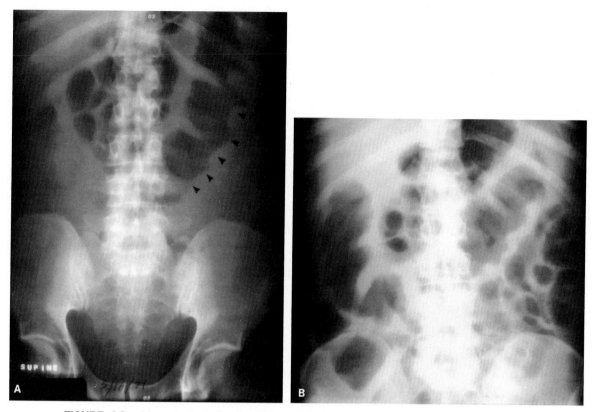

FIGURE 4-3. Mesenteric ischemia (ileus). This patient was admitted to the emergency department because of the sudden onset of abdominal pain, distention, weakness, and low-grade fever. **A:** On the first plain radiograph of the abdomen, the right colon and transverse colon are distended with gas and demonstrate a scalloped margin (*arrowheads*) and thickened edematous haustra. Acute ischemic enterocolitis was suspected. After 2 days of observation, the general condition deteriorated and more abdominal distention was observed clinically. **B:** The follow-up radiograph reveals similar but more pronounced findings. An emergency operation confirmed the diagnosis of thromboembolic occlusion of the ileocolic branches of the superior mesenteric artery, resulting in necrosis of the distal 35 cm of ileum and proximal colon, including the right four fifths of the transverse colon.

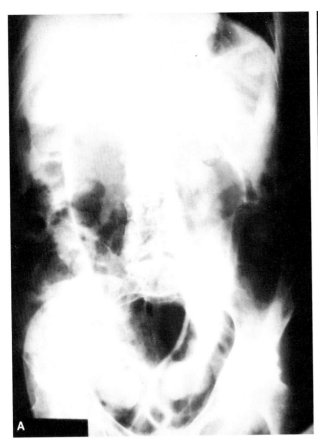

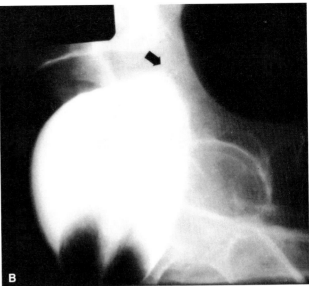

FIGURE 4-4. Sigmoid volvulus. **A:** The plain abdominal radiograph shows a markedly distended loop of colon overlying the spine. This so-called coffee bean sign is the characteristic appearance of sigmoid volvulus. Barium enema examination was ordered for both confirmatory and therapeutic purposes. **B:** Barium did not pass beyond the tapered narrowing ("beaking") where the colon is twisted (*arrow*). Operation confirmed the diagnosis of sigmoid volvulus without necrosis.

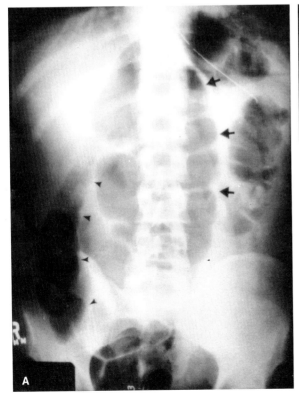

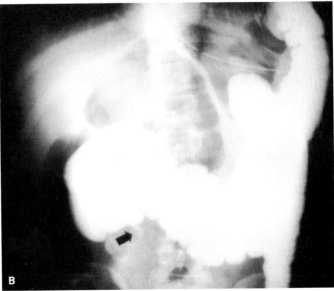

FIGURE 4-5. Cecal volvulus. **A:** An enormously distended cecum (*arrows*) and a long segment of dilated ileum (*arrowheads*) are demonstrated on this radiograph of an acutely ill patient. **B:** A characteristic feature of cecal volvulus; however, for therapeutic purposes a barium enema study was performed. No release of the obstruction was obtained, but beaking of the twisted site is demonstrated (*arrow*). At operation, surgical resection was performed of a gangrenous cecum and distal ileum resulting from compromised vascular flow.

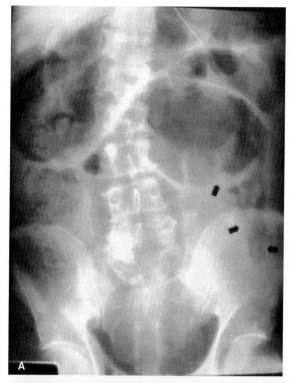

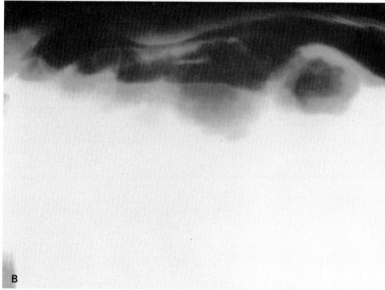

FIGURE 4-6. Toxic megacolon and perforated viscus. A patient with a history of ulcerative colitis suddenly became ill and had nausea, vomiting, and abdominal cramping pain. This was accompanied by progressive abdominal distention. **A:** Plain radiograph of the abdomen shows distended colon with absence of normal haustra. The mucosal surface is nodular (*arrows*). Toxic megacolon was suspected. **B:** Four hours later, the patient's condition suddenly deteriorated. The follow-up lateral decubitus radiograph reveals a large amount of free air collected in the right paracolic gutter. Emergency operation confirmed the radiographic diagnosis. Perforation was found in the diseased cecum, and total colectomy was performed.

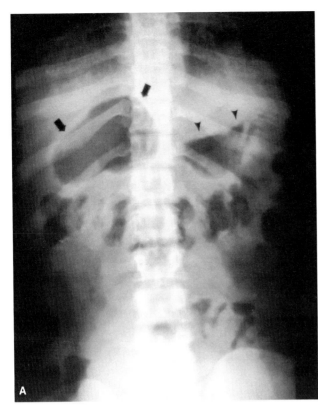

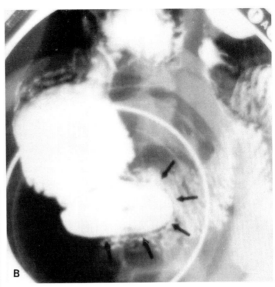

FIGURE 4-7. Duodenal obstruction. A 19-year-old man had frequent epigastric pain and bilious vomiting after meals. **A:** Plain supine abdominal radiograph demonstrates a dilated proximal duodenum (*arrows*) and air collection in the gastric antrum (*arrowheads*); this is routinely called the double bubble sign. It is characteristic of obstruction of the second portion of the duodenal loop. **B:** Barium meal study of the upper gastrointestinal tract discloses a duplication cyst in the inferior flexure of the duodenal loop (*arrows*).

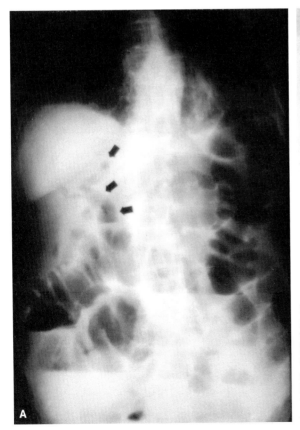

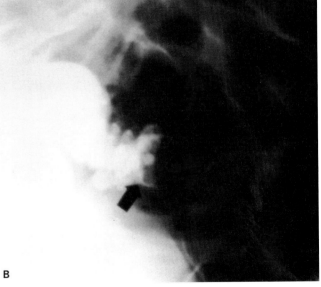

FIGURE 4-8. Gallstone obstruction. **A:** A collection of air is present in the biliary tree (*arrows*) of this acutely ill patient with gaseous distention, obstipation, and occasional cramping abdominal pain. Gallstone obstruction in the distal part of the colon was suspected. **B:** Barium enema study discloses an impacted stone (*arrow*) in the midsigmoid colon. The stone had eroded through the gallbladder into the adjacent hepatic flexure of the colon.

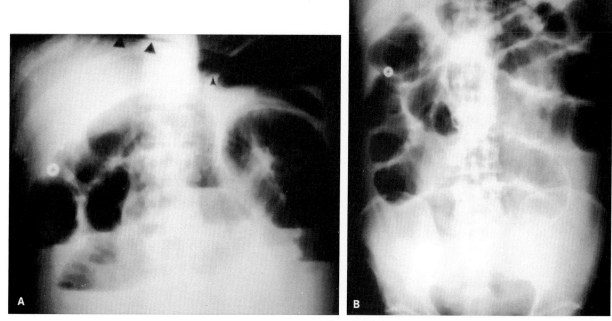

FIGURE 4-9. Ileus caused by peritonitis. A young woman had a 3-day history of abdominal pain associated with fever and vomiting. These plain abdominal radiographs show free air in both subphrenic apices (*arrowheads*) (**A**) and a large amount of gas distending the ileum (**B**), suggesting a perforated viscus. Emergency operation disclosed a perforated appendix and peritonitis.

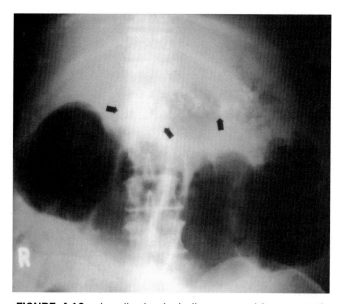

FIGURE 4-10. Localized colonic ileus caused by pancreatitis. This plain abdominal radiograph reveals diffuse calcifications of the pancreas (*arrows*), indicating chronic pancreatitis. The markedly distended transverse colon abruptly ends at the splenic flexure ("colon cut-off sign"). This finding and an elevated serum amylase level strongly suggest the diagnosis of an acute exacerbation of pancreatitis with functional colonic obstruction (localized ileus).

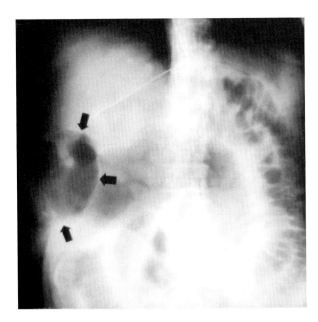

FIGURE 4-11. Closed-loop right colonic obstruction caused by incisional hernia. This patient underwent cholecystectomy 25 years ago, and intermittent protrusion of a hernia had been observed in the incision site for the last 5 to 6 years. The patient suddenly experienced crampy abdominal pain and abdominal distention. The plain radiograph demonstrates the presence of surgical sutures within a herniated segment of colon in the incisional hernia (*arrows*). The cecum and a long segment of ileum are distended by gas. Also present is nodularity of the cecal mucosa, which suggests edema of the intestinal loop proximal to the mechanical obstruction. The hernia was repaired surgically, but it was not necessary to resect any of the involved intestine.

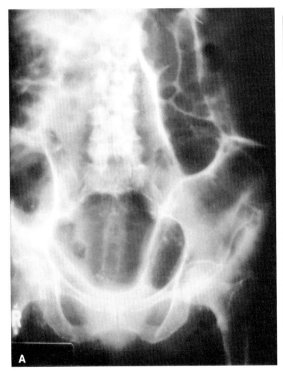

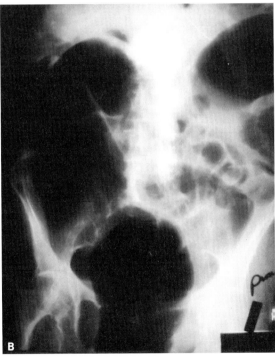

FIGURE 4-12. Pseudoobstruction of the colon. Heavily medicated patients from long-term care institutions or psychiatric hospitals often have bouts of severe distention, commonly from gas in the colon. It is necessary to differentiate this from fecal impaction or organic obstruction. In many instances the problem may be most simply resolved by changing the patient's position during the procedure, especially from the prone position, and repeating the radiograph. **A:** Plain radiograph of the abdomen in the supine position was obtained on this patient from a long-term care institution because of progressive abdominal distention. **B:** To rule out mechanical obstruction of the distal colon, an additional prone recumbent radiograph was obtained. A huge gas-distended rectum makes mechanical obstruction unlikely if the rectal examination is normal.

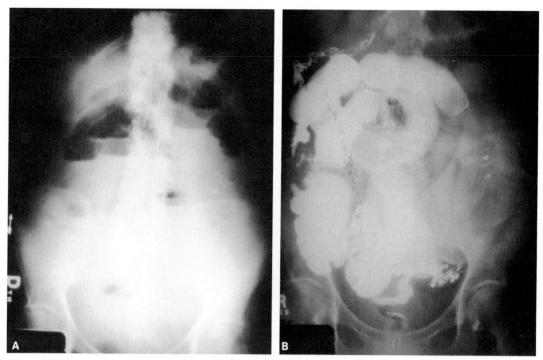

FIGURE 4-13. Chronic pseudoobstruction of the intestine. The differential diagnosis between adynamic ileus and mechanical obstruction is frequently a challenge to both clinicians and radiologists. Multiple air-fluid levels in a "stepladder" pattern were once believed to be specific for mechanical obstruction. However, such findings also are seen among patients with adynamic ileus or visceral myopathy. Spinal and upright radiographs of abdomen were obtained on this patient believed to have had recurrent episodes of obstructive symptoms since childhood. **A:** The upright radiograph appears to have multiple air-fluid levels in a "stepladder" pattern in the distended small bowel. **B:** Barium enema study was performed, and a large amount of barium refluxed into the small intestine. No obstruction was found at any level. The diagnosis of pseudoobstruction from idiopathic visceral myopathy was made from a surgical specimen.

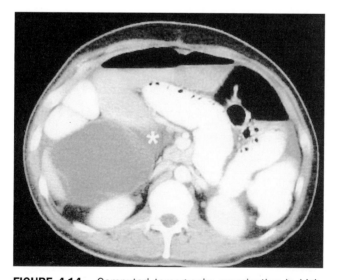

FIGURE 4-14. Computed tomography examination in high-grade obstruction of the small bowel by mesenteric spread of gastric cancer. Note the contrast-filled loops of small bowel are moderately dilated. However, contrast has not yet passed to the point of obstruction (*asterisk*), where small bowel loops are fluid-filled and massively dilated. (Courtesy of Dr. Bruce Brown.)

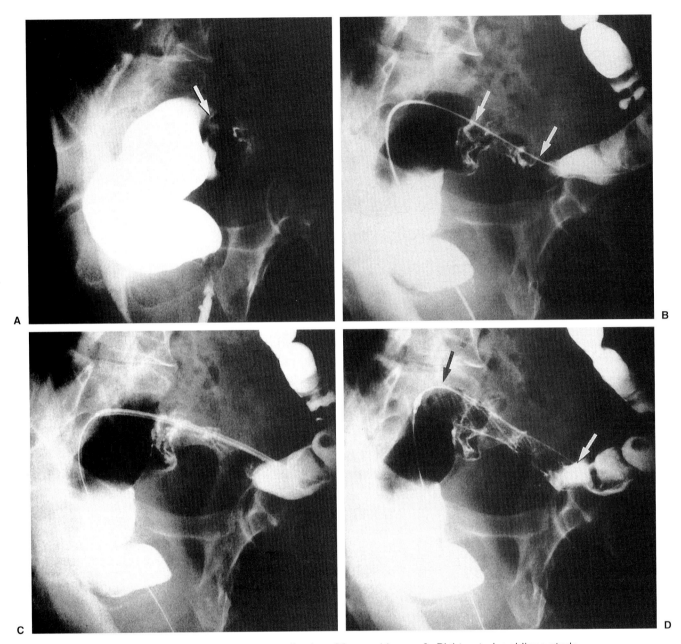

FIGURE 4-15.   Barium enema studies in a 69-year-old man. **A:** Right anterior oblique study shows a tight colorectal stenosis (*arrow*). **B:** After the hydrophilic guidewire and an angiographic catheter were guided through the area of occlusion, nonionic contrast material was injected to define the anatomy of the proximal and distal regions of the lesion (*arrows*) and to rule out colonic perforation. **C:** The guidewire is replaced by an Amplatz stiff guidewire, and the delivery system has been introduced. **D:** Radiograph reveals deployment of the stent (*arrows*), which is fully expanded.

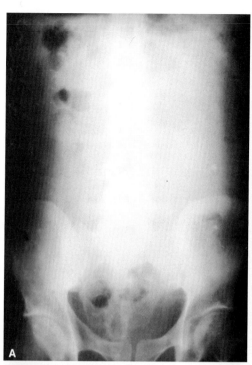

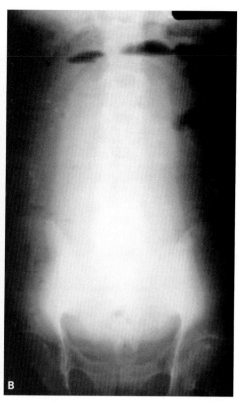

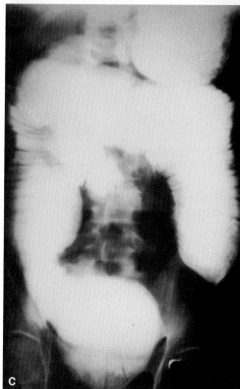

FIGURE 4-16. Obstruction of the small intestine caused by Crohn's disease. In chronic small-intestinal obstruction, plain radiographs of the abdomen occasionally show only a small amount of air in distended bowel loops because of the accumulation of a large amount of fluid within the lumen. Plain abdominal radiographs were ordered because of progressive abdominal distention and other signs of intestinal obstruction in this young woman with a long history of ileal Crohn's disease. **A:** In the supine view a large amount of fluid has accumulated in the dilated small intestine lumen, giving it a ground glass appearance. An erroneous interpretation may be "no evidence of obstruction." **B:** Multiple, small air-fluid levels are demonstrated in the upright position. **C:** Barium meal study revealed an enormously dilated jejunum and proximal ileum. A barium meal study 2 years earlier had revealed a segment of narrowed ileum with mild proximal dilation. A severely stenotic segment of ileum was resected at laparotomy.

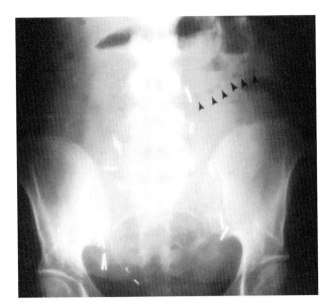

FIGURE 4-17. Obstruction of the small intestine caused by metastatic disease. If a string of beads sign occurs within larger gas bubbles, this finding is diagnostic of mechanical obstruction. This occurs when gas bubbles are trapped in the recesses of valvulae conniventes in the upright or decubitus position while a large amount of fluid is retained in these dilated loops. This 32-year-old woman had a previous pelvic operation for uterine leiomyosarcoma that was followed by radiation therapy. A typical string of beads sign (*arrowheads*) is present on this upright radiograph. Numerous metastases at multiple levels from the distal jejunum to the proximal ileum were found at a subsequent operation to be causing high-grade obstruction of the small intestine.

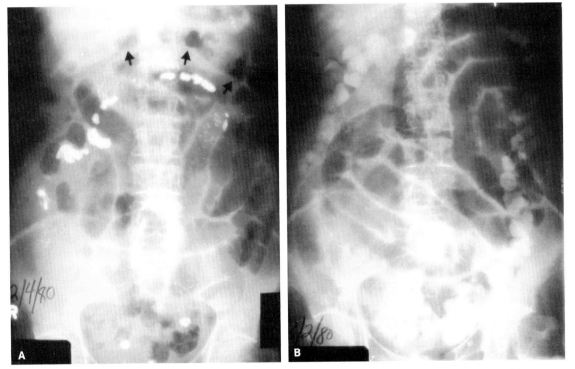

FIGURE 4-18. Small-intestinal obstruction caused by ileocecal carcinoma. An 82-year-old woman had intermittent cramping, abdominal pain, and progressive abdominal distention. **A:** Plain abdominal radiograph obtained 1 month earlier reveals the small intestine to be distended with gas and a small amount of barium. Colonic gas is scanty and scattered (*arrows*). **B:** The admission radiograph shows increased accumulation of gas in the entire small intestine to the terminal ileum. The barium retained in the colon is from a normal-appearing barium enema examination 1 day earlier. These findings indicate ileocecal obstruction. At operation the patient was found to have cancer of the ileocecal valve.

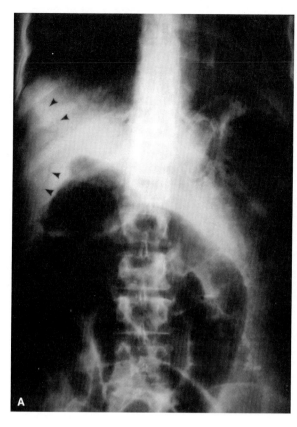

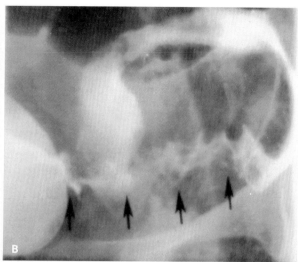

FIGURE 4-19. Colonic obstruction caused by sigmoid carcinoma. **A:** Plain supine abdominal radiograph shows a large amount of liquid stool throughout the colon. The ileum is dilated, but the diameter is less than that of the transverse colon. An incidental finding was the presence of gas in the portal venous system of the liver (*arrows*). This is believed to occur when severe dilation from an obstructing lesion causes compromise of the mucosal blood supply, mucosal necrosis, and pneumatosis. Gas in the portal venous blood is then transported to the liver. **B:** Follow-up barium enema examination showed obstructing sigmoid cancer (*arrows*).

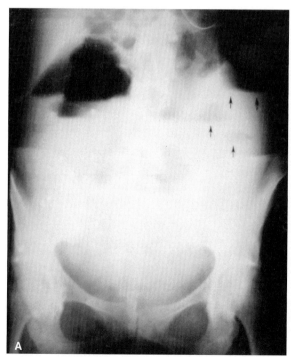

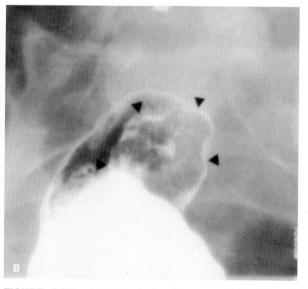

FIGURE 4-20. Colonic obstruction caused by sigmoid carcinoma. **A:** This upright abdominal radiograph reveals multiple air-fluid levels (*arrows*) in the dilated left hemicolon with no gas distally. **B:** Barium enema reveals complete obstruction of the sigmoid colon by a concentric cancer (*arrowheads*). Air-fluid levels in the distal colon are almost always caused by mechanical obstruction if they are not caused by recent cleansing enemas.

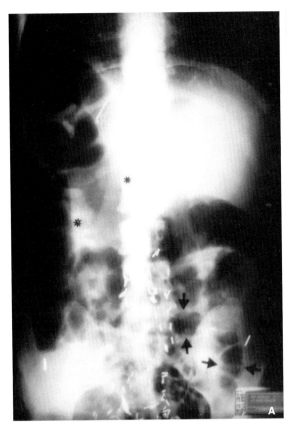

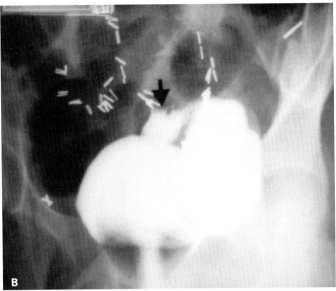

FIGURE 4-21. Colonic obstruction caused by sigmoid carcinoma. **A:** Plain abdominal radiograph reveals dilated small intestine and colon. The diameter of the small bowel (*arrows*) remains smaller than that of the transverse colon (*asterisks*). Fluid levels are present in the descending colon. Surgical clips in the lower lumbar and pelvic region are from a previous operation for ovarian cancer. **B:** Barium enema study reveals simple adhesion (*arrow*) at the level of the distal sigmoid. No tumor recurrence was found at subsequent laparotomy.

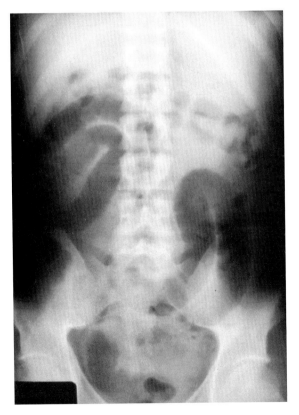

FIGURE 4-22. Mechanical obstruction of the small intestine. This supine radiograph of the abdomen was taken of a 29-year-old man with a 12-hour history of severe periumbilical pain. Multiple dilated loops of the small intestine are almost as large as the transverse colon, suggesting the diagnosis of mechanical obstruction of the small intestine. At operation, a large Meckel diverticulum filled with vegetable matter had undergone torsion, causing mechanical obstruction. No perforation was present.

APPROACH TO THE PATIENT WITH DIARRHEA

DON W. POWELL

Diarrheal diseases have quite different prevalences and outcomes in developed and developing countries (Figs. 5-1 through 5-3). Infant and child mortality rates decreased in developing nations from 5 million a year in 1987 to 3.5 million a year in 1995. The infant mortality rate from diarrheal diseases in the United States is stable at 300 to 500 deaths per year over the same period. In the United States, the death rate from diarrhea among persons older than 74 years is nearly ten times that of infants, children, and younger adults.

Diarrhea (stool volumes greater than 200 mL/24 h) results from alterations in water and electrolyte transport mediated through changes in intracellular messengers (Figs. 5-4 and 5-5) or from unabsorbed osmotic solutes that retain fluid within the intestinal lumen. Inflammatory diarrhea causes systemic symptoms through the release of cytokines (Fig. 5-6).

Acute diarrhea is defined as that less than 2 to 3 weeks in duration. The most common causes are infections (Table 5-1). The incidence of diarrhea is high in daycare centers (Table 5-2) and hospitals (Table 5-3). Consolidation of the food industry, the increased number of and use of fast-food restaurants and a change in eating habits in industrialized nations has led to a marked increase in food-borne illness and diarrheal disease. The illnesses may be caused by ingestion of toxins (Tables 5-4 through 5-6) or infection with microorganisms (Fig. 5-7). Various algorithms have been made to guide physicians in the investigation and management of acute diarrhea (Fig. 5-8). A key feature in most diagnostic algorithms is the presence or absence of fecal leukocytes (Table 5-7). Management of diarrhea can be symptomatic and primarily involves rehydration (Tables 5-8 and 5-9); in specific instances, antimicrobial therapy may be used (Tables 5-10 and 5-11). The various bacteria are most sensitive to specific antibiotics; however, trimethoprim-sulfamethoxazole and fluoroquinolones are effective management of most enteric organisms. *Campylobacter* infections require erythromycin. Traveler's diarrhea (Fig. 5-9; Table 5-12) and acquired immunodeficiency syndrome diarrhea (Fig. 5-10; Table 5-13) are special forms of diarrheal disease that require a different approach.

Chronic diarrhea is that which lasts longer than 3 to 6 weeks. It may be caused by malabsorption, intestinal secretory states, or intestinal inflammation. The classic example of a malabsorptive disease is celiac sprue (Table 5-14). In infancy and childhood, the manifestations are recognized with chronic severe malnutrition and include abnormal hair growth as seen in the eyelashes (Fig. 5-11). The diagnosis of celiac disease will be facilitated by new serologic tests, especially antiimmunoglobulin A (IgA) and anti-IgG tests against tissue transglutaminase (tTG), which promises to make the antigliadin (AGA) and antiendomysial antibody tests (AEA) obsolete (Table 5-15). Treatment of celiac disease is the strict dietary exclusion of gluten, which may be difficult (Tables 5-16 and 5-17). Celiac disease support groups are useful to educate patients with this disease (Table 5-18). Despite attempted gluten exclusion, some patients do not respond and must be further evaluated (Fig. 5-12). Whipple disease is another malabsorptive disease. Like celiac sprue, it has an inflammatory component that causes many systemic symptoms, including arthritis (Table 5-19). The infectious agent of Whipple disease can invade the central nervous system and cause severe and drastic complications (Table 5-20). Treatment of Whipple disease is depicted in Fig. 5-13. The steatorrhea of celiac sprue sometimes can be differentiated from that of pancreatic exocrine insufficiency on clinical grounds alone (Table 5-21). Steatorrhea is the clinical hallmark of malabsorption (Fig. 5-14). Abnormal qualitative stool-fat findings, if the examination is properly performed (Figs. 5-15 and 5-16) lead the physician to initiate an evaluation for malabsorption. Severe diarrhea of any type (e.g., secretory diarrhea or osmotic diarrhea from MgOH ingestion) can cause mild steatorrhea and mislead the clinician to a diagnosis of generalized malabsorption (Fig. 5-17). Endoscopic duodenal biopsy (Fig. 5-18) may be the best way to differentiate intestinal from pancreatic malabsorption. A D-xylose absorption test is much less frequently used in adult medicine because of the various factors that affect its interpretation (Table 5-22). Radiography of the small intestine is of only limited value in the diagnosis of intestinal malabsorptive diseases (Fig. 5-19).

Malabsorption of carbohydrate alone causes watery diarrhea. The most common cause of carbohydrate malabsorption is lactose intolerance, a condition prevalent throughout the world (Fig. 5-20). The use of the nonabsorbable carbohydrate sorbitol to sweeten dietetic chewing gum and candy also can cause diarrhea (Tables 5-23 and 5-24). Sorbitol also is present in some fruits (see Table 5-23) and medicines (Table 5-25). Diarrhea caused by the high sorbitol content of liquid medicine is called *elixir diarrhea*. Fructose is the primary sugar in fruit juice and is often used as a sweetener for soft drinks; some persons also malabsorb fructose.

Secretory diarrhea may be caused by activation of various endogenous regulating systems (Fig. 5-21), factitious ingestion of laxatives, use of drugs, or endocrine tumors. Factitious diarrhea is the most common of the secretory type and may be recognized with several characteristic clinical features (Tables 5-26 and 5-27), including the finding of melanosis coli at sigmoidoscopy (Fig. 5-22). When secretory diarrhea is suspected, a cathartic screening test should be performed on the stool specimen. Such screening tests lead to a search for the agents listed in Table 5-28 and for magnesium and PO_4. The docusates (dioctyl sodium sulfosuccinate) may not be available in the screen, and phenolphthalein is off the market now in the United States. Neuroendocrine tumors are fairly rare, but they result in devastating, high-volume secretory diarrhea because of the elaboration of secretory hormones (Tables 5-29 and 5-30). Pancreatic endocrine tumors that secrete vasoactive intestinal polypeptide (VIP) are a cause of secretory diarrhea. Suspicion of these tumors can be confirmed with various blood and urine tests (Table 5-31). Octreotide therapy can be useful to control symptoms, pending surgical intervention (Fig. 5-23).

Stool electrolyte measurements and the response to fast often are helpful in sorting out the cause of diarrhea (Fig. 5-24). Secretory diarrheas generally do not decrease on fast to volumes less than 200 mL/24 h unless the secretory state is mild, as in collagenous or microscopic colitis. Determination of the osmotic gap in the stool can be useful in differentiating secretory from osmotic diarrhea. Fermentation of nonabsorbed carbohydrate by intestinal bacteria increases the osmolality of stool after it is passed into the container and during storage before testing (Table 5-32). Because of their effect on colonic bacteria, antibiotics also alter stool electrolyte content. Stool sodium concentrations less than 50 mEq/L with osmotic gaps more than 100 mOsm are characteristic of osmotic diarrhea, whereas stool sodium concentrations greater than 100 mEq/L and osmotic gaps less than 50 to 100 mOsm are classic for secretory diarrhea (Table 5-33). Specific congenital diarrhea can be suspected in infants and children because of changes in stool chloride or sodium content (Table 5-34). Congenital secretory diarrheas, e.g., microvillus inclusion disease (Fig. 5-25), may cause stool electrolyte excretion like that of the adult pancreatic cholera syndrome. Inflammatory diarrhea may be caused in part by ulceration of the mucosa, malabsorption caused by crypt hyperplasia, and intestinal secretion stimulated by inflammatory mediators (Fig. 5-26).

Many causes of diarrhea can be diagnosed on the basis of history, physical examination, and routine blood tests (Fig. 5-27). A stool examination for microorganisms, blood, and fat and a colonic biopsy bring the diagnostic yield to 75% to 80%. The remaining 20% of cases are elusive diarrheas that necessitate hospitalization and extensive testing.

The management of mild diarrhea is best accomplished with drugs, such as opiates, that alter intestinal motility. The somatostatin analog octreotide has been shown to be useful in the management of neuroendocrine tumors. Somatostatin inhibits secretion of peptide hormones by the tumor (Fig. 5-28), and this is accompanied by marked reduction in the secretory diarrhea (Fig. 5-29).

(figures begin on page 64)

TABLE 5-1

Clinical Presentations and Likely Causes of Acute Diarrheal Disease in an Outpatient Setting

CLINICAL TYPE	APPROXIMATE PERCENTAGE OF PATIENTS	LIKELY CAUSE	
		Industrialized Countries	*Less-developed Countries*
Watery diarrhea	90	Rotavirus, other viruses	Rotavirus, ETEC, EPEC, *Campylobacter jejuni*
Dysentery	5–10	*Shigella*, EIEC, *C jejuni*	*Shigella*, EIEC, *C jejuni*, *Entamoeba histolytica*
Protracted diarrhea (>14 d)	3–4	EPEC, *Giardia*, *Yersinia*	EPEC, *Giardia*
Severe purging with rice-water stool	1 (higher in cholera-endemic areas)	*Salmonella*, ETEC	*Vibrio cholerae*, ETEC
Hemorrhagic colitis	<1?	EHEC	EHEC

EIEC, enteroinvasive *Escherichia coli*; EHEC, enterohemorrhagic *E coli*; EPEC, enteropathogenic *E coli*; ETEC, enterotoxigenic *E coli*.

From DiJohn D, Levine MR. Treatment of diarrhea. Infect Dis Clin North Am 1988;2:719.

TABLE 5-2
Causes of Diarrhea in Day-care Centers in the United States

ORGANISM	ATTACK RATE (%)	SECONDARY ATTACK RATE* (%)
Rotavirus	71–100	15–79
Shigella	33–73	26–46
Campylobacter jejuni	20–50	?
Clostridium difficile	32	?
Giardia lamblia	17–90	12–50
Cryptosporidium sp	to 50–65	14

*Among family members.

From Guerrant RL, Hughes JM, Lima NL, Crane J. Diarrhea in developed and developing countries: magnitude, special settings, and etiologies. Rev Infect Dis 1990;12 [Suppl 1]:541.

TABLE 5-3
Causes of Nosocomial Diarrhea

ORGANISM	PERCENTAGE OF PATIENTS STUDIED WITH INDICATED DIARRHEAL CAUSE	
	Marrow Transplant Patients*	Medical Pediatric Patients†
Clostridium difficile	15% (12/78)	52% (11/21)
Salmonella	0	3% (1/30)
Rotavirus	12% (9/78)	38% (3/8)
Adenovirus	15% (12/78)	ND
Coxsackievirus	5% (4/78)	ND

ND, not done.

*At Johns Hopkins Hospital.

†At University of Virginia Hospital.

From Guerrant RL, Hughes JM, Lima NL, Crane J. Diarrhea in developed and developing countries: magnitude, special settings, and etiologies. Rev Infect Dis 1990;12 [Suppl 1]:541.

TABLE 5-4
Clinical Diagnosis of Food–borne Illness by Incubation Period and Symptoms

PREDOMINANT SYMPTOM	INCUBATION PERIOD			
	<2 h	1–7 h	8–14 h	>14 h
Upper intestinal, nausea/ vomiting	Heavy metals, chemicals, mushrooms	Staphylococcus aureus, Bacillus cereus, Anisakis	Anisakis	Norwalk agent
Noninflammatory, diarrhea, no fecal leukocytes Inflammatory, ileocolitis			Clostridium perfringens, B cereus	Enterotoxigenic Escherichia coli, Vibrio cholerae, Giardia lamblia, Norwalk agent Salmonella, Shigella sp, Campylobacter sp, invasive E coli, Vibrio parahaemolyticus, Entamoeba histolytica
Extragastrointestinal, neurologic	Insecticides, mushroom and plant toxins, monosodium glutamate, shellfish, scombroid	Shellfish, ciguatera	Botulism	

From Aucott JN. Food poisoning. In: Blaser MJ, et al., eds. Infections of the gastrointestinal tract. New York: Raven Press, 1995:237.

TABLE 5-5
Naturally Occurring Fish and Shellfish Toxins

POISONING	TOXIN	CLINICAL SYNDROME
Ciguatera	Dinoflagellate toxin from reef algae ingested by tropical fish: amberjack, snapper, grouper, and barracuda	Gastrointestinal (diarrhea, nausea, vomiting, abdominal pain) and neurological symptoms (hot-cold inversion, muscle aches, perioral numbness and tingling, metallic taste, weakness, paresthesias, dizziness, and sweating
Diarrhetic shellfish poisoning	Okadaic acid, in certain marine phytoplankton ingested by bivalve mollusks (mussels, clams, oysters, scallops) in Japan, Spain, and Chile	Gastrointestinal symptoms (diarrhea, nausea, vomiting, abdominal pain)
Paralytic shellfish poisoning	Dinoflagellates ingested by bivalve "mollusks" in New England waters and Alaska, Washington, and California	Neurological symptoms as above but more severe and possibly proceeding to respiratory paralysis and death
Neurotoxic shellfish poisoning	Brevetoxin in red tide algae in Gulf of Mexico	Neurological symptoms as above but milder and transient (hours or days)
Estuarine toxin or *Pfiesteria piscicida* poisoning	Toxin of the dinoflagellate *Pfiesteria piscicida* ingested by fish in the Albemarle-Pamlico estuary of the southeastern United States	Neurological symptoms as above. Effects on humans only now (1998) being clarified
Puffer fish poisoning	Tetrodotoxin contained in puffer fish eaten predominantly in Japan	Neurological symptoms as above. May cause respiratory paralysis and death (20–200 deaths per year)

Adapted from Ahmed FE, ed. Seafood safety. Washington, DC: National Academy Press, 1991, and Morris JG Jr. Natural toxins associated with fish and shellfish. In: Blaser MJ, et al., eds. Infections of the gastrointestinal tract. New York: Raven Press, 1995:251.

TABLE 5-6
Toxin–related Food Poisoning

CAUSE	FOOD	INCUBATION PERIOD	DURATION	VOMITING	DIARRHEA	FEVER
Preformed toxin						
Staphylococcus aureus	Meat, egg salad, pastries	1–6 h	<12 h	Present	Rare	Rare
Bacillus cereus (emetic)	Fried rice	1–6 h	<12 h	Present	Rare	Rare
Toxin production in vivo						
B cereus (diarrheal)	Meat, vegetables	6–24 h	<24 h	Rare	Present	Rare
Clostridium perfringens	Meat, gravy	6–24 h	<24 h	Rare	Present	Rare
Vibrio cholerae	Shellfish	16–72 h	5–7 d	Rare	Present	Absent
ETEC	Vegetables, meat	16–72 h	3–5 d	Rare	Present	Rare
EHEC	Meat, dairy products	1–8 d	3–6 d	Rare	Present	Rare

EHEC, enterohemorrhagic *Escherichia coli*; ETEC, enterotoxigenic *E coli*.

From Afgani B, Stutman HR. Toxin-related diarrheas. Pediatr Ann 1994;23:549.

TABLE 5-7
Fecal Leukocytes in Intestinal Infections

PRESENT	VARIABLE	ABSENT
Shigella sp	*Salmonella* sp	*Vibrio cholerae*
Campylobacter sp	*Yersinia* sp	Toxigenic *Escherichia coli*
Invasive *E coli*	*Vibrio parahaemolyticus*	Enteropathogenic *E coli*
	Clostridium difficile (antibiotic-associated colitis)	Adenovirus (enteric)
		Rotavirus
		Coronavirus
		Norwalk virus
		Astrovirus
		Giardia lamblia
		Entamoeba histolytica
		Staphylococcus aureus
		Clostridium perfringens
		Bacillus cereus

From Thorne GM. Diagnosis of infectious diarrheal diseases. Infect Dis Clin North Am 1988;2:747.

TABLE 5-8
Signs and Symptoms of Dehydration Among Patients with Diarrhea

	OUTCOME		
EXAMINATION	No Signs of Dehydration	Some Dehydration	Severe Dehydration
Look at			
Mental status	Well, alert	Restless, irritable*	Lethargic or unconscious; floppy infant*
Eyes	Normal	Sunken	Very sunken and dry
Tears	Present	Absent	Absent
Mouth, tongue	Moist	Dry	Very dry
Thirst	Drinks normally, not thirsty	Thirsty, drinks eagerly*	Drinks poorly or not able to drink*
Feel			
Skin pinch	Goes back rapidly	Goes back slowly*	Goes back very slowly*
Pulse	Normal	Faster than normal*	Very fast, weak, or nonpalpable*
Fontanelle	Normal	Sunken	Very sunken
Decide degree of dehydration	No signs of dehydration, <2.5% of body weight	If two or more of these signs exist, including at least one important* sign, then there is *some* dehydration, 2.5%–10% of body weight	If two or more of these signs exist, including at least one important sign, then there is *severe* dehydration, >10% of body weight

*Important signs and symptoms for assessment of dehydration.
Adapted from Swerdlow DL, Ries AA. Cholera in the Americas. JAMA 1992;267:1495.

TABLE 5-9
Composition of Some Currently Available and Experimental Oral Rehydration Solutions

SOLUTION	Na$^+$ (mmol/L)	K$^+$ (mmol/L)	Cl$^-$ (mmol/L)	HCO$_3^-$ (mmol/L)	CITRATE (mmol/L)	GLUCOSE (mmol/L)	RICE DERIVATIVE OR GLUCOSE POLYMER	OSMOLALITY (mOsm/Kg)
WHO (formula C)*	90	20	80	—	10	111	—	311
WHO (formula B)*	90	20	80	30	—	111	—	331
BP 1993[†]	90	20	80	—	10	111	—	311
USP 23[†]	90	20	80	—	10	111	—	311
Diocalm Junior‖ (SmithKline Beecham, Philadelphia)	60	20	50	—	10	111	—	251
Dioralyte‖ (Rhone-Poulenc Rorer, Collegeville, PA)	60	20	60	—	10	90	—	240
Elecrolade‖ (Searle, Chicago, IL)	50	20	40	30	—	111	—	251
Gluco-Lyte‖ (Eastern, Smithtown, PA)	35	20	37	18	—	200	—	310
Infalyte¶ (Cupal, U.K.)	50	25	45	—	34	—	30[††]	200
Pedialyte¶ (Mead Johnson, Princeton, NJ)	45	20	35	—	30	139	—	269
Rapolyte‖ (Jannsen, U.K.)	60	20	50	—	10	111	—	251
Rehidrat‖,# (Searle, U.K.)	50	20	50	20	9	91	—	336
Rehydralyte¶ (Ross)	75	20	65	—	30	139	—	329
Resol¶ (Wyeth-Ayerst, Philadelphia)	50	20	50	—	34	111	—	265
Experimental rice-based solution**	60	20	60	—	10	—	17.4‖‖	140
Experimental glucose polymer-based solution[††]	60	20	60	—	10	—	18¶¶	168

UNICEF, United Nations International Children's Emergency Fund; WHO, World Health Organization.

*WHO/UNICEF universal solution.

[†]From the British Pharmacopeia.

[†]From the U.S. Pharmacopeia/National Formulary.

‖Currently available in the United Kingdom (British National Formulary 1996).

¶Currently available in the United States.

#Also contains sucrose (94 mmol/L) and fructose (2 mmol/L).

**Rice-based experimental polymer oral rehydration solution used by Thillainayagam et al.

[††]An experimental polymeric oral rehydration solution used by Thillainayagam et al.

[††]Rice syrup solids (g/L).

‖‖Ground rice powder (g/L).

¶¶A defined glucose polymer of mean chain length five glucose molecules (mmol/L).

From Thillainayagam AV, Hunt JB, Farthing MJE. Enhancing clinical efficacy of oral therapy: is low osmolality the key? Gastroenterology 1998;114:197.

TABLE 5-10

Relative Indications for Use of Antimicrobial Agents in Diarrheal Disease of Established Cause

CLEARLY INDICATED	INDICATED IN SOME SITUATIONS	NOT INDICATED
Shigellosis	Nontyphoidal salmonellosis (in infants	Rotavirus infection
Cholera	<12 wk of age and	Other viral infections
Traveler's diarrhea*	immunocompromised hosts)	Nontyphoidal salmonellosis
Amebiasis	EPEC (nursery outbreaks)	Cryptosporidiosis
Giardiasis	EIEC	
	Campylobacter infection (early	
	treatment of dysentery)	
	Clostridium difficile colitis	
	(Protracted *Yersinia* infection)	
	Noncholera *Vibrio* infection	

*Enterotoxigenic *Escherichia coli* is the most common cause of acute traveler's diarrhea, and certain antibiotics are highly effective.

EIEC, enteroinvasive *E coli;* EPEC, enteropathogenic *E coli.*

From DiJohn D, Levine MR. Treatment of diarrhea. Infect Dis Clin North Am 1988;2:719.

TABLE 5-11

Patients Who Receive Antimicrobial Therapy for Infections Accompanied by Diarrhea

No one with mild disease or improving
All who are debilitated:
    Leukemia and lymphoma
    Malignancies, especially those receiving chemotherapy
    Immunosuppressed (AIDS, congenital, steroids, transplant)
    Abnormal cardiovascular system (valve prosthesis or disease, aneurysms or vascular grafts)
    Orthopedic prostheses
    Hemolytic anemia
    Extremes of age (old or young)
Prolonged symptoms or relapse

AIDS, acquired immunodeficiency syndrome.

TABLE 5-12
Pharmacologic Self-therapy for Traveler's Diarrhea Based on Clinical Features

CLINICAL SYNDROME	PROBABLE CAUSE	AGENT RECOMMENDED
Watery diarrhea (no blood in stool or fever)	Bacteria	Antibacterial drug* plus (for adults) 4 mg of loperamide initially, then 2 mg after each unformed stool, not to exceed 8 mg/d (over-the-counter dose) or 16 mg/d (prescription dose)
Dysentery (passage of bloody stools) or fever (temperature >37.8°C [>100°F])	Invasive bacteria	Antibacterial drug*
Vomiting, minimal diarrhea	Viruses; preformed toxin (food poisoning)	Bismuth subsalicylate (for adults): 30 mL or 2 tables (262 mg/tablet or 15 mL) every 30 min for five doses; may be repeated on day 2
Diarrhea in infants (<2 y old)	Bacteria	Fluids and electrolytes
Diarrhea in pregnant women	Bacteria	Fluids and electrolytes, can consider attapulgite: 3 g initially, repeated after unformed stools or every 2 h (whichever comes first), for total dosage of 9 g/d
Diarrhea despite trimethoprim-sulfamethoxazole prophylaxis	Unknown, possibly drug-resistant bacteria	Fluoroquinolone, with loperamide (see dose above) if no fever or blood in stool
Diarrhea despite fluoroquinolone prophylaxis	Unknown	Bismuth subsalicylate (see dose above) for mild-to-moderate disease; consult physician for moderate-to-severe disease or if disease persists

*The recommended antibacterial drugs are as follows: trimethoprim (160 mg) and sulfamethoxazole (800 mg) for inland Mexico during the summer and norfloxacin (400 mg), ciprofloxacin (500 mg), ofloxacin (300 mg), or fleroxacin (400 mg) for other areas in other seasons. The drugs should be taken in these doses twice daily for 3 days for more severe illness, particularly that associated with fever or the passage of bloody stools. For milder illness, single-dose therapy is effective. All patients should take oral fluids (e.g., Pedialyte [Mead Johnson, Princeton, NJ], Lytren) or flavored mineral water plus saltine crackers.

From DuPont HL, Erricsson CD. Prevention and treatment of traveler's diarrhea. N Engl J Med 1993;328:1821.

TABLE 5-13
Diarrhea in AIDS

All biopsies show intestinal inflammation
Pathogens found in 75%. *If* you culture stool and blood, look for ova and parasites, and obtain a biopsy specimen of the intestine for light and electron microscopic examination
75% improve with special therapy
Diarrhea more frequent in homosexual (80%) than among heterosexual patients (60%)
Multiple infections common (25%)
Bacteremia common (40%)
Some infections persist and necessitate continual treatment (*Salmonella* and *Campylobacter*)

AIDS, acquired immunodeficiency syndrome.

TABLE 5-14
Characteristics of Celiac Disease by Age Group

Children
    0–5 y   Common presentation
                                Poor growth
                                Proximal muscle wasting
                                Abdominal distention
                                Irritability
                                Abnormal stools
    5–15 y   Nutritional deficiencies
                                  Anemia
                                Glossitis, mouth ulcers
                                Tetany
Adults
                              Insidious features
                                Nutritional deficiencies
                                Delayed puberty
                              Acute features
                                Diarrhea
                                Weight loss
                                Vomiting, anorexia
                                Anemia
                                Hypoproteinemia
                                Tetany

From Stevens FA. Celiac disease: clinical manifestations. Pract Gastroenterol 1980;4:10.

TABLE 5-15
Serologic Testing in Celiac Disease

TEST	SENSITIVITY	SPECIFICITY	PPV	NPD
AGA IgG	57–100	42–98	20–95	41–88
AGA IgA	53–100	65–100	28–100	65–100
AEA IgA*	75–98	96–100	98–100	80–95
Guinea pig tTg[†]	90.2	95		
Human tTg[†]	98.5	98		

AEA, antiendomysial antibody; AGA, antigliadin antibody; NPD, negative predictive value; PPV, positive predictive value.

*Patients older than 2 y.

[†]IgG + IgA antibodies.

Adapted from Fasano A, Catassi C. Current approaches to diagnosis and treatment of celiac disease: an evolving spectrum. Gastroenterology 2001;120:636.

> ### TABLE 5-16
> **Frequently Overlooked Items That May Contain Gluten**

Broth	Malt, malt flavoring, vinegar
Breading	Modified food starch
Brown rice syrup	Nondairy creamer
Coating mixes	Pastas
Couscous	Peanut butter
Crouton	Processed meats and poultry
Caramel color	Salad dressings
Cereal products	Sausage products
Catsup and mustard	Sauces
Candy bars	Some brands of ice cream
Cheese spreads	Soup bases
Chip and dip mixes	Soy sauce
Flavoring in meat products	Stuffings
Hydrolyzed meat protein	Tomato sauce
Hot chocolate mixes or cocoa	Vegetable gum
Imitation bacon or seafood marinades	Vegetable protein (thickener)
Instant coffee and tea	Yogurts with fruit

From Abdulkarim AS, Murray JA. Celiac disease. Curr Treat Options Gastroenterol 2002;5:27.

> ### TABLE 5-17
> **Companies That Make Gluten-free Products**

Dietary Specialties, Inc. P. O. Box 227 Rochester, NY 14601 (800) 544-0099	Kingsmill Foods Company, Ltd. 1399 Kennedy Road, Unit 17 Scarborough, ON M1P 2L6 CANADA (416) 755-1124
Ener-G Foods, Inc. P. O. Box 84487 Seattle, WA 98124 (800) 331-5222	Med-Diet, Inc. 3050 Ranchview Lane Plymouth, MN 55447 (800) 633-3438
Fearn Natural Foods P. O. Box 09398 Milwaukee, WI 53209 (414) 352-3333	Miss Ruben's P. O. Box 1434 Frederick, MD 21702 (800) 891-0083
Gluten-Free Delights P. O. Box 284 Cedar Falls, IA 50613 (319) 266-7167	Pamela's Products, Inc. 335 Allerton Avenue South San Francisco, CA 94080 (650) 952-4546
The Gluten-Free Pantry, Inc. P. O. Box 840 Glastonbury, CT 06033 (860) 633-3826	Sterk's Bakery 3866 23rd Street Vineland, ON LOR 2C0 CANADA (800) 608-4501

From Abdulkarim AS, Murray JA. Celiac disease. Curr Treat Options Gastroenterol 2002;5:27.

TABLE 5-18

Celiac Disease Support and Resource Groups in the United States and Canada

American Celiac Society
58 Musano Court
West Orange, NJ 07052
(973) 325-8837

Canadian Celiac Association
190 Britannia Road East, Unit 11
Mississauga, ON L4Z 1W6 CANADA
(905) 507-6208

Celiac Disease Foundation
13251 Ventura Blvd., #1
Studio City, CA 91604
(818) 990-2354

www.celiac.com[*]

Celiac Sprue Association/USA, Inc.
P. O. Box 31700
Omaha, NE 68131
(402) 558-0600
URL: www.csaceliacs.org

Midwest Gluten Intolerance Group
4007 Forest Road
St. Louis Park, MN 55416
(612) 925-6136

Gluten Intolerance Group of North America
P. O. Box 23053
Seattle, WA 98102
(206) 325-6980
URL: www.celiac.org

www.celiacdatabase.org[†]

[*]Comprehensive website with many links and useful information for the experienced patient with celiac disease (CD). May overwhelm patients with newly diagnosed CD.

[†]Useful website where a food product's gluten-free status can be checked using the UPC code or EAN code.

From Abdulkarim AS, Murray JA. Celiac disease. Curr Treat Options Gastroenterol 2002;5:27.

TABLE 5-19

Causes of Enteropathic Arthritis

Whipple disease
Ulcerative colitis
Crohn's disease
Shigellosis
Salmonellosis
Yersinia enterocolitis
Campylobacter colitis
Post–small intestine bypass (for obesity)

From Feldman M. Southwestern Internal Medicine Conference: Whipple's disease. Am J Med Sci 1986;291:59.

TABLE 5-20
Central Nervous System Symptoms and Signs in Whipple Disease

SYMPTOMS	SIGNS
Mental and personality changes	Dementia
Lethargy, coma	Papilledema
Headache	Ophthalmoplegia
Convulsions	Hemiparesis
Motor weakness	Sensory loss
Numbness	Myoclonus
Slurred speech	Hyperreflexia ($\pm$ positive Babinski sign)
Visual difficulties (diplopia, blurring)	Ataxia
Incoordination	Pupillary abnormalities
Dizziness	Nystagmus
Tinnitus	Ptosis
Hearing loss	Muscle rigidity
Muscular jerks and twitches	Loss of vibratory and position sense
Stiff neck	Hearing loss
Facial pain	
Sleep disorders	
Polydipsia	

From Feldman M. Southwestern Internal Medicine Conference: Whipple's disease. Am J Med Sci 1986;291:59.

TABLE 5-21
Comparison of Clinical Features of Malabsorption Caused by Mucosal Disease (Celiac Sprue) with Impaired Intralumenal Digestion (Chronic Pancreatic Insufficiency)

CLINICAL MANIFESTATIONS	CELIAC SPRUE	PANCREATIC INSUFFICIENCY
Symptom or sign		
Sex	F > M (2:1)	M > F (3:1)
Age at onset (%)	<3; 20–40	30–60
Diarrhea (%)	70–90	70–90
Weight loss (%)	60–90	90
Flatulence and bloating (%)	40	0
Weakness and lethargy (%)	95	4
Anorexia (%)	30–50	0
Oral aphthous ulcers, recurrent (%)	60	0
Severe abdominal pain (%)	0	64
Increased appetite (%)	15	70
Oil separated from stool (%)	0	57
Extraintestinal symptoms		
Tetany, bone pain, hemorrhagic diathesis, edema or ascites, nocturnal polyuria (%)	20–50	0–10
Laboratory tests		
Stool fat, g/24 h	25 (range 3.5–87)	48 (range 8–180)
Stool fat concentration, g/100 g stool (%)	<9.5	>9.5
Total serum protein <6 g/dL (%)	71	14
Anemia (%)	21	0

Adapted from Evans WB, Wollaeger EE. Incidence and severity of nutritional deficiency states in chronic exocrine pancreatic insufficiency: comparison with nontropical sprue. Am J Dig Dis 1966;11:594; and Bo-Linn GW, Fordtran JS. Fecal fat concentration in patients with steatorrhea. Gastroenterology 1984;87:319.

TABLE 5-22
Dietary Factors, Disease States, and Drugs Affecting Standard Oral D-xylose Tests

FACTOR	5-H URINE EXCRETION OF D-XYLOSE	1-H SERUM LEVEL OF D-XYLOSE
Delayed gastric emptying	May decrease	May decrease
Dietary fiber or glucose	May decrease	May decrease
Meat	May increase	May Increase
Renal disease		
Not requiring dialysis	Decreases	No decrease
Requiring dialysis		Decreases
Portal hypertension	Decreases	Decreases
Ascites	Decreases	May decrease
Myxedema	Decreases	No decrease
Drugs		
Aspirin and indomethacin	May decrease	May decrease
Neomycin	May decrease	May decrease
Glipizide	May decrease	May decrease

From Craig RM, Atkinson AJ. D-Xylose testing: a review. Gastroenterology 1988;95:223.

TABLE 5-23
Sorbitol Content of "Sugar-free" Products and Various Foods

FOOD	SORBITOL CONTENT
"Sugar-free" gum	1.3–2.2 g/piece
"Sugar-free" mints	1.7–2.0 g/piece
Pears	4.6 g[*]
Prunes	2.4 g[*]
Peaches	1.0 g[*]
Apple juice	0.3–0.9 g[*]

[*]Expressed as grams of sorbitol per 100 g dry matter or per 100 g juice. Dry weight equals approximately 15% of fresh weight.

From Hyams JS. Sorbitol intolerance: an unappreciated cause of functional gastrointestinal complaints. Gastroenterology 1983;84:30.

TABLE 5-24
Symptoms Associated with Sorbitol and Lactulose Ingestion

| SYMPTOM | DOSE OF SORBITOL (g)[*] | | | LACTULOSE (g) |
	5	10	20	10
Gas	3/7	5/7	5/7	5/7
Bloating	3/7	5/7	5/7	5/7
Cramps	0/7	1/7	4/7	2/7
Diarrhea	0/7	1/7	4/7	2/7

[*]No. patients with symptom/no. patients tested.

From Hyams JS. Sorbitol intolerance: an unappreciated cause of functional gastrointestinal complaints. Gastroenterology 1983;84:30.

TABLE 5-25
Two References Containing Extensive Tables of Sorbitol Content in Various Commonly Used Oral Liquid Medications

Lutomski DM, Gora ML, Wright SM, Martin JE. Sorbitol content of selected oral liquids. Ann Pharmacother 1993;27:269

Johnston KR, Govel LA, Andritz MH. Gastrointestinal effects of sorbitol as an additive in liquid medications. Am J Med 1994;97:185

TABLE 5-26
Common Features and Symptoms of Patients with Factitious Diarrhea

Features
   Predominantly women (>90%)
   Multiple previous examinations
   Exploratory laparotomies
   Psychological abnormalities

Symptoms
   Severe, chronic, watery diarrhea
   Abdominal pain
   Weight loss
   Nausea and vomiting
   Peripheral edema
   Generalized weakness and hypokalemia

From Ewe K, Karbach U. Factitious diarrhea. Clin Gastroenterol 1986;15:723.

TABLE 5-27
Findings Suggestive of Factitious Diarrhea

INVESTIGATION	CHARACTERISTIC FINDINGS	CAUSE
Sigmoidoscopy	Melanosis coli	Anthraquinones
Barium enema	"Cathartic" colon	Diphenolic laxatives and anthraquinones
Stool electrolytes and osmolality (if volume >500 mL/d and other causes are excluded)	$(Na^+ + K^+) \times 2 <$ osmolality	Osmotic laxatives, urine contamination
	$(Na^+ + K^+) \times 2 =$ osmolality	Secretory laxatives (anthraquinone and diphenolic laxatives)
	Osmolality < 200 mOsm/L	Addition of water to stool

From Ewe K, Karbach U. Factitious diarrhea. Clin Gastroenterol 1986;15:723.

TABLE 5-28
Composition of Laxatives Commonly Used in the United States

TRADE NAME	DDS DOCUSATES	DIPHENOLS		ANTHRAQUINONES				OIL
		Phenolphthalein	Bisacodyl	Aloe	Cascara	Danthron	Senna	Mineral Oil
Agoral		x						
Black-Draught		x		x				
Carter's Little Pills	x						x	
Colace	x							
Correctol	x	x						
Dialose	x							
Doxidan	x					x		
Ducolax			x					
Evac-U-Gen		x						
Ex-Lax		x						
Extra Gentle Ex-Lax	x	x						
Feen-a-Mint	x	x						
Haley's MO								x
Modane						x		
Modane Plus	x					x		
Nature's Remedy				x	x			
Peri-Colace	x				x			
Petrogalar								x
Senokot							x	
Surfak	x							
Unilax	x					x		
X-Prep							x	
Yellolax		x						

DDS, dioctyl sodium sulfosuccinate.

Adapted from Sekas G. The use and abuse of laxatives. Pract Gastroenterol 1987;11:33.

TABLE 5-29
Hormones Produced by Carcinoid Tumors and Medullary Thyroid Carcinoma

HORMONE	CARCINOID TUMORS	MEDULLARY THYROID CARCINOMA	STIMULATORY EFFECT ON INTESTINAL FLUID SECRETION AND/OR MOTILITY
Serotonin	+	+	+
5-Hydroxytryptophan	+		+
Histamine	+		+
Kallikrein → bradykinin	+	+	+
Calcitonin	+	+	+
Noncalcitonin peptide		+	?
Calcitonin gene-related peptide		+	?
Katacalcin		+	?
Motilin	+	+	+
Substance P	+	+	+
Tachykinin-like immunoreactivity	+		+
Neurotensin	+	+	+
Bombesin and gastrin-releasing peptide	+	+	+
Glucagon, enteroglucagon	+		+
Gastrin	+		+
Prostaglandins E and $F_{2\alpha}$	+		+
Dopamine	+		−
Norepinephrine	+		−
Peptide YY	+		−
Somatostatin	+	+	−
β-Endorphin		+	−
Nerve growth factor		+	?
γ-Trace		+	?
Helodermin		+	?

From Rambaud JC, Hautefeuille M, Ruskone A, Jacquenod P. Diarrhoea due to circulating agents. Clin Gastroenterol 1986;15:603.

TABLE 5-30
Hormone Products Found in Carcinoid Tumors

Serotonin	Somatostatin
Tachykinins	Adrenocorticotrophic hormone
Histamine	Growth hormone
Substance P	Gastrin-releasing peptide
Substance K	Gastrin
Pentagastrin	Insulin
Pancreatic polypeptide	Melanocyte-stimulating hormone

From O'Neil BH, Venook AP. Carcinoid tumors and the carcinoid syndrome. Clin Perspect Gastroenterol 2001:279.

TABLE 5-31

Tests Used in the Examination of Patients with Endocrine Diarrhea

Gastrinoma
　Gastric acid secretion
　Plasma gastrin
　Secretin provocative test

VIPoma
　Gastric acid secretion
　Serum calcium
　Fasting plasma glucose, glycosuria
　Plasma VIP and calcitonin
　Plasma and urinary catecholamines and metabolites

Somatostatinoma
　Gastric and exocrine pancreas secretions
　Fasting plasma glucose, glycosuria
　Plasma somatostatin

Carcinoid syndrome
　Blood serotonin
　Urinary 5-HIAA

Medullary thyroid carcinoma
　Plasma calcitonin
　Serum carcinoembryonic antigen

Hyperthyroidism
　Plasma triiodothyronine, thyroxine, and thyroid-stimulating hormone

5-HIAA, 5-hydroxyindoleacetic acid; VIP, vasoactive intestinal polypeptide; VIPoma, vasoactive intestinal polypeptide-secreting tumor.

From Rambaud J-C, Hautefauille M, Ruskone A, Jacquenod P. Diarrhoea due to circulating agents. Clin Gastroenterol 1986;15:603.

TABLE 5-32

Factors Affecting Stool Electrolyte and Osmolality Measurements

	TEMPERATURE (°C)	TIME AFTER COLLECTION (H)	OSMOLALITY (mOsm)	SODIUM (mEq/L)	POTASSIUM (mEq/L)	OSMOTIC GAP* (mOsm)
Storage temperature	25	0	281	54	115	−57
		24	417	54	115	79
	25	0	300	40	101	18
		24	453	40	101	153
	25	0	291	76	38	63
		24	389	77	43	149
Antibiotics						
Oral neomycin	25	0	285	3	20	239
	25	48	281	3	22	231
Triple therapy	25	0	305	5	19	257
	25	48	304	5	18	258

*Osmotic gap = measured osmolality $-2 \times$ (Na + K).

From Shiau Y-F, Feldman GM, Resnick MA, Coff PM. Stool electrolyte and osmolality measurements in the evaluation of diarrheal disorders. Ann Intern Med 1985;102:773.

TABLE 5-33

Characteristics of Patients with Secretory and Osmotic Diarrhea and Results of Stool Osmolality and Electrolyte Measurements

PATIENT	DIAGNOSIS OR TREATMENT	EFFECT OF FASTING ON DIARRHEA	OSMOLALITY (mOsm)	SODIUM (mEq/L)	POTASSIUM (mEq/L)	OSMOTIC GAP* (mOsm)
1	Carcinoid syndrome	Persisted	320	98	90	−56
	Carcinoid syndrome[†]	Persisted	345	135	54	−33
2	Acute diarrhea	Persisted	281	54	115	−57
3	Idiopathic pseudoobstruction	Persisted	285	139	14	−21
4	Secretory diarrhea	Persisted	284	47	108	−26
5[†]	Secretory diarrhea	Persisted	300	40	101	18
6	Diabetic diarrhea	Persisted	330	82	24	118
7[‖]	Diabetic diarrhea	Persisted	348	115	25	68
8	Pseudomembranous colitis	Persisted	285	92	15	71
9	Pancreatic insufficiency	Resolved	291	76	38	63
10	Two days after discontinuation of lactulose		298	45	49	110
	Taking lactulose[¶]	Resolved	285	3	20	239
11	Taking lactulose	Resolved	285	21	38	167
12[¶]	Taking lactulose	Resolved	305	5	19	257

*Osmotic gap = measured osmolality $-2 \times$ (Na + K).

[†]Serum Na concentration was 167 mEq/L.

[†]Measurements were done 4 hours after stool collection.

[‖]Serum Na, 144 mEq/L; blood urea nitrogen, 80 mg/dL; and glucose, 360 mg/dL.

[¶]Patients were receiving antibiotic agents.

From Shiau Y-F, Feldman GM, Resnick MA, Coff PM. Stool electrolyte and osmolality measurements in the evaluation of diarrheal disorders. Ann Intern Med 1985;102:773.

TABLE 5-34

Fecal Electrolyte Composition, Osmolality, and pH In Congenital Chloride Diarrhea Compared with Normal State and with Different Types of Secretory Diarrhea (Values Are Mean ± SEM)

	VOLUME (mL)	Na$^+$ (mmol/L)	K$^+$ (mmol/L)	Cl$^-$ (mmol/L)	HCO$_3^-$ (mmol/L)	OSMOLALITY (mOsm/kg)	pH
Normal adults		31 ± 2	75 ± 2	16 ± 1	40 ± 2	376 ± 8	7.0 ± 0.1
Congenital chloride diarrhea	943 ± 86	60 ± 3	40 ± 3	140 ± 5	3 ± 0.5	307 ± 6	5.9 ± 0.1
Congenital sodium diarrhea	1470 ± 159	104 ± 3	57 ± 4	46 ± 2	59	291 ± 2	7.1 ± 0.9
Pancreatic cholera syndrome	2764 ± 745	76 ± 10	54 ± 8	47 ± 13	66	284 ± 6	7.7
Cholera		126 ± 1	19 ± 1	94 ± 1	47 ± 1		

Note: Values are given at age 6 to 12 years for congenital chloride diarrhea and 6 to 8 years for congenital sodium diarrhea; all other values are for adults.

SEM, standard error of the mean.

From Holmberg C. Congenital chloride diarrhea. Clin Gastroenterol 1986;15:58.

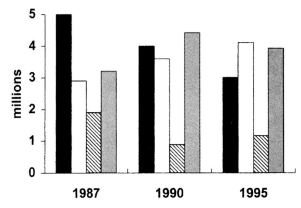

FIGURE 5-1. Diarrheal disease death rates (■) among children younger than 5 years, compared with death rates from acute respiratory infections (□), measles (▨), and other causes (▧).

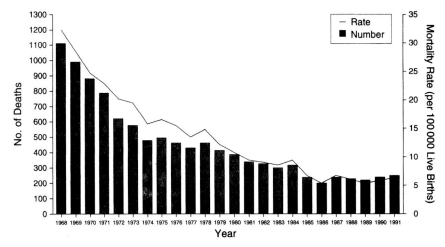

FIGURE 5-2. Diarrheal disease death rates (*solid line*) and annual number (*bar*) among U.S. infants.

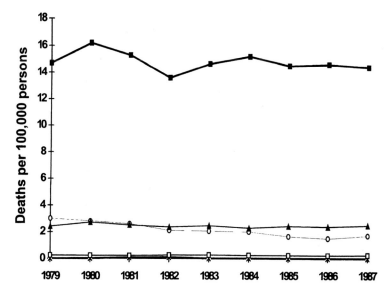

FIGURE 5-3. Diarrheal death rates in the United States. O, age less than 4 years; ∗, age 5 to 24 years; □, age 25 to 54 years; ▲, age 55 to 74 years; ■, age greater than 74 years.

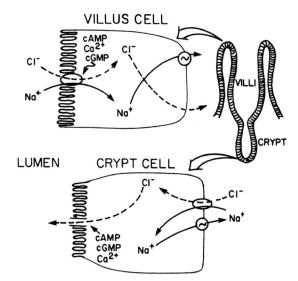

FIGURE 5-4. Intestinal absorption of sodium (Na⁺) and secretion of chloride (Cl⁻) both are regulated by the following intracellular messengers: cyclic adenosine monophosphate (*cAMP*), ionized calcium (*Ca²⁺*), and cyclic guanosine monophosphate (*cGMP*). Diarrhea may result from inhibition of NaCl absorption and stimulation of Cl⁻ secretion.

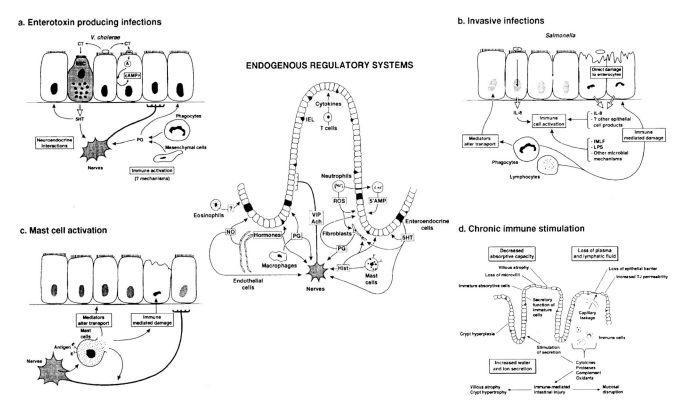

FIGURE 5-5. Endogenous regulatory systems involved in intestinal ion transport (**central figure**). Enteroendocrine cells in the crypt release mediators such as serotonin (*5-HT*) across the basolateral membrane to regulate adjacent epithelial cells (paracrine regulation). If released in large enough quantities in the bloodstream, these mediators have endocrine actions (hormones). Peptides such as vasoactive intestinal peptide (*VIP*) or neurotransmitters such as acetylcholine (*ACh*) are released from the nerve endings of neurons to regulate epithelial cells (neurocrine regulation). Substances including reactive oxygen species (*ROS*), 5′ adenosine monophosphate (*5'AMP*), prostaglandins (*PG*), and histamine (*hist*) released from activated immune cells such as phagocytes, mast cells, and lymphocytes also can regulate epithelial cells (immune regulation). Other mesenchymal cells, particularly myofibroblasts, release mediators (e.g., *PG*) that alter epithelial ion transport. In addition to directly stimulating epithelial cells, immune-mesenchymal and neurohormonal mediators also may act on nerves, immune cells, fibroblasts, and smooth muscle (not depicted). Only key aspects of these complex interactions are depicted in this schematic. *IEL*, intraepithelial lymphocytes; *NO*, nitric oxide. **a–d:** Mechanisms of altered intestinal ion transport. Schematic of the complex mechanisms that lead to altered fluid and electrolyte secretion in various diarrheal conditions. **a:** Enterotoxins such as *Vibrio cholerae* toxin (*CT*) stimulate secretion and inhibit absorption by a receptor-mediated process in which cyclic nucleotide levels are increased. CT also releases 5-HT from intestinal enteroendocrine cells (*EEC*), which acts on nerves to stimulate alterations of ion transport. **b:** Invasive organisms such as *Salmonella* organisms may directly induce epithelial damage, but they also activate immune-mesenchymal cells through bacterial (e.g., formylmethionylleucylphenylalanine [*f-MLF*], lipopolysaccharide (*LPS*), or perhaps through epithelial cell products (e.g., *IL-8*) to alter transport through receptor-mediated actions on enterocytes or by means of damaging the epithelium further. **c:** Mast cell activation by means of antigen or nonimmune mechanisms releases mediators that act directly and indirectly to stimulate secretion, whereas others lead to epithelial damage. **d:** Chronic stimulation of the immune system in celiac disease and other disorders can lead to the development of villous atrophy and crypt hyperplasia (**left**) associated with a reduced absorptive capacity, and enhanced secretion caused by increased numbers of crypt cells and the secretory effects of immune cell mediators. Activation of inflammatory cells also disrupts epithelial barrier function, which in addition to endothelial injury, leads to the loss of plasma and lymphatic fluid (**right**).

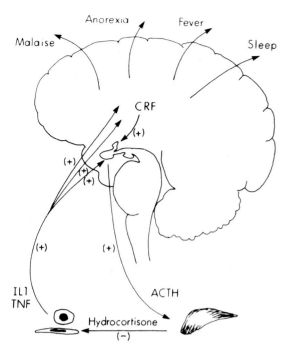

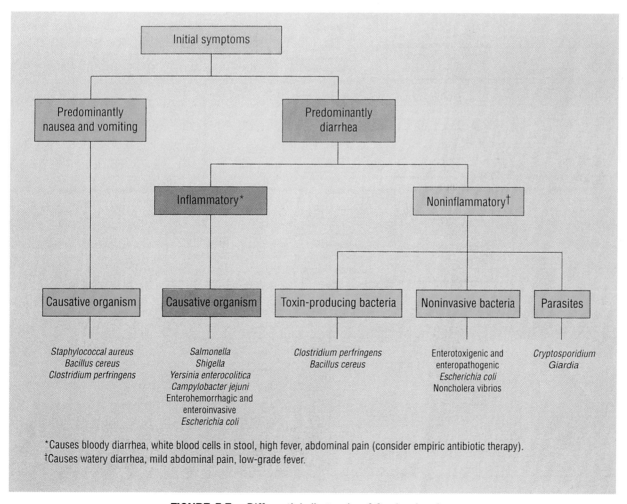

FIGURE 5-6. The systemic manifestations of severe intestinal inflammation are caused primarily by release of interleukin-1 (*IL-1*) and tumor necrosis factor (*TNF*), which have effects in the central nervous system. These agents also stimulate the pituitary-adrenal axis and initiate the glucocorticoid stress response. Glucocorticoids, through a negative feedback action, down-regulate the inflammatory cells in the lamina propria and decrease IL-1 and TNF release. *ACTH*, adrenocorticotropic hormone; *CRF*, corticotropin-releasing factor.

FIGURE 5-7. Differential diagnosis of food poisoning.

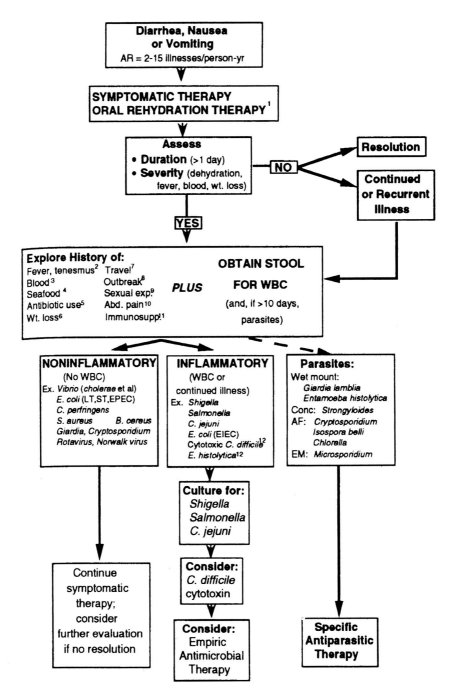

FIGURE 5-8. Approach to the diagnosis and management of infectious diarrhea.

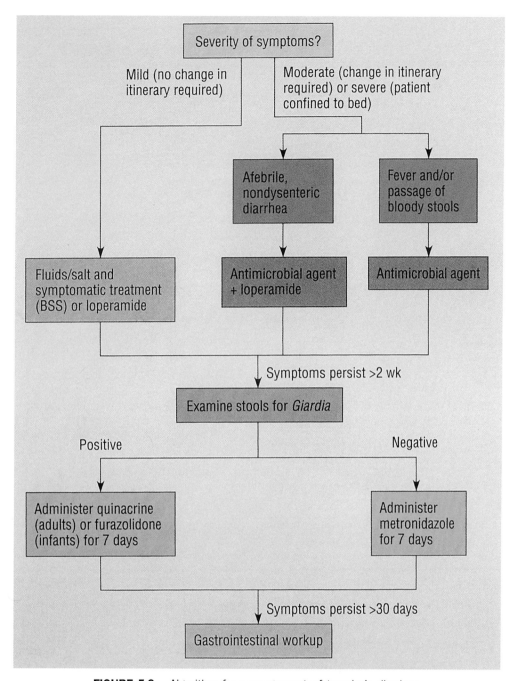

FIGURE 5-9. Algorithm for management of traveler's diarrhea.

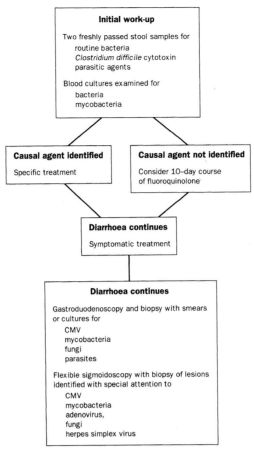

FIGURE 5-10. Algorithm for the evaluation of acquired immunodeficiency syndrome diarrhea.

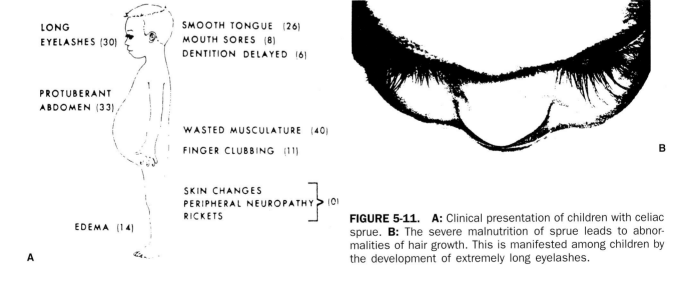

FIGURE 5-11. **A:** Clinical presentation of children with celiac sprue. **B:** The severe malnutrition of sprue leads to abnormalities of hair growth. This is manifested among children by the development of extremely long eyelashes.

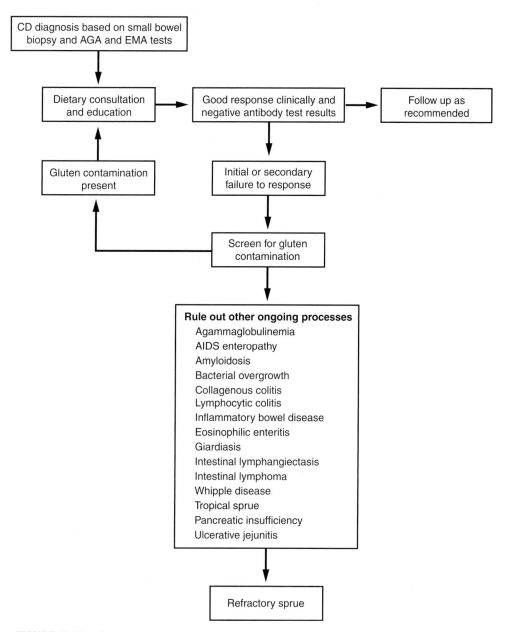

FIGURE 5-12. Suggested diagnostic algorithm for patients with nonresponsive celiac disease. AGA, antigliadin antibody; EMA, endomysial antibody.

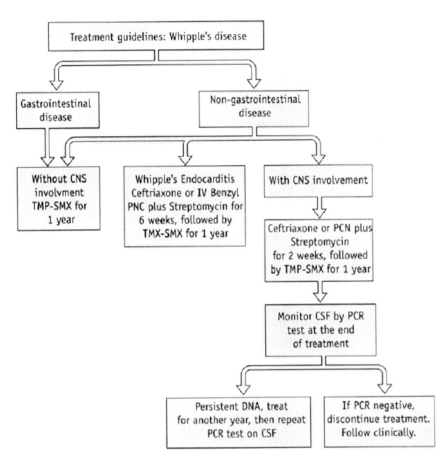

FIGURE 5-13. Treatment guidelines: Whipple disease.

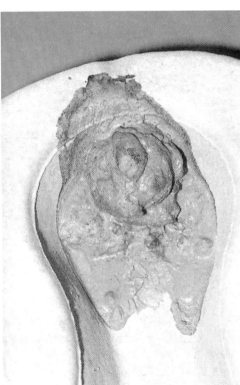

FIGURE 5-14. This steatorrheic stool is not easily confused with watery diarrhea. The first step in diagnosing the cause of diarrhea is to look at the stool.

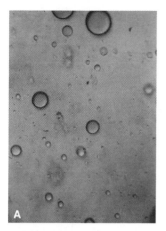
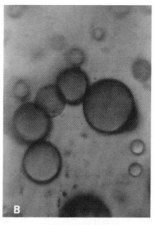

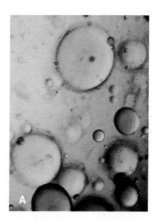
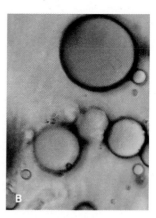

FIGURE 5-15. The hallmarks of abnormal findings at qualitative fecal fat examination are an increase in the number and, more important, an increase in the size of fat droplets. **A:** This specimen has 1% triglyceride and is equivalent to a quantitative stool fat level of 5 to 6 g/24 h. **B:** This specimen has 5% triglyceride and is equivalent to a quantitative stool fat level of 10 g/24 h.

FIGURE 5-16. When fatty acids are present at usual stool pH, they are either ionized or in the form of soaps and will not readily take up Sudan stain. **A:** At pH 5.6, fatty acids do not stain well with Sudan stain. **B:** After acidification with two drops of acetic acid, the fatty acid droplets readily take up Sudan stain.

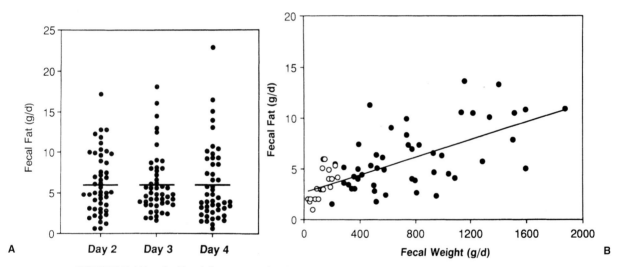

FIGURE 5-17. **A:** Fecal fat output for healthy persons among whom diarrhea has been induced with MgOH₂ plus phenolphthalein (combined osmotic plus secretory diarrhea) can exceed 6 g/24 h. **B:** Fecal fat output exceeds this value among more than 50% of persons if the diarrhea is severe; that is, fecal weight is more than 800 g/24 h.

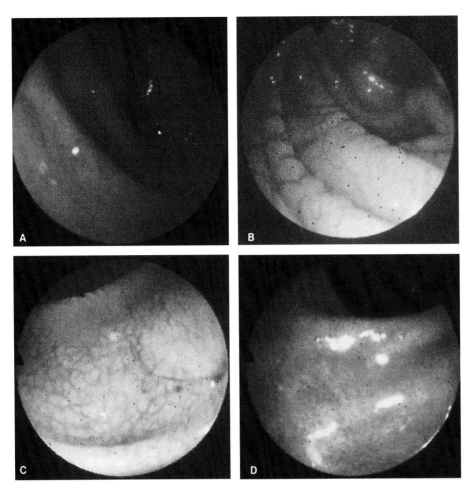

FIGURE 5-18. Duodenal biopsy specimen obtained means of upper gastrointestinal endoscopy can be diagnostic for intestinal causes of malabsorption. One disease that can be diagnosed on the basis of gross endoscopic appearance is celiac sprue. **A:** Normal duodenal mucosa is smooth, velvety, and reddish. **B:** Scalloped valvulae conniventes in the duodenum of a patient with celiac sprue. **C:** Mosaic pattern of visible vasculature and scalloped valvulae conniventes is seen best on the edge of the valvula. **D:** Mucosal appearance of the duodenal mucosa in a patient treated for sprue has returned toward normal with revision.

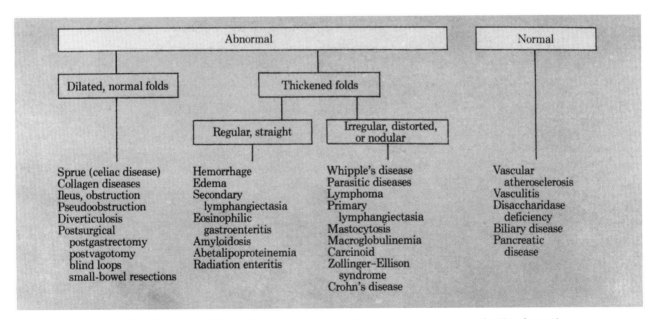

FIGURE 5-19. A small-intestinal radiograph should not be a primary examination for malabsorption, but may reveal changes that can lead to diagnosis of the cause.

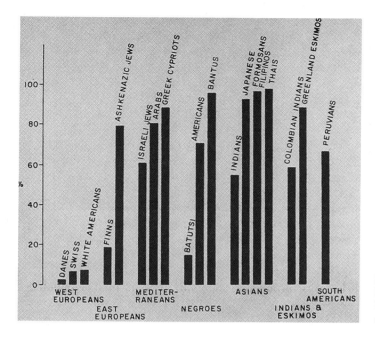

FIGURE 5-20. The prevalence of low lactase levels or lactose intolerance in various populations ranges from less than 10% among western Europeans and their descendants to 80% to 90% in other races and countries.

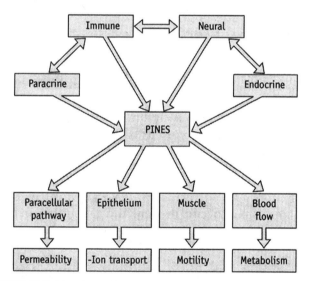

FIGURE 5-21. Interplay among the paracrine, immune, neural, and endocrine systems (PINES): the pathophysiology of secretory diarrhea.

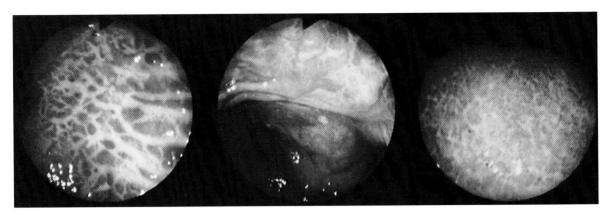

FIGURE 5-22. Melanosis coli develops from chronic use of anthracene cathartic agents. The endoscopic appearance of melanosis coli can be quite varied.

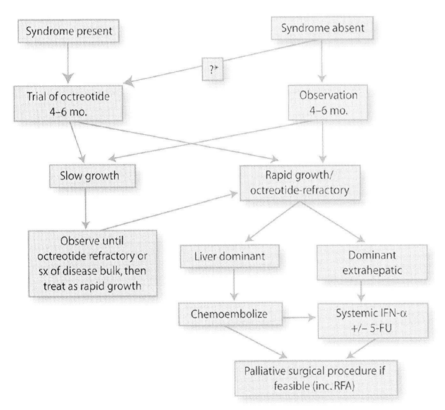

FIGURE 5-23. Algorithm for treatment of unresectable metastatic carcinoid-carcinoid syndrome. (*sx*, symptoms; *IFN*; interferon; *5-FU*, 5-fluorouracil; *inc.*, including; *RFA*, radio frequency ablation.)

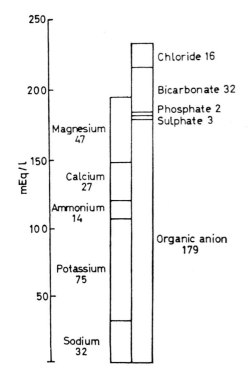

FIGURE 5-24. Human stool electrolyte concentrations obtained by means of fecal dialysis.

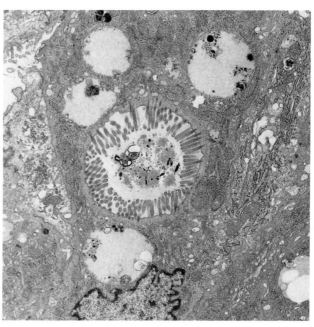

FIGURE 5-25. Microvillus inclusion disease is an autosomally transmitted recessive disorder in which the epithelial cells of the small intestine, colon, and gallbladder display intracytoplasmic vacuoles that contain brush borders that are not expressed on the apical surface of the absorbing epithelial cells. The epithelial cells may have rudimentary microvilli, as in this specimen. In some epithelial cells, however, the microvilli are closer to normal than shown here. These patients have severe secretory diarrhea and need parenteral fluid replacement if they are to live beyond infancy.

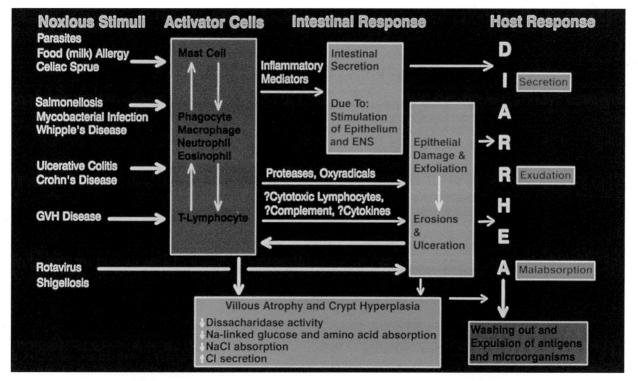

FIGURE 5-26. The pathophysiological sequence of inflammatory diarrhea.

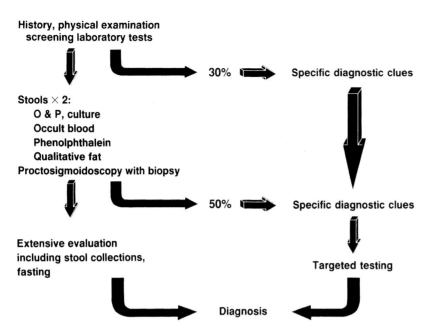

FIGURE 5-27. Evaluation of chronic diarrhea. *O & P,* ova and parasites.

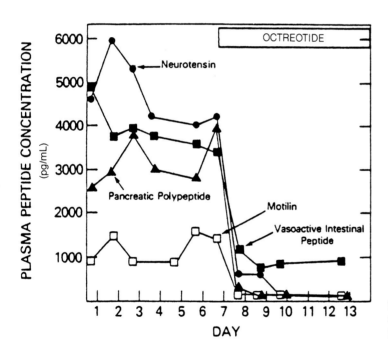

FIGURE 5-28. The somatostatin analog octreotide significantly reduces tumor secretion of various hormones.

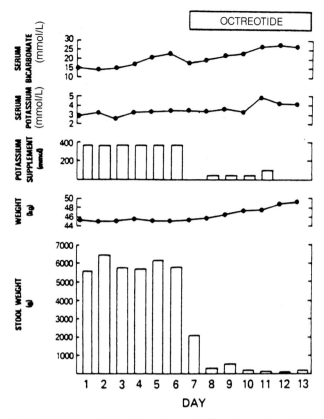

FIGURE 5-29. Octreotide also significantly reduced the diarrhea of this patient with a neuroendocrine tumor. This reduction in diarrhea is largely caused by the ability of the somatostatin analog to reduce hormone secretion by the tumor.

APPROACH TO THE PATIENT WITH CONSTIPATION

ARNOLD WALD

Constipation is a symptom rather than a disease and therefore represents a patient's subjective interpretation of a real or imaginary somatic disturbance. Although no single definition is applicable to all patients with constipation, for clinical purposes one may use difficulty during defecation either alone or in conjunction with frequency of defecation of less than three times per week, especially if this represents a distinct change in regular bowel habits.

Constipation may be regarded conceptually as disordered movement through the colon or anorectum. From a pathophysiological standpoint, this can occur because of a primary motor disorder, in association with various diseases, or as a side effect of many drugs.

The classical example of neurogenic constipation is Hirschsprung disease, which results from a developmental arrest of caudal migration of neural crest cells from the notochord during embryonic development. This is characterized by colonic dilation proximal to a contracted nonpropulsive segment of distal bowel, which can be seen at barium enema examination (Fig. 6-1). In these patients, the internal anal sphincter does not relax after rectal distention (Fig. 6-2). Because this finding is universal in all forms of Hirschsprung disease, demonstration at anorectal manometry of the rectosphincteric inhibitory reflex excludes the disease from consideration. On occasion, Hirschsprung disease presents itself as involvement of only a short segment of distal colon. In such cases, diagnosis may be delayed into adolescence or adulthood. Barium radiographs may be similar to those of children who have idiopathic constipation with megacolon (Fig. 6-3). Manometry should be performed, and the diagnosis can be confirmed by examination of rectal biopsy specimens to prove the absence of intramural ganglion cells in the distal rectum.

Most patients with constipation have no obvious cause to explain their symptoms, but can be categorized into several broad groups on the basis of age at presentation, studies of colonic transit and anorectal sensorimotor function, and in some instances, psychological profile. Studies of colonic transit are performed by having the patient ingest radiopaque markers and by following transit of the markers through the colon with serial abdominal radiographs (KUB). Markers are counted in the right, left, and rectosigmoid regions of the colon, as defined by certain anatomic landmarks (Fig. 6-4). In such studies, approximately 30% of adults with infrequent defecation refractory to therapy have normal transit. The other patients have slow transit as defined by transit times in excess of normal values (Fig. 6-5) and may exhibit a pattern of delayed transit through the proximal colon (colonic inertia) or have a pattern in which stagnation of markers is confined to the rectosigmoid colon (outlet obstruction). The latter is not specific and occurs in a variety of conditions.

One possible cause of outlet obstruction is rectosphincteric dyssynergia, in which ineffective defecation is associated with failure to relax or with inappropriate contraction of the puborectalis and external anal sphincter muscles. This condition can be diagnosed with radiography, electromyography recordings, or anorectal manometry (Fig. 6-6).

The pathogenesis of this disorder is uncertain, but it may represent an acquired, learned dysfunction. Biofeedback techniques have been used to normalize defecation patterns of both children and adults with this abnormality (Fig. 6-7).

Functional studies are usually reserved for patients with severe idiopathic constipation who fail to respond to simple therapeutic measures (Fig. 6-8).

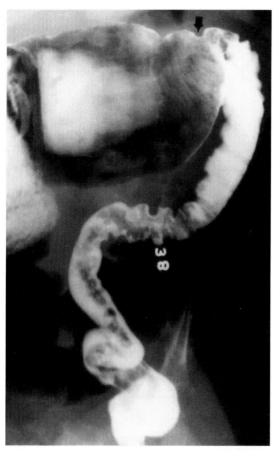

FIGURE 6-1. Barium enema radiograph of a child with Hirschsprung disease. A narrow section extends to the splenic flexure (*arrow*) with proximal dilation of the bowel. (Courtesy of the Department of Radiology, Children's Hospital of Pittsburgh.)

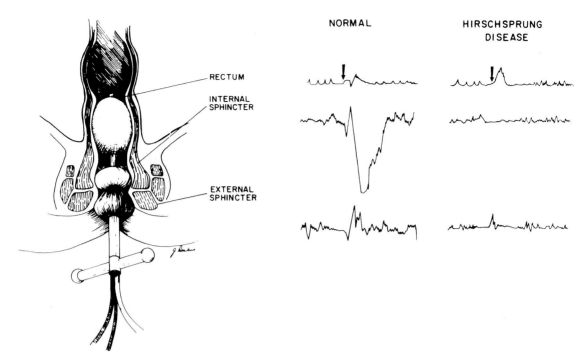

FIGURE 6-2. Anorectal manometric patterns of a healthy person (**left**) and of a child with Hirschsprung disease (**right**). The technique used to record anorectal reflexes consists of arranging air-filled balloons in series and connecting them to a recording machine. Rectal distention with air (*arrows*) normally results in temporary relaxation of the internal anal sphincter. Patients with Hirschsprung disease have no sphincter relaxation.

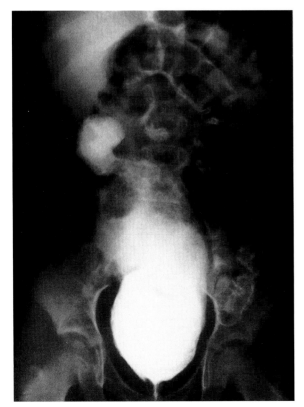

FIGURE 6-3. Barium enema radiograph of an 11-year-old boy with constipation since 2 years of age and fecal soiling for approximately 3 years. The rectum and sigmoid colon are dilated above the anal verge, consistent with idiopathic childhood constipation. However, anorectal manometry did not demonstrate internal sphincter relaxation. Rectal biopsy revealed absence of ganglion cells for a distance of 1 cm above the internal anal sphincter. The patient responded well to rectal myotomy. (Courtesy of the Department of Radiology, Children's Hospital of Pittsburgh.)

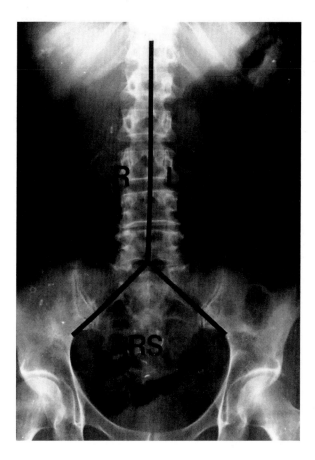

FIGURE 6-4. Plain radiograph of the abdomen (KUB) of a person with constipation who had swallowed 20 ring-shaped markers and 20 linear markers. Lines drawn through bony landmarks divide the colon into right (*R*), left (*L*), and rectosigmoid (*RS*) segments. The markers are equally distributed and show no outlet obstruction. With the use of two different markers administered 24 hours apart, radiographs may be taken at 48-hour intervals with a maximum of four radiographs during the 8-day study.

	Hinton	Arhan	Metcalf	Consensus
Day 1	24 Markers	24 Markers	24 Markers	24 Markers
Day 2		KUB	24 Markers	24 Markers
Day 3		KUB	24 Markers	24 Markers
Day 4		KUB	KUB	24 Markers
Day 5	KUB	KUB		24 Markers
Day 6		KUB		24 Markers
Day 7		KUB	KUB	KUB
Day 8		KUB		
Transit	--	$T = n_1+n_2...$	$T = n_4+n_7$	$T = n_7$
Normal	<20% retention	<70 Hr	<70 Hr	<70 Hr

$$T = \frac{\text{KUB Interval (Hr)}}{\text{No. of Markers}}$$

n = number of markers
T – are expressed in hours

FIGURE 6-5. Different published methods used to determine colonic transit times.

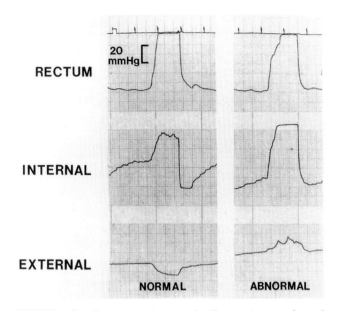

FIGURE 6-6. Pressure changes in the rectum and anal canal during attempted expulsion of manometer. Normal defecation pattern is characterized by increased intrarectal pressure reflected in rectal and internal sphincter balloons and decreased pressure in the external sphincter balloon. Rectosphincteric dyssynergia pattern is characterized by increased pressure in the external sphincter balloon.

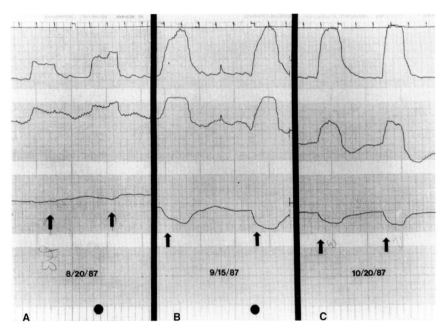

FIGURE 6-7. Manometric patterns during attempted expulsion of manometer (*arrows*) by a patient with rectosphincteric dyssynergia before and after biofeedback therapy. **A:** Before biofeedback therapy there is no decrease in pressure on external balloon. **B:** During biofeedback therapy patient has successfully achieved normal relaxation of the external anal sphincter, first with and then without visual feedback. **C:** During follow-up examination patient continues to exhibit normal defecation pattern.

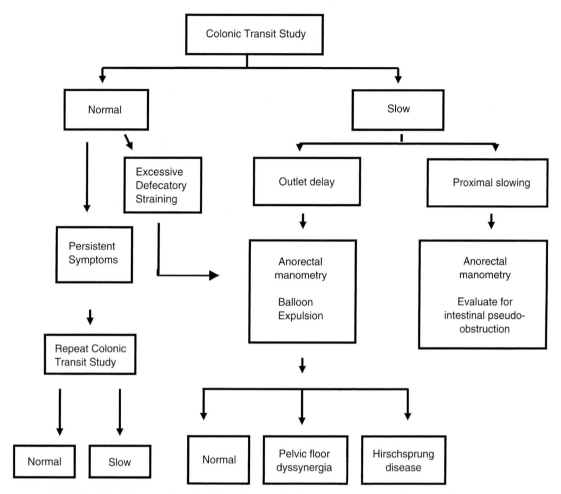

FIGURE 6-8. Diagnostic algorithm for evaluation of severe constipation that has not responded to simple therapeutic measures.

APPROACH TO THE PATIENT WITH JAUNDICE

RAPHAEL B. MERRIMAN ◼ V. RAMAN MUTHUSAMY ◼ MARION G. PETERS

Jaundice is the yellow discoloration of skin, sclera, and mucous membranes caused by the excessive accumulation of bilirubin pigments, and is clinically apparent when total bilirubin exceeds 3 mg/dL. Hyperbilirubinemia can result from a disorder in bilirubin metabolism, hepatic function, or biliary disease, or a combination of those processes. Unconjugated bilirubin is formed by the degradation of the heme group. Bilirubin is rendered more soluble by conjugation in the liver, thereby permitting its hepatic excretion. In clinical medicine, the optimal management of the jaundiced patient demands the precise localization of the site of disordered bilirubin handling. Cholestasis results from the failure of adequate amounts of bile to reach the duodenum and is characterized by the accumulation in blood of conjugated bilirubin, bile salts, and cholesterol.

When first evaluating a patient with jaundice, key questions must be asked:

1. Is the hyperbilirubinemia predominantly unconjugated or conjugated?
2. In unconjugated hyperbilirubinemia, is it caused by increased production or impaired conjugation?
3. In conjugated hyperbilirubinemia, is the disorder intrahepatic or extrahepatic?
4. Is the process acute or chronic?

The answers to these questions are best obtained through a systematic approach that fully uses the patient's history, physical examination, and laboratory and radiologic tests to pinpoint the cause of jaundice. A quick assessment of the urgency of the condition must be first ascertained. Fever, leukocytosis, and hypotension may point to ascending cholangitis. Asterixis, confusion, or stupor may indicate severe hepatocellular dysfunction or fulminant hepatic failure.

Focused history taking always provides important clues to the possible cause of hyperbilirubinemia and will also guide the subsequent diagnostic evaluation. Table 7-1 illustrates the important questions that should be asked of the jaundiced patient.

The physical examination should include a thorough search for evidence of acute and chronic liver disease and extrahepatic disease manifestations as outlined in Table 7-2.

Laboratory tests can confirm or refute clinical suspicions formed by the history and physical examination. Hyperbilirubinemia is classified as an excess of either conjugated or unconjugated bilirubin (Fig. 7-1). A pure increase in unconjugated bilirubin is usually indicative of defective conjugation, and Gilbert syndrome is by far the most common cause. Hemolysis and ineffective erythropoiesis cause a mild unconjugated hyperbilirubinemia. Hyperbilirubinemia that is predominantly conjugated may be due to congenital, familial, or acquired causes, the latter constituting the largest group by far (Table 7-3). Congenital causes of conjugated hyperbilirubinemia are very rare and are associated with isolated mild hyperbilirubinemia. Familial causes of conjugated hyperbilirubinemia result in intermittent or persistent hepatocellular cholestasis associated with other specific clinical, biochemical, genetic, and histological features. In cases of suspected acquired conjugated hyperbilirubinemia, appropriate hepatobiliary imaging will usually distinguish between extrahepatic and intrahepatic causes (Fig. 7-2). Hyperbilirubinemia may accompany both acute or chronic hepatocellular disease, especially when severe or end stage such as acute viral hepatitis and alcoholic liver disease, respectively; the latter two conditions constitute the most common causes of intrahepatic cholestasis. Occasionally, the evaluation of intrahepatic cholestasis may point toward a subtle extrahepatic cause requiring further radiologic evaluation (see Fig. 7-2).

In conjugated hyperbilirubinemia, aminotransferases and alkaline phosphatase should also be measured. These tests help determine if hepatocellular or cholestatic disease predominates. Aminotransferases are usually more elevated with acute hepatitis and less elevated with cholestasis (especially if extrahepatic). Bilirubin levels consistently below 5 mg/dL are not seen in extrahepatic biliary obstruction, unless the condition is in the early stages, but they are common in patients with cirrhosis. Bilirubin levels greater than 20 mg/dL, especially in the elderly, should raise suspicion for malignant biliary obstruction. If the alkaline phosphatase level is normal, extrahepatic obstruction is unlikely except in early acute obstruction. If the alkaline phosphatase level is more than three times normal, cholestasis probably exists. The level of alkaline phosphatase may be elevated disproportionately compared to bilirubin in partial biliary obstruction or early intrahepatic cholestasis (e.g., primary sclerosing cholangitis [PSC] and primary biliary cirrhosis [PBC], respectively). If both the alkaline phosphatase and bilirubin levels are markedly elevated, a common bile duct stone should be excluded. Indeed overall, alkaline phosphatase level is a more sensitive test for biliary obstruction than bilirubin level. In suspected cholestasis with an isolated elevated alkaline phosphatase, other tests (e.g., γ-glutamyltransferase, 5′-nucleotidase, leucine aminopeptidase) may confirm the hepatic source. Further disease-specific laboratory tests, with or without the aid of a liver biopsy, will usually define the etiology of suspected intrahepatic cholestasis. Evidence of disease chronicity may be suggested by hypoalbuminemia, and a prolonged prothrombin time.

Ultrasound is the preferred initial screening test to detect extrahepatic biliary obstruction. Variability in sensitivity reflects operator experience, overlying fat and bowel gas, site and size of the stones, and the stage of evolution of ductal dilation. Computed tomography (CT) scanning is similarly sensitive and is not impeded by adipose tissue, but is more costly and often requires intravenous contrast. Magnetic resonance imaging (MRI) is more sensitive and specific than contrast CT for the detection and evaluation of focal hepatic lesions. Magnetic resonance cholangiopancreatography (MRCP) (Figs. 7-5–7-6) is especially useful for detecting bile duct calculi, permitting imaging of the biliary tree both proximal and distal to the site of obstruction. This is particularly valuable after inadequate or unsuccessful endoscopic retrograde cholangiopancreatography (ERCP), although its use is more difficult to justify if there is a high probability that therapeutic intervention will be required. ERCP can localize the site of extrahepatic obstruction in more than 90% of patients, and both ERCP and percutaneous transhepatic cholangiography (PTC) permit concomitant therapeutic intervention (Figs. 7-7–7-19). ERCP also permits tissue and cytologic specimen collection, and imaging of the pancreatic ductal system and sphincter of Oddi manometry.

Endoscopic ultrasound (EUS) is superior to ultrasound and CT for diagnosing bile duct stones (Fig. 7-20), and is also useful for evaluating potential pancreatic causes of bile duct obstruction (Fig. 7-21). If available, EUS should be considered, particularly if there is a contraindication to ERCP or if prior ERCP was unsuccessful. The decision to pursue ERCP, PTC, or EUS depends on the presumed site of obstruction, the presence of coagulopathy, and available local expertise. Cost may be a consideration. If high-grade extrahepatic obstruction has been excluded or hepatic parenchymal disease is strongly suspected, a liver biopsy should be performed. The decision tree that the clinician follows depends to a great extent on pretest probability. Judgment that is based upon the patient's history and physical examination is dependable in the initial evaluation of patients with jaundice.

(figures begin on page 91)

TABLE 7-1
Clinical History in the Jaundiced Patient

Jaundice: speed of onset, duration, evolution, contact with jaundiced individuals, stool and urine color changes
Age at onset of symptoms
Constitutional upset: fatigue, weight loss, anorexia, fever, chills, rigors, confusion, sleep pattern alterations
Bleeding, especially gastrointestinal, symptoms of anemia
Abdominal pain: site, severity, frequency, radiation
Pruritus: onset, duration, site, severity
Alcohol use—both recent and lifetime, alcohol-associated illnesses, abbreviated CAGE questionnaire
Sexual history: number of sexual contacts, sexual practices, high-risk sexual contacts, STDs, HIV status
Country of origin and travel history to areas of endemic hepatitis
Blood product transfusion or infusion history: including history of operative, dental, and other procedures that may have involved use of
    transfusions or infusions, especially pertaining to serious trauma and childbirth
Behaviors involving needle use: tattoos, acupuncture, occupational
Environmental hepatotoxin exposure
Nutrition and dietary history including recent food ingestion (especially shellfish), obesity, rapid weight gain or loss
Symptoms of fat-soluble vitamin deficiency, hepatic osteodystrophy
Medical history: especially renal, cardiac, and neoplastic disorders; diabetes mellitus and thyroid disorders; hyperlipidemia; rheumatologic
    disease; dermatologic conditions diagnosed or without a specific diagnosis; hematologic disorders including thrombophilia; inflammatory
    bowel disease
Abdominal surgery history, especially pancreaticobiliary and gastrointestinal
Pregnancy history: current stage, prior or family history of jaundice in pregnancy
Occupational history: including exposure to needlestick risk, exposure to human waste matter, employment involving alcohol, incarceration
Family history of jaundice, liver, and pancreaticobiliary disease
Medication history: prescription, preoperative, nonprescription, substances of abuse, nutritional or herbal supplements, and folk or
    traditional remedies
Allergic symptoms and medication allergy history

CAGE, cut down, annoyed by criticism, guilty about drinking, eye-opener drinks; HIV, human immunodeficiency virus; STDs, sexually transmitted diseases.

TABLE 7-2
Physical Signs in the Jaundiced Patient

General appearance
   Scleral icterus, pallor
   Pigmentation: slate-grey, melanin
   Muscle wasting (+/− muscle tenderness)
   Edema
   Excoriation
   Behavioral changes (confusion, euphoria)
   Fever/hypothermia
   Scant body hair

Extremities
   Palmar erythema
   Dupuytren contracture
   Clubbing
   Leukonychia
   Koilonychia
   Tattoos
   Needle tracks
   Hyperreflexia
   Rashes, bullae, atrophic scars
   Arthropathy
   Xanthomata
   Ecchymoses
   Purpura (+/− palpable)

Head, neck, and thorax
   Xanthelasma
   Kayser-Fleischer rings
   Corneal arcus
   Parotid enlargement
   Xerostomia
   Fetor hepaticus
   Cyanosis
   Asterixis
   Constructional apraxia
   Lymphadenopathy
   Jugular venous distention
   Spider nevus
   Gynecomastia

Abdomen
   Hepatomegaly: smooth or irregular, pulsatile, tender
   Splenomegaly
   Ascites, everted umbilicus
   Palpable, +/− tender gallbladder, Murphy sign
   Operative scars
   Abdominal vein distention and direction of venous flow
      Outward from umbilicus: caput medusae (portal hypertension)
      Upward: Budd-Chiari syndrome or IVC obstruction
   Bruits, venous hums (hepatic, splenic, umbilical)
   Testicular atrophy
   Rectal examination (stool color, presence of blood)

IVC, inferior vena cava.

TABLE 7-3
Causes of Conjugated Hyperbilirubinemia

Congenital conjugated hyperbilirubinemias
  Rotor syndrome
  Dubin-Johnson syndrome

Intrahepatic cholestasis
  Familial and congenital
    PFIC-1, 2, 3
    BRIC
    Cholestasis of pregnancy
    Choledochal cysts
    Caroli disease
    Congenital biliary atresia
  Acquired
    Hepatocellular
      Alcohol
      Viral hepatitis
      Autoimmune disease
      Cirrhosis
      Drugs
      Wilson disease
      Hereditary hemochromatosis
    Infiltrative
      Granulomatous
      Carcinoma
      Hematologic malignancy
      Amyloidosis
    Cholangiopathies
      Primary biliary cirrhosis
      Idiopathic adult ductopenia
    Infections
      Bacterial
      Fungal
      Parasitic
      HIV-related
    Miscellaneous causes
      Postoperative sepsis
      Pregnancy
      Total parenteral nutrition
      Post–liver transplant cholestasis

Extrahepatic cholestasis
  Within bile ducts
    Calculi
    Parasites

  Bile duct wall
    Stricture
    Cholangiocarcinoma
    Sclerosing cholangitis
    Choledochal cysts

  Outside bile ducts
    Tumor in porta hepatis
    Tumor in porta hepatis
    Tumor in pancreas
    Tumor at ampulla of Vater
    Pancreatitis, acute or chronic

BRIC, benign recurrent intrahepatic cholestasis; HIV, human immunodeficiency virus; PFIC, progressive familial intrahepatic cholestasis.

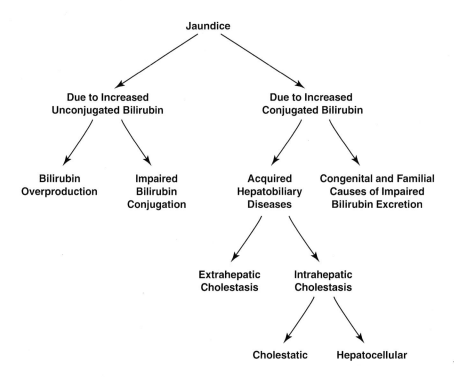

FIGURE 7-1. Differential diagnosis of the jaundiced patient.

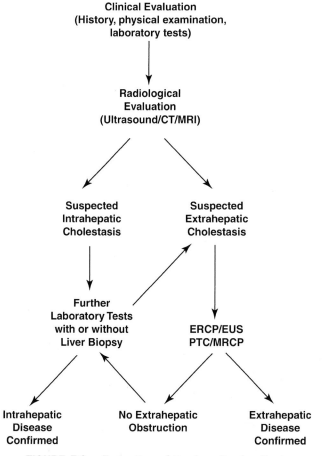

FIGURE 7-2. Evaluation of the jaundiced patient.

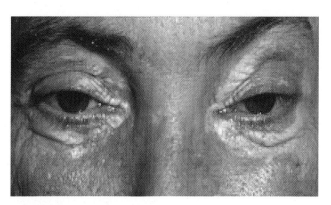

FIGURE 7-3. Numerous xanthelasma in a woman with primary biliary cirrhosis.

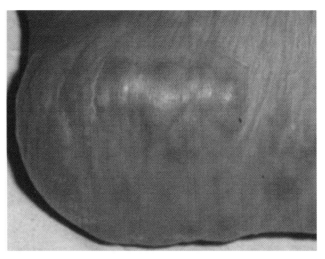

FIGURE 7-4. Tuberous xanthomas on the extensor surface of the foot in a patient with chronic cholestasis.

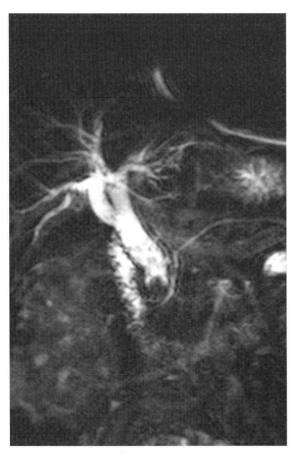

FIGURE 7-5. This magnetic resonance cholangiopancre-atography image shows a dilated biliary tree with several small calculi in the distal common bile duct.

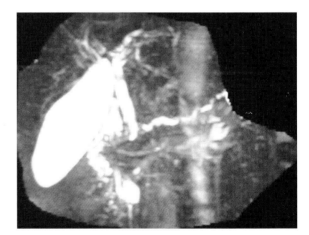

FIGURE 7-6. A magnetic resonance cholangiopancreatog-raphy image illustrating the double-duct sign: the pancreatic duct and the common bile duct are both dilated (the gall-bladder is also dilated). This elderly patient was later con-firmed to have unresectable pancreatic adenocarcinoma of the head of the pancreas.

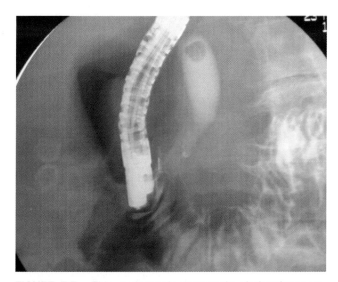

FIGURE 7-7. This endoscopic retrograde cholangiopancreatography image indicates endoscopic cannulation of the common bile duct, revealing biliary obstruction with common bile duct dilation secondary to choledocholithiasis. Gallbladder calculi are also noted.

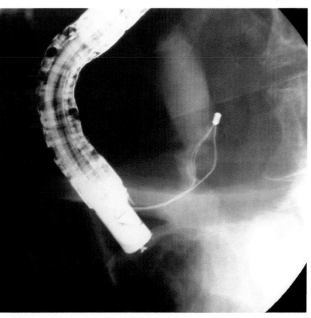

FIGURE 7-8. An endoscopic retrograde cholangiopancreatography image demonstrating the technique of basket extraction of common bile duct stones in a patient who presented with symptoms consistent with ascending cholangitis.

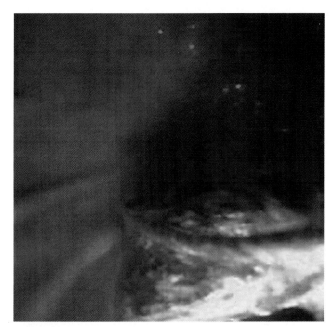

FIGURE 7-9. This endoscopic photograph shows a large stone removed via basket extraction after endoscopic sphincterotomy. Adequate sphincterotomy is essential prior to such techniques to avoid entrapment of the basket and stone at the level of the ampulla of Vater.

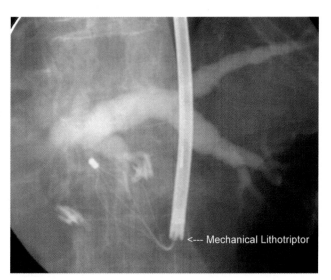

<--- Mechanical Lithotriptor

FIGURE 7-10. Mechanical lithotripsy may be necessary when large, hard stones are present as shown in this endoscopic retrograde cholangiopancreatography image. These stones, often composed primarily of calcium bilirubinate, are often too large for balloon retrieval or basket extraction, despite the presence of an adequate sphincterotomy. Once the stones are fragmented with lithotripsy, they may be removed safely.

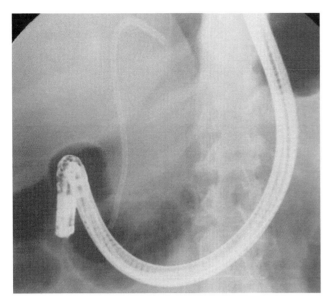

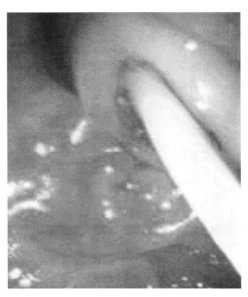

FIGURE 7-11. This endoscopic retrograde cholangiopancreatography image shows a Cotton-Leung stent extending from the duodenal lumen proximally into the left intrahepatic ductal system.

FIGURE 7-12. This endoscopic view provides the lumenal confirmation of successful transpapillary endoscopic stent placement. Nonmetallic biliary stents are susceptible to reocclusion and should be exchanged after several weeks if long-term stenting is anticipated.

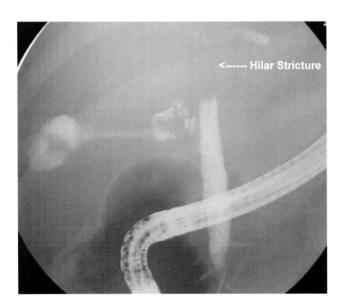

FIGURE 7-13. A large hilar stricture is seen in this endoscopic retrograde cholangiopancreatography image with some proximal dilation of the intrahepatic ductal system. As contrast is injected, preferential filling of the gallbladder, rather than the intrahepatic ductal system, is observed because of flow resistance in the common hepatic duct created by the stricture. Cytologic brushings subsequently confirmed the diagnosis of cholangiocarcinoma.

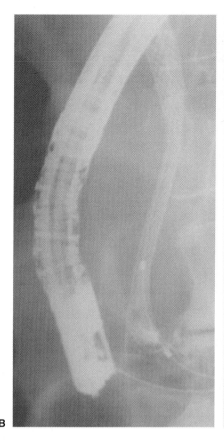
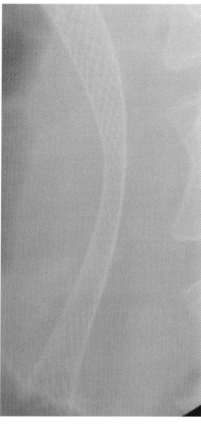

A, B

FIGURE 7-14. A: Endoscopic common bile duct metal stent (Wallstent, Boston Scientific, Natick, MA) placement with endoscopic retrograde cholangiopancreatography in a patient with unresectable pancreatic cancer and jaundice. **B:** The waist of the stent gradually expands after deployment.

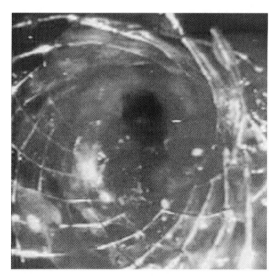

FIGURE 7-15. Endoscopic view of a common bile duct metal stent placed for the palliation of malignant biliary obstruction, with successfully reestablished lumenal patency.

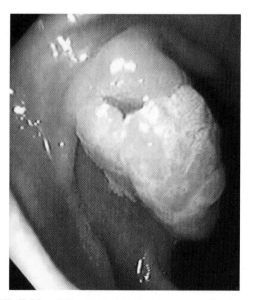

FIGURE 7-16. Biliary obstruction may result from neoplasms of the ampullary region. This endoscopic image shows an ampullary adenoma (confirmed by histology) that was identified during an endoscopic retrograde cholangiopancreatography examination performed for the evaluation of jaundice.

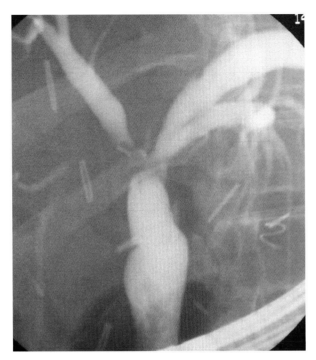

FIGURE 7-17. This endoscopic retrograde cholangiopan-creatography image shows a discrete hilar stricture with prox-imal intrahepatic ductal dilation, likely resulting from ductal ischemia in a patient who underwent an orthotopic liver transplantation several months previously. Serial balloon dila-tions and sequential stenting have been shown to be bene-ficial in the management of such strictures.

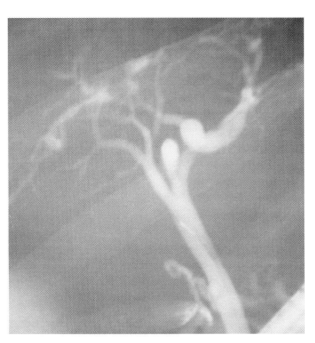

FIGURE 7-18. This cholangiogram exhibits the typical fea-tures of cirrhosis. The extrahepatic biliary tree is relatively normal, but marked attenuation of the intrahepatic system is noted. The left intrahepatic duct has the appearance of being displaced, a finding often caused by the nodular parenchyma found in cirrhosis.

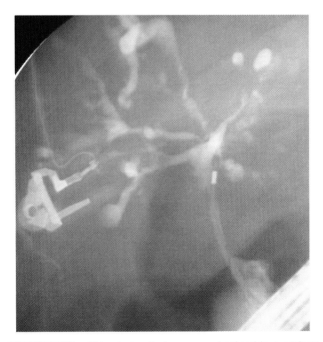

FIGURE 7-19. This cholangiogram was obtained in a patient with long-standing ulcerative colitis and new-onset jaundice due to primary sclerosing cholangitis. Marked stricturing of the extrahepatic biliary tree is seen. The intrahepatic system shows the more classic "chain of lakes" appearance with areas of stricturing and proximal saccular dilation.

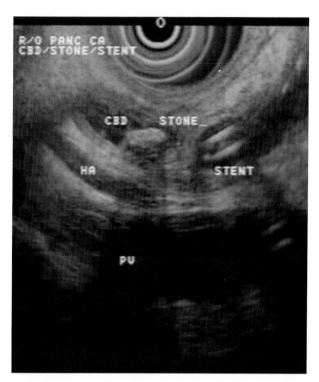

FIGURE 7-20. This image by radial endoscopic ultrasound shows a small stone, confirmed by the presence of post-acoustic shadowing, present proximal to a previously placed biliary stent for biliary obstruction of uncertain etiology in this elderly patient. The hepatic artery (*HA*) and portal vein (*PV*) are seen adjacent to the common bile duct (*CBD*). A subsequent endoscopic retrograde cholangiopancreatography with endoscopic sphincterotomy and balloon sweep allowed the extraction of two small stones and resolution of jaundice. There was no sonographic evidence of a pancreatic mass lesion.

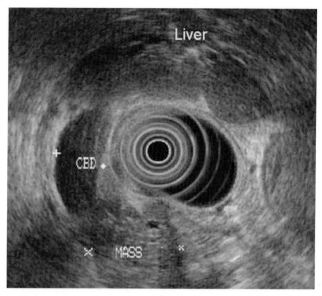

FIGURE 7-21. Radial endoscopic ultrasound examination of the pancreatic head reveals a pancreatic head lesion leading to obstruction and dilation of the common bile duct (*CBD*). (Courtesy of the Digestive Disease Center Web site, Medical University of South Carolina, *www.ddc.musc.edu.*)

APPROACH TO THE PATIENT WITH ABNORMAL LIVER CHEMISTRIES

RICHARD H. MOSELEY

Since the advent of routine automated serum testing, a common problem in gastroenterology has been the determination of the cause, and thus the importance, of abnormalities in liver chemistries. At first, such evaluations may be frustrating because of the lack of any well-defined diagnostic algorithms. However, armed with an understanding of the diverse panel of available measurements of liver function and serum markers of hepatobiliary disease, and knowledge of the patterns by which specific hepatobiliary disorders typically present themselves, the clinician can usually approach these diagnostic challenges in an orderly and selective manner. The normal values of certain laboratory tests that either lead to or assist in diagnosis are listed in Table 8-1, with ranges or reference intervals in traditional units and Système International d'Unités (SI).

Drug-induced abnormalities in liver chemistries are frequently encountered. Although familiarity with the hepatic side effects of all drugs used is not possible, knowledge of the potential for and clinical pattern of hepatotoxicity associated with commonly used agents is extremely useful. Representative drugs and their typical pattern of hepatic injury are listed in Table 8-2. Scales for scoring the probability of drug-induced hepatotoxicity have been developed, such as the Council for International Organizations of Medical Sciences (CIOMS) system (Table 8-3).

The use of alternative medicine, particularly herbal medicines, is increasing and hepatotoxicity is a recognized complication of these preparations. A representative list of these remedies and their reported hepatotoxicity is provided in Table 8-4.

A thorough occupational history may provide important clues to an otherwise cryptic case of abnormal liver chemistries. A representative list of industrial and environmental hepatotoxins is provided in Table 8-5.

Elevated serum aminotransferase levels can be observed among patients with any type of liver disease, and among patients with cardiac and skeletal muscle disorders. All too commonly, serum aminotransferase elevations are incorrectly ascribed to alcoholic liver injury. Alternative diagnoses, such as autoimmune hepatitis, viral and drug-induced hepatitis, nonalcoholic steatohepatitis, hemochromatosis, Wilson disease, and α_1-antitrypsin deficiency, should always be considered (Fig. 8-1). The highest elevations of serum aminotransferases are seen in patients with viral, toxin-induced, and ischemic hepatitis. In alcoholic liver disease, serum aspartate aminotransferase (AST; SGOT) and alanine aminotransferase (ALT; SGPT) levels are typically less than 300 units/L, and the ratio of AST to ALT is greater than 2. In the case of acetaminophen hepatotoxicity involving a patient with alcoholism, this ratio is maintained. In this setting, the serum aminotransferase elevation is striking, reaching and often exceeding levels typically associated with toxic, ischemic, or viral injury. Diagnosis of acute viral hepatitis requires appropriate application of serologic tests (Table 8-6). The typical course of chronic hepatitis B and chronic hepatitis C infection is illustrated in Figs. 8-2 and 8-3, respectively.

Elevation of serum alkaline phosphatase levels occurs primarily in cholestatic disorders, but the degree of elevation does not help one differentiate extrahepatic from intrahepatic causes. In the face of findings inconsistent with extrahepatic obstruction, intrahepatic cholestasis, whether drug-induced or from disorders such as primary biliary cirrhosis, as well as infiltrative processes, such as tuberculosis, sarcoidosis, and metastatic carcinoma, should be considered (Fig. 8-4). The differential diagnosis of granulomatous processes involving the liver that may present with infiltrative features is quite extensive. A partial listing of some of these disorders is provided in Table 8-7.

(figures begin on page 103)

TABLE 8-1
Normal Values of Laboratory Tests Used in the Approach to the Patient with Abnormal Liver Chemistries

TEST	REFERENCE INTERVAL		CONVERSION FACTOR
	Present	*SI*	
Alanine aminotransferase	0–35 U/L	0–0.58 μkat/L	0.01667
Albumin	4.0–6.0 g/dL	40–60 g/L	10.0
Alkaline phosphatase	30–120 U/L	0.5–2.0 μkat/L	0.01667
α_1-Antitrypsin	150–350 mg/dL	1.5–3.5 g/L	10.0
α-Fetoprotein	0–20 ng/mL	0–20 μg/L	1.00
Ammonia (venous)	10–80 μg/dL	5–50 μmol/L	0.5872
Aspartate aminotransferase	0–35 U/L	0–0.58 μkat/L	0.01667
Bile acids, total	Trace–3.3 μg/mL	Trace–8.4 μmol/L	2.547
Cholate	Trace–1.0 μg/mL	Trace–2.4 μmol/L	2.448
Chenodeoxycholate	Trace–1.3 μg/mL	Trace–3.4 μmol/L	2.547
Deoxycholate	Trace–1.0 μg/mL	Trace–2.6 μmol/L	2.547
Lithocholate	Trace	Trace	2.656
Bilirubin, total	0.1–1.0 mg/dL	2–18 μmol/L	17.10
Bilirubin, conjugated	0–0.2 mg/dL	0–4 μmol/L	17.10
Ceruloplasmin	20–35 mg/dL	200–350 mg/L	10.0
Copper, serum	70–140 μg/dL	11.0–22.0 μmol/L	0.1574
Ferritin	18–300 ng/mL	18–300 μg/L	1.00
γ-Glutamyltransferase	0–30 U/L	0–0.50 μkat/L	0.01667
Iron, serum			
Men	80–180 μg/dL	14–32 μmol/L	0.1791
Women	60–160 μg/dL	11–29 μmol/L	0.1791
Iron-binding capacity	250–460 μg/dL	45–82 μmol/L	0.1791

Note: The Système International d'Unités (SI) was adopted by the World Health Organization in 1977 in an attempt to bring international uniformity to laboratory measurements. The table lists the normal range or reference intervals of laboratory values in traditional units and the multiplication factor necessary to convert to SI units. Certain values listed are method dependent and therefore verification of the reference interval for a given clinical laboratory may be necessary.

TABLE 8-2

Partial List of Drug-Induced Abnormalities in Liver Chemistries

Hepatocellular injury (aminotransferase elevations)
    Acetaminophen
    α-Methyldopa
    Amiodarone
    Ampicillin
    Clozapine
    Dantrolene
    Dapsone
    Diclofenac
    Disulfiram
    Etoposide
    Fluconazole
    Glyburide
    Heparin
    Isoniazid
    Ketoconazole
    Labetalol
    Lovastatin
    Methotrexate
    Nicotinic acid
    Nitrofurantoin
    Propylthiouracil
    Rifampin
    Tacrine
    Terbutaline
    Trazodone
Cholestatic injury (bilirubin or alkaline phosphatase elevations)
    Androgenic anabolic steroids (e.g., methyltestosterone, danazol)
    Amoxicillin/clavulanic acid
    Atenolol
    Captopril
    Chlorpropamide
    Ciprofloxacin
    Cyclosporine
    Dicloxacillin
    Erythromycin
    Estrogenic steroids
    Flurazepam
    Floxuridine
    Gold salts
    Griseofulvin
    Haloperidol
    Imipramine
    Methimazole
    Penicillin
    Phenothiazines
    Piroxicam
    Propafenone
    Thiabendazole
    Ticlopidine
    Tolazamide
    Tolbutamide
    Trimethoprim-sulfamethoxazole
    Warfarin
Mixed hepatocellular and cholestatic injury
    Azathioprine
    Flutamide
    Phenylbutazone
    Phenytoin
    Sulfonamides
    Terbinafine
    Valproic acid
Granulomatous infiltration (alkaline phosphatase elevation)
    Allopurinol
    Carbamazepine
    Diltiazem
    Phenytoin

	HEPATOCELLUAR TYPE		CHOLESTATIC OR MIXED TYPE		ASSESSMENT
1. TIME TO ONSET					
Incompatible	Reaction occurred before starting the drug or more than 15 days after stopping the drug (except for slowly metabolized drugs)		Reaction occurred before starting the drug or more than 30 days after stopping the drug (except for slowly metabolized drugs)		UNRELATED
Unknown	When information is not available to calculate time to onset, then the case is				Insufficient data
	Initial Treatment	Subsequent Treatment	Initial Treatment	Subsequent Treatment	Score
From the initiation of the drug					
Suggestive	5 to 90 days	1 to 15 days	5 to 90 days	1 to 90 days	+ 2
Compatible	< 5 or > 90 days	> 15 days	< 5 or > 90 days	> 90 days	+ 1
From cessation of the drug					
Compatible	≤ 15 days	≤ 15 days	≤ 30 days	≤ 30 days	+ 1
2. COURSE	Difference between the peak of ALT and upper limit of normal values		Difference between the peak of alk. phos. (or TB) and upper limit of normal values		
After cessation of the drug					
Highly suggestive	Decrease ≥ 50% within 8 days		Not applicable		+ 3
Suggestive	Decrease ≥ 50% within 30 days		Decrease ≥ 50% within 180 days		+ 2
Compatible	Not applicable		Decrease < 50% within 180 days		+ 1
Inconclusive	No information or decrease ≥ 50%, after the 30th day		Persistance or increase or no information No situation		0
Against the role of the drug	Decrease < 50%, after the 30th day or recurrent increase		Not applicable		- 2
If the drug is continued					
Inconclusive	All situations		All situations		0
3. RISK FACTORS	Ethanol		Ethanol or Pregnancy		
Presence					+ 1
Absence					0
Age of the patient ≥ 55 years					+ 1
Age of the patient < 55 years					0
4. CONCOMITANT DRUG(S)					
None or no information or concomitant drug with incompatible time to onset					0
Concomitant drug with compatible or suggestive time to onset					- 1
Concomitant drug known as hepatotoxin and with compatible or suggestive time to onset					- 2
Concomitant drug with evidence for its role in this case (positive rechallenge or validated test)					- 3
5. SEARCH FOR NON DRUG CAUSES					
Group 1 (6 causes) = RECENT VIRAL INFECTION WITH HAV (IgM anti-HAV antibody) or HBV (IgM anti-HBc antibody) or HCV (anti-HCV antibody) and circumstantial arguments for non A-non B hepatitis); BILIARY OBSTRUCTION (ultrasonography); ALCOHOLISM (AST/ALT ≥ 2); ACUTE RECENT HYPOTENSION HISTORY (particularly if underlying heart disease)	All causes – groups I and II – reasonably ruled out				+ 2
	The 6 causes of group I ruled out				+ 1
	5 or 4 causes of group I ruled out				0
	Less than 4 causes of group I ruled out				- 2
	Non drug cause highly probable				- 3
Group II = Complications of underlying disease(s); Clinical and/or biological context suggesting CMV, EBV or Herpes virus infection					
6. PREVIOUS INFORMATION ON HEPATOTOXICITY OF THE DRUG					
Reaction labelled in the product characteristics					+ 2
Reaction published but unlabelled					+ 1
Reaction unknown					0
7. RESPONSE TO READMINISTRATION					
Positive	Doubling of ALT with the drug alone		Doubling of AP (or TB) with the drug alone		+ 3
Compatible	Doubling of ALT with the drugs already given at the time of the 1st reaction		Doubling of AP (or TB) with the drugs already given at the time of the 1st reaction		+ 1
Negative	Increase of ALT but less than N in the same conditions as for the first administration		Increase of AP (or TB) but less than N in the same conditions as for the first administration		- 2
Not done or not interpretable	Other situations		Other situations		0
				TOTAL (add the encircled figures)	

Scores may range from −5 to 14: <0, relationship excluded; 1–2, unlikely; 3–5, possible; 6–8, probable; >8, highly probable.

Adapted from Danan G, Benichou C. Causality assessment of adverse reactions to drugs—I: a novel method based on the conclusions of international consensus meetings: application to drug-induced liver injuries. J Clin Epidemiol 1993;46:1323–1330, and Benichou C, Danan G, Flahault A. Causality assessment of adverse reactions to drugs—II: an original model for validation of drug causality assessment methods: case reports with positive rechallenge. J Clin Epidemiol 1993;46:1331–1336.

TABLE 8-4
Herbal Hepatotoxins

AGENT	LIVER INJURY PATTERN
Greater celandine (*Chelidonium majus*)	Cholestatic hepatitis
Hydrazine sulfate	Submassive bridging necrosis
Chaparral (*Larrea tridentata*)	Cholestatic hepatitis
Jin Bu Huan (*Lycopodium serratum*)	Hepatitis with microvesicular steatosis
Germander (*Teucrium chamaedrys*)	Hepatitis
Pyrrolizidine alkaloids	
Comfrey tea (*Symphytum* species)	Venoocclusive disease
Crotalaria	
Senecio	
Heliotropium	

TABLE 8-5
Occupational and Environmental Hepatotoxins

AGENT	SETTING	LIVER INJURY PATTERN
Dimethylformamide	Organic solvent; used in many industrial applications including manufacture of polyurethane products and acrylic fibers	Hepatocellular
2-Nitropropane	Organic solvent; used in many industrial applications including manufacture of water-resistant coatings, printing inks, and adhesives	Hepatocellular
1,1,1-Trichloroethane	Organic solvent; widely used in industry	Hepatocellular
Trichloroethylene	Organic solvent; widely used in industry, including dry cleaning	Hepatocellular
Vinyl chloride	Polyvinyl chloride production	Infiltrative
Beryllium	Used in the manufacture of electrical equipment	Infiltrative

TABLE 8-6
Serologic Tests in Acute Viral Hepatitis

Hepatitis A	IgM anti-HAV
Hepatitis B	HBsAg and IgM anti-HBc
Hepatitis C	HCV RNA
Hepatitis D	HBsAg and anti-HDV

HAV, hepatitis A virus; HBc, hepatitis B core; HBsAg, hepatitis B surface antigen; HCV, hepatitis C virus; HDV, hepatitis D virus; IgM, immunoglobulin M; RNA, ribonucleic acid.

TABLE 8-7
Hepatic Granulomas

Infectious processes
   Tuberculosis
   Atypical mycobacterial infections
   Brucellosis
   Coccidioidomycosis
   Histoplasmosis
   Candidiasis
   Q fever
   Syphilis
Hepatobiliary disorders
   Primary biliary cirrhosis
Miscellaneous disorders
   Drugs
   Berylliosis
   Sarcoidosis

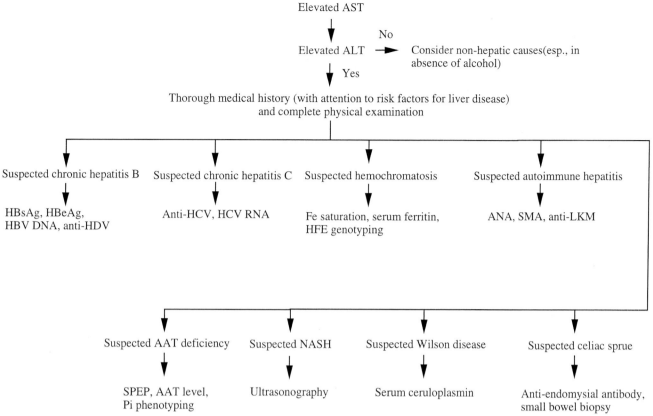

FIGURE 8-1. Algorithm for diagnosing the patient with elevated serum aminotransferase levels. Liver biopsy should be considered in most cases to confirm suspected disorders. *AST*, aspartate aminotransferase; *ALT*, alanine aminotransferase; *ANA*, antinuclear antibody; *SMA*, smooth muscle antibody; *anti-LKM*, antibody to liver kidney microsomes; *AAT*, α_1-antitrypsin; *SPEP*, serum protein electrophoresis; *NASH*, nonalcoholic steatohepatitis.

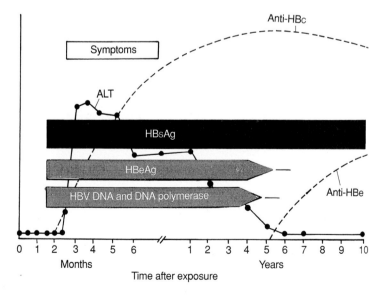

FIGURE 8-2. Typical course of chronic hepatitis B infection.

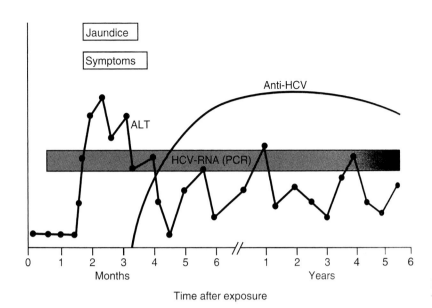

FIGURE 8-3. Typical course of chronic hepatitis C infection.

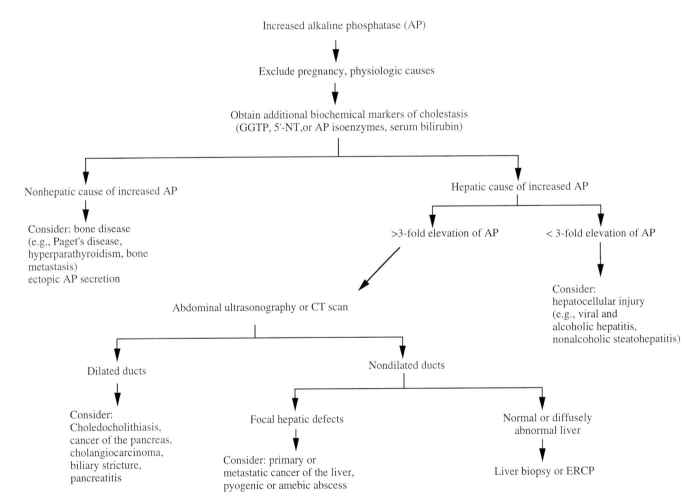

FIGURE 8-4. Algorithm for diagnosing the patient with elevated serum alkaline phosphatase levels. *CT,* computed tomography; *ERCP,* endoscopic retrograde cholangiopancreatography; *GGTP,* serum γ-glutamyltransferase; *5'NT,* 5'-nucleotidase.

APPROACH TO THE PATIENT WITH ASCITES

BRUCE A. RUNYON

The ancient Greeks around 400 B.C. first recognized that ascites was associated with liver disease. Abdominal paracentesis is one of the oldest medical procedures; the first report of this procedure is dated about 20 B.C. Yet the bulk of the literature regarding the diagnosis and management of ascites and the details of paracentesis has been published only since 1980.

The causes of ascites in the United States have changed during the last 100 years. At the turn of the century, patients with ascites were usually found to have cardiac or renal failure. Now more than 80% of patients with ascites seen by general internists and gastroenterologists-hepatologists have chronic parenchymal liver disease, that is, cirrhosis or alcoholic hepatitis. Heart failure and malignancy cause ascites in most of the remaining patients.

A detailed history, physical examination, careful analysis of ascitic fluid, and abdominal ultrasound (Tables 9-1 through 9-6) provide the diagnosis of the cause of ascites in most patients. Diagnostic paracentesis is a very important procedure to perform early in the evaluation of these patients (see Table 9-6). Despite selective intestinal decontamination of patients at high risk for spontaneous infections, spontaneous bacterial peritonitis remains a common complication of ascites (see Table 9-5). Early detection and early treatment of this reversible cause of deterioration of patients with cirrhosis and ascites maximize survival. Routine admission paracentesis has become the standard at many institutions for rapid assessment of the cause of ascites formation and early detection of infection.

The serum-ascites albumin gradient (SAAG) has replaced ascitic fluid total protein concentration (AFTP) in the classification of ascites (see Table 9-3). Ascites is characterized as high albumin gradient (≥ 1.1 g/dL) or low albumin gradient (< 1.1 g/dL) rather than transudative or exudative (see Table 9-4). The efficacy of treatment of patients with ascites has been found to depend in large part on the cause of ascites formation. Patients with high-albumin-gradient (e.g., cirrhotic or cardiac) ascites respond to sodium restriction and diuretics, whereas patients with low-albumin-gradient ascites (e.g., peritonitis or ovarian peritoneal carcinomatosis) do not respond to diuretics and need specific therapy.

Diagnostic ultrasound is more cost effective than a computed tomographic scan in the evaluation of the patient with ascites. Diagnostic ultrasound involves no iodinated contrast or need for intravenous access. Diagnostic ultrasound frequently provides information confirming the presence of cirrhosis (nodularity of the liver, abnormal portal venous size or flow pattern, and splenomegaly) and assists in screening for hepatocellular carcinoma. It is useful for the radiologist to provide the maximum dimension of the spleen. If this dimension is greater than 12 cm, the patient probably has portal hypertension.

Patients who seek medical attention late in the course of disease or who have disease refractory to medical management may have abdominal hernias from the weight of the fluid or even rupture of the hernia and leakage of ascitic fluid (Figs. 9-1 through 9-4).

In recent years, therapeutic abdominal paracentesis has been investigated scientifically and has been found to be safe and effective in the management of ascites. However, because about 90% of patients with ascites respond to diuretics and because chronic therapeutic paracentesis is highly consumptive of physician hours, therapeutic paracentesis is reserved for patients with tense ascites who need urgent decompression and for patients with ascites refractory to diuretic therapy. Therapeutic paracentesis can be performed relatively rapidly with semirigid tubing (e.g., a blood collection set) and vacuum bottles or a peristaltic pump.

If there is no reversible component to the liver injury (e.g., alcoholic-related injury), cirrhosis usually progresses over time such that patients with diuretic-sensitive ascites become diuretic-resistant. If they survive long enough, their renal function usually deteriorates further, and they may develop functional renal failure, otherwise known as hepatorenal syndrome (Fig. 9-5). Without successful treatment of hepatorenal syndrome, death is expected. Treatment options include liver transplantation, octreotide and midodrine, and transjugular intrahepatic portosystemic stent shunt.

(figures begin on page 109)

TABLE 9-1
When to Perform a Diagnostic Paracentesis

New-onset ascites
At the time of hospitalization
At the time of clinical deterioration
  Abdominal pain
  Fever
  Confusion

TABLE 9-2
Laboratory Data to Be Obtained for Patients with Ascites

MANDATORY	OPTIONAL	UNUSUAL
Ascitic fluid		
Cell count	Lactate dehydrogenase	Tuberculosis smear and culture
Albumin	Glucose	Cytologic testing
Culture in blood culture bottles	Gram stain	Triglyceride
	Amylase	Bilirubin
Total protein		
Simultaneous serum		
Albumin	Glucose	Bilirubin
	Lactate dehydrogenase	α-Fetoprotein
	Amylase	Alkaline phosphatase

Adapted from Runyon BA. Approach to the patient with ascites. In Yamada T, et al., eds. Textbook of gastroenterology, 4th ed. Philadelphia: Lippincott Williams & Wilkins, 2003.

TABLE 9-3

Classification of Ascites by Serum-Ascites Albumin Concentration Gradient

HIGH GRADIENT (≥1.1 g/dL)	LOW GRADIENT (<1.1 g/dL)
Cirrhosis	Peritoneal carcinomatosis
Alcoholic hepatitis	Tuberculosis (without cirrhosis)
Cardiac ascites	Pancreatic ascites (without cirrhosis)
Massive liver metastases	Biliary ascites (without cirrhosis)
Fulminant hepatic failure	Nephrotic syndrome
Budd-Chiari syndrome	Ascites in patients with connective tissue disease
Portal venous thrombosis	Ascites due to intestinal obstruction or infarction
Venoocclusive disease	
Acute fatty liver of pregnancy	
Myxedema	
Mixed ascites	

From Runyon BA. Approach to the patient with ascites. In: Yamada T, et al., eds. Textbook of gastroenterology, 4th ed. Philadelphia: Lippincott Williams & Wilkins, 2003.

TABLE 9-4

Accuracy of Ascitic Fluid Parameters

PARAMETER	ACCURACY (%)
SAAG ≥ 1.1 g/dL in detection of portal hypertension	96.7
AFTP > 2.5 g/dL in detection of exudate	55.6
Ascitic fluid LDH, ascitic fluid/serum LDH, ascitic fluid/serum total protein in detection of exudate	57.0

AFTP, ascitic fluid total protein concentration; LDH, lactate dehydrogenase; SAAG, serum-ascites albumin concentration gradient.

TABLE 9-5

Classification of Infected Ascites

CATEGORY	ASCITIC FLUID ANALYSIS
Spontaneous bacterial peritonitis	PMN ≥ 250/mm^3, single organism
Culture-negative neutrocytic ascites	PMN ≥ 250/mm^3, negative culture
Secondary bacterial peritonitis	PMN ≥ 250/mm^3, usually multiple organism
Monomicrobial bacterascites	PMN < 250/mm^3, single organism
Polymicrobial bacterascites	PMN < 250/mm^3, multiple organisms

PMN, polymorphonuclear leukocytes.

TABLE 9-6
Characteristics of Ascitic Fluid

CONDITION	SAAG (g/dL)	CELL COUNT (PER mm^3) PMN	WBC	TOTAL PROTEIN (g/dL)	GLUCOSE (mg/dL)	LDH (IU/L)	MISC.
Cirrhosis	1.7 ± 0.3 100% ≥ 1.1	37 ± 46	250 ± 25	1.8 ± 0.8 0.9–6.0	130 ± 30 0% < 50	60 ± 20 0% > 225	
Spontaneous bacterial peritonitis	1.8 ± 0.5 100% ≥ 1.1	7800	9300	0.7 ± 0.5 76% < 1.0	128 ± 63 0% < 50	170 ± 230 12% > 225	Monomicrobial
Intestinal perforation	1.4 ± 0.6 65% ≥ 1.1	8300	9400	2.5 ± 1.1 17% < 1.0	36 ± 47 67% < 50	850 ± 600 100% > 225	Polymicrobial
Cardiac disease	1.4 ± 0.3 100% ≥ 1.1	40 ± 60	480 ± 490	3.9 ± 1.1	149 ± 57 0% < 50	110 ± 44 0% < 225	
Tuberculous peritonitis	0.9 ± 0.4 50% ≥ 1.1	450 ± 860 30% > 250	1500 ± 1400 80% > 500	4.2 ± 2.1 67% > 2.5	85 ± 17 78% < 100	265 ± 178 50% > 225	50% cirrhotic
Nephrogenous disorder	1.1 ± 0.3 50% ≥ 1.1	10 ± 16	348 ± 227 25% > 500	4.6 ± 0.5	115 ± 8	94 ± 27	50% cirrhotic
Fulminant hepatic failure	2.3 ± 0.2 100% ≥ 1.1	319 ± 300	390 ± 360	0.5 ± 360 100% < 1.0	117 ± 20	23 ± 1	25% have spontaneous bacterial peritonitis
Lymphatic tear	1.6 ± 0.4	15 ± 6	480 ± 350 50% > 500	3.5 ± 1.2 50% > 2.5	130 ± 30	50 ± 11	Triglycerides 1465 ± 435 mg/dL
Pancreatic*	1.1 ± 0.3	3520	4240	3.15 ± 0.3	188 ± 135	1558 ± 1745	Amylase 1957 ± 1093 U/L
Biliary*	1.2 ± 0.5	2985	3403	2.6 ± 0.2	87 ± 84	2552 ± 154	Ascitic fluid bilirubin > 3.0 mg/dL, 50% infected
Peritoneal carcinomatosis	0.8 ± 0.4	110 ± 119	2800 ± 5500 75% > 500	3.6 ± 1.4 83% > 2.5	82 ± 44 71% < 100	901 ± 1833 74% > 225	100% positive cytologic results, 17% with cirrhosis
Massive liver metastases	1.9 ± 0.6	58 ± 76	297 ± 350	2.2 ± 0.7	102 ± 20	179 ± 84	100% alkaline phosphatase > 350 U/L
Peritoneal carcinomatosis and massive liver metastases	1.7 ± 0.2	550 ± 700	1890 ± 2180	2.2 ± 1.0	137 ± 31	214 ± 162	100% alkaline phosphatase > 350 U/L
Hepatocellular carcinoma	1.6 ± 0.5	992 ± 1956	1685 ± 2586	1.7 ± 0.8	135 ± 24	164 ± 160	High serum AFP
Nephrotic syndrome	0.7	5	130	0.6	105	38	

Note: Data expressed as mean ± SD except where specified differently (e.g., range, %, or < or > a cutoff).

AFP, α-fetoprotein; LDH, lactate dehydrogenase; PMN, polymorphonuclear leukocytes; SAAG, serum-ascites albumin concentration gradient; WBC, white blood cell.

*Approximately 50% of patients with pancreatic and biliary ascites have underlying cirrhosis and therefore mixed ascites.

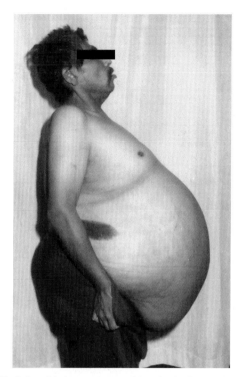

FIGURE 9-1. Male patient with alcoholic cirrhosis and ascites that was so massive it caused a gait disturbance. (Courtesy of T.B. Reynolds.)

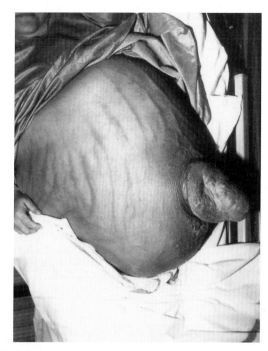

FIGURE 9-2. Female patient with cryptogenic cirrhosis who did not seek medical attention until her umbilical hernia almost touched the floor when she was sitting. (Courtesy of T.B. Reynolds.)

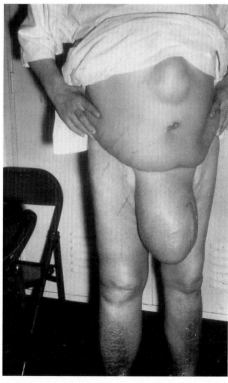

FIGURE 9-3. Male patient with large umbilical hernia and massive inguinal hernia. (Courtesy of T.B. Reynolds.)

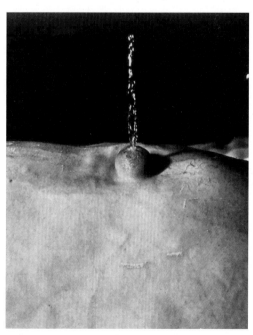

FIGURE 9-4. Ruptured umbilical hernia—one of the most feared complications of ascites. (Courtesy of T.B. Reynolds.)

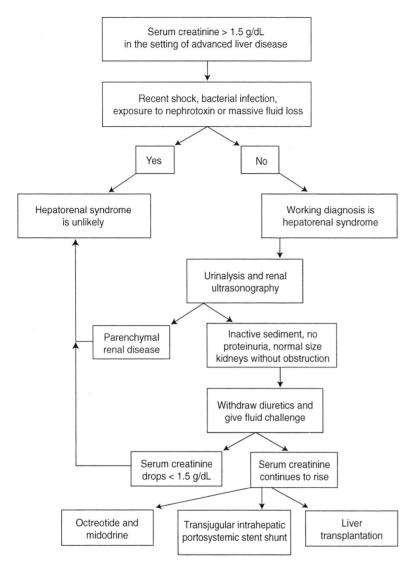

FIGURE 9-5. Algorithm for diagnosis and treatment of hepatorenal syndrome.

APPROACH TO THE PATIENT WITH A LIVER MASS

UMAPRASANNA S. KARNAM ■ K. RAJENDER REDDY

Liver masses are being increasingly detected on imaging studies—either in patients with abdominal symptoms or following surveillance in patients with chronic liver disease. These lesions may be benign or malignant, symptomatic or incidental, and single or multiple. The approach to a patient with a liver mass is steered by the pattern of patients' symptoms, findings on laboratory or imaging studies, and in a few cases by biopsy or surgical resection. A brief description of the individual entities is presented, followed by Tables 10-1 through 10-3 and a simplified algorithm for evaluation of a patient with a liver mass.

HEMANGIOMA

Hemangioma is the most common benign hepatic lesion, with a prevalence ranging from 3% to 20%. The lesion generally presents in women in their middle age as an *incidentaloma*. Larger lesions (>10 cm) (Fig. 10-1) may cause symptoms that include pain, which may be due to intralesional hemorrhage, localized thrombosis, or distention of the Glisson capsule. The T2 magnetic resonance imaging (MRI) scan is characteristic (Fig. 10-2). Most hemangiomas follow a benign course and most persons *live and die with the lesion rather than of it.* Treatment is not indicated for asymptomatic lesions that are less than 5 cm in diameter. Enucleation or resection is reserved for symptomatic lesions, rapidly enlarging lesions, and lesions that are greater than 15 cm in diameter at initial presentation.

FOCAL NODULAR HYPERPLASIA

Like hepatic hemangiomas, focal nodular hyperplasias (FNHs) also rarely cause symptoms and most often are discovered during an evaluation for abdominal pain. FNH is a nodular hyperplastic lesion that has a large female predominance (female to male ratio of 6 to 8:1) and the average age of presentation is between 30 and 50 years. A central scar is characteristic (Figs. 10-3 and 10-4). Although surgery is not recommended for asymptomatic FNH lesions, enucleation or resection is undertaken in symptomatic patients or those with rapidly enlarging lesions.

NODULAR REGENERATIVE HYPERPLASIA

Nodular regenerative hyperplasia (NRH) is a benign proliferative process in which the normal hepatic parenchyma is replaced by diffuse regenerative nodules of hepatocytes. NRH is relatively common and autopsy studies show a prevalence of 2%. The nodules vary in size from 0.1 to 1 cm. NRH has been associated with lymphoproliferative disorders, rheumatoid arthritis, primary biliary cirrhosis, bone marrow transplantation, anabolic steroids, Budd-Chiari syndrome, liver and renal transplantation, polyarteritis nodosa, hereditary hemorrhagic telangiectasia, systemic mastocytosis, amyloidosis, toxic oil exposure, partial hepatectomy, Felty syndrome, hepatocellular carcinoma, and other conditions. The clinical presentation of patients with NRH varies from an incidental finding in asymptomatic patients at one end of the spectrum to hepatic failure at the other extreme. Portal hypertension may evolve and ascites and esophageal varices develop in some patients.

HEPATIC ADENOMA

Hepatic adenoma (HA) is a lesion characterized by the benign proliferation of hepatocytes. HA is found predominantly in young or middle-aged women. These lesions are usually solitary in two thirds of the patients (Figs. 10-5 through 10-7). Few have multiple lesions and up to one third of lesions are larger than 10 cm. Although the annual incidence of HA is 1 to 1.3 per million in women who had never used oral contraceptives (OCPs), it increases exponentially to 34 per million in long-term users of OCPs. HA is also associated with glycogen storage disease, diabetes mellitus, pregnancy, and use of androgens. HA is frequently symptomatic, with the most common symptom being that of epigastric or right upper quadrant pain. Severe and sudden pain may be the presenting symptom and may be due to intralesional or intraperitoneal rupture. Although rare, catastrophic intraperitoneal bleeding is a well-recognized manifestation. Risk of malignancy and symptomatic complications mandate surgical removal of hepatic adenomas. In patients taking OCPs, a period of observation after removal of estrogens may be prudent because the lesions have been reported to decrease in size after discontinuation of OCPs. However, surgical resection is often favored, particularly in a solitary and surgically accessible lesion, because of the concern about complications.

BILIARY CYSTADENOMA

Biliary cystadenoma and its malignant counterpart, cystadenocarcinoma, are the most commonly encountered primary cystic neoplasms of the liver. It is more common in women, and can occur at extremes of age, although the mean age of presentation is usually in the fourth decade. The most common presenting symptom is right upper quadrant discomfort. Malignant transformation to cystadenocarcinoma has been described in up to 25% of cases and no imaging modality can clearly distinguish the benign from the malignant form. Hence, complete surgical excision is the treatment of choice.

SOLITARY HEPATIC CYST

Usually discovered incidentally in women (female to male ratio of 4:1), solitary hepatic cysts are commonly found in the right hepatic lobe. The most common and overt clinical presentation is right upper quadrant pain, which usually occurs in cysts larger than 5 cm in diameter. Intracystic hemorrhage, infection, and neoplasia are some of the reported complications. Asymptomatic solitary hepatic cysts are best managed conservatively. Laparoscopic fenestration of the cyst is the procedure of choice for a symptomatic cyst, and open surgical therapy is seldom needed. Ultrasound or computed tomography (CT) guided aspiration of symptomatic cysts has a high rate of recurrence, although it does provide symptomatic relief and also helps in establishing a relationship between the symptom of pain and the cystic lesion.

FOCAL FATTY INFILTRATE

Focal fatty infiltrate is an ill-defined lesion on an imaging study and is due to macrovesicular steatosis involving contiguous acini with no distortion of acinar architecture. Abnormalities due to focal fatty infiltration may be single or multiple and may mimic a malignancy. Focal fatty infiltrate is associated with alcoholism, obesity, malnutrition, total parenteral nutrition, chemotherapy, hypertriglyceridemia, diabetes mellitus, and acquired immunodeficiency syndrome (AIDS). Nonspecific abnormalities in hepatic biochemical tests have been reported. A liver biopsy may be needed to definitively rule out malignancy. Resolution of the lesions on correction of the underlying medical problem has been reported.

INFLAMMATORY PSEUDOTUMOR

Inflammatory pseudotumor represents less than 1% of all benign focal lesions of the liver and presents primarily in middle-aged men with fever, jaundice, weight loss, abdominal pain, and malaise. Although cultures of the lesion are negative, this entity is thought to result from a localized infection. Leucocytosis, elevated erythrocyte sedimentation rate (ESR), and normal α-fetoprotein help in differentiating inflammatory pseudotumor from a neoplastic process. Spontaneous regression has been reported in a few instances. When there is any doubt about the diagnosis, resection is in order.

CLINICAL APPROACH TO A LIVER MASS

The approach to a liver mass predicates on several factors such as the age and gender of the patient, mode of presentation, methods used in diagnosis, presence of underlying liver disease, and the degree of certitude desired by the clinician and the patient. The diagnosis and therapy of a liver mass has to be tailored to every case, and rigid adherence to any protocol might be detrimental. In some situations, referral to a tertiary care center would be prudent and in the best interest of the patient.

Advances in imaging technology have increased the precision of establishing a definitive diagnosis. However, exceptions to rules do occur, and histology—either by a needle biopsy or wedge resection—may ultimately be needed prior to a definitive procedure. Laparoscopy is an important investigative tool in select cases and contributes to a higher diagnostic yield. A simplified algorithm for evaluation of focal liver masses is presented in Fig. 10-8. The laparoscopic appearance of some lesions is shown in Figs. 10-9 through 10-11.

(figures begin on page 115)

TABLE 10-1
Classification of Hepatic Tumors

ORIGIN	BENIGN	MALIGNANT
Hepatocellular	Adenoma	Hepatocellular carcinoma
	Regenerating nodules	Fibrolamellar carcinoma
	Focal nodular hyperplasia	Hepatoblastoma
Cholangiocellular	Bile duct adenoma	Cholangiocarcinoma
	Biliary cystadenoma	Cystadenocarcinoma
Mesenchymal	Hemangioma	Angiosarcoma
	Lipoma	Primary lymphoma
Heterotopic	Adrenal/pancreatic	Metastases

TABLE 10-2
Characteristics of Hepatic Mass Lesions

	HEMANGIOMA	FNH	ADENOMA	CYST	HCC	METASTASES
Age (y)	30–50	20–40	20–40	All ages	50–70	40–70
Sex	F > M	F ≫ M	F ≫ M	F > M	M > F	M = F
US	Hyperechoic	Varied	Varied	Anechoic	Varied	Varied
CT	Strong enhancement	Scar	Capsule	Hypodense	Varied	Varied
MRI	CSF intensity	Liver intensity	Liver intensity	CSF intensity	Liver intensity	Spleen intensity
AG	Hypervascular	Hypervascular	Hypervascular	Avascular	Hypervascular	Varied
SS	RBC uptake	Uptake	Uptake	Cold	Cold	Cold
Scar	No	Yes	Occasional	No	Occasional	No
Cal	Yes	No	No	Occasional	Rare	Rare
Rupture	Rare	No	Yes	Rare	Yes	No

AG, angiogram; Cal, calcification; CSF, cerebrospinal fluid; CT, computed tomography; FNH, focal nodular hyperplasia; HCC, hepatocellular carcinoma; MRI, magnetic resonance imaging; RBC, red blood cell; SS, scintiscan; US, ultrasonography.

Adapted from Weissleder R, Pieumont MJ, Wittenberg J. Primer of diagnostic imaging, 2nd ed. St. Louis: CV Mosby, 1997.

TABLE 10-3
Radiologic Differential Diagnosis of Hepatic Lesions

HYPERVASCULAR HEPATIC LESIONS*	HYPOVASCULAR HEPATIC LESIONS*
Benign	
Hemangioma	Simple hepatic cyst
Focal nodular hyperplasia	Mesenchymal hamartoma
Hepatocellular adenoma	Bile duct hamartoma
Malignant	
Primary	
Hepatocellular carcinoma	Hepatoblastoma
	Fibrolamellar carcinoma
Metastases	
Renal cell carcinoma	Cervical carcinoma
Choriocarcinoma	Pancreas
Breast carcinoma	Lymphoma
Melanoma	Lung (adenocarcinoma)
Pheochromocytoma	Nasopharyngeal carcinoma
Thyroid carcinoma	
Sarcoma	
Carcinoid	
Ovarian cystadenocarcinoma	
Colon carcinoma	
Islet cell tumor	

*In general, hypervascular lesions are hyperdense on computed tomography scan with enhancement and hypovascular lesions are hypodense.

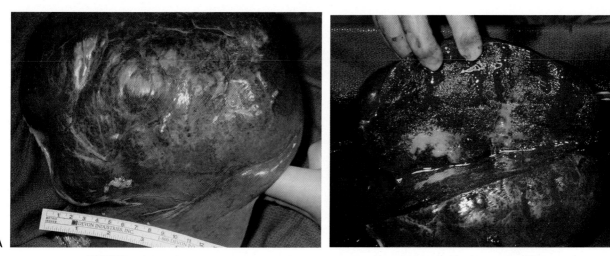

FIGURE 10-1. Gross specimen of a large hepatic hemangioma (**A**). The spongiform appearance of this lesion can be seen when the tumor is cut (**B**).

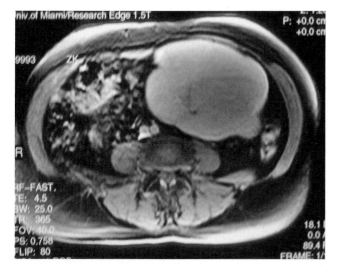

FIGURE 10-2. T2 magnetic resonance imaging scan shows characteristic features of hemangioma.

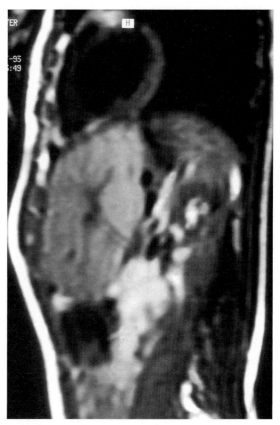

FIGURE 10-3. Characteristic central scar of focal nodular hyperplasia (magnetic resonance imaging).

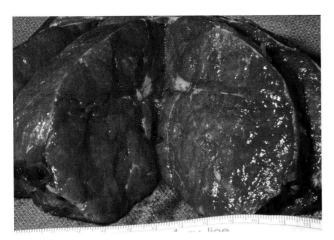

FIGURE 10-4. Gross appearance of focal nodular hyperplasia.

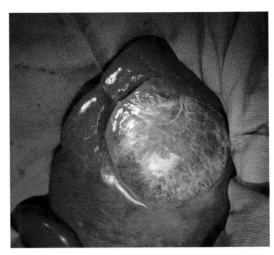

FIGURE 10-5. Gross specimen of hepatic adenoma. Note the well-encapsulated nature of the lesion.

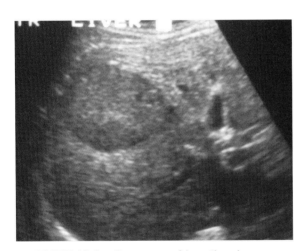

FIGURE 10-6. Sonogram of hepatic adenoma.

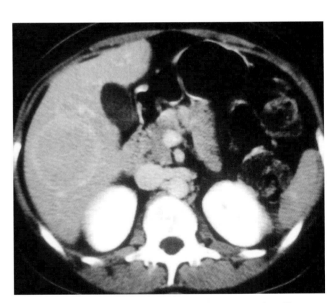

FIGURE 10-7. Computed tomography image of well-encapsulated hepatic adenoma.

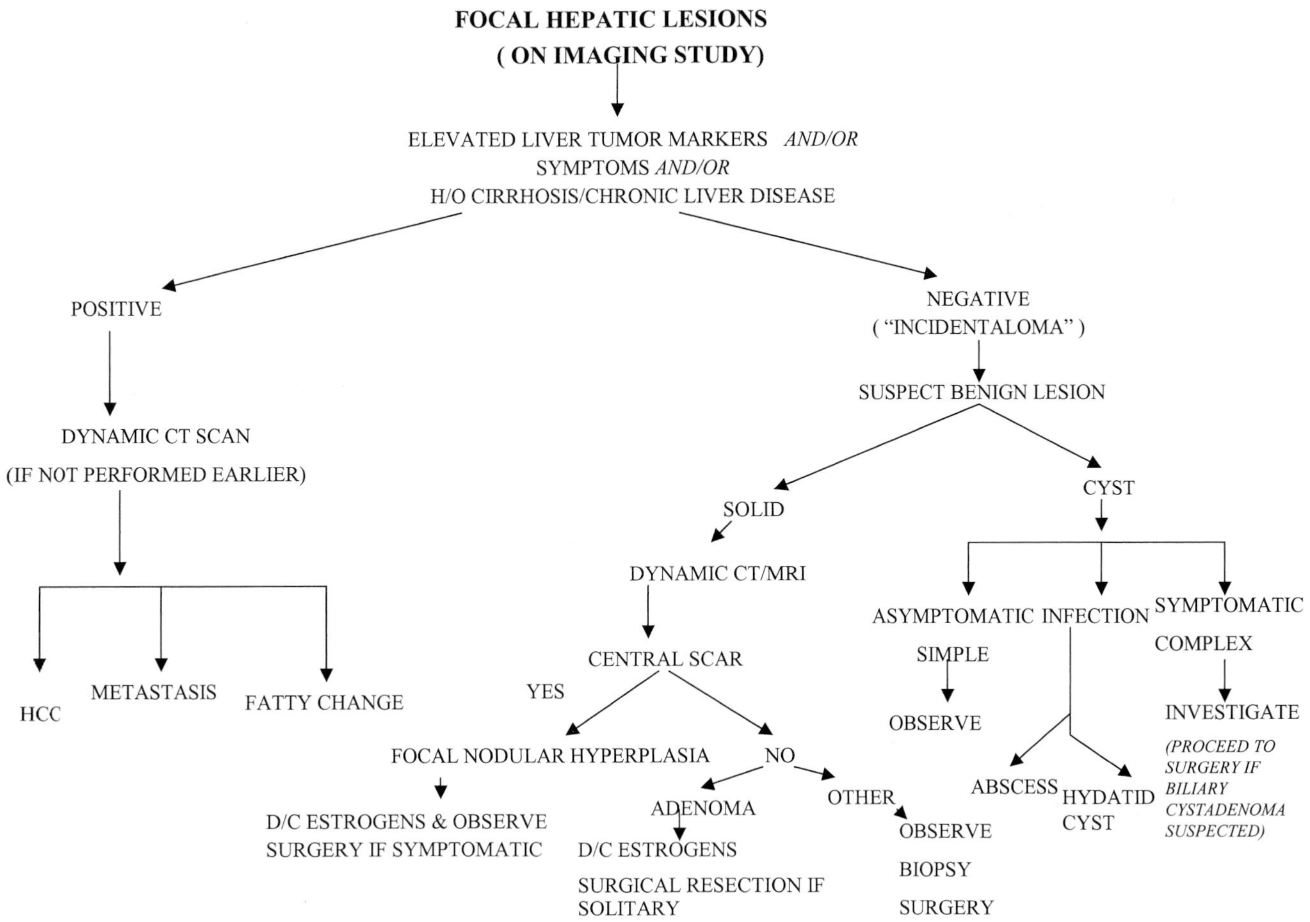

FOCAL HEPATIC LESIONS
(ON IMAGING STUDY)

ELEVATED LIVER TUMOR MARKERS *AND/OR*
SYMPTOMS *AND/OR*
H/O CIRRHOSIS/CHRONIC LIVER DISEASE

POSITIVE

NEGATIVE
("INCIDENTALOMA")

SUSPECT BENIGN LESION

DYNAMIC CT SCAN
(IF NOT PERFORMED EARLIER)

SOLID

CYST

DYNAMIC CT/MRI

ASYMPTOMATIC   INFECTION   SYMPTOMATIC

SIMPLE

COMPLEX

HCC

METASTASIS

FATTY CHANGE

CENTRAL SCAR

YES

OBSERVE

INVESTIGATE

FOCAL NODULAR HYPERPLASIA   NO

OTHER

ABSCESS
HYDATID
CYST

*(PROCEED TO
SURGERY IF
BILIARY
CYSTADENOMA
SUSPECTED)*

D/C ESTROGENS & OBSERVE
SURGERY IF SYMPTOMATIC

ADENOMA

D/C ESTROGENS

SURGICAL RESECTION IF
SOLITARY

OBSERVE

BIOPSY

SURGERY

FIGURE 10-8. A simplified algorithm for evaluation of a patient with a liver mass. See text for detailed description.

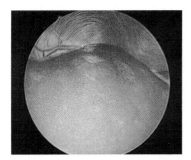

FIGURE 10-9. Laparoscopic view of a nodular lesion with central indentation consistent with focal nodular hyperplasia.

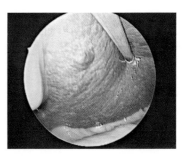

FIGURE 10-10. Laparoscopic demonstration of a purplish-blue lesion on the surface of the liver, which is characteristic of a hemangioma.

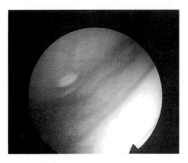

FIGURE 10-11. A white, partly umbilicated lesion consistent with metastatic adenocarcinoma.

APPROACH TO THE PATIENT WITH FULMINANT (ACUTE) LIVER FAILURE

PETER C. HAYES ■ KENNETH J. SIMPSON

Fulminant liver failure is a consequence of severe hepatic injury that results in a sudden deterioration in hepatocellular function and a characteristic clinical syndrome with hepatic encephalopathy, multiorgan failure, and death in severe cases. Fulminant hepatic failure (FHF) has many causes, which vary in relative frequency in different parts of the world. Supportive therapy allows both functional and structural regeneration of the liver in surviving patients, without the development of chronic liver disease. In selected cases, the prognosis is so grave that emergency liver transplantation is indicated. Such cases may become less common with the development and refinement of bioartificial liver systems, hepatocyte transplantation, and gene therapy.

The original clinical syndrome of FHF was defined more than 30 years ago as "a potentially reversible condition as a consequence of severe liver injury in which the onset of hepatic encephalopathy is within 8 weeks of the first symptoms of illness, in the absence of preexisting liver disease." Subsequently, there have been several attempts to refine the definition to take into account the common causes, complications, and prognosis. For example, the most recent modification proposed replacing FHF with the term *acute liver failure*, subcategorized into three groups: hyperacute liver failure, when the interval between jaundice and encephalopathy is 7 days or less; acute liver failure, for cases where the interval is between 7 and 28 days; and subacute liver failure, when the interval is between 5 and 12 weeks. However, many clinicians continue to use the original definition proposed by the Fulminant Hepatic Failure Surveillance Study as described above, and this definition is used throughout this chapter.

Prediction of those patients with severe liver damage who will subsequently deteriorate allows the earliest referral to a specialist center for consideration of liver transplantation and other supportive therapy and avoids the known dangers of transferring patients with encephalopathy. This "preencephalopathy" stage of FHF has been defined as "severe acute hepatic failure," and "impending" or "incipient" FHF. Many specialist centers have provided guidelines about which patients might be appropriate for transfer (Table 11-1), but prognostic studies on patients with impending FHF are lacking.

The main differential diagnosis when considering FHF is decompensation of chronic liver disease. The constellation of clinical and biochemical features including

118

hepatic encephalopathy, jaundice, transaminitis, and coagulopathy often determines the diagnosis of FHF. However, patients with a prolonged clinical course might be difficult to differentiate from those with decompensated chronic liver disease, especially when other complications such as ascites have developed. Careful review of all the patient's records may reveal previous evidence of a liver abnormality or identify alcohol abuse causing alcoholic hepatitis, which may simulate FHF, although in the latter clinical condition significant elevation of serum aminotransferases does not occur. The presence of cutaneous stigmata of chronic liver disease, clinical or radiological detection of splenomegaly, or the endoscopic appearance of esophageal varices is more suggestive of chronic liver disease in patients who have been jaundiced for less than 2 weeks. Occasionally, a liver biopsy is required and because of the universal coagulopathy, this is most safely performed by the transjugular route. At the same time, measurement of hepatic venous pressure gradient may suggest the presence of portal hypertension. A transjugular liver biopsy can exclude cirrhosis and may provide some prognostic information. In addition, potential information may be provided by the liver biopsy about the cause of FHF. Very rarely, other extrahepatic conditions may be confused with FHF, including severe intra-abdominal sepsis, acute pancreatitis, and tropical diseases.

The relative causes of FHF differ in different parts of the world (Table 11-2). Worldwide viral hepatitis is the most common cause of FHF, but in western countries toxic drug reactions and acetaminophen poisoning are the most common causes and are increasing in frequency.

ACETAMINOPHEN TOXICITY

Acetaminophen poisoning is the most common cause of FHF in the United States (36% of cases), but this frequency is much lower than in the United Kingdom, where up to 80% of cases may be secondary to acetaminophen poisoning. In the United Kingdom, the majority of these patients have taken acetaminophen during attempted suicide. In contrast, in the United States, most patients report accidental ingestion of large quantities of acetaminophen over a relatively short period or ingestion of therapeutic doses (so-called therapeutic misadventure). Fatal ingestion of therapeutic doses may also occur in patients taking enzyme-inducing drugs, such as anticonvulsants, and those who have been fasting or consume excessive amounts of alcohol. The diagnosis of acetaminophen-induced FHF is suggested by the presence of markedly elevated serum aminotransferases (>100 times normal), early development of acute renal failure secondary to acute tubular necrosis, metabolic acidosis, and hypophosphatemia. As liver failure progresses, acetaminophen metabolism is inhibited, therefore acetaminophen may still be detectable in the blood many hours after ingestion. Spontaneous rates of survival are higher in acetaminophen poisoning compared with other etiologies of FHF. Figure 11-1 shows typical centrilobular coagulative necrosis, and Fig. 11-2 provides the algorithm for acetaminophen levels used to decide risk of serious toxicity (high risk has a lower threshold).

ACUTE VIRAL HEPATITIS

Acute viral hepatitis is responsible for 10% of cases of FHF in the United States and the United Kingdom, but is more common in France and causes the majority of cases in Africa, Japan, and India. The most common cause of acute viral hepatitis is hepatitis B virus (HBV). The frequency of acute HBV causing FHF is decreasing, perhaps because of the widespread introduction of vaccination. FHF can also occur with reactivation of HBV following immunosuppressive or cytotoxic chemotherapy, during seroconversion to anti–hepatitis B early antigen (anti-HBe) positivity, or following coinfection or superinfection with hepatitis D virus (HDV). In patients with suspected acute viral hepatitis leading to FHF, the presence of immunoglobulin M (IgM) anti-HBV core antibody at high titer is diagnostic. Very rarely in patients with occult FHF, HBV-DNA has been detected by the polymerase chain reaction in liver tissue. The presence of HDV-RNA, IgM anti-HDV, or HDV antigen suggests super or coinfection with the HDV. A reasonable expectation of survival is associated with FHF secondary to HBV.

Both hepatitis A virus (HAV) and hepatitis E virus (HEV) can cause FHF, but the relative frequency is much less than HBV infection. The development of fulminant liver failure following HAV infection is more common in patients older than 40 years of age and those with preexisting liver disease. Detection of IgM antibody against HAV is diagnostic and the prognosis in such patients is relatively good. HEV has a more restricted geographic distribution compared with HAV. Epidemics of HEV infection occur in the Indian subcontinent, and pregnant women particularly appear at risk of developing FHF. Usually patients in developed areas such as North America and Europe have a history of having traveled to endemic areas within the previous 1 to 2 months. The finding of IgM anti-HEV antibody in the serum is diagnostic of acute HEV infection, and the mortality is similar to that of HAV infection. The risk of developing FHF following infection with hepatitis C virus HCV is not clear. Geographic areas with a high frequency of HCV infection have reported that HCV causes 40% to 50% of cases of FHF, but in western countries such as France, United Kingdom, and United States, such cases are very uncommon.

Many other viruses have been associated with FHF, including herpes simplex virus, varicella zoster, cytomegalovirus, Epstein-Barr virus, human herpesvirus 6, human parvovirus B19, and the RNA viruses, which are responsible for viral hemorrhagic fevers. In most reported series, a significant proportion of patients with FHF have no identifiable cause. Patients with non-A through E hepatitis have a worse prognosis compared with those infected with HBV or HAV.

IDIOSYNCRATIC DRUG REACTIONS

Severe hepatotoxicity resulting in FHF is an uncommon complication of drug treatment (excluding acetaminophen poisoning), but a wide range of drugs can cause severe liver injury and rarely, FHF develops. The relative contribution of idiosyncratic drug reactions to other causes of FHF varies relative to the geographic distribution; these reactions are responsible for 16% to 17% of FHF cases in the United States. Idiosyncratic drug reactions causing FHF are generally associated with a poor prognosis compared with other causes.

Reye syndrome is characterized by rapidly progressive hepatic encephalopathy with cerebral edema and hepatic steatosis. This syndrome, most commonly described in children, is strongly associated with the use of salicylates. The ingestion of herbal remedies, available without prescription, and other over-the-counter remedies may also lead to the development of FHF. FHF may also result from illicit drug ingestion. The consumption of cocaine or ecstasy has been associated with FHF, which in the latter case may or may not be associated with a hyperpyrexia syndrome. Industrial solvents such as carbon tetrachloride and heavy metals can also cause FHF. Amanita mushroom consumption has also been reported to cause FHF in both continental Europe and the United States. This produces a characteristic clinical syndrome with severe vomiting and diarrhea lasting 1 to 4 days, followed by massive elevation of the aminotransferases and the development of FHF.

OTHER CAUSES

FHF may occur during pregnancy either because of acute fatty liver of pregnancy or as part of the hemolysis, elevated liver enzymes, and low platelet count (HELLP) syndrome. Such patients often also suffer with hypertension or preeclampsia. Other causes of FHF, including potentially useful diagnostic tests of all causes of FHF, are detailed in Table 11-3.

MANAGEMENT

Early Pre-Intensive Care Unit (ICU) Management

Cardiovascular

FHF is characterized by a hyperdynamic circulation, with tachycardia, hypotension, increased cardiac output, and low peripheral vascular resistance. This clinical picture resembles that seen in sepsis and the two conditions often coexist. Monitoring of the cardiovascular system with measurements of pulse, blood pressure, and urine output is appropriate in the very early clinical stages (preencephalopathy), but measurement of the central venous pressure or pulmonary artery wedge pressure is usually required. The former is often undertaken before the development of encephalopathy. The latter allows more information to be gained regarding systemic vascular resistance, cardiac output, and left ventricular filling pressure, but may only be available in the ICU setting. Maintenance of adequate central venous pressure with both crystalloid and colloid is essential and may be the most effective method of preventing further renal injury secondary to hypotension. Inotropic support may be necessary, is usually provided in the ICU, and is discussed in the Late ICU Management section below.

Metabolic

The most important and potentially serious metabolic complication of FHF is hypoglycemia, which occurs because of reduced hepatic synthesis. Frequent blood glucose testing should be carried out (every 2 hours) and dextrose (10%–20% solutions) administered as a prophylactic measure. Treatment of hypoglycemia uses bolus 50% dextrose, which may have to be administered by continuous infusion. Acidosis is common in patients with acetaminophen poisoning and has prognostic significance. A pH of less than 7.3 ($H^+ > 50$ nmol/L) in patients who have been fully resuscitated is associated with a greater than 90% mortality (Table 11-4). Hypokalemia and hypophosphatemia may occur and require correction.

Renal

Renal failure is common in FHF, particularly in acetaminophen poisoning because this drug is also directly toxic to the kidneys. Close monitoring of urine output is required. Measurement of serum creatinine gives a better indication of renal function, because blood urea is dependent on hepatic synthesis and may be misleadingly low. An elevated serum creatinine also is a marker of poor prognosis in patients with acetaminophen-induced FHF (see Table 11-4).

Hematologic

The prothrombin time is a readily available test and perhaps one of the best markers of hepatic synthetic function (Table 11-4). Because prothrombin time is such a valuable marker of prognosis, it is advisable to avoid administering fresh frozen plasma or clotting factors prophylactically unless there is clinical evidence of significant bleeding. In a series of patients with FHF studied from King's College Hospital, London, a prothrombin time of more than 50 seconds in non–acetaminophen-induced FHF and more than 100 seconds in acetaminophen-induced cases were markers of poor prognosis (i.e., mortality rates of >90%). Furthermore, an increase in the prothrombin time between days 3 and 4 following ingestion of a single overdose and a single prothrombin time of more than 180 seconds have also been reported to carry a poor prognosis in acetaminophen-induced FHF. Thrombocytopenia is common in FHF but platelet transfusion should be avoided unless the patient has active bleeding, because clotting factors are contained within the replacement packs and might affect the prothrombin time. In general, patients are administered proton pump inhibitors, H_2-blockers, or sucralfate to prevent gastrointestinal hemorrhage.

Infection

Sepsis is a common and often fatal complication of FHF. Once encephalopathy has developed, the prophylactic administration of antibiotics such as ciprofloxacin is recommended. Frequent and rigorous screening for both bacterial and fungal infection is essential. Because of the inherent delay in receiving confirmation of infection, many specialist units advocate both prophylactic antibacterial and antifungal measures.

Neurological

Encephalopathy is the cardinal feature of FHF and should be actively and frequently sought. Traditionally encephalopathy is divided into four grades (Table 11-5). This four-point grading system is important, because more severe grades of hepatic encephalopathy have prognostic significance following acetaminophen poisoning. Patients who have developed grade 3 encephalopathy cannot protect their airways and therefore are transferred to ICU for assisted ventilation. Occasionally, patients with grade 2 hepatic encephalopathy become very aggressive and agitated, making invasive monitoring and other management difficult. These patients also require sedation and mechanical ventilation. With increasing severity of encephalopathy, there is an increasing risk of developing cerebral edema and increased intracranial pressure. This complication can still occur in patients with mild encephalopathy and may be heralded by bradycardia, hypertension, dilated or unequal pupils, and decerebrate posturing.

N-Acetylcysteine

N-acetylcysteine (NAC) is a highly effective antidote for acetaminophen poisoning and is widely used intravenously in the United Kingdom. Oral administration of NAC or methionine also reduces the risk of liver failure after acetaminophen poisoning, but the vomiting that frequently occurs reduces its efficacy. A randomized clinical trial suggested that late administration of NAC in patients with acetaminophen-induced FHF was effective in reducing the progression of hepatic encephalopathy and the development of other complications. Some studies have suggested that NAC may also be beneficial in non–acetaminophen-induced FHF, perhaps by improving tissue oxygen delivery. However, recent data have not confirmed this finding and clinical trials are continuing.

Late ICU Management

Cardiovascular

Hypotension is often present by the time patients with FHF reach the ICU. Invasive monitoring for this complication is generally undertaken as described above. The presence of a systolic blood pressure less than 100 mm Hg and a mean arterial pressure of less than 70 mm Hg are indicators for inotropic support. Norepinephrine is the most widely employed inotrope, with the dose titrated to reach a mean arterial pressure of greater than 80 mm Hg.

Ventilation

Pulmonary problems in patients with FHF are common and include aspiration, pneumonia, noncardiogenic neurogenic pulmonary edema, and the development of the adult respiratory distress syndrome (ARDS) as part of the multiorgan failure syndrome. The onset of such respiratory complications is highly problematic and may contraindicate hepatic transplantation in certain patients.

Intracranial Pressure

As discussed above, the development of increased intracranial pressure and cerebral edema is more common as hepatic encephalopathy progresses. The clinical features of increased intracranial pressure or cerebral edema described above are late features. In many ICUs, an intracranial extradural pressure monitor will be inserted in the patient (Figs. 11-3 and 11-4). Although this procedure carries some risk of intracranial hemorrhage, no increased mortality has been reported in clinical trials. On the other hand, no benefits in survival have been reported. Before insertion of such transducers, abnormal coagulation requires correction. The detection of an intracranial pressure greater than 20 mm Hg for longer than 10 minutes is an indicator for treatment. Perhaps of more value is the recording of cerebral perfusion pressure (mean arterial pressure minus intracranial pressure). Maintaining the cerebral perfusion pressure (CPP) greater than 60 mm Hg is one of the goals of ICU treatment. A CPP of less than 40 mm Hg for longer than 60 minutes is, in some units, a contraindication to liver transplantation.

Treatment of increased intracranial pressure initially depends on mannitol infusion. Repeated administration may be required, but the efficacy of this treatment decreases with time. A recognized complication of repeat administration of mannitol is hyperosmolality; plasma osmolality should therefore be measured during repeated administration. Mannitol treatment acts by inducing an osmotic diuresis. Therefore, mannitol treatment in patients with renal failure is problematic and requires the early intervention with renal support therapy, as discussed below. If the increased intracranial pressure becomes resistant to mannitol therapy, second-line treatment with thiopentone may be started, but has not shown to be beneficial in randomized trials. Other treatments include the induction of moderate hypothermia or explantation of the liver with the hope of transplantation as a two-stage procedure. An additional important neurological complication of FHF is epileptic seizures, which may be masked by sedation and occur subclinically. A recent study advocated prophylactic phenytoin treatment with continuous electroencephalogram (EEG) monitoring to avoid this complication.

Renal

As discussed, renal failure is common in patients with FHF and the majority of patients in the ICU will require renal support. Continuous venovenous hemofiltration or arteriovenous hemofiltration is preferable to intermittent filtration or dialysis, which can lead to uncontrollable increases in intracranial pressure. Prostacyclin is often used in preference to heparin as an anticoagulant in the hemofiltration system, although in certain cases no anticoagulant may be necessary. Because of the acidosis, lactate buffers are chosen over bicarbonate buffers for filtration. Following recovery of hepatic synthetic function or liver transplantation, continued renal support may be required for several weeks.

Transplantation

It is generally in the ICU that liver function deteriorates to such a degree that the prognosis is considered grave. In such patients, liver transplantation may be considered (Table 11-4). In the United Kingdom, the most commonly used criteria for determining prognosis were derived from a series of patients managed at King's College Hospital, London. An acute physiology and chronic health evaluation II

(APACHE II) score of greater than 15 soon after admission to the ICU may also be useful in identifying a poor prognosis. APACHE II has an advantage over the King's College criteria in that ICU physicians are familiar with its use. However, the predictive power of the two scoring systems is similar. Survival figures of approximately 60% are often quoted for patients with FHF compared with 80% or higher for those transplanted with cirrhosis.

Liver Support Devices

Over several decades studies have reported the use of liver support devices designed to detoxify the blood of patients with FHF or provide undefined, liver-derived factors. The former includes hemofiltration, charcoal hemoperfusion and plasmapheresis, but none of these have proven to be of value in clinical practice. Extracorporeal hepatic perfusion has also been attempted. More recently, bioreactors have been developed that have included liver cells incorporated into a filtering system containing a framework physically supportive to the cells. Many different bioreactors are at various stages of clinical development and some have entered trials, but the reports of these are still awaited, and liver transplantation remains the mainstay for treatment of severely affected individuals.

(figures begin on page 126)

TABLE 11-1

Clinical Features of FHF that Suggest Discussion with a Specialist Liver Center

Prothrombin time > 20 s
INR > 2.0
Hypoglycemia
Encephalopathy
Developing renal failure
Bilirubin > 100 μmol/L

FHF, fulminant hepatic failure; INR, international normalized ratio.

TABLE 11-2

Etiological Distribution of FHF in Different Countries

	UNITED STATES	UNITED KINGDOM	FRANCE	INDIA
Acetaminophen	20	73	3	—
Drug reaction	13	3	17	6
Non-A, non-B hepatitis	15	8	20	66
Hepatitis B	10	3	32	29
Hepatitis A	6	3	4	3
Hepatitis D	—	—	—	13
Wilson disease	5	3	3	3
Pregnancy	1	2	—	—

Note: Data presented as frequency of total cases (percent). FHF, fulminant hepatic failure.

TABLE 11-3
Fulminant Liver Failure: Causes and Helpful Diagnostic Investigations

Acetaminophen poisoning	Acidosis, early renal failure, very high aminotransferases (5000 IU), detectable acetaminophen
Idiosyncratic drug reactions	Positive serology
Budd-Chiari syndrome	Ultrasound, CT scan, MRI, hepatic venogram
Wilson disease	Slitlamp examination, hemolytic anemia, relatively normal aminotransferases, reduced ceruloplasmin, elevated urinary and serum copper
Hepatitic malignancy	Ultrasound scan, CT scan, MRI, transjugular biopsy
Autoimmune hepatitis	Immunoglobulins, positive antinuclear factor or anti–smooth muscle antibody
Viral hepatitis	
Hepatitis A	IgM anti-HAV
Hepatitis B	IgM anti-HBc
Hepatitis D	HDV, RNA, IgM and anti-HDV, HDV antigen

CT, computed tomography; HAV, hepatitis A virus; HBc, hepatitis B core; HDV, hepatitis D virus; IgM, immunoglobulin M; MRI, magnetic resonance imaging; RNA, ribonucleic acid.

TABLE 11-4
Indicators of Poor Prognosis in FHF

Acetaminophen poisoning
    Arterial pH < 7.3 ($H^+ > 50$ nmol/L) or
    Three of the following
        Prothrombin time > 100 s
        Serum creatinine > 300 μmol/L
        Encephalopathy grade 3 or 4

Non–acetaminophen group
    Prothrombin time > 100 s or
    Three of the following
        Unfavorable cause (e.g., idiosyncratic drug reaction, non-A through E hepatitis)
        Jaundice for > 7 d before encephalopathy
        Age < 10 or > 40 y
        Prothrombin time > 50 s
        Serum bilirubin > 300 μmol/L

FHF, fulminant hepatic failure.

TABLE 11-5
Clinical Grading of Hepatic Encephalopathy

CLINICAL GRADE	CLINICAL SIGNS
Grade 1	Poor concentration, slurred speech, slow mentation, disordered sleep rhythm
Grade 2	Drowsy but easily rousable, occasional aggressive behavior, lethargic
Grade 3	Marked confusion, drowsy, sleepy but responds to pain and voice, gross disorientation
Grade 4	Unresponsive to voice, may or may not respond to painful stimuli, unconscious

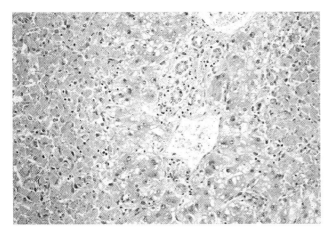

FIGURE 11-1. Microscopic appearance of the liver following acetaminophen poisoning.

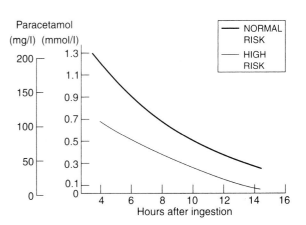

FIGURE 11-2. Acetaminophen venous blood concentrations following overdose. The high-risk group includes patients abusing alcohol and those taking enzyme-inducing drugs.

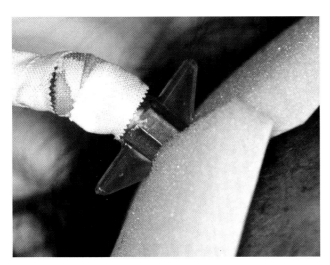

FIGURE 11-3. Intracranial pressure monitor inserted into the nondominant frontal hemisphere to allow the early diagnosis of increased intracranial pressure.

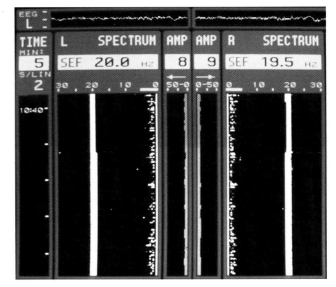

FIGURE 11-4. Cerebrotrack monitor (Neurosciences, United Kingdom) tracing in patient with acute liver failure.

12

SKIN LESIONS ASSOCIATED WITH GASTROINTESTINAL DISEASES

MICHELLE L. BENNETT ■ ELIZABETH F. SHERERTZ ■ JOSEPH L. JORIZZO

Skin lesions may be a presenting sign of conditions involving the gastrointestinal tract or liver, as in the case of pyoderma gangrenosum, dermatitis herpetiformis, or the skin changes of cryoglobulinemia. Primary skin diseases occasionally may involve the gastrointestinal tract directly, as in the case of blistering diseases. In some situations, examination of the skin during evaluation of gastrointestinal symptoms may help provide an important clue to internal diseases. On the other hand, it is important to maintain an objective, morphologic approach to diagnosis of skin lesions for such patients. Do not assume an association between cutaneous and gastrointestinal signs.

The keys to diagnosis of some of the conditions shown here are to

- take the time to listen to the patient's possible incidental concerns
- perform a thorough examination of the skin
- recognize disease associations or common skin and gastrointestinal pathological conditions and
- perhaps most important, have the cutaneous diagnosis confirmed by a dermatologist.

Figures 12-1 through 12-75 illustrate examples of occasional and rare cutaneous involvement of disease processes.

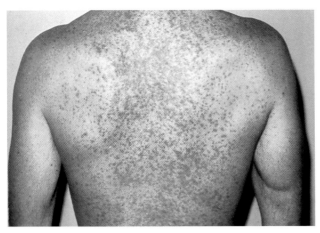

FIGURE 12-1. Generalized morbilliform erythema caused by penicillin allergy.

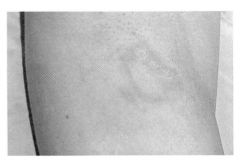

FIGURE 12-2. Erythema annulare centrifugum without identified precipitant.

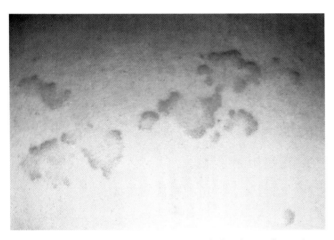

FIGURE 12-3. Urticaria. Note the variation in configuration. Each lesion resolved within 24 hours.

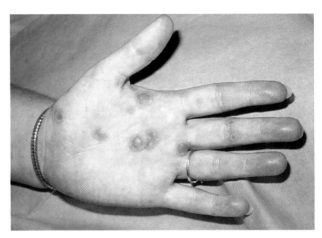

FIGURE 12-4. Erythema multiforme. Typical target lesions.

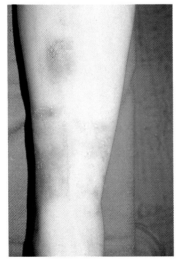

FIGURE 12-5. Erythema nodosum. These tender nodules occurred in association with ulcerative colitis.

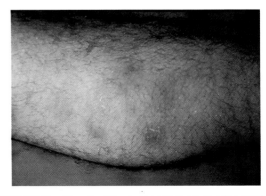

FIGURE 12-6. Panniculitis presenting as tender erythematous nodules on a patient with pancreatitis.

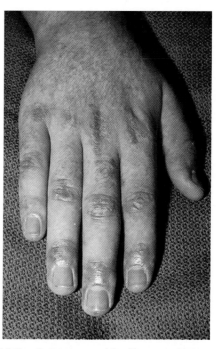

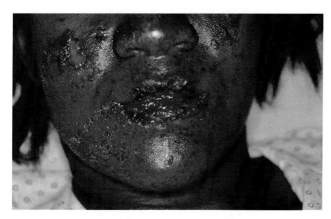

FIGURE 12-7.   Stevens-Johnson syndrome. Note crusted lip involvement.

FIGURE 12-8.   Dermatomyositis. Note erythematous shiny papules involving the knuckles (Gottron sign).

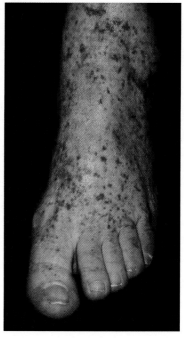

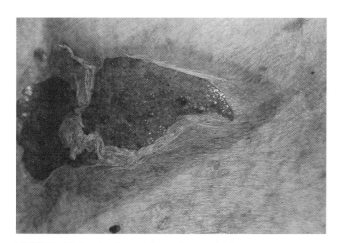

FIGURE 12-9.   Toxic epidermal necrolysis caused by allopurinol reaction.

FIGURE 12-10.   Necrotizing venulitis (i.e., small-vessel leukocytoclastic vasculitis), which was idiopathic in this patient and confined to the skin.

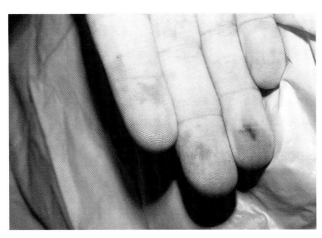

FIGURE 12-11.   Polyarteritis nodosum. Note the necrotizing changes in multiple digits.

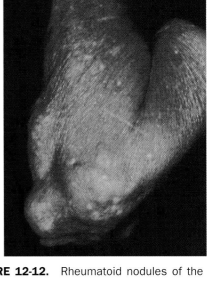

FIGURE 12-12.   Rheumatoid nodules of the elbow.

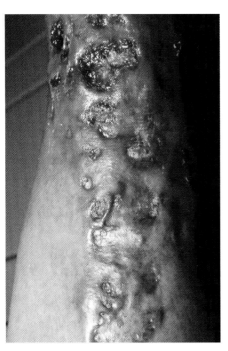

FIGURE 12-13.   Superficial ulcerating necrobiosis in a patient with severe rheumatoid arthritis.

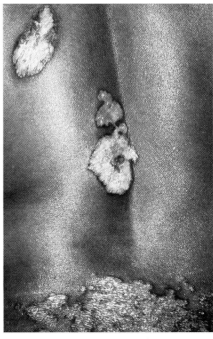

FIGURE 12-14.   Chronic cutaneous lupus erythematosus. Note the typical discoid lesions that are well marginated and show central scarring.

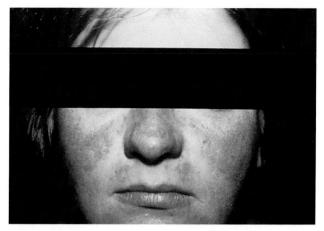

FIGURE 12-15. Systemic lupus erythematosus. Note the malar poikiloderma (i.e., hyperpigmentation and hypopigmentation, telangiectasia, and epidermal atrophy).

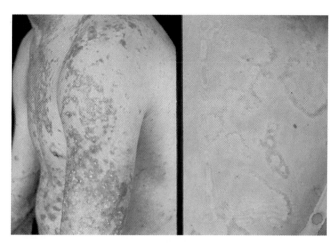

FIGURE 12-16. Subacute cutaneous lupus erythematosus. Note both the annular and the papulosquamous forms of the disease. (Courtesy of Dr. Richard Sonthelmer.)

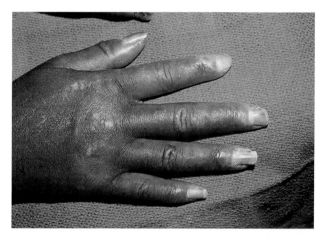

FIGURE 12-17. Scleroderma—CREST (calcinosis, Raynaud phenomenon, esophageal dysfunction, sclerodactyly, telangiectasia) type. Note "salt and pepper" dyspigmentation over sclerotic areas.

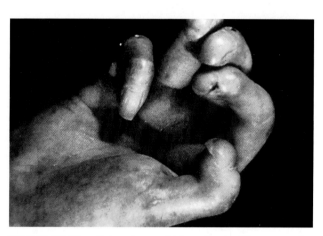

FIGURE 12-18. Scleroderma. This patient with progressive systemic scleroderma had a truncal pattern of onset and associated severe deformity of the hands.

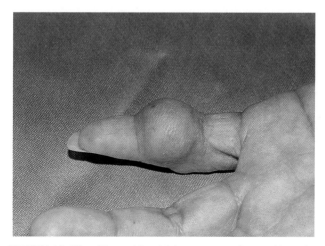

FIGURE 12-19. Blue rubber bleb nevus syndrome. Note the large vascular malformation.

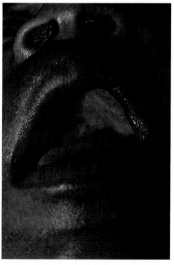

FIGURE 12-20. Typical telangiectasia of Osler-Weber-Rendu disease.

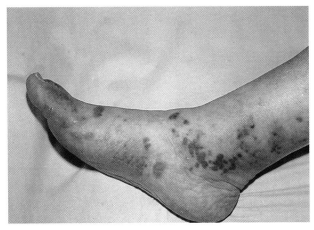

FIGURE 12-21. Kaposi sarcoma—classic type. Note the vascular tumors in a typical dependent site.

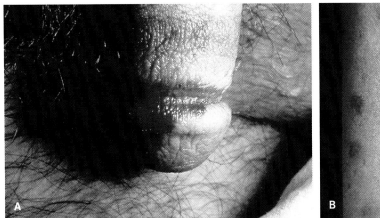

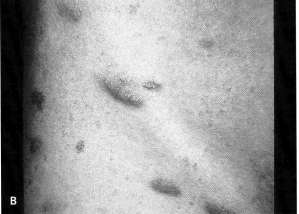

FIGURE 12-22. A, B: Kaposi sarcoma of patients with acquired immunodeficiency syndrome.

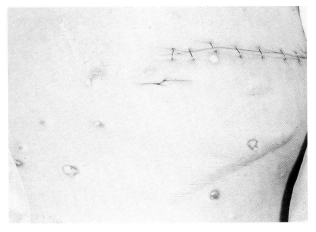

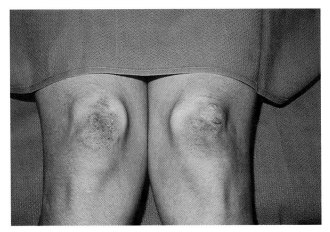

FIGURE 12-23. Degos disease. Note the typical cutaneous lesions with "porcelain" centers and the scars from management of gastrointestinal bleeding.

FIGURE 12-24. Ehlers-Danlos syndrome. Note the "fish mouth" scars and "pseudotumors" on the knees. This patient died of aortic rupture during her pregnancy.

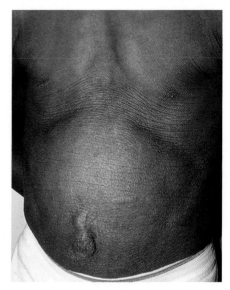

FIGURE 12-25. Cutis laxa. Note the skin "too large for the body" of this young boy.

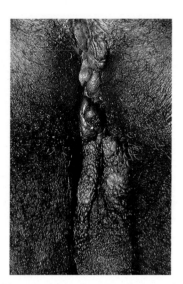

FIGURE 12-26. Amyloidosis. Note the perirectal amyloid nodules of this patient with multiple myeloma.

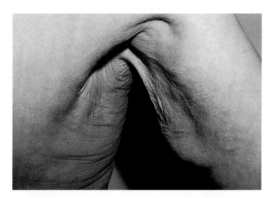

FIGURE 12-27. Pseudoxanthoma elasticum. Note the "chicken skin" appearance of the axillary skin.

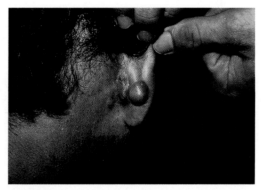

FIGURE 12-28. Gardner syndrome. Note the typical epidermal inclusion cyst. This patient had multiple other cystic nodules, particularly on the scalp.

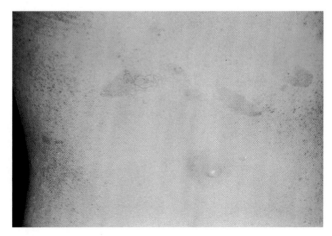

FIGURE 12-29. Neurofibromatosis, Note the café-au-lait macules and neurofibroma on this patient's back.

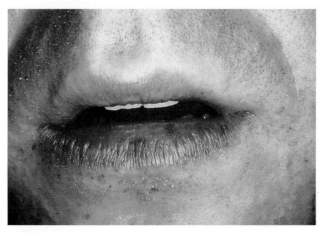

FIGURE 12-30. Peutz-Jeghers syndrome. Note pigmented macules on the lips that cross the vermilion border. (Courtesy of Dr. Jeffrey P. Callen.)

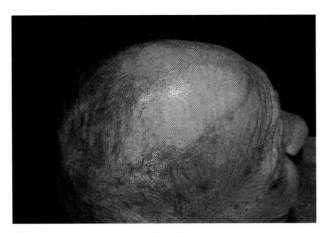

FIGURE 12-31.   Cronkhite-Canada syndrome. Note alopecia and hyperpigmentation.

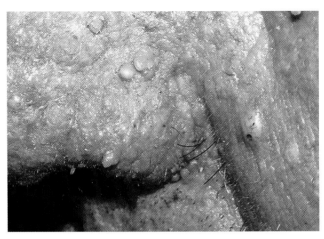

FIGURE 12-32.   Cowden disease (multiple hamartoma syndrome). Note multiple tricholemmomas on the nose. (Courtesy of Dr. Jeffrey P. Callen.)

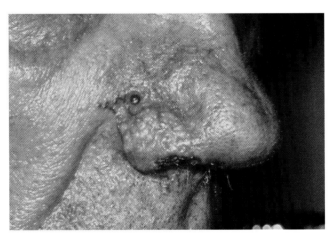

FIGURE 12-33.   Muir-Torre syndrome. Note sebaceous adenomas of the nose. (Courtesy of Dr. Jeffrey P. Callen.)

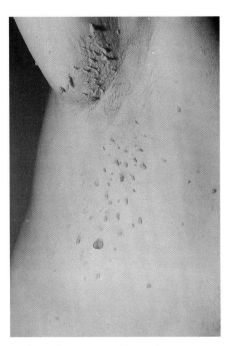

FIGURE 12-34.   Skin tags. Note the numerous typical lesions near the axilla.

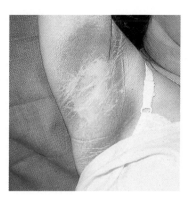

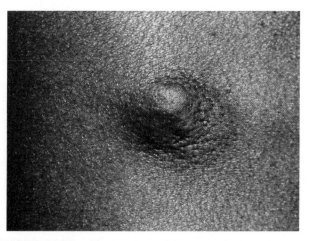

FIGURE 12-35.   Acanthosis nigricans in a nonobese adult patient.

FIGURE 12-36.   Metastatic nodule with primary adenocarcinoma of the colon.

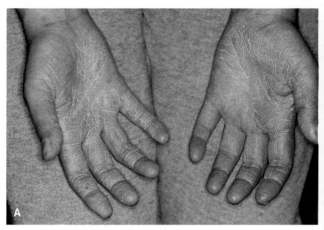

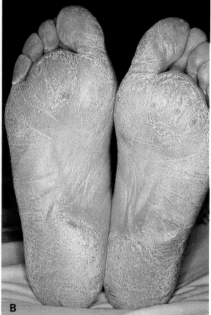

FIGURE 12-37. A, B: Acquired palmar-plantar keratoderma of a patient found to have carcinoma of the esophagus.

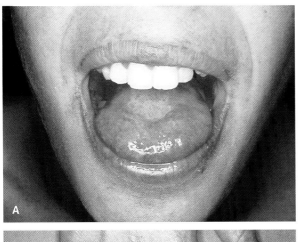

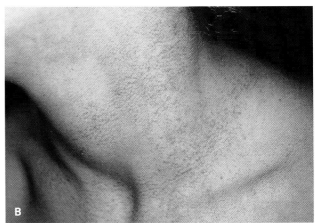

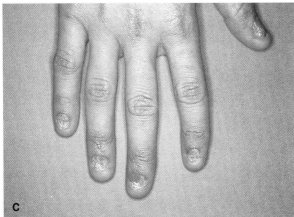

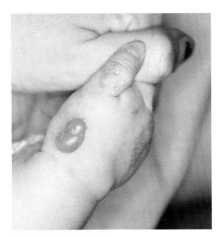

FIGURE 12-38. A–C: Dyskeratosis congenita. White keratotic lesions of the tongue, reticulated neck pigmentation, and dystrophic nails of a boy.

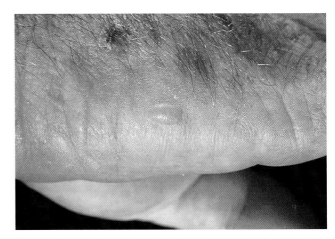

FIGURE 12-39. Epidermolysis bullosa, dystrophic type. Note scarring on thumb and dorsal hand of this infant.

FIGURE 12-40. Epidermolysis bullosa acquisita. The bullous lesion is not inflamed.

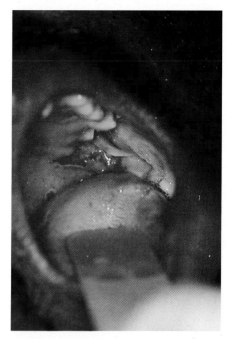

FIGURE 12-41. Pemphigus vulgaris. Oral erosions may be the initial manifestation.

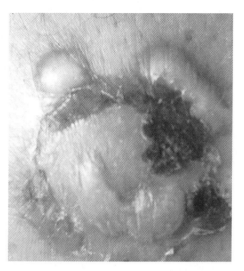

FIGURE 12-42. Pemphigus vulgaris. Note multiple bullous lesions and crusted erosions.

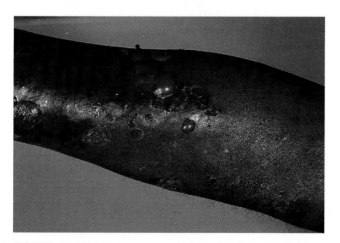

FIGURE 12-43. Bullous pemphigoid. The large bullae are tense and leave circular healing sites.

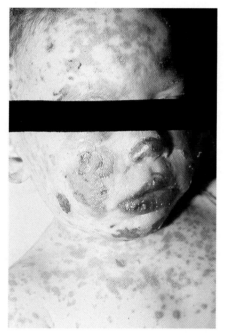

FIGURE 12-44. Erythema multiforme (Stevens-Johnson syndrome). Lip crusting is typical.

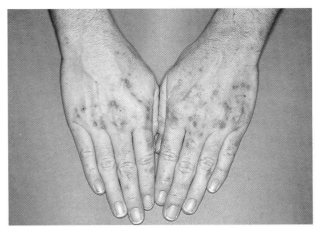

FIGURE 12-45. Variegate porphyria. Scarring and erosions in sun-exposed sites may be more prominent than intact blistering. The clinical features are the same as those of porphyria cutanea tarda.

FIGURE 12-46. Angiokeratoma. The patient has Fabry disease.

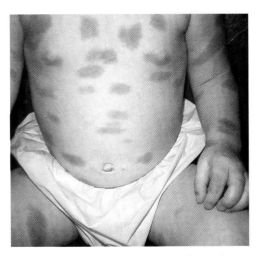

FIGURE 12-47. Urticaria pigmentosum form of mastocytosis in an infant.

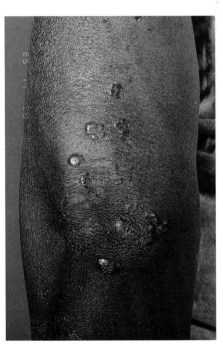

FIGURE 12-48. Eruptive xanthoma. New onset of multiple shiny papules over extensor surfaces of diabetic patient with a triglyceride level greater than 50 mmol/L.

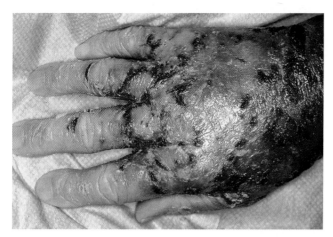

FIGURE 12-49. Pellagra. Erosions and crusting on sun-exposed site of a patient with chronic ethanol intake and poor nutrition.

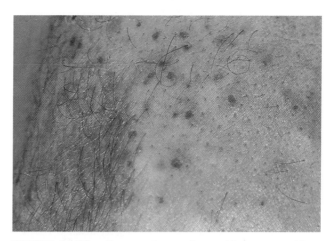

FIGURE 12-50. Scurvy of a patient with poor nutrition. Note perifollicular hemorrhage.

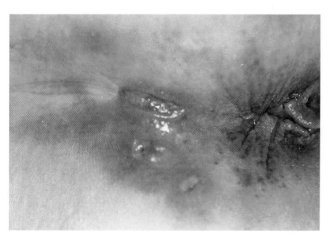

FIGURE 12-51. Herpes simplex. Persistent perianal erosions that were culture positive. Patient is immunosuppressed.

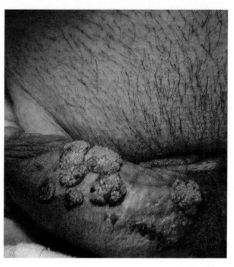

FIGURE 12-52. Condyloma acuminatum. Typical verrucous papules and nodules in the genital area.

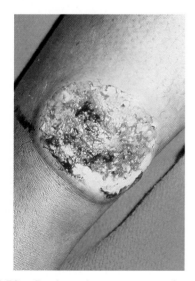

FIGURE 12-53. Pyoderma gangrenosum of a patient with Crohn's disease.

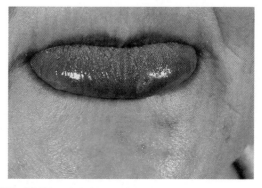

FIGURE 12-54. Aphthous ulcer involving the tongue of a patient with Behçet disease.

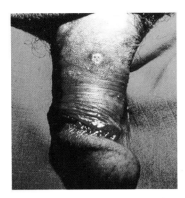

FIGURE 12-55. Behçet disease. Note early genital aphtha showing features of pustular vasculitis.

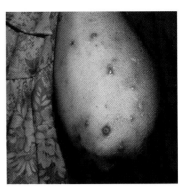

FIGURE 12-56. Bowel-associated dermatosis-arthritis syndrome. Pustular vasculitis lesions on a patient with a blind loop after Billroth II operation.

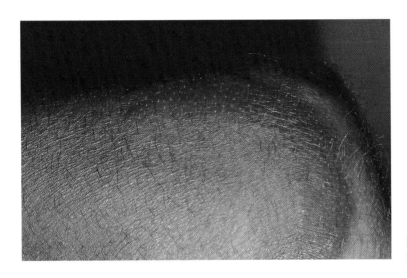

FIGURE 12-57. Typical lesions over joints of a patient with erythema elevatum diutinum.

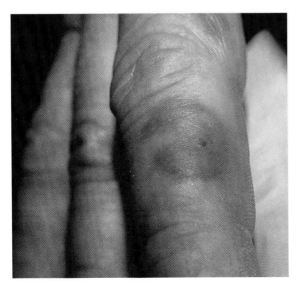

FIGURE 12-58. Tender erythematous papules and plaques on the upper extremities of a patient with Sweet syndrome.

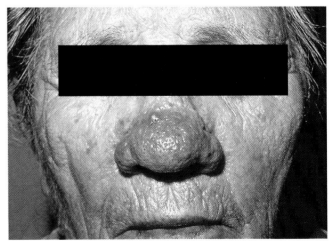

FIGURE 12-59. Characteristic telangiectasia, acneiform papules, and rhinophyma of a patient with rosacea.

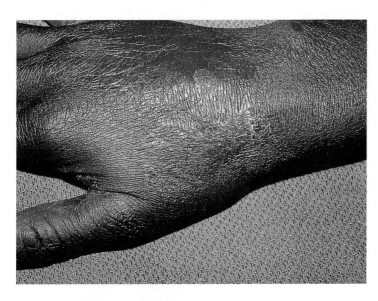

FIGURE 12-60. Scaling and thickened leathery skin of a patient with pellagra.

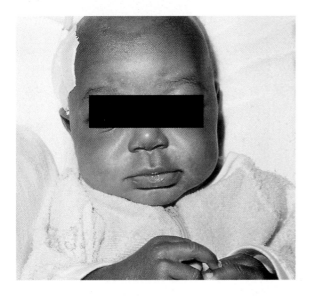

FIGURE 12-61. Patches of dry, scaly, eczematous skin of a young patient with acrodermatitis enteropathica.

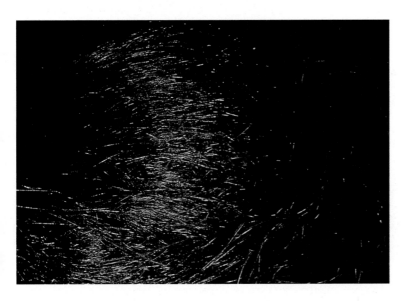

FIGURE 12-62. Flag sign in kwashiorkor.

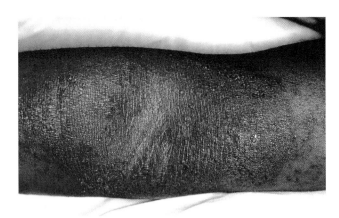

FIGURE 12-63. Pruritus of liver disease. Chronic scratching produces hyperpigmentation and lichenification.

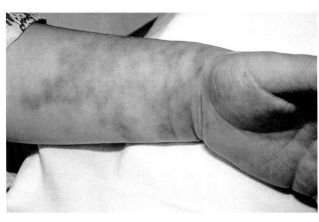

FIGURE 12-64. Polyarteritis nodosa. Livedo reticularis and tender subcutaneous nodules are characteristic.

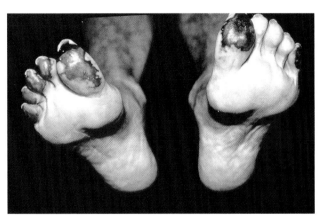

FIGURE 12-65. Cryoglobulinemia produces acral vasculitic infarcts. Hepatitis C is a leading cause.

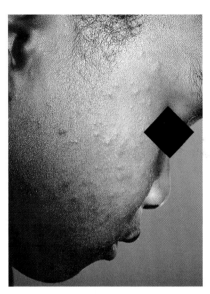

FIGURE 12-66. Papular acrodermatitis of childhood (Gianotti-Crosti syndrome) produces asymptomatic papules on the face and extremities of children. It was first noted in association with hepatitis B infection.

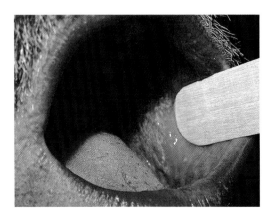

FIGURE 12-67. Lichen planus produces lacy mucosal plaques and pruritic papules on the skin. Patients should be evaluated for hepatitis C infection.

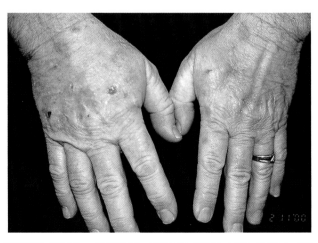

FIGURE 12-68. Porphyria cutanea tarda, with bullae, erosions, and scarring on the hands, can occur with many forms of liver disease.

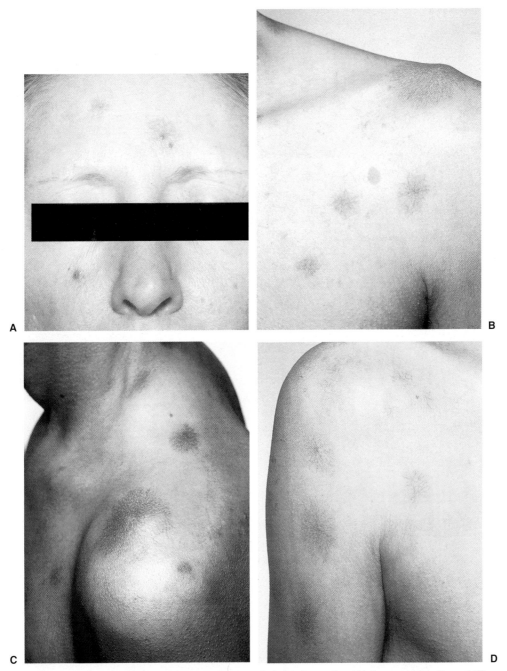

FIGURE 12-69. Cutaneous spider angiomas of cirrhosis on the (**A**) face and (**B, C,** and **D**) upper torso. (Courtesy of Dr. Telfer Reynolds.)

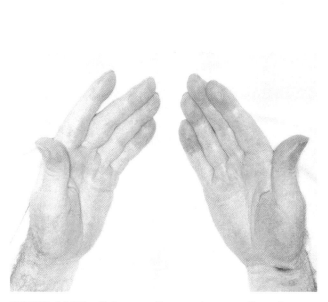

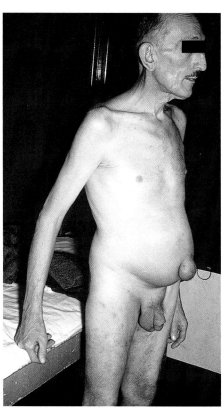

FIGURE 12-70. Palmar erythema of severe liver disease. (Courtesy of Dr. Telfer Reynolds.)

FIGURE 12-71. Severe muscle atrophy and malnutrition of chronic liver disease. The patient also has moderate ascites and a small umbilical hernia. (Courtesy of Dr. Telfer Reynolds.)

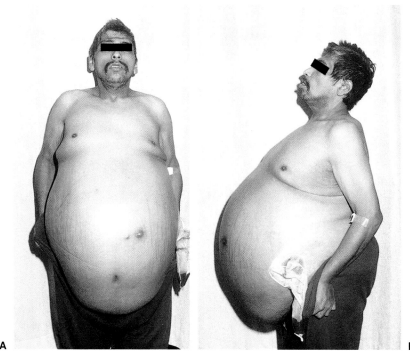

A

B

FIGURE 12-72. **A:** Anterior and (**B**) side view of a cirrhotic patient with massive ascites. (Courtesy of Dr. Telfer Reynolds.)

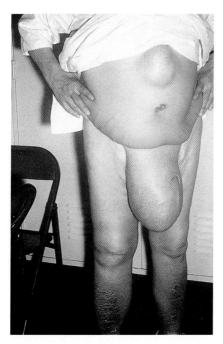

FIGURE 12-73. This patient demonstrates three not-uncommon findings in cirrhosis with ascites: abdominal distention, umbilical hernia, and scrotal edema. (Courtesy of Dr. Telfer Reynolds.)

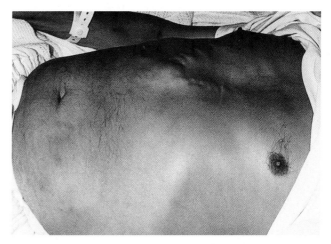

FIGURE 12-74. The caput medusae of cirrhosis with portal hypertension. (Courtesy of Dr. Telfer Reynolds.)

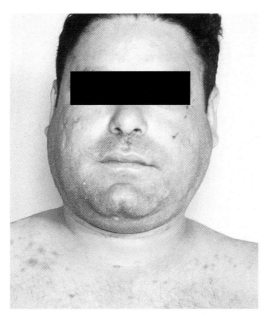

FIGURE 12-75. Parotid hypertrophy may be a clue to chronic alcoholism. (Courtesy of Dr. Telfer Reynolds.)

ORAL MANIFESTATIONS OF GASTROINTESTINAL DISEASES

JOHN C. RABINE* ■ **TIMOTHY T. NOSTRANT**

In patients with gastrointestinal symptoms, the oropharynx can provide diagnostic clues in disease processes ranging from rare hereditary syndromes such as familial polyposis to more frequently encountered entities such as inflammatory bowel disease and gastroesophageal reflux. Oral manifestations of gastrointestinal disease may be secondary to vitamin deficiencies caused by accompanying malabsorption or poor dietary intake, caused by recurrent exposure of the oropharynx to gastric contents, or as a result of susceptibility to oropharyngeal infections in immunodeficiency states. In other cases, oropharyngeal features may be a primary manifestation of the gastrointestinal disorder such as the mucocutaneous lesions in Peutz-Jeghers syndrome or hereditary hemorrhagic telangiectasias.

Although often merely a cosmetic nuisance, oral lesions may impair mastication and swallowing, be a source of bleeding, or predispose to infectious processes and premature tooth decay. Figures 13-1 through 13-18 are illustrations of oral lesions seen in association with disease processes affecting the gut.

*The views expressed in this article are those of the author and do not reflect the official policy or position of the U.S. Air Force, Department of Defense, or the U.S. Government.

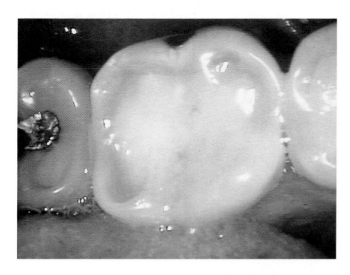

FIGURE 13-1. Dental erosion. Circumscribed yellowish regions correspond to exposed dentin in areas of enamel loss from repeated exposure to gastric contents secondary to chronic gastroesophageal reflux.

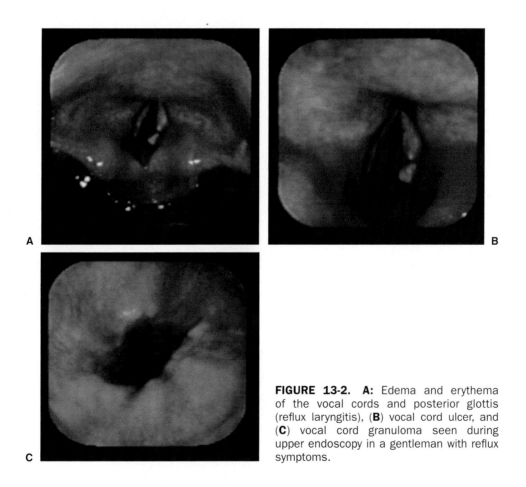

FIGURE 13-2. A: Edema and erythema of the vocal cords and posterior glottis (reflux laryngitis), (**B**) vocal cord ulcer, and (**C**) vocal cord granuloma seen during upper endoscopy in a gentleman with reflux symptoms.

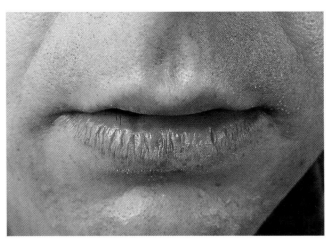

FIGURE 13-3. Melanin spots in a young male with Peutz-Jeghers syndrome.

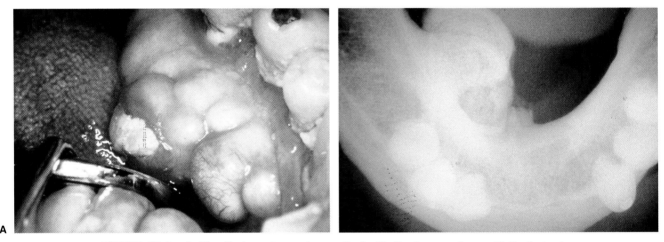

FIGURE 13-4. **A:** Mandibular osteoma in a patient with Gardner syndrome. **B:** Radiograph of the mandible in this patient.

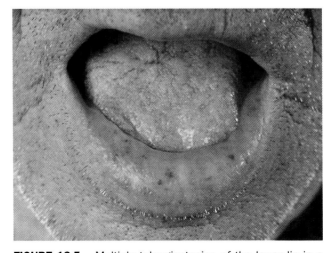

FIGURE 13-5. Multiple telangiectasias of the lower lip in a man with Osler-Weber-Rendu syndrome.

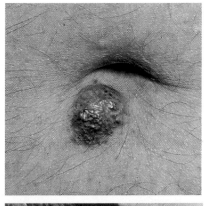

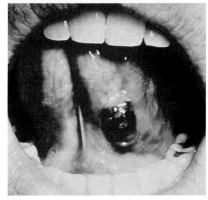

FIGURE 13-6.   A: Hemangioma of the oral cavity in a patient with blue rubber bleb nevus syndrome. The blue rubbery appearance is characteristic of the hamartomatous growths, which may be seen at any mucocutaneous site in this unusual disorder **(A, B)**.

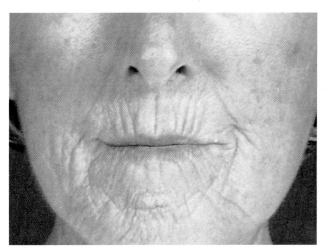

FIGURE 13-7.   Degenerative changes and fibrosis of the perioral skin limit mobility of the mouth in progressive systemic sclerosis. Oral hygiene may be compromised in this setting.

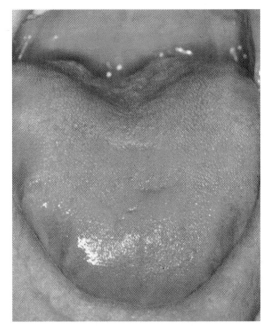

FIGURE 13-8.   Macroglossia due to infiltration of the tongue in a patient with primary amyloidosis. Evidence of repeated tongue-biting is illustrated in this photograph.

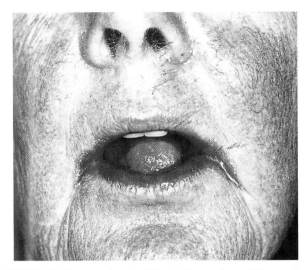

FIGURE 13-9. Angular cheilitis. Inflammation at the angles of the mouth is commonly associated with deficiencies of B vitamins such as riboflavin (B$_2$), niacin (B$_3$), and pyridoxine (B$_6$). Secondary infection with *Candida* or staphylococci may occur.

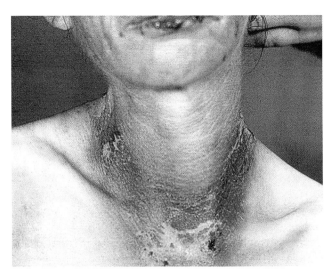

FIGURE 13-10. Pellagra develops from niacin and tryptophan deficiencies (because the latter can be synthesized into niacin) and is typically seen in alcoholism and severe malabsorption states. Dermatitis (usually in sun-exposed areas), diarrhea, dementia, and death are the classical sequelae of pellagra. The tongue and oral cavity may be painful and swollen.

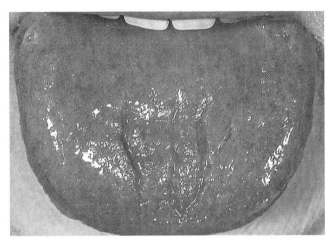

FIGURE 13-11. A raw, fissured tongue, especially in the setting of peripheral neuropathy, should raise the suspicion of vitamin B$_{12}$ deficiency. In later stages, the tongue may appear more atrophic with a bald, glistening surface.

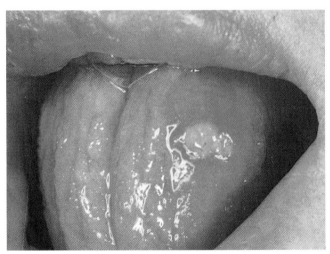

FIGURE 13-12. Aphthous ulcer. Aphthae appear as minute, shallow white ulcers distributed along mucous membranes. Although observed in normal individuals, multiple or persistent lesions mandate exclusion of an underlying disease process such as inflammatory bowel disease or Behçet disease.

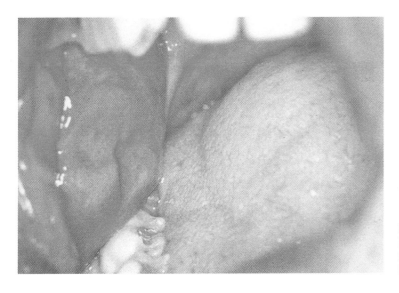

FIGURE 13-13. Orofacial granulomatosis diagnosed by biopsy from a patient with painful swelling of the mouth. This buccal abnormality is uncommonly seen in patients with Crohn's disease.

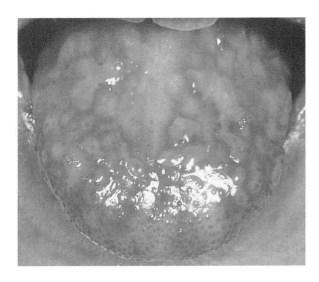

FIGURE 13-14. Ulcerated tongue in a patient with graft versus host disease following bone marrow transplantation. This phenomenon, whereby mature donor lymphocytes attack the recipient's tissues, consists of a tetrad of painful oral mucositis, enteritis, dermatitis, and hepatic dysfunction.

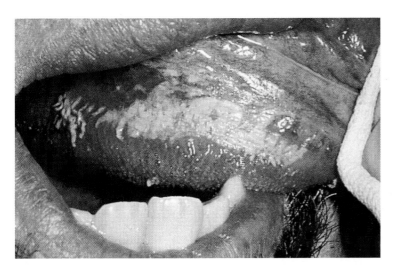

FIGURE 13-15. Oral hairy leukoplakia in a patient with acquired immunodeficiency syndrome. Painless whitish, verrucous excrescences along the lateral aspects of the tongue, that harbor the Epstein-Barr virus, are characteristic of this entity.

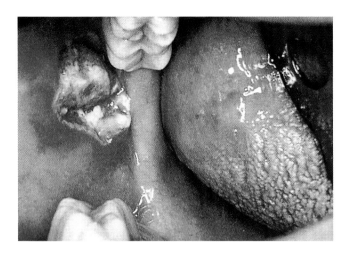

FIGURE 13-16. Necrotizing stomatitis. This is the most severe form of periodontal disease in the acquired immunodeficiency syndrome population, with extension of inflammation and necrosis from the gingiva and underlying bone to adjacent soft tissue and nonalveolar bone.

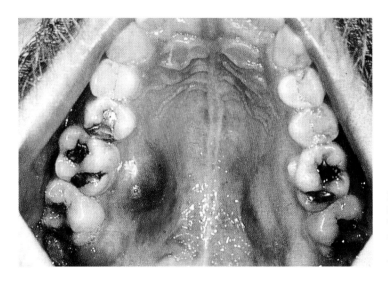

FIGURE 13-17. Kaposi sarcoma of the palate in an acquired immunodeficiency syndrome patient. These vascular tumors initially present as oval, poorly demarcated, rust-colored or violaceous plaques that rapidly progress to bulky lesions, which may affect mastication and swallowing.

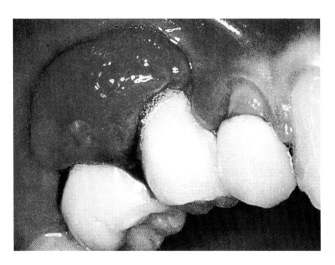

FIGURE 13-18. Oral lymphoma in an acquired immunodeficiency syndrome patient. These aggressive tumors typically present as firm, painless masses which progress to elevated, ulcerated regions marked by rapid proliferation.

14

ADVICE TO TRAVELERS

SAMUEL L. STANLEY JR.

The successful prevention of illnesses among travelers to developing countries and the recognition and diagnosis of disease among returning travelers requires the physician to stay up-to-date on disease patterns worldwide. Information on vaccines, disease outbreaks, unstable political situations, and other information critical to safe travel is provided by a number of government agencies and private sources. Table 14-1 is a selected list of these sources for physicians and travelers. Many of the listed sources contain referrals or, in the case of World Wide Web locations, links to other useful resources. Among the listed resources, the Centers for Disease Control and Prevention (CDC) book *Health Information for International Travel* is singled out as an especially valuable reference for the prevention of disease among travelers. The information that follows is designed to supplement the information provided in Chapter 56 of the *Textbook of Gastroenterology,* 4th edition. The reader is referred to that chapter for detailed information on these and other topics related to advising travelers.

Yellow fever is the only disease for which countries can, under international health regulations, require proof of vaccination before allowing entry into the country. The disease is found only in Central and South America and Africa. A detailed list of the requirements of different countries regarding yellow fever vaccination is available in *Health Information for International Travel* and can also be found at the World Health Organization (WHO) World Wide Web site listed in Table 14-1. The maps in Fig. 14-1 indicate regions of South America and Africa where yellow fever is endemic. Although yellow fever endemic zones are no longer included in international health regulations, many countries design their vaccination requirements on the basis of these zones. Thus, these maps provide a resource for determining the need of a given traveler for yellow fever vaccine.

Dengue fever represents a growing threat to travelers to a variety of destinations. Although disease among travelers (manifest usually as fever, frontal headache, myalgia, and occasionally rash) is generally benign and self-limited, convalescence may be prolonged, and persons with the infection are at risk for development of dengue hemorrhagic fever, which can be fatal. As shown in Fig. 14-2, dengue virus is now endemic in most tropical countries, and it has become the most common arbovirus infection worldwide. Since 1982, major epidemics have occurred in many countries, including Brazil, Costa Rica, Panama, Venezuela, Saudi Arabia, Kenya, China, and Taiwan. The presence of dengue fever in Mexico and the Caribbean—common tourist destinations for travelers from the United States—suggests physicians will be seeing more of this disease in the near future. There is no specific therapy for dengue fever, and prevention of the disease is based on the avoidance of *Aedes aegypti* mosquito bites.

Meningococcal disease is a medical problem in the United States and in developing countries. Epidemics of meningococcal disease are rare in the United States, but they are frequent in developing countries, especially in an area of sub-Saharan Africa that has been called the "meningitis belt." As shown in Fig. 14-3, this region extends from Gambia and Mali eastward to Ethiopia, encompassing a number of countries. Disease is most common in the dry season (from December to June), and all travelers to this region should be vaccinated against meningococcal disease. Most outbreaks of disease have been caused by group A or group C meningococci. Infection with either organism can be prevented with quadrivalent A/C/Y/W-135 vaccine. It is important to emphasize that epidemics of meningococcal disease can arise in areas outside this belt (recent epidemics have included Burundi, Tanzania, and Mongolia), and physicians need to rely on the sources listed in Table 14-1 to make sure they have up-to-date information on risk for meningococcal disease worldwide.

Tables 14-2 through 14-4 are designed to provide a concise summary of some current recommendations for preventing travel-related diseases through the use of vaccinations and chemoprophylaxis. These tables do not deal with important components of these recommendations, such as avoiding contaminated food and water and mosquito bites. Details on those factors are available in Chapter 56 of the *Textbook of Gastroenterology*, 4th edition, and in the sources listed in Table 14-1.

(figures begin on page 158)

TABLE 14-1
Selected Sources of Information on Travel Medicine for Physicians and Travelers

Health Information for International Travel—Available through Superintendent of Documents, US Government Printing Office, Washington, DC, 20402, (202) 783-3238
The "yellow book" provides country by country information on malaria and other health risks, and general information on travel-related diseases and other infectious diseases. It is updated yearly or every 2 years, and represents an authoritative source in the field. With the purchase of the yellow book one receives the future updates, and also the "blue sheets" which provide biweekly information about the activity of yellow fever and plague around the world, information on disease outbreaks worldwide, and periodic updates on information in the yellow book. No one interested in travel medicine should be without this resource.

Centers for Disease Control and Prevention (CDC) Travel Information—www.cdc.gov/travel
An outstanding World Wide Web site that contains much useful information, including access to recommendations from the yellow book (see above) and the health updates provided by the blue sheets (see above). An Adobe Acrobat version of the yellow book is available on site. In addition, summaries of sanitation reports from cruise ships are available, along with sections on current worldwide disease outbreaks, and sections that provide detailed information on a variety of subjects including the HIV+ traveler, preventing food-borne illness, malaria in pregnancy, and others.

CDC Hotline, (404) 332-4555
An automated service that provides information by either phone messages or by fax transmission. Multiple travel-related topics are covered, including malaria and yellow fever, and information is provided in a clear and concise manner. Transfer to a CDC physician is available during business hours for many of the topics.

CDC Summary of Sanitation Inspections of International Cruise Ships
Published every 2 weeks, the "green sheets" provide information on the results of inspections by the CDC's Vessel Sanitation Program (VSP), and should be required reading for travelers contemplating a cruise. Cruise ships are scored for a number of sanitation and food-handling categories—the higher the number, the better the level of sanitation on the ship. The green sheets are available to the public via fax-back services [(404) 332-4565, request document 510051], by writing to the VSP, National Center for Environmental Health, Centers for Disease Control and Prevention, 1015 North American Way, Room 107, Miami, FL, 33132, or on the World Wide Web at www.cdc.gov/travel/cruiships.htm.

IAMAT—www.sentex.net/~iamat/
The International Association for Medical Assistance to Travelers is a nonprofit organization that provides a number of benefits, including a comprehensive list of medical care providers around the world. They also feature publications on several topics of interest to travelers. Their address is IAMAT, 417 Center Street, Lewiston, NY 14092, (716) 754-4883.

Shoreland's Travel Health Online—www.tripprep.com
Another very good World Wide Web site with country by country profiles for disease and a list of travel medicine providers.

World Health Organization (WHO) International Travel and Health Page—www.who.int/ith/english/
This site is based on the WHO's book on advice for travelers (also a yellow book), and features a list of the vaccination requirements for a number of countries worldwide, as well as information on malaria within those countries.

HIV, human immunodeficiency virus.

TABLE 14-2
Vaccines Recommended for Prevention of Disease Among Travelers

VACCINE	AGE	DOSAGE	VOLUME/ROUTE	NO. OF DOSES	SCHEDULE	COMMENTS
Hepatitis A					Months	Both are inactivated virus—no special precautions for immunocompromised individuals. Safety in pregnancy not established; theoretically, risk is low. Duration of protection probably at least 10 y.
Havrix	2–18 y	720 EL.U.	0.5 mL IM	2	0, 6–12	
	>18 y	1440 EL.U.	1.0 mL IM	2	0, 6–12	
Vaqta	2–17 y	25 U.	0.5 mL IM	2	0, 6–18	
	>17 y	50 U.	1.0 mL IM	2	0, 6	
Hepatitis B					Months	Both are recombinant antigen-based vaccines. No special precautions in immunocompromised individuals. Safe in pregnancy and during lactation. Long-lived protection. No current recommendations for booster immunization. A special 40-μg dose is available for immunocompromised or dialysis patients. This is administered as 40-μg dose on the three-dose schedule for Recombivax, or as 80-μg dose on the four-dose schedule for Energix-B.
Recombivax	<11 y	2.5 μg	IM	3	0, 1, 7	
	11–19 y	5 μg	IM	3	0, 1, 7	
	>19 y	10 μg	IM	3	0, 1, 7	
Energix-B	<11 y	10 μg	IM	3 or 4	0, 1, 7 or 0, 1, 2, 12	
	11–19 y	10 μg	IM	3 or 4	0, 1, 7 or 0, 1, 2, 12	
	>19 y	20 μg	IM	3 or 4	0, 1, 7 or 0, 1, 2, 12	
Yellow Fever Vaccine	>9 mo		0.5 mL IM	1		Live virus vaccine. Contraindicated in children and infants younger than 9 mo. Contraindicated in immunocompromised individuals and pregnant women unless chance of yellow fever exposure is high. Contraindicated in individuals with hypersensitivity to eggs. Booster dose after 10 y.
Rabies Preexposure Immunization					Days	HDCV can be administered using the IM or ID schedule. Intradermal vaccination is less immunogenic and should not be used in immunocompromised patients or individuals taking medications (antimalarials) that reduce the immune response. RVA and PCEC rabies vaccines are administered only by the IM route. Booster is a single dose of HDCV, RVA, or PCEC.
HDVC	All ages		1.0 mL IM	3	0, 7, 21 or 28	
			0.1 mL ID	3	0, 7, 21 or 28	
RVA	All ages		1.0 mL IM	3	0, 7, 21 or 28	
PCEC	All ages		1.0 mL IM	3	0, 7, 21 or 28	
Rabies Postexposure Prophylaxis If Previously Vaccinated						Previously vaccinated individuals receiving postexposure prophylaxis do not require RIG. Individuals never previously vaccinated should receive 20 IU RIG/kg body weight with half the dose infiltrated at the wound site, and the remainder IM.
HDVC	All ages		1.0 mL IM	2	0, 3	
RVA	All ages		1.0 mL IM	2	0, 3	
PCEC	All ages		1.0 mL IM	2	0, 3	
Rabies Postexposure Prophylaxis If Not Previously Vaccinated						
HDVC	All ages		1.0 mL IM	5	0, 3, 7, 14, 28	
RVA	All ages		1.0 mL IM	5	0, 3, 7, 14, 28	
PCEC	All ages		1.0 mL IM	5	0, 3, 7, 14, 28	
Japanese Encephalitis Vaccine	1–2 y		0.5 mL SC	3	0, 7, 30	Inactivated virus preparation. Vaccination during pregnancy should be avoided unless the risk for disease is high. There have been significant allergic reactions with this vaccine. Duration of protection is not clearly established. A booster dose of 1.0 mL SC can be given at > 36 mo after completion of the primary series.
	>3 y		1.0 mL SC	3	0, 7, 30	
Poliomyelitis–Previously Vaccinated						
Enhanced potency inactivated poliovirus vaccine (IPV)				1		A one-time booster dose of IPV is indicated for previously vaccinated individuals. IPV should also be used in immunocompromised individuals. For unvaccinated adults, a primary

(continued)

TABLE 14-2. *(Continued)*

VACCINE	AGE	DOSAGE	VOLUME/ROUTE	NO. OF DOSES	SCHEDULE	COMMENTS
Oral poliovirus vaccine (OPV)				1		series of three doses of IPV, with the second dose administered 4–8 wk after the first dose, and the third dose administered 6–12 mo after the second dose should be used. Alternative regimens for individuals who cannot complete a full schedule are in reference.
Typhoid Fever						
Oral TY-21a	6 y			4	Every 48 h	Capsules must be kept refrigerated, all four doses should be taken. Contraindicated in immunosuppressed individuals; generally avoided in pregnancy. Should not be taken simultaneously with antibiotics. Booster should be given every 5 y.
Vi capsular polysaccharide	2 y		0.5 mL IM	1		No general contraindications to use. Booster every 2 y.
Meningococcal						
Quadravalent A/C/Y/W-135	All ages		As indicated by manufacturer SC	1		Polysaccharide capsular-based vaccine that may not be protective in children younger than 2 y. Vaccine is safe in immunocompromised individuals, but should be used in pregnancy only if the risk of infection is high. Booster is given > 3 y after primary dose.
Tetanus, Diphtheria–Not Previously Vaccinated						
DTP	<7 y			4	See comments	For previously unvaccinated children, the first three doses of DTP are given at 4- to 8-wk intervals, the fourth dose is given 6–12 mo after third dose. A booster dose is given if the fourth dose was given before the child's fourth birthday. The booster can be the new DTaP vaccine, which contains the acellular pertussis vaccine. Td (tetanus diphtheria toxoid for adult use) is given to children older than 7 y and adults who were never vaccinated against tetanus or diphtheria. The first two doses are given at 4–8 wk apart, and the third dose is given 6–12 mo after the second dose.
Td	>7 y			3		
Tetanus, Diphtheria–Previously Vaccinated						
Td				1		
						A booster dose should be administered every 10 y. In some cases a booster dose every 5 y may be indicated.
Cholera Vaccine	6 mo to 4 y		0.2 mL (IM or SC)	2	1 wk to 1 mo	Vaccine is of limited efficacy. Should not be administered within 3 wk of yellow fever vaccine. Booster is a single dose given every 6 mo. Safety in pregnancy not established.
	5–10 y		0.3 mL (IM or SC)	2	1 wk to 1 mo	
	>10 y		0.5 mL (IM or SC)	2	1 wk to 1 mo	

DTaP, diphtheria-tetanus-acellular pertussis; DTP, diphtheria-tetanus-pertussis; ID, intradermally; IM, intramuscularly; HDCV, human diploid cell vaccine; PCEC, purified chick embryo cell; RIG, rabies immunoglobulin; RVA, rabies vaccine absorbed; SC, subcutaneously; Td, tetanus-diphtheria toxoid.

From Centers for Disease Control and Prevention, Health Information for International Travel, DHHS, Atlanta Georgia, 1997;145.

TABLE 14-3
Prevention of Malaria by Means of Administration of Chemoprophylaxis

DRUG	USAGE	ADULT DOSAGE	PEDIATRIC DOSAGE
Mefloquine (Lariam)	Areas where chloroquine-resistant malaria has been reported	228 mg base (250 mg salt) orally, once/wk beginning 1–2 wk prior to travel to area and continuing for 4 wk after leaving malarious area	<15 kg, 4.6 mg/kg base (5 mg/kg salt) 15–19 kg, 1/4 tab/wk 20–30 kg, 2 tab/wk 31–45 kg, 3/4 tab/wk >45 kg, 1 tab/wk Same dosing schedule as adults
Doxycycline	Areas where mefloquine resistance has been reported, or for individuals with a contraindication to mefloquine use	100 mg orally, once/d. Begin 1–2 d prior to travel to malarious area, continue daily while there, and continue for 4 wk after leaving malarious area	>8 y, 2 mg/kg orally/d with a maximum dosage of 100 mg/d Same dosing schedule as adults
Atovaquone/proguanil (Malarone)	Individuals who cannot take mefloquine or doxycycline.	1 tablet (250 mg atovaquone/100 mg proguanil hydrochloride) daily. Begin 1–2 d before travel, continue daily during travel, and for 7 d after leaving the malarious area	11–20 kg, 1 pediatric tablet (62.5 atovaquone/25 mg proguanil HCl) daily 21–30 kg, 2 pediatric tablets daily 31–40 kg, 3 pediatric tablets daily >40 kg, 1 adult tablet daily
Chloroquine (Aralen)	Only in areas where chloroquine resistance has not been reported.	300 mg base (500 mg salt) orally, once/wk, beginning 1–2 wk prior to travel to malarious area and continuing for 4 wk after leaving malarious area	5 mg/kg base (8.3 mg/kg salt), orally, once/wk, maximum dose 300 mg Same dosing schedule as adults

Adapted from Centers for Disease Control and Prevention, Health Information for International Travel 1999–2000, DHHS, Atlanta, GA, 1999.

TABLE 14-4
Drugs Used for the Management and Prevention of Travelers' Diarrhea

DRUG	DOSAGE	COMMENTS
Drugs Used for Self-Treatment of Travelers' Diarrhea		
Fluoroquinolones		Fluoroquinolones are currently drugs of choice for self-treatment of travelers' diarrhea, except in areas where infection with quinolone-resistant *Campylobacter* organisms is a prominent problem (areas of Southeast Asia). The doses listed are those shown to be effective in clinical trials; it is likely that single-dose or single-day treatment may be effective for all the quinolones, but this has not yet been tested. Fluoroquinolones should not be used by children or pregnant women. Side effects include insomnia, restlessness, tendonitis, dizziness, and headaches.
Ciprofloxacin	500 mg bid × 5 d	
Norfloxacin	400 mg bid × 3–5 d	
Ofloxacin	300 mg bid × 3–5 d	
Fleroxacin	400 mg qd × 1–2 d	
Enoxacin	400 mg bid × 5 d	
Macrolides		Useful in areas where *Campylobacter jejuni* is a major cause of travelers' diarrhea. Effective against other enteric pathogens. Side effects are rare; most frequent are gastrointestinal disturbances.
Azithromycin	500 mg qd × 5 d	
Sulfa drugs		Less effective than quinolones because of TMP-SMX resistance in many areas. Most common problem is allergic reaction to the sulfa component.
Trimethoprim-sulfamethoxazole (TMP-SMX, 160 mg TMP/800 mg SMX)	1 tablet bid × 5 d	
Drugs Used for Prophylaxis of Travelers' Diarrhea		Many authorities do not recommend prophylaxis for travelers' diarrhea, and prefer the self-treatment regimens listed above. For short-duration stays, or persons at high risk, the use of prophylactic medication may be indicated.
Fluoroquinolones		
Norfloxacin	400 mg qd	
Ciprofloxacin	500 mg qd	
Ofloxacin	300 mg qd	
Bismuth subsalicylate	Two 262-mg tablets chewed 4 times/d	Less effective than antimicrobials, but avoids resistance issues. Contraindicated for persons taking aspirin or other salicylate-containing drugs. Turns tongue and stool black.

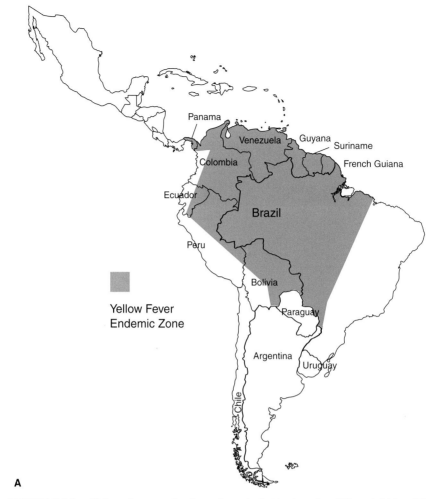

A

FIGURE 14-1.   Yellow fever endemic regions in Latin America (**A**) and Africa (**B**).

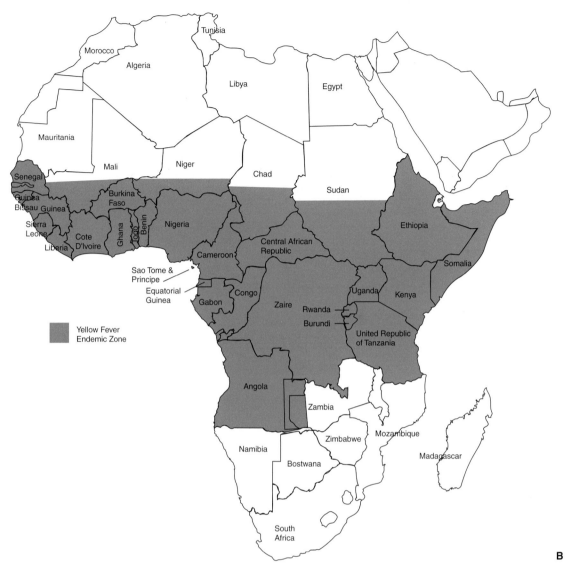

Yellow Fever
Endemic Zone

B

FIGURE 14-1. (Continued)

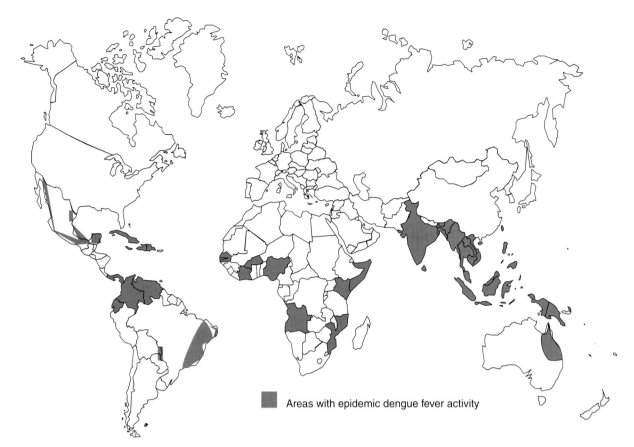

FIGURE 14-2. Distribution of dengue fever worldwide.

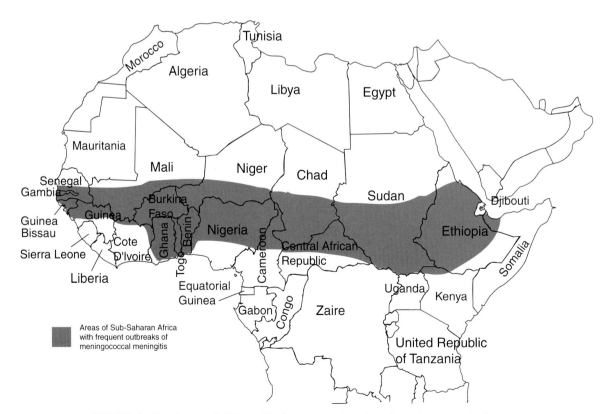

FIGURE 14-3. Areas of Africa with frequent outbreaks of meningococcal disease.

PART TWO

GASTROINTESTINAL DISEASES

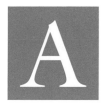
15

ESOPHAGUS: Anatomy and Structural Anomalies

H. WORTH BOYCE JR. ■ GREGORY A. BOYCE

A thorough knowledge of normal esophageal anatomy is essential as a basis for the diagnosis of pathological conditions of the esophagus. Structural anomalies, both congenital and acquired, may be considered as part of the spectrum of normality because most are asymptomatic. Figures 15-1 through 15-3 demonstrate the usual normal anatomy and Figs. 15-4 through 15-16 demonstrate several structural anomalies. These conditions are recognized clinically by means of one or more methods: radiography, endoscopy, endoscopic ultrasonography, or direct observation during an operation or at postmortem examination. Computed tomography is usually of little help. Endoscopic ultrasonography is helpful to demonstrate the features of intramural and paraesophageal lesions.

Some structural anomalies such as heterotopic gastric mucosa and webs in the cervical esophagus may have an etiologic relationship (Figs. 15-5 and 15-7A, B, C). Congenital esophageal stenosis may be associated with structural alterations similar to the so-called "ringed" esophagus, which in some patients is associated with eosinophilic esophagitis and/or gastroesophageal acid reflux disease (Fig. 15-11).

The nonspecific symptoms produced by structural anomalies make their diagnosis, or even a reasonable suspicion of their presence, difficult at best. The appearance of structural anomalies such as diverticula (Figs. 15-8A, B through 15-10) is so fascinating at times that it may lead to a failure to completely evaluate the esophagus and ultimately to make what proves to be an impertinent diagnosis related to a diverticulum. A mild to moderate degree of stenosis from inflammation or neoplasm may be the cause of dysphagia. It can be missed unless a barium esophagram with bolus challenges and endoscopy are used to supplement the standard barium esophagram.

The more rare esophageal disorders such as vascular anomalies (Fig. 15-12) and intramural cysts (Fig. 15-13) typically cause no symptoms and therefore are discovered during examinations for other conditions. They may, however, create diagnostic or therapeutic dilemmas.

163

Endoscopic ultrasonography is used to study mural alterations in the esophagus. This method is effective for staging of invasive malignant tumors and of alterations of the esophageal wall either by intramural and paraesophageal lesions or by contiguous organs. Endoscopic ultrasonography is substantially more sensitive than computed tomography in the evaluation of intramural and paraesophageal disorders. Figure 15-16*A*, *B* demonstrates endoscopic and ultrasound images that confirm the morphologic features of a submucosal lesion typical of a duplication cyst at the esophagogastric junction.

Clinicians should take every opportunity to study the range of anatomic presentations offered by the excellent diagnostic modalities described herein. Specialists are expected to recognize and properly manage even the rarest of conditions. A lifetime of experience with some of the rare entities may include only one or two patients. Consequently, careful study of atlas presentations such as these can provide a knowledge base for future diagnosis.

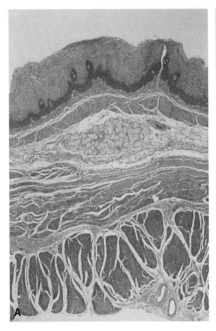
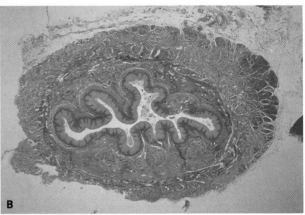

FIGURE 15-1 **A:** Longitudinal section of esophageal wall (H&E stain; original magnification ×10). **B:** Cross section of esophageal wall (H&E stain; original magnification ×2.5). (Courtesy of Dr. Rodger Haggitt.)

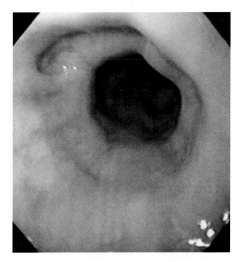

FIGURE 15-2. A normal esophagus with nonperistaltic tertiary contractions in the distance.

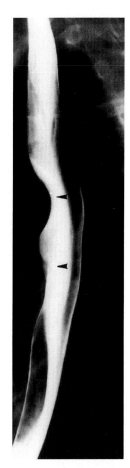

FIGURE 15-3. Barium esophagram shows normal indentations of esophageal wall by aorta (*top arrow*) and left mainstream bronchus (*bottom arrow*).

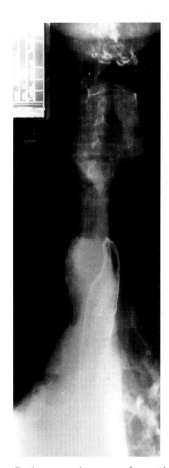

FIGURE 15-4. Barium esophagram of a patient with Kartagener syndrome shows esophageal compression by the right-sided aortic arch and dextrocardia.

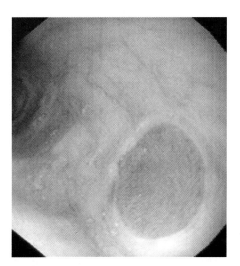

FIGURE 15-5. Heterotopic gastric mucosa in the cervical esophagus (so-called inlet patch) is found in as many as 5% of patients who have a careful endoscopic examination of the cervical esophagus. This gastric columnar mucosa is the typical salmon color and sharply contrasts with the surrounding squamous mucosa. Inlet patches are often multiple and frequently contain oxyntic cells that secrete and that may be associated with formation of cervical webs.

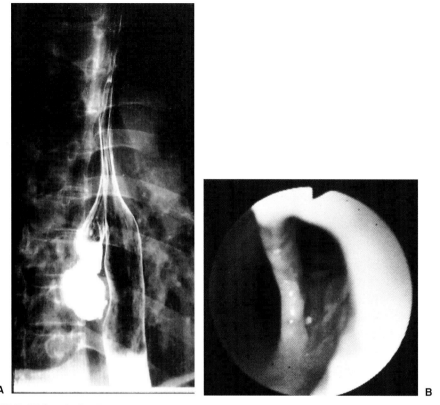

FIGURE 15-6.   A: Radiograph shows tubular duplication of the esophagus. **B:** Endoscopic view shows opening to tubular duplication (*right*) and esophageal lumen (*left*).

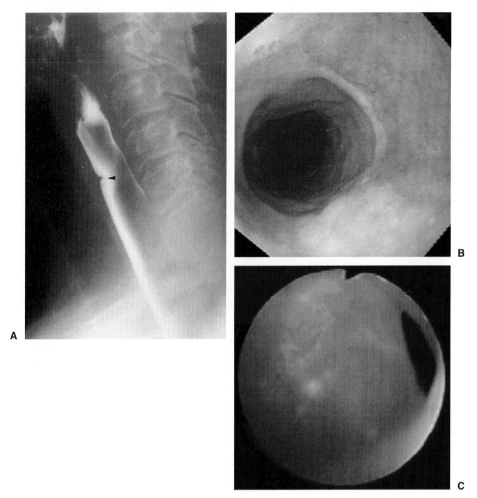

FIGURE 15-7. A: Barium contrast radiograph shows partial mucosal web in the cervical esophagus. Small webs of this type usually cause no symptoms. Some are associated with and adjacent to heterotopic gastric mucosa in the cervical esophagus. **B:** Certain portions of the junction between patches of heterotopic gastric mucosa and squamous epithelium may protrude into the lumen when it is distended by air or barium and present as a small web as shown in **A. C:** Webs in the cervical esophagus are a typical feature of the now rare Plummer-Vinson or Paterson-Kelly syndrome (cervical webs, iron deficiency anemia, koilonychias, and glossitis). In some patients, webs seen in association with heterotopic gastric mucosa are believed to be related to acid secretion by the oxyntic cells in this columnar mucosa. This web produced an eccentric lumen opening (*right center*) and dysphagia. The blue-grey coloration of the web at *top-center* is indicative of the thinness of the web and the darker lumen beyond.

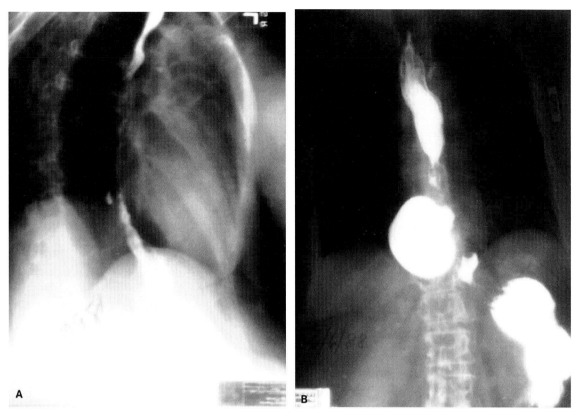

FIGURE 15-8. **A:** Esophagram of a 75-year-old woman obtained in 1981 shows a tiny barium-filled diverticulum projecting to the right side in the distal third of the esophagus. **B:** By 1989, there was a massive increase in the size of the diverticulum. The patient had symptoms of postprandial chest discomfort and dysphagia at this time.

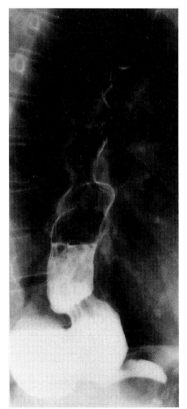

FIGURE 15-9. Barium esophagram of large epiphrenic diverticulum projecting from right wall of esophagus of a patient who also has achalasia. Such large pouches usually are symptomatic. Among patients without achalasia, the diverticular opening moves into the direct lumenal axis of the esophagus proximal to it and fills with food, producing dysphagia, chest pain, and regurgitation, either singly or in combination. In this patient with achalasia, there was no clinical indication of this lesion other than its finding on this study.

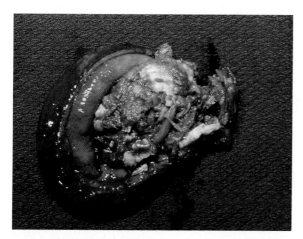

FIGURE 15-10. Surgical specimen of a resected esophageal diverticulum in which a bezoar had formed. (Courtesy of Dr. Thomas W. Rice.)

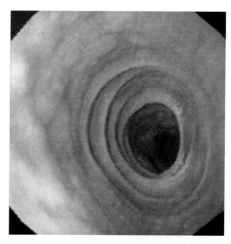

FIGURE 15-11. Congenital esophageal stenosis represents one cause of a "ringed" esophagus producing a mid-esophageal narrowing. Patients often give a history of dysphagia to solid foods dating to childhood. These lesions are not difficult to dilate, but carry an increased risk for mucosal tears, perforation, and pain when rapid dilation to large diameters is performed.

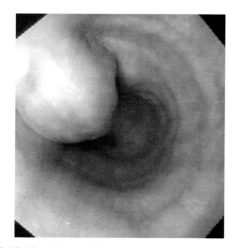

FIGURE 15-12. Congenital venous malformations as shown here may also be called primary varices because no secondary cause such as portal hypertension can be identified. Rarely, they may bleed spontaneously or unfortunately following an inappropriate biopsy attempt. Endosonography confirmed a conglomerate of venous channels in this lesion.

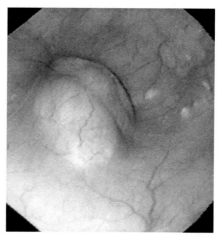

FIGURE 15-13. Small intramural cysts such as the bilobate type shown here are not symptomatic and are typically identified by barium esophagram or endoscopy done for some other indication. Endosonography confirms the site of origin in the wall and the cystic nature of the lesion. The most common differential diagnosis is leiomyoma or varix.

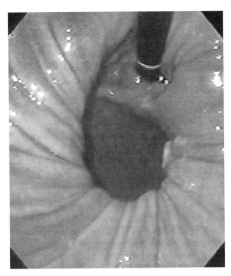

FIGURE 15-14. Retrograde view from the stomach into a combined hiatal hernia. The direct portion of the hernia is toward the *top* with the shaft of the endoscope coming through the lower esophageal sphincter, which is shown closed around the instrument. Toward the *bottom* is an opening into a large paraesophageal hernia. The intact angle of His separates the two portions of the hernia. The gastric wall is forced into many linear folds as it crosses over the diaphragmatic margin. The greater curvature aspect of the gastric wall is toward the *bottom* of this view.

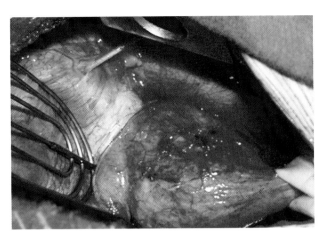

FIGURE 15-15. Large hiatal hernia (*lower center*) demonstrated during an antireflux operation. The superior surface of the diaphragm (*left*) and the phrenic nerve (*top left*) are shown. A Penrose drain retracts the distal esophagus just proximal to the hernia (*lower right*). (Courtesy of Dr. Thomas W. Rice.)

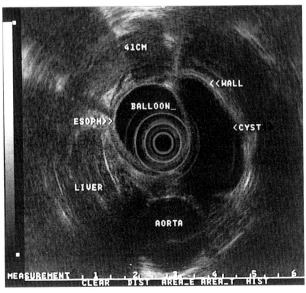

A

B

FIGURE 15-16. **A:** Endoscopic retrograde view of a submucosal lesion at the gastroesophageal junction protruding into the proximal stomach. Such submucosal lesions cannot be accurately evaluated without resection, except by means of endosonography. There are no abnormalities of the overlying mucosa. The surface of the lesion is slightly irregular. The patient has no symptoms related to this lesion. **B:** Endoscopic ultrasonography revealed this anechoic cystic lesion to be a duplication cyst in the submucosa of the esophagogastric junction with intact surrounding mucosal layers. The gastroesophageal junction and stomach are the least common sites of duplication cysts. Formation of duplication cysts is believed to be caused by invagination and fusion of the longitudinal epithelial folds during fetal organogenesis. More than 80% of these lesions are diagnosed in patients younger than 12 years of age. The ratio of women to men is 8:1. This lesion measured 4.1×1.5 cm, remained unchanged in size, and was asymptomatic at repeated examinations after 18 months. Total surgical excision has been the usual approach when therapy is indicated. Endoscopic drainage by means of making incisions with a needle knife or aspiration under endoscopic ultrasound control have been successful. Malignant transformation has been reported. Other congenital anomalies such as esophageal duplication cysts, aberrant pancreas and vertebral abnormalities are reported to be associated findings in 35% to 50% of cases.

16

MOTILITY DISORDERS OF THE ESOPHAGUS

IKUO HIRANO ■ JOHN E. PANDOLFINO ■ PETER J. KAHRILAS

Oropharyngeal dysphagia can be thought of as resulting from propulsive or structural abnormalities. Propulsive defects can result from the dysfunction of control mechanisms of the central nervous system, peripheral nerves, or intrinsic musculature, whereas structural defects may arise from congenital anomalies, neoplasm, surgery, or trauma. In the esophagus, the physiological correlate of dysphagia, unrelated to intrinsic or extrinsic lumenal narrowing, is a peristaltic defect. Failure of the propulsive mechanism may be intermittent or continuous and may result from dysfunction of deglutitive inhibition and/or propagated excitation from motor disorders such as achalasia or esophageal spasm.

Refinements in the methodology for measuring intralumenal pressure, advancements in radiologic imaging, and improved computer technology have vastly enhanced our understanding of these disorders. This chapter summarizes the pathophysiology, clinical manifestations, and diagnostic studies deemed most important to the comprehension and evaluation of these problems.

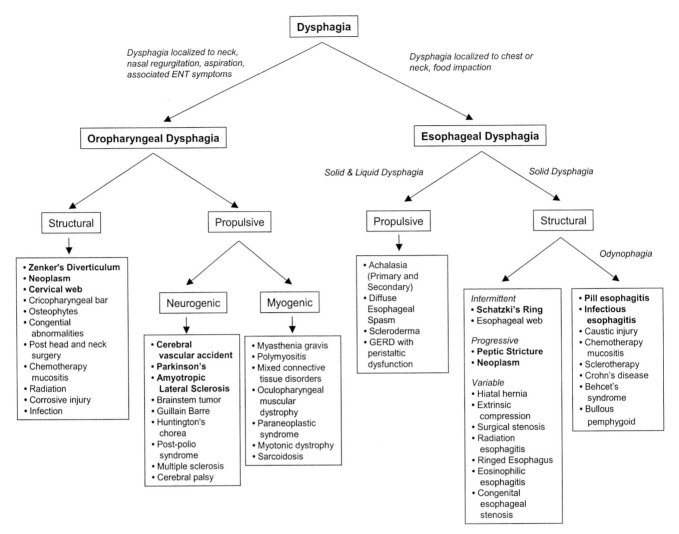

FIGURE 16-1. Algorithm for the conceptualization of dysphagia. More common etiologies are highlighted in bold.

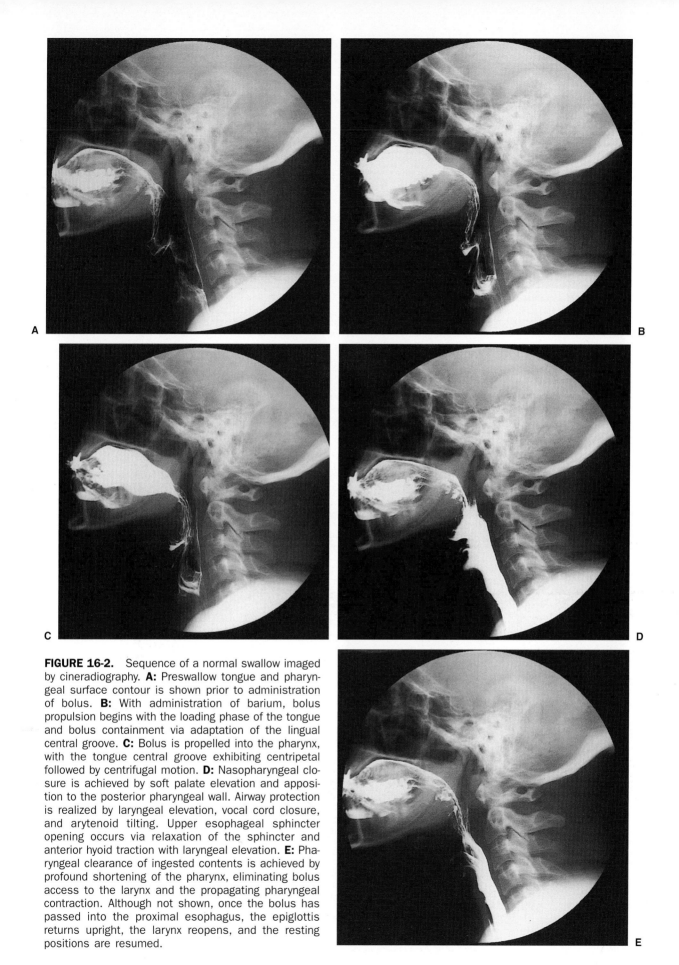

FIGURE 16-2. Sequence of a normal swallow imaged by cineradiography. **A:** Preswallow tongue and pharyngeal surface contour is shown prior to administration of bolus. **B:** With administration of barium, bolus propulsion begins with the loading phase of the tongue and bolus containment via adaptation of the lingual central groove. **C:** Bolus is propelled into the pharynx, with the tongue central groove exhibiting centripetal followed by centrifugal motion. **D:** Nasopharyngeal closure is achieved by soft palate elevation and apposition to the posterior pharyngeal wall. Airway protection is realized by laryngeal elevation, vocal cord closure, and arytenoid tilting. Upper esophageal sphincter opening occurs via relaxation of the sphincter and anterior hyoid traction with laryngeal elevation. **E:** Pharyngeal clearance of ingested contents is achieved by profound shortening of the pharynx, eliminating bolus access to the larynx and the propagating pharyngeal contraction. Although not shown, once the bolus has passed into the proximal esophagus, the epiglottis returns upright, the larynx reopens, and the resting positions are resumed.

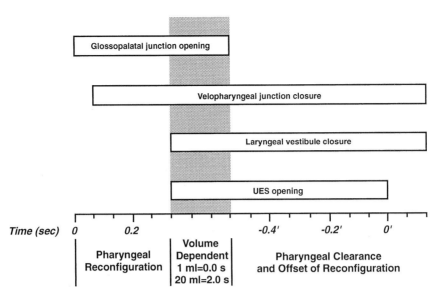

FIGURE 16-3. Time line showing the coordination and volume-induced modifications in the timing of events within the pharyngeal swallow. The *horizontal lines* depict the period during which each of the oropharyngeal valves is in its swallow configuration as opposed to its respiratory configuration. Note that events at the onset and offset of pharyngeal reconfiguration bear a fixed time relationship to each other regardless of swallow bolus volume. The stereotypy of these phases is demonstrated by referencing onset events from time 0 and counting forward or referencing offset events from time 0 and counting backward. This timing scheme defines the middle portion of the time line (*shaded*) as the volume-dependent section, which has a value of 0 seconds for 1-mL swallows and 0.2 seconds for 20-mL swallows. Therefore, the alteration in the timing of the swallow response with large-volume swallows occurs by prolonging the persistence of pharyngeal reconfiguration without changing the synchrony of events at the onset or offset.

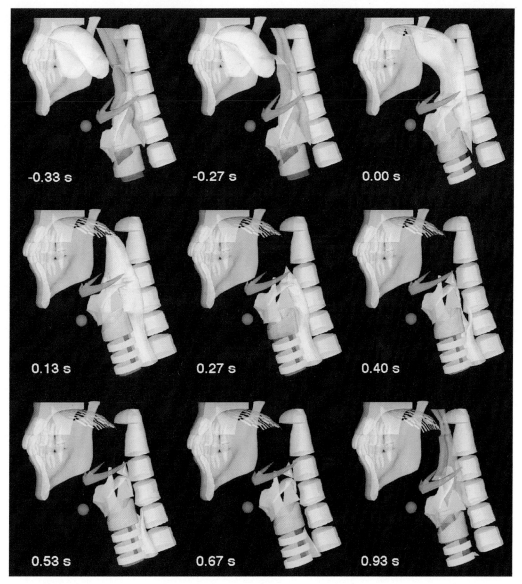

FIGURE 16-4. Three dimensional modeling of the oropharynx during swallowing. This figure shows the reconstructions of nine representative pharyngeal configurations during a 10-mL swallow. In each image the bolus chamber is shown in *white,* the supraglottic airway is *blue,* the infraglottic airway is *purple,* the vertebrae are *light tan,* the hyoid is *orange,* the epiglottis is *yellow,* the arytenoid cartilage is *dark green,* the cricoid cartilage is *dark pink,* the tracheal rings are *light blue,* and the hemisected thyroid cartilage is *light green.* The times next to the images are referenced to the upper esophageal sphincter (UES) opening (time 0.0 seconds). Many mechanical events are encompassed during the act of deglutition. The *preswallow configuration* (−0.33 seconds) is characterized by the bolus chamber being dissociated from the airway by the sealed glossopalatal junction. At the time of *velopharyngeal closure* (−0.27 seconds), the nasopharynx is sealed from the bolus chamber by elevation of the soft palate and the bolus chamber expands to include the retrolingual space as the glossopalatal junction opens. The central groove of the tongue blade has deepened and the posterior oral portion of the pharyngeal propulsive chamber is forming. The larynx has begun elevating and the arytenoid is tilting toward the base of the epiglottis. At the instant of *UES opening* (0.00 seconds) the laryngeal vestibule has been obliterated by contact of the arytenoid against the epiglottic base. Note that the UES (at the inferior aspect of the cricoid cartilage) has elevated relative to its preswallow position and that the pharyngeal bolus chamber is fully formed. During *lingual bolus propulsion* (0.13 seconds), the volume of the bolus chamber is reduced by the centrifugal motion of the tongue surface and bolus expulsion results in full distention of the UES and proximal esophagus. The epiglottis is folded over the arytenoid and there is maximal pharyngeal shortening. The next 4 reconstructions, *early pharyngeal clearance* (0.27 seconds), *midpharyngeal clearance* (0.40 seconds), *late pharyngeal clearance* (0.53 seconds), and *UES closure* (0.67 seconds), show the caudal progression of the pharyngeal contraction stripping the residua from the oropharynx into the esophagus. Ultimately, with *airway reopening* (0.93 seconds) the pharynx commences its return to the respiratory configuration as the larynx descends, the epiglottis flips up, and the velopharyngeal junction reopens.

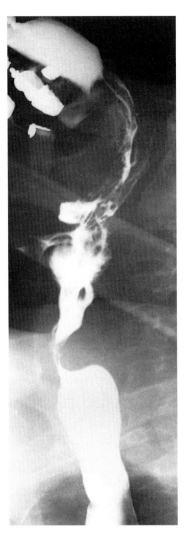

FIGURE 16-5. Cricopharyngeal bar in a patient with oropharyngeal dysphagia. This term refers to an impingement of the pharyngoesophageal junction seen at the level of C4 or C5 and is caused by a noncompliant cricopharyngeus muscle.

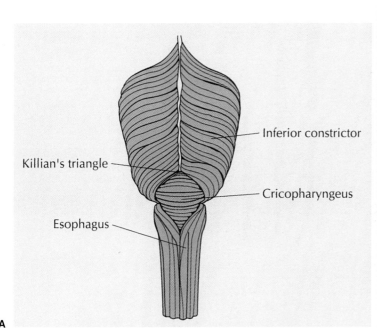

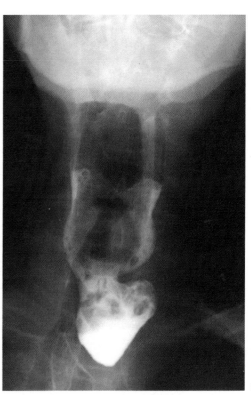

A

B

FIGURE 16-6. Zenker diverticulum. Diverticula can occur throughout the hypopharynx, but when they are located posteriorly between the intersection of the transverse fibers of the cricopharyngeus and obliquely oriented fibers of the inferior pharyngeal constrictors (Killian dehiscence) (**A**), they are called Zenker diverticula (**B**). Note the barium-filled outpouching of the pharynx.

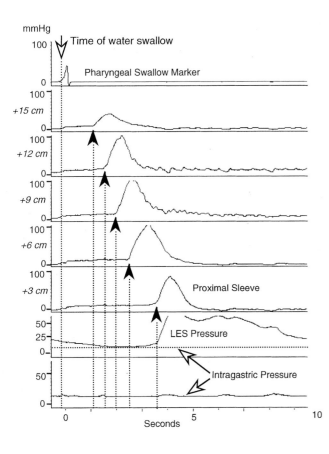

FIGURE 16-7. Normal esophageal manometric recording during a water swallow. The recording was obtained using an eight-lumen manometric assembly with a sleeve sensor. The sleeve sensor is positioned in the lower esophageal sphincter (*LES*), and the center of the sleeve for each side hole sensing site is indicated by *italicized numbers* to the left of the pressure calibrations. The timing of the swallow is indicated by the *first vertical dotted line*. The timing of the onset of the peristaltic contraction at each site is indicated by the *filled arrows* under the manometric tracings. Prior to swallowing, the esophageal body is quiet. Relaxation of the LES to intragastric pressure occurs with the onset of the peristaltic contraction and persists until arrival of the peristaltic wave.

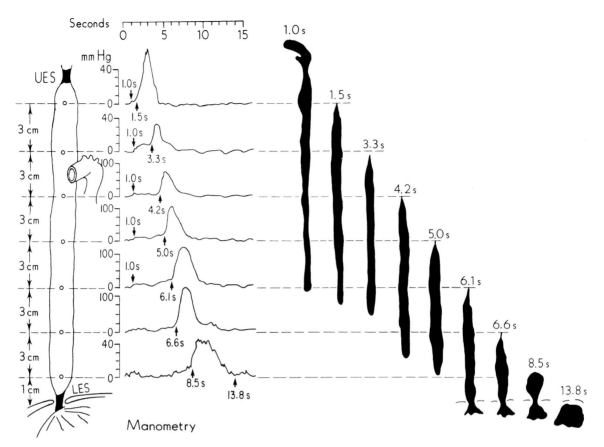

FIGURE 16-8. The single peristaltic sequence that completely clears the barium bolus from the esophagus is illustrated using concurrent manometric and videofluoroscopic imaging during 5-mL liquid barium swallows. The tracings from the video images of the fluoroscopic sequence on the *right* show the distribution of the barium column at times indicated on the individual tracings and by *arrows* on the manometric recording. Pharyngeal injection of barium into the esophagus occurs at 1.0 seconds. The entry of barium causes a slight distention and a slight increase in intralumenal pressure, indicated by the *downward pointing arrow.* Following this, esophageal peristalsis is initiated. During esophageal peristalsis, the tail of the barium bolus, which is equated to lumenal closure, passes each recording site concurrent with the onset of the manometric pressure wave. Therefore, at 1.5 seconds, the peristaltic contraction has reached the proximal recording site and barium has been stripped from the esophagus proximal to that point. Similarly, at 4.2 seconds, the peristaltic contraction has reached the third recording site and the tail of the barium bolus is located at the third recording site. After completion of the peristaltic contraction (at time 13.8 seconds), all of the barium has been cleared into the stomach.

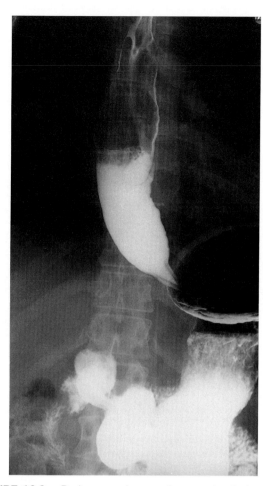

FIGURE 16-9. Barium esophagram in an untreated patient with achalasia. Note the classical radiologic features of a dilated esophagus, retained barium, and an intralumenal air-fluid level with smooth tapering of the esophagogastric junction.

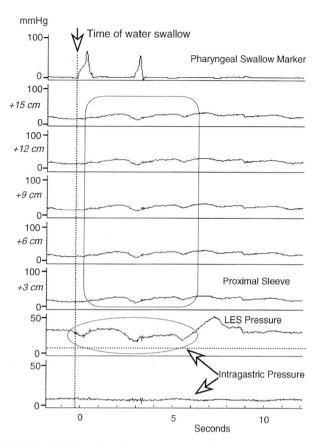

FIGURE 16-10. Esophageal manometric recording in a patient with achalasia. This recording was obtained using the same manometric assembly as in Figure 16-7. The rectangle surrounds an area with an absence of peristaltic activity with elevated intraesophageal pressures. In this part of the recording, the five recording sites demonstrate isobaric wave forms contained within a "common cavity" sealed from above and below by higher-amplitude, lumen-obliterating contractions. The area highlighted by the *ellipse* demonstrates an elevated resting lower esophageal sphincter (*LES*) pressure of 30 mm Hg relative to intragastric pressure with incomplete relaxation during swallow.

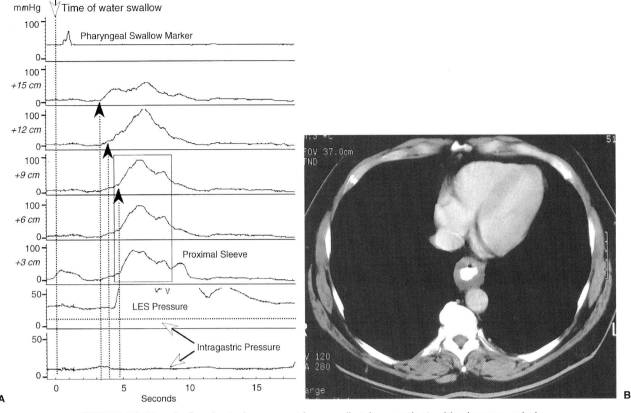

FIGURE 16-11. A: Esophageal manometric recording in a patient with vigorous achalasia. This recording was obtained using the same manometric assembly as in Fig. 16-7. The rectangle surrounds a section of the tracing from three esophageal recording sites. In this period of the recording, simultaneous high-amplitude contractions (>60 mm Hg) are evident. The basal lower esophageal sphincter (*LES*) pressure is 20 mm Hg relative to intragastric pressure, yet shows no deglutitive relaxation. **B:** Thoracic computed tomograph scan of a patient with vigorous achalasia demonstrating marked thickening of the distal esophageal wall. The esophageal lumen is not dilated although it is filled with contrast material.

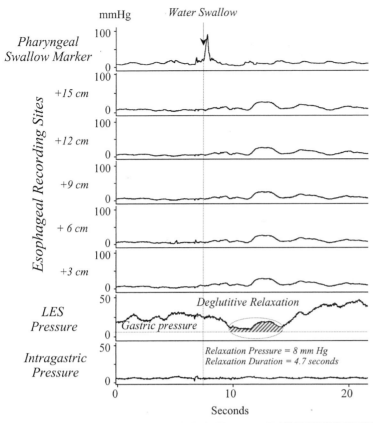

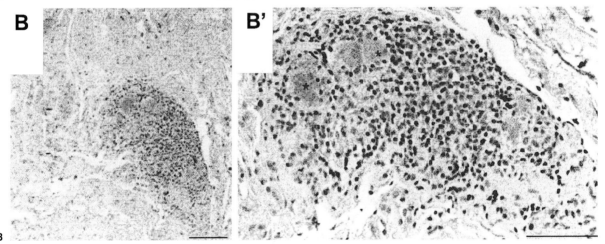

FIGURE 16-12. A: Recording from a patient with a manometric variant of idiopathic achalasia. The recording demonstrates complete esophageal aperistalsis that is typical for classical achalasia. Atypical, however, is the finding of preserved deglutitive relaxation following a water swallow. The relaxation lower esophageal sphincter (*LES*) pressure was 8 mm Hg. **B:** Histological sections of the myenteric plexus of this patient. Low (*B*) and high (*B'*) power views of a myenteric ganglion show nitric oxide synthase-immunoreactive neurons (*). Numerous lymphocytes infiltrate this region, suggesting ongoing chronic inflammatory activity of the myenteric plexus. Such inflammation may lead to the eventual destruction of the myenteric neurons that characterizes the pathophysiology of achalasia.

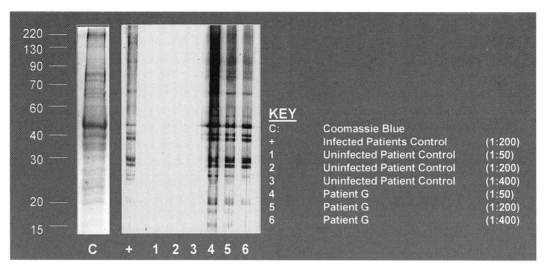

FIGURE 16-13. Western blot confirming the diagnosis of Chagas disease in a patient with clinical manifestations indistinguishable from idiopathic achalasia. Serologic testing is important in patients with achalasia from areas of the world where Chagas disease is endemic. Achalasia is a delayed complication of the infection caused by *Trypanosoma cruzii* and typically presents many years after inoculation by the reduviid bug. (Courtesy of David Engman, M.D.)

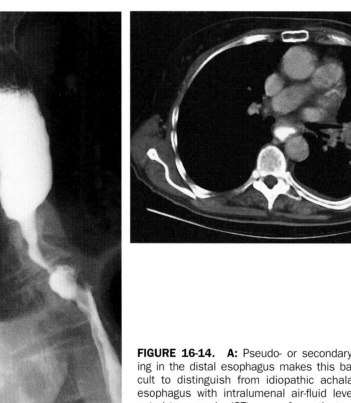

FIGURE 16-14. **A:** Pseudo- or secondary achalasia. The tapering in the distal esophagus makes this barium esophagram difficult to distinguish from idiopathic achalasia. Note the dilated esophagus with intralumenal air-fluid level. **B:** Abdominal computed tomography (CT) scan of a patient with pseudo- or secondary achalasia. This CT image demonstrates a stellate pulmonary mass originating in the left lung invading the gastroesophageal junction.

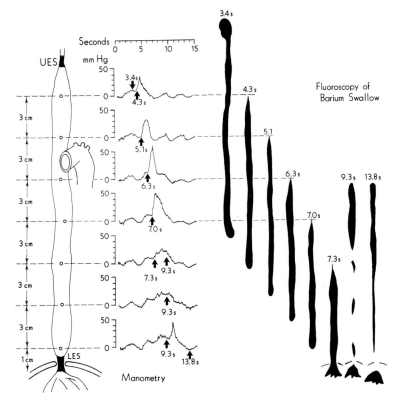

FIGURE 16-15. Simultaneous manometry and fluoroscopy showing minimal esophageal volume clearance with failed peristalsis and simultaneous contractions. As described in Fig. 16-8, the tracings from the video images of the fluoroscopic sequence on the *right* show the distribution of the barium column at times indicated on the individual tracings and by *arrows* on the manometric recording. Pharyngeal injection of barium into the esophagus occurs at 3.4 seconds. Following this, esophageal peristalsis is initiated. At 7.0 seconds, the peristaltic contraction has stripped the barium from the esophagus proximal to that point. However, at 9.3 seconds, there is failed peristalsis and simultaneous contraction at the three distal sites. This results in impaired esophageal volume clearance and the appearance of retained barium at multiple locations in the esophagus which remain at 13.8 seconds.

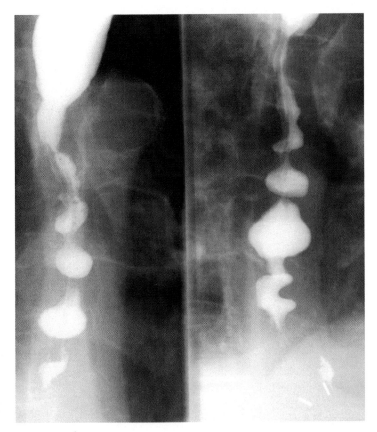

FIGURE 16-16. Barium esophagram demonstrating esophageal spasm. The corkscrew appearance results from simultaneous nonpropulsive contractions of the esophagus occurring at multiple levels.

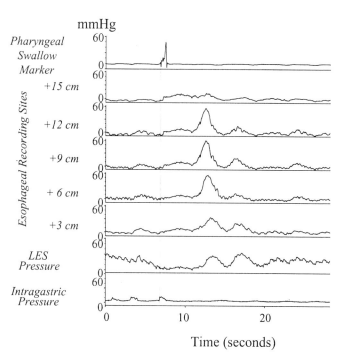

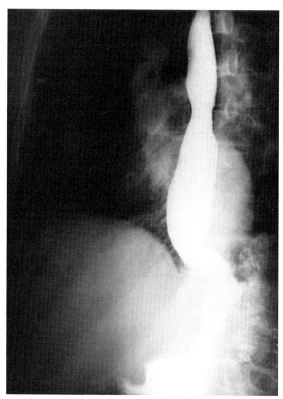

FIGURE 16-17. Manometric recording in a patient with diffuse esophageal spasm. This recording was obtained using the same manometric assembly as in Fig. 16-7. The recording demonstrates simultaneous esophageal contractions at several recording sites with normal basal lower esophageal sphincter pressures and relaxation.

FIGURE 16-18. Barium esophagram in a patient with scleroderma. Note the dilated atonic esophagus yet patulous gastroesophageal junction.

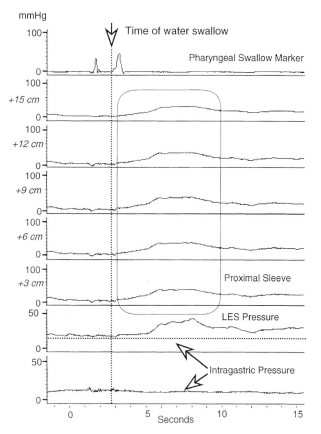

FIGURE 16-19. Manometric recording demonstrating a scleroderma-like pattern. This recording was obtained using the same manometric assembly as in Fig. 16-7. The *rectangle* surrounds a section of the tracing demonstrating an absence of peristaltic activity in five esophageal recording sites. The basal lower esophageal sphincter pressure is hypotonic and approximates intragastric pressure.

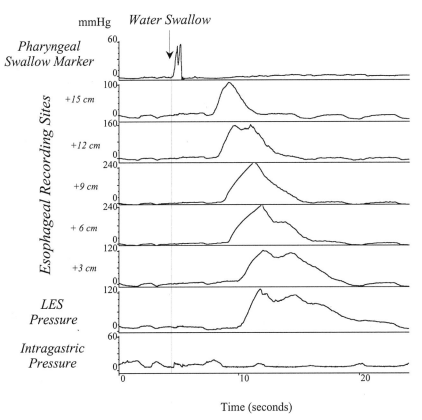

FIGURE 16-20. Esophageal manometry in a patient with "nutcracker esophagus." The recording depicts peristaltic esophageal contractions in response to a water swallow. The amplitudes of the esophageal contractions in channels 4 and 5 are quite high (237 and 248 mm Hg, respectively). There is poor correlation between symptoms of chest pain and the manometric abnormalities in patients with this entity.

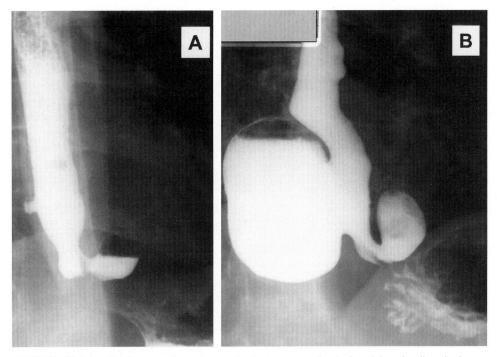

FIGURE 16-21. Barium swallow demonstrating an esophageal epiphrenic diverticulum. Panel (**A**) was taken 10 years prior to panel (**B**) and illustrates the enlargement of the diverticulum, over time. Such outpouchings are typically associated with an underlying esophageal motility disorder such as diffuse esophageal spasm or achalasia.

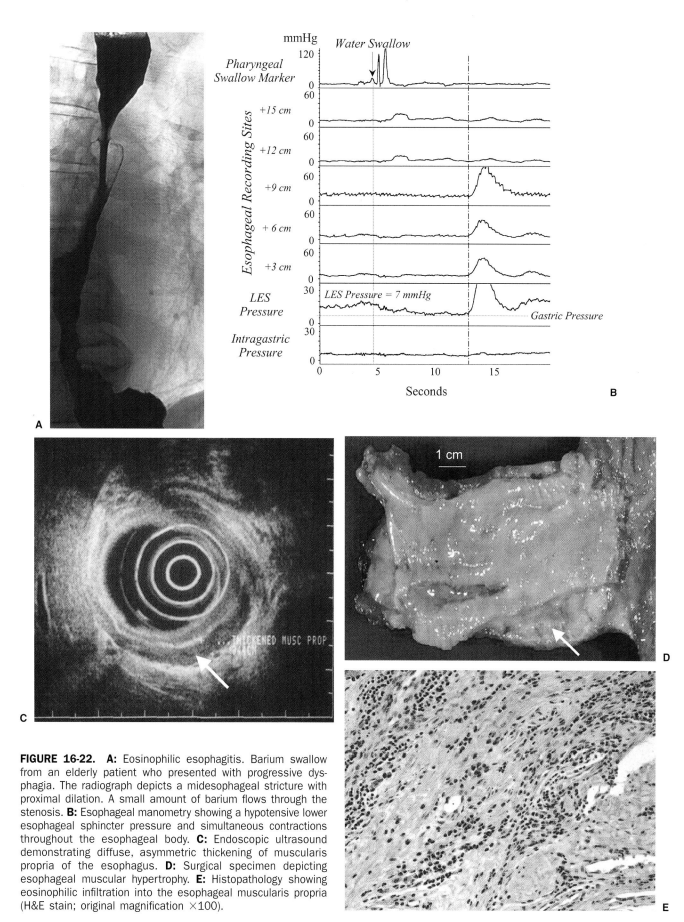

FIGURE 16-22. **A:** Eosinophilic esophagitis. Barium swallow from an elderly patient who presented with progressive dysphagia. The radiograph depicts a midesophageal stricture with proximal dilation. A small amount of barium flows through the stenosis. **B:** Esophageal manometry showing a hypotensive lower esophageal sphincter pressure and simultaneous contractions throughout the esophageal body. **C:** Endoscopic ultrasound demonstrating diffuse, asymmetric thickening of muscularis propria of the esophagus. **D:** Surgical specimen depicting esophageal muscular hypertrophy. **E:** Histopathology showing eosinophilic infiltration into the esophageal muscularis propria (H&E stain; original magnification ×100).

GASTROESOPHAGEAL REFLUX DISEASE

JOEL E. RICHTER

Gastroesophageal reflux disease (GERD) is due to the failure of the normal antireflux mechanism to protect against frequent and abnormal amounts of gastroesophageal reflux; that is, the effortless movement of gastric contents from the stomach into the esophagus. GERD is a common problem. In a survey from Olmsted County Minnesota, the prevalence of heartburn and acid regurgitation in the past 12 months was 42% and 45%, respectively. Frequent symptoms (at least weekly) were reported by 20% of the respondents with an equal gender distribution across all ages (Fig. 17-1).

The pathophysiology of GERD is complex. It results from an imbalance between *defensive factors* protecting the esophagus, including the antireflux barrier, particularly the lower esophageal sphincter, hiatal hernia, lumenal clearance mechanisms (gravity, peristalsis, salivary bicarbonate) and tissue resistance, and *aggressive factors* from the stomach contents, including gastric acidity, volume, and duodenal contents (Fig. 17-2) (Table 17-1).

GERD is recognized clinically by the development of classical symptoms of heartburn or acid regurgitation. Less common symptoms include dysphagia, water brash, odynophagia, burping, hiccups, nausea, and vomiting. Extraesophageal manifestations of GERD include chest pain; pulmonary; and ear, nose, and throat complaints. These latter symptoms result from either a vagally mediated reflex between the esophagus and bronchopulmonary tree or from microaspiration of acid (Fig. 17-3).

Multiple tests are available for evaluating the patient with suspected GERD or its complications. Upper endoscopy is the most sensitive and specific test in assessing tissue injury from reflux esophagitis. It is the best test for identifying reflux esophagitis (Fig. 17-4), peptic stricture (Fig. 17-5), Barrett esophagus (Fig. 17-6) or Barrett esophagus with associated adenocarcinoma (Fig. 17-7). Biopsies from the esophagus help confirm the presence of esophagitis (Fig. 17-8), especially when there is no erosive disease, and are required to make the diagnosis of specialized intestinal metaplasia characteristic of Barrett esophagus (Fig. 17-9). The barium esophagram helps in the evaluation of reflux patients with dysphagia. Good distention of the distal esophagus will bring out subtle strictures and rings (Fig. 17-10). Prolonged esophageal pH monitoring is helpful before antireflux surgery and among patients with difficult to manage typical or extraesophageal symptoms in whom the endoscopy is normal (Table 17-2).

The treatment of GERD involves the relief of symptoms, healing of esophagitis, and the prevention of relapses and complications. Lifestyle modifications are especially helpful in patients with mild symptoms or nocturnal complaints (Table 17-3). Patients with symptoms and no esophagitis can be treated with over-the-counter antacids, Gaviscon, histamine-2 receptor antagonists (H_2RAs), or prokinetic drugs. Patients with severe symptoms, esophagitis, or complications will need proton pump inhibitor therapy or should be considered for antireflux surgery.

TABLE 17-1

Components of Tissue Resistance Against Acid Injury to the Esophagus

Preepithelial defenses
   Mucous layer
   Unstirred water layer
   Surface bicarbonate ion concentration

Epithelial defenses
   Structures
      Cell membrane
      Intercellular junctional complexes (tight junctions, glycoconjugates or lipid)
   Functions
      Epithelial transport
         Na^+/H^+ exchanger
         Na^+-dependent Cl^-/HCO_3^- exchanger
      Intracellular buffers
      Cell replication

Postepithelial defenses
   Blood flow
   Tissue acid-base status

From Orlando RC. Esophageal epithelial defenses against acid injury. Am J Gastroenterol 1994;89:S48.

TABLE 17-2

Guidelines for the Clinical Use of Esophageal pH Monitoring

Definite indications
   To document abnormal esophageal acid exposure in an endoscopy-negative patient
      prior to antireflux surgery
   To evaluate patients after antireflux surgery who are suspected of having persistent or
      recurring reflux symptoms
   To evaluate patients with either normal or equivocal endoscopic findings and reflux
      symptoms refractory to PPIs

Possible indications
   To evaluate patients for suspected extraesophageal symptoms of GERD

Not indicated
   To detect or verify reflux esophagitis, which is best done by endoscopy with biopsies

---

GERD, gastroesophageal reflux disease; PPI, proton pump inhibitor.

From Kahrilas PJ, Quigley EMM. Clinical esophageal pH recording: a technical review of practice guideline development. Gastroenterology 1996;110:1982.

TABLE 17-3

Lifestyle Factors Aggravating GERD and Their Proposed Mechanisms for Heartburn

LOW LES PRESSURE	DIRECT MUCOSAL IRRITANT	INCREASED INTRA-ABDOMINAL PRESSURE	OTHERS
Certain foods	Certain foods	Bending over	Supine position
Fats	Citrus products	Lifting	Lying on right side
Sugar	Tomato-based products	Straining at stool	Red wine
Chocolate	Spicy foods	Exercising	Emotions
Onions	Coffee		
Carminatives	Tea		
Coffee	Cola drinks		
Alcohol	Medications		
Cigarettes	Aspirin		
	NSAIDs		
Medications	Tetracycline		
Progesterone	Quinidine		
Theophylline	Aldreonates		
Anticholinergics	Potassium tablets		
Diazepam	Iron salts		
Nitrates			
Calcium channel blockers			

GERD, gastroesophageal reflux disease; LES, lower esophageal sphincter; NSAIDs, nonsteroidal antiinflammatory drugs.

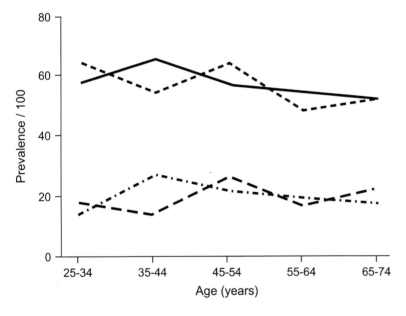

FIGURE 17-1. Age and gender-specific prevalence rates (per 100) for any episodes of either heartburn or acid regurgitation and for at least weekly episodes among Olmsted County, MN, residents aged 25 to 74 years. (Men any ▪▬▬▪; weekly ▬ ▬ ▬; women any ▬▬▬▬; weekly ▪▬▪▬▪▪.)

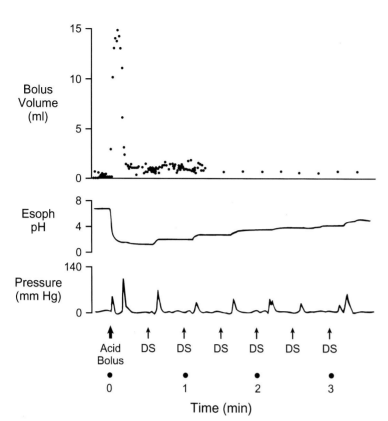

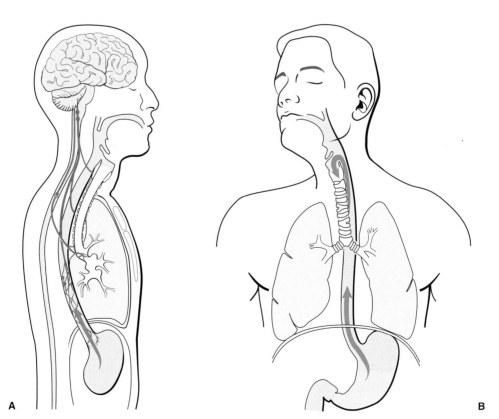

FIGURE 17-2. Relationship between esophageal peristalsis, distal esophagus pH, esophageal volume, and esophageal acid clearance in a healthy volunteer. Acid reflux is replicated by infusing radiolabeled 0.1 N HCl into the esophagus and scanning over the chest. The first peristaltic contraction clears all but about 1 mL of the infused fluid, but the esophageal pH remains unchanged. Stepwise increase in distal esophageal pH occurs with subsequent swallows secondary to bicarbonate-enriched saliva.

FIGURE 17-3. Proposed mechanisms for extraesophageal symptoms of gastroesophageal reflux disease. **A:** Vagally mediated reflex arc between distal esophagus and bronchopulmonary tree. **B:** Microaspiration of gastric acid.

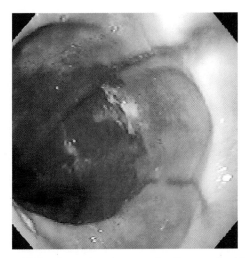

FIGURE 17-4. Los Angeles grade B esophagitis with mucosal breaks greater than 5 mm on multiple esophageal folds. These changes would be compatible with Savary-Miller and Hetzel grade II esophagitis.

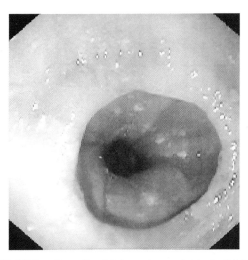

FIGURE 17-5. Smooth, thickened esophageal stricture at the squamocolumnar junction just above a hiatal hernia. No esophagitis is seen.

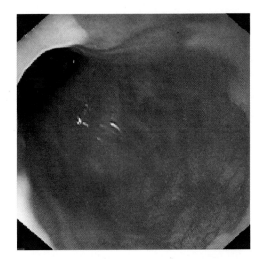

FIGURE 17-6. Long-segment Barrett esophagus measuring 4 cm above the hiatal hernia. The specialized intestinal metaplasia has a distinct reddish pink appearance in contrast to the glossy white squamous mucosa of the esophagus.

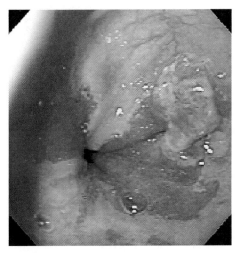

FIGURE 17-7. Barrett esophagus with an early adenocarcinoma identified on surveillance endoscopy.

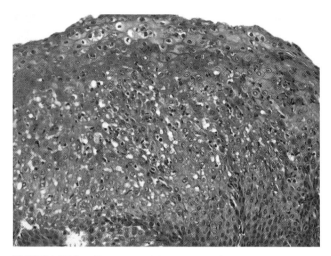

FIGURE 17-8. Esophageal biopsy of reflux esophagitis with increased neutrophils and eosinophils in the squamous mucosa.

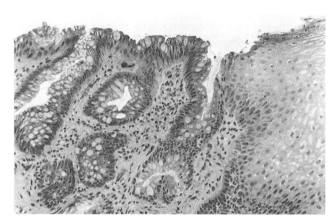

FIGURE 17-9. Esophageal biopsy at the new squamo-columnar junction in a Barrett esophagus patient. Specialized intestinal metaplasia with goblet cells (*left*). The normal squamous mucosa (*right*).

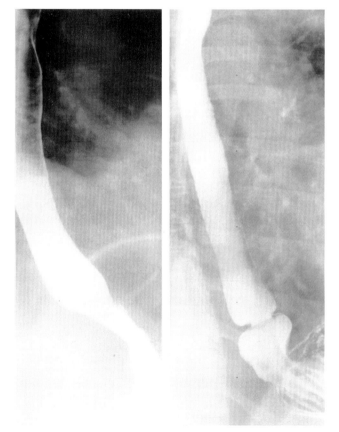

FIGURE 17-10. Barium esophagram in a patient with dysphagia. **Left:** The x-ray suggests a possible subtle stricture. **Right:** Good esophageal distention by the Valsalva maneuver brings out a Schatzki ring with a small hiatal hernia.

18

ESOPHAGEAL INFECTIONS AND DISORDERS ASSOCIATED WITH ACQUIRED IMMUNODEFICIENCY SYNDROME

C. MEL WILCOX

A number of factors are responsible for the upsurge in esophageal infections witnessed over the last two decades. These include further applications of organ transplantation and immunosuppressive therapy, more potent chemotherapeutic regimens for the treatment of neoplasms, the acquired immunodeficiency syndrome (AIDS) epidemic, and the ability to diagnose these disorders more effectively through improvements in endoscopic and microbiologic techniques. A timely and accurate diagnosis of esophageal infections is important because therapy is available for essentially all of these disorders. Furthermore, despite the immunocompromised condition of these patients, antimicrobial therapies are highly efficacious.

Esophageal infections can be categorized by the infecting organism. *Candida* species are the most common fungal pathogens; aspergillosis, histoplasmosis, and blastomycosis are very rare. After fungi, viruses are the most common cause of infection; herpes simplex virus (HSV) and cytomegalovirus (CMV) are most frequent. Additional causes of esophagitis include bacteria and mycobacteria, and rarely, parasites. Odynophagia is the most common symptom of esophageal infection; dysphagia is reported less frequently. Chest pain or back pain may be reported when the disease is severe. Rarely, the presenting manifestation of esophageal infection is a complication such as bleeding, stricture, or fistula. Although barium esophagography is helpful in suggesting the presence of infectious esophagitis, these studies are rarely diagnostic. Endoscopy provides the highest diagnostic sensitivity and specificity.

Candida albicans is the most common pathogen causing esophageal infection. Classically, barium radiographs of esophageal candidiasis reveal a "shaggy" appearance resulting from diffuse plaque material that coats the esophageal mucosa and mimics ulceration (Fig. 18-1). The endoscopic appearance of *Candida* is well recognized and is essentially pathognomonic. The severity can be graded as follows:

- Grade 1—scattered plaques involving less than 50% of the esophageal mucosa
- Grade 2—scattered plaques involving more than 50% of the esophageal mucosa (Fig. 18-2).

- Grade 3—confluent plaque material circumferentially coating at least 50% of the esophageal mucosa
- Grade 4—findings of grade 3 plus impingement of the plaque material into the esophageal lumen despite air insufflation (Fig. 18-3).

Candida rarely causes true ulceration; thus, the presence of esophageal ulcer associated with *Candida* esophagitis suggests an additional esophageal process (Fig. 18-4). Esophageal brushings have the highest diagnostic yield for candidal infection. Mucosal biopsies will be diagnostic when more severe disease (grades 2–4) is present, and should be performed in the presence of ulceration. Fungal cultures are not widely available and provide no additional information over the endoscopic and histological findings unless fungi other than *Candida* are suspected.

Other fungi rarely cause esophageal disease. *Histoplasma* is the most frequent fungal pathogen reported to involve the esophagus, usually from mediastinal involvement (Fig. 18-5).

In contrast to *Candida* esophagitis, barium radiographs of viral esophagitis demonstrate ulceration. The ulcers are usually well circumscribed but may coalesce to form a superficial esophagitis. Ulcers associated with HSV infection typically are small and well circumscribed, whereas those associated with CMV have a greater propensity to form larger, well-circumscribed longitudinal or linear lesions. A diffuse viral esophagitis may result in a cobblestone or shaggy mucosal appearance similar to that observed in esophageal candidiasis (Fig. 18-6). Endoscopically, HSV ulcers correspond to the radiographic features appearing as well-circumscribed shallow ulcers (Fig. 18-7); occasionally when multiple and small, the lesions may mimic esophageal candidiasis (Fig. 18-8). Although esophageal ulcers caused by CMV may resemble HSV (Fig. 18-9), in general, CMV causes larger lesions that are often very deep in patients with AIDS (Figs. 18-10 and 18-11). Multiple biopsies of the ulcer with careful histological examination of biopsy material should reveal the intranuclear (Cowdry type A) or cytoplasmic inclusions characteristic of HSV or CMV infection (Fig. 18-12), respectively. The viral cytopathic effect of HSV is typically located in squamous epithelium, whereas CMV resides in granulation tissue (endothelial and mesenchymal cells). Therefore, biopsies of the ulcer edge are most appropriate to diagnose HSV infection and biopsies of the ulcer base best identify CMV.

Radiographic findings in esophageal tuberculosis are nonspecific but may show ulceration, stricture, or fistulae extending from the esophagus to the trachea, bronchi, or mediastinal lymph nodes (Fig. 18-13). The endoscopic findings are nonspecific. Appropriate stains of biopsy specimens taken from these lesions may reveal acid-fast organisms that may grow in culture. In AIDS, mediastinal tuberculous lymphadenopathy can also extend to involve the esophagus. As a result, transmural lesions such as esophagoesophageal fistulae may occur (Fig. 18-14). Esophageal infections caused by other bacteria such as *Treponema pallidum* are exceedingly rare and are not associated with characteristic radiographic or endoscopic findings. An interesting disorder of the pathogenesis which is not well defined is the human immunodeficiency virus (HIV)-associated idiopathic esophageal ulcer. Characteristically, these lesions become manifest when immunodeficiency is severe (CD4 lymphocyte count $<100/mm^3$). The clinical, radiographic, and endoscopic manifestations are indistinguishable from CMV (Figs. 18-15 through 18-17). Other esophageal diseases seen in patients with AIDS include parasites and rarely neoplasms (Kaposi sarcoma and non-Hodgkin lymphoma).

In summary, in most cases of infectious esophagitis, determination of the specific infection and institution of appropriate therapy will result in mucosal healing and relief of symptoms. Endoscopy is the most sensitive and specific technique for establishing the etiology of esophageal infections.

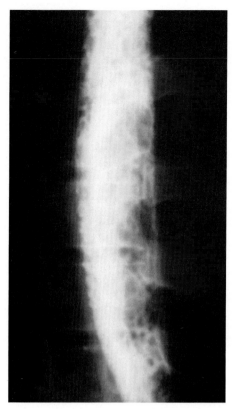

FIGURE 18-1. Barium esophagram shows multiple filling defects with irregularity of the mucosal surface resulting in a "shaggy" appearance caused by esophageal candidiasis.

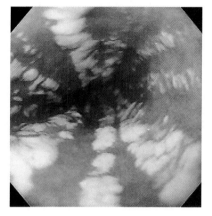

FIGURE 18-2. Multiple raised white plaques involving the esophagus with normal intervening mucosa. This would be classified as grade 2 *Candida* esophagitis.

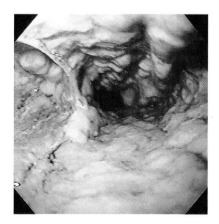

FIGURE 18-3. Exuberant yellow plaque material encroaching on the esophageal lumen is typical of severe *Candida* esophagitis (grade 4).

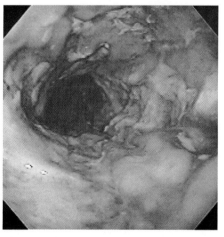

FIGURE 18-4. Diffuse ulceration with a serpiginous appearance with overlying candidal debris. This patient with acquired immunodeficiency syndrome has cytomegalovirus esophagitis and *Candida* coinfection.

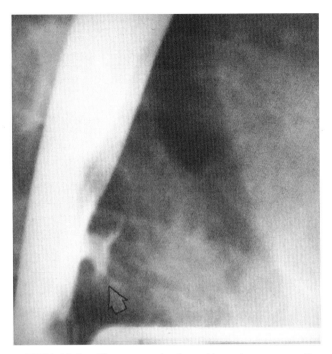

FIGURE 18-5. Ulcer seen in the midesophagus near the bronchus (*arrow*) caused by an infected lymph node from *Histoplasma capsulatum*. (Courtesy of Robert Koehler, M.D.)

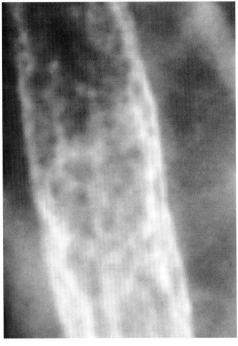

FIGURE 18-6. Barium esophagram showing diffuse mucosal irregularity resembling *Candida* esophagitis. This patient with acquired immunodeficiency syndrome had diffuse erosive esophagitis caused by herpes simplex virus.

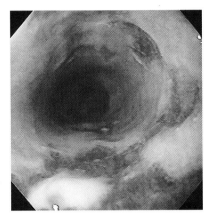

FIGURE 18-7. Multiple, well-circumscribed, shallow esophageal ulcers caused by herpes simplex virus esophagitis.

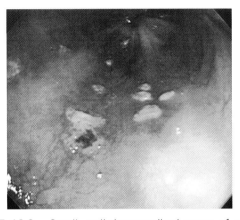

FIGURE 18-8. Small, well-circumscribed areas of exudate resembling *Candida*. This is a classical appearance of mild herpes simplex virus esophagitis. This patient had neutropenia.

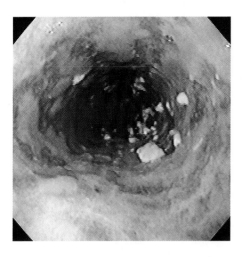

FIGURE 18-9. Shallow, irregular ulceration with intervening areas of preserved but edematous squamous mucosa caused by cytomegalovirus. Note also the candidal plaques in the distal esophagus. This endoscopic appearance is also compatible with herpes simplex virus esophagitis.

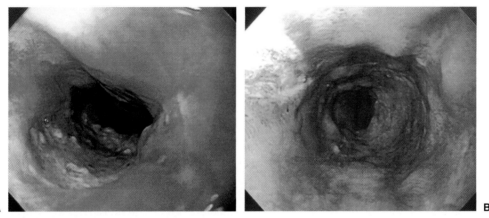

A   B

FIGURE 18-10. A: Large, deep ulceration in the proximal esophagus caused by cytomegalovirus in a patient with acquired immunodeficiency syndrome. **B:** Ulcerations in the distal esophagus are smaller, more linear, and not as deep. Ulceration may not be uniform in the same patient.

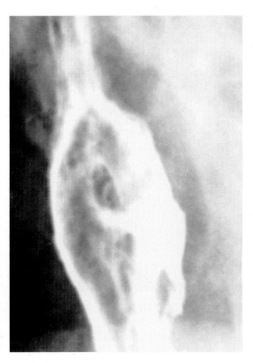

FIGURE 18-11. Barium esophagram shows large esophageal ulceration caused by cytomegalovirus esophagitis in a patient with acquired immunodeficiency syndrome.

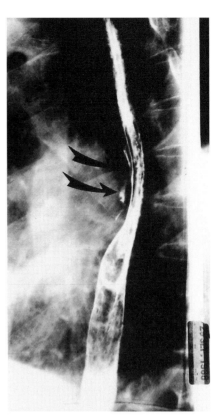

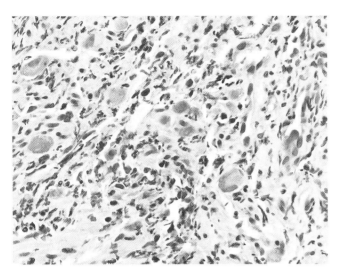

FIGURE 18-12. Multiple large cells with both intranuclear and intracytoplasmic inclusions typical of cytomegalovirus viral cytopathic effect.

FIGURE 18-13. Barium esophagram reveals diffuse mucosal irregularity and a fistulous tract (*arrows*) to mediastinal lymph nodes in a patient with acquired immunodeficiency syndrome. This patient has tuberculosis. Endoscopy showed Candidiasis and an ulcer at the opening of the fistulous tract. (Courtesy of Dr. R. DeSilva.)

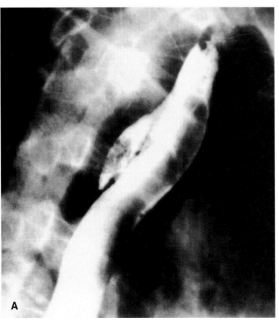

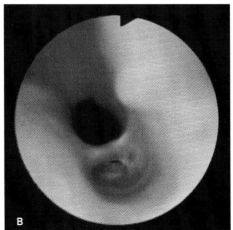

FIGURE 18-14. Barium esophagram (**A**) and endoscopic photograph (**B**) of an esophageal fistula caused by *Mycobacterium tuberculosis* in a man with acquired immunodeficiency syndrome. (Courtesy of Dr. J.P. Raufman.)

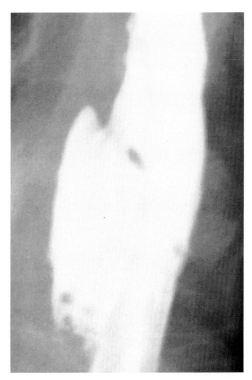

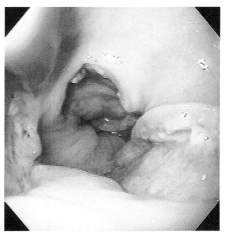

FIGURE 18-15. Barium esophagram shows large solitary ulceration in the midesophagus that was idiopathic in a patient with acquired immunodeficiency syndrome.

FIGURE 18-16. Three large, deep ulcerations (idiopathic) in the distal esophagus in a patient with acquired immunodeficiency syndrome.

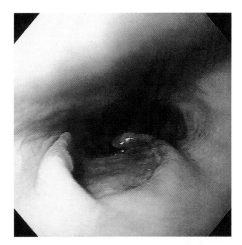

FIGURE 18-17. Solitary, large, well-circumscribed ulceration with a heaped-up appearance typical of idiopathic esophageal ulceration of acquired immunodeficiency syndrome.

ESOPHAGEAL NEOPLASMS

ANIL K. RUSTGI

The most common malignant esophageal neoplasms are squamous cell carcinoma and adenocarcinoma, the latter typically arising in Barrett epithelium. Although esophageal squamous cell carcinoma is the more common of the two worldwide, adenocarcinoma is more frequent in the United States. Frequent symptoms resulting from lumenal masses include dysphagia, odynophagia, and weight loss, which require diagnosis by means of fiberoptic endoscopy with biopsy and cytology. On establishment of diagnosis, preoperative staging is needed before selection of therapy.

Esophageal squamous cell carcinoma occurs predominantly in lower socioeconomic groups within the United States, with predilection for African-American males. Risk factors include tobacco and alcohol use, although in high-incidence areas of the world (northern China, India, Iran, southern Russia, South Africa, and some parts of South America), other factors appear more critical, such as exposure to nitrosamines and concomitant nutritional (minerals and vitamins) deficiencies. Clinical suspicion of squamous cell carcinoma merits performance of a barium esophagography. This may reveal an early cancer manifest by as a plaque-like lesion (Fig. 19-1) or alternatively, advanced cancer with an ulcerated polypoid lesion (Fig. 19-2) or a circumferential annular lesion (Figs. 19-3 and 19-4). Endoscopy with biopsies may demonstrate various stages: dysplasia, carcinoma in situ, or carcinoma (Fig. 19-5). Preoperative staging is necessary with endoscopic ultrasound to determine esophageal wall invasion and lymph node involvement (Fig. 19-6). A computerized tomography (CT) (Fig. 19-7) scan will exclude regional and distant metastases. Although surgical resection with esophagectomy and gastric interposition is preferred for cure of patients who are appropriate candidates, neoadjuvant therapy with chemotherapy and radiation therapy followed by surgery has shown promise. Palliation is needed for patients who cannot undergo potentially curative therapy (Fig. 19-8).

Esophageal adenocarcinoma invariably develops in the setting of Barrett esophagus (Fig. 19-9A). An important factor in the development of Barrett esophagus is gastroesophageal reflux, although other unidentified factors may be important. Because Barrett esophagus may progress from metaplasia to low-grade dysplasia and high-grade dysplasia with eventual adenocarcinoma, endoscopic surveillance with a systematic protocol for biopsies is warranted. Initial suspicion and diagnosis of Barrett dysplasia and esophageal adenocarcinoma require barium esophagography (Fig. 19-10) and fiberoptic endoscopy (Fig. 19-9B). Pathology may reveal Barrett esophagus with varying degrees of dysplasia (Fig. 19-11) and adenocarcinoma (Fig. 19-12). As with squamous cell carcinoma, preoperative staging entails endoscopic ultrasound (Fig. 19-13) and

CT scanning. Therapy may be surgical or multimodal (neoadjuvant chemotherapy and radiation therapy followed by surgery) if the patient is an appropriate candidate. Otherwise, palliative therapy is provided. It should be noted that both esophageal neoplasms could have associated complications such as fistula formation (Fig. 19-14).

There are many other epithelial and nonepithelial esophageal neoplasms, both benign and malignant, but they are generally quite rare. An example of a benign nonepithelial tumor is leiomyoma, which is typically silent and patients are generally asymptomatic (Fig. 19-15). Rare malignant esophageal neoplasms include carcinosarcoma, metastatic cancer (melanoma, breast cancer), neuroendocrine tumors, and various sarcomas (Fig. 19-16).

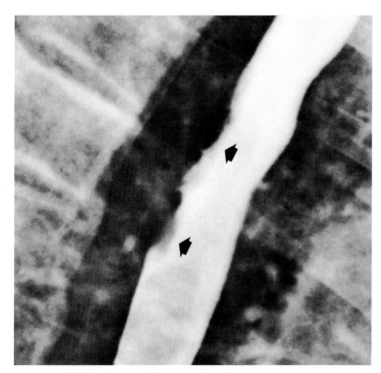

FIGURE 19-1. Early squamous cell carcinoma of the esophagus presenting as a plaque-like lesion (*arrows*) on the posterior wall.

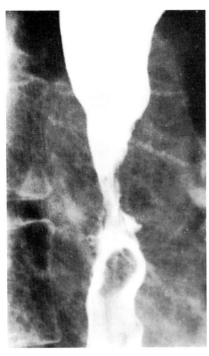

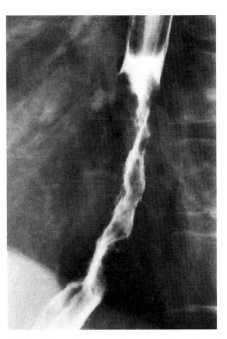

FIGURE 19-2. Ulcerated circumferential apple core–type squamous cell carcinoma.

FIGURE 19-3. Esophagram shows extensive infiltrative lesion of the distal esophagus.

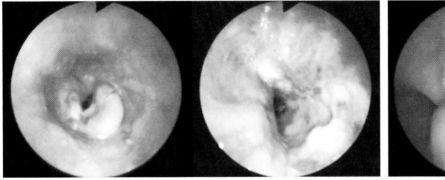

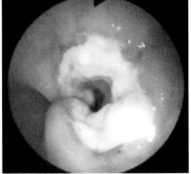

FIGURE 19-4. Endoscopic appearance of infiltrating squamous cell carcinoma. These three carcinomas have variously occluded the lumen and would present as dysphagia.

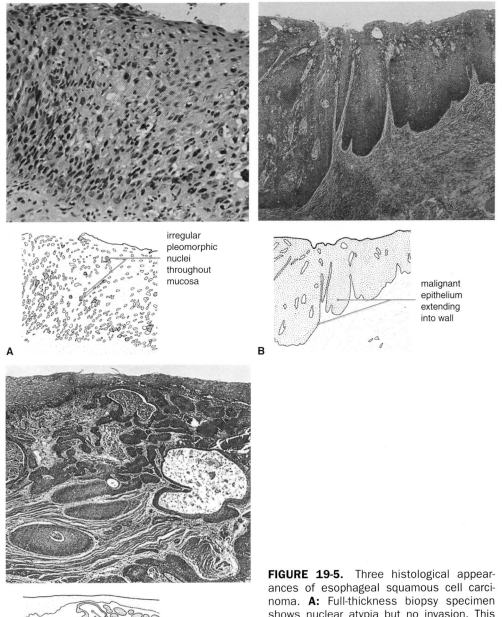

irregular
pleomorphic
nuclei
throughout
mucosa

A

malignant
epithelium
extending
into wall

B

islands of
malignant
epithelium
penetrating
wall

muscle
coat

C

FIGURE 19-5. Three histological appearances of esophageal squamous cell carcinoma. **A:** Full-thickness biopsy specimen shows nuclear atypia but no invasion. This is carcinoma in situ. **B:** Specimen shows early invasive squamous cell carcinoma with downward extension of the tumor into the submucosa. **C:** Established infiltrating, well-differentiated carcinoma. There are islands of malignant tissue under essentially normal squamous epithelium.

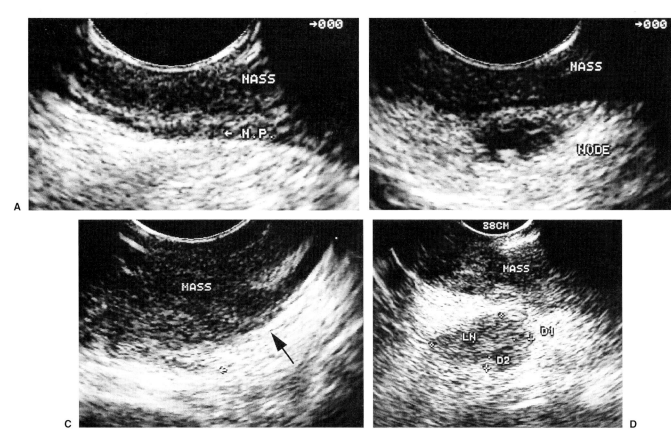

FIGURE 19-6.   A–D: Endoscopic ultrasound images of different stages of esophageal cancer. (Courtesy of William Brugge, M.D.)

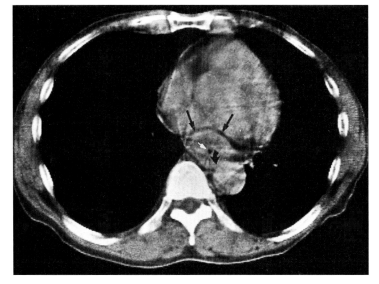

FIGURE 19-7. Use of computed tomographic (CT) scanning for staging esophageal carcinoma. CT scan shows bulky carcinoma (*straight black arrows*) essentially occluding the esophageal lumen (*white arrow*) and obliterating the fat plane adjacent to the aorta (*curved black arrow*). This obliteration of tissue planes indicates mediastinal extension of the lumen.

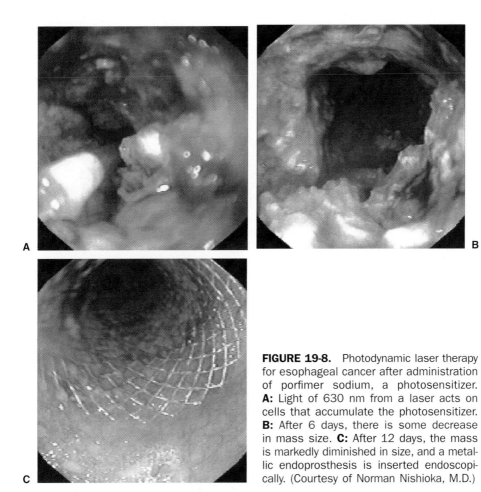

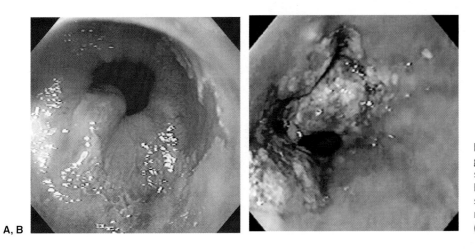

FIGURE 19-8. Photodynamic laser therapy for esophageal cancer after administration of porfimer sodium, a photosensitizer. **A:** Light of 630 nm from a laser acts on cells that accumulate the photosensitizer. **B:** After 6 days, there is some decrease in mass size. **C:** After 12 days, the mass is markedly diminished in size, and a metallic endoprosthesis is inserted endoscopically. (Courtesy of Norman Nishioka, M.D.)

FIGURE 19-9. Barrett esophagus. **A:** Upper endoscopy reveals shortsegment Barrett esophagus. **B:** Upper endoscopy reveals long-segment esophagus with inflammation and possible early cancer. (Courtesy of David Katzka, M.D.)

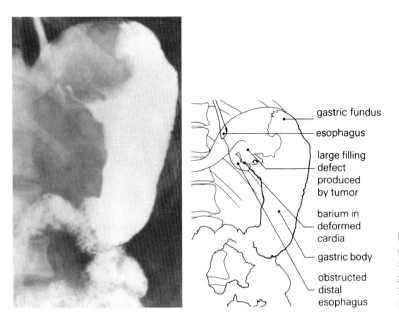

gastric fundus
esophagus
large filling defect produced by tumor
barium in deformed cardia
gastric body
obstructed distal esophagus

FIGURE 19-10. Adenocarcinoma of the distal esophagus may be difficult to differentiate from squamous cell carcinoma on the basis of radiographic appearance. However, as shown here, when the tumor extensively involves the fundus of the stomach, the diagnosis is more certain.

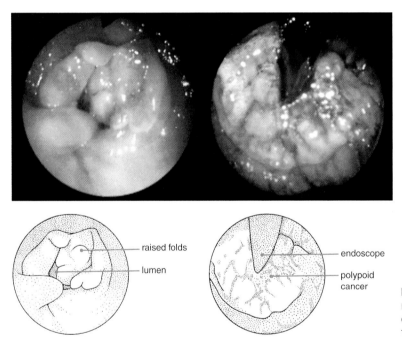

raised folds
lumen

endoscope
polypoid cancer

FIGURE 19-11. At endoscopy, adenocarcinoma may be difficult to differentiate from squamous cell carcinoma. Retroflexed views of the tumor from the stomach may help.

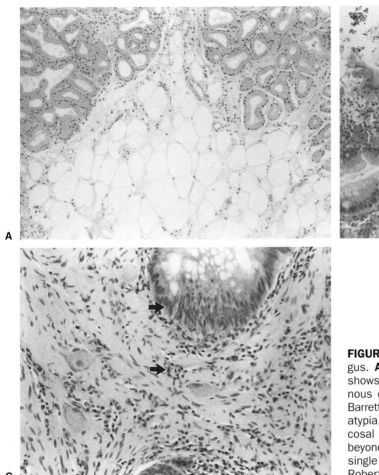

A

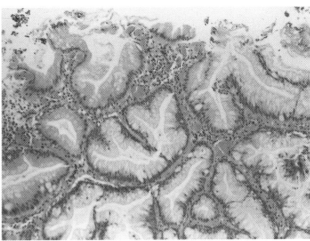

B

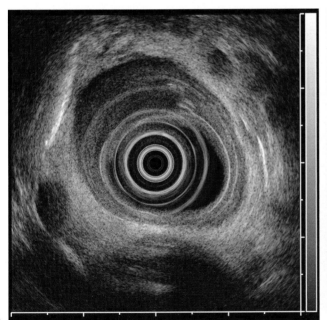

C

FIGURE 19-12. Histological appearance of Barrett esophagus. **A:** Specialized-type Barrett esophagus. The epithelium shows intestinal-type absorptive cells, goblet cells, and mucinous cells in a villiform pattern. **B:** High-grade dysplasia in Barrett esophagus. Epithelium shows architectural complexity, atypia, pleomorphism, and nuclear stratification. **C:** Intramucosal adenocarcinoma in Barrett esophagus. Tumor invasion beyond the basement membrane is present in the form of single cells, small glands, or sheets of cells. (Courtesy of Robert Odze, M.D.)

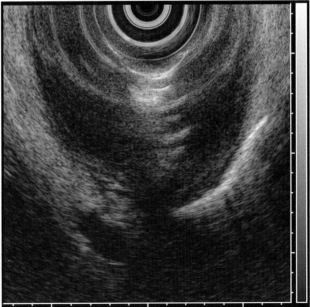

A

B

FIGURE 19-13. Endoscopic ultrasound (EUS). **A:** EUS demonstrates a T2N1 esophageal adenocarcinoma. **B:** The lesion is invading the right pleura. (Courtesy of Michael Kochman, M.D.)

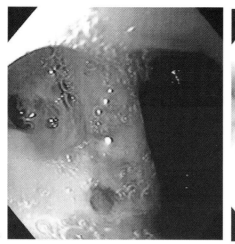 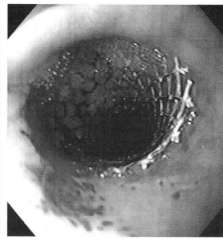

A, B

FIGURE 19-14. A: Esophageal fistula complication of esophageal cancer. **B:** Stent inserted to seal the fistula. (Courtesy of Michael Kochman, M.D.)

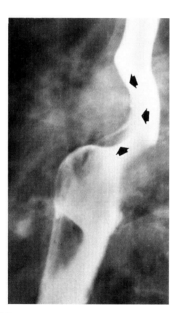

FIGURE 19-15. Leiomyoma usually presents itself as a smooth, rounded intramural defect (*arrows*) that encroaches on the barium column.

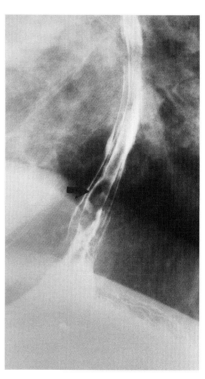

FIGURE 19-16. Kaposi sarcoma of the esophagus represented by dumbbell-shaped submucosal mass (*arrow*) with superficial ulceration. (Courtesy of Deborah Hall, M.D.)

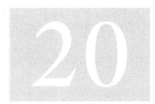

MISCELLANEOUS DISEASES OF THE ESOPHAGUS: Systemic and Dermatologic Disease, Foreign Bodies, and Physical Injury

DOUGLAS O. FAIGEL

Because of its function, location, and squamous lining, the esophagus may be subject to trauma, obstruction by foreign bodies and food, and involvement by systemic and dermatologic diseases. This chapter highlights the miscellaneous disorders that involve the esophagus.

The normal function of the esophagus is to transport food from the pharynx to the stomach. Motor abnormalities, unusual shapes (pointed ends), or structural narrowing may result in impaction of the swallowed material. Sharp objects such as fish bones (Fig. 20-1) may lodge anywhere in the esophagus, whereas blunt objects (Fig. 20-2) and food impaction (Fig. 20-3) usually occurs in the distal portion at the site of peptic strictures or esophageal rings. These objects usually pass spontaneously or can be removed endoscopically (see Fig. 20-3), but recurrence is common unless the underlying stricture, ring, or motility disorder is managed.

Mucosal injury to the esophagus may be medication induced. Pills such as nonsteroidal antiinflammatory drugs, tetracycline, quinidine, and potassium can produce focal erosions and ulceration (Fig. 20-4) by means of either a direct toxic effect or a systemic effect. During healing of pill-induced injury, stricture formation may occur (Fig. 20-4*D*) and result in dysphagia and food impaction. Therapy for pill esophagitis is discontinuation of the offending agent. Prevention depends on the patient swallowing medications in the full upright position and the use of adequate fluid to ensure passage of the pill into the stomach.

Ingestion of strong alkali or acids, either accidentally (usually by children) or deliberately (suicide attempts) can result in a spectrum of esophageal injury ranging from none to mild or moderate (Fig. 20-5*A, B*) to severe injury with necrosis (see Fig. 20-5*C*) and perforation. Caustic injury to the esophagus, if severe, can result in stricture formation (Fig. 20-6) or fistulization into the mediastinum or respiratory tract (Fig. 20-7).

Trauma to the esophagus may occur from rapid increases in intra-abdominal pressure such as during vomiting or retching or from instrumentation. Mallory-Weiss tears are mucosal tears usually located on the gastric side of the squamocolumnar junction along the lesser curvature (Fig. 20-8). If the tear involves a blood vessel, bleeding may be seen and can be severe. Treatment is directed at the bleeding site and avoidance of further trauma to the esophagus by means of controlling nausea and vomiting. Intramural hematoma of the esophagus (esophageal apoplexy) can also occur as a result of vomiting or retching, and usually is related to coagulation defects (hypoprothrombinemia or thrombocytopenia). The hematoma may be large (Fig. 20-9) and obstruct the lumen, resulting in pain and dysphagia. The wall of the esophagus may be disrupted during passage of an endoscope or with esophageal dilation. The diagnosis can be made at the time of the procedure with recognition of the defect in the wall of the esophagus (Fig. 20-10*A*) or later with demonstration of the perforation on radiographs (see Fig. 20-10*B*). Spontaneous rupture of the esophagus (Boerhaave syndrome) is rare but can occur during retching. The diagnosis usually is made when a barium swallow examination (Fig. 20-11) demonstrates extravasation of contrast material into the pleural space.

The esophagus may be involved in systemic disease processes. Crohn's disease may affect the tubular gastrointestinal tract from mouth to anus. Multiple shallow ulcers can be seen endoscopically (Fig. 20-12) or observed with contrast studies of the esophagus (Fig. 20-13). More severe involvement results in formation of nodules, deeper ulceration, intramural sinus tracts (Fig. 20-14), or fistulization to adjacent structures. Other systemic inflammatory diseases may involve the esophagus. Behçet disease is characterized by mucosal ulceration of the esophagus (Fig. 20-15) and other mucosal surfaces, such as the genital tract. Graft versus host disease following bone marrow transplantation can affect the esophagus and manifest as minor mucosal edema or rings (Fig. 20-16), or in more severe forms that cause stricture formation (Fig. 20-17).

Diseases that affect the squamous epithelium of the skin also affect the esophagus. Pemphigus vulgaris is a chronic blistering autoimmune disease of older adults that may cause esophageal blistering and ulceration (Fig. 20-18). Epidermolysis bullosa dystrophica is a rare genetic disorder that also causes bullae formation (Fig. 20-19) and severe strictures (Fig. 20-20).

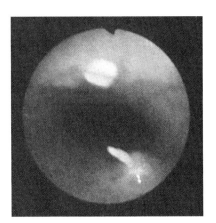

FIGURE 20-1. Endoscopic view of a fish bone lodged in the proximal esophagus after the patient sought treatment with severe neck pain after swallowing the bone. A contralateral ulcer is present in the 12 o'clock position.

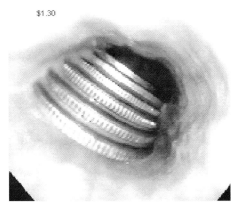

FIGURE 20-2. Endoscopic view of coins lodged in the distal esophagus in a psychiatric patient. (Photo courtesy of Drs. Anna Sasaki and Daniel Zovich.)

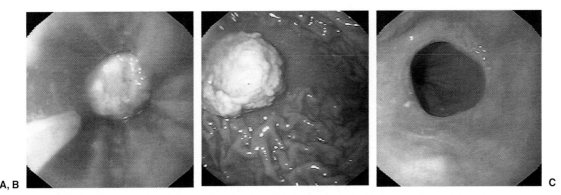

A, B   C

FIGURE 20-3.   A: Food impaction in the distal esophagus. **B:** When cleared by advancing the bolus into the stomach, a Schatzki ring (**C**) is evident.

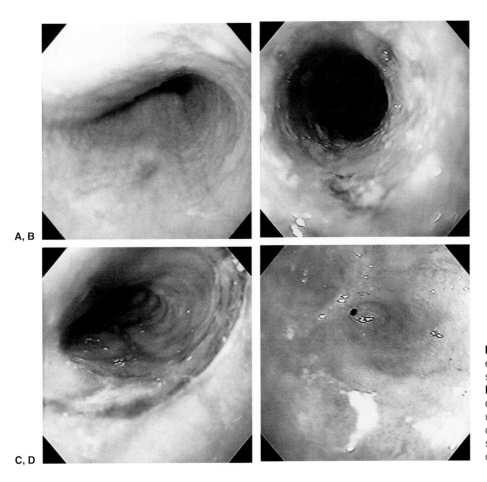

A, B

C, D

FIGURE 20-4.   A: Midesophageal erosion in a patient taking nonsteroidal antiinflammatory drugs. **B:** Midesophageal erosion caused by quinidine. **C:** Proximal esophageal ulceration in a patient taking quinidine. **D:** Pill-induced esophageal stricture in a patient taking quinidine.

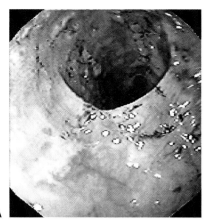

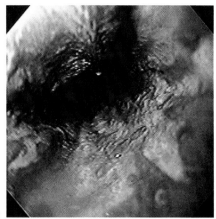

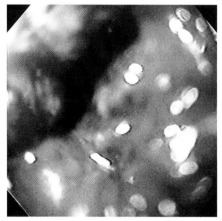

FIGURE 20-5. The endoscopic spectrum of the effect of alkali ingestion on the esophagus. **A:** Mild to moderate injury. **B:** Ulceration and exudate, which indicate more severe mucosal injury. **C:** Mucosal necrosis after alkali ingestion.

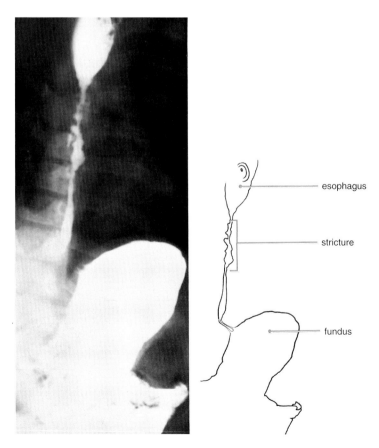

FIGURE 20-6. Esophageal stricture caused by caustic injury to the esophagus.

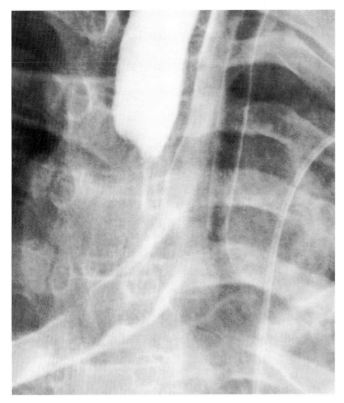

FIGURE 20-7. Esophageal-respiratory fistula 1 month after caustic injury to the esophagus.

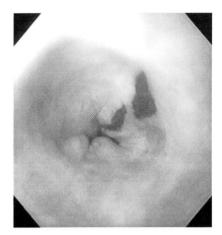

FIGURE 20-8. Endoscopic view of a Mallory-Weiss tear. A nonpenetrating mucosal laceration occurred as a result of retching in a 53-year-old woman.

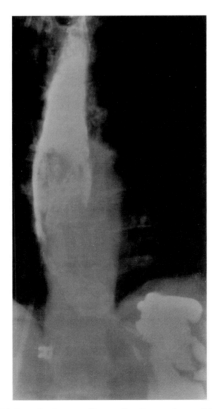

FIGURE 20-9. Barium radiograph of a patient with leukemia demonstrates esophageal hematoma with obstruction.

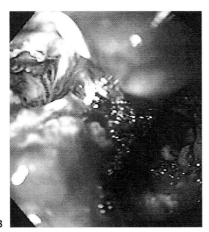

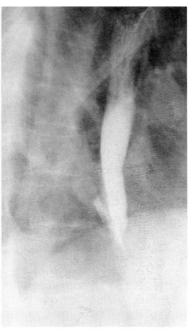

A, B

FIGURE 20-10. Endoscopic and radiographic demonstration of esophageal perforation after bougie dilation of the esophagus 2 days earlier. **A:** Endoscopic view of the perforation between the 10 and 11 o'clock positions. **B:** Barium swallow demonstrates contained perforation.

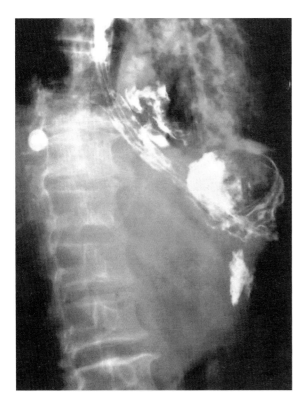

FIGURE 20-11. Barium swallow image of a patient with Boerhaave syndrome demonstrates extravasation of contrast material from a distal esophageal perforation.

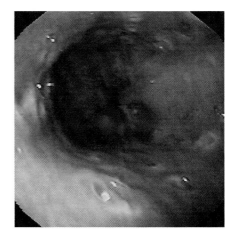

FIGURE 20-12. Esophageal involvement with Crohn's disease demonstrated by the endoscopic finding of multiple esophageal ulcers.

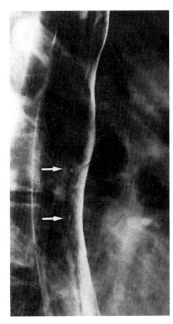

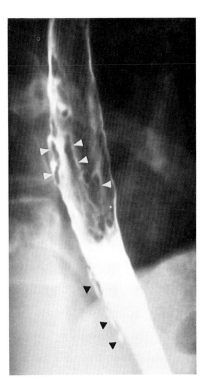

FIGURE 20-13. Barium swallow radiograph demonstrates aphthoid ulcers (*white arrows*) of the midesophagus with a central collection of barium and a peripheral halo.

FIGURE 20-14. Radiograph demonstrates severe esophageal involvement with Crohn's disease. Mucosal nodularity, ulceration (*white arrowheads*), and intramural sinus tracts (*black arrowheads*) are present.

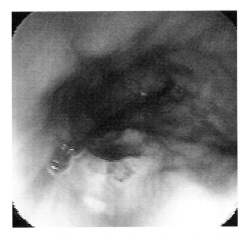

FIGURE 20-15. Endoscopic view of esophageal ulceration in a patient with Behçet disease.

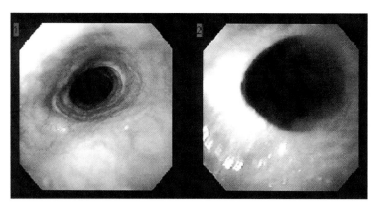

FIGURE 20-16.   Graft versus host disease. Multiple fine mucosal webs are present in the esophagus.

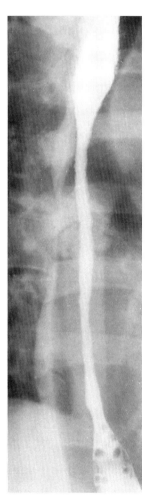

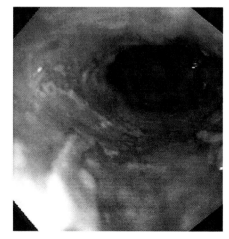

FIGURE 20-17.   Long, tight stricture of the mid-distal esophagus in a patient with graft versus host disease involving the esophagus.

FIGURE 20-18.   Desquamated mucosa in a patient with pemphigus vulgaris.

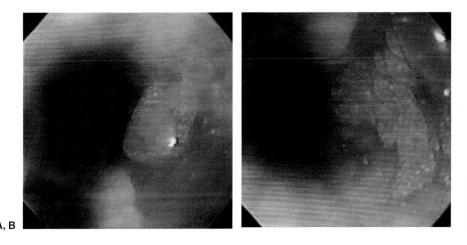

A, B

FIGURE 20-19.   A, B: Endoscopic views of the bulla found in the esophagus of a patient with epidermolysis bullosa.

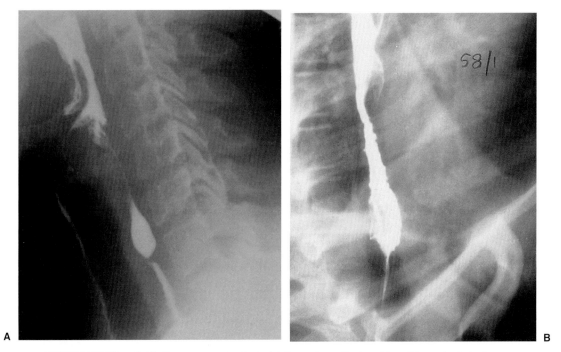

A   B

FIGURE 20-20.   A, B: Severe esophageal strictures in patients with epidermolysis bullosa.

Acknowledgment

Dr. M. Brian Fennerty's assistance in preparing this chapter is gratefully acknowledged.

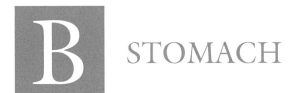

B STOMACH

STOMACH: Anatomy and Structural Anomalies

JEAN-PIERRE RAUFMAN

NORMAL GASTRIC AND DUODENAL ANATOMY

The tubular esophagus abruptly joins the sack-like stomach at the gastroesophageal junction (Fig. 21-1A). The cardiac region (Fig. 21-1B) and fundus (Fig. 21-1C) of the stomach abut the gastric side of the gastroesophageal junction. Like an accordion, the folds of the gastric body (Fig. 21-1D) permit distention of the stomach when full and contraction when empty. The smooth distal antrum (Fig. 21-1E) leads to the pyloric channel (Fig. 21-1F). The first portion or bulb of the duodenum (Fig. 21-1G) takes a turn into the tubular second and third portions (Fig. 21-1H) of the duodenum.

VAGAL INNERVATION AND LYMPHATICS OF THE STOMACH

Vagal fibers provide parasympathetic innervation to the stomach (Fig. 21-2). The branches of the anterior gastric nerve from the anterior vagal trunk innervate the cardia and provide a branch running to the right of the lesser curvature known as the anterior nerve of Latarjet. The hepatic nerve, also a branch of the anterior vagus, innervates the liver, gallbladder, pylorus of the stomach, and proximal duodenum. The posterior vagal trunk divides into a celiac branch, which innervates the pancreas and other abdominal viscera, and posterior gastric branches, which innervate both surfaces of the stomach and form the posterior nerve of Latarjet. The anterior and posterior nerves of Latarjet course along the lesser curvature, give off branches to the fundus and body, and terminate in a "crow's foot" neural distribution to the antrum and pylorus (see Fig. 21-2). The gastric lymphatics (see Fig. 21-2) have a similar pattern to that of the arterial supply (Fig. 21-3) although flow is in the opposite direction. Lymph from the stomach drains into the celiac and gastric lymph nodes.

VASCULATURE OF THE STOMACH AND DUODENUM

The stomach and duodenum derive their blood supply primarily from the celiac axis (see Fig. 21-3) and the superior mesenteric artery (Fig. 21-4). The celiac artery gives off the splenic, left gastric, and hepatic arteries (see Fig. 21-3). Branches from these vessels, including the right gastric and gastroduodenal artery from the hepatic artery and the short gastric arteries and left gastroepiploic artery from the splenic artery, form a dense anastomotic network that encircles the stomach. The right gastric artery and superior pancreaticoduodenal artery, which also arise from the hepatic artery (see Fig. 21-3), supply the duodenum. In concert with the superior mesenteric artery, these vessels provide a rich blood supply to the stomach and duodenum.

The superior mesenteric artery derives from the aorta 3 to 4 cm below the celiac artery, just behind the body of the pancreas and the third to fourth parts of the duodenum (Figs. 21-4 and 21-5). The inferior pancreaticoduodenal branch of the superior mesenteric artery supplies the distal stomach and the duodenum. Corresponding veins course with the arteries and ultimately drain into the portal vein (see Fig. 21-4).

GASTRIC MUCOSAL CELLS

The organizational units of the glandular stomach (fundus and body) are the gastric glands that empty their contents into the gastric lumen through pits that stud the mucosal surface. These contents comprise an aqueous mixture of secretions primarily from mucous, parietal, and chief cells.

Mucous cells, which line the gastric surface, and, in larger number, mucous neck cells are the most common cell type in the upper third of the gastric glands (Fig. 21-6). The main secretory product of these cells is the glycoprotein mucin, which helps to protect the gastric epithelium from acid, pepsin, and other endogenous and exogenous injuriants. Parietal (oxyntic) cells, which secrete hydrochloric acid, are found predominantly in the midportion of the gastric glands. These cells are readily identified because of their concentric nuclei, abundant mitochondria, and eosinophilia (Fig. 21-7). Chief cells, which secrete the proenzyme pepsinogen, are found largely at the base of gastric glands. These polar, basophilic cells are filled with zymogen granules at their apical poles. Numerous endocrine cells, such as the histamine-secreting enterochromaffin-like cells and somatostatin-secreting D cells are scattered throughout the lower two thirds of the gastric glands close to their cellular targets.

Stimulation of parietal cells causes translocation of H^+, K^+-adenosine triphosphatase to the membrane of the expanded canaliculi. Activation of this enzyme, the so-called "proton pump," results in secretion of acid into the glandular lumen. Stimulation of chief cells results in movement of zymogen granules to the apical membrane, fusion of granule membranes with the apical membrane, and extrusion of pepsinogen into the glandular lumen. Hydrostatic forces "pump" glandular contents into the gastric lumen, where the acid environment catalyzes the hydrolysis of pepsinogen to the active acid protease pepsin.

EMBRYOLOGY

The primitive foregut gives rise to the stomach and proximal duodenum. The distal duodenum, from the middle of the second part onward, is formed from the cephalic end of the midgut. During the fourth week of development, the stomach consists of a fusiform dilation in the foregut that over subsequent weeks rotates 90° clockwise around its longitudinal axis. The stomach ends with the left side anterior and the right side posterior (Fig. 21-8). The result of this rotation is that the left vagus nerve supplies the anterior wall of the stomach and the right vagus nerve supplies the posterior wall (see Fig. 21-1). The left wall of the stomach grows faster than the right, resulting in formation of the greater (left) and lesser (right) curvatures. Rotation of the developing stomach pulls the dorsal mesentery (mesogastrium) left to form the omental bursa (lesser sac) of the peritoneum (see Fig. 21-8). The ventral mesentery attaches the stomach and duodenum to the liver and antral wall. During gastric development, the duodenum enlarges rapidly to form a loop that projects ventrally, rotates right, and ends as a retroperitoneal organ.

CONGENITAL ABNORMALITIES OF THE STOMACH AND DUODENUM

Congenital abnormalities of the stomach include atresia, mucosal membranes, diverticula, duplication, teratoma, microgastria, and hypertrophic pyloric stenosis. Atresia and mucosal membranes in the antrum or pylorus probably result from failure of recanalization of the lumen, which is temporarily obstructed by the epithelium during normal embryogenesis. Membranes that contain either squamous or columnar epithelium encircle but generally do not occlude the lumen. Plain abdominal radiographs usually do not show mucosal membranes, but barium studies may demonstrate delayed emptying of contrast material and a sharply defined, bandlike defect in the prepyloric antrum that simulates a second duodenal bulb (Fig. 21-9). Gastric duplications, which contain mucosa, submucosa, and muscle, share a common wall and may communicate with the stomach (Fig. 21-10).

Intestinal malrotation, the most common cause of duodenal obstruction, may result in mesenteric bands or compression of the ligament of Treitz on the second or third parts of the duodenum (Fig. 21-11). Developmental abnormalities of adjacent organs, such as annular pancreas, preduodenal portal vein, or superior mesenteric artery syndrome, may obstruct the duodenum (Fig. 21-12).

In the superior mesenteric artery syndrome, this artery compresses the third portion of the duodenum against fixed retroperitoneal structures (see Fig. 21-12). This may result from acute angulation of the superior mesenteric artery with the abdominal aorta associated with rapid childhood growth, weight loss, and immobilization, but the cause is not clear.

Plain abdominal radiography of a patient with duodenal obstruction is unlikely to reveal the cause. Nevertheless, duodenal obstruction is suggested on these radiographs by a "double-bubble" sign (Fig. 21-13). In general, gastrointestinal barium contrast studies are more helpful in defining the abnormality. These radiographs typically show an abrupt cutoff of barium at the obstruction and proximal dilation (see Fig. 21-12). However, instillation of barium into the obstructed stomach or duodenum carries risk for aspiration of contrast medium. The stomach must be completely decompressed before administration of small, incremental amounts of barium, or a less risky modality, such as ultrasonography, should be used first. In superior mesenteric artery syndrome, abdominal aortograms in the lateral view may show narrowing of the angle between the superior mesenteric artery and the aorta.

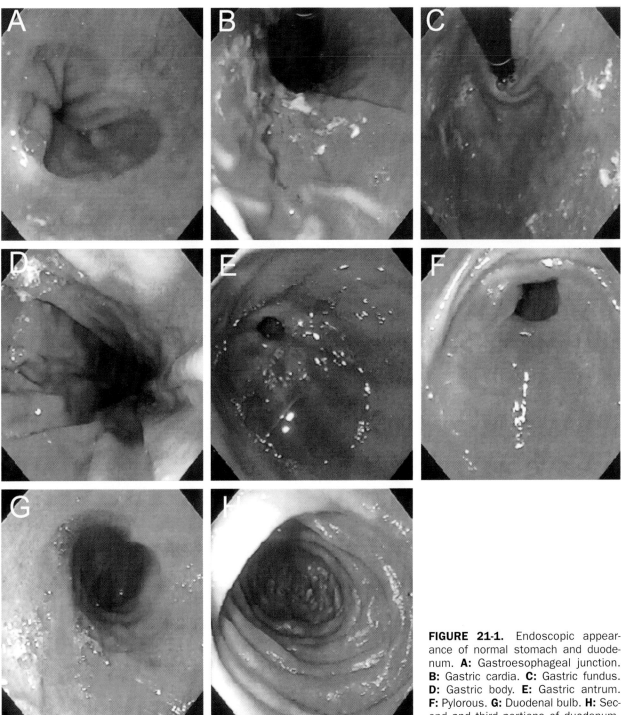

FIGURE 21-1. Endoscopic appearance of normal stomach and duodenum. **A:** Gastroesophageal junction. **B:** Gastric cardia. **C:** Gastric fundus. **D:** Gastric body. **E:** Gastric antrum. **F:** Pylorous. **G:** Duodenal bulb. **H:** Second and third portions of duodenum.

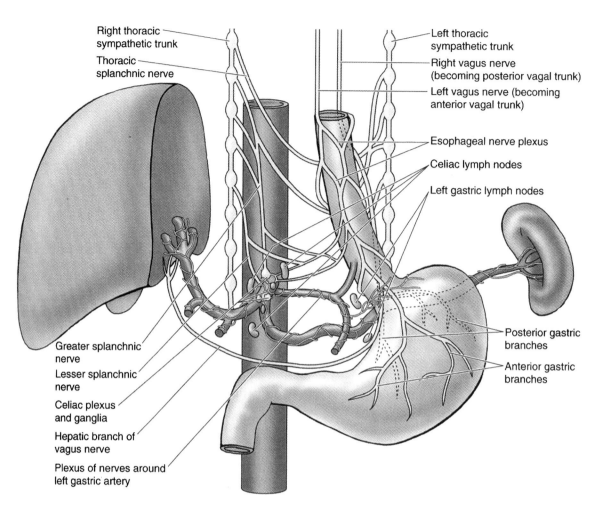

Right thoracic sympathetic trunk
Thoracic splanchnic nerve

Left thoracic sympathetic trunk
Right vagus nerve (becoming posterior vagal trunk)
Left vagus nerve (becoming anterior vagal trunk)
Esophageal nerve plexus
Celiac lymph nodes
Left gastric lymph nodes

Greater splanchnic nerve
Lesser splanchnic nerve
Celiac plexus and ganglia
Hepatic branch of vagus nerve
Plexus of nerves around left gastric artery

Posterior gastric branches
Anterior gastric branches

FIGURE 21-2. Vagal innervation and lymphatics of the stomach.

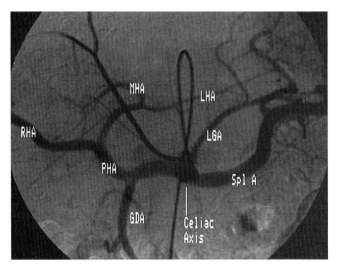

FIGURE 21-3. Celiac artery angiogram shows proper hepatic artery (*PHA*), right hepatic artery (*RHA*), left hepatic artery (*LHA*), left gastric artery (*LGA*), splenic artery (*Spl A*), gastroduodenal artery (*GDA*), and middle hepatic artery (*MHA*). The short gastric arteries are to the right behind the splenic artery. (Courtesy of Dr. David McFarland.)

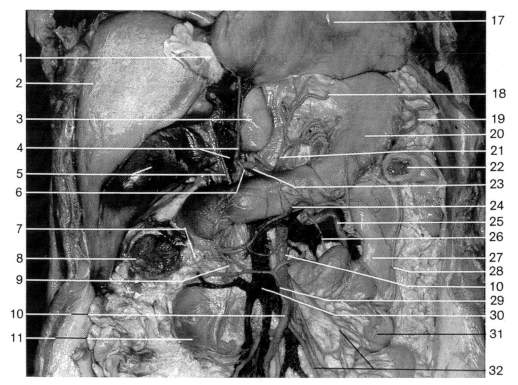

FIGURE 21-4. Vasculature of stomach and duodenum. *Red*, arteries; *blue*, veins; *1*, ligamentum teres; *2*, liver; *3*, caudate lobe of liver; *4*, proper hepatic artery and portal vein; *5*, gallbladder and common bile duct; *6*, right gastric artery; *7*, pancreas; *8*, right colic flexure; *9*, gastroduodenal artery; *10*, superior mesenteric artery; *11*, duodenum; *17*, left lobe of liver; *18*, cardioesophageal branch of left gastric artery; *19*, left gastroepiploic artery; *20*, stomach; *21*, left gastric artery; *22*, left colic flexure; *23*, common hepatic artery; *24*, right gastroepiploic artery; *25*, renal artery; *26*, left testicular artery; *27*, left kidney; *28*, left colic artery; *29*, middle colic artery; *30*, superior mesenteric vein; *31*, jejunum; *32*, jejunal arteries.

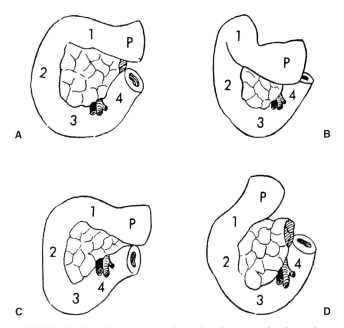

FIGURE 21-5. Normal variations in shape and orientation of the duodenum. *P,* Pylorus; *1–4*, first through fourth portions of the duodenum. Anatomic distinctions between the four parts of the duodenum become less distinct as one progresses from **A** to **D.**

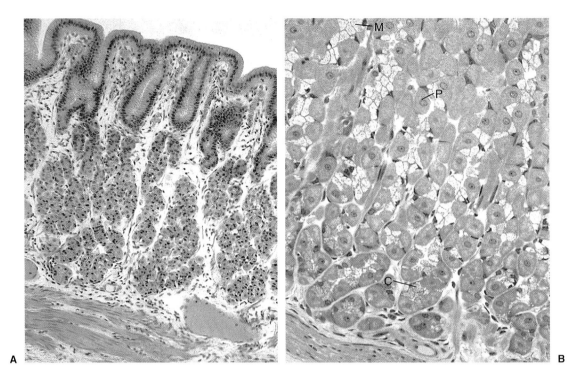

FIGURE 21-6. A: Photomicrograph (original magnification × 132) of the mucosa of the fundic stomach. **B:** Photomicrograph (original magnification × 270) of fundic glands. *M,* Mucous neck cell; *P,* parietal cell; *C,* chief cell.

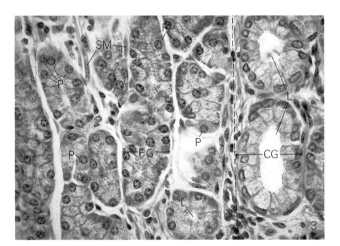

FIGURE 21-7. Comparison of fundic (*FG*) and cardiac (*CG*) gastric glands. Cardiac glands have larger lumens. Parietal cells (*P*) are eosinophilic with concentric nuclei. Unlabeled cells with more basophilic cytoplasm and basal nuclei are chief cells. Smooth muscle cells (*SM*) extend into the lamina propria from the muscularis mucosae. *L,* Gland lumen.

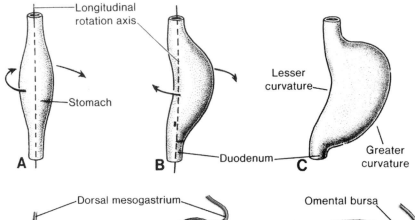

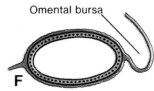

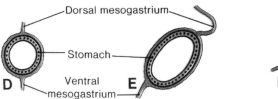

FIGURE 21-8. Development of the stomach and omental bursa (lesser sac). Fusiform dilation of the foregut during the fourth week enlarges and rotates clockwise around its longitudinal axis over subsequent weeks so that the original left side faces anteriorly and right side faces posteriorly.

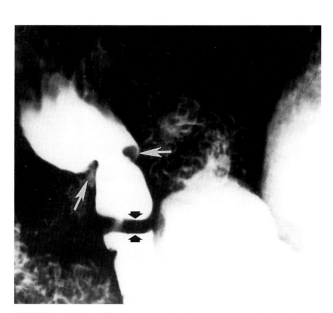

FIGURE 21-9. Barium contrast upper gastrointestinal series shows antral mucosal membrane (*black arrows*). *White arrows* point to the normal pylorus.

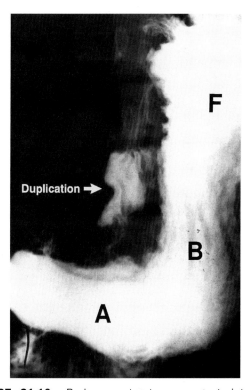

FIGURE 21-10. Barium contrast upper gastrointestinal series shows gastric duplication (*arrow*, rugal folds are present) communicating with the stomach (*F*, fundus; *B*, body; *A*, antrum). (Courtesy of Dr. Timothy Carter.)

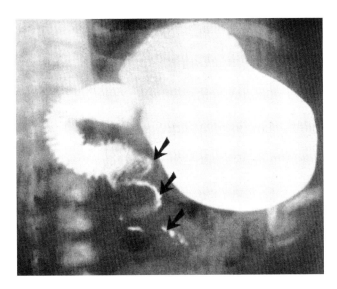

FIGURE 21-11. Barium contrast upper gastrointestinal series demonstrates midgut volvulus in intestinal malrotation. This results in dilation of the duodenal bulb and proximal duodenum, which terminates in a cone-shaped narrowing (*upper arrow*) and a "corkscrew" pattern of the distal duodenum and proximal jejunum (*lower arrows*).

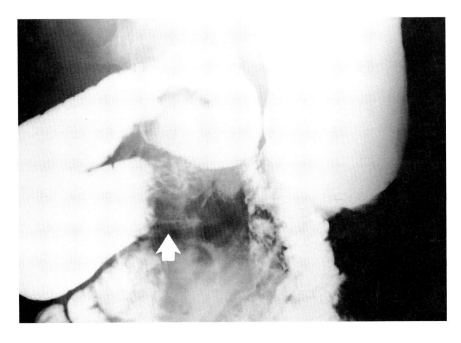

FIGURE 21-12. Barium contrast upper gastrointestinal series shows cutoff (*arrow*) in the third part of the duodenum consistent with obstruction by the superior mesenteric artery.

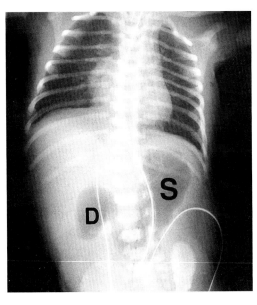

FIGURE 21-13. "Double bubble" sign on plain radiograph of the abdomen of an infant with duodenal atresia. Upper, larger "bubble" (S) represents gas in the stomach. Lower bubble (D) represents gas in the dilated duodenum proximal to the obstruction. (Courtesy of Dr. Timothy Carter.)

DISORDERS OF GASTRIC EMPTYING

HENRY P. PARKMAN ■ ROBERT S. FISHER

GASTRIC MOTILITY

Gastric motility plays a role in accommodating and storing the ingested meal, grinding down or triturating solid particles, and then emptying the meal in a regulated fashion into the duodenum (Fig. 22-1). The motor activity of the stomach is generated by two different anatomic regions of the stomach (the proximal fundus and distal antrum), each with different motility patterns. Gastric emptying is a highly regulated process reflecting coordination between the propulsive forces of proximal fundic tone and distal antral contractions, and relaxation of the pylorus. Potential sites for pathophysiological mechanisms include relaxation (compliance) of the fundus, antral contractility, pyloric tone, and antropyloroduodenal coordination.

Gastric emptying scintigraphy of a solid meal remains the test of choice for evaluating patients to detect delayed gastric emptying. Conventionally, the test has been performed for 2 hours after ingestion of a radiolabeled meal. However, the yield in detecting delayed gastric emptying is higher if the gastric emptying test is extended to 4 hours, with determination of the percent gastric retention at both 2 and 4 hours (Fig. 22-2). Clinical factors in dyspeptic patients that suggest gastroparesis include female gender, postprandial fullness, and vomiting.

Two technical advances in scintigraphic imaging—regional gastric scintigraphy and dynamic antral scintigraphy—provide more information on proximal and distal gastric function during gastric emptying scintigraphy. Regional gastric scintigraphy can assess intragastric meal distribution and movement within the proximal and distal portions of the stomach. Rapid proximal gastric transit caused by impaired fundic accommodation with resultant antral distention occurs in many patients with functional dyspepsia and may be responsible for the symptom of early satiety (Fig. 22-3). Slow proximal gastric emptying with proximal gastric distention may trigger transient lower esophageal sphincter relaxations in patients with gastroesophageal reflux disease. Dynamic antral scintigraphy with frequent 1-second imaging over several minutes can be used to noninvasively evaluate antral wall motion and contractility (Fig. 22-4).

New diagnostic tests to evaluate gastric motor function include the ^{13}C-octanoic acid breath test and electrogastrography. Both of these are now being used in some centers: electrogastrography for clinical evaluation and the breath test usually for pharmaceutical studies. Additional tests that assess gastric motility, but are still solely research techniques, include magnetic resonance imaging (MRI), ultrasonography, and single photon emission computed tomography.

227

Electrogastrography is the cutaneous recording of myoelectric activity of the gastric smooth muscle by means of superficial abdominal wall electrodes overlying the stomach. The recorded signal is called an electrogastrogram (EGG) and usually consists of a 3 cycles per minute (cpm) signal reflecting gastric slow-wave (pacemaker) activity and the subsequent gastric contractions (Figs. 22-5, 22-6, and 22-7). Abnormalities in the EGG signal have been demonstrated in patients with gastroparesis and functional dyspepsia. A significant percentage of these patients may have very rapid, slow-wave frequencies (tachygastria) or very slow, slow-wave frequencies (bradygastria) (Fig. 22-8). Thus, the EGG may provide clues that the stomach dysfunction is involved in a variety of upper gastrointestinal symptoms. Electrogastrography equipment has recently been approved by the U.S. Food and Drug Administration for patient evaluation and CPT (current procedural technology) codes have been generated.

Recently, multichannel EGG recording has been suggested as a way to assess gastric electrical slow-wave propagation velocity and to detect electromechanical uncoupling (Fig. 22-9). In this technique, the EGG is recorded using electrodes placed at different positions overlying the stomach. Multichannel electrogastrography may enhance the diagnostic utility of the test compared to traditional one-channel recording in detecting abnormalities such as ectopic gastric pacemaker and abnormal coupling of the electrical slow waves. In an initial study, patients with functional dyspepsia were found to have inconsistencies in the frequency and regularity of the gastric slow wave as well as impaired slow-wave propagation and coupling (Fig. 22-10).

Breath tests employing stable nonradioactive isotopes offer an attractive alternative to scintigraphic techniques for the measurement of gastric emptying. The ^{13}C-octanoate breath test (OBT) has been developed to measure solid-phase gastric emptying. Octanoic acid is a naturally occurring eight-carbon fatty acid typically found in butter as an ester. This and other medium-chain fatty acids (MCFAs) are efficiently absorbed by the small intestine and rapidly transported to the liver bound to serum albumin. In the liver, MCFAs are efficiently oxidized to CO_2, which is then excreted in the lungs (Fig. 22-11A). Gastric emptying is the rate-limiting step for the pulmonary excretion of $^{13}CO_2$ derived from ^{13}C-octanoic acid. Thus, measurement of $^{13}CO_2$ in breath samples is an indirect measurement of gastric emptying. With the OBT test, a test meal is labeled with ^{13}C-octanoate and administered after an overnight fast. Breath samples are collected at 15-minute intervals over several hours using a breath collection device. Mathematical analysis of the $^{13}CO_2$ appearance in breath can be used to estimate gastric emptying parameters $T_{1/2}$, which is the time required for 50% of the test meal to be emptied from the stomach. The OBT result has been shown to correlate with scintigraphically determined gastric emptying (Fig. 22-11B).

GASTROPARESIS

The pathogenesis of gastroparesis is multifactorial. In a study of 146 patients with gastroparesis, Soykan and colleagues (1998) reported the etiology of gastroparesis was idiopathic in 36%, diabetes mellitus in 29%, and postgastric surgery in 14% (Fig. 22-12). Of interest, idiopathic gastroparesis was suspected of being associated with a previous viral infection in 23% of cases.

Gastroparesis is a well-recognized complication of diabetes mellitus. Diabetic gastroparesis is clinically important because it causes gastrointestinal symptoms, alterations in glycemic control, and changes in oral drug absorption. It is most commonly associated with long-standing, insulin-dependent diabetes mellitus (IDDM) with the complications of retinopathy, nephropathy, and peripheral neuropathy. Recent longitudinal studies, however, suggest that delayed gastric emptying of solid or nutrient liquid meals is common, not only in 30% to 50% of patients with long-standing type 1 diabetes, but in patients with type 2 diabetes as well. In addition, it is not always associated with other complications of diabetes.

Rapid gastric emptying has been described in type 2 diabetes mellitus (Fig. 22-13). Usually this occurs early in the disease. This may be related to a lack of a fundic receptive relaxation response, normally mediated by the vagus nerve.

Hyperglycemia, itself, may reversibly affect gastric motility by decreasing antral contractility, reducing antral phase III migrating motor complex activity, increasing pyloric contractions, stimulating gastric dysrhythmias (primarily tachygastria), and thus delaying gastric emptying (Figs. 22-14 and 22-15). Normalization of serum glucose in hyperglycemic patients has been shown to improve gastric myoelectric activity, accelerate gastric emptying, and restore antral phase III activity in some patients. In addition, hyperglycemia reduces the effect of prokinetic agents (Fig. 22-16). The mechanism by which hyperglycemia adversely affects gastric motility has not been elucidated. Hyperglycemia in healthy subjects appears to cause a reversible impairment of vagal efferent function as evidenced by reduced pancreatic polypeptide secretion, which is under vagal cholinergic control. Glucose-responsive neurons have been identified in the central nervous system that may modify vagal efferent activity. Prostaglandins may also be involved; indomethacin can reverse abnormal gastric electrical rhythms that occur during hyperglycemia (see Fig. 22-14).

In addition to abnormalities in gastric emptying, subjects with IDDM have an increased perception of gastric distention produced with a gastric barostat, perhaps resulting in exaggerated nausea, bloating, and upper abdominal pain (Fig. 22-17). Increased sensitivity of the proximal stomach may be responsible for dyspeptic symptoms in the postprandial period in which the proximal stomach is distended by a meal. This phenomenon has been shown during euglycemia, is heightened during hyperglycemia, and has been shown in normal subjects as well as patients with IDDM. Thus, in some patients with diabetic gastroparesis, there is visceral hypersensitivity similar to that described in functional dyspepsia. There is also an overlap between idiopathic gastroparesis and functional dyspepsia, in that delayed gastric emptying has been described in approximately 35% of patients with functional dyspepsia (Fig. 22-18). In these cases, one might be able to treat the gastroparesis with prokinetic agents and/or the dyspeptic symptoms with sensory modulating agents.

Changes of gastric motility may also significantly affect postprandial blood glucose concentrations. In some diabetic patients, delayed gastric emptying may contribute to poor glucose control because of unpredictable delivery of food into the duodenum. Impaired gastric emptying with continued administration of exogenous insulin may also produce hypoglycemia. Conversely, acceleration of emptying has been reported to cause hyperglycemia. Problems with blood sugar control may be the first indication that a diabetic patient is developing a gastric motility disorder. Interestingly, in some of these patients, gastroparetic symptoms may be mild or absent.

Prokinetic agents enhance the motility of the upper gastrointestinal tract and accelerate the aboral movement of the intralumenal contents. In general, prokinetic agents increase gastric antral contractility, correct gastric dysrhythmias, and improve antroduodenal coordination (Fig. 22-19). Current prokinetic agents for treatment include oral agents metoclopramide and erythromycin. Cisapride (Propulsid) was taken off the market in 2000 because of cardiac side effects. Domperidone is not available in the United States, although it is available in Canada, Mexico, and Europe. Intravenous agents currently used to treat hospitalized patients include metoclopramide and erythromycin. New pharmacological agents are being tested for gastroparesis, including 5-HT$_4$ receptor agonists, dopamine receptor antagonists, and motilin receptor agonists.

Gastric electrical stimulation with an implanted neurostimulator is an emerging therapy for treatment of refractory gastroparesis. It has been intensely investigated over the last two decades. Only in the last 5 years, however, have promising results been reported. There are several ways to electrically stimulate the stomach. First is gastric electrical pacing. Here, the goal is to entrain and pace the gastric slow waves at a higher rate than the patient's normal 3.0 cpm. Pacing at 10% higher than the basal rate has been shown to accelerate gastric emptying and improve dyspeptic symptoms (Fig. 22-20). Second is neuromodulation using high-frequency stimulation at four times the basal rate (12 cpm). With these stimulation parameters, there may be improvement in symptoms with little change in gastric emptying. It has been suggested that this type of stimulation activates sensory afferent nerves to suppress symptoms. Finally, early studies in animals have used sequential circumferential direct muscle stimulation employing bursts of very high frequency stimulation to sequentially induce direct muscle stimulation in a peristaltic fashion and accelerate gastric emptying.

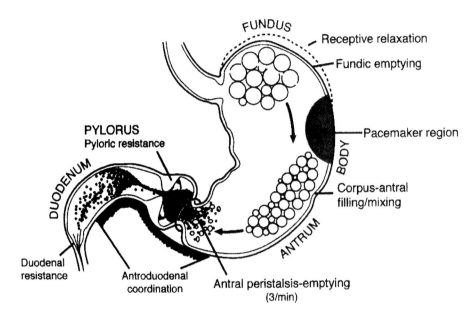

FIGURE 22-1. Postprandial gastric motility. Normal events involved in gastric emptying include fundic receptive relaxation to accommodate the ingested food, and gastric peristaltic contractions in the corpus and antrum for mixing and emptying the chyme into the duodenum. Gastric peristalsis occurs at approximately 3 cpm. Antroduodenal coordination is important for efficient emptying.

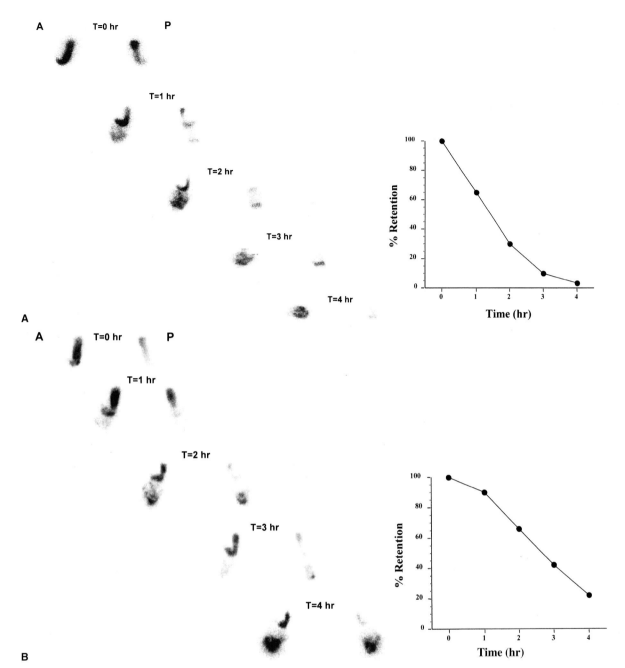

FIGURE 22-2. Gastric emptying scintigraphy. **A:** Normal gastric emptying of solids using an egg sandwich meal with water. Anterior (A) and posterior (P) images at each time point are shown on the **left**. Time activity curves for each patient are shown on the **right**. There is 30% percent gastric retention at 2 hours after meal ingestion (normal <50%), 10% at 3 hours (normal <25%), and 3% at 4 hours (normal <10%). **B:** A patient with abnormal gastric emptying. Abnormal retention is present at 2 hours (66% retention), 3 hours (42%), and 4 hours (22%) postprandially. The next two figures illustrate the value of extending gastric emptying from 2 to 4 hours. *(Continued)*

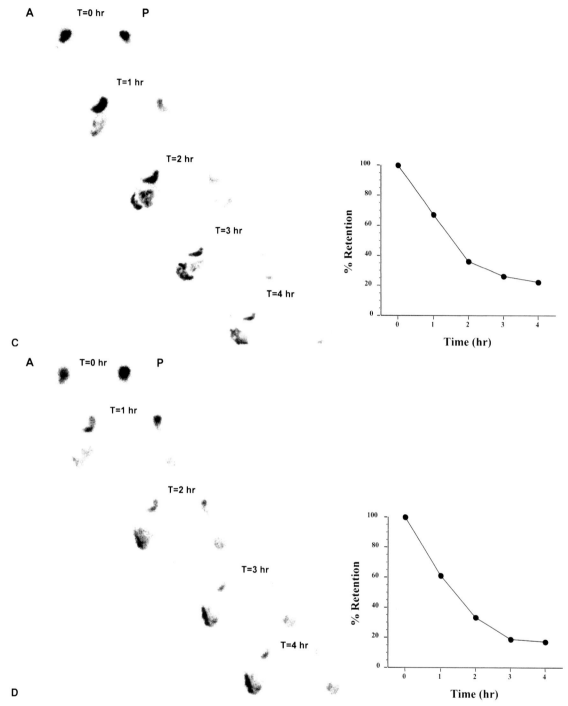

FIGURE 22-2. **(Continued) C:** Normal retention at 2 hours (36% retention), but abnormal at 3 hours (26%) and 4 hours (22%). **D:** Normal retention at 2 hours (33%) and 3 hours (19%), but abnormal at 4 hours (18%). *(Continued)*

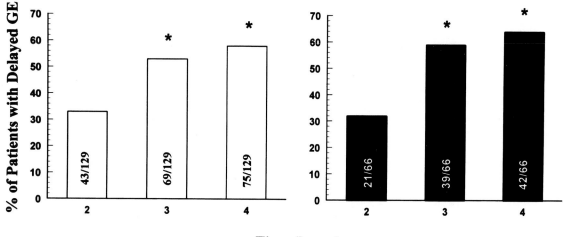

Time (hours)

E

FIGURE 22-2. **E:** The incremental value of extending the gastric emptying scintigraphy from 2 to 3 and 4 hours in patients undergoing gastric emptying scintigraphy for clinical evaluation. The percentage of patients with a delayed gastric emptying test at 2 hours was 33%. This value increased to 53% if the examination was extended to 3 hours, and 58% if the test was extended to 4 hours. On the **right** are the values for patients with functional dyspepsia. The percentage of functional dyspeptic patients with delayed gastric emptying with the conventional 2-hour test was 32%. Extending gastric emptying scintigraphy to 4 hours increased the percentage of dyspeptic patients with delayed gastric emptying to 64%. These data indicate that the proportion of patients with functional dyspepsia who have gastroparesis may be underestimated when only a 2-hour gastric emptying test is used.

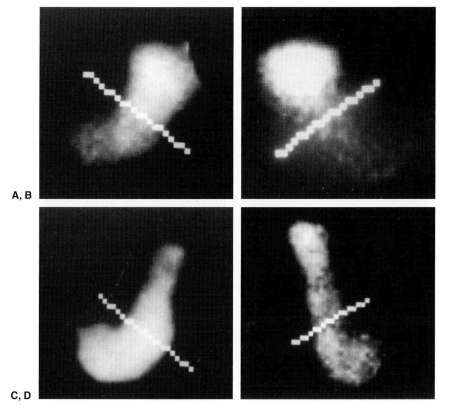

FIGURE 22-3. Regional gastric emptying abnormalities in functional dyspepsia. Images **A** and **B** are anterior and posterior views taken immediately after food ingestion from a normal subject, whereas images **C** and **D** are anterior and posterior views from a dyspeptic patient. In controls, food remained predominantly in the proximal half of the stomach after ingestion and then redistributed to the distal half over time. In the dyspeptic patients, initial activity in the proximal half was lower and distributed quickly to the distal portion of the stomach.

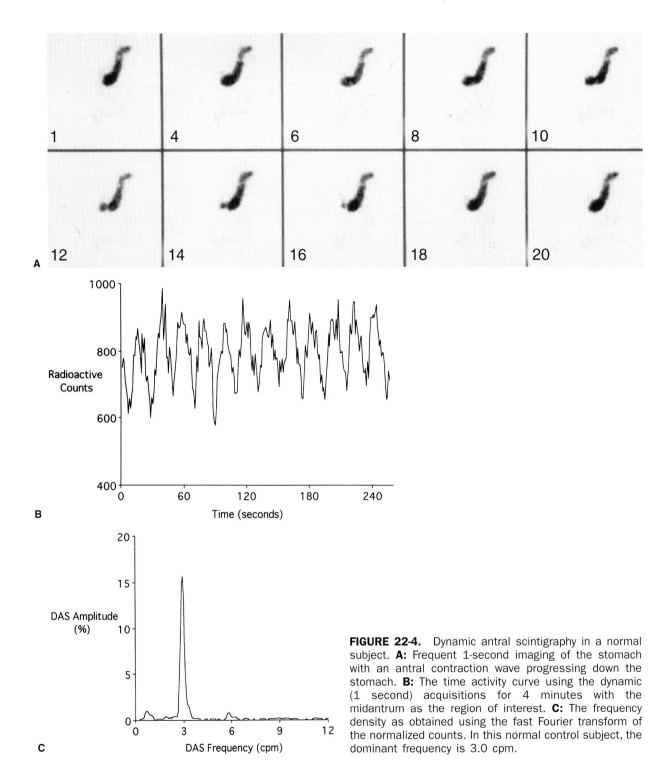

FIGURE 22-4. Dynamic antral scintigraphy in a normal subject. **A:** Frequent 1-second imaging of the stomach with an antral contraction wave progressing down the stomach. **B:** The time activity curve using the dynamic (1 second) acquisitions for 4 minutes with the midantrum as the region of interest. **C:** The frequency density as obtained using the fast Fourier transform of the normalized counts. In this normal control subject, the dominant frequency is 3.0 cpm.

FIGURE 22-5. Electrogastrogram (EGG) tracing and analysis. **A:** EGG tracing from a normal subject. The top tracing is a portion of the EGG from the fasting and postprandial state from a normal subject. During both periods, there is a 3 cpm signal. There is an increase in amplitude of the EGG signal in the postprandial period. **B:** Running spectral analysis of the EGG recording of a normal individual. The power (or relative strength) of the dominant frequencies for 4-minute time segments is shown for both the preprandial state (**left** portion of the figure) and in the postprandial state (**right** portion of the figure). In this normal volunteer, the dominant frequencies for nearly all of the time intervals in both the preprandial and postprandial states were in the normal range of 2 to 4 cpm. **C:** Power-frequency spectrum of the 1-hour fasting period (**left** portion of the figure) and 1-hour postprandial period (**right** portion of the figure). The overall dominant frequency is the frequency with the highest power. In the postprandial period, the dominant frequency is ~3 cpm; smaller peaks at the harmonics of this normal 3-cpm signal are also seen at 6 and 9 cpm.

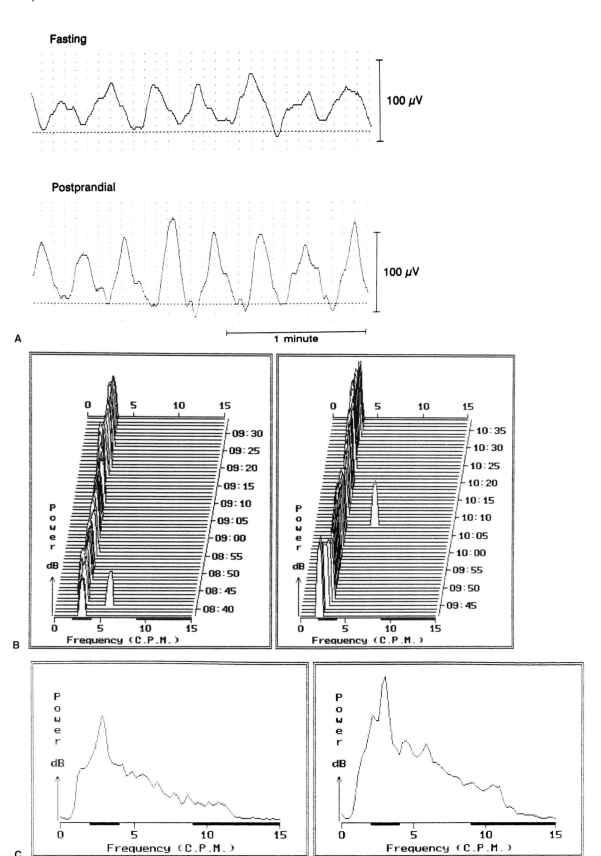

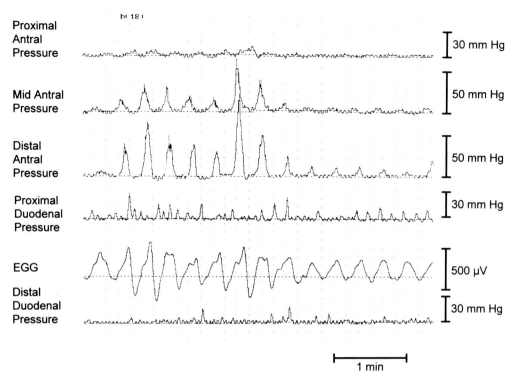

FIGURE 22-6. Electrogastrogram (EGG) and antral contractility. Simultaneous antroduodenal manometry and EGG recording. Manometric pressures from the proximal, mid-, and distal antrum, and the proximal and distal duodenum are shown. In addition, the EGG signal is recorded simultaneously. This tracing, taken during the postprandial pattern, shows prominent 3-cpm antral contractile activity and 3-cpm EGG activity. The EGG amplitude correlates with the amplitude of the antral contractions.

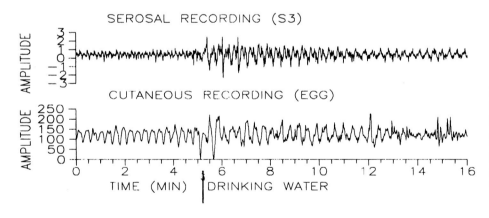

FIGURE 22-7. Simultaneous serosal and cutaneous electrogastrogram (EGG) recordings in patients with gastroparesis. There is an increase in the amplitude of both the cutaneous and serosal recordings after the patient drinks water.

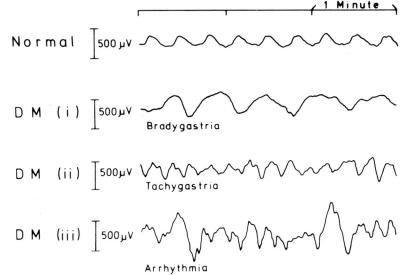

FIGURE 22-8. Gastric dysrhythmias recorded from electrogastrograms (EGGs) from diabetic patients. The top tracing shows a normal 3 cpm EGG recording from a normal subject. The next tracings show examples of bradygastria, tachygastria, and an arrhythmia (tachy-bradygastria).

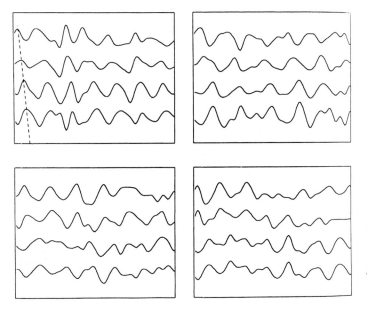

FIGURE 22-9. Multichannel electrogastrogram (EGG) recordings in normal subjects. Two-minute portions of EGG recordings obtained from four different normal subjects are shown. In each subject, propagation of the gastric slow wave from the proximal channel (**top tracing**) to the distal channel (**bottom tracing**) can be seen.

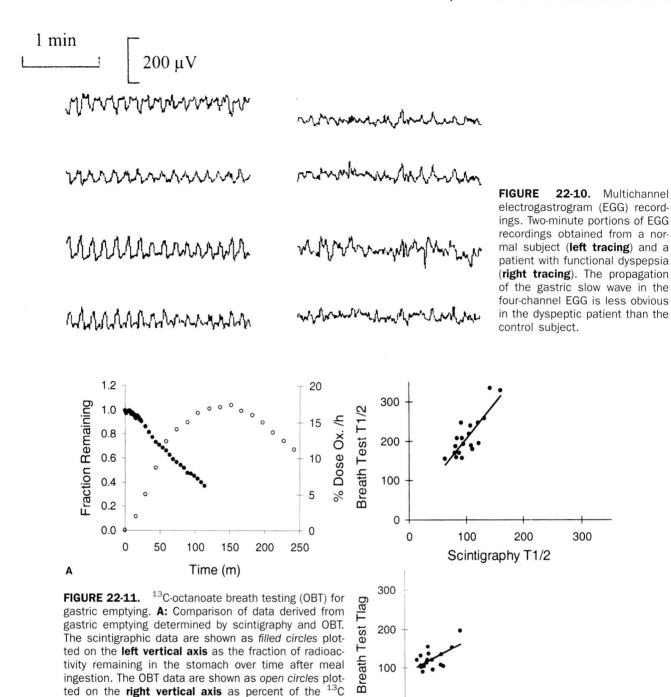

FIGURE 22-10. Multichannel electrogastrogram (EGG) recordings. Two-minute portions of EGG recordings obtained from a normal subject (**left tracing**) and a patient with functional dyspepsia (**right tracing**). The propagation of the gastric slow wave in the four-channel EGG is less obvious in the dyspeptic patient than the control subject.

FIGURE 22-11. ^{13}C-octanoate breath testing (OBT) for gastric emptying. **A:** Comparison of data derived from gastric emptying determined by scintigraphy and OBT. The scintigraphic data are shown as *filled circles* plotted on the **left vertical axis** as the fraction of radioactivity remaining in the stomach over time after meal ingestion. The OBT data are shown as *open circles* plotted on the **right vertical axis** as percent of the ^{13}C dose oxidized (Ox) per hour. **B:** Correlation of simultaneously performed OBT and scintigraphy for gastric emptying using a muffin meal labeled with technetium-99m and ^{13}C-octanoate. The **top panel** shows the half emptying times. There is a good correlation ($r = 0.83$) between the two tests. The values for $T_{1/2}$ for OBT are greater than the $T_{1/2}$ for scintigraphy; this represents postgastric emptying processing of the ^{13}C, which includes small intestinal absorption, liver metabolism, and pulmonary excretion. The **bottom panel** shows the correlation of the lag times in minutes ($r = 0.63$).

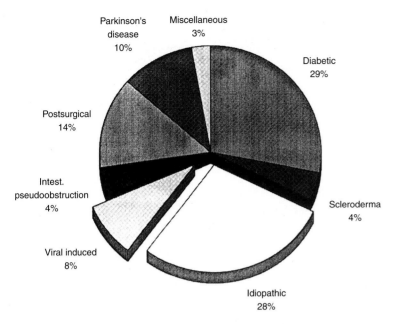

FIGURE 22-12. Etiology of gastroparesis. The causes of gastroparesis among 143 patients seen at a tertiary motility center are shown. Diabetic gastroparesis was present in 29% of the patients and postsurgical causes in 14%. In this series, postviral gastroparesis was believed to be present in 12 (8%) of the total 143 patients. The viral gastroparesis group is usually included in the idiopathic group; this would increase the idiopathic category to a total of 36%.

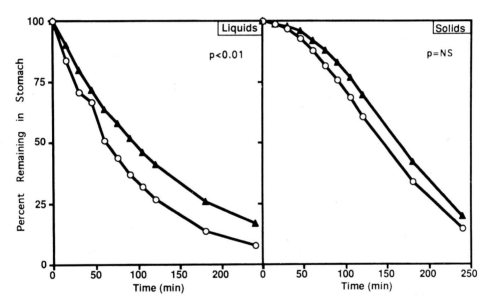

FIGURE 22-13. Rapid gastric emptying in non–insulin-dependent diabetes mellitus (NIDDM). Computer-generated plots of gastric emptying curves for liquids and solids in NIDDM (*open circles*) and healthy controls (*filled triangles*). Emptying of liquids is significantly faster in patients with NIDDM than in healthy volunteers. The difference between emptying of solids was not statistically significant.

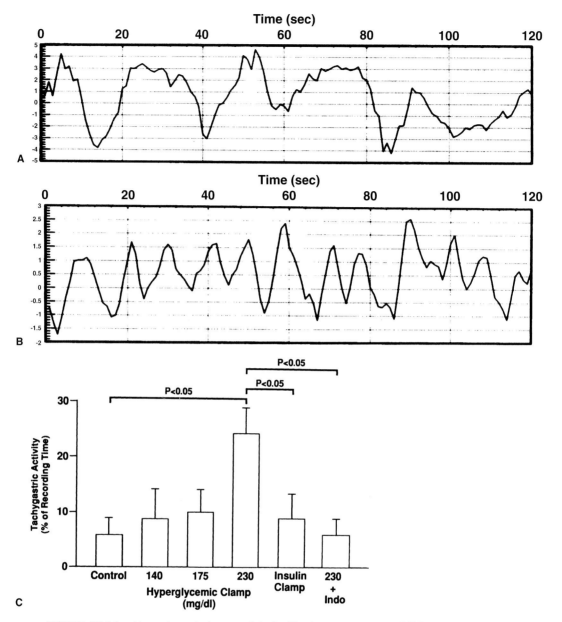

FIGURE 22-14. Hyperglycemia is associated with electrogastrogram (EGG) dysrhythmias in normal subjects. **A:** A sample EGG result from a healthy volunteer under control conditions. The raw slow-wave signal shows a rhythmic, high-amplitude oscillation at 3 cpm. **B:** A sample EGG from a healthy volunteer during hyperglycemia with glucose clamping at 230 mg/dL. The raw slow-wave signal is rapid at approximately 6 cpm, irregular, and of low amplitude. **C:** The tachygastric activity as a percent of recording time in the postprandial period. Hyperglycemic clamping leads to a significant increase in tachygastria at plasma glucose levels of 230 mg/dL. In contrast, euglycemic, hyperinsulinemic clamping to insulin levels that reproduce those observed at the highest plasma glucose levels do not disrupt slow-wave frequency. In this study, pretreatment with indomethacin prevents induction of tachygastria by hyperglycemic clamping to 230 mg/dL. This suggests that induction of dysrhythmias is dependent on endogenous prostaglandin synthesis.

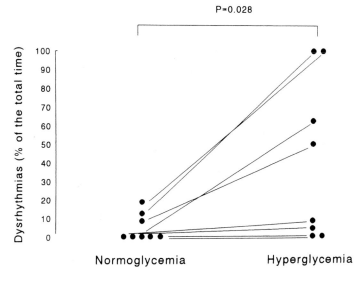

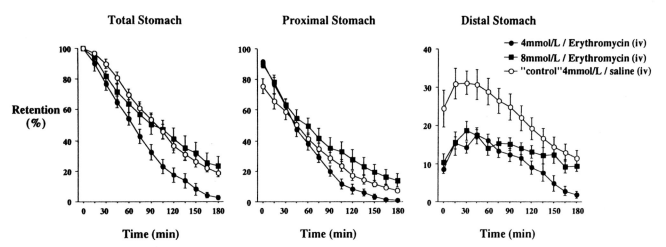

FIGURE 22-15. Hyperglycemia causes electrogastrogram (EGG) dysrhythmias in patients with diabetes mellitus. The duration of dysrhythmias (primarily tachygastrias), expressed as the percentage of the total duration of the study, was significantly longer during hyperglycemia than during normoglycemia (41% and 7% of the total duration, respectively).

FIGURE 22-16. Hyperglycemia prevents the prokinetic effects of erythromycin. Total, proximal, and distal stomach retention values over time are shown for saline infusion and erythromycin infusion with the blood glucose levels maintained at 4 mmol/L (72 mg/dL). Erythromycin caused an acceleration of gastric emptying from the whole stomach and both the proximal and distal portions. In contrast, when the glucose was maintained at higher levels (8 mmol/L; 144 mg/dL), the prokinetic effect of erythromycin was not present. This suggests that the effect of erythromycin on gastric emptying is modified by elevations in the blood glucose concentration. Even plasma glucose concentrations within the normal postprandial physiological range can affect gastric motility.

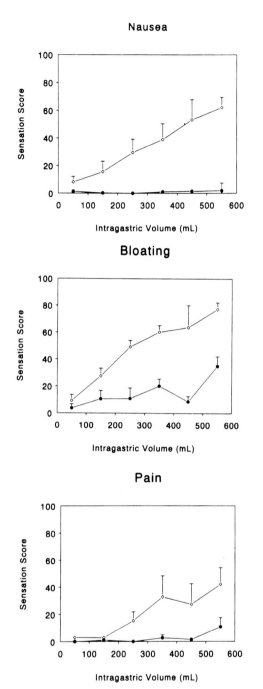

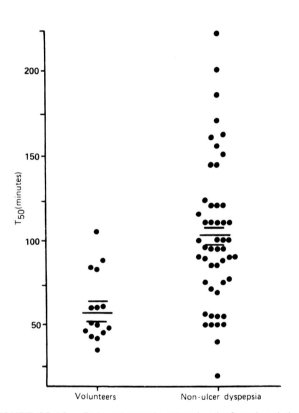

FIGURE 22-17. Visceral hypersensitivity in diabetes mellitus. Sensation scores for nausea, bloating, and upper abdominal pain during distention of the proximal stomach in diabetic patients (*open diamonds*) and healthy volunteers (*solid dots*). There are significantly higher sensation scores for nausea, bloating, and abdominal pain in the diabetic patients than in the healthy volunteers.

FIGURE 22-18. Delayed gastric emptying in functional dyspepsia. The half emptying times (T_{50}) of solid meal gastric emptying were generally greater for patients with nonulcer dyspepsia (mean value of 102 minutes) than in normal volunteers (mean value of 64 minutes). Delayed gastric emptying was identified in 21 of 50 patients (42%).

Month   Electrogastrograms (EGG)

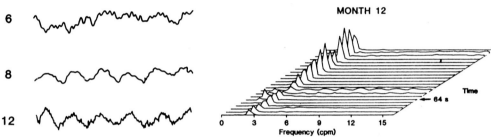
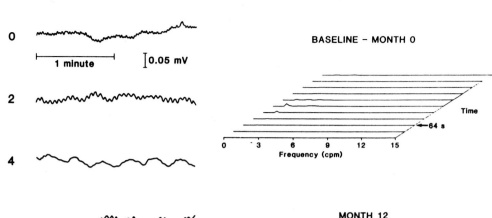

FIGURE 22-19. Improvement in gastric myoelectric activity with prokinetic therapy. Serial electrogastrograms (EGGs) are shown on the **left** in a symptomatic patient with type I diabetes mellitus and gastroparesis. Bradygastria is seen at month 0 prior to treatment. During treatment with the prokinetic agent, domperidone, the bradygastria disappeared and the EGG normalized to 3 cpm activity. The patient's symptoms of nausea and vomiting also disappeared. On the **right**, the running spectral analysis of the EGG signal recorded at month 0 and month 12 illustrates the change from no clear frequencies in the EGG signal at month 0 to clear peaks at 3 cpm at month 12.

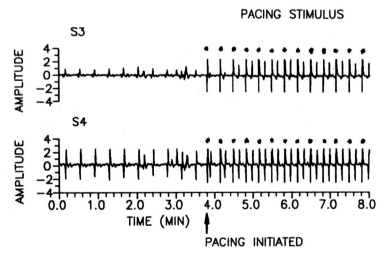

FIGURE 22-20. Gastric electrical pacing. Gastric slow waves before and during gastric pacing at two gastric recording leads (S3, S4) are shown. The *dots* indicate pacing stimulus. Entrainment can be appreciated as the slow waves are phase-locked at an increased frequency with the pacing stimulus about 2 minutes after the initiation of pacing.

23

ACID PEPTIC DISORDERS

JOHN DEL VALLE ■ **JAMES M. SCHEIMAN**

Acid peptic disorders of the gastrointestinal tract comprise a common group of pathological states that affect millions of persons in the United States each year. This group of disorders includes gastritis, gastric ulcers, and duodenal ulcers. A break in the mucosal integrity of the stomach or duodenum is the common thread unifying these entities. The past several decades have served witness to a geometric expansion in our knowledge regarding the pathogenesis and treatment of this heterogeneous group of disorders. Extensive investigative efforts have provided substantial insight into the pathways leading to the altered mucosal integrity typical of peptic ulcer disease. This chapter is a pictorial representation of several key issues regarding the pathogenesis and diagnosis of peptic ulcer disease.

An important step toward elucidating the pathogenesis of peptic ulcer disease has been understanding the physiological mechanisms responsible for protecting or maintaining mucosal integrity of the stomach and duodenum (Fig. 23-1). These protective factors are numerous, and include the mucous gel layer, which through its physicochemical properties provides the first level of protection against injury. Additional important components of the mucosal protective barrier include membrane hydrophobicity of the epithelial cells, bicarbonate secretion, and mucosal blood flow. Each of these constituents of the mucosal barrier is regulated to varying degrees by important chemical mediators of mucosal protection, such as prostaglandins, gastrointestinal hormones, and growth factors. Multiple aggressive factors can disrupt the delicate balance provided by these protective factors and result in the formation of mucosal lesions that can vary from superficial damage (subepithelial hemorrhage and erosion), to frank ulceration.

It is clear that gastric acid plays a critical role in disrupting mucosal integrity; therefore the old dictum by Schwartz, "No acid no ulcer," still holds true to a considerable degree. Exogenous factors are also critically important in the pathogenesis of peptic ulcer disease. The bacterium *Helicobacter pylori* and nonsteroidal antiinflammatory drugs (NSAIDs) are the two most important agents responsible for the disruption of mucosal integrity that leads to peptic ulcer disease. Poor mucosal perfusion or ischemia can also play a role in the development of peptic ulcer in select cases.

The discovery by Marshall and Warren that *H pylori* is of central importance in the pathogenesis of acid peptic disorders has revolutionized the diagnostic and therapeutic approaches to this disease process. The organism is associated with several pathological processes including chronic gastritis, peptic ulcer disease, and gastric malignancy. The outcome of infection with this organism is dictated by multiple

244

bacterial and host factors (Fig. 23-2). How this array of factors interacts toward a final pathological state is unclear. Although *H pylori* organisms reside in the mucous layer of the gastric antrum, ulcerations most often occur in the duodenal mucosa. The mechanism by which this organism results in the downstream untoward effects on duodenal mucosal integrity is unclear. Figure 23-3 is a partial summary of the potential pathophysiological mechanisms hypothesized to participate in *H pylori*–mediated duodenal ulceration. A local mucosal inflammatory response to the bacteria, with concomitant release of lipopolysaccharides, cytotoxic factors from the bacteria, and proinflammatory cells are important in the local disruption of mucosal integrity that leads to chronic active gastritis. These same factors may also alter expression of hormonal mediators that are important in regulating gastric acid secretion. Some investigators have observed that patients infected with *H pylori* have increased basal acid secretion, which has been thought to be secondary to diminished antral somatostatin expression and a relative increase in gastrin levels. The exact role of these alterations in the pathogenesis of duodenal ulceration is speculative at this time.

Figures 23-4 and 23-5 are representative microscopic views of normal fundic and antral gland histology respectively. As Fig. 23-4 shows, the fundic (body) portion of the gastric mucosa consists of shallow pits. Glands that contain chief cells (basophilic staining) are found primarily near the base of the gland, and parietal cells (pale staining) are located primarily in the midgland region. The antral mucosa (Fig. 23-5) on the other hand, contains deep pits without chief or parietal cells. The predominant cell type in this region is the mucin-producing mucous cell.

H pylori organisms often escape detection on routine histological staining of antral biopsies. In an effort to increase the sensitivity of detecting this organism in tissue sections, special stains such as the one illustrated in Fig. 23-6 are used. The method of silver staining markedly enhances the visualization of these rod shaped organisms. A closer look at *H pylori* (Fig. 23-7) clearly illustrates its rod-like morphology and the presence of flagella.

Documentation or demonstration of gastric or duodenal ulcer requires a structural study of the gastrointestinal tract. Traditional radiographic studies, such as a barium meal examination, are useful for detecting gastric and duodenal lesions (Fig. 23-8). Barium pooling in a distinct crater, surrounded by a radiolucent halo corresponding to mucosal edema is a typical finding suggestive of a benign ulcer. Barium studies are particularly useful for detecting infiltrative disorders, strictures, or masses of the gastroduodenal area. Figures 23-9 and 23-10 demonstrate examples of a gastric carcinoma and a benign duodenal stricture, respectively.

Endoscopic examination of the stomach and duodenum provides a sensitivity and specificity of greater than 95% for detecting gastric and duodenal lesions. It also allows tissue diagnosis of suspicious lesions and documentation of the presence of *H pylori* organisms. Figures 23-11 and 23-12 demonstrate examples of benign gastric ulcers. Endoscopy also provides a greater sensitivity than barium meal examinations for detecting small superficial erosions. Figure 23-13 illustrates an endoscopic view of NSAID-induced erosion and erythema.

Great strides have been made toward understanding NSAID-induced gastrointestinal mucosal damage. One advance in the field has been elucidating the pathways by which prostaglandins are synthesized and processed (Figs. 23-14 and 23-15). Two types of cyclooxygenase (COX) enzymes (types 1 and 2) are essential in the conversion of arachidonic acid into prostaglandins. Prostaglandins derived from COX-1 are primarily involved in housekeeping functions such as maintenance of gastrointestinal tract mucosal integrity, whereas prostaglandins derived from COX-2 play a key role in mediating inflammation and regulating cell proliferation. Recent studies have demonstrated differential expression of these two enzymes (Fig. 23-15). As shown in Fig. 23-15, COX-1 is found primarily in platelets, endothelium, stomach, and kidney, whereas COX-2 is found in macrophages, leukocytes, fibroblast, and endothelial cells.

On the basis of these important discoveries regarding prostaglandin synthesis, extensive effort has been directed at the development of selective NSAIDs. NSAIDs that block COX-2 while leaving COX-1 unaltered would give the benefit of an anti-inflammatory agent while sparing toxicity to sites such as the gastrointestinal tract and the kidney. Recent studies have demonstrated that the selective COX-2 inhibitors lead to a substantially lower incidence of gastric and duodenal ulceration than nonselective NSAIDs such as naproxen and ibuprofen (Fig. 23-16).

NSAIDs can induce gastrointestinal mucosal damage through direct toxicity. Figure 23-17 summarizes the mechanism for NSAID-induced mucosal damage by ionic trapping. A summary of the different pathways by which NSAIDs induce gastric and duodenal mucosal damage is outlined in Fig. 23-18.

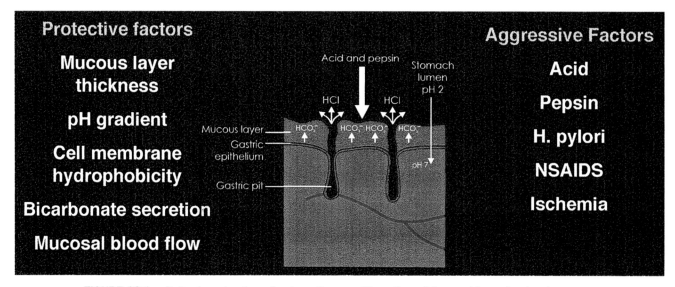

FIGURE 23-1. Pathogenesis of peptic ulcer disease. Ulceration of the gastric or duodenal mucosa results from disruption of a fine balance between a series of protective and aggressive factors. The former includes the mucous layer, pH gradient, cell membrane hydrophobicity, bicarbonate secretion, and mucosal blood flow. Aggressive factors can be either endogenous, such as gastric acid or pepsin, or exogenous such as *H pylori* and nonsteroidal antiinflammatory drugs.

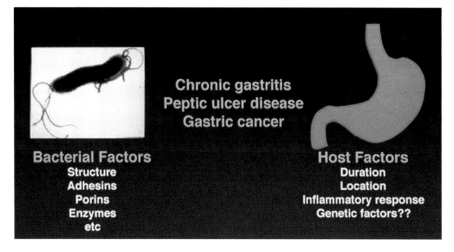

FIGURE 23-2. *H pylori*–induced pathology is determined by the interaction of multiple bacterial and host factors.

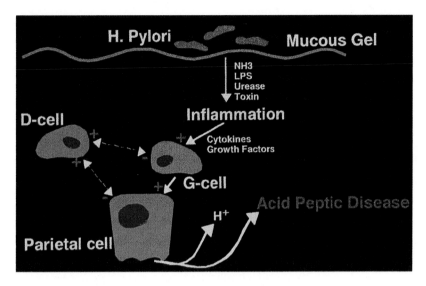

FIGURE 23-3. Potential pathogenetic mechanisms for *H pylori*–induced peptic ulcer disease. Pathways by which this organism can alter the factors important in regulating gastric acid secretion are illustrated.

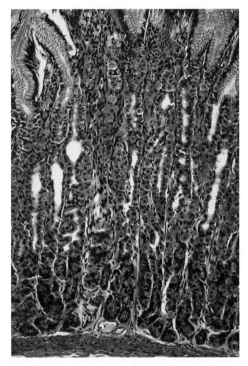

FIGURE 23-4. Normal fundic (body) gland histology.

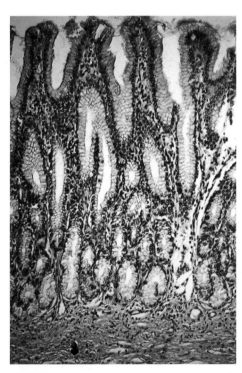

FIGURE 23-5. Normal pyloric (antral) gland histology.

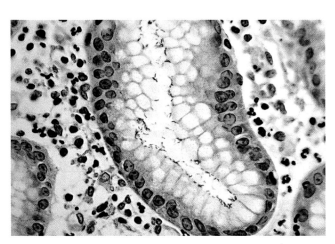

FIGURE 23-6. Silver stain of antral biopsy demonstrating *H pylori* organisms. Initial efforts to visualize *H pylori* organisms were enhanced by the addition of special staining procedures, such as the one shown here. This often difficult to observe bacteria is clearly visualized as a rod-shaped organism in the mucous layer of the stomach. (Courtesy of H. Appelman, M.D., Department of Pathology, University of Michigan Medical School.)

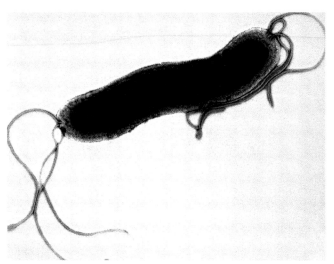

FIGURE 23-7. *H pylori*, high-power view. This detailed micrograph illustrates the rod-shaped flagellated organism established as a chief aggressive factor in the pathogenesis of peptic disease of the stomach and duodenum.

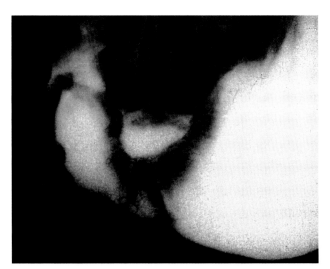

FIGURE 23-8. Barium study illustrating a benign antral ulcer crater. The pooling of barium in a crater-like defect surrounded by the radiolucent halo typical of mucosal edema is a radiographic characteristic of a benign ulcer.

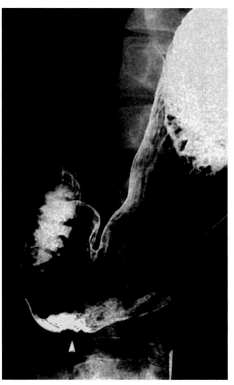

FIGURE 23-9. Barium study illustrating a gastric carcinoma. Barium studies are particularly useful in identifying infiltrating disorders of the stomach and duodenum, as illustrated in this view of a gastric carcinoma (*arrow*).

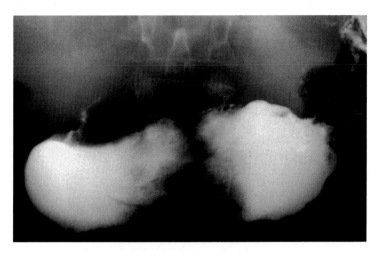

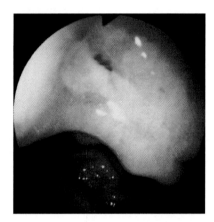

FIGURE 23-10. Barium study of a benign duodenal stricture showing a distinct narrowing of the duodenum accompanied by gastric distention with retained barium in the stomach.

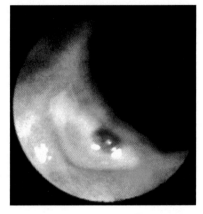

FIGURE 23-11. Endoscopic view of a benign antral ulcer. Well-demarcated smooth margins delineating a clean-based crater are typical characteristics of a benign ulcer. A visible vessel is shown at the margin of the crater.

FIGURE 23-12. Endoscopic view of a benign gastric ulcer.

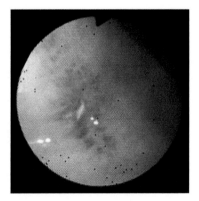

FIGURE 23-13. Endoscopic view of nonsteroidal antiinflammatory drug–induced mucosal injury.

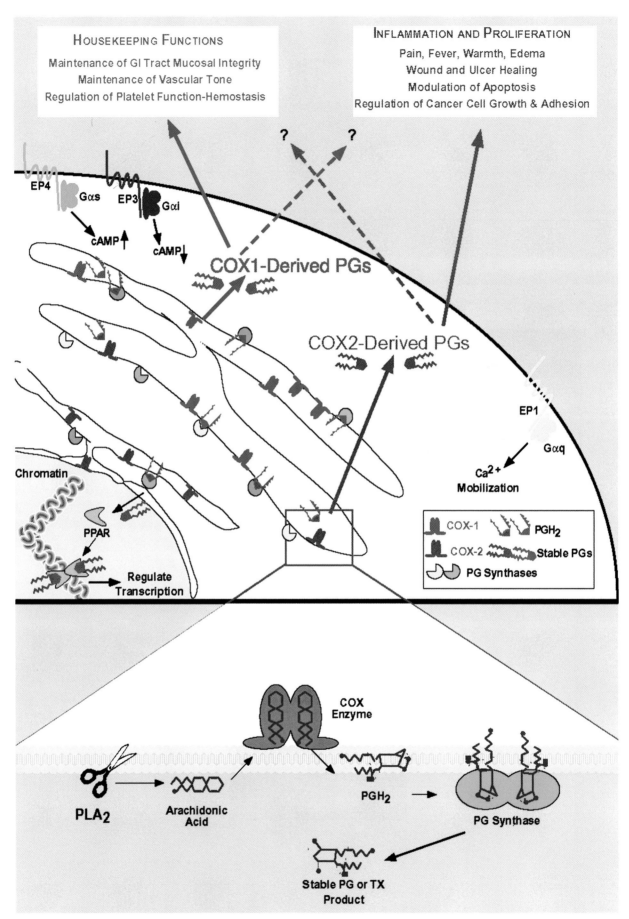

FIGURE 23-14. Biosynthesis of prostaglandins.

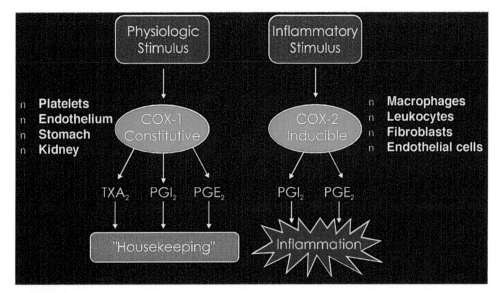

FIGURE 23-15. Cyclooxygenase isoenzymes and their corresponding distribution and function.

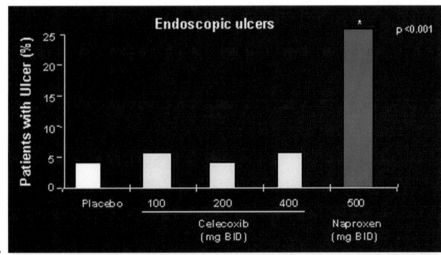

A

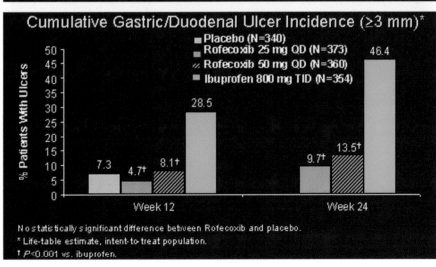

B

FIGURE 23-16. Incidence of peptic ulcers in patients using selective cyclooxygenase-2 inhibitors versus nonselective nonsteroidal antiinflammatory drugs. **A:** Comparison between celecoxib and naproxen for ulcer formation in patients with rheumatoid arthritis. **B:** Comparison between rofecoxib and ibuprofen for ulcer formation in patients with osteoarthritis.

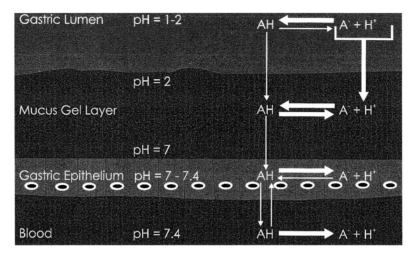

FIGURE 23-17. Direct nonsteroidal antiinflammatory drug (NSAID)–induced mucosal damage by ion trapping. NSAIDs are weak organic acids with ionization constants (pK$_a$) in the range of 3 to 5 and are soluble at the low pH of the stomach lumen. In the strongly acidic environment of gastric juice (pH < 2.5), these lipidic drugs are nonionized and freely diffuse across cell membranes into mucosal cells. Once the drug is inside the cell, the elevated intracellular pH favors dissociation of the H$^+$ ion and trapping of the negatively charged acid moiety. Because the nonionized form remains in equilibrium across the cell membrane, the total intracellular drug concentration (ionized plus nonionized) will be much higher than outside the cell. Ion trapping allows direct cellular injury caused by the toxicity of high intracellular levels of the NSAID.

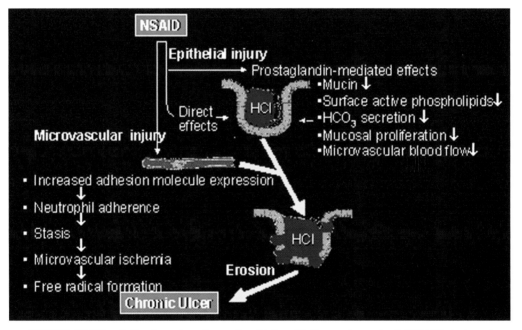

FIGURE 23-18. Pathogenesis of nonsteroidal antiinflammatory drug (NSAID)–induced ulcers. A summary of the pathogenetic mechanisms by which NSAIDs induce mucosal damage are outlined.

Acknowledgments

I am grateful to Pamela Glazer for typing this manuscript. The manuscript was supported by NIH Grant R01 DK34306 and funds from the Michigan Gastrointestinal Peptide Research Center (NIH Grant P30-DK34933).

24

GASTRITIS AND GASTROPATHY

ISMAEL MAGUILNIK ■ DAVID Y. GRAHAM ■ ROBERT M. GENTA

AUTOIMMUNE GASTRITIS

Autoimmune gastritis is a corpus-restricted chronic atrophic gastritis usually associated with serum anti–parietal cell and anti–intrinsic factor antibodies and with intrinsic factor deficiency, with or without pernicious anemia.

Clinical Aspects

Most clinical manifestations of autoimmune gastritis result from the loss of parietal and chief cells of the oxyntic mucosa, and only become apparent in the florid or end-stage phases of the disease. Major effects include achlorhydria, hypergastrinemia, loss of pepsin and pepsinogens, iron deficiency with macrocytic anemia, vitamin B_{12} deficiency with megaloblastic anemia, and increased risk of gastric neoplasms.

Endoscopic Appearance

Because this disease is limited to the mucosa, no abnormalities are found in the gastric wall other than submucosal congestion. In the corpus, the mucosa is usually thinner than normal (Fig. 24-1); this explains why few folds are left and fine submucosal vessels are easily recognized at endoscopic examination, especially in advanced disease (Fig. 24-2). The antral mucosa is reported to be endoscopically normal in the majority of cases. Figure 24-3 shows the appearance of an atrophic antrum.

Histopathological Aspects

The main histopathological features of advanced autoimmune gastritis are the diffuse involvement of the oxyntic mucosa by chronic atrophic gastritis with moderate intestinal metaplasia and a normal gastric antrum. The oxyntic mucosa is greatly reduced in thickness and may show foveolar hyperplasia with loss or metaplastic change of virtually all oxyntic glands (pyloric, pseudopyloric, pancreatic acinar, or intestinal metaplasia) (Fig. 24-4). Thus, neither parietal nor peptic cells are detectable.

Enterochromaffin-like cell hyperplasia and dysplasia (Fig. 24-5), and multiple carcinoids are commonly found in association with an end-stage histopathological

253

pattern. In the majority of patients the antral mucosa is either normal or there are only focal areas of chronic inflammation with intestinal metaplasia, similar in degree and extension to what is observed in the general asymptomatic population. However, hyperplasia of gastrin cells, secondary to achlorhydria, is often seen.

INTESTINAL METAPLASIA

Intestinal metaplasia is the replacement of the mucous cells that line the normal gastric mucosa with an epithelium similar to that of the small intestine. Intestinal metaplasia is found more frequently in *Helicobacter pylori*–positive subjects, despite the tendency for stomachs with extensive metaplasia to lose *H pylori*, and in patients with autoimmune atrophic gastritis. Small foci of intestinal metaplasia may be found in the antrum of apparently normal subjects and in individuals with associated chemical gastritis, particularly as a result of bile reflux. The clinical significance of intestinal metaplasia is related to its ability to progress to dysplasia and adenocarcinoma.

Endoscopic Appearance

Experienced endoscopists are often able to correctly predict that a characteristic appearance of the gastric mucosa will show the histopathological features of intestinal metaplasia. The endoscopic features most commonly associated with intestinalization are an irregular surface with patchy pink and pale areas (Figs. 24-6 and 24-7). The pale areas often have a velvety appearance and appear to be elevated compared to the pink areas. The pink areas can vary from light to dark and the unwary endoscopist might mistake dark pink areas for erosions. Histologically, both pale and pink areas appear similar. A technique that has encountered much favor in Japan, but has not been found to be very reliable in either North America or Europe, is the spraying of the gastric mucosa with indigo carmine, toluidine blue, or methylene blue. After the metaplastic mucosa sample is washed with saline, it maintains the characteristic blue color and may be differentiated from the nonmetaplastic areas.

Histopathological Features

Some metaplastic areas look like normal small intestinal epithelium with an absorptive brush border and goblet cells that produce acidic mucins (Fig. 24-8); other areas are lined by a disorderly mixture of irregularly shaped goblet cells and immature intermediate cells that produce a wide spectrum of sialo- and sulfomucins. The most often-used classification was proposed by Jass and Filipe: type I (brush border and no sialomucins); type II (no brush border, rare sulfomucins); type III (no brush border, cellular disarray, abundant sulfomucins). The distinction was thought to be important because metaplasia with sulfated mucins may represent a greater risk for adenocarcinoma. Follow-up studies have shown that repeat biopsy in the same area often shows a different type. Typing of metaplasia does not seem to have clinical utility. The presence of extensive intestinal metaplasia is essentially diagnostic of atrophic gastritis.

FOLLICULAR GASTRITIS CAUSED BY *H PYLORI*

Chronic *H pylori* gastritis is often viewed as a condition rather than a disease, with few if any distinctive clinical aspects. The extraordinary importance of this condition is mostly related to its consequences, which include increased risk for duodenal and gastric ulcer, gastric cancer, and lymphoma.

Endoscopic Appearance

Hyperemia, erosions, ulcerations, hypertrophy, and atrophy may coexist in various combinations in the same stomach, juxtaposed to one another and to apparently normal areas, and none of these features has been proven useful for predicting the presence or absence of chronic *H pylori* gastritis. Although there is no distinct endoscopic pattern of chronic *H pylori* gastritis, the pattern of follicular gastritis (Fig. 24-9) is almost invariably associated with this infection.

Histopathology

The most distinctive features of the gastric mucosa infected by *H pylori* are

- the infiltration of the gastric epithelium by polymorphonuclear neutrophils
- a mixed infiltrate in the lamina propria, consisting of neutrophils, lymphocytes, plasma cells, and variable amounts of eosinophils
- the formation of mucosal lymphoid follicles.

Lymphoid follicles are virtually always found in infected stomachs; the greatest density is in the region of the *incisura angularis* and the lowest density is in the proximal greater curvature (Fig. 24-10). Follicular gastritis is the endoscopic entity that corresponds to a particularly florid lymphoid follicle response in the mucosa (Fig. 24-11). Because of the univocal association between lymphoid follicles and *H pylori* infection, the Sydney system does not consider this particular endoscopic aspect as a separate entity.

CHEMICAL GASTROPATHY

The collection of endoscopic and histological features caused by chemical injury to the gastric mucosa is known as chemical gastropathy. In clinical practice, it is found almost exclusively in patients who use aspirin and other nonsteroidal antiinflammatory agents (NSAIDs). Other rare causes of this type of gastric mucosal damage include alcohol and chemicals ingested accidentally or for suicidal purposes.

Reactive gastropathy has been documented (endoscopically or histologically) in 10% to 45% of long-term users of NSAIDs. No relationship between the appearance of the mucosa and dyspeptic symptoms has been recognized. Bleeding, however, is associated with visible erosions or ulcers.

Pathogenesis

Prostaglandins exert their cytoprotective effects in the gastric mucosa by regulating the mucosal blood flow, increasing secretion of mucus and bicarbonate ions, and protecting the epithelial cells against cytotoxic injury. NSAIDs reduce prostaglandin synthesis, which results in inadequate cytoprotection.

Endoscopic Appearance

The mucosa of chronic NSAID users, unless they have gastric ulcers or erosions, has no distinctive appearance. NSAID erosions are typically found in the antrum, often on the tops of folds. The erosions are generally multiple, and are characterized by a central depression with or without a necrotic floor, a red rim, and prominent reaction in the surrounding mucosa. Most are small (2–4 mm), but they can be more than 1 cm in diameter. NSAID-associated lesions ranging from very superficial erosions to ulcer are represented in Figs. 24-12 through 24-15.

Histopathology

The histopathological diagnosis of chemical gastropathy remains a challenging problem. Several mucosal changes have been associated with reactive gastropathy, including foveolar hyperplasia, prominent smooth muscle fibers, edema, glandular and foveolar dilation, hemorrhage, and focal atrophy. However, the specificity and predictive value of any of these features is low: Some normal subjects with no history of NSAIDs use and many patients with *H pylori* infection have one or more of these histological features (Fig. 24-16). Superficial erosions without surrounding inflammation (Fig. 24-17) are almost always caused by chemical injury, whereas the etiology of multiple inflamed erosions (Fig. 24-18) is virtually impossible to determine. Thus, the pathologist can suspect chemical gastropathy, but a firm diagnosis can only be made when supportive clinical data are available and no confounding factors (e.g., *H pylori* infection) are present.

BILE-REFLUX GASTROPATHY

Postgastrectomy bile reflux may present with a syndrome characterized by burning midepigastric pain unresponsive to antacids and aggravated by eating and recumbency. Bilious vomiting, anemia, and weight loss may occur. Endoscopic confirmation of bile reflux and documentation of the characteristic histopathological findings support the diagnosis, and corrective surgery (e.g., creation of a 40- to 50-cm Roux-en-Y gastrojejunostomy) is successful in about half of all cases.

Pathogenesis

In patients with a gastric stump anastomosed to the proximal jejunum (Billroth II), small intestinal contents (with alkaline pancreaticoduodenal secretions, acids, bile salts, and lysolecithin) regurgitate into the gastric cavity, disrupt the mucus barrier, and damage the gastric surface epithelium. The resulting accelerated regeneration of the epithelium causes the characteristic histopathological appearance.

Endoscopic Appearance

The gastric mucosa at the anastomotic site may have a polypoid appearance with congestion, edema, and friability (Fig. 24-19). Superficial erosions may also be present in more proximal areas of the gastric stump.

Histopathology

The most characteristic changes include evidence of epithelial regeneration, extreme foveolar hyperplasia, edema of the lamina propria, and expansion of the smooth muscle fibers into the upper third of the mucosa (Figs. 24-20 and 24-21). The enhanced epithelial proliferation may cause the foveolar cells to have increased nuclear-cytoplasmic ratio and mild to moderate architectural disarray. These findings (known to pathologists as "atypia") may be incorrectly interpreted as dysplasia or neoplasia.

Partial Gastrectomy and Carcinoma

The polypoid appearance of the distal portions of the gastric stump in postgastrectomy patients has been referred to as *gastritis cystica polyposa*. Several European and Japanese studies have reported a high prevalence of low-grade dysplasia in these polypoid areas, as well as an increased incidence of gastric adenocarcinoma two to three decades after gastrectomy. These findings have not been confirmed in North America.

WATERMELON STOMACH

Watermelon stomach, or gastric antral vascular ectasia (GAVE syndrome), is a rare condition of unknown etiology that is frequently associated with gastric atrophy and autoimmune and connective tissue disorders, particularly systemic sclerosis. More than 70% of reported cases have occurred in older women. Occult bleeding is seen at presentation in almost 90% of the cases; melena or hematemesis is seen in 60% of the cases. In most patients, the chronic blood loss causes iron deficiency anemia.

Endoscopic Appearance

Watermelon stomach was so named because of the "longitudinal antral folds seen converging on the pylorus, containing visible and ectatic vessels resembling the stripes on a watermelon" (Fig. 24-22). In other metaphors, the prominent dilated vessels have been compared to "a large, flat mushroom" or a "honeycomb."

Histopathology

In the antrum, the lamina propria is due to smooth muscle proliferation and fibrosis, and contains markedly dilated mucosal capillaries (Fig. 24-23). Fibrin thrombi are often found within the dilated capillaries (Fig. 24-24).

Management

Therapeutic endoscopy with obliteration of the dilated vessels by argon plasma coagulation is the accepted treatment of choice because of its feasibility and satisfactory long-term results. Endoscopic treatment has greatly reduced the need for antrectomy, which used to be the most effective treatment option.

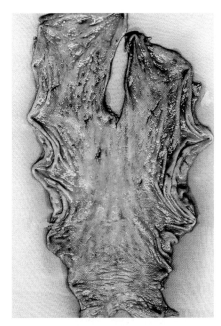

FIGURE 24-1. Total gastrectomy performed in a patient with end-stage autoimmune atrophic gastritis and multiple carcinoid tumors. The mucosa of the corpus is completely devoid of *rugae,* whereas the antrum maintains its normal anatomy.

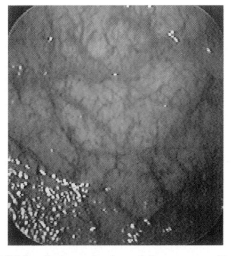

FIGURE 24-2. Endoscopic view of the corpus with severe atrophy. The mucosa appears thin and the underlying vasculature is prominent.

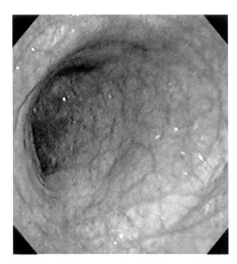

FIGURE 24-3. An endoscopic picture from a case similar to that depicted in figure 24-2 with clearly visible mucosal and submucosal vessels is seen in a patient with antral atrophy. The bluish discoloration in the *upper left corner* is the shade of the liver seen through the thin distended gastric wall.

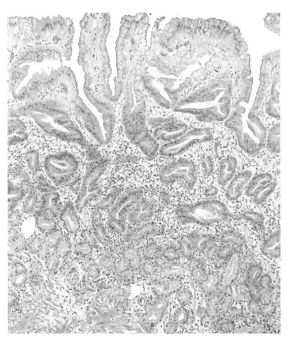

FIGURE 24-4. The mucosa of the corpus has completely lost its normal appearance: The normal tightly packed acid-secreting oxyntic glands have been progressively destroyed by the autoimmune inflammatory process and are replaced by mucous-secreting glands similar to those found in the distal antrum. The phenomenon is known as pyloric (or pseudopyloric) metaplasia.

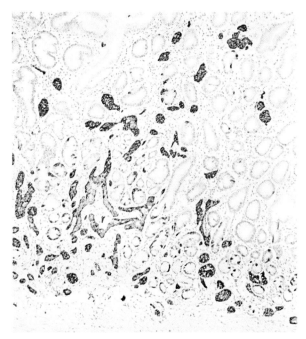

FIGURE 24-5. Chromogranin stain of the fundic mucosa shows severe enterochromaffin-like (ECL) cell hyperplasia and dysplasia. This is a consequence of the stimulus caused by the hypergastrinemia the patients develop in response to the low or absent acid content of the atrophic stomach. Both ECL cell hyperplasia and dysplasia are considered to be a precursor of carcinoid tumors, which frequently arise in the corpus of patients with autoimmune atrophic gastritis.

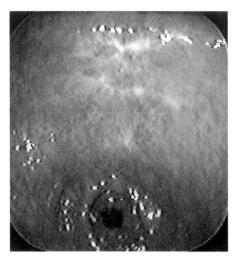

FIGURE 24-6. Intestinal metaplasia is usually difficult to diagnose endoscopically. Histopathological examination of biopsy specimens obtained from the flat yellowish areas visible in this antrum, originally interpreted as either metaplastic or fibrotic areas (scars), showed diffuse intestinal metaplasia.

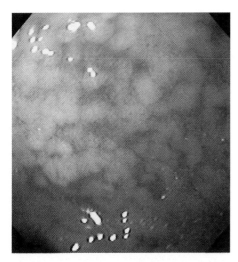

FIGURE 24-7. Large area of intestinal metaplasia in the antral mucosa. The appearance is characteristically pale and velvety.

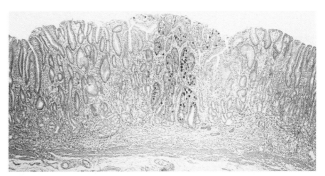

FIGURE 24-8. Antral mucosa with a small focus of intestinal metaplasia. Goblet cells are best visualized when Alcian blue at pH 2.5 is added to the traditional hematoxylin and eosin stains. Intestinal metaplasia is a precursor of dysplasia and adenocarcinoma. The larger the area of the gastric mucosa affected by metaplasia, the greater the risk for gastric cancer.

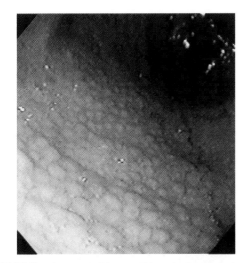

FIGURE 24-9. Innumerable small hemispherical elevations, many with a slightly depressed or umbilicated center, are characteristic of follicular gastritis.

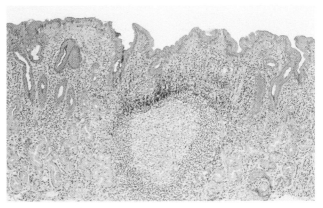

FIGURE 24-10. In most subjects infected with *H pylori*, small lymphoid follicles develop in the gastric mucosa. When their diameter is smaller than the mucosal thickness, they are not visible endoscopically.

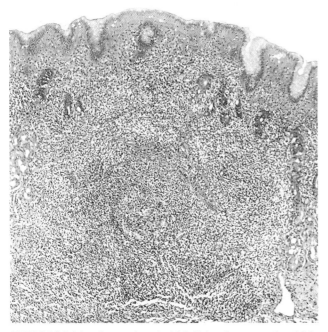

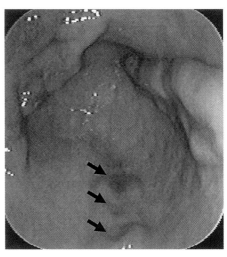

FIGURE 24-11. Larger lymphoid follicles increase the thickness of the mucosa and create endoscopically detectable elevations. When follicles are extremely numerous and most are large, the mucosal appearance is that of follicular gastritis.

FIGURE 24-12. Superficial antral erosions (*arrows*) in a patient using nonsteroidal antiinflammatory drugs.

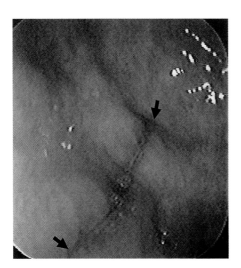

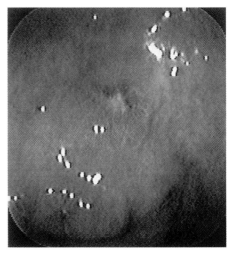

FIGURE 24-13. Characteristic of aspirin-induced linear erosion (*extending between the two arrows*).

FIGURE 24-14. Large, deep erosion or superficial ulcer in a patient using nonsteroidal antiinflammatory drugs.

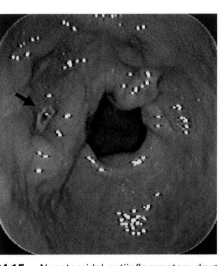

FIGURE 24-15. Nonsteroidal antiinflammatory drug–induced small ulcer.

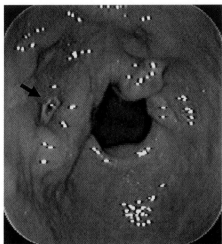

FIGURE 24-16. Foveolar hyperplasia is generally believed to be a characteristic histopathological finding in chemical gastropathy. This mucosal change, however, simply reflects increased epithelial turnover caused by superficial damage, and may occur in other conditions, including *H pylori* infection. In this patient with both *H pylori* gastritis and a history of nonsteroidal antiinflammatory drug use, the etiology of the foveolar alterations cannot be determined.

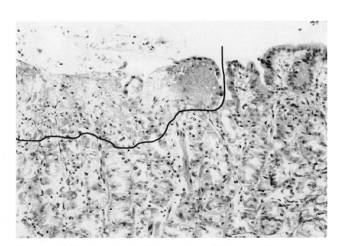

FIGURE 24-17. Superficial erosion of the oxyntic mucosa. The mucosa to the *right and below the red line* is completely normal and without inflammation. The affected portion shows hemorrhage, necrosis, and epithelial regeneration. This association of normal mucosa with an abrupt limited hemorrhagic and necrotic lesion is characteristic of chemical injury. The absence of inflammation all but excludes *H pylori* infection.

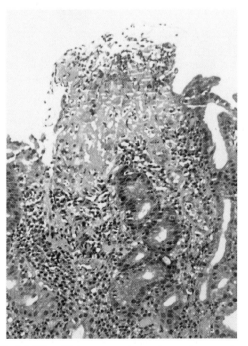

FIGURE 24-18. High-power view of a microerosion. The epithelium has disappeared and the uppermost part of the mucosa contains fibrin and inflammatory cells projected toward the lumen in a fashion that has been likened to a minuscule eruption.

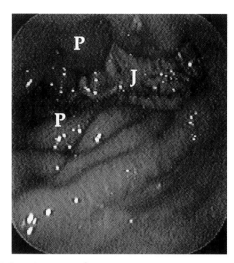

FIGURE 24-19. Polypoid appearance of the gastric mucosa (*P*) at the anastomotic site in a patient with Billroth II gastrojejunostomy. A portion of the jejunum (*J*) is visible, surrounded by thickened gastric mucosa.

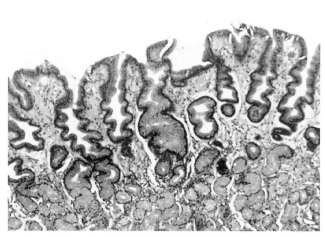

FIGURE 24-20. Foveolar hyperplasia without inflammation is likely caused by chemical injury.

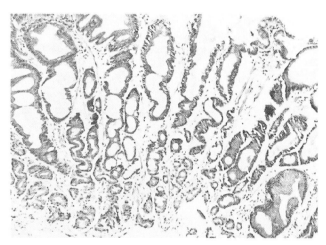

FIGURE 24-21. Extreme foveolar hyperplasia and dilation in a biopsy specimen from the gastric stoma in a patient with Billroth II gastrectomy. This degree of foveolar hyperplasia accounts for the juicy, polypoid aspect of the area immediately juxtaposed to the anastomotic site.

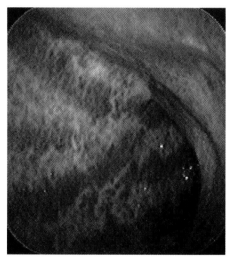

FIGURE 24-22. Hemorrhagic hyperemic streaks apparently converging toward the pylorus, in the antrum of a middle-aged woman with scleroderma and progressive anemia. The appearance of the streaks has been compared to the stripes of a watermelon, hence the term watermelon stomach.

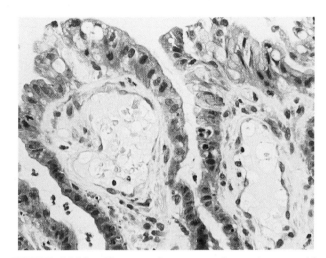

FIGURE 24-23. The antral mucosa shows innumerable dilated subepithelial capillaries.

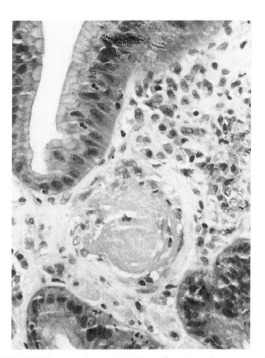

FIGURE 24-24. A characteristic—if not pathognomonic—finding in watermelon stomach is the presence of thrombi in the dilated superficial capillaries.

25

TUMORS OF THE STOMACH

WAI K. LEUNG ■ JOSEPH J.Y. SUNG

Gastric cancer is the second most common cause of death from cancer worldwide. In 1990, it was estimated that more than 600,000 people died from this malignancy and 60% of the deaths occurred in developing countries. There are considerable geographic differences in the incidence of this malignancy. The highest rate is observed in eastern Asia, where the age-standardized rate in men is more than 40 per 100,000. The incidence rates in Japanese and Chinese men are approximately 35 per 100,000. By contrast, North America, northern Europe, Africa, and southeast Asia have lower gastric cancer incidences. In the United States and many other developed countries, there is a progressive decline in the incidence of this disease (Fig. 25-1). This largely reflects the decline in cancer of the distal stomach with intestinal-type histology. Nonetheless, the total number of new cases in the world is increasing because of the growth of elderly population and the preferential population growth in developing countries with high background gastric cancer incidences.

Adenocarcinomas comprise of more than 90% of stomach cancers (Fig. 25-2) and the rest are predominantly lymphoma and stromal tumors. Detailed World Health Organization (WHO) classification of gastric tumors is presented in Table 25-1. Adenocarcinoma can be broadly categorized into intestinal and diffuse type as proposed by Lauren. Intestinal-type carcinoma is characterized by the presence of cohesive neoplastic cells forming glandular tubular structures, whereas diffuse-type cancer shows sheets of epithelial cells or cells scattered in a stromal matrix without evidence of gland formation (Fig. 25-3). The carcinogenesis of gastric cancer, particularly the intestinal type, is generally believed to be a multi-step development from chronic gastritis, which is usually triggered by chronic *Helicobacter pylori* infection, to atrophic gastritis, intestinal metaplasia, dysplasia, and carcinoma. Numerous genetic alterations have been demonstrated in this histological progression, including cyclooxygenase-2 overexpression, *p53* mutation, and microsatellite instability.

Radiologic examination was once the investigation of choice for gastric diseases, but its role has been largely replaced by endoscopy. Diminished distensibility of the stomach on barium meal examination suggests a diffusely infiltrative cancer. In addition, the presence of an asymmetric ulcer crater eccentrically located on an irregular mass with distortion or obliteration of normal mucosal fold strongly suggests malignant ulcer (Fig. 25-4). However, the definite diagnosis of malignancy is impossible without tumor biopsy obtained through endoscopic examination. Another advantage of endoscopy is the direct visualization of subtle mucosal changes found in early gastric cancer (Fig. 25-5). With the use of chromoendoscopy and magnifying endoscopes, the ability to detect early gastric cancer can be enhanced.

The revised primary tumor node metastasis (TNM) staging of gastric cancer is given in Table 25-2. The T-staging remains unchanged (Fig. 25-6), but major modifications have been made in the classification of regional lymph nodes, which is now determined by the number instead of the anatomic location of the involved lymph nodes. Because the mainstay of treatment for gastric cancer is surgery, the importance of accurate pre-operative staging cannot be over-emphasized. The extent of surgical resection, especially the extent of lymph node dissection, is still a matter of debate. Because of the delay in presentation, not all gastric cancers could undergo curative resection.

Despite the advances in imaging techniques, no single imaging modality is sensitive or specific enough to detect local or distant metastasis. Approximately 10% to 20% of patients being explored for potentially curative resection are found to have peritoneal seeding at the time of surgery. Because of the poor visualization of stomach wall, computerized tomography (CT) appears to be only useful in demonstrating local or distant invasion (Fig. 25-7). Even with the use of helical CT scan, about 25% to 50% of tumor invasion into colon or pancreas may be missed. On the other hand, the extent of local invasion, in particular the T staging, is better delineated with the use of endoscopic ultrasound (EUS) (Fig. 25-8). The overall accuracy of EUS in T staging was 78%. However, because of the poor penetration of high-frequency ultrasound, the role of EUS in assessing distant metastasis is limited. The use of EUS and CT scan may be complementary in assessing local invasion and distant metastasis. Diagnostic accuracy can be further improved by the use of preoperative laparoscopy that detects unexpected peritoneal and liver metastasis (Fig. 25-9), which is particularly useful in patients with locally advanced disease.

Lymphoma accounts for about 10% of all gastric malignancies. The gastrointestinal tract is the most common extranodal site for non-Hodgkin lymphoma. The majority of gastric lymphomas are B-cell lymphomas, including high-grade lymphoma and low-grade mucosa-associated lymphoid tissue (MALT) lymphomas. MALT lymphoma is a special entity that is closely linked to *H pylori* infection. Histologically, MALT lymphoma mimics that of normal MALT with marginal zone B-cell immunophenotypes (Fig. 25-10). The typical lymphoepithelial lesions are characterized by infiltration of the glandular epithelium by clusters of neoplastic lymphoid cells with associated destruction of gland architecture and morphologic changes within the cells. Eradication of *H pylori* alone has been shown to produce complete regression of low-grade MALT lymphoma. In this context, EUS may help to identify those who would respond to antibacterial treatment; that is, patients with stage I_{E1} disease (confined to mucosa and submucosa) (Fig. 25-11).

Most gastric mesenchymal neoplasms are gastrointestinal stromal tumors (GIST) or smooth muscle types (Figs. 25-12 through 25-17). Although the term GIST was originally reserved for tumors that are neither leiomyomas nor schwannomas, GIST has been loosely used to describe the majority of mesenchymal tumors. The cellular origin of GIST has been proposed to be the interstitial cell of Cajal and most malignant GIST harbor mutations in the *c-kit* gene, which would result in constitutive activation of the tyrosine kinase. In this context, immunoreactivity against c-KIT (CD117) was found to be present in 80% to 100% of GIST (Fig. 25-13*F*). In general, tumors greater than 5 cm in size and with high mitotic counts (>10 mitoses/10 high-power field) are considered to be of higher malignant potential (Fig. 25-15).

TABLE 25-1
WHO Histological Classification of Gastric Tumors

EPITHELIAL TUMORS	NONEPITHELIAL TUMORS
Intraepithelial neoplasia or adenoma	Leiomyoma
Carcinoma	Schwannoma
Adenocarcinoma	Granular cell tumor
Intestinal type	Glomus tumor
Diffuse type	Leiomyosarcoma
Papillary adenocarcinoma	GI stromal tumor
Tubular adenocarcinoma	Benign
Mucinous adenocarcinoma	Uncertain malignant potential
Signet-ring cell carcinoma	Malignant
Adenosquamous carcinoma	Kaposi sarcoma
Squamous cell carcinoma	Others
Small cell carcinoma	Malignant lymphomas
Undifferentiated carcinoma	Marginal zone B-cell lymphoma of MALT type
Others	Mantle cell lymphoma
Carcinoid (well-differentiated endocrine neoplasm	Diffuse large B-cell lymphoma
	Others
	Secondary tumors

GI, gastrointestinal; MALT, mucosa-associated lymphoid tissue; WHO, World Health Organization.

TABLE 25-2
The Fifth Edition of the UICC/AJCC TNM Classification of Gastric Carcinoma

---

A. TNM CLASSIFICATION

T: Primary Tumor
TX   Primary tumor cannot be assessed
T0   No evidence of primary tumor
Tis   Carcinoma in situ; intraepithelial tumor without invasion of lamina propria
T1   Tumor invades lamina propria or submucosa
T2   Tumor invades muscularis propria or subserosa
T3   Tumor penetrates serosa (visceral peritoneum) without invasion of adjacent structures
T4   Tumor invades adjacent structures

N: Regional Lymph Node
NX   Regional lymph nodes cannot be assessed
N0   No regional lymph node metastasis
N1   Metastasis in 1–6 regional lymph nodes
N2   Metastasis in 7–15 regional lymph nodes
N3   Metastasis in more than 15 regional lymph nodes

M: Distant Metastasis
MX   Distant metastasis cannot be assessed
M0   No distant metastasis
M1   Distant metastasis

B. STAGE GROUPING

STAGE	T	N	M
0	Tis	N0	M0
IA	T1	N0	M0
IB	T1	N1	M0
	T2	N0	M0
II	T1	N2	M0
	T2	N1	M0
	T3	N0	M0
IIIA	T2	N2	M0
	T3	N1	M0
	T4	N0	M0
IIIB	T3	N2	M0
IV	T4	N1–3	M0
	T1–3	N3	M0
	Any T	Any N	M1

AJCC, American Joint Commission for Cancer; TNM, primary tumor, regional nodes, metastasis; UICC, International Union Against Cancer.

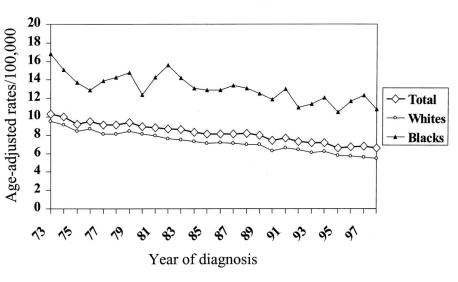

FIGURE 25-1. The age-adjusted incidence rates of gastric cancer in the United States (1973–1998). A progressive decline in cancer incidences in both the Caucasian and African American population during the last 25 years was noted.

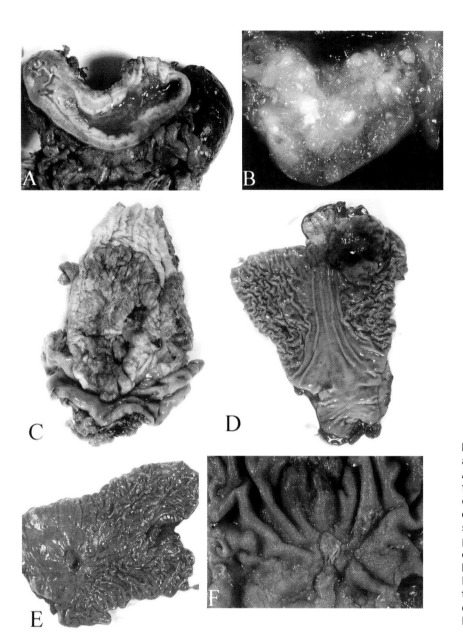

FIGURE 25-2. Macroscopic appearances of gastric adenocarcinoma. **A:** Linitis plastica. The gastric wall is diffusely thickened and the spleen and omentum were removed en bloc in radical gastrectomy. **B:** Mucoid carcinoma of stomach demonstrating multiple mucin pools. **C:** An ulcerative tumor at the cardia. **D:** A polypoid tumor at the cardia. **E:** A malignant ulcer located in the lesser curve. **F:** An early gastric cancer that resembles a benign ulcer. (Courtesy of Dr. K.F. To, Prince of Wales Hospital, Hong Kong.)

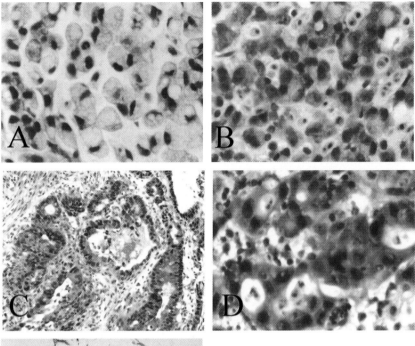

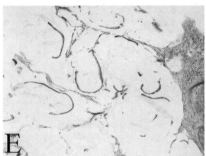

FIGURE 25-3. Histological subtypes of gastric adenocarcinoma. **A:** Diffuse-type adenocarcinoma with signet ring (H&E stain; original magnification ×400). **B:** Diffuse-type adenocarcinoma with discohesive sheets of carcinoma cells and moderate amount of pale eosinophilic cytoplasm (H&E stain; original magnification ×400). **C:** Intestinal-type adenocarcinoma that was arranged in a tubular glandular pattern with invasion into the desmoplastic stroma (H&E section, ×200). **D:** Intestinal-type adenocarcinoma with irregular fused small glandular pattern (H&E stain; original magnification ×400). **E:** Mucinous adenocarcinoma (H&E stain; original magnification ×100). (Courtesy of Dr. K.F. To, Prince of Wales Hospital, Hong Kong.)

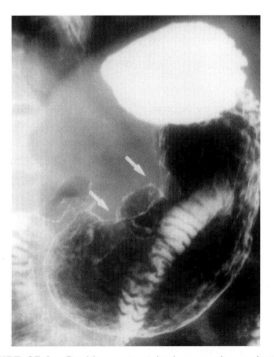

FIGURE 25-4. Double contrast barium meal examination demonstrating an ulcerative tumor in the angular incisura (*arrows*).

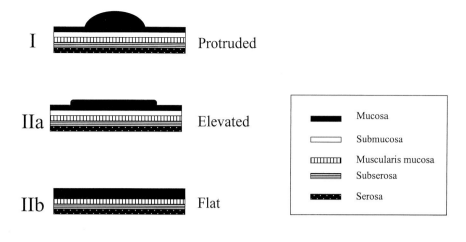

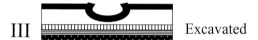

FIGURE 25-5. Classification of early gastric cancer. Type I is an exophytic lesion, type II is flat (or superficial), and type III is an ulcerated or depressed lesion. Type II is further divided into three subtypes depending on whether it is elevated (IIa), flat (IIb), or depressed (IIc).

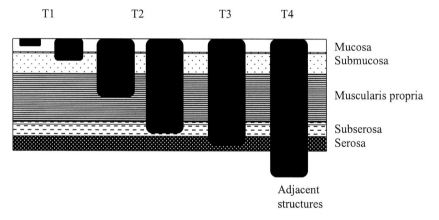

FIGURE 25-6. T-classification of gastric carcinoma. (Primary tumor node metastasis staging system.)

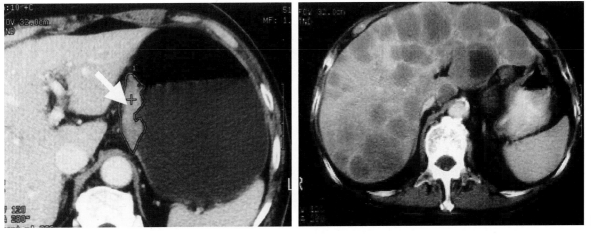

FIGURE 25-7. Computerized tomography of gastric cancer. **A:** Primary gastric carcinoma as illustrated by the *arrow*. **B:** Multiple liver metastasis from primary gastric carcinoma as shown by the hypodense lesions.

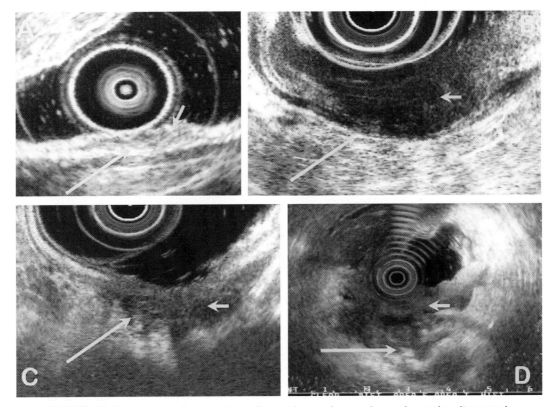

FIGURE 25-8. Preoperative staging of gastric carcinoma by endoscopic ultrasound. **A:** Intramucosal early gastric cancer (Tis) with focal mucosal thickening (*short arrow*) and intact lamina propria (*long arrow*). **B:** T2 gastric cancer (*short arrow*) invaded into the muscularis layer with intact serosa (*long arrow*). **C:** Small gastric cancer (*short arrow*) invaded through the serosa (T3) (*long arrow*). **D:** Large T4 gastric cancer (*short arrow*) invaded into the neck of pancreas (*long arrow*). (Courtesy of Dr. Y.T. Lee, Prince of Wales Hospital, Hong Kong.)

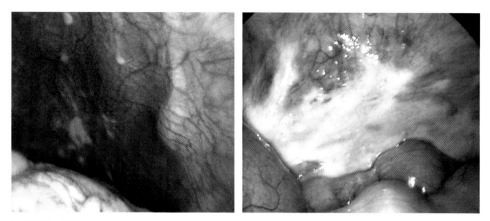

FIGURE 25-9. Laparoscopic views of peritoneal seeding from gastric adenocarcinoma. (Courtesy of Dr. Enders Ng, Prince of Wales Hospital, Hong Kong.)

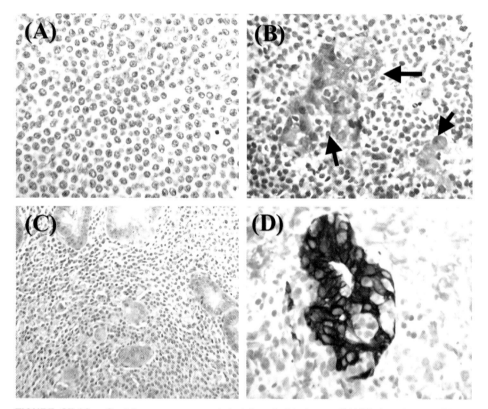

FIGURE 25-10. Gastric mucosa-associated lymphoid tissue (MALT) lymphoma. Characteristic features of low-grade MALT lymphoma: (**A**) centrocyte-like cells (H&E stain; original magnification ×200); (**B**) lymphoepithelial lesions (marked by *arrows*) (H&E stain; original magnification ×200); (**C**) plasmacytic differentiation (H&E stain; original magnification ×100); and (**D**) lymphoepithelial lesions (immunostain for cytokeratin; original magnification ×200). (Courtesy of Dr. Wing Y. Chan, the Chinese University of Hong Kong, Prince of Wales Hospital, Hong Kong.)

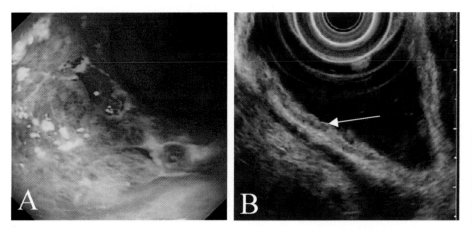

FIGURE 25-11. Mucosa-associated lymphoid tissue (MALT) lymphoma. **A:** Endoscopic appearance of MALT lymphoma. **B:** Thickened gastric mucosa without submucosa involvement (*arrow*) as shown by endoscopic ultrasonography (stage I_{E1}).

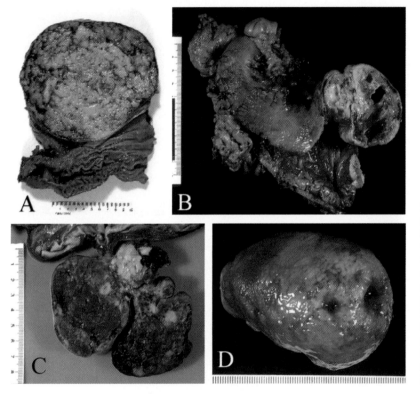

FIGURE 25-12. Gross appearances of gastric mesenchymal tumors. **A:** A huge gastric stromal tumor arising from the gastric wall and protruding into the serosal surface. The tan-colored solid tumor was punctuated with areas of hemorrhage. **B:** Another example of gastric stromal tumor that mainly protruded into the gastric lumen and exhibited cystic degeneration. **C:** A gastric stromal tumor that was attached to the gastric wall by a narrow pedicle. **D:** The surface of this tumor was covered by gastric mucosa with typical central umbilication. (Courtesy of Dr. K.F. To, Prince of Wales Hospital, Hong Kong.)

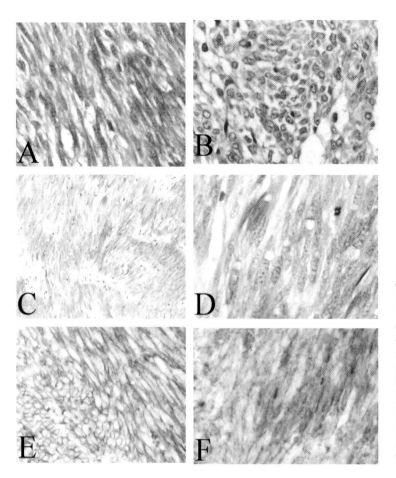

FIGURE 25-13. Microscopic appearances of gastric stromal tumors. (Courtesy of Dr. K.F. To, Prince of Wales Hospital, Hong Kong.) **A–D:** Gastric stromal tumors have a wide range of histological and cytological patterns. **A:** Fascicular pattern with spinal cell morphology (H&E stain; original magnification ×200). **B:** Sheet-like pattern with epithelioid appearance (H&E stain; original magnification ×200). **C:** Palisade pattern with resemblance to nerve sheet tumor (H&E stain; original magnification ×100). **D:** Juxta-nuclear vacuolation suggestive of smooth muscle cells. **E, F:** Strong immunoreactivity against CD34 (**E**) and CD117/c-KIT (**F**) in gastric stromal tumor. (Courtesy of Dr. K.F. To, Prince of Wales Hospital, Hong Kong.)

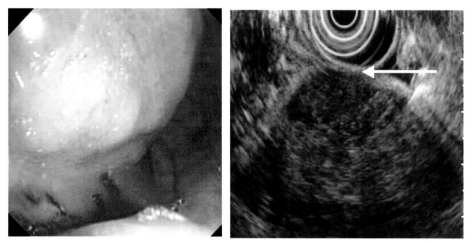

FIGURE 25-14. Gastric leiomyosarcoma. **Left:** Endoscopic examination showed a huge mass in the greater curve of the stomach with normal mucosa. **Right:** Endoscopic ultrasound examination (7.5 MHz, Olympus GF-UM240, Japan) revealed a 10-cm heterogeneous tumor arising from the muscularis layer with normal mucosa and submucosa (*arrow*). There were cystic changes within the parenchyma, whereas the pancreas was normal. (Courtesy of Dr. Y.T. Lee, Prince of Wales Hospital, Hong Kong.)

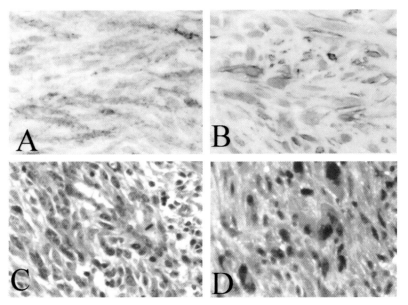

FIGURE 25-15. Smooth muscle tumor. **A, B:** Smooth muscle origin was supported by the positive immunoreactivity against smooth muscle actin (**A:** original magnification ×200) and desmin (**B:** original magnification ×200). **C, D:** Potential malignant smooth muscle tumor demonstrates cytologic atypia and high mitotic activity. (Courtesy of Dr. K.F. To, Prince of Wales Hospital, Hong Kong.)

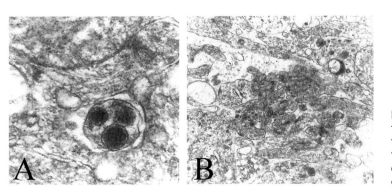

FIGURE 25-16. Gastrointestinal autonomic nerve tumor (GANT). The reconciliation of GANT relies on the typical ultrastructure appearances of interdigitating cell processes (**A**) and presence of neurosecretory granules (**B**). (Courtesy of Dr. K.F. To, Prince of Wales Hospital, Hong Kong.)

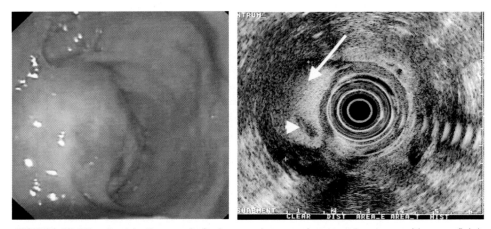

FIGURE 25-17. Gastric lipoma. **Left:** large submucosal mass at antrum with superficial ulceration on endoscopic examination. **Right:** Endoscopic ultrasound examination (7.5 MHz, Olympus GF-UM240) showed a smooth regular hyperechoic mass (*long arrow*) situated in the submucosal layer with deep ulceration (*short arrow*). The muscularis and mucosal layers were normal. (Courtesy of Dr. Y.T. Lee, Prince of Wales Hospital, Hong Kong.)

26

SURGERY FOR PEPTIC ULCER DISEASE AND POSTGASTRECTOMY SYNDROMES

NEAL E. SEYMOUR ■ DANA K. ANDERSEN

The role of the surgeon in the management of peptic ulcer disease has been dramatically altered with improved understanding of ulcer pathogenesis and new therapies that address the underlying causes of gastroduodenal mucosal injury. Despite these developments, it is vital to understand that surgical science continues to contribute to the care of patients with peptic ulcers, particularly patients with complicated disease. Clinicians must be familiar with the various methods of surgical management of duodenal and gastric ulcers and must be able to appreciate the implications of these treatments for patients who have undergone them in the past.

VAGOTOMY FOR DUODENAL ULCER

Disruption of vagal control of gastric acid secretion is the physiological basis for elective surgical management of peptic ulcer. Vagal fibers to the stomach can be interrupted at different levels relative to the parietal cells to spare or ablate extragastric and pyloroantral vagal effects. Highly selective vagotomy has proved to be both effective and well tolerated. It is generally favored over other operations for peptic ulcer, which may be associated with complications of less-selective vagotomy or alterations in the gastroduodenal conduit.

GASTRIC DRAINAGE

Truncal and selective vagotomy must be performed in conjunction with a gastric drainage procedure to circumvent problems related to gastric stasis and impaired pyloric relaxation. A variety of methods have been described to achieve gastric drainage, all of which are associated with accelerated emptying of liquid gastric contents and dumping syndrome. Although it is infrequently performed, in selected circumstances (particularly bleeding duodenal ulcer) vagotomy with gastric drainage remains a valuable procedure.

ANTRECTOMY

Truncal or selective vagotomy with antrectomy must be considered the standard of operations for duodenal ulcer if recurrence rate alone is taken as the ultimate measure of success of the procedure. The potential complications of this procedure have made it a less well-received alternative to highly selective vagotomy when elective surgical therapy for duodenal ulcer is deemed necessary. Although truncal vagotomy with antrectomy is very infrequently performed, the ulcer recurrence rate after the procedure is less than 2%.

ULCER RECURRENCE AFTER OPERATIONS FOR PEPTIC ULCER

Ulcer recurrence rates after operations for duodenal ulcer vary depending on the type of operation performed, the characteristics of the individual instance of the disease, and specific technical issues pertaining to the operation. Although it is certainly important to achieve low recurrence rates after any operation for peptic ulcer, this goal must be balanced with patient tolerance of the procedure. Duodenal ulcer recurrence rates tend to be higher after HSV than after truncal vagotomy and antrectomy. However, highly selective vagotomy has achieved greater worldwide acceptance because of an excellent degree of patient tolerance.

LAPAROSCOPIC MANAGEMENT OF PEPTIC ULCERS

Reports of successful laparoscopic vagotomy have generated interest in the use of this procedure to manage peptic ulcer disease. The benefits of laparoscopic abdominal operations include shorter hospital stay, decreased use of narcotic analgesics, and earlier return to work and other activities. However, the indications for operative management of peptic ulcer remain quite circumscribed despite the potential benefits.

SURGICAL MANAGEMENT OF GASTRIC ULCERS

Operative strategies in the management of gastric ulcer differ from those described for duodenal ulcer. Surgical therapy generally is offered when the ulcer is refractory to medical therapy or complicated by bleeding or perforation. The type of procedure offered depends largely on the location of the ulcer. Resection of the ulcer, either alone or with a segment of stomach, is the most appropriate treatment. Vagotomy is appropriate only in selected instances in which the ulcer can be predicted to demonstrate clinical behavior similar to that of duodenal ulcers.

SURGICAL MANAGEMENT OF BLEEDING ULCERS

Despite the effectiveness of medical therapy for peptic ulcer, bleeding remains a common presentation of this disease and is the most frequent indication for surgical management of duodenal ulcer. Therapeutic endoscopic measures can control most instances of ulcer bleeding. However, early recognition of the need for operative intervention is vital to minimize the mortality rate, particularly among patients who may have poor tolerance of ongoing hemorrhage (e.g., the elderly and patients with serious comorbid conditions).

SURGICAL MANAGEMENT OF PERFORATED ULCERS

Perforation is a potential initial presentation of peptic ulcer, particularly anterior ulcers of the first portion of the duodenum. Pain associated with perforation is frequently very acute in onset. Patients may present with frank peritonitis, and approximately half have pneumoperitoneum. Most patients undergo immediate abdominal exploration with repair of the perforation. Some patients have a more insidious presentation and may be considered for nonoperative treatment with nasogastric decompression and antibiotics after demonstration of contained perforation by means of a water-soluble contrast study.

COMPLICATIONS OF OPERATIONS FOR PEPTIC ULCER

Despite the relative rarity of elective operations for peptic ulcer, complications of these procedures may be encountered in clinical practice. Recognition of complications depends on familiarity with the postsurgical anatomical and physiological alterations produced by such procedures. Suspicion of gastric stasis, efferent loop obstruction after a Billroth II procedure, and dumping syndrome may be prompted by the clinical history. Recurrent ulcer, alkaline reflux, gastric remnant cancer, and afferent loop problems may be more difficult to diagnose. A clear understanding of the previous operation and an accurate interpretation of the clinical history should prompt the appropriate investigations.

TABLE 26-1
Physiologic Consequences of Truncal Vagotomy

Stomach	*Pancreas*
Secretory	Decreased basal enzyme secretion
85% reduction in basal acid secretion	Loss of cephalic and gastric phases of
50% reduction in maximal acid output	pancreatic secretion
80% reduction in basal and stimulated	*Gallbladder*
pepsin secretion	Defective gallbladder contraction
Basal and postprandial hypergastrinemia	Loss of gastrocholecystic reflex
Motor	*Small intestine*
Loss of fundic receptive relaxation	Loss of regulated absorptive,
Loss of pyloric sphincter relaxation	secretory, and propulsive activity
Defective antral grinding function	Development of poorly understood
	"postvagotomy diarrhea"

From Debas HT, Orloff SL. Surgery for peptic ulcer disease and postgastrectomy syndromes. In: Yamada T, Alpers DH, Powell DW, Owyang C, Silverstein FE, eds. *Textbook of gastroenterology,* 2nd ed. Philadelphia: JB Lippincott, 1995:1523.

TABLE 26-2
Ulcer Recurrence Rates after Operations for Peptic Ulcer

OPERATION	RECURRENCE RATE (%)	REMARKS
75% gastric resection	2–5	Of historical interest
Vagotomy and drainage	10–15	Pyloroplasty most frequent drainage procedure
Vagotomy and antrectomy	0–2	Lowest recurrence rates
Highly selective vagotomy	10–17	Operator dependent

Adapted from McFadden DW, Zinner MJ. Reoperation for recurrent peptic ulcer disease. Surg Clin North Am 1991;71:77.

TABLE 26-3
Recurrent Ulcer Rate after Highly Selective Vagotomy

AUTHOR	YEAR	NO. OF PATIENTS	RECURRENCE RATE (%)	FOLLOW-UP PERIOD (Y)
Blackett	1981	233	10.7	5–12
Enskog	1986	326	13.8	1–10
Byrne	1988	223	11.2	1–14
Soper	1989	396	14	5–13
Jordan	1989	424	9.7	2–16
Macintyre	1990	283	17.3	5–12
Johnston	1991	305	15	>10

From Seymour NE, Andersen DK. Surgery for peptic ulcer disease and postgastrectomy syndromes. In: Yamada T, Alpers DH, Laine L, Owyang C, Powell DW, eds. Textbook of gastroenterology, 3rd ed. New York: Lippincott Williams & Wilkins, 1999.

TABLE 26-4
Factors Predictive of Mortality in Bleeding Duodenal Ulcer

Transfusion requirement > 5 units
Age > 60 y
Shock on presentation
Concomitant medical illnesses

Adapted from Branicki FJ, Boey J, Fok PJ, et al. Bleeding duodenal ulcer. A prospective evaluation of risk factors for rebleeding and death. Ann Surg 1990; 211:411.

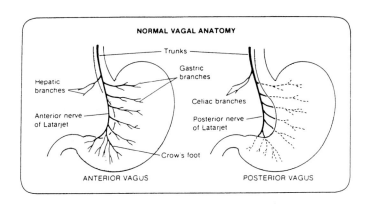

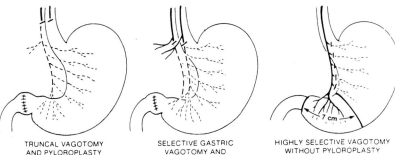

FIGURE 26-1. Normal vagal anatomy and types of vagotomy. In *truncal vagotomy* (a) nerve trunks are divided above the celiac and hepatic branches; (b) the cholinergic drive to gastric acid production is removed and parietal cell sensitivity to gastrin is reduced; (c) loss of normal pyloroantral motor function necessitates a gastric drainage procedure (pyloroplasty shown). In *selective vagotomy* (a) anterior and posterior nerves are divided distal to the celiac and hepatic branches; (b) extragastric innervation of the gastrointestinal tract is preserved and risk for gallstone formation and diarrhea theoretically are reduced; (c) a gastric drainage procedure is required. In *highly selective vagotomy* (a) individual branches of the anterior and posterior nerves of Latarjet to the body of the stomach are divided, and the terminal branches to the pylorus and antrum (crow's foot are spared); (b) pyloroantral motor function is preserved, and gastric drainage is unnecessary.

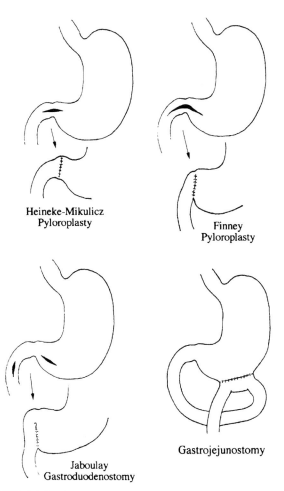

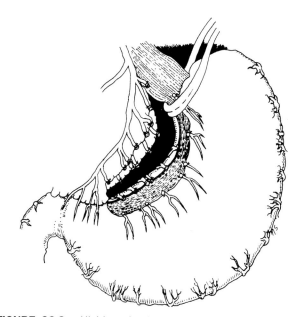

FIGURE 26-2. Methods of gastric drainage after vagotomy. *Heineke-Mikulicz pyloroplasty* is the simplest method of gastric drainage. It is most frequently used to manage duodenal ulcer bleeding, because the transpyloric incision needed to expose the bleeding ulcer can be closed easily in a transverse orientation. *Finney pyloroplasty and Jaboulay gastroduodenostomy* historically have been performed if the duodenal bulb is badly deformed by chronic ulcer scar. *Gastrojejunostomy* may be performed if access to the pyloroduodenal area is limited.

FIGURE 26-3. Highly selective vagotomy. Selective denervation of the parietal cell mass is achieved by means of careful division of all proximal anterior and posterior vagal branches distally to a point 6 to 7 cm from the pylorus. All surrounding tissues are dissected from a 5- to 6-cm segment of esophagus proximally. Antropyloric innervation must be carefully preserved to prevent postoperative gastric stasis. The bare area on the lesser curvature can be closed with seromuscular sutures, but more typically is left undisturbed.

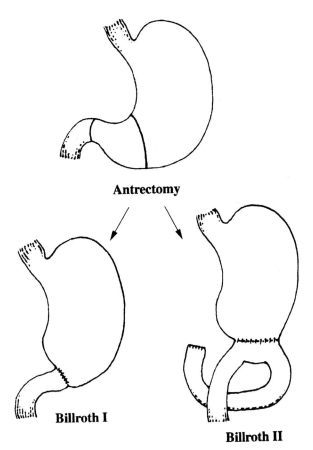

FIGURE 26-4. Reconstruction after antrectomy—Billroth I (gastroduodenostomy) and Billroth II (loop gastrojejunostomy). The Billroth I is the preferred reconstruction after gastrectomy for benign disease because it avoids the complications associated with duodenal stump closures and afferent intestinal loops.

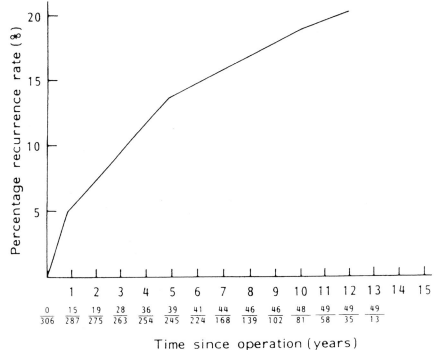

FIGURE 26-5. Ulcer recurrence rate after highly selective vagotomy increases with time after operation. Fractions below the x-axis represent the ratio of patients with recurrent ulcer to patients available for study at that postoperative time point.

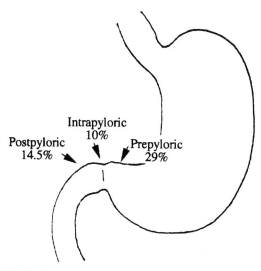

FIGURE 26-6. Ulcer recurrence rate after highly selective vagotomy according to preoperative site of ulcer. Data reported by Schafmayer and colleagues reflect a 5-year follow-up study with 392 patients. Prepyloric ulcer location appears to be associated with a higher risk for ulcer recurrence than duodenal or intrapyloric location.

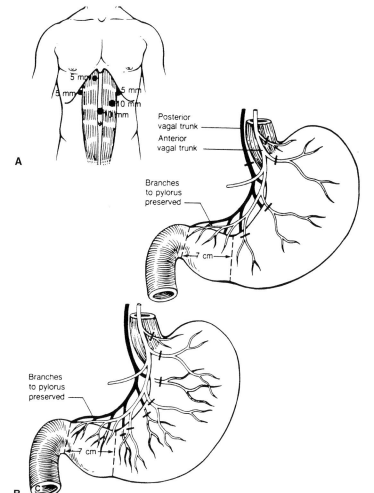

FIGURE 26-7. Laparoscopic operations for peptic ulcer. Procedures typically require five upper abdominal operative ports. Parietal cell denervation is accomplished as follows. **A:** Anterior seromyotomy and posterior truncal vagotomy (Taylor procedure) to interrupt the branches of the anterior nerve of Latarjet within the wall of the stomach. **B:** Formal highly selective vagotomy to interrupt the branches of the posterior nerve of Latarjet.

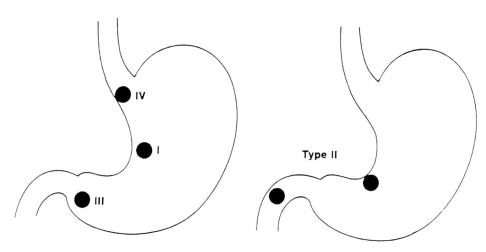

FIGURE 26-8. Gastric ulcer classification and selection of operation. Type I ulcer—antrectomy (Billroth I reconstruction); type II—highly selective vagotomy (with or without ulcer excision); type III—vagotomy and antrectomy; type IV—gastrectomy and Roux-en-Y esophagogastrojejunostomy (Csendes procedure).

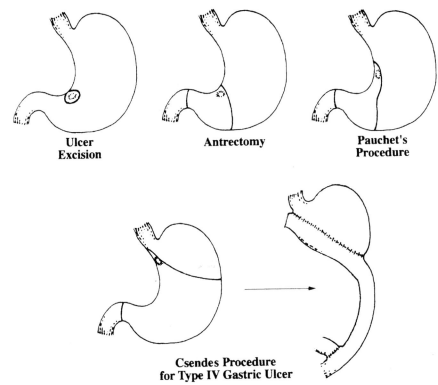

Ulcer
Excision

Antrectomy

Pauchet's
Procedure

Csendes Procedure
for Type IV Gastric Ulcer

FIGURE 26-9. Operations for benign gastric ulcer. Although ulcer excision may be technically feasible, ulcer recurrence is minimized by means of removing the ulcer en bloc with the gastric antrum. Ulcers in a more proximal location (type IV) present formidable technical challenges. Resection with esophagogastrojejunostomy reconstruction is an effective alternative to antrectomy alone, which leaves the ulcer in situ (Kelling-Madlener procedure).

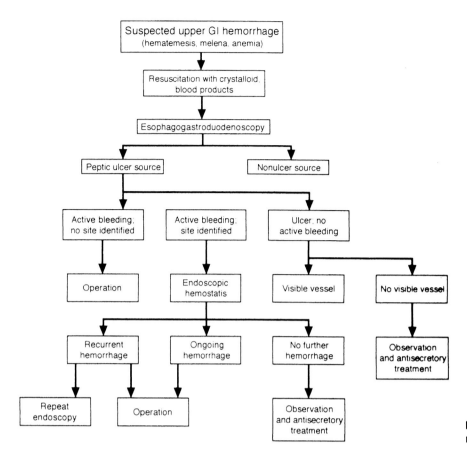

FIGURE 26-10. Algorithm for management of bleeding peptic ulcer.

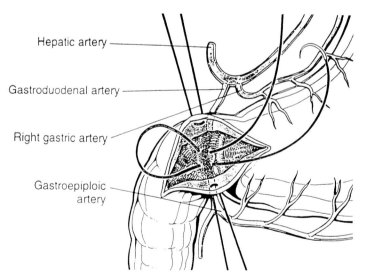

FIGURE 26-11. Suture control of bleeding posterior duodenal ulcer. Exposure is with longitudinal gastroduodenotomy. The bleeding point in the gastroduodenal artery is undersewn with nonabsorbable monofilament suture. Additional transfixing sutures along the course of the vessel above and below this point provide more secure hemostasis.

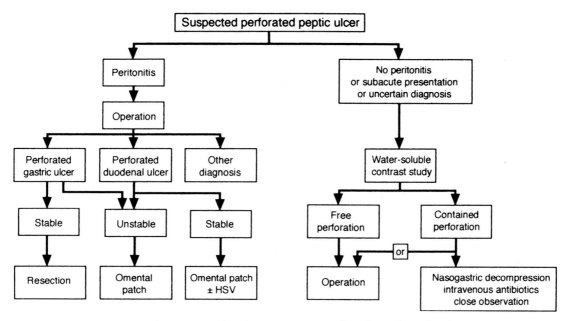

FIGURE 26-12. Algorithm for management of perforated peptic ulcer.

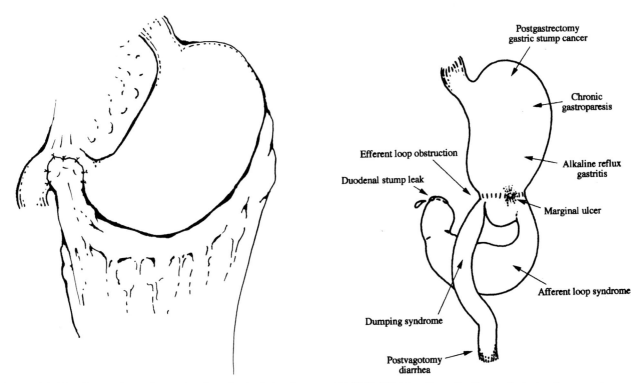

FIGURE 26-13. Omental patch repair of perforated duodenal ulcer. If no omentum is available, falciform ligament may be similarly used to patch the perforation.

FIGURE 26-14. Complications of gastrectomy and operations for peptic ulcer.

MISCELLANEOUS DISEASES OF THE STOMACH

JOHN C. RABINE* ■ TIMOTHY T. NOSTRANT

HIATAL HERNIAS

Under normal circumstances, the stomach is held in position by the gastrophrenic, gastrohepatic, gastroduodenal, and gastrosplenic ligaments. Furthermore, the phrenoesophageal membrane helps to prevent herniation through the diaphragmatic hiatus. This membrane attaches near the squamocolumnar junction and extends approximately 1 cm above the junction. During swallowing and longitudinal esophageal muscle contraction, there is "physiological" herniation of the gastric cardia through the diaphragmatic hiatus. The phrenoesophageal membrane has a recoil action to pull the squamocolumnar junction back into its normal anatomic position. When these mechanisms are defective, true herniation can develop. The most common type of hernia is the sliding, or type I, hernia. This herniation is often transient and asymptomatic, but larger hernias are often nonreducing and predispose to gastroesophageal reflux. Plain radiographs may suggest a hiatal hernia by demonstrating the presence of a large air bubble behind the cardiac silhouette (Fig. 27-1). The cardia, identified by gastric folds, will be seen extending above the diaphragmatic impression, and the gastroesophageal junction is also displaced cephalad (Fig. 27-2).

Approximately 5% of hiatal hernias are types II through IV—the paraesophageal hernias. Unlike type I hernias, these hernias are associated with fundic herniation into the thoracic cavity (i.e., alongside the gastroesophageal junction); the gastroesophageal junction may or may not be displaced as well (Figs. 27-3, 27-4, and 27-5). Although relatively uncommon, these hernias are associated with severe complications such as gastric volvulus and strangulation. In type II hernias, there is a localized phrenoesophageal membrane defect allowing the gastric fundus to become the lead point of a herniation. The gastroesophageal junction is still in proper anatomic attachment to preaortic fascia and the phrenoesophageal membrane. As more fundus herniates into the thoracic cavity, in part because of gastrocolic and gastrosplenic ligament laxity, gastric rotation can develop along the longitudinal axis

*The views expressed in this article are those of the author and do not reflect the official policy or position of the U.S. Air Force, Department of Defense, or the U.S. Government.

of the stomach. This organoaxial volvulus results in the greater curve lying anterior to the lesser curve. Type II hernias can also result in a mesenteroaxial volvulus where rotation is along the transverse axis, but this is much less common. Type III hernias are a combination of types I and II; the fundus herniates through the hiatus, but stretching of the phrenoesophageal membrane results in displacement of the gastroesophageal junction above the diaphragm as well. Type IV hernias are rare and involve a massive hiatal defect that results in herniation of abdominal organs (colon, small bowel, spleen, and pancreas) into the thoracic cavity.

GASTRIC VOLVULUS

A volvulus of the stomach occurs when one portion of the stomach twists around another. If the twist occurs around an imaginary line between the pylorus and the gastroesophageal junction, it is an organoaxial volvulus (Figs. 27-6A and 27-7). Typically, the greater curve spins upward such that the stomach appears "upside-down" with the true posterior wall lying anteriorly. The antrum rotates anteriorly and superiorly while the fundus is displaced posteriorly and inferiorly. Alternatively, a mesenteroaxial volvulus develops when the distal stomach twists around an imaginary line between the center of the greater curve and the porta hepatis (see Fig. 27-6B). The antrum and distal body twist to the right (anteriorly and superiorly) such that the posterior wall again becomes anterior in placement.

GASTRIC BEZOARS

Bezoars are collections of foreign material that are retained most frequently within the stomach but have also been found in the esophagus and rectum (Figs. 27-8 and 27-9). Such matter may include plant and vegetable debris (phytobezoar), hair (trichobezoar), medications (pharmacobezoar), and persimmons (diospyrobezoar). Concretions are a type of bezoar that are typically very hard. Shellac, furniture polish, and concrete are classical components of such a bezoar, and surgery may be necessary to remove concretions; other therapies are generally ineffective. The formation of bezoars is likely multifactorial, and altered gastric motility and emptying are the primary etiologies. The size and digestibility of swallowed material are factors as well. Prior gastric surgery, whether pyloroplasty, antrectomy, or partial gastrectomy, clearly places patients at risk for phytobezoar or fungus ball formation. In addition to surgery, gastric stasis and bezoars have been linked to diabetic gastroparesis, mixed connective tissue disease, hypothyroidism, and myotonic dystrophy.

HETEROTOPIC PANCREAS

Heterotopic pancreatic tissue, also termed a "pancreatic rest," can be found in the stomach, duodenum, or jejunum. Typically, these rests are asymptomatic, but abdominal pain, nausea, vomiting, and rarely bleeding have been attributed to rests located in the stomach. These lesions typically appear as 2- to 4-cm submucosal masses in the prepyloric region, and it is not unusual that central umbilication is noted (Fig. 27-10). The nodules are firm and may have a yellow appearance.

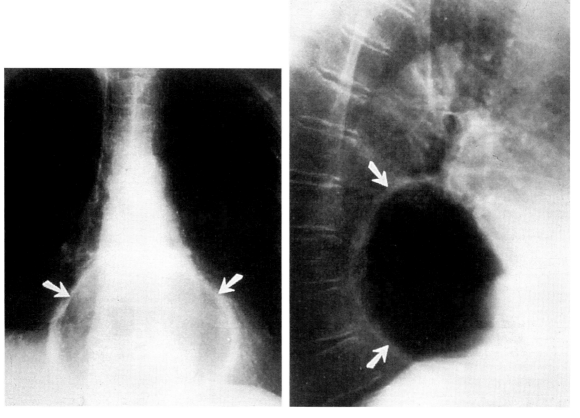

FIGURE 27-1. Appearance of a large hiatal hernia (*arrows*) on a routine chest radiograph.

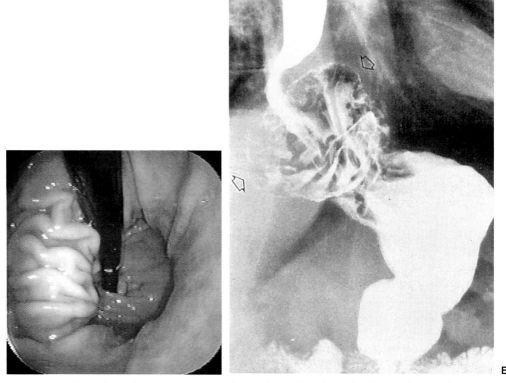

FIGURE 27-2.   A: Endoscopic view of a type I hiatal hernia while in gastric retroflexion.
B: Appearance of a large hiatal hernia on a barium examination.

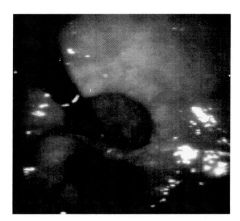

FIGURE 27-3. Endoscopic view of a paraesophageal hernia while in gastric retroflexion. The fundus is herniating into the thoracic cavity alongside a concomitant type I hernia.

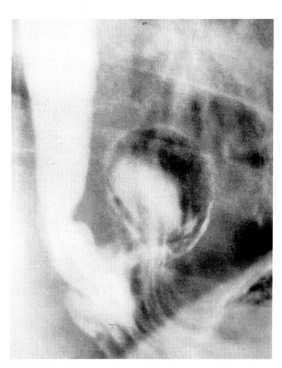

FIGURE 27-4. Paraesophageal hernia on barium radiograph.

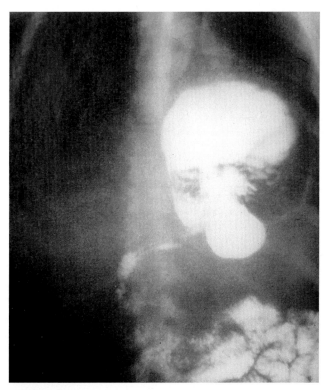

FIGURE 27-5. Type II paraesophageal hernia where the gastroesophageal junction remains below the diaphragm. The entire stomach has herniated into the chest, illustrating an "upside-down" appearance.

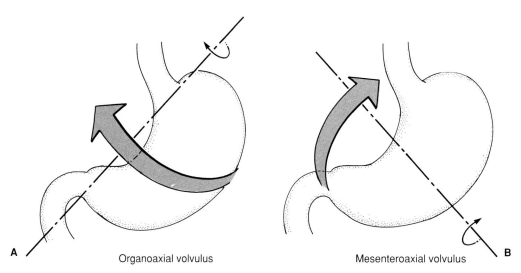

Organoaxial volvulus   Mesenteroaxial volvulus

FIGURE 27-6. Schematic representation of organoaxial volvulus (**A**) and mesenteroaxial volvulus (**B**).

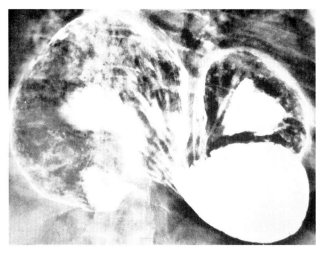

FIGURE 27-7. Organoaxial volvulus associated with a large hiatal hernia.

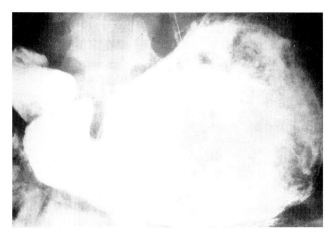

FIGURE 27-8. Large gastric bezoar.

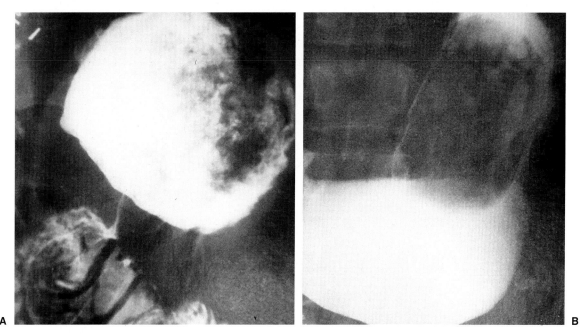

FIGURE 27-9. **A:** Gastric phytobezoar on barium examination. **B:** Glue concretion in a model airplane builder.

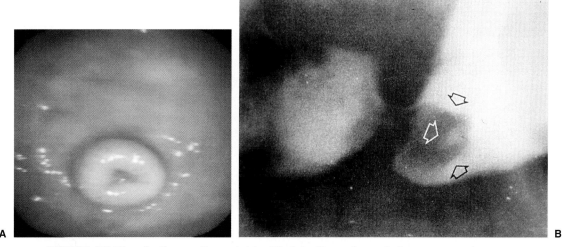

FIGURE 27-10. **A:** Pancreatic rest identified in the antrum during upper endoscopy. **B:** Radiographic appearance of a pancreatic rest with an antral filling defect (*black arrows*), and the *white arrow* denotes central filling with barium.

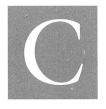

C SMALL INTESTINE

28

SMALL INTESTINE: Anatomy and Structural Anomalies

DEBORAH C. RUBIN ■ **JACOB C. LANGER**

EMBRYOLOGY OF THE SMALL INTESTINE

The primitive human gut forms when the dorsal part of the yolk sac is incorporated into the embryo at 4 weeks of development, giving rise to the foregut, midgut, and hindgut. The foregut is the progenitor of the esophagus, stomach, duodenum up to the biliary duct ampulla, pharynx, respiratory tract, liver, pancreas, and biliary tract. The midgut gives rise to the duodenum distal to the common bile duct, jejunum, ileum, cecum, appendix, ascending colon, and one half to two thirds of the transverse colon. The rest of the colon and superior anal canal are derived from the hindgut.

The gut endoderm is the precursor of the gastrointestinal tract epithelium. Its endothelium arises from the ectoderm of the stomodeum and proctodeum as well as the endoderm. The splanchnic mesenchyme supplies the muscular and connective tissue components of the gastrointestinal tract. The midgut first freely communicates with the yolk sac and then narrows to be connected by the omphalomesenteric or vitelline duct. The primitive gut forms a U-shaped loop that grows so rapidly compared with the embryo that it herniates into the umbilical cord at the sixth week of gestation (Fig. 28-1). The proximal limb of the loop elongates into multiple intestinal loops, whereas the distal limb simply develops into the cecal diverticulum. The first stage of rotation is 90° counterclockwise around the superior mesenteric artery axis. At 10 weeks, the intestines return into the abdominal cavity and rotate a further 180° counterclockwise in the second stage. Finally, the cecum and appendix descend from the right upper quadrant to the right lower quadrant, and the proximal part of the colon elongates to form the hepatic flexure and ascending colon (third stage of rotation). Fixation occurs as the ascending colonic mesentery fuses with the parietal peritoneum and becomes fixed retroperitoneally. The mesentery of the small intestine attains a broad-based attachment to the posterior abdominal wall and extends from the duodenojejunal junction to the ileocecal region. The end result of this process is the normal location of the small and large intestines.

CONGENITAL ANOMALIES

A brief review of the main features of the common congenital anomalies is presented and illustrated with pictures of surgical specimens.

Meckel Diverticulum

Meckel diverticulum is the most common congenital anomaly of the gastrointestinal tract. It results from failure of the vitelline duct to be completely resorbed (Fig. 28-2). Large autopsy series indicate a 2% to 3% prevalence of Meckel diverticulum in the general population. Meckel diverticula are true diverticula, containing all layers of the bowel from serosa to mucosa. Heterotopic tissue is present approximately 50% of the time and includes gastric mucosa, pancreatic tissue, and less commonly, colonic mucosa, Brunner glands, and jejunal or hepatobiliary tissue. The presence of heterotopic mucosa correlates with increased risk for symptomatic, complicated Meckel diverticulum.

The complications of Meckel diverticulum include bleeding, intestinal obstruction, diverticulitis, perforation, and carcinoma. The frequency of specific complications varies between adult and pediatric patients. Among children, the most common complications are gastrointestinal bleeding and obstruction. For adults, intestinal obstruction is by far the most frequent complication, and gastrointestinal bleeding is rare.

The diagnosis of Meckel diverticulum remains a challenge. Sodium pertechnetate technetium 99m radionuclide scanning is particularly useful in the care of children. This isotope is taken up into gastric mucosal cells and can help detect Meckel diverticula that contain ectopic gastric mucosa. Other examinations include enteroclysis and angiography, which may show the vitelline artery.

Management of complicated Meckel diverticulum is surgical. The management of asymptomatic Meckel diverticulum that is an incidental finding remains controversial, although prophylactic removal seems to be safe and produces low morbidity and mortality rates.

Duplications

Duplications of the gastrointestinal tract are rare congenital cystic anomalies attached to the intestinal mesenteric border (Fig. 28-3). Duplications may occur anywhere along the gastrointestinal tract, although those of small bowel origin are usually found in the ileum. Most duplications are diagnosed during infancy and early childhood, but duplications are occasionally newly discovered in adults. Symptoms in childhood include abdominal pain, obstructive symptoms, and hemorrhage. Adults frequently have no symptoms or have mild abdominal symptoms. Intussusception, gastrointestinal hemorrhage, or carcinoma occasionally develops in adults. Detection may be difficult. Small bowel follow-through shows a duplication only if the lumen of the normal intestine communicates with the duplication. Ultrasonography or computed tomographic scanning is valuable for detecting a cystic mass. Duplications are managed surgically.

Intestinal Atresia and Stenosis

Intestinal atresia is a condition in which segments of the lumen contain areas of total occlusion (Figs. 28-4 and 28-5). Atresia is one of the common causes of intestinal obstruction among neonates. Atresia may be single or multiple and is found from esophagus to rectum. The prevalence is from 1 in 3000 to 1 in 5000 live births. In type I atresia, a membranous septum or diaphragm of mucosa and submucosa obstructs the lumen, but the intestinal wall and mesentery are intact. Type II is characterized by two blind bowel ends connected by a fibrous cord with intact mesentery in between (see Fig. 28-4). In type IIIa lesions (see Fig. 28-5), two blind bowel ends are separated by a mesenteric gap. Type IIIb is "apple peel" atresia, in which there is proximal atresia in the small intestine and absence of the distal superior mesenteric artery (less than 5% of all instances of atresia). In this case, the bowel distal to the atresia is foreshortened and coiled, and receives retrograde blood supply from the ileocolic, right colic, or inferior mesenteric artery. Type IV denotes multiple areas of atresia throughout the small bowel, which have the appearance of a string of sausages; the atresia may be type I, II, or IIIa.

Polyhydramnios is frequently detected in proximal gastrointestinal atresia, but amniotic fluid may be normal in distal atresia. Bilious vomiting soon after birth is a characteristic symptom of proximal atresia, whereas abdominal distention, later vomiting, and failure to pass meconium are found in distal atresia. Diagnosis may be made by means of prenatal ultrasonography followed by plain radiography, and cautious contrast radiography after birth and before surgical intervention.

Gastroschisis and Omphalocele

Gastroschisis occurs when there is a small defect in the abdominal wall through which there is massive evisceration of the intestines (Fig. 28-6). The bowel has no membranous covering, has been exposed to amniotic fluid in utero, is thickened, and is covered with adhesions. Omphalocele occurs when the abdominal viscera herniate through the umbilical ring and persist outside the body covered by a membranous sac but not by skin (Fig. 28-7). Omphalocele is associated with a variety of other anomalies of chromosomal origin. The diagnosis of an abdominal wall defect is suggested by the presence of a high maternal serum α-fetoprotein level. Prenatal ultrasonography also is a sensitive method of prenatal diagnosis. Prenatal detection allows for obstetric planning so that the patient can be at a tertiary care facility for delivery. Treatment is surgical by means of primary closure, or use of a silo or polymeric silicone sac.

Volvulus

Volvulus is abnormal twisting of the intestine around the axis of its own mesentery, resulting in obstruction of the more proximal bowel (Fig. 28-8). The twisting of the mesentery may involve the mesenteric vessels and make the involved loop particularly susceptible to strangulation and gangrene. In the United States, volvulus of the small intestine is usually caused by a preexisting defect such as an anomaly of rotation and fixation, postoperative adhesion, or congenital bands. Patients have symptoms of obstruction of the small intestine and an acute abdomen. The severity of pain may be out of proportion to the physical findings, which include abdominal distention, rebound tenderness, guarding and rigidity, and a palpable abdominal mass. The diagnosis is made with plain abdominal radiographs, which may demonstrate distended bowel with air-fluid levels consistent with obstruction or free air from a perforation. Barium studies can be useful in depicting disorders of rotation. A typical corkscrew-like appearance of barium in the distorted duodenum and jejunum also is diagnostic. Angiography may reveal twisting of the branches of the superior mesenteric artery. Rapid recognition of volvulus and prompt surgical intervention are the keys to decreasing the fatality rate associated with this condition.

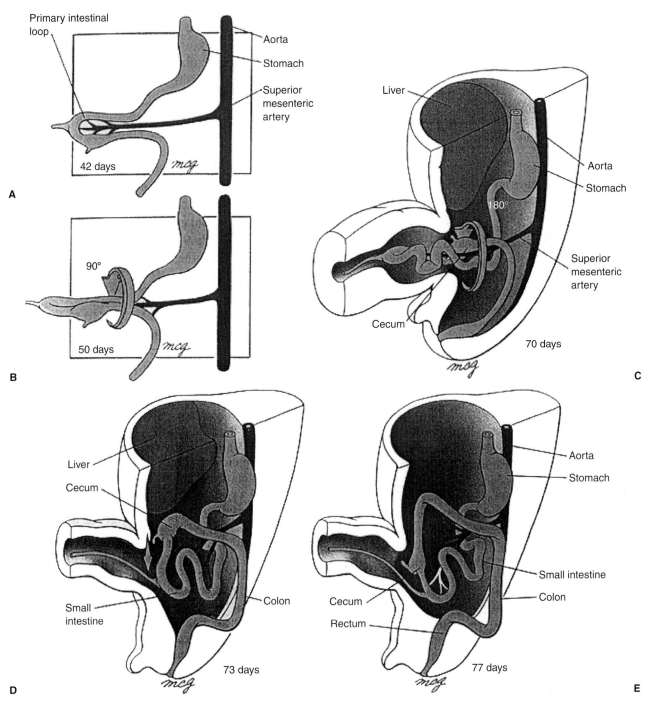

FIGURE 28-1. Herniation and rotation of the intestine. **A, B:** At the end of the sixth week, the primary intestinal loop herniates into the umbilicus, rotating through 90° counterclockwise (in frontal view). **C:** The small intestine elongates to form jejunal-ileal loops, the cecum and appendix grow, and at the end of the 10th week, the primary intestinal loop retracts into the abdominal cavity rotating an additional 180° counterclockwise. **D, E:** During the 11th week, the retracting midgut completes this rotation as the cecum is positioned just inferior to the liver. The cecum is then displaced inferiorly, pulling down the proximal hindgut to form the ascending colon. The descending colon is simultaneously fixed on the left side of the posterior abdominal wall. The jejunum, ileum, and transverse and sigmoid colons remain suspended by mesentery.

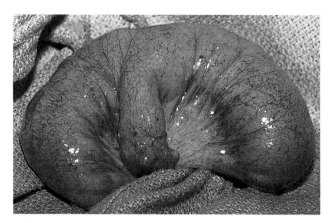

FIGURE 28-2. Meckel diverticulum. These true diverticula contain all layers of the intestinal wall. Ectopic gastric mucosa may appear as small, red nodules.

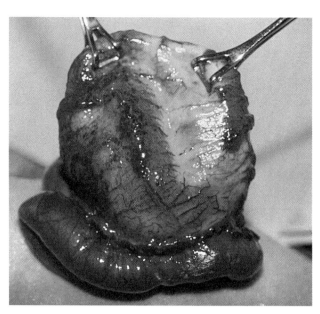

FIGURE 28-3. Jejunal duplication. Duplications are present on the mesenteric border and share a common blood supply with the adjacent bowel.

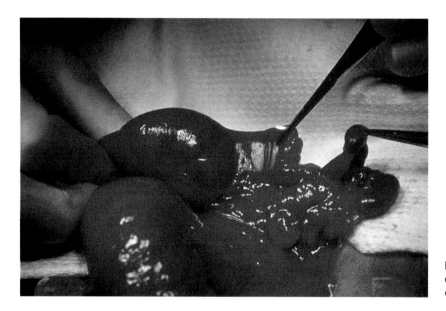

FIGURE 28-4. Jejunal atresia, type II. A cordlike fibrous segment connects the two ends of intestine.

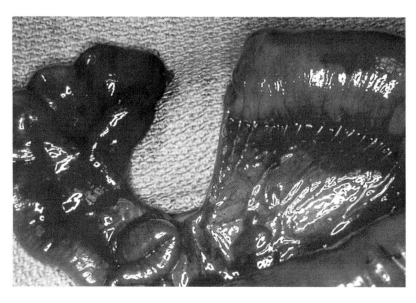

FIGURE 28-5. Atresia of the small intestine, type IIIa. There is complete separation of the blind ends of the small bowel and a mesenteric gap.

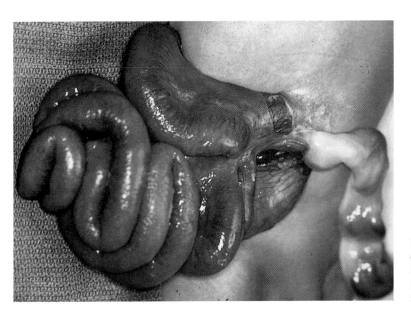

FIGURE 28-6. Gastroschisis. Multiple loops of exteriorized small intestine are depicted. The bowel is often dilated, edematous, and thickened, presumably because of direct exposure to amniotic fluid.

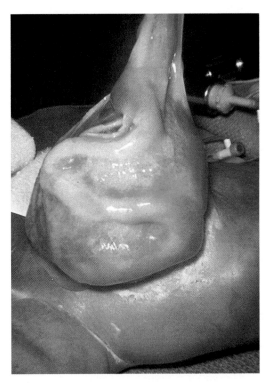

FIGURE 28-7. Omphalocele. Loops of intestine sit in a thin-walled sac composed of umbilical cord coverings.

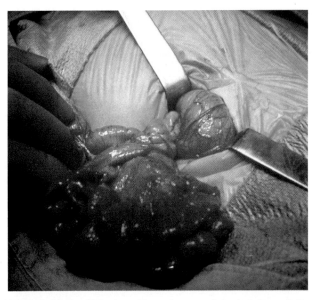

FIGURE 28-8. Volvulus. There is complete twisting of the small bowel around the axis of its mesentery. Although in this case the loops of small intestine appear normal, ischemia or frank necrosis of the intestine may be present.

29

DYSMOTILITY OF THE SMALL AND LARGE INTESTINE

MICHAEL CAMILLERI ■ SILVIA DELGADO-AROS

Motility of the digestive tract is the result of the myoelectric activity, contractile activity, tone, compliance, and transit. The correct function of all of these components of the motility of the small intestine ensures the appropriate absorption of the nutrients, propels the bolus through the intestine, and prevents bacterial overgrowth. Properly functioning colonic motility is particularly important to prevent diarrhea and constipation.

Motility is controlled by the enteric nervous system (ENS), which is modified by extrinsic nerves as well as gastrointestinal hormones. The effects of these neurons on the gut muscle rely partly on interstitial cells of Cajal (ICC). Dysfunctions in any of these components may cause intestinal or colonic dysmotility (Fig. 29-1).

Diseases that affect gastrointestinal smooth muscle include primary visceral myopathies, collagen diseases, muscular dystrophies, amyloidosis, and thyroid disease (Table 29-1). Enteric nerve dysfunction occurs in primary visceral neuropathies, Hirschsprung disease, diabetes mellitus, Chagas disease, ganglioneuromatosis, paraneoplastic visceral neuropathy, and Parkinson disease. Small intestine and colonic dysmotility may be also caused by drugs (such as phenothiazines, tricyclic antidepressants, ganglionic blockers, and narcotics) and occurs among patients with jejunoileal bypass and celiac disease. The effect of gastrointestinal hormones on the motility of the small and large intestine is manifested clinically by diarrhea in patients with carcinoid syndrome and irritable bowel syndrome. These syndromes are associated with elevated circulating serotonin levels and rapid intestinal transit that may partly reflect abnormal motor function and/or abnormal intestinal secretion.

Regardless of the underlying causes, patients with dysmotility of the small intestine and colon may have a wide range of clinical manifestations. Patients may be asymptomatic, or at the other end of the spectrum, they may present with chronic intestinal pseudoobstruction. Between the two extremes, patients may have dyspeptic symptoms, including intermittent postprandial epigastric or periumbilical abdominal pain, bloating, nausea, vomiting, and diarrhea or constipation. Intestinal bacterial overgrowth occurs in severe cases of intestinal dysmotility and results in steatorrhea and sometimes diarrhea. Symptoms tend to occur in the postprandial period. Extraintestinal manifestations of the underlying disease may be detected among patients with the secondary causes of small intestine and colonic dysmotility.

Small intestine dysmotility seems to occur less frequently in comparison with colonic dysmotility. However, the lack of validated tests to evaluate small intestine motility makes it difficult to precisely estimate the prevalence. Novel techniques are being developed to improve measurements of the motor function of the small intestine that may help to diagnose and better estimate the prevalence of these dysfunctions. In contrast, constipation affects 12% to 15% of the population and Hirschsprung disease; the prototypic congenital colonic dysmotility affects 1 in 5000 births. This chapter reviews primary and secondary causes of small intestine and colon motility diseases.

PRIMARY CAUSES

Visceral Myopathies

Familial Visceral Myopathies

Familial visceral myopathies (FVMs) are a group of genetic diseases characterized by degeneration and fibrosis of the gastrointestinal smooth muscle and, in certain types, the urinary smooth muscle. There are at least three reported types of FVM based on gross lesions of the gastrointestinal tract and the pattern of inheritance (Table 29-2). Well-documented mitochondrial and gene alterations exist in type II FVM, also called mitochondrial neurogastrointestinal encephalomyopathy syndrome (MNGIE). On routine pathological examination, the histological findings in all three types of FVM are similar and are characterized by degenerated muscle cells and fibrosis. Recognition of milder lesions may be facilitated by use of trichrome stain (Fig. 29-2). Intestinal manometric studies on patients with FVM reveal low-amplitude (usually less than 20 mm Hg and on average less than 10 mm Hg) intestinal contractions (Fig. 29-3). Recent advances in type II FVM or MNGIE warrant a more detailed discussion of this entity.

Type II FVM (MNGIE)

This entity forms part of a heterogeneous group of disorders that result from structural, biochemical, or genetic derangements of mitochondria. MNGIE has an autosomal recessive inheritance and it is characterized by gastrointestinal dysmotility, ophthalmoplegia, peripheral neuropathy, and on skeletal muscle biopsy, ragged red fibers demonstrated best on Gomori trichrome stain (Fig. 29-4). Additional clinical features include lactic acidosis, increased cerebrospinal fluid protein, and leukodystrophy, which is identified by magnetic resonance imaging of the brain. The ubiquity of mitochondria explains the association of neuromuscular, gastrointestinal, and other nonneuromuscular symptoms that are characteristic of this syndrome. Some patients have been found to have multiple mitochondrial DNA deletions in skeletal muscle. Mitochondrial DNA contains genes that encode polypeptides that are components of the cellular oxidative phosphorylation system. Nuclear genes, however, also encode for components of this system. It is believed that mutations of nuclear DNA genes that control the expression of the mitochondrial genome are the underlying genetic defect of this syndrome. It was proposed that a unique gene located in the long arm of chromosome 22 (22q13.32-qter), distal to locus D22S1161, is responsible for this syndrome.

Childhood Visceral Myopathies

Two distinct forms of childhood visceral myopathies (CVM) have been recognized (Table 29-3); the second is identified by the phenotype of megacystis-microcolon-intestinal hypoperistalsis. These two diseases differ from FVM in their clinical manifestations and modes of inheritance. Degeneration and fibrosis of gastrointestinal and urinary smooth muscle can be detected in both types of CVM and result in bowel dilation (Fig. 29-5), ureteropelvicaliectasis (Fig. 29-6), or megacystis, which results from bladder degeneration (Fig. 29-7).

Nonfamilial Visceral Myopathies

It is unclear whether cases of nonfamilial visceral myopathy among adults represent sporadic cases or unrecognized variants of FVM with a recessive pattern of inheritance. There is no histological difference between the familial and the nonfamilial forms of visceral myopathy, and both show low-amplitude contractions when investigated with intestinal manometry.

Visceral Neuropathies

The ENS is a vast network of ganglionated plexuses located in the wall of the gastrointestinal tract and it is in close contact with ICC. Normal migration, differentiation, and subsequent survival or maintenance of the precursor cells of the ENS derived from the neural crest has been demonstrated to be crucial for the normal function of the intestine. Different genetic defects in migration, differentiation, and maintenance of enteric neurons have been identified in several causes of gut dysmotility (Table 29-4). These include abnormalities of RET, the gene that encodes for the tyrosine kinase (Trk) receptor; the endothelin B system (which tends to retard development of neural elements, thereby facilitating colonization of the entire gut from the neural crest), Sox-10 (a transcription factor that enhances maturation of neural precursors), and c-Kit, which is a marker for ICCs. Disturbances in these mechanisms result in syndromic dysmotilities such as Hirschsprung disease, Waardenburg syndrome (pigmentary defects, piebaldism, neural deafness, and megacolon), and idiopathic hypertrophic pyloric stenosis. Figure 29-8 demonstrates some of the mutations in the Trk receptor that have been reported in gut dysmotility associated with familial or sporadic medullary carcinoma of the thyroid, multiple endocrine neoplasia type 2A or B (Fig. 29-9), and Hirschsprung disease.

The effects of motor neurons on the gastrointestinal and colonic muscle cells are relayed at least in part via the ICCs, which are electrically coupled to the muscle (Figs. 29-10 and 29-11). They have receptors for the inhibitory transmitters vasoactive intestinal peptide (VIP) and nitric oxide (NO) and for the excitatory tachykinin transmitters. The protooncogene c-*kit* encodes a transmembrane TrK receptor c-Kit. Activation of this receptor is responsible for the development of the ICCs. Disruption of ICCs by treatment of neonatal rats with antibodies to c-Kit receptor impairs excitatory and inhibitory transmission to the circular muscle of the small and large intestine. ICCs have also been recognized as the pacemaker cells of the gut because they generate physiological slow waves in the gastrointestinal tract. Slow waves are the rhythmic oscillations of the membrane potential that characterize the electrical activity of gut muscle. Slow waves are the rate-limiting step for contractile function in the smooth muscle cells. Contraction typically occurs when there is superimposition of spike bursts on the slow waves. The relevance of these functions of ICCs as neuromodulators and "pacemakers" of the gut is highlighted by the several examples of gut motility dysfunction associated with anomalous ICCs. A smaller number of ICCs were found in slow-transit constipation (Figs. 29-12 and 29-13), and abnormal distribution of these cells has been found in Hirschsprung disease. Variants of enteric neuropathic dysmotility, such as hypoganglionosis, immature ganglia, neuronal intestinal dysplasia, and infantile pyloric stenosis, as well as in chronic and transient intestinal pseudoobstruction, also have been observed. A diminished number, altered networks, and altered ultrastructural features of gastric ICCs have been demonstrated in diabetic mice with gastroparesis (Fig. 29-14).

Visceral neuropathy may result in bowel dilation (Fig. 29-15), although this is generally less frequent or less severe than in visceral myopathy. In Hirschsprung disease, the aganglionic segment is permanently contracted, causing dilation proximal to it (Fig. 29-16). Intestinal manometry is characterized by normal-amplitude contractions with evidence of incoordination in, for example, the propagation of fasting migrating motor complexes (MMCs), or recurrence of MMC-like activity in the first postprandial hour.

Familial Visceral Neuropathies

Familial visceral neuropathies (FVNs) are a group of genetic diseases characterized by degeneration of the enteric nervous system. Two distinct phenotypes, I and II, have been distinguished, which are summarized in Table 29-5.

Hirschsprung Disease (Congenital Megacolon)

Aganglionosis is caused by arrest of the caudal migration of cells from the neural crest, which is destined to develop as the gut's intramural plexuses. In Hirschsprung disease, the aganglionic segment always extends from the internal anal sphincter for a variable distance proximally; in most instances, it stays within the rectum and sigmoid colon ("classical type"), although involvement of very short segments and longer segments or the entire colon have also been described. The genetic disorders resulting in altered development of the neural crest in Hirschsprung disease have been discussed in detail above (see Table 29-4). The defect occurs once in each 5000 live births and is in some cases familial, with an overall incidence of 3.6% among siblings of index cases. Although most children have major manifestations before the second month of life, very short segment aganglionosis may not cause severe symptoms until after infancy. Mucosal suction biopsy can rule out the disease if submucosal ganglia are present. However, the absence of ganglion cells does not establish the diagnosis, and a deep or full-thickness biopsy from at least 3 cm proximal to the pectinate line should be obtained. Ganglia may be absent from the deep and superficial submucosal layers for even longer distances, and myenteric ganglia may also be absent in normal infants over that distance proximal to the internal sphincter. A very short aganglionic segment may be missed by biopsy and x-ray films. In these cases, the absence of internal sphincter relaxation in response to rectal distention may help to confirm the diagnosis. However, distention of a balloon in a dilated rectum (that is, for chronic constipation or megarectum) may be associated with a false-positive result, because the intrarectal balloon may not sufficiently distend the rectum to elicit the reflex relaxation of the internal anal sphincter.

Idiopathic Nonfamilial Visceral Neuropathies (Chronic Neuropathic Intestinal Pseudoobstruction of Idiopathic Variety)

Damage to the myenteric plexus can occur for a variety of different reasons, including chemical exposure, drug use, and viral infections. Patients with idiopathic nonfamilial visceral neuropathy may have dysmotility at any level of the gastrointestinal tract present with features of chronic intestinal pseudoobstruction, and a useful screening test is a solid-phase gastric emptying test. The intestine may be dilated but shows active, nonperistaltic contractions. Histological examination of the myenteric plexus shows a reduction in the total number of neurons; the remaining neurons may be enlarged with thick, clubbed processes. An increase in the number of Schwann cells and hypertrophy of the muscularis propria may also be observed. In colonic inertia patients, the ICCs are reduced in number and are morphologically abnormal. The precise mechanism and neurotransmitter deficiencies of this disorder are unclear. Table 29-6 summarizes information from a number of studies in the literature regarding histological changes that have been found in patients with slow transit constipation severe enough to warrant subtotal colectomy. In less severe cases, differentiation from constipation-predominant irritable bowel syndrome may be difficult, especially when the gut is not dilated. Features of intestinal manometry mimic those of familial and secondary neuropathies (Fig. 29-17). In slow-transit constipation, colonic manometry shows a reduction in high-amplitude peristaltic waves.

SECONDARY CAUSES

Several systemic diseases may involve the digestive tract and result in intestinal dysmotility, although gastrointestinal manifestations rarely are the presenting feature. These secondary dysmotilities include diseases involving the intestinal smooth muscle; that is, collagen diseases (such as scleroderma, dermatomyositis, systemic lupus erythematosus, and mixed connective tissue disease) (Fig. 29-18), muscular dystrophy, and amyloidosis. Secondary intestinal dysmotility may also occur in diseases with associated neurological derangement (diabetic neuropathy, Chagas disease, Parkinson disease, neurofibromatosis, and paraneoplastic visceral neuropathy), endocrine disorders (diabetes mellitus, thyroid and parathyroid disease), drug-induced conditions (by phenothiazines, tricyclic antidepressants, antiparkinsonian drugs, ganglionic blockers, and narcotics), and miscellaneous diseases (celiac disease, radiation enteritis, immunoproliferative disorders, jejunoileal bypass, and postgastrointestinal viral infection) (see Figs. 29-17 and 29-19).

(figures begin on page 305)

TABLE 29-1
Causes of Gut Dysmotility

Primary causes
Visceral myopathies
   Familial visceral myopathies: type I, II (MNGIE), III
   Childhood visceral myopathies: type I, II (megacystis-microcolon-intestinal hypoperistalsis)
   Nonfamilial visceral myopathies
Visceral neuropathies
   Familial visceral neuropathies: type I, II
   Hirschsprung disease
   Idiopathic nonfamilial visceral neuropathies
Secondary causes
Disease involving the intestinal smooth muscle
   Collagen diseases (e.g., scleroderma, dermatomyositis, systemic lupus erythematosus, mixed connective tissue disease)
   Muscular dystrophies (e.g., myotonic dystrophy, Duchenne muscular dystrophy)
   Amyloidosis
Neurological diseases
   Chagas disease, ganglioneuromatosis of the intestine, paraneoplastic neuropathy, Parkinson disease, spinal cord injury
Endocrine disorders
   Diabetes mellitus, thyroid disease (i.e., hyperthyroidism, hypothyroidism), hypoparathyroidism
Pharmacologic agents
   Phenothiazines, tricyclic antidepressants, anti-parkinsonian medications, ganglionic blockers, clonidine, narcotics (morphine and meperidine)
Miscellaneous intestinal disorders
   Celiac disease
   Radiation enteritis
   Diffuse lymphoid infiltration of the small intestine
   Jejunoileal bypass
   Postgastrointestinal viral infection

MNGIE, mitochondrial neurogastrointestinal encephalomyopathy syndrome.

TABLE 29-2
Classification of Familial Visceral Myopathies

CHARACTERISTICS	TYPE I	TYPE II (MNGIE)	TYPE III
Mode of transmission	Autosomal dominant	Autosomal recessive; isolated cases	Autosomal recessive
Gross lesions	Esophageal dilation, megaduodenum, redundant colon, and megacystis	Gastric dilation, slight dilation of the entire small intestine with numerous diverticula	Marked dilation of the entire digestive tract from the esophagus to the rectum
Microscopic changes	Degeneration and fibrosis of both muscle layers	Gastric dilation, slight dilation of the entire small intestine with numerous diverticula	Marked dilation of the entire digestive tract from the esophagus to the rectum
Clinical manifestations			
Age at onset	After the first decade	Teens	Middle age
Percentage symptomatic	<50%	>75%	>75%
Symptoms of CIP	Variable severity	Severe plus pain	Classic CIP
Extra-GI manifestations	Megacystis, uterine inertia, and mydriasis	Ptosis and external ophthalmoplegia, muscle pain, peripheral neuropathy, and deafness	None observed
Treatment, prognosis	Prognosis good ± surgery	No effective medical or surgical treatment; prognosis poor	No effective medical or surgical treatment; prognosis poor

CIP; chronic intestinal pseudoobstruction; GI, gastrointestinal; MNGIE, mitochondrial neurogastrointestinal encephalomyopathy syndrome.

TABLE 29-3
Classification of Childhood Visceral Myopathies

CHARACTERISTICS	TYPE I	TYPE II (MEGACYSTIS-MICROCOLON-INTESTINAL HYPOPERISTALSIS)
Mode of transmission	Autosomal recessive (?)	Autosomal recessive (?)
Gross lesions	Dilation of entire GI tract	Short, malrotated small intestine and malfixation of microcolon
Microscopic changes	Degeneration and fibrosis of GI and urinary smooth muscle cells	Vacuolar degeneration of GI and urinary smooth muscle cells
Clinical manifestations		
Age of onset	Infancy and young childhood	Infancy
Gender	Both	Predominantly female
Symptoms	Constipation, distention ± CIP	Obstipation, intestinal pseudoobstruction
Extra-GI manifestations	Megacystis and mega-ureters	Megacystis and mega-ureters
Treatment, prognosis	No effective medication; prognosis poor	No effective Rx; prognosis poor

CIP, chronic intestinal pseudoobstruction; GI, gastrointestinal.

TABLE 29-4

Genetic Defects Identified in Different Causes of Gut Dysmotility

GENETIC DEFECT	PHENOTYPE	ASSOCIATED NON-GI DISEASE	DYSMOTILITY: PREVALENCE IN PHENOTYPE
RET/GDNF	Hirschsprung	None in humans	20%–50% *RET*, 5% *GDNF*
ET-3/ET-B	Hirschsprung or megacolon	Waardenburg-Shah	5%–10% Hirschsprung
SOX-10	Hirschsprung	Waardenburg-Shah	?
c-kit	?CIP/Hirschsprung	None	?

CIP, chronic intestinal pseudoobstruction; GI, gastrointestinal.

TABLE 29-5

Classification of Familial Visceral Neuropathies

CHARACTERISTICS	TYPE I	TYPE II
Mode of transmission	Autosomal dominant	Autosomal recessive
Gross lesions	Dilation of lengths of small intestine, often distal small bowel; megacolon; gastroparesis in ~25% of patients	Hypertrophic pyloric stenosis, dilated short small intestine, malrotation of small intestine
Microscopic changes	Degeneration of argyrophilic neurons and decreased numbers of nerve fibers	Deficiency of argyrophilic neurons and increased neuroblasts
Clinical manifestations		
Age of onset	Any age	Infancy
Percentage symptomatic	>75%	100%
Symptoms	~67% CIP	All CIP
Extra-GI manifestations	None	± Malformation of CNS, patent ductus arteriosus
Treatment, prognosis	No effective medical or surgical treatment; prognosis fair	No effective medical or surgical treatment; prognosis poor

CIP, chronic intestinal pseudoobstruction; CNS, central nervous system; GI, gastrointestinal.

TABLE 29-6

Colonic Neuropathology in Slow Transit Constipation

Histological and immunohistochemical findings

    Decreased number or abnormal appearance of silver staining neurons or axons; increased number of variably sized nuclei within ganglia

    Decreased colonic VIP nerves

    Decreased neurofilament staining in myenteric plexus in 75% of patients; 17/29 entire colon affected; 12/29 segmental involvement

    Increased number of PGP 9.5 reactive nerve fibers in muscularis layer of ascending and descending colon

    Decreased total nerve density in myenteric plexus; decreased VIP and increased NO positive neurons

    Decreased substance P nerves in 7/10 patients; decreased VIP nerves in 4/7 patients

    Decreased substance P in mucosa and submucosa of rectal biopsies

    Increased VIP, substance P and galanin in ascending colon; increased VIP and galanin in transverse colon; increased VIP and neuropeptide Y in descending colon myenteric plexus; decreased VIP in submucosa

    Decreased tachykinin (substance P) and enkephalin fibers in circular muscle

    Decreased colonic total neuron density; decreased VIP and NO neurons in myenteric, decreased VIP neurons in submucous plexus

    Decreased enteroglucagon and 5-HT cells in mucosa; decreased cell secretory indices of enteroglucagon and somatostatin cells

    Decreased volume of interstitial cells of Cajal and neurons in circular muscle

NO, nitric oxide; PGP 9.5, protein gene product 9.5; VIP, vasoactive intestinal polypeptide.

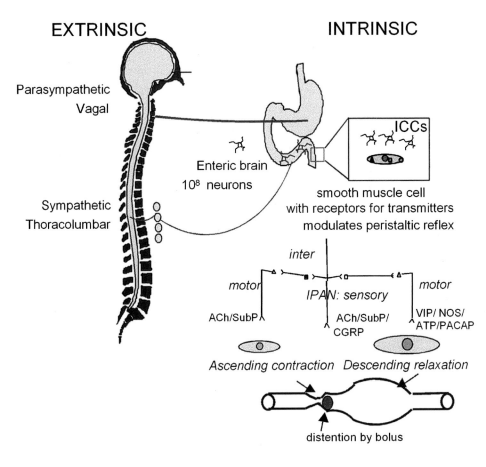

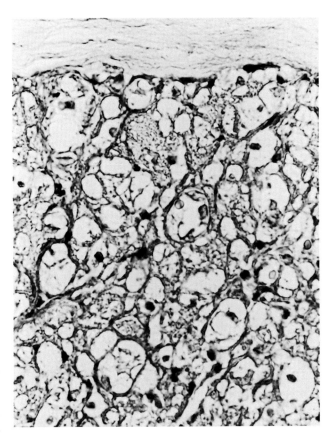

FIGURE 29-1. Extrinsic and enteric control of gut motility. The enteric nervous system (ENS) controls stereotypical motor functions such as the migrating motor complex and the peristaltic reflex; enteric control is modulated by the extrinsic parasympathetic and sympathetic nerves, which respectively stimulate and inhibit nonsphincteric muscle. *IPAN,* intrinsic primary afferent neuron. (*ACh,* acetylcholine; *ATP,* adenosine triphosphate; *CGRP,* calcitonin gene-related peptide; *ICCs,* interstitial cells of Cajal; *NOS,* nitric oxide synthase; *PACAP,* pituitary adenylate cyclase-activating polypeptide; *SubP,* substance P; *VIP,* vasoactive intestinal polypeptide.)

FIGURE 29-2. Characteristic vacuolar change with collagen fibers encircling spaces filled by fragmented muscle cells. Patient has familial visceral myopathy (trichrome stain; original magnification ×470).

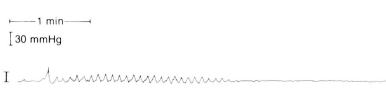

I

II

III

IV

V

FIGURE 29-3. Jejunal manometric record of a patient with type I familial visceral myopathy reveals weak contractions (amplitude < 30 mm Hg) of phase 3. Five tracings are shown and each is 5 cm apart. Phase 3 contractions were detected in only tracings I and II but not at other locations because of the weakness of contractions at these locations.

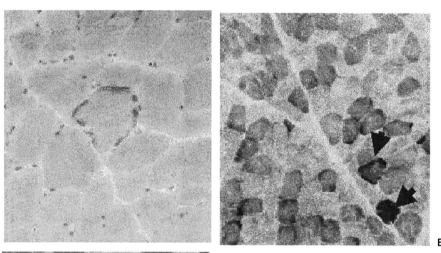

A

B

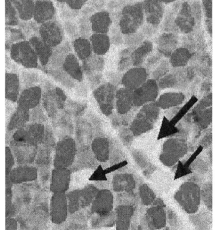

C

FIGURE 29-4. Histological and histochemical studies of skeletal muscle biopsy from a patient with mitochondrial myopathy. **A:** Note the ragged red fibers characterized by the subsarcolemmal location of giant mitochondria in a few fibers, and the paucity of mitochondria in other fibers. **B:** On histochemical analysis, a few fibers are succinate dehydrogenase positive (ragged blue appearance [**arrowheads**]) **C:** The same fibers do not express cytochrome c oxidase (*arrows*), suggesting a defect in the respiratory enzyme chain that results in mitochondrial dysfunction and systemic acidosis.

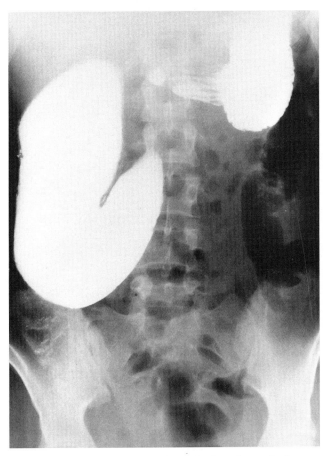

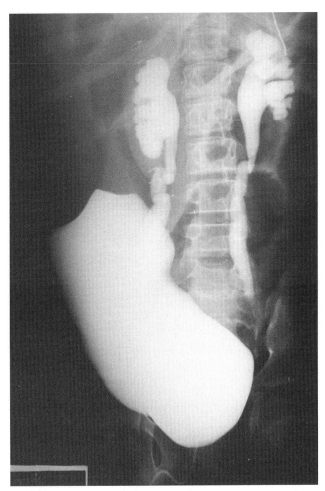

FIGURE 29-5. Upper gastrointestinal radiograph from a patient with type I familial visceral myopathy demonstrates severe megaduodenum.

FIGURE 29-6. An intravenous pyelogram of a child with type I childhood visceral myopathy shows megacystis and bilateral ureteral pyelocaliectasis.

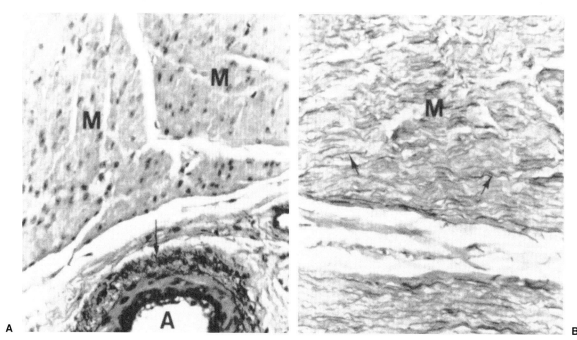

FIGURE 29-7. **A:** Bladder muscularis from a control specimen demonstrates elastic fibers (*arrow*) in the adventitia of a small artery (*A*). No elastic fibers are present within muscle bundles (*M*). **B:** Bladder muscularis from a type I childhood visceral myopathy patient demonstrates numerous, parallel, coarse, wavy, elastic fibers (*arrows*) within muscle bundles (*M*). (Verhoeff-van Gieson stain; original magnification ×325.)

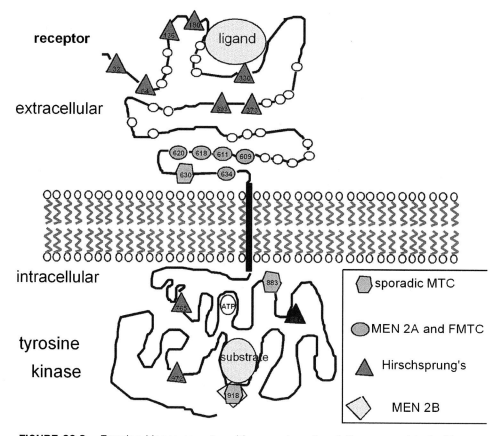

FIGURE 29-8. Tyrosine kinase receptor with examples of mutations associated with specific genetic disorders (*ATP,* adenosine triphosphate; *[F] MTC,* [familial] medullary carcinoma of the thyroid; *MEN,* multiple endocrine neoplasia).

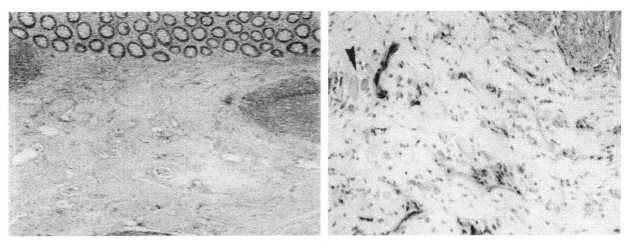

FIGURE 29-9. In multiple endocrine neoplasia (MEN) IIB, intestinal pathology shows transmural intestinal ganglioneuromatosis filling the submucosa (**left panel**), and the myenteric plexus (**right panel**). Note thick nerve trunks embedded with mature neurons (*arrowhead*).

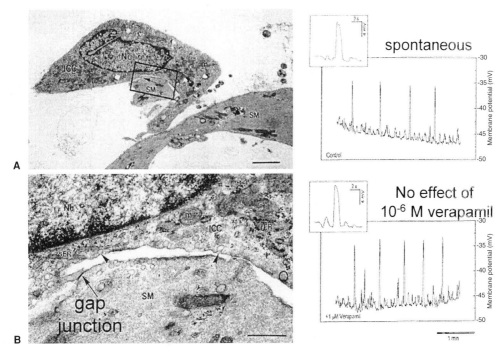

FIGURE 29-10. Gap junctions between interstitial cells of Cajal (ICCs) and smooth muscle cells; note spontaneous electrical oscillations of the resting membrane potential of ICCs (**A**) and lack of inhibition by the L-type calcium channel blocker, verapamil (**B**). (*m*, mitochondria; *Nu*, nucleus; *RER*, rough endoplasmic reticulum; *SER*, smooth endoplasmic reticulum; *SM*, smooth muscle.)

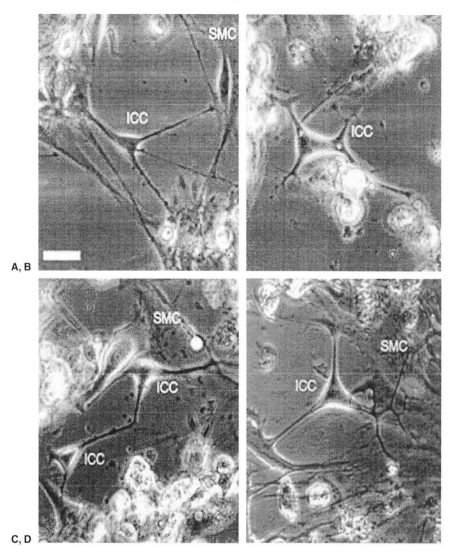

FIGURE 29-11.   A–D: In short-term culture, interstitial cells of Cajal (*ICC*) take a triangular shape, and have three to four branches that establish contact with cultured smooth muscle cells (*SMC*).

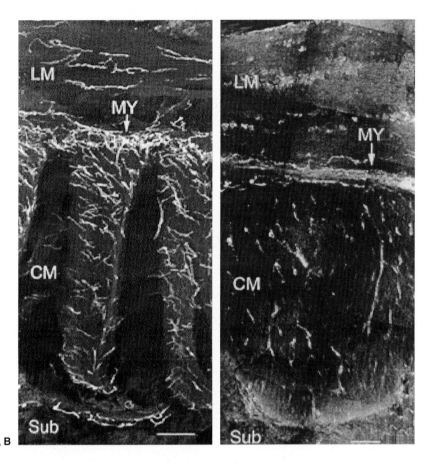

A, B

FIGURE 29-12. Distribution of interstitial cells of Cajal in whole transverse mounts of the sigmoid colon in a normal-appearing disease-control section of the sigmoid colon (**A**) and the sigmoid colon of a patient with slow-transit constipation (**B**).

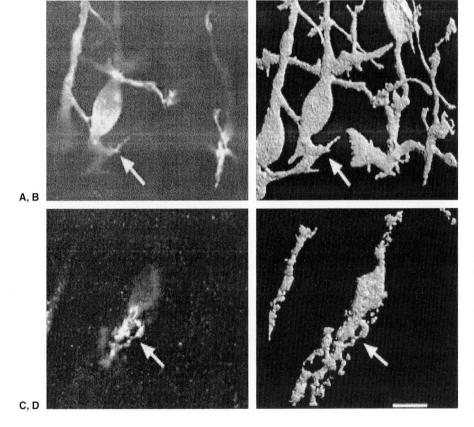

A, B

C, D

FIGURE 29-13. High-magnification confocal microscopy of the interstitial cells of Cajal (ICCs) from human sigmoid colon. **A** and **C** are single slices; **B** and **D** are reconstructions of 20 consecutive single slices. **A** and **B** are from healthy-appearing disease-control colon; note multiple fine processes and the network of interconnecting ICCs. **C** and **D** are from a patient with slow-transit constipation. Note the irregular markings and loss of fine processes (bar equals 10 μm).

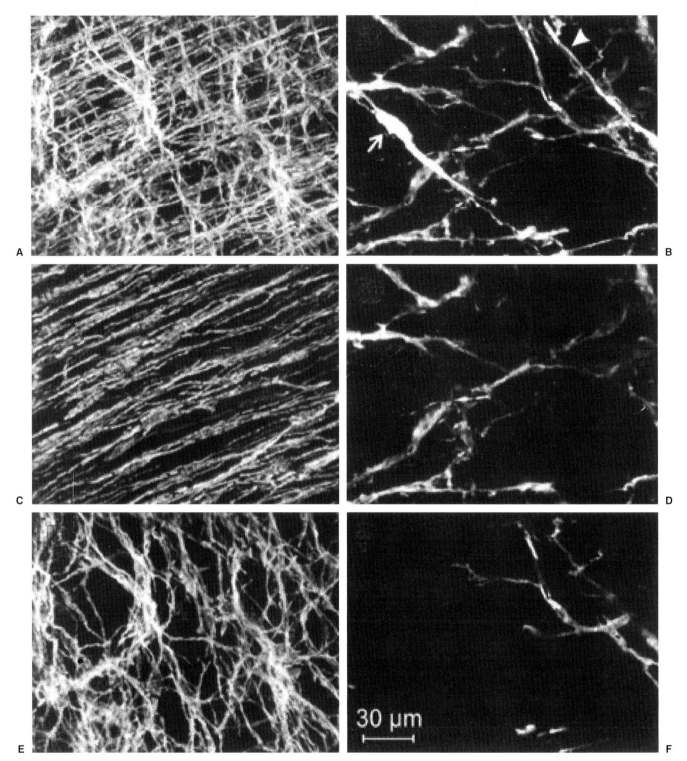

FIGURE 29-14. Effects of diabetes on gastric antral interstitial cells of Cajal (ICC) networks: Kit-like immunoreactivity in the proximal antrum of nondiabetic (**A**, **C**, and **E**) and diabetic (**B**, **D**, and **F**) mice. Confocal images representing the entire thickness of the tunica muscularis (**A** and **B**), the thickness of the circular muscle (**C** and **D**), and the myenteric region (**E** and **F**) are shown. Note the profound reduction in ICC number in the tunica muscularis of the diabetic animal. The *arrow* and *arrowhead* in **B** indicate a cell body and process of an ICC, respectively. Scale bar applies to all panels.

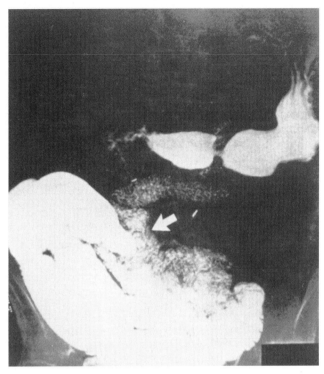

FIGURE 29-15. Small bowel radiograph from a patient with type I familial visceral neuropathy shows a normal stomach, duodenum, and proximal jejunum, but a dilated distal small bowel (*arrow*).

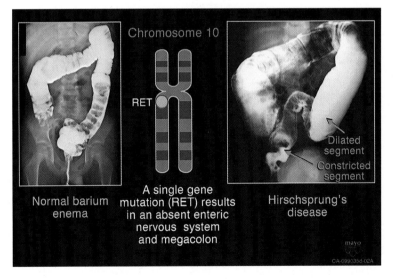

FIGURE 29-16. Barium enema in a normal child contrasted with megacolon and narrow segment of Hirschsprung disease.

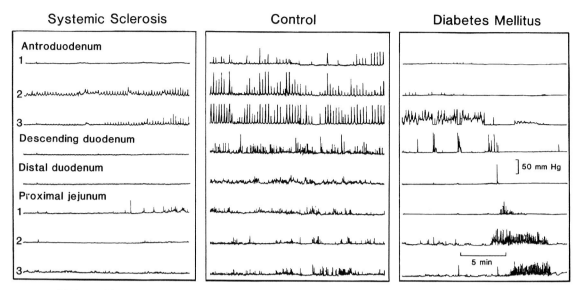

FIGURE 29-17. Altered postprandial intestinal manometric tracing in a patient with scleroderma (**left**) and in a patient with diabetes mellitus (**right**). Note the low amplitude of contractions typical of a myopathic disorder in the **left panel**, and the normal amplitude but abnormal pattern typical of a neuropathic disorder in the **right panel**. The antral hypomotility, excessive pyloric tonic and phasic pressure activity, and the persistence of the migrating motor complex during the postprandial period are typical features of enteric nerve dysfunction.

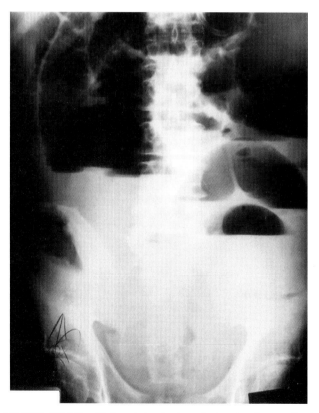

FIGURE 29-18. Plain abdominal radiograph of a patient with scleroderma and intestinal pseudoobstruction demonstrates dilated loops of small bowel with air-fluid levels.

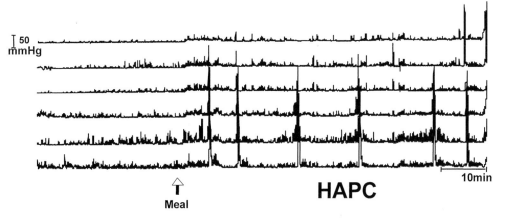

FIGURE 29-19. High-amplitude pressure contractions recorded in the left side of the colon after a meal in a patient with diarrhea caused by extrinsic neuropathy.

SMALL INTESTINE: Infections with Common Bacterial and Viral Pathogens

HARRY B. GREENBERG ■ **SUZANNE M. MATSUI** ■ **MARK HOLODNIY**

The small intestine serves a myriad of important functions that are not fully appreciated in the normal, healthy state. It is not until the protective barrier provided by the small intestine is breached by bacterial, viral, or protozoal infection (or other chronic illnesses) that its critical role in nutrient absorption and maintenance of fluid and electrolyte balance is realized. As discussed in the *Textbook of Gastroenterology*, 4th edition (see Chapter 74), bacterial and viral pathogens that infect the small intestine have evolved a variety of mechanisms to take advantage of this rich and unique environment. Figures 30-1 through 30-9 highlight some of the important clinical and pathogenetic features of intestinal infection that can best be conveyed through images.

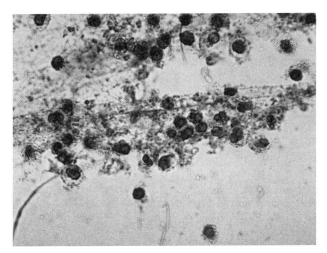

FIGURE 30-1. Fecal leukocytes (original magnification ×450). For patients with severe or protracted cases of diarrhea, examination of the stool for fecal leukocytes can help to narrow the differential diagnosis. Fecal leukocytes are most abundant in inflammatory diarrhea caused by such colonic pathogens as *Shigella* sp, *Campylobacter* sp, *Clostridium difficile,* and invasive *Escherichia coli* (enteroinvasive and enterohemorrhagic types). *Salmonella, Yersinia, Vibrio parahaemolyticus, Aeromonas,* and *Plesiomonas* infections are sometimes associated with the presence of fecal leukocytes. Absence of fecal leukocytes is typical of small-bowel infections caused by viruses, *Giardia*, and enterotoxigenic bacteria. Shedding of fecal leukocytes is not restricted to infectious diarrhea and can be observed in other conditions such as inflammatory bowel disease. To test for fecal leukocytes, a simple smear of fresh stool, or mucus, is stained with methylene blue, Wright stain, or Gram stain and examined by light microscopy under high power. The test is considered positive if three or more leukocytes are identified in each of four or more high-power fields.

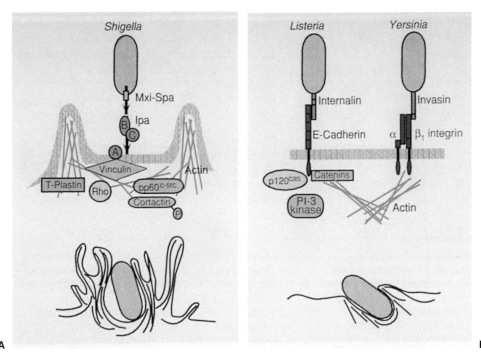

FIGURE 30-2. Mechanisms of bacterial invasion. Studies with modern techniques of cellular and molecular biology continue to advance and enhance our knowledge of microbial pathogenesis. These studies have been successful in identifying common pathways that determine pathogenicity of distinctly different bacteria. For example, it is recognized that bacteria that invade host intestinal cells do so by one of two mechanisms. **A:** *Salmonella* and *Shigella* organisms enter intestinal epithelial cells by means of a trigger mechanism— *Salmonella* organisms through the apical surface and *Shigella* organisms through the basolateral surface. These bacteria express secretion and effector protein complexes that trigger activation of host cell signaling pathways, resulting in substantial rearrangement of cellular actin and membrane ruffling. Bacteria are taken up in membrane-bound vacuoles that are formed in this process. **B:** *Yersinia* and *Listeria* organisms use a zipper mechanism to invade cells. Specific bacterial outer surface proteins interact with host cell receptor proteins and stimulate modest local cytoskeletal rearrangements that cause the host cell membrane to zipper around the bacteria.

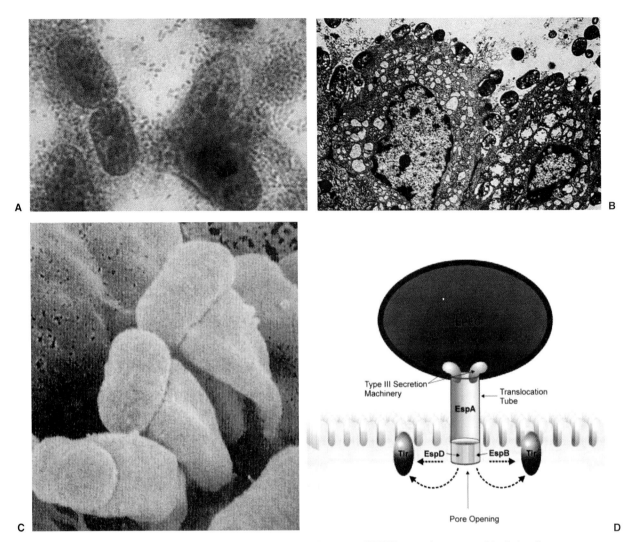

FIGURE 30-3. Adherence of enteropathogenic *E coli* (EPEC) organisms to epithelial cells. EPEC is not an invasive organism, but it interacts intimately with host epithelial cells. **A:** At light microscopic examination (oil; original magnification ×1000), numerous EPEC organisms can be seen adhering to the surface of intestinal mucosal cells. **B:** Electron micrograph (original magnification ×10,000) shows that EPEC adheres to the intestinal mucosal cell surface but does not enter the cell. **C:** Scanning electron micrograph shows EPEC on HeLa cell pedestals. In these attaching and effacing lesions, there is focal effacement of microvilli that damages the surface of absorptive intestinal cells and is associated with dramatic local cytoskeletal rearrangements that induce pedestal formation. **D:** Upon binding to host cells, EPEC uses its type III secretion system (or "molecular syringe") to first establish with EPEC-secreted proteins (EspA, EspB, and EspD) a pore into the host cell membrane through which other bacterial effector proteins, such as Tir, are translocated. These bacterial virulence factors induce cytoskeletal changes, as well as interfere with critical cellular functions, including signal transduction pathways, and lead to disease.

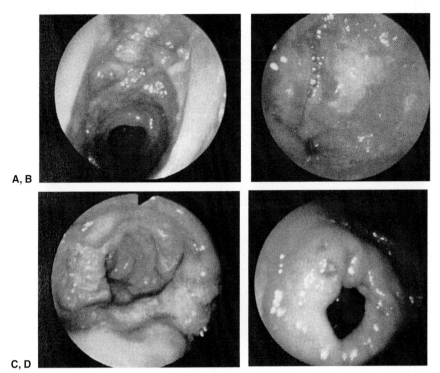

A, B

C, D

FIGURE 30-4. Endoscopic findings of *Yersinia* enterocolitis. In a study of Japanese patients infected with *Yersinia enterocolitica* serotype O:3, the following endoscopic findings were observed: multiple round or oval elevations, possibly caused by hyperplasia of Peyer patches in the terminal ileum, with erosions **(A)**; shallow ulcers with irregular margins, large **(B)** and small **(C),** in the terminal ileum of two separate patients; and small ulcers of the ileocecal valve **(D)** of the patient in **A**. In this study, abnormal endoscopic findings were limited to the terminal ileum (*n* = 8 of 8 patients), cecum (*n* = 6), ileocecal valve (*n* = 5), and ascending colon (*n* = 2). The remainder of the colon was not affected. More distal colonic involvement with mucosal changes mimicking pseudomembranous colitis has been reported with non–serotype O:3 *Y enterocolitica* infections.

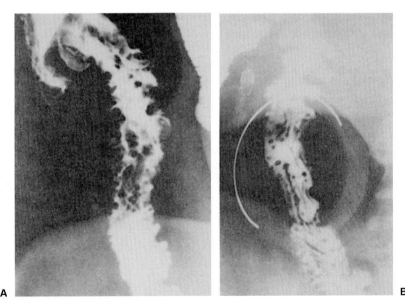

A   B

FIGURE 30-5. Radiographic findings of *Yersinia* enteritis. Most patients who have gastrointestinal symptoms caused by *Yersinia* infection have mucosal abnormalities at barium studies. **A:** The earliest and most common findings are those of diffuse thickening of folds and a nodular mucosal pattern in the terminal ileum. In nearly half of the patients examined, ulcers (ranging from aphthoid to oval and longitudinal) also were discernible. **B:** Radiographic abnormalities generally resolve after symptoms subside, but in a few cases, follicular ileitis (a pattern of small, 1- to 2-mm diameter filling defects) may persist for several months in patients who no longer have symptoms.

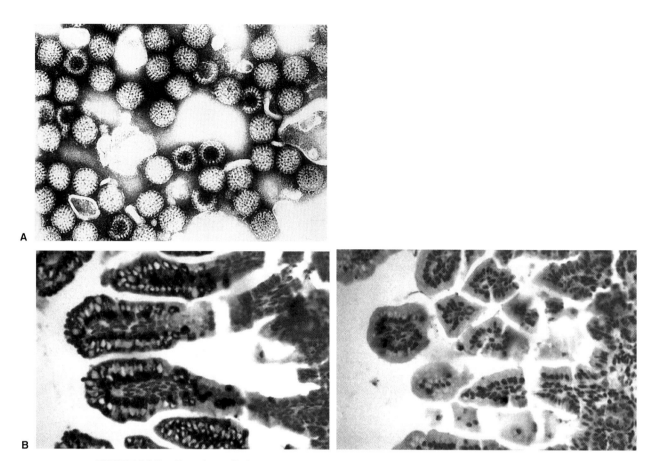

FIGURE 30-6. Rotavirus. Globally, group A rotaviruses constitute the single most important cause of severe dehydrating diarrhea of early childhood. **A:** Negatively stained electron micrograph of human rotavirus particles (approximately 75 nm in diameter), recovered from an infant with acute gastroenteritis demonstrates the characteristic wheel-with-spokes structure for which the virus was named (Latin, *rota,* "wheel"). In recent years, cryoelectron microscopy has provided a more refined ultrastructural map of the virion: a triple-layered capsid with icosahedral symmetry decorated with spike-like projections of the outer capsid protein VP4. The viral genome consists of 11 segments of double-stranded RNA and is enclosed within the triple-layered capsid. **B:** Immunostained sections of loops of intestine of a newborn mouse demonstrate that murine rotavirus EW preferentially infects villous tip cells (**left panel**). In a similar section, the simian rotavirus RRV infects only a small number of mouse intestinal cells, indicating the inefficiency of heterologous infection caused by marked host range restriction (**right panel**). Host range restriction forms the basis for attenuation of rotavirus vaccines. (Courtesy of Drs. J.E. Ludert and H.B. Greenberg.)

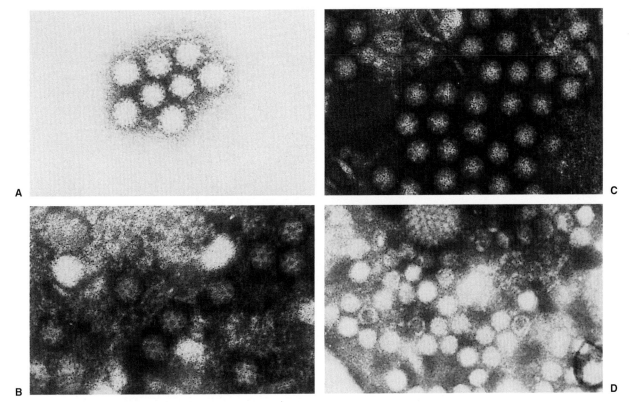

FIGURE 30-7. Negatively stained electron micrographs of other viral pathogens. **A:** Cluster of Norwalk virus particles (approximately 30 nm in diameter) from the feces of an infected patient. For years, this fastidious agent, an important cause of food-borne gastroenteritis, eluded study and was classified morphologically as a small, round-structured virus, because of its amorphous surface features. Molecular characterization of the viral RNA genome in the early 1990s, combined with knowledge of its capsid protein profile, led to the inclusion of Norwalk and related viruses in the family *Caliciviridae.* **B:** Human caliciviruses (approximately 30–35 nm in diameter) with typical morphologic features are shown here for comparison with Norwalk virus **(A)**. These viral particles demonstrate the characteristic cup-like (Latin, *calyx*) surface depressions and the six-pointed star-of-David configuration of caliciviruses. In developed countries, Norwalk virus infection is more common among older children and adults, whereas human caliciviruses with classic morphologic features typically cause diarrhea among infants and young children. **C:** Human astroviruses (approximately 30 nm in diameter) are now classified into a unique family of RNA viruses, the *Astroviridae.* Astroviruses were named for the distinctive five- to six-pointed star on their surface, as is evident in this micrograph. Recent ultrastructural studies have demonstrated short peg-like spikes emanating from the surface of these viral particles. Although first identified among newborn infants with diarrhea, astroviruses are also known to cause illness in institutional settings (e.g., nursing homes, day-care centers) and among immunocompromised persons. **D:** A single particle of enteric adenovirus (approximately 80 nm in diameter) among adeno-associated parvoviruses in feces. Adenoviruses, unlike the viruses shown in **A, B** and **C**, have a DNA genome. Enteric adenoviruses typically cause infection among infants and young children. (Courtesy of Dr. C.R. Madeley.)

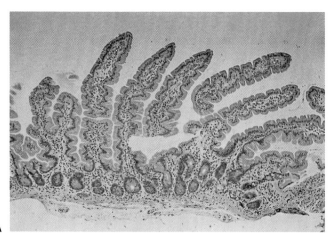

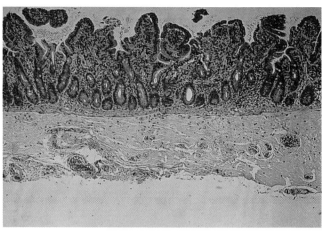

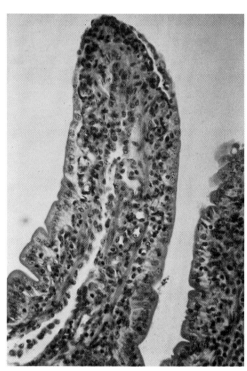

FIGURE 30-8. Histopathological features of Norwalk virus infection. Light micrographs (H&E stain) of peroral intestinal biopsies from human volunteers who were administered a safety-tested inoculum of Norwalk virus. **A:** Intestinal biopsy specimen from the level of the ligament of Treitz of a volunteer before administration of the viral inoculum demonstrates normal villous architecture and cellular pattern (original magnification ×100). **B:** Intestinal biopsy of the same volunteer during the acute phase of illness shows flattening and broadening of the villi (original magnification ×100). **C:** Intestinal biopsy specimen of another ill volunteer shows epithelial cells with vacuoles containing non–lipid staining material (oil immersion, original magnification ×1000). Electron micrographs of biopsy specimens from the ill patients revealed abnormalities, including dilation of the rough and smooth endoplasmic reticulum, an increase in multivesiculate bodies, and shortening of microvilli. No viral particles were identified with certainty within these cells. Biopsy specimens obtained during convalescence showed complete resolution of these histological and ultrastructural changes.

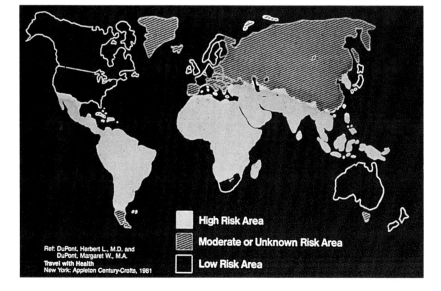

FIGURE 30-9. Relative risk for acquiring traveler's diarrhea. Each traveler incurs a certain amount of risk for traveler's diarrhea according to destination. In general, the risk is highest in developing countries in Africa, South America, and parts of Asia and lowest in more developed countries, including the United States, Canada, countries of northern Europe, Australia, and South Africa. Travelers should be mindful of safe eating practices as a first line of defense in preventing traveler's diarrhea at any destination.

31

CHRONIC INFECTIONS OF THE SMALL INTESTINE

GEORGE T. FANTRY ■ LORI E. FANTRY ■ STEPHEN P. JAMES ■ DAVID H. ALPERS

There are four chronic infections of the small intestine that occur in immunocompetent hosts: Whipple disease, tropical sprue, tuberculosis, and histoplasmosis. Other chronic infections of the small intestine are seen primarily among immunocompromised hosts and include mycotic infections such as aspergillosis, candidiasis, and mucormycosis and *Mycobacterium avium* complex (MAC) occurring among patients with acquired immunodeficiency syndrome (AIDS). The latter infection may mimic the histopathologic findings of Whipple disease.

Whipple disease is a rare syndrome caused by infection with *Tropheryma whippelii*. The most important step in the evaluation of Whipple disease is to have a high degree of suspicion in the appropriate clinical settings. The challenge is to establish the correct diagnosis while avoiding the temptation to overdiagnose the disease. The diagnostic procedure of choice is endoscopic small intestine mucosal biopsy. The disease is usually diffuse but can be patchy; therefore, multiple (four to six) biopsy specimens should be obtained. The characteristic duodenal appearance consists of thickened mucosal folds coated with a yellow granular material or 1- to 2-mm yellow plaques that may be diffuse or patchy (Fig. 31-1).

The appearance with periodic acid–Schiff (PAS) staining often is sufficient to establish the diagnosis of Whipple disease for most patients (Figs. 31-2 through 31-5); however, it can be confirmed with electron microscopic demonstration of the bacilli (Fig. 31-6). Occasional macrophages are found in the normal intestinal lamina propria. These macrophages usually stain faintly PAS-positive, but the inclusions are not sickle-shaped as in Whipple disease. There are three clinical entities in which the presence of numerous PAS-positive macrophages in the intestinal lamina propria may be misleading: AIDS with MAC infection, systemic histoplasmosis, and macroglobulinemia. These diseases can be differentiated from Whipple disease because of the faintly staining, homogeneously PAS-positive macrophages of macroglobulinemia and the large, PAS-positive, rounded, encapsulated *Histoplasma* organisms. More care must be taken to differentiate the histopathological findings in the intestinal mucosa of patients with Whipple disease from those of patients with AIDS and MAC infection. In MAC infection, the lamina propria is packed with macrophages containing MAC, which when stained with hematoxylin and eosin and PAS stain, clearly resemble those seen in Whipple disease. However, MAC bacilli are acid fast, easily cultured, and have an electron microscopic appearance quite different from that of Whipple bacilli (Fig. 31-7). The diagnosis of MAC is easily established among persons with human immunodeficiency virus (HIV) infection. *T whippelii* infection has not been reported among persons with HIV infection. Studies have suggested that polymerase chain reaction may be a helpful confirmatory test for patients believed to have Whipple disease.

In very rare instances, the diagnosis of Whipple disease has been established in the absence of intestinal involvement. In these cases, the diagnosis was established with electron microscopic demonstration of bacilli in cerebrospinal fluid, brain biopsy specimens, or peripheral lymph nodes.

Considerable caution is required in the interpretation of gastric and rectal biopsy findings. PAS-positive macrophages frequently are present in the normal gastric and rectal mucosa, and in many diseases of the stomach and rectum. The stomach often contains faintly PAS-positive, lipid-containing macrophages (lipophages), whereas the rectal mucosa usually contains strongly PAS-positive muciphages and pigment-containing macrophages (Fig. 31-8). Electron microscopic demonstration of Whipple bacilli in these tissues usually is necessary to establish the diagnosis.

Barium studies of the small intestine usually are abnormal in Whipple disease and may reveal a characteristic but nonspecific finding of marked thickening of the mucosal folds (Fig. 31-9). These findings usually are more prominent in the duodenum and proximal jejunum and less prominent in the distal jejunum; the ileum is spared. In addition to marked thickening of the proximal small bowel, abdominal computed tomographic scanning often reveals marked mesenteric, paraaortic, and retroperitoneal adenopathy (Fig. 31-10).

Three specific chronic bacterial infections of the small intestine are due to *Yersinia* (*Y. enterocolitica* and *Y. pseudotuberculosis*), *Mycobacterium tuberculosis*, and *Histoplasma capsulatum*. Yersinia penetrates the lamina propria and causes submucosal thickening that can mimic Crohn's disease (Fig. 31-11). Histologically, there are massively enlarged lymphoid follicles with prominent germinal centers (Fig. 31-12).

Intestinal tuberculosis is most common in patients with active pulmonary disease, and is caused by swallowed organisms that cross the mucosa of the bowel segments rich in lymphoid tissue, i.e., ileum and cecum. Figure 31-13 shows tuberculosis in the ileocecal region, where nearly all gastrointestinal infections occur. The tissue response can be either hypertrophic (Fig. 31-13*B*), ulcerative (Fig. 31-13*C*), or a combination of both. When tuberculosis becomes disseminated (miliary tuberculosis), tubercles are found on the serosal surface of the bowel (Fig. 31-14).

Histoplasmosis is originally a pulmonary infection that most often becomes generalized as in immunocompromised patients. The organism can affect both the small or large intestine and liver, although symptoms are most often attributed to small bowel disease (crampy abdominal pain, diarrhea, anemia, malabsorption). Figure 31-15*A* shows nodular ulcerated lesions. This ulceration is accompanied by intense mononuclear cell infiltrate, possibly with granuloma formation (Fig. 31-15*B*), in those patients who are immunocompetent enough to mount a response.

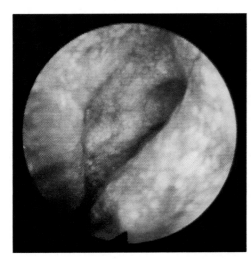

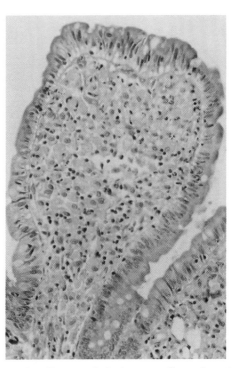

FIGURE 31-1. Characteristic duodenoscopic appearance of the duodenum of an untreated patient with Whipple disease. The folds are thickened and are covered with small yellowish-white plaques. This endoscopic appearance may be the first clue to the diagnosis.

FIGURE 31-2. Characteristic hematoxylin and eosin staining appearance of an intestinal villus in Whipple disease. The macrophages, although abundant throughout the lamina propria, are rather inapparent (original magnification ×200). (Courtesy of Dr. John E. Stone.)

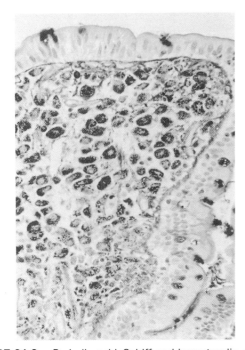

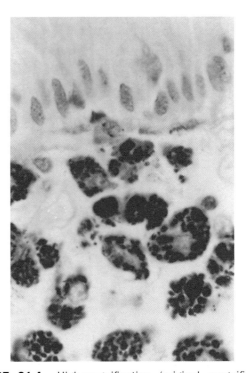

FIGURE 31-3. Periodic acid–Schiff and hematoxylin stain of the same villus as in Fig. 31-2 shows prominence of the macrophages with this stain (original magnification ×200). (Courtesy of Dr. John E. Stone.)

FIGURE 31-4. High-magnification (original magnification ×1000) photograph of macrophages stained periodic acid–Schiff in the intestinal mucosa in Whipple disease. Note the characteristic rounded and sickle-shaped inclusions in the macrophages. This appearance alone is highly suggestive of the diagnosis.

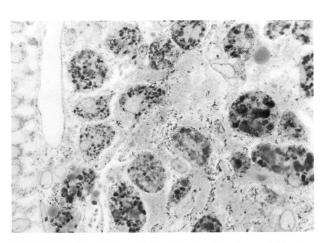

FIGURE 31-5. High-magnification (original magnification ×750) photograph of toluidine blue–stained section of plastic-embedded specimen of intestinal mucosa in Whipple disease. Characteristic macrophage inclusions and numerous extracellular bacilli are present throughout the lamina propria.

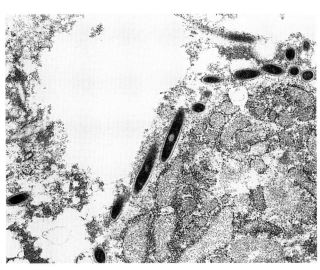

FIGURE 31-6. Electron micrograph of duodenal biopsy specimen from a patient with Whipple disease shows the cytoplasm of a macrophage, with positive results at periodic acid–Schiff staining, and its surrounding extracellular space. Note the numerous bacilli with a characteristic cell wall and pale central nuclei just outside the macrophage.

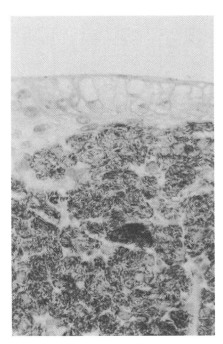

FIGURE 31-7. High-magnification (original magnification ×1000) photograph of acid-fast–stained intestinal villus in *Mycobacterium avium* complex infection in acquired immunodeficiency syndrome. Exclusively intracellular, very large bacilli are present. Whipple bacilli are much smaller, largely extracellular, and not acid fast. (Courtesy of Dr. Wilfred M. Weinstein.)

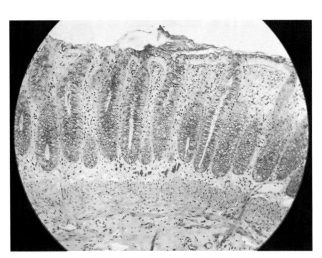

FIGURE 31-8. Periodic acid–Schiff and hematoxylin stain of rectal biopsy specimen of a healthy person. Prominent macrophages are just below the crypts and above the muscularis mucosae. This finding is a frequent cause of confusion; however, the rectum and colon are very rarely involved in Whipple disease (original magnification ×100).

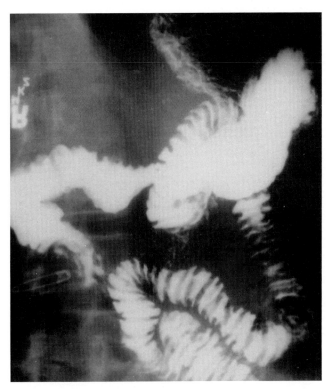

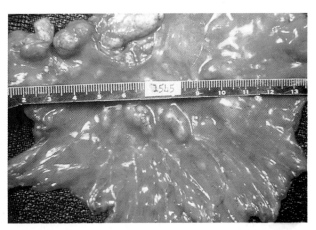

FIGURE 31-9. Radiograph shows coarsened folds in the duodenum and jejunum of an untreated patient with Whipple disease. (Courtesy of Dr. John E. Stone.)

FIGURE 31-10. Autopsy image of the mesentery and nodes of a patient with Whipple disease shows marked thickening of the mesentery and a striking degree of adenopathy.

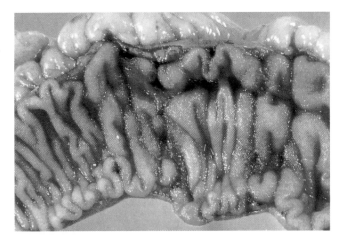

FIGURE 31-11. *Yersinia.* Gross appearance in a patient with culture-proven *Yersinia* infection. The mucosal folds are unduly prominent because of the granulomatous inflammation that extends into the submucosa.

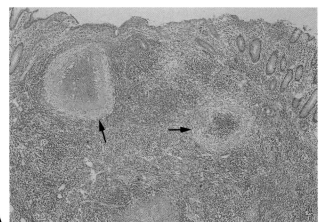

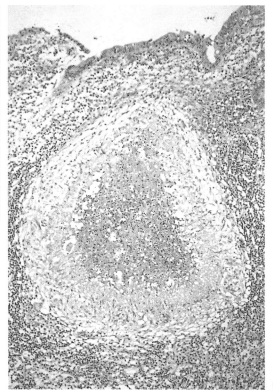

FIGURE 31-12. *Yersinia* enterocolitis. **A** and **B** demonstrate the presence of the prominent necrotizing granulomas that characterize *Yersinia* when it presents in a typical fashion. **A:** Contains two granulomas (*arrows*). The overlying epithelium appears atrophic and ulcerated. **B:** Higher magnification showing palisading histiocytes without foreign body giant cells. The entire granuloma is surrounded by a prominent cuff of lymphocytes.

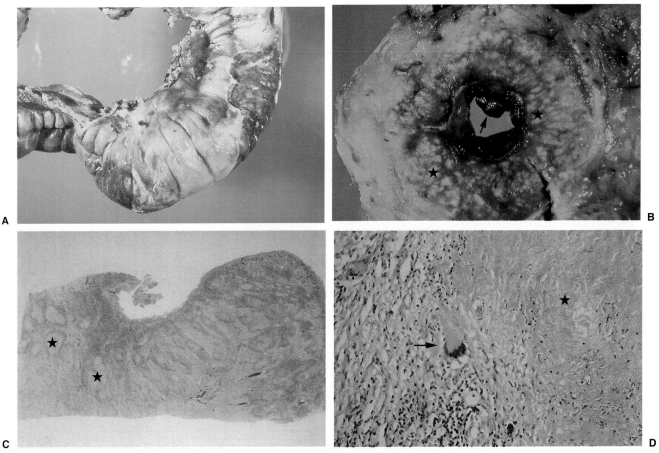

FIGURE 31-13. Ileocecal tuberculosis. **A:** Gross photograph of the resection specimen demonstrating the presence of an ileocolectomy with transmural inflammation. It is difficult to delineate the exact ileocecal valve area. The serosal tissues are markedly congested and edematous, and show fibrinous adhesions. **B:** Cross section through the specimen demonstrating transmural necrosis and replacement of the intestinal wall by numerous granulomas, several of which are indicated by *stars.* The intestinal lumen is severely compromised and narrowed. A hypertrophic lesion protrudes into the lumen (*arrow*). **C:** Low-magnification photograph of the wall demonstrating the presence of the granulomas, some of which are indicated by *stars.* Granulomas appear centrally pale and are surrounded by a bluer rim. **D:** Higher-magnification photograph showing a portion of a granuloma with central caseous necrosis (*star*) and a surrounding giant cell (*arrow*).

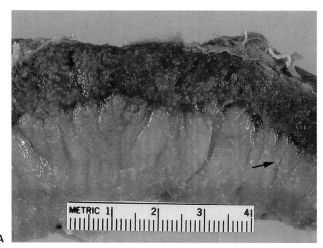
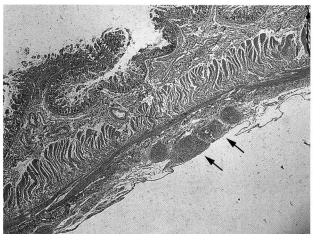

A   B

FIGURE 31-14. Miliary tuberculosis. Gross and microscopic features of miliary tuberculosis. **A:** Gross resection specimen demonstrates numerous whitish nodules on the mucosal surface representing tubercles within the Peyer patches. The fat in the surrounding bowel also demonstrates large numbers of 1- to 2-mm whitish nodules, one of which is indicated by an *arrow*. Fine adhesions are also seen. **B:** Histological section through several of the serosal tubercles (*arrows*). Mucosal and submucosal tubercles are not seen in this photograph.

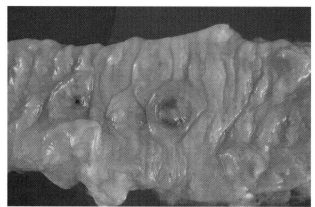
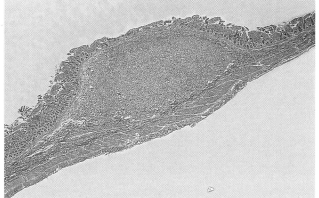

A   B

FIGURE 31-15. **A:** Histoplasmosis. Intestinal resection specimen showing nodular ulcerated lesions diffusely throughout the bowel wall obliterating the normal mucosal fold pattern. **B:** Histological section of the lesion shown in **A** indicating the presence of a submucosal granuloma.

32

CELIAC DISEASE

PAUL J. CICLITIRA

Celiac disease or gluten-sensitive enteropathy is a defined condition in which abnormal jejunal mucosa improves morphologically when treated with a gluten-free diet and relapses when gluten is reintroduced. The condition, commonly called *celiac sprue* or *gluten-sensitive enteropathy* in the United States, was previously called *nontropical sprue, celiac syndrome, idiopathic steatorrhea,* or *primary malabsorption.* A typical adult patient is shown in Fig. 32-1, and a child before diagnosis and after 6 months of a gluten-free diet is shown in Fig. 32-2. Patients frequently have steatorrhea.

Dermatitis herpetiformis is a related condition in which an itchy, blistering skin eruption frequently affects the knees, elbows, buttocks, and back with deposition of granular immunoglobulin A (IgA) at the dermoepidermal junction, including uninvolved skin. An example of a typical blister on the elbow is shown in Fig. 32-3, and the immunohistochemical staining pattern for IgA in a skin biopsy specimen is shown in Fig. 32-4.

Celiac disease is known to be associated with various other disorders (Table 32-1), particularly those linked to histocompatibility antigen HLA-DQ2. The age at the time of diagnosis among a group of patients is shown in Fig. 32-5.

Diagnosis involves taking a history and examining the patient. The radiographic appearance (dilation of the intestine, flocculation, and segmentation of barium) at small bowel follow-through examination of an untreated patient with celiac disease is shown in Fig. 32-6. It should be noted that as many as 25% of untreated patients with celiac disease have no detectable abnormalities at radiography of the small intestine. If the diagnosis is suspected, it is therefore crucial either to perform a biopsy of the small intestine or at the very least to screen for the condition with a serologic test such as an antiendomysial antibody test. If serologic screening is undertaken, it is critical that it be performed in a laboratory experienced in this technique. Otherwise, the normal sensitivity of 97% is reported to fall to 50%.

The jejunal mucosa in celiac disease may be flat and featureless, but usually it has a mosaic pattern caused by interaction of deep depressions bearing elevated mounds. Each mound has 8 to 40 crypt openings. The diagnosis of celiac disease depends on the finding of abnormal small intestine mucosa. The dissecting microscopic appearances of a normal jejunal mucosal biopsy specimen are shown in Fig. 32-7A. This compares with the dissecting microscopic appearance of a flat jejunal mucosa from an untreated patient with celiac disease in Fig. 32-7B.

The histological appearance of the jejunal mucosa from a healthy person is shown in Fig. 32-8A, in which normal, tall, slender villi are depicted. This compares with the appearance of the jejunal mucosa from an untreated patient with celiac disease—loss of the normal villous architecture, an inflammatory cell infiltrate (particularly in the lamina propria), an increase in intraepithelial lymphocyte count, and a decrease in surface enterocyte height are observed (see Fig. 32-8*B*).

It is customary for the diagnosis of celiac disease to be made with endoscopic biopsy specimens obtained during upper gastrointestinal endoscopy. However, should there be difficulty with the diagnosis because of interpretation of the histological findings after endoscopic duodenal biopsy, the previously used method of obtaining tissue with a Crosby or Watson suction biopsy capsule (Fig. 32-9) should be considered.

Monitoring management of celiac disease involves advice for patients to eat a gluten-free diet in which wheat, rye, triticale, barley, and oats are avoided. The relation of these cereals to those that are nontoxic, including rice and maize, is shown in Fig. 32-10. The toxicity of oats remains controversial. However, because most commercially available oat flour is contaminated with wheat flour during commercial milling, persons with celiac disease should avoid oat-containing products. The constituents of a grain of wheat are shown in Fig. 32-11. Early investigators showed that the endosperm, or flour, contains the active constituent. However, it should be noted that other fractions of the wheat grain are invariably heavily contaminated with the flour, and therefore should be avoided by persons with celiac disease.

Wheat proteins derived from gluten are classified according to their relative solubility characteristics (Fig. 32-12). The domain structure and the amino acid sequence of A-gliadin, a type of α-gliadin, are shown in Figs. 32-13 and 32-14, respectively. To investigate celiac disease, Frazer made a physiological peptic tryptic digest of wheat gluten, termed *Frazer's fraction III*, the details of which are shown in Fig. 32-15.

It has been shown that celiac disease is closely linked to certain human leucocyte antigen (HLA) class II genes, in particular *HLA-DQ2* encoded by the alleles A1*0501 and B1*0201. A peptide corresponding to amino acids 31 through 49 of A-gliadin stimulated a T-cell clone obtained from the peripheral blood of a patient with celiac disease. This result provided evidence for the involvement of gluten-sensitive T cells in the pathogenesis of the condition. This same peptide was subsequently shown to be toxic to celiac small intestine biopsy specimens cultured in vitro and to exacerbate celiac disease in vivo among treated patient volunteers with celiac disease. The binding of this peptide to HLA-DQ2 (α1*0501, β1*0201) was studied in a cellular binding assay using truncated and conservative point-substituted analogs of peptide A. The results have led to a computer model of the binding characteristics of this peptide to HLA-DQ2, an example of which is shown in Fig. 32-16. Combined use of these approaches should allow investigators to unravel the pathogenesis of this fascinating condition.

It should be noted that a small percentage of patients eventually have complications such as ulcerative jejunitis. As many as 15% of untreated patients with celiac disease later have T-cell lymphoma of the small intestine (Fig. 32-17).

(figures begin on page 334)

TABLE 32-1

Factors and Diseases Associated with Celiac Disease

DISEASE	APPROXIMATE REPORTED INCIDENCE (%)
First-degree relative of patient with celiac disease	10
Dermatitis herpetiformis	80
Immunoglobulin A deficiency	20
Hyposplenism	100
Aphthous ulceration	5
Cow's milk protein intolerance	10
T-cell lymphoma of the small intestine	6
Thyroid disease	U
Diabetes mellitus	U
Cutaneous vasculitis	U
Fibrosing alveolitis	U
Sjögren syndrome	U
Polyarteritis	U
Addison disease	U
Systemic lupus erythematosus	U
Ulcerative colitis	U
Rheumatoid arthritis	U
Idiopathic pulmonary hemosiderosis	U
Glomerulonephritis	U
Schizophrenia	U
Sarcoidosis	U
Histocompatibility antigens HLA-B8 and DR3	U

U, incidence unknown.

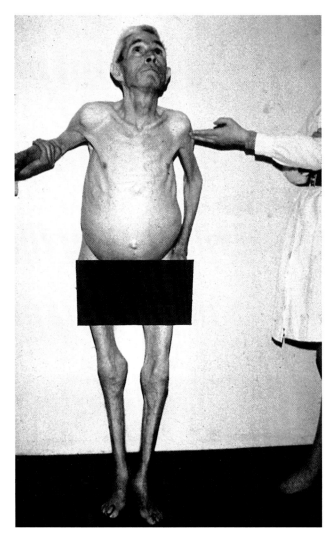

FIGURE 32-1.   Adult presentation of celiac disease.

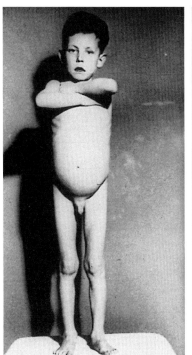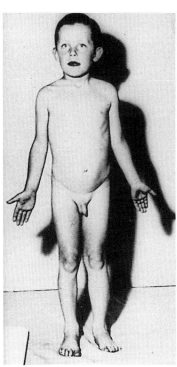

A, B

FIGURE 32-2.   Child before diagnosis (**A**) and after introduction of a gluten-free diet (**B**).

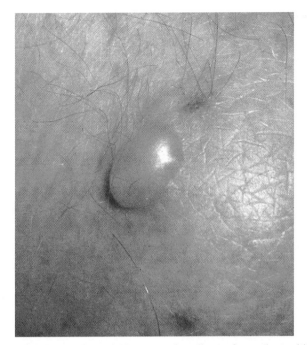

FIGURE 32-3. Typical blister on the elbow of a patient with dermatitis herpetiformis.

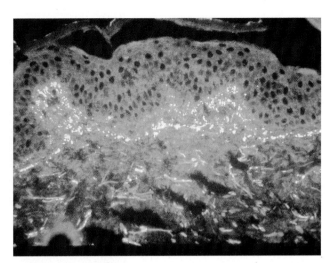

FIGURE 32-4. Immunohistochemical staining of a skin biopsy specimen from a patient with dermatitis herpetiformis shows the granular pattern of immunoglobulin A deposition at the dermoepidermal junction.

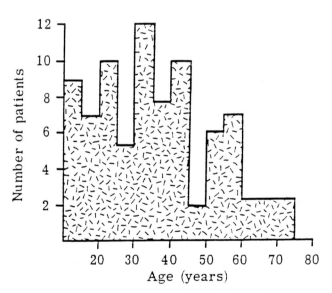

FIGURE 32-5. Age at diagnosis of celiac disease by means of jejunal biopsy among 84 adults.

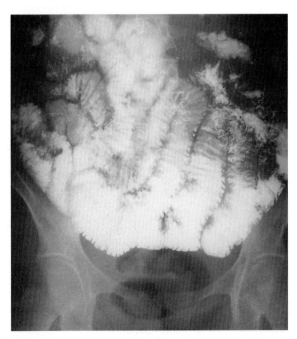

FIGURE 32-6. Small bowel follow-through image of dilated loop of jejunum with characteristic appearance of untreated celiac disease.

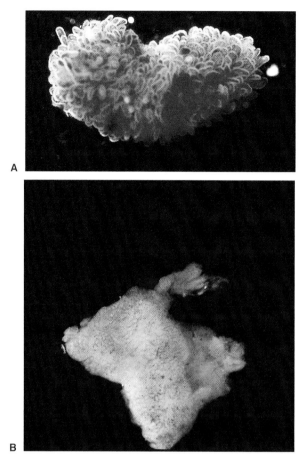

FIGURE 32-7. A: Dissecting microscopic appearance of normal jejunal mucosa. **B:** Dissecting microscopic appearance of flat jejunal mucosa from an untreated patient with celiac disease.

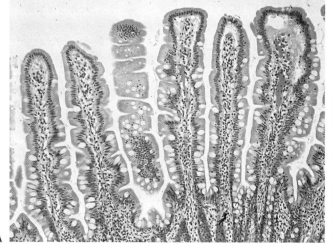
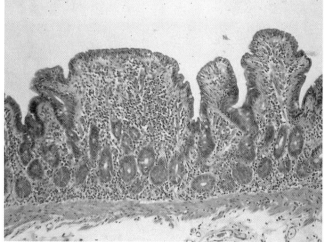

FIGURE 32-8. A: Histological appearance of jejunal mucosa from a healthy person. **B:** Histological appearance of the jejunal mucosa of an untreated patient with celiac disease.

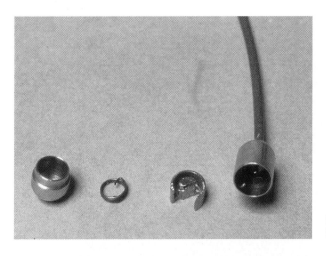

FIGURE 32-9. Photograph shows a Watson jejunal biopsy suction capsule, knife blade, and top.

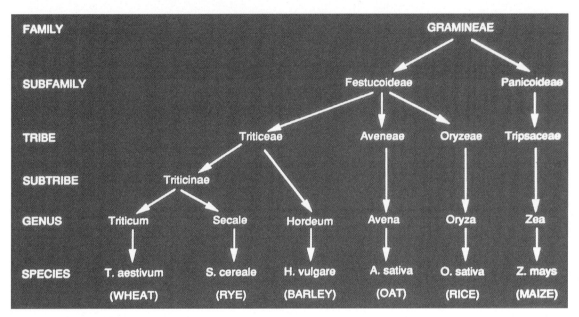

FIGURE 32-10. Taxonomy of celiac disease: relations among principal cereal grains.

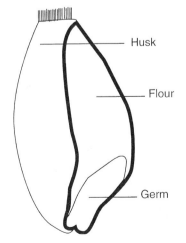

FIGURE 32-11. Constituents of a grain of wheat.

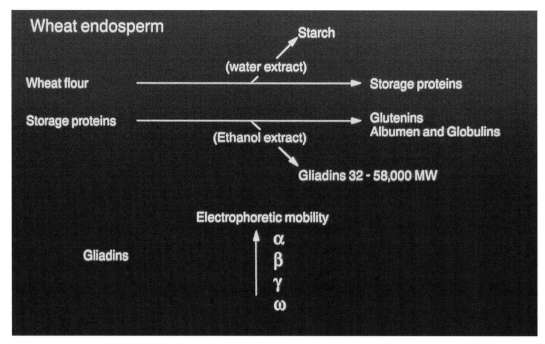

FIGURE 32-12. Cereal chemistry of celiac disease: classification of wheat proteins.

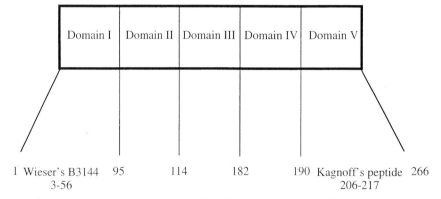

FIGURE 32-13. The domain structure of A-gliadin. A-gliadin is divided into five domains according to amino acid residues: domain 1, repairing sequence; domain 2, polyglutamine; domain 3, unique sequence; domain 4, polyglutamine; domain 5, unique sequence.

V - R - V - P - V - P - Q - L - Q- P$_{10}$ - Q - N - P - S - Q - Q - Q - P - Q   -E$_{20}$ - Q - V - P - L - V - Q - Q - Q- F$_{30}$

- L - G - Q - Q - Q - P - F - P - P - Q$_{40}$ - Q - P - Y - P - Q - P - Q - P - F - P$_{50}$ - S - Q - Q - P - Y - L - Q - L - Q - P$_{60}$

- F - P - Q - V - Q - L - P - Y - S - Q$_{70}$ - P - Q - P - F - R - P - Q - Q - P - Y$_{80}$ - P - Y - P - Q - P - Q - Y - S - Q- P$_{90}$

- Q - Q - P - I - S - Q - Q - Q - Q- Q$_{100}$ - Q - Q - Q - Q - Q- Q - Q - Q - Q - Q$_{110}$ - Q - Q - Q - I - L - Q - Q - I - L - Q$_{120}$

- Q - Q - L - I - F - C - M - D - V - V$_{130}$ - L - Q - Q - H - N - I - A - H - G - R$_{140}$ - S - Q - V - L - Q - Q - S - T - Y - Q$_{150}$

- L - L - Q - L - L - C - C - Q - H- L$_{160}$ - W - Q - I - P - E - Q - S - Q - C - Q$_{170}$ - A - I - H - V - V - V - H - A - C - I$_{180}$

- L - H - Q - Q - Q - K - Q - Q - Q- Q$_{190}$ - P - S - S - Q - V - S - F - Q - Q - P$_{200}$ - L - Q - Q - Y - P - L - G - Q - G - S$_{210}$

- F - R - P - S - Q - Q - N - P - Q- A$_{220}$ - Q - G - S - V - Q - P - Q - Q - L - P$_{250}$ - Q - F - E - E - I - R - N - L - A- L$_{240}$

- Q - T - L - P - A - M - C - N - V - Y$_{250}$ - I - A - P - Y - C - T - I - A - P - F$_{280}$ - G - I - F - G - T - N -

FIGURE 32-14. The amino acid structure of A-gliadin. Domain 1, residues 1 through 95; domain 2, residues 96 through 113; domain 3, residues 114 through 182; domain 4, residues 183 through 190; domain 5, residues 191 through 266.

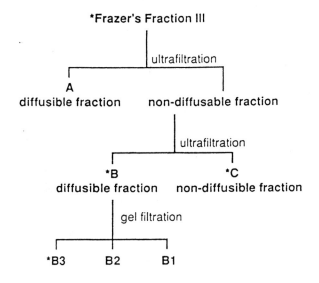

* Toxic fractions

FIGURE 32-15. Frazer's fractionation of wheat proteins.

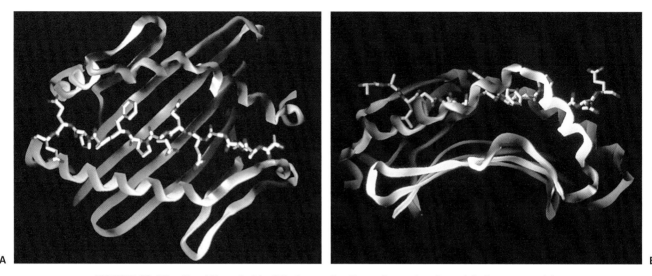

FIGURE 32-16. Top (**A**) and side (**B**) views of a three-dimensional model show a peptide corresponding to amino acids 31 through 49 bound within the HLA-DQ2 (A1*0501, B1*0201) binding cleft. This provides further evidence of the role of this gluten peptide in the pathogenesis of celiac disease.

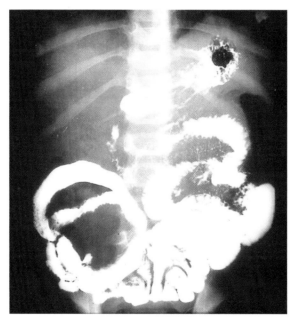

FIGURE 32-17. Small bowel lymphoma complicating celiac disease with a mass in the right iliac fossa.

33

SPECIFIC MUCOSAL PROTEIN DEFICIENCY STATES

RICHARD J. GRAND ■ MARK L. LLOYD ■ WARD A. OLSEN

Most inherited disorders of proteins involved in nutrient transport in the small intestine are rare. Two exceptions are lactase deficiency and cystic fibrosis. Lactase deficiency is the norm among mammals and most humans after weaning from breast-feeding and is not, strictly speaking, a disease. Enzyme activities are regulated at the level of lactase mRNA transcription. However, the symptoms that arise from carbohydrate malabsorption must be differentiated from those caused by other intestinal disorders. The simplest screening test to identify lactose intolerance is withdrawal of dietary milk products. Should this maneuver produce confusing results, the next screening test can be breath hydrogen greater than 10 ppm over baseline after ingestion of a lactose load (Fig. 33-1).

Cystic fibrosis is the most commonly occurring lethal genetic disorder in the western continents. With modern treatment programs, more children are surviving to early adulthood and are experiencing symptoms involving extrapulmonary organs, including the intestine. Intestinal symptoms are caused by the presence of thick mucus produced by altered chloride secretion (Fig. 33-2) with prominent goblet cells and luminal retention of mucus (Fig. 33-3). These pathophysiological changes produce intestinal pseudoobstruction (Figs. 33-4 and 33-5) or actual mechanical obstructions. Colonic mucosa also shows the effects of abnormal mucus production (Fig. 33-6).

Much less common conditions include abetalipoproteinemia (Fig. 33-7) and sucrase-isomaltase deficiency. Of all the disorders of congenital carbohydrate absorption, the altered cellular events associated with sucrase-isomaltase deficiency have been best characterized. Studies have suggested that this condition may arise as a result of several different biosynthetic defects (Table 33-1).

The symptoms are characteristic of carbohydrate malabsorption. A presumptive diagnosis of sucrase deficiency can be made after a clinical response to sucrose exclusion from the diet. The diagnosis can be confirmed by means of breath hydrogen testing after administration of 2g/kg body weight (maximum 25 g) oral sucrose (Fig. 33-8), or by means of mucosal disaccharidase assays that show low sucrase activity in biopsy specimens with normal mucosal histological features. Some patients with this condition lack any isomaltase activity. The associated decreased maltase activity is attributable to the fact that sucrase-isomaltase accounts for a substantial amount of normal maltose hydrolysis.

Two of eight patients with sucrase-isomaltase deficiency in the series reported by Naim and colleagues (1988) showed exclusive synthesis of the high-mannose precursor and demonstrated accumulation of the protein in the Golgi apparatus at immunoelectron microscopic examination (Table 33-1). Other subjects had immunoreactive sucrase-isomaltase of a size that suggested that trimming reactions associated with the endoplasmic reticulum had failed to occur. A set of twins had identifiable sucrase-isomaltase in the brush border membrane that was catalytically inactive. These studies suggest that mutations leading to small changes in the primary structure of the sucrase-isomaltase gene product can have profound influences on the processing, intracellular transport, and function of the molecule. To date, no studies that have incorporated the technique of metabolic labeling have demonstrated complete absence of identifiable sucrase-isomaltase in this condition.

TABLE 33-1
Types of Sucrase-Isomaltase Deficiency

	TYPE I	TYPE II	TYPE III
Forms of sucrase-isomaltase detected	High mannose (M_r = 212,000) +/− complex (M_r = 245,000) in reduced amounts	High mannose (M_r = 210,000)	High mannose (M_r = 210,000) Complex (M_r = 245,000) Sucrase (M_r = 145,000) Isomaltase (M_r = 151,000)
Immunolocalization defect	Not studied Incomplete trimming reaction in endoplasmic reticulum	Golgi Transport arrested in Golgi apparatus	Brush border Sucrase enzymatic active site altered

M_r, relative molecular mass.

Adapted from Naim HY, Roth J, Sterchi EE, et al. Sucrase-isomaltase deficiency in humans: different mutations disrupt intracellular transport, processing and function of an intestinal brush border enzyme. J Clin Invest 1988;82:667.

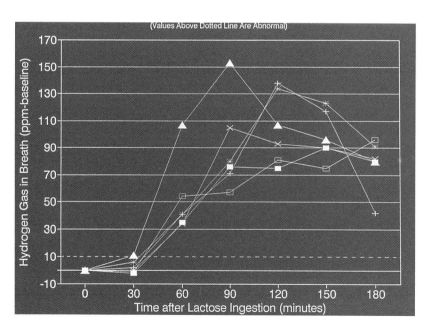

FIGURE 33-1. Lactose breath hydrogen tests in four persons with lactose intolerance. Values above the *dotted line* are abnormal. After an overnight fast, a basal breath sample is obtained, and lactose (2 g/kg body weight) is administered in water. Breath is sampled every 30 minutes for 3 hours and analyzed for hydrogen content in a dedicated gas chromatograph (in this study, a Quinton instrument [Quinton Instruments, Bothell, WA] was used). The peak in breath hydrogen occurs at 90 to 120 minutes, and remarkably similar curves are seen for all four subjects. It is customary to obtain a concomitant symptom chart to correlate breath hydrogen excretion with subjective symptoms.

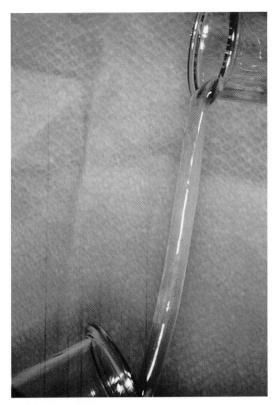

FIGURE 33-2. Duodenal mucus from a patient with cystic fibrosis obtained by means of intraduodenal intubation. Extremely viscid mucus retains its elastic properties even when poured from flask to flask.

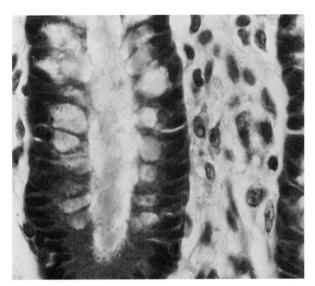

FIGURE 33-3. Ileal biopsy specimen from a patient with cystic fibrosis at operation for distal intestinal obstruction syndrome (periodic acid–Schiff stain). Prominent and enlarged goblet cells and retained mucus are present in the crypt lumen. This appearance is virtually pathognomonic of cystic fibrosis.

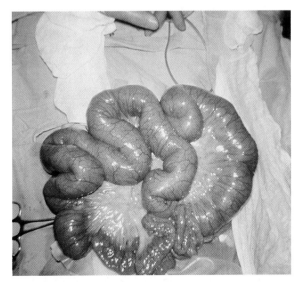

FIGURE 33-4. Photograph obtained at operation shows distal intestine of an adolescent patient with cystic fibrosis and distal intestinal obstruction. Terminal ileum is enlarged with impacted retained mucoid material, which failed to pass with nonoperative therapy. When surgical intervention is necessary, it is often sufficient to milk the retained intestinal contents distally. It is usually unnecessary to perform enterotomy or resection.

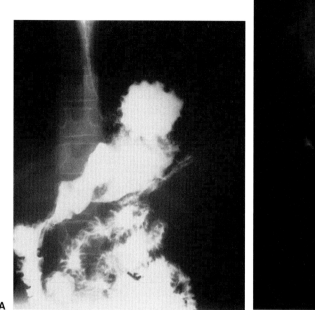
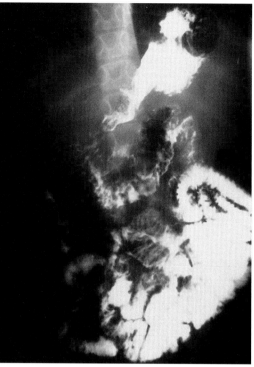

A   B

FIGURE 33-5. Upper gastrointestinal barium series with small bowel follow-through shows a 9-year-old patient with newly diagnosed cystic fibrosis. **A:** The gastric and duodenal mucosa are nodular, thickened, and irregular. **B:** The small intestine has a thickened, irregular mucosa with scattered nodularity.

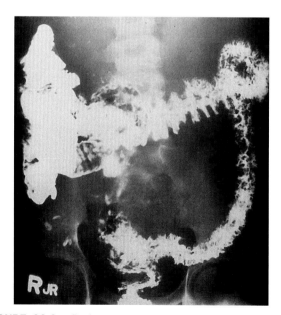

FIGURE 33-6. Barium enema radiograph of a 9-year-old patient with newly diagnosed cystic fibrosis. Spiculations, thickening, and irregularity of the mucosa are depicted. The nodularity is readily visible.

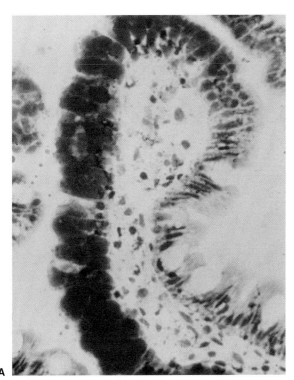
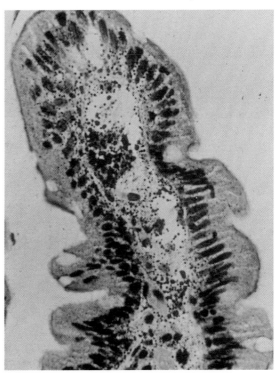

FIGURE 33-7. Small intestine biopsy specimens after lipid feeding of a patient with abetalipoproteinemia (**A**) and a healthy subject (**B**). Frozen sections were stained with oil-red-O. Among patients with abetalipoproteinemia, lipid cannot be transported out of the enterocyte, and it accumulates intracellularly in large droplets, here stained *red*. Among healthy persons, lipid is transported into the lymphatic vessels, where it exists in small droplets.

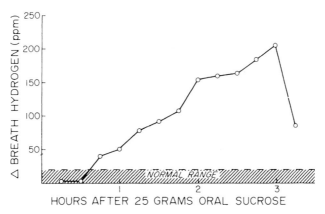

FIGURE 33-8. Breath hydrogen response to sucrose of a patient with sucrase-isomaltase deficiency. A marked increase in breath hydrogen level follows ingestion of 25 g sucrose. The hydrogen production reflects colonic fermentation of the unabsorbed disaccharide.

34

SHORT-BOWEL SYNDROME

RICHARD N. FEDORAK ▪ LEAH M. GRAMLICH

The term *short-bowel syndrome* is used to refer to the clinical consequences and pathophysiological disorders associated with a malabsorptive state resulting from the removal of a large portion of the small and/or large intestine. The degree of nutrient and nonnutrient malabsorption that occurs in a patient with extensive intestinal resection is a consequence of a number of factors: the extent and site of the resected intestine; the presence or absence of an ileal cecal valve, the condition of the remaining intestine, and the degree of adaptation of the residual small intestine (Table 34-1). It is thus possible that the removal of similar lengths of small intestine might cause short-bowel syndrome to develop in one person, but not in another.

Diarrhea is inevitable for patients who have had intensive small intestinal resection and have developed short-bowel syndrome. Diarrhea and fluid and electrolyte loss is multifactorial and often involves one or more of the following multiple causes: reduction of absorptive surface area, decreases in intestinal transit time, hormone-mediated intestinal hypersecretion, increases in the osmolality of intestinal contents, and bacterial overgrowth. Rational and judicious use of varying antidiarrheal therapies can significantly limit fluid and electrolyte losses and reduce or even eliminate the requirements for parenteral nutrition (Table 34-2).

In addition to the severe losses of fluid and electrolytes, micronutrient deficiencies (Fig. 34-1) and systemic complications such as gallstones (Fig. 34-2), enteric hyperoxaluria, renal calculi (Fig. 34-3 and Table 34-3), and bacterial overgrowth are likely to occur. Almost all patients with short-bowel syndrome at one time or another need parenteral nutrition or intravenous fluid and electrolyte therapy. Although the parenteral nutrition and/or electrolyte therapy may be transient, intermittent, or both, it is often life-sustaining therapy (Fig. 34-3).

Tables 34-4 through 34-10 provide examples of total parenteral nutrition order forms, component composition, and suggested blood work and additive routines for the adult population. Tables 34-11 through 34-15 provide similar information for pediatric patients.

Once parenteral nutrition is initiated for short-bowel syndrome patients, it often becomes life sustaining, requiring lifetime home parenteral nutrition therapy. The complication rates of home parenteral nutrition therapy tend to be related to the central venous catheter (Table 34-16). Indeed, a minority of patients are susceptible to recurrent problems and many patients have very few complications. Quality of life for patients receiving home parenteral nutrition is generally reasonable and seems to plateau after 3 to 5 years (Table 34-17). The 1-year survival rate of patients receiving home parenteral nutrition is approximately 95% for the young Crohn's disease patient; however, this survival rate decreases dramatically in the elderly patient and over time (Table 34-18).

Intestinal transplantation has become a life-saving treatment that can be considered for patients with irreversible intestinal failure who cannot be maintained on parenteral nutrition. Figure 34-4 describes an algorithm for patients with intestinal failure and describes the management that should be considered in defining those individuals for intestinal transplantation. Figure 34-5 represents intestinal transplant graft and patient survival data by era of transplant from the intestinal transplant registry. Centers performing large numbers of intestinal transplants are reporting 1-year graft and patient survival as 90% and 70%, respectively.

(figures begin on page 358)

TABLE 34-1
Factors Influencing Short-Bowel Syndrome

Extent of intestine removed
Site of intestine removed
Presence of an ileocecal valve
Extent of intestinal adaptation

TABLE 34-2
Antidiarrheal Therapies

DRUG	DOSAGE	ADVERSE EFFECTS	COMMENTS
Opiate agonists			
opium and belladonna suppository	1 q12h prn	Sedation, potentially addictive, nausea, dry mucous membranes	60–65 mg opium, 15–16 mg belladonna
Opium (Diban)	1 q4h prn	Sedation, nausea, potentially addictive	Capsule: 12 mg opium, 52 g hyoscyamine, 10 g atropine, 3 g scopolamine, 300 mg attapulgite, 71 mg pectin
Opium camphor (paregoric)	Varies depending on concentration	Sedation, nausea, potentially addictive	May not be generally available
Codeine	30–60 mg q4h prn	Sedation, nausea, potentially addictive	Tablet: 15 or 30 mg Solution: 30 or 60 mg/mL
Diphenoxylate atropine sulfate (Lomotil, generics)	5 mg initially then 2.5 mg after each loose bowel movement to a maximum of 20 mg/d	Sedation, abdominal cramps, dry skin and mucous membranes (from atropine), some addiction potential	Capsule: 2.5 mg diphenoxylate, 0.025 mg atropine
Loperamide (Imodium, generics)	2 mg after each loose bowel movement to a maximum of 16 mg/d	Sedation, abdominal cramps	Capsule: 2 mg Solution: 2 mg/10 mL after oral administration, absorption is poor, ~40% excreted unabsorbed in feces
α_2-Adrenergic agonists			
Clonidine (Catapres, generics)	0.1–0.6 mg q12h	Centrally medicated sedation and hypotension	Tablet: 0.1 and 0.2 mg
Somatostatin			
Octreotide (Sandostatin)	50–500 mcg q8–12h	Pain at injection site, diarrhea, abdominal pain	Ampules: 50, 100, 500 mcg Multidose vial: 200, 1000 mcg/mL
Sandostatin LAR depot	10–30 mg q4 wk intragluteally	Pain at injection site, diarrhea, abdominal pain	Ampules: 10, 20, 30 mg
Bulking agents			
Psyllium (Fibrepur, Metamucil, generics)	1 tsp (5–6 g) q12h	Inhaled psyllium powder may cause allergic reaction	Products where psyllium has been mixed with laxatives need to be avoided
Cholestyramine resin (Questran, generics)	4 g q12h	Nausea, fat-soluble vitamin deficiency with long-term use, may bind other drugs in GI tract	1 packet: 4 g; should not be taken dry, must be mixed with fluids; no oral drugs 1 h before or 4 h after

GI, gastrointestinal.

TABLE 34-3
Foods That Contain High Oxalate Concentrations

Beets
Green beans
Spinach
Collard greens
Mustard greens
Turnip greens
Asparagus
Brussel sprouts
Cabbage
Carrots
Cranberries
Concord grapes
Oranges
Rhubarb
Tea
Cola
Chocolate
Celery
Peas
Tomatoes
Potatoes
Apples
Bananas
Cherries
Strawberries
Peaches
Pears
Plums

TABLE 34-4
Total Parenteral Nutrition Orders: Adult

Copy to be received in the Pharmacy Department no later than 1100 hours.
Orders received after this time will be processed the following day.

Patient Dry Weight _____ kg

☐ central administration   ☐ peripheral administration

Components	Recommended Requirements	24 hour intake (g)	Energy Provided (kcal)	24 hour volume (mL)	Rate (mL/hr)	Pharmacy Use only
Amino acids (as 10%)	1-1.5 g/kg/24 hrs				█	
Dextrose (as D70W)	2 -4 mg/kg/min				█	
Additional volume	150 mL minimum	█	█		█	
Total Amino Acid Dextrose Solu (mL)	█	█	█			
Lipid (as 20%)	1 g/kg/24 hours					
Total Fluid Volume	30 mL/kg/24hours	█	█		█	
Total Energy (kcal)	25-30 kcal/kg/24hrs	█		█	█	

1. Volume for additives and/or free water.

Additives [5]	Recommended Requirements	Total 24 -hour Intake
Sodium (mmol) [1]	60-150 mmol/day	
Potassium (mmol) [1]	30-80 mmol/day	
Calcium (mmol)	5-15 mmol/day	
Magnesium (mmol)	4-8 mmol/day	
Phosphate (mmol)	15-30 mmol/day	
Acetate (mmol)	as required	
Multiple Vitamin soln [3]	10 mL/day	
Vitamin K (mg)	10 mg/week	
Trace Element soln [4]	1 mL/day	
Zinc (mg)	additional as required	
Folic Acid (mg)	additional as required	
Ranitidine/Famotidine (circle one)	as required	
Heparin (units)	as required	
Insulin, Human Regula (units) Novolin/Humulin (circle one)	as required	
Other (specify)		

1. Sodium and potassium will be added as chloride salts unless otherwise indicated.   4. See Table 4
2. Patient must reach glucose hemostatsis for at least 48 hours.   5. See Table 2
3. See Table 3

*Cycled Administration (if appropriate)
Cycle over _____ hours at _____ mL/hr Start Time _____ Stop Time _____ Decrease rate to_____mL/hr Start time _____ Stop Time _____
Flush line per protocol, device dependent.

Duration of order: *Maximum 96 hours.*
Date Ordered _____   Date to be reordered _____

Nutritions Support Service Signature _____   Physician Signature _____

Bag Number				
Nursing Initials				
Date				

TABLE 34-5

Additive Equivalents for Use in Both Adult and Pediatric Total Parenteral Nutrition Solutions

Calcium gluconate 1 mEq = 0.5 mmol Ca^{2+} = 216 mg Ca^{2+}
Potassium chloride 1 mEq = 1 mmol K^+
Magnesium sulfate 1 mEq = 0.5 mmol Mg^{2+} = 125 mg Mg^{2+}
Sodium acetate 1 mEq = 1 mmol Na^+
Potassium acetate 1 mEq = 1 mmol K^+
Potassium phosphate 1 mL = 4.4 mmol K^+ and 3 mmol P
Sodium phosphate 1 mL = 4 mmol Na^+ and 3 mmol P
1 g nitrogen = 6.25 g protein
1 g protein = 4 kcal
1 g fat = 9 kcal
1 g dextrose = 3.4 kcal
20% lipid 1 mL = 2 kcal
Amino acid = 100 mOsm/g
Dextrose = 50 mOsm/g

TABLE 34-6

Intravenous Multiple Vitamin: 12-Component Composition for Use by Adults

COMPONENT	AMOUNT PER 10 mL
Vitamin A (IU)	3300
Vitamin B_1, thiamine (mg)	3.0
Vitamin B_2, riboflavin (mg)	3.6
Vitamin B_6, pyridoxine (mg)	4.0
Vitamin B_{12}, cyanocobalamin (μg)	5.0
Niacinamide (mg)	40
Vitamin C (mg)	100
Vitamin D (IU)	200
Vitamin E (IU)	10
D-panthenol (mg)	15
Biotin (μg)	60
Folic acid (mg)	0.4

TABLE 34-7

Intravenous Trace Element Composition for Use by Both Adults and Children

COMPONENT	AMOUNT PER 1 mL
Zinc	5 mg
Copper	1 mg
Manganese	0.5 mg
Chromium	10 μg
Selenium	60 μg

TABLE 34-8

Suggested Routine Bloodwork for Adults and Children (6 mo to 14 y) on Total Parenteral Nutrition

Initial: CBC, electrolytes, magnesium, phosphorus, calcium, albumin, PT (INR), PTT, creatinine, urea, glucose
Biweekly: CBC, sodium, potassium, CO_2, creatinine, urea, glucose
Weekly (as appropriate): alkaline phosphatase, albumin, ALT, bilirubin, magnesium, phosphorus, calcium, PT (INR), PTT
Others as needed: 24-h urine for electrolytes and nitrogen balance, cholesterol, triglycerides

ALT, alanine aminotransferase; CBC, complete blood count; INR, international normalized ratio; PT, prothrombin time; PTT, partial thromboplastin time.

TABLE 34-9
Suggested Daily Intravenous Intake of Vitamins for Adults

VITAMIN	RDA ADULT RANGE
Ascorbic acid (mg)	45
Biotin (μg)	150–300*
Folacin (μg)	400
Niacin (mg)	12–20
Pantothenic acid (mg)	6–10*
Riboflavin (mg)	1.1–1.8
Thiamin (mg)	1.0–1.5
Vitamin A (IU)	4000–5000†
Vitamin B_8 (pyridoxine) (mg)	1.6–2.0
Vitamin B_{12} (cyanocobalamin) (μg)	3
Vitamin D (IU)	400
Vitamin E (IU)	12–15

Note: Results do not include requirements of pregnancy or lactation.

*Recommended daily allowance (RDA) not established; amount considered adequate in usual dietary intake.

†Assumes 50% intake as carotene, which is less available than Vitamin A.

TABLE 34-10
Suggested Daily Intravenous Intake of Trace Elements for Adults

TRACE ELEMENT	STABLE ADULT	ADULT IN ACUTE CATABOLIC STATE*	STABLE ADULT WITH INTESTINAL LOSSES*
Zinc	2.5–4.0 mg	Additional 2.0 mg	Add 17.1 mg/kg of stool or ileostomy output
Copper	0.5–1.5 mg		
Manganese	0.15–0.8 mg		
Chromium	10–15 μg		
Selenium	40–80 μg		

*Frequent monitoring of blood levels for these patients is essential to provide proper dosage.

TABLE 34-11
Total Parenteral Nutrition Orders: Pediatric (6 months to 14 years)

Copy to be received in the Pharmacy Department no later than 1100 hours.
Orders received after this time will be processed the following day.

Patient Weight _____ kg   Height _____ cm

☐ central administration   ☐ peripheral administration
                                                  (Maximum 12.5% dextrose concentration)

Components	24 hour intake (g)	Energy Provided (kcal)	24 hour volume (mL)	Rate (mL/hr)	Pharmacy Use only
Amino acids (as 10%)				■	
Dextrose (as D70W)				■	
Additional volume	■			■	
Total Amino Acid - Dextrose Soln (mL)	■				
Lipid (as 20%)					
Total Energy (kcal)	■		■	■	
Total Volume	■			■	

1. Volume for additives and/or free water.

Additives [4]	Recommended Requirements	Total 24 -hour Intake
Sodium (mmol) [1]	2-3 mmol/kg/day	
Potassium (mmol) [1]	1-3 mmol/kg/day	
Calcium (mmol)	0.5-1 mmol/kg/day	
Magnesium (mmol)	0.3-0.5 mmol/kg/day	
Phosphate (mmol)	0.5-1 mmol/kg/day	
Acetate (mmol)	for correction of acidemia	
Multiple Vitamin soln, Pediatric [2]	5 mL/day	
Trace Element soln [3]	0.02 mL/kg to a maximum of 1 mL/day	
	Other (specify)	
Heparin (units)	as required	

1. Sodium and potassium will be added as chloride salts unless otherwise indicated
2. See Table 9
3. See Table 4
4. See Table 2

Duration of order: *Maximum 96 hours.*
Date Ordered _____   Date to be reordered _____

Nutritions Support Service Signature _____   Physician Signature _____

Bag Number				
Nursing Initials				
Date				

TABLE 34-12
Intravenous Multiple Vitamin Composition for Use by Children 6 Mo to 14 Y

COMPONENT	AMOUNT PER 5 ML
Vitamin A (IU)	2300
Vitamin B_1, thiamine (mg)	1.2
Vitamin B_2, riboflavin (mg)	1.4
Vitamin B_6, pyridoxine (mg)	1
Vitamin B_{12}, cyanocobalamin (μg)	1
Niacinamide (mg)	17
Vitamin C (mg)	80
Vitamin D (IU)	400
Vitamin E (IU)	7
D-panthenol (mg)	5
Biotin (μg)	20
Folic acid (mg)	0.14
Vitamin K (μg)	200

IU, international units.

TABLE 34-13
Suggested Protein, Fat, and Energy Requirements for Children

AGE	GENDER	PROTEIN REQUIREMENTS (g/kg/d)	FAT REQUIREMENT (g/kg/d)	ENERGY REQUIREMENTS*
0–2 mo	Both	2.2		100–200 kcal/kg/d
3–4	Both	1.5	1–3 (initiate at 1 g/kg/d)	95–100 kcal/kg/d
6–8	Both	1.4		95–97 kcal/kg/d
9–11	Both	1.4		97–99 kcal/kg/d
1–3 y	Both	1.2		13.5 kcal/cm/d
4–6	Both	1.1		17 kcal/cm/d
7–9	M	1.0	1–3 (initiate at 1 g/kg/d)	17.5 kcal/cm/d
	F	1.0		15 kcal/cm/d
10–12	M	1.0		17.5 kcal/cm/d
	F	1.0		15.5 kcal/cm/d
13–15	M	1.0		17.5 kcal/cm/d
	F	0.9	2 (initiate at 1 g/kg/d)	14 kcal/cm/d
16–18	M	0.9		18.5 kcal/cm/d
	F	0.9		13 kcal/cm/d

*Actual energy requirements may vary 20% to 30% depending on stress and activity factors.

TABLE 34-14

Suggested Daily Intravenous Intake of Vitamins for Children

VITAMIN	TERM INFANTS AND CHILDREN DOSE PER DAY
Lipid soluble	
A (μg)*	700
E (mg)*	7
K (μg)	200
D (μg)*	10
Water soluble	
Ascorbic acid (mg)	80
Biotin (μg)	20
Folate (μg)	140
Niacin (mg)	17
Pantothenate (mg)	5
Pyridoxine (mg)	1.0
Riboflavin (mg)	1.4
Thiamin (mg)	1.2
Vitamin B_{12} (μg)	1.0

*700 μg vitamin A = 2300 international units (IU); 7 mg α-tocopherol = 7 IU; 10 μg vitamin D = 400 IU.

TABLE 34-15

Suggested Daily Intravenous Intake of Trace Elements in Children

ELEMENT	INFANTS ($\mu g/kg^{-1}/d^{-1}$)		CHILDREN ($\mu g/kg^{-1}/d^{-1}$)
	Preterm	Term	
Zinc	400	250 < 3 mo	50 (5000)
		100 > 3 mo	
Copper*	20	20	20 (300)
Chromium[†]	0.20	0.20	0.20 (5)
Manganese*	1.0	1.0	1.0 (50)
Selenium[†]	2.0	2.0	2.0 (30)
Molybdenum*	0.25	0.25	0.25 (5)
Iodide	1.0	1.0	1.0 (70)

Note: Value in parentheses is maximum micrograms per day.

*Omit for patients with obstructive jaundice.

[†]Omit for patients with renal dysfunction.

TABLE 34-16

Complications of Home Parenteral Nutrition (episodes per catheter year, unless indicated)

STUDY (AUTHOR AND PUBLICATION YEAR)	CATHETER SEPSIS (95% CI)	CATHETER SEPSIS (PATIENTS PER CATHETER YEAR) (95% CI)	CATHETER OCCLUSION (95% CI)	CENTRAL VEIN THROMBOSIS (95% CI)	LIVER/BILIARY PROBLEMS (95% CI)	METABOLIC BONE DISEASE (95% CI)	OTHER
Beers, 1990	—	—	—	0.04 (0.02, 0.07)	—	—	—
Bisset, 1992	—	—	—	—	—	—	Sepsis 0.73
Bowyer, 1985	—	—	—	—	15% (7%, 27%) liver problems 3% (0.4%, 12%) deaths	—	—
Buchman, 1994(a)	—	—	0.07 (0.06, 0.09)	0.02 (0.01, 0.03)	—	—	—
Buchman, 1994(b)	0.23 (0.2, 0.27) not possible to calculate rates for children	0.23 (0.2, 0.26)	—	—	—	—	—
Buchman, 1993	—	—	—	—	—	—	Low plasma-free choline levels are prevalent, associated with elevated serum aminotransferases
Buchman, 1993	—	—	—	—	—	—	Fall in renal function of 3.5 ± 6.3%/y
Burnes, 1992	0.27 (0.2, 0.35)	—	—	—	—	—	—
DePotter, 1992	0.40 (0.33, 0.49)	0.23	0.04 (0.02, 0.07)	—	0.03 (0.01, 0.05)	—	—
Dollery, 1994	—	—	—	16 episodes of major thrombosis in 12 of 34 patients	—	—	—
Dudrick, 1984	0.39 (0.26, 0.54)	0.15 (0.08, 0.26)	—	—	—	—	—
Folders, 1990	—	—	—	—	—	90% (56%, 99%)	—
Galandiuk, 1990	0.27 (0.19, 0.38)	—	—	—	—	—	—
Gouttebel, 1987	0.70 (0.49, 0.97)	0.42 (0.26, 0.4)	—	—	—	—	—
Herfindal, 1992	0.46 (0.3, 0.7)	0.14 (0.06, 0.29)	0.22 (0.12, 0.39)	—	0.42 (0.27, 0.63)	0.05 (0.01, 0.15)	Metabolic complications 0.61
Howard, 1993	—	—	—	—	—	—	Total complication rate is higher for those younger than 18 y
Howard, 1986	0.37 (0.33, 0.42)	—	—	—	—	0.013 (0.005, 0.025)	—
Hurley, 1990	0.30 (0.17, 0.49)	—	0.02 (0.06, 0.47)	—	—	—	—
Johnston, 1993	0.16 (0.05, 0.47)	—	—	0.28 (0.06, 0.47)	—	—	Total complications: cancer 2.22 (1.4, 3.4), benign 0.89 (0.64, 1.2) P < 0.01
King, 1993	0.54 (0.22, 1.11)	?	—	—	—	—	—
Manji, 1989	—	—	—	—	Symptomatic gallstones in 100%	—	—

(Continued)

355

TABLE 34-16. *(Continued)*

STUDY (AUTHOR AND PUBLICATION YEAR)	CATHETER SEPSIS (95% CI)	CATHETER SEPSIS (PATIENTS PER CATHETER YEAR) (95% CI)	CATHETER OCCLUSION (95% CI)	CENTRAL VEIN THROMBOSIS (95% CI)	LIVER/BILIARY PROBLEMS (95% CI)	METABOLIC BONE DISEASE (95% CI)	OTHER
Messing, 1989	0.38 (0.30, 0.48)	?	0.18	0.07	—	—	—
Mukau, 1992	0.2 (0.1, 0.35)	?	—	0.07 (0.02, 0.17)	—	—	—
Nightingale, 1995	24 fungal infections; total no. of lines not given	—	—	—	—	—	Four developed eye infections; two had recurrent infection
O'Hanrahan, 1992	0.47 (0.38, 0.58)	—	0.44 (0.36, 0.55)	0.06 (0.03, 0.11)	—	—	Metabolic complications 0.12 (0.08, 0.18)
Perl, 1981	—	—	—	—	—	—	Depression 80% (44, 98)
Pironi, 1993	0.12 (0.03, 0.3)	—	0.03 (0, 0.16)	0.09 (0.02, 0.26)	0.15 (0.05, 0.34)	—	—
Robb, 1983	0.42 (0.25, 0.68)	—	0.1 (0.03, 0.24)	—	—	—	—
Roslyn, 1983	—	—	—	—	Symptomatic gallstones in 23% (15%, 32%)	—	—
Schmidt-Sommerfeld, 1990	0.71 (0.5, 0.97)	—	0.29 (0.17, 0.47)	0.07 (0.02, 0.19)	—	—	—
Shike, 1986	—	—	—	—	—	67% (35%, 90%)	—
Shike, 1980	—	—	—	—	—	75% (48%, 93)	—
Singer, 1991	A 0.43 (0.05, 1.55) C 0.2 (0.07, 1.43) H 0.1 (0.04, 0.22)	—	A 0.21 (0.05, 1.2) C 0.03 (0, 0.18) H 0.06 (0.02, 0.16)	—	—	—	Metabolic distribution A 0.43 (0.05, 1.55) C 0.49 (0.28, 0.81) H 0.17 (0.08, 0.3)
Staun	—	—	—	—	—	4% decrease in bone mineral content/y	—
Steiger, 1983	—	—	—	—	—	—	Percent of hospitalized days Crohn's, 24%; radiation enteritis, 13%
Vargas, 1987	0.37 (0.29, 0.46)	0.20 (0.15, 0.28)	—	—	Any 0.06 (0.03, 0.1) Severe 0.024 (0.008, 0.057)	—	—
Weiss, 1982	0.2 (0.01, 1.11)	0.2 (0.01, 1.11)	—	—	—	—	—

?, Data in the study not sufficient for calculation of rates; 95% CI, 95% confidence interval; A, acquired immunodeficiency syndrome; C, cancer; H, home parenteral nutrition.

TABLE 34-17
Quality of Life for Patients Receiving Home Parenteral Nutrition

STUDY (AUTHOR AND PUBLICATION YEAR)	WHOSE VALUES?	INSTRUMENT USED	PROFILE OR INDEX	INDEX SCORES	BEST QOL OR OUTCOME	WORST QOL OR OUTCOME	COMMENTS
Carlson, 1995	Patient	Nonvalidated questionnaire	Index	0.64 (0–1 scale*)	—	—	QOL independent of variables tested; younger patients keen on intestinal transplantation
Detsky, 1986	Patient	Category scaling, time trade-off plus one other	Index	0.73 (0–1 scale*)	Scores improve with time and peak at 4–5 y	Lowest scores seen in the first year of HPN	Scores were measured for 37 and estimated for 36; no subgroup analysis was performed
Duclaux, 1993	Doctor	Nonvalidated simple questionnaire	Profile	—	—	—	QOL much improved at home; development and psychological well-being much improved
Galandiuk, 1990	Patient plus doctor	QOL score, social activity score, psychological score	Index	Pre-HPN, 7.1 Receiving HPN, 5.3†	—	—	Index scores were better when receiving HPN; pre-HPN QOL was significantly worse (P < 0.01); all patients in this study had Crohn's disease
Herfindal, 1989	Patient	Multiple-validated instruments	Profile	—	Long duration (>6 mo)	Duration < 6 mo	HPN patients had lower (worse) scores than renal transplant recipients and normal U.S. population
Ladefoged, 1981	Patient	Nonvalidated questionnaire	Profile	—	Acceptable in two thirds of cases	—	QOL parameters were independent of all variables, but not enough data to test
Messing, 1989	Doctor	Functional assessment	—	—	Age < 65 y, benign	Age > 65 y, malignancy, pseudo-obstruction	Simple four-stage rehabilitation profile; stage decided by physician, not the patient
O'Hanrahan, 1992	Doctor	Functional assessment	Profile	—	Crohn's disease	All other diagnostic groups	Same four-point scale used
Pironi, 1993	Doctor	Functional assessment	Profile	—	—	—	Two thirds in the upper two groups
Richards, 1995	Patient	SF-36 and Euro QOL	Both	0.51	Age < 45 y	Age > 55 y, narcotic addiction	No significant difference between disease subgroups, stomas, recent hospitalization, and duration of HPN
Smith, 1993	Patient	Multiple-validated instruments	Profile	—	Stable relationship	Long duration of HPN, poor income	Loss of friends, loss of employment, and depression were noted in two thirds of families

*Scale 0 to 1, 0 = death, 1 = best possible QOL.
†Scale 3 to 9, 9 = severe disablement and 3 = best possible QOL.

QOL, quality of life; HPN, home parenteral nutrition; SF, symptomatic function.

357

Survival When Receiving Home Parenteral Nutrition

STUDY (AUTHOR AND PUBLICATION YEAR)	BENIGN UNDERLYING DISEASE	MALIGNANT UNDERLYING DISEASE (INCLUDING AIDS)
August, 1991	—	Average months survived: cancer ovary, 1.3; cancer colon, 3; cancer appendix, 6
Grabowski, 1989	Scleroderma: 3 of 4 died at 12, 14, and 17 mo	—
Howard, 1991	1-y mortality rates: Crohn's disease, 5%; vascular occlusion, 20% (4% thereafter); pseudoobstruction, 20%	1-y mortality rates: cancer, 75%; AIDS, 93%
Howard, 1993	1-y survival: Crohn's disease, 95%; radiation enteritis, 76%	1-y survival: cancer, 30%
Howard, 1986	50% survival at 36 mo, 15% survival at year 8	50% survival at 6 mo, 15% at 1 y, all dead by 23 mo
Howard, 1995	1-y survival > 90% (age 0–55 y), 1-y survival ~ 65% (age > 55 y)	—
King, 1993	—	Gynecological malignancy: median survival, 2 mo (range 0–26)
Messing, 1995	1-y survival 91%, 2-y survival 70%, 3-y survival 62%	—
Van Gossum, 1995	6-mo mortality rates: Crohn's disease, 0%; vascular occlusion, 8%; miscellaneous, 13%; radiation enteritis, 7%	6-mo mortality rates: cancer, 71%; AIDS, 88%

AIDS, acquired immunodeficiency syndrome.

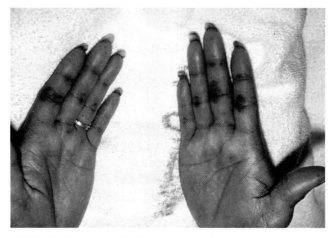

FIGURE 34-1. Acral skin lesions of a patient receiving home total parenteral nutrition without supplemental zinc.

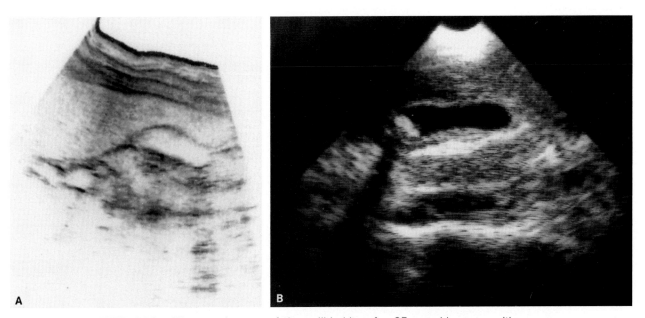

FIGURE 34-2. Ultrasound scans of the gallbladder of a 35-year-old woman with severe short-bowel syndrome after multiple resections for Crohn's disease. **A:** Ultrasound scan before home total parenteral nutrition (TPN) shows no stones. **B:** Ultrasound scan after 2 years of home TPN demonstrates stones and sludge. The patient needed a cholecystectomy for symptomatic cholelithiasis.

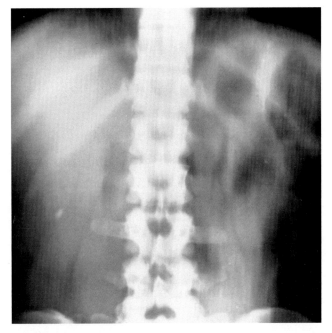

FIGURE 34-3. Nephrotomogram of a patient after resection of all but 100 cm of small intestine because of midgut volvulus with infarction, showing bilateral renal calculi. The patient had hyperoxaluria (urinary oxalate excretion 70 mg/d). Analysis of a surgically extracted stone showed that it was composed of calcium oxalate.

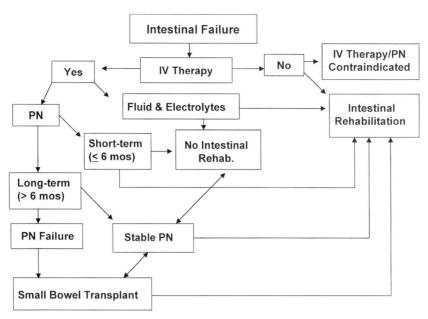

FIGURE 34-4. Algorithm for intestinal failure. PN, parenteral nutrition; IV, intravenous.

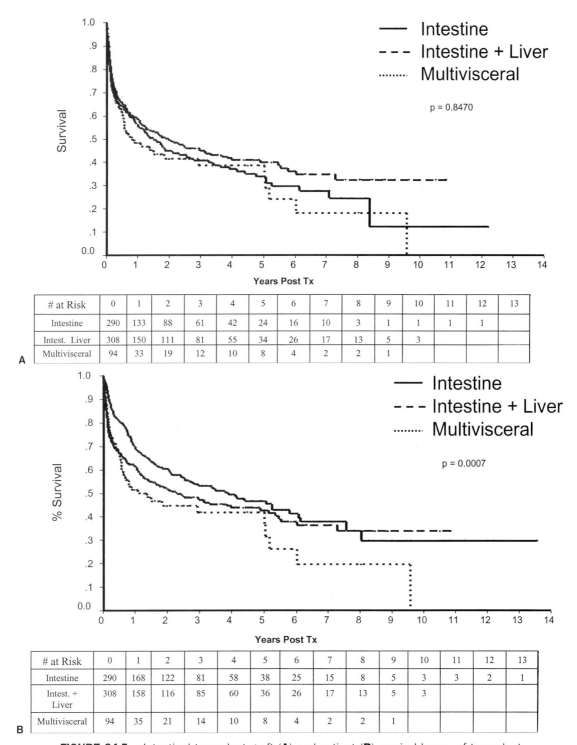

FIGURE 34-5. Intestinal transplant graft (**A**) and patient (**B**) survival by era of transplant.

35

TUMORS OF THE SMALL INTESTINE

ROBERT S. BRESALIER ■ **M. PETER LANCE**

Small intestinal tumors (tumors of the duodenum, jejunum, and ileum) are uncommon in comparison with those occurring elsewhere in the gastrointestinal tract. Although the small intestine is approximately 20 ft long, comprising 75% of the length of the gastrointestinal tract and 90% of its mucosal surface area, less than 2% of malignant gastrointestinal tumors are derived from this organ. Nonetheless, primary small intestinal tumors are diverse in nature because they are derived from both epithelial and mesenchymal components of the small bowel (Table 35-1). The most frequent primary histological types of malignant tumors include adenocarcinomas, carcinoids, lymphomas, and sarcomas (most are now classified as gastrointestinal stromal tumors). Approximately 5300 new cases of small intestinal cancer are expected in the United States in 2002 (equally distributed between men and women), with 1100 estimated cancer deaths. The relative frequency of primary tumors reported in the literature show primary adenocarcinoma (24%–52%), malignant carcinoid (17%–41%), lymphoma (12%–29%), and sarcomas (11%–20%) as the most frequently described tumors. In a recent review of the U.S. National Cancer Data Base for the years 1985 to 1995, the relative frequencies by histological type was adenocarcinoma (35.1%), carcinoid (27.6%), lymphoma (20.8%), sarcoma (10.1%), and other (6.4%). This is similar to the histological distribution in other population-based studies. The pattern of distribution of tumors in the small intestine is dependent on histological type. In western countries, adenocarcinomas are most commonly found in the duodenum. In the setting of Crohn's disease, adenocarcinomas may occur distally in the ileum, reflecting the distribution of the underlying inflammatory bowel disease. Carcinoids and primary lymphomas occur predominantly in the ileum and jejunum. Sarcomas are found more evenly distributed throughout the small intestine. Metastases to the small bowel account for approximately 50% of all small bowel tumors. Metastases may arise from several sources including a variety of carcinomas and sarcomas.

Adenocarcinoma of the small intestine represents the most common primary malignancy of this organ in most series, but the overall incidence is low in comparison to malignancies of the colon. The incidence per million of small bowel adenocarcinoma ranges between 3.0 and 6.5 in population-based studies. Adenocarcinomas represent approximately 40% of primary small bowel tumors in most population-based studies (range 24%–42%), and between 20% and 69% in selected case studies. Small bowel adenocarcinoma accounts for approximately 2% of gastrointestinal tumors and 1% of gastrointestinal cancer deaths. In a recent analysis of the U.S. National Cancer Data Base, a joint project of the American College of

Surgeons Commission on Cancer and the American Cancer Society, there were 4995 small bowel adenocarcinomas reported between 1985 and 1995. Fifty-five percent occurred in the duodenum, 18% in the jejunum, 13% in the ileum, and 14% in nonspecified sites. Fifty-three percent of those with small bowel adenocarcinomas were male and 47% were female. The overall 5-year survival was 30.5%, with a median survival of 19.7 months.

Adenocarcinomas arise from adenomas or dysplastic changes of the small intestine. Adenomas and adenocarcinomas of the small intestine, and especially of the duodenum and ampulla of Vater, are most frequently encountered in the setting of familial adenomatous polyposis (FAP). Duodenal adenomas have been reported in up to 90% of FAP patients, but the potential for malignant degeneration and natural history have not been studied in detail. Adenocarcinomas of the small bowel are also associated with hereditary nonpolyposis colorectal cancer (HNPCC), hamartomatous polyposis syndromes (especially the Peutz-Jeghers syndrome), Crohn's disease, bile diversion (previous cholecystectomy), and gluten-sensitive enteropathy. Other conditions that have been associated with adenocarcinoma of the small intestine include urinary diversion to the small bowel (ileal loop conduits), and long-standing ileostomies and ileal pouches in patients with inflammatory bowel diseases and FAP.

Adenomas in the small intestine display the same gross and microscopic features as those in the large intestine. They may be pedunculated or sessile. Tubular adenomas tend to be small, whereas those with villous architecture tend to be larger. The presence of multiple duodenal adenomas or adenomatous changes in the ampulla of Vater suggests the diagnosis of FAP. Small intestinal adenocarcinomas may appear grossly as flat, stenosing, ulcerative, infiltrating, or polypoid lesions. Most are moderately differentiated tumors with gland formation and variable degrees of mucin secretion. Adenocarcinomas invade the muscularis propria and bowel wall to invade veins, lymphatics, and nerves, and metastasize to regional lymph nodes and distant sites such as the liver and lungs. Tumors often invade adjacent structures and the retroperitoneum, including the pancreas.

The mean age of presentation for adenocarcinomas is approximately 65 years of age, with a wide range of age at presentation. Less than 1% of tumors occur before age 30 years, and approximately 85% occur after age 50 years. Symptoms relate to tumor size, location, and blood supply. Small tumors are asymptomatic or may present with anemia secondary to chronic blood loss, but for the most part are indolent and difficult to diagnose. Abdominal pain and other obstructive symptoms such as nausea and vomiting are common late symptoms as tumors obstruct because of infiltration with lumenal narrowing, or mass effect. Anorexia and weight loss are also common symptoms.

Endoscopy may be used to examine the duodenum where a lesion is suspected or in families with FAP. Small bowel follow-through (SBFT) is an extension of the conventional barium study in which oral contrast is ingested and followed through the small bowel. SBFT has been reported to be 70% to 80% accurate for detection of duodenal lesions. This accuracy can be improved by the use of hypotonic duodenography. Barium studies, however, are not as accurate in detecting tumors that are more distal. Enteroclysis involves intubation of the duodenum and instillation of dilute barium into the small intestine. In a study comparing the sensitivity and tumor detection rate of enteroclysis and SBFT, the SBFT had a sensitivity of 61% and enteroclysis had a sensitivity of 95%. Computerized tomography (CT) is being used increasingly in demonstrating small bowel tumors and their complications. Endoscopic ultrasonography has emerged as an important tool for diagnosing and staging tumors of the gastrointestinal tract. A high-frequency transducer placed at the tip of the endoscope is used to obtain high-resolution transmural sonographic images of the intestinal wall and surrounding structures. Surgical resection is the treatment of choice for adenocarcinoma of the small intestine.

Carcinoid tumors (or argentaffinoma) belong to a family of rare neuroendocrine neoplasms known also as amine precursor uptake and decarboxylation tumors. This entire family of neoplasms has in common the ability to secrete amines and polypeptides, which produce the characteristic clinical syndromes with which they sometimes present. Seventy-four percent of carcinoid tumors occur in the gastrointestinal tract. The majority appear in the appendix, followed in frequency by the small bowel and rectum. Most of the clinically significant carcinoid tumors are located in the small bowel. Eighty-seven percent of small bowel tumors are in the ileum; 40% of these can be found within 2 ft of the ileocecal valve. Carcinoid tumors are malignant, despite their sometimes-indolent course. Small bowel carcinoids, in particular, are associated with local-regional spread or metastases at the time of diagnosis. The tumors are usually intramucosal, and rarely ulcerate to the lumen of the bowel. Small bowel carcinoids spread locally through the muscularis propria, toward the serosa. When serosal breach has occurred, an intense local fibroblastic reaction is commonly seen. The desmoplastic reaction is responsible for many of the clinical findings in patients with small bowel carcinoid.

Patients with small bowel carcinoids can present with nonspecific gastrointestinal symptoms, small bowel obstruction, intestinal ischemia, intussusception, gastrointestinal hemorrhage, hepatomegaly, or symptoms of the carcinoid syndrome. Many of the signs and symptoms of small bowel carcinoids are due to the intense desmoplastic reaction of the mesentery in proximity to the tumor. The fibrosis initially causes intestinal buckling or kinking, which leads to partial small bowel obstructions and nonspecific gastrointestinal symptoms. Patients with liver metastases from carcinoids may exhibit symptoms and signs of the carcinoid syndrome. Flushing of the face and neck may be episodic or permanent, and is usually a deep red, or purple color. Diarrhea manifests as intermittent episodes of explosive, watery diarrhea caused by intestinal hypermotility. Abdominal cramping may accompany the diarrhea episodes, and is the third most common symptom of the syndrome. Dyspnea can be due to advanced carcinoid heart disease, or less frequently from bronchoconstriction and asthma. Two thirds of patients with carcinoid syndrome will present with a large liver or an abdominal mass. Forty percent will have heart valve abnormalities than can be auscultated at presentation. Other less common signs include cyanosis, peripheral edema, arthritis, and pellagra.

Conventional barium studies of the small intestine may identify the primary lesion as a smooth, semilunar filling defect in the lumen. Scintigraphy has long been used for detecting neuroendocrine tumors. Octreotide-labeled scintigraphy is useful not only as a diagnostic modality, but may also be used to predict who will respond to octreotide therapy, and to locate tumors prior to surgical debulking. Small bowel carcinoids have been detected endoscopically in the duodenum, proximal jejunum, and terminal ileum. The tumors generally appear as nodular, submucosal protuberances with a yellowish, shiny appearance. Duodenal carcinoids can also be diagnosed by endoscopic ultrasound.

Neoplasms of mesenchymal origin are uncommon in the gastrointestinal tract, accounting for less than 1% of all gastrointestinal malignancies. A multitude of tumors that occur in the small intestine have been described on the basis of their appearance at light microscopy. The most common variant is the mesenchymal spindle-cell tumor. Some mesenchymal tumors represent clear-cut diagnostic entities (e.g., lipoma, ganglioneuroma), whereas most are more difficult to classify into any specific cell lineage. Tumors may share overlapping features of several diagnostic entities. They may also be histologically heterogeneous, with features of different tumor types in different areas of the same tumor. Given the uncertainty about the histogenesis and behavior of these tumors, the general term *gastrointestinal stromal-cell tumors* (GISTs) was coined to describe the group. Malignant GISTs are gut-specific sarcomas and represent 11% to 12.7% of all small bowel malignancies. GISTs of the small bowel occur most frequently in the jejunum, followed by the ileum, and then the duodenum. GISTs mostly arise from the muscularis propria and generally tend to grow extramurally. Small bowel GISTs generally have a spindle-cell–like appearance, but infrequently can appear epithelioid.

GISTs of the small bowel tend to invade locally, and frequently present with peritoneal seeding or direct invasion to adjacent organs. The most useful indicators of survival and the risk of metastases are the size of the tumor at presentation and the mitotic index (the number of mitotic figures per 50 high-power fields). In addition, histological evidence of tumor invasion into the bowel lamina propria is a consistently poor prognostic indicator. More than 50% of patients with tumors greater than 5 cm will have either a palpable abdominal mass or gastrointestinal hemorrhage. Perhaps the greatest advance in endoscopic diagnosis of submucosal gastrointestinal tumors is endoscopic ultrasound. GISTs appear as hypoechoic masses arising from the fourth echo layer (muscularis propria). Surgical resection is the treatment of choice for GISTs.

Involvement of the intestine with lymphomatous neoplasms can occur in several settings. The following criteria should be met to designate a primary small bowel lymphoma:

- the absence of palpable peripheral lymphadenopathy
- a normal peripheral leukocyte count and differential
- no mediastinal lymphadenopathy on a chest x-ray
- involvement of only the organs of the gastrointestinal tract and proximal regional lymph nodes
- no involvement of the liver or spleen, unless by direct extension from the primary gastrointestinal tumor.

Small bowel lymphomas represent 1% to 10% of all extranodal lymphomas. Small bowel lymphomas account for 7% to 25% of all small bowel tumors. Primary small bowel lymphomas (PSBL) occur most often in the ileum, followed by the jejunum, and then the duodenum. They are generally localized to one segment of the bowel, except in the case of mantle-cell lymphoma—otherwise known as multiple lymphoid polyposis.

The tumors have many different appearances. They may be large exophytic masses, polyp-like, ulcer-like, or appear as nodularity and inflammation. Tumor growth and extension is frequently intramural for a prolonged period of time before intralumenal ulceration or extralumenal invasion occurs. Involvement of regional lymph nodes is present in approximately 50% of patients with most types of PSBL. In contrast to PSBL, immunoproliferative small intestinal disease (IPSID) tends to be a very diffuse disease and most often involves the jejunum. Gross findings can range from thickened folds to discrete masses. Although the macroscopic appearance of IPSID is generally less impressive than that of PSBL, the disease affects a significant portion of the intestine in a contiguous fashion. The great majority of small bowel lymphomas are B-cell derived.

The symptoms of PSBL are usually nonspecific, and may continue for 4 to 18 months before a diagnosis is rendered. Abdominal pain is reported in 65% to 87% of patients with PSBL. Weight loss is seen in approximately 50% of patients with PSBL. The symptoms of IPSID differ from those of PSBL. Nearly all patients with IPSID will have diarrhea, weight loss, anorexia, and abdominal pain. Emesis and fever occur in 50% of patients. If a small bowel lymphoma is suspected, the diagnosis can be achieved by radiologic, endoscopic, or surgical means. The mainstay of treatment for PSBL is surgical resection. PSBL that cannot be completely resected is usually treated by chemotherapy and sometimes with the addition of radiotherapy. IPSID is less amenable to surgical resection than PSBL because of the diffuse nature of the tumor, and the low performance status of patients at the time of presentation.

Metastatic tumors represent the commonest tumors involving the small intestine in many series. Grossly secondary tumors often present as submucosal nodules or plaques, and may grow to form intramural masses, which cause obstruction, intussusception, or perforation. Tumors often present as stenotic lesions or infiltrative lesions that simulate Crohn's disease. Metastases from melanoma, and carcinomas of the lung, testes, adrenal, ovary, stomach, large intestine, uterus, cervix, liver, and kidney to the small intestine have all been reported.

The benign tumors that are most often encountered clinically are adenoma, leiomyoma, Brunner gland hamartoma, and lipoma. Adenocarcinoma of the small intestine probably arises from adenoma. The incidence of periampullary adenocarcinoma is greatly increased among persons with familial adenomatous polyposis.

The histological nature of a tumor of the small intestine is usually not apparent from the clinical features. Intermittent, partial obstruction of the small intestine is the most common way for both benign and malignant small bowel tumors to present themselves. Benign small bowel tumors are the most common cause of intussusception among adults. Occult blood loss and weight loss each are features in about 50% of cases of malignant tumors of the small intestine. Most patients with periampullary adenocarcinoma have jaundice. The diagnosis of a small bowel tumor is often not made before laparotomy.

TABLE 35-1
Classification of Small Intestinal Tumors

Benign epithelial tumors
  Brunner gland lesions*
  Benign intestinal epithelial polyps
    Adenomas
    Hamartomas (Peutz-Jeghers syndrome, Cronkhite Canada syndrome,
      juvenile polyposis, Cowden disease, Bannayan-Riley-Ruvalcaba syndrome)

Malignant epithelial lesions
  Primary adenocarcinomas
  Secondary carcinomas (metastases)
  Carcinoid tumors (neuroendocrine tumors)

Lymphoproliferative disorders
  B-cell
    Diffuse large cell lymphoma
    Small non–cleaved-cell lymphoma
    Malt cell lymphoma
    Mantle cell lymphoma (multiple lymphomatous polyposis)
    Immunoproliferative small intestinal disease
  T-cell
    Enteropathy-associated T-cell lymphoma

Mesenchymal tumors†
  Gastrointestinal stromal tumors (benign and malignant)
  Fatty tumors (lipoma, liposarcoma)
  Neural tumors (gut autonomic tumors, Schwannomas, neurofibromas,
    ganglioneuromas, granular cell tumors)
  Paragangliomas
  Smooth muscle tumors (leiomyoma, leiomyosarcoma)
  Vascular tumors (hemangioma, angiosarcoma, lymphangioma, Kaposi sarcoma)

Note: This is a partial list of tumors found in the small intestine. Although the overall incidence of small intestinal tumors is low, a wide variety of benign and malignant lesions have been described in this organ.

*It is unclear whether these lesions should be classified as hyperplasias, neoplasias, hamartomas, or adenomatous proliferations.

†Some mesenchymal tumors represent clear-cut diagnostic entities, whereas many are more difficult to classify into any specific cell lineage. The latter are designated as gastrointestinal stromal tumors.

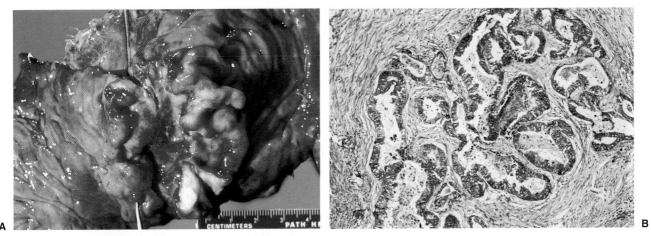

FIGURE 35-1. Small intestinal adenocarcinomas. **A:** Gross specimen. Opened section of duodenum with stenosing, infiltrating lesion. (Courtesy of Dr. Chan Ma.) **B:** Histological section demonstrating typical gland formation in this moderately differentiated adenocarcinoma.

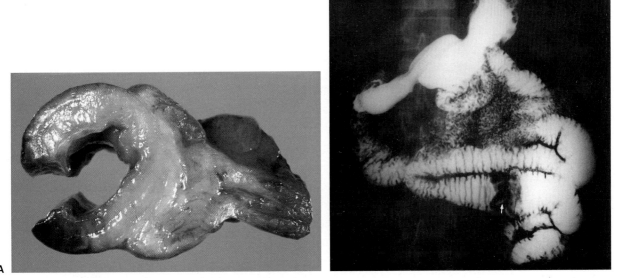

FIGURE 35-2. Small intestinal adenocarcinoma. Annular constricting lesion of the jejunum. (Courtesy of Dr. Chan Ma.) **A:** Gross specimen. **B:** Upper gastrointestinal barium study demonstrating "apple core" lesion (*arrow*).

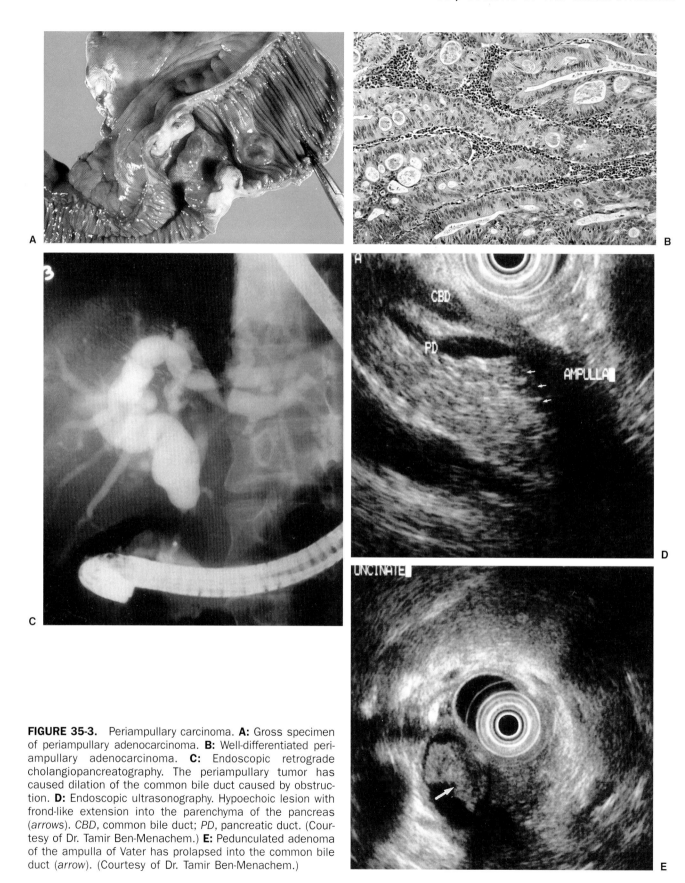

FIGURE 35-3. Periampullary carcinoma. **A:** Gross specimen of periampullary adenocarcinoma. **B:** Well-differentiated periampullary adenocarcinoma. **C:** Endoscopic retrograde cholangiopancreatography. The periampullary tumor has caused dilation of the common bile duct caused by obstruction. **D:** Endoscopic ultrasonography. Hypoechoic lesion with frond-like extension into the parenchyma of the pancreas (*arrows*). *CBD*, common bile duct; *PD*, pancreatic duct. (Courtesy of Dr. Tamir Ben-Menachem.) **E:** Pedunculated adenoma of the ampulla of Vater has prolapsed into the common bile duct (*arrow*). (Courtesy of Dr. Tamir Ben-Menachem.)

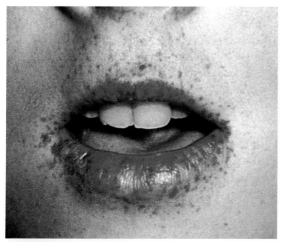

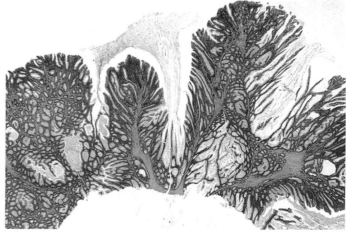

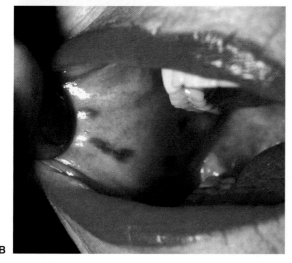

FIGURE 35-4. Peutz-Jeghers syndrome. **A, B:** Characteristic buccal and perioral pigment spots characteristic of this syndrome. **C:** Distinctive polyp with arborizing pattern of growth of the muscularis mucosae extending into the branching fronds of the polyp.

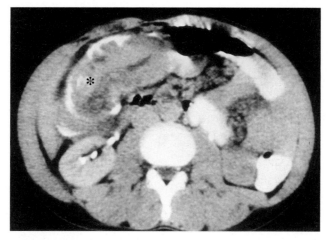

FIGURE 35-5. Computed tomography scan demonstrating intussusception in the terminal ileum caused by a small intestinal carcinoma (*asterisk*).

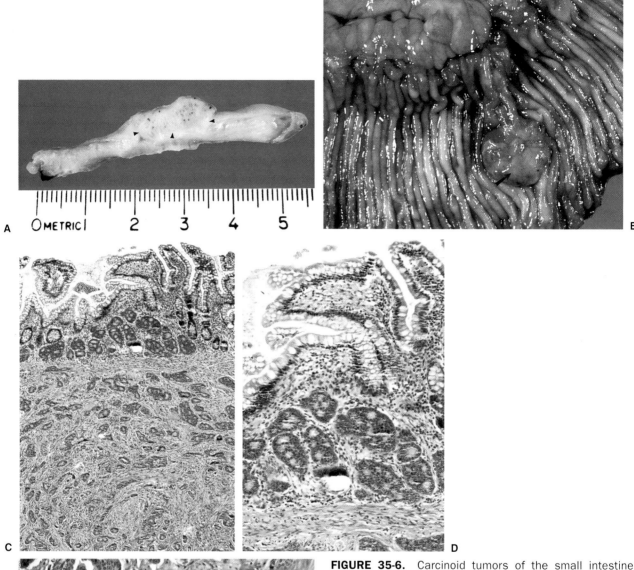

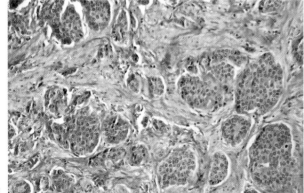

FIGURE 35-6. Carcinoid tumors of the small intestine. Carcinoid tumors develop deep in the mucosa and grow slowly, extending into the underlying submucosa and the overlying mucosa. They form firm intramural nodules that grossly appear tan or yellow. **A:** Gross specimen of small intestinal carcinoid appearing as tan nodular tumor. **B:** Small nodular carcinoid (*arrow*) can be distinguished in unfixed opened specimen of this ileal resection. **C, D, E:** Histological sections show small intestinal carcinoid tumors characterized by closely packed, round, regular, and monomorphous cell masses, buds, and islands. Lumena and rosette-like structures are present in **C** and **D**. (Courtesy of Dr. Raouf Nakhleh.) **C** demonstrates the desmoplastic reaction responsible for many of the clinical findings of small intestinal carcinoid tumors.

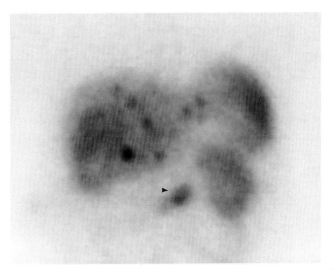

FIGURE 35-7. Octreotide scan, which demonstrates small intestinal carcinoid (*arrow*) and numerous hepatic metastases. (Courtesy of Dr. K. Karvelis.)

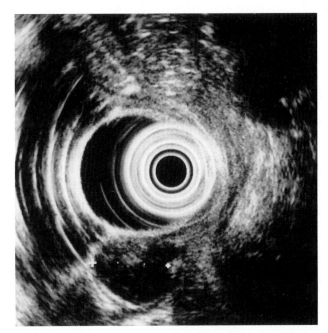

FIGURE 35-8. Carcinoid tumor. Endoscopic ultrasound demonstrating small noninvasive lesion arising in the third echo-layer (submucosa) of the duodenum (marked by *cursor +*). (Courtesy of Dr. Tamir Ben-Menachem.)

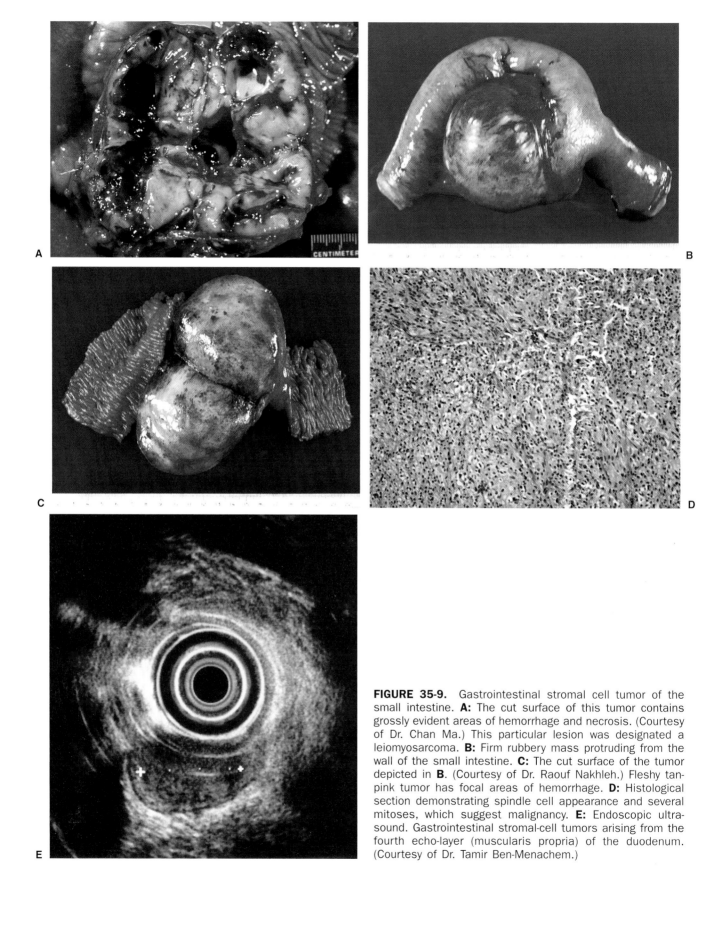

FIGURE 35-9. Gastrointestinal stromal cell tumor of the small intestine. **A:** The cut surface of this tumor contains grossly evident areas of hemorrhage and necrosis. (Courtesy of Dr. Chan Ma.) This particular lesion was designated a leiomyosarcoma. **B:** Firm rubbery mass protruding from the wall of the small intestine. **C:** The cut surface of the tumor depicted in **B**. (Courtesy of Dr. Raouf Nakhleh.) Fleshy tan-pink tumor has focal areas of hemorrhage. **D:** Histological section demonstrating spindle cell appearance and several mitoses, which suggest malignancy. **E:** Endoscopic ultrasound. Gastrointestinal stromal-cell tumors arising from the fourth echo-layer (muscularis propria) of the duodenum. (Courtesy of Dr. Tamir Ben-Menachem.)

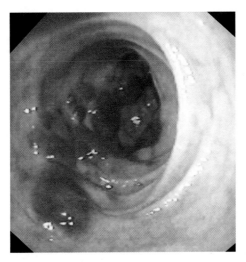

FIGURE 35-10. Kaposi sarcoma. Violaceous nodules in the duodenal mucosa seen at endoscopy in a patient with acquired immunodeficiency syndrome. (Courtesy of Dr. Tamir Ben-Menachem.)

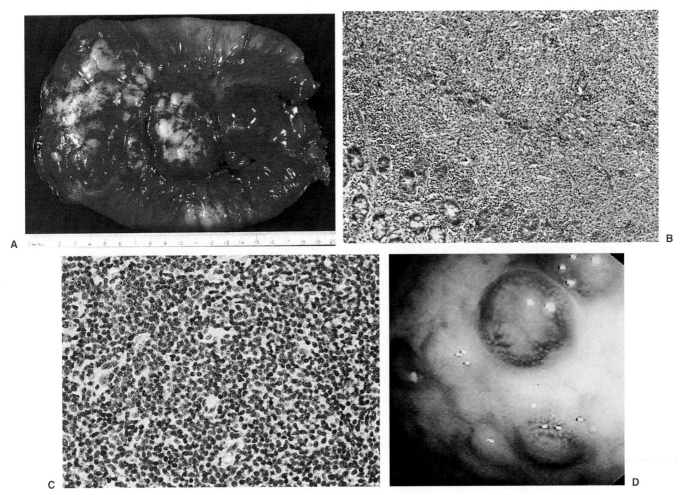

FIGURE 35-11. Primary small intestinal lymphomas. **A:** Gross specimen of primary lymphoma extensively involving the small intestine. (Courtesy of Dr. Raouf Nakhleh.) **B:** Low-power photomicrographs of diffuse B-cell lymphoma of the small intestine. **C:** High-power photomicrograph of intestinal B-cell lymphoma of the terminal ileum. **D:** Mantle cell lymphomatous polyposis of the intestine seen endoscopically. The mucosa is studded with elevated polypoid nodules. *(Continued)*

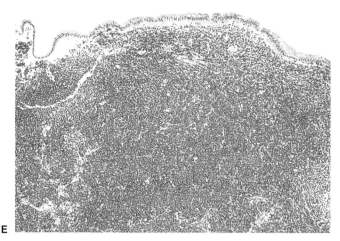

E

FIGURE 35-11. (Continued) E: Low-power photomicrograph of polypoid lymphoma.

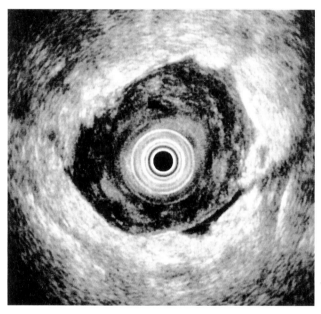

FIGURE 35-12. Endoscopic ultrasound demonstrating primary small bowel lymphoma of the duodenum. Characteristic irregular hypoechoic mass disrupts the architecture. All echo-layers in the duodenum are obliterated, which suggests involvement of the entire duodenal wall. (Courtesy of Dr. Tamir Ben-Menachem.)

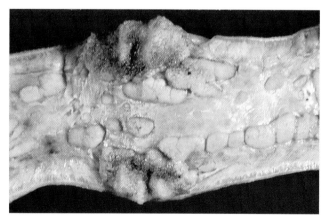

FIGURE 35-13. Fixed specimen of ileum demonstrating denuded and nodular mucosa characteristic of Crohn's disease, with small bowel lymphoma arising in this setting. (Courtesy of Dr. Raouf Nakhleh.)

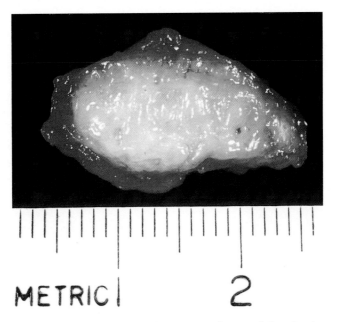

FIGURE 35-14. Gangliocytic paraganglioma of the duodenum. This is a rare submucosal polypoid tumor. Tumors contain proliferating neurites and Schwann cells, ganglion cells with Schwann cells, or proliferations of clear epithelioid cells resembling carcinoid tumors. (Courtesy of Dr. Raouf Nakhleh.)

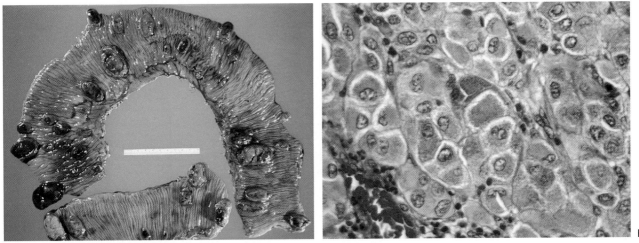

FIGURE 35-15. Metastatic melanoma. **A:** Multiple submucosal metastases appear as plaques and nodules with "target-like" appearance throughout this section of small intestine. **B:** Pleomorphic pigmented neoplastic cells account for the black gross appearance seen in **A**. (Courtesy of Dr. Chan Ma.)

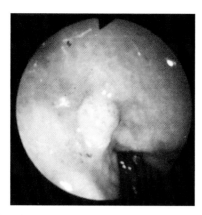

FIGURE 35-16. Adenomatous polyp of duodenum. Endoscopic view of a polyp at the junction of the bulb and descending duodenum in a patient with familial polyposis coli.

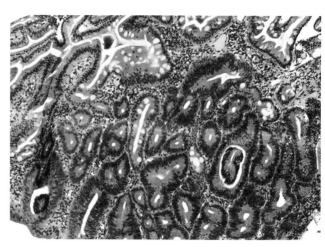

FIGURE 35-17. Tubular adenoma of the duodenum. In the **lower part** of this section, characteristic densely packed tubules are present in which the cells have hyperchromatic nuclei. A transition between these tubules and less abnormal glands that contain goblet cells is present in the **upper part** of the section. (Courtesy of Dr. S.K. Satchidanand.)

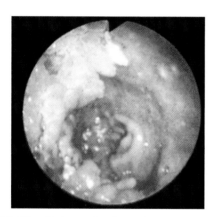

FIGURE 35-18. Endoscopic view of duodenal villous adenoma. The polyp is multilobular and has a velvety surface.

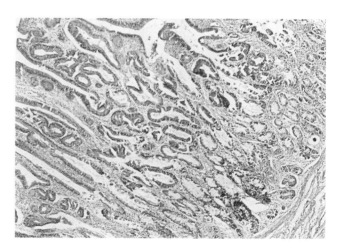

FIGURE 35-19. Villous adenoma of the duodenum. Muscularis mucosae are present (**bottom right**). Finger-like projections of lamina propria surrounded by a layer of epithelial cells extend toward the bowel lumen. (Courtesy of Dr. S.K. Satchidanand.)

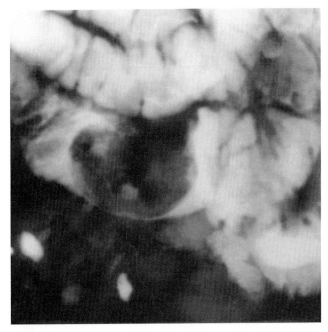

FIGURE 35-20. Leiomyoma of proximal ileum. The tumor appears as an intralumenal filling defect. Barium fills ulcerated areas on the surface of the filling defect. (Courtesy of Dr. M.L. Andres.)

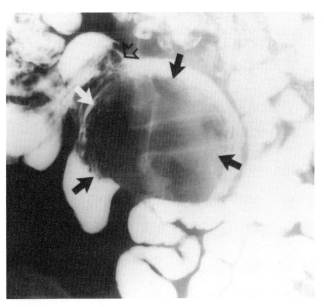

FIGURE 35-21. Leiomyoma of terminal ileum. The tumor appears as an extralumenal mass (*solid arrows*) compressing the intestine immediately proximal to the ileocecal valve (*open arrow*). (Courtesy of Dr. M.L. Andres.)

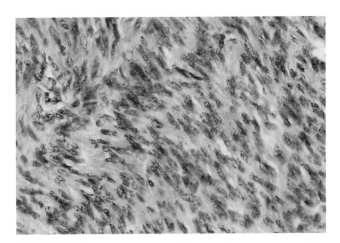

FIGURE 35-22. Leiomyoma of ileum. The tumor consists of bundles of spindle cells. The absence of mitoses differentiates this tumor from leiomyosarcoma. (Courtesy of Dr. S.K. Satchidanand.)

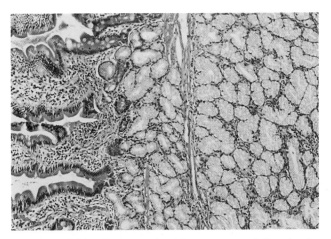

FIGURE 35-23. Brunner gland hamartoma of the duodenum. An excess of Brunner gland tissue, predominantly below the muscularis mucosae, forms a small tumor. There is no cellular atypia. The presence of Paneth cells identifies this tumor as hamartoma. (Courtesy of Dr. S.K. Satchidanand.)

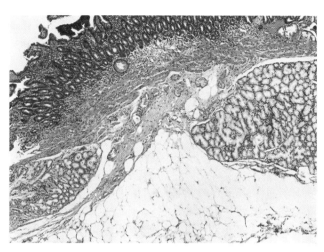

FIGURE 35-24. Duodenal lipoma. Submucosal adipose tissue contracts with Brunner glands (**right**). (Courtesy of Dr. S.K. Satchidanand.)

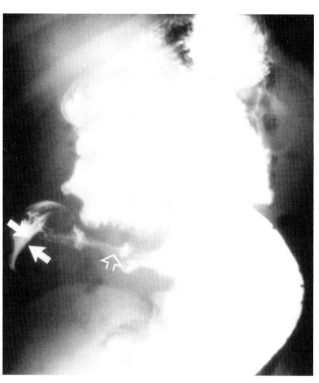

FIGURE 35-25. Intussusception of the ileum. The intussuscipiens (*white arrows*) was a juvenile polyp. Compression in the intussusceptum is depicted as a narrow column of barium (*open arrow*). (Courtesy of Dr. M.L. Andres.)

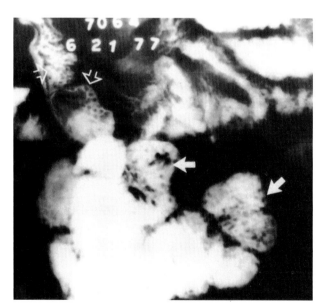

FIGURE 35-26. Nodular lymphoid hyperplasia. Involvement of the terminal ileum (*open arrows*) may occur among healthy persons. A lesion in the midportion of the ileum (*white arrows*), as in this immunocompromised patient with giardiasis, is regarded as abnormal. (Courtesy of Dr. M.L. Andres.)

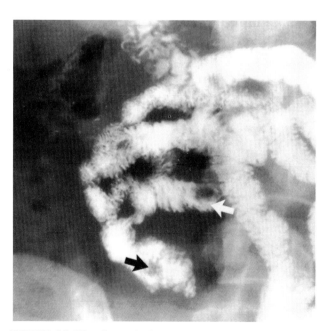

FIGURE 35-27. Peutz-Jeghers syndrome. Two polyps are depicted as filling defects in the midjejunum of this patient with the syndrome. (Courtesy of Dr. M.L. Andres.)

MISCELLANEOUS DISEASES OF THE SMALL INTESTINE

CHANDRA PRAKASH ■ **MARC S. LEVIN**

ULCERS OF THE SMALL INTESTINE

There are many causes of ulcers of the small intestine (Table 36-1). Primary (idiopathic) small bowel ulcers are diagnosed when other identifiable causes of small bowel ulcers are eliminated. Seventy-five percent are located in the middle to distal ileum. Symptomatic complications include bleeding, perforation, and obstruction. The ulcers vary in size from 0.3 to 5 cm and usually have sharp, demarcated borders. The diagnosis sometimes is made with radiologic studies, such as small bowel barium studies (Fig. 36-1) and enteroclysis, or small bowel enteroscopy, but most symptomatic idiopathic ulcers are first diagnosed at exploratory laparotomy. Therapy is dictated by the severity of complications. Perforation and bleeding usually necessitate surgical resection. Intraoperative enteroscopy may be a useful adjunct in the operative diagnosis.

Many medications have been known to cause ulcers and strictures of the small intestine (Table 36-2), and among them nonsteroidal antiinflammatory drugs (NSAIDs) are recognized as common causes. Although the exact pathogenesis is unknown, increased intestinal permeability is believed to increase susceptibility to lumenal macromolecules, bacteria, and toxins. NSAID-mediated cyclooxygenase inhibition is not believed to play an important role in the pathogenesis. NSAID-associated intestinal injury primarily affects the distal small intestine, which leads to diagnostic confusion with Crohn's disease. Therapy includes discontinuation of the offending agent whenever possible. Surgical intervention may be needed for symptomatic strictures or intestinal perforation. When an acceptable alternative medication is unavailable, use of prodrugs such as sulindac or nabumetone may lessen intestinal toxicity.

Other medications implicated as ulcerogens include enteric-coated potassium chloride, ferrous salts (Fig. 36-2), digoxin, corticosteroids, cytarabine and other chemotherapeutic agents, and clofazimine. Parenteral gold therapy has been associated with enterocolitis characterized by edema and ulceration of the ileum. Ischemic damage can result from drugs that interfere with autonomic regulation of vascular supply to the bowel (see Table 36-2; Fig. 36-3), or with the coagulation process, resulting in intravascular thrombus formation (Fig. 36-4). On the other hand, anticoagulants can cause ulceration from intramucosal and transmural hematoma formation with mucosal pressure necrosis (Fig. 36-5). Drug smugglers sometimes ingest packets of illicit drugs for transport to avoid detection (body packer, Fig. 36-6), the rupture of which can result in overwhelming toxicity from the drug and often death of the smuggler.

Behçet syndrome is associated with intestinal ulceration among less than 1% of patients. These patients have multiple deep ulcers, often bleeding or penetrating, in the ileocecal region. Microthrombosis and vasculitis with intestinal ischemia can result in intestinal ulceration in systemic lupus erythematosus. Mesenteric vasculitis with small-bowel ischemia and stricture formation has been reported in rheumatoid arthritis, scleroderma, polyarteritis nodosa (Fig. 36-7), Henoch-Schönlein purpura, Wegener granulomatosis (Fig. 36-8), giant cell arteritis, Churg-Strauss syndrome, and Sézary syndrome. Spasm of the mesenteric arteries (see Fig. 36-3), sometimes induced by drugs such as ergot or cocaine, can cause mesenteric ischemia and result in ulceration if prolonged. Thrombosis of the mesenteric veins resulting from many conditions, including hypercoagulable states and collagen vascular diseases, can cause transmural hemorrhage, mucosal ulceration, or even perforation of the bowel (see Fig. 36-4). Angiodysplasia consists of ectatic submucosal blood vessels with a thin, overlying mucosal layer (Fig. 36-9), the erosion or rupture of which can result in ulceration and gastrointestinal bleeding. Radiation damage to the intestine can result in fibrosis of the submucosal layers and vascular insufficiency with the formation of intraepithelial telangiectasia (Fig. 36-10). Stricture formation can result in bowel obstruction, sometimes necessitating surgical intervention.

Chronic ulcerative jejunoileitis (CUJ) is a rare clinical syndrome. It occurs among patients with long-standing gluten-sensitive enteropathy in the sixth or seventh decade of life. It is characterized by malabsorption, abdominal pain, and multiple nonmalignant ulcers of the small intestine. Villous atrophy, which is believed to be related to infiltration by activated T cells, usually is present. Mucosal ulceration, crypt hyperplasia, and an inflammatory cell infiltrate also occur and result in malabsorption and protein-losing enteropathy. Other symptoms include midepigastric pain, weight loss, and complications of ulceration, including small bowel obstruction, bleeding, and perforation. The diagnosis should be considered in the care of patients with long-standing gluten-sensitive enteropathy with worsening malabsorption despite continued compliance with a gluten-free diet. Biopsies of the small intestine are essential to establish the diagnosis. Although oral steroids and surgical resection of severely affected bowel have been tried, no specific therapy has been shown to modulate the course of CUJ. Data suggest that CUJ may be an important risk factor for the development of enteropathy-associated T-cell lymphoma (Fig. 36-11).

NECROTIZING ENTEROCOLITIS

Acute jejunitis is largely a disease of nonindustrialized nations. Outbreaks are most frequent in communities in which protein deprivation and poor food hygiene are prevalent. *Clostridium perfringens* type C has been established as the causative organism. The illness is characterized by bloody diarrhea, fever, and abdominal pain. Nonocclusive small-intestinal ischemia results in necrosis of varying severity. Successful treatment involves early recognition, antibiotics, and surgical resection of severely affected bowel segments.

Neonatal necrotizing enterocolitis (NEC) is a disorder of unknown causation. It affects premature infants and low-birth-weight neonates. It is characterized by focal or diffuse small intestine ulceration and necrosis (Fig. 36-12). Pathogenic etiologic factors implicated include prematurity, intestinal ischemia, infectious agents, and initiation of enteral nutrition. There is a high prevalence among infants whose mothers used cocaine during pregnancy, suggesting a pathogenic role of hypoxic and ischemic injury. Although no organism has been consistently identified with NEC, a pathogenic role for bacteria is suggested by the occurrence of epidemics within intensive care units.

PROTEIN-LOSING GASTROENTEROPATHY

The defining characteristic of protein-losing gastroenteropathy (PLGE) is hypoproteinemia resulting from gastric or intestinal loss of plasma proteins in abnormal amounts. A number of intestinal disorders have been implicated in the pathogenesis (Table 36-3; Figs. 36-13 and 36-14; see Fig. 36-11). The diagnosis is established with documentation of excessive intestinal protein losses by means of measuring fecal α_1-antitrypsin clearance. There is no specific therapy for PLGE, and management of the primary condition is the only effective remedy.

TABLE 36-1
Causes of Small Intestine Ulceration

Infectious	Tuberculosis, typhoid, cytomegalovirus infection, syphilis, parasitic infestation, strongyloidosis hyperinfection, *Campylobacter* infection, yersiniosis
Toxic	Acute jejunitis (β-toxin–producing *Clostridium perfringens*), arsenic
Inflammatory	Crohn's disease, systemic lupus erythematosus with high serum antiphospholipid levels, diverticulitis
Mucosal lesions	Gluten-sensitive enteropathy (jejunoileitis)
Tumors	
Primary	Malignant histiocytosis, lymphoma
Secondary	Adenocarcinoma, melanoma, Kaposi sarcoma
Vascular	Mesenteric insufficiency, giant cell arteritis, vasculitis, vascular abnormality, amyloidosis (ischemic lesion)
Metabolic	Uremia
Drugs	Potassium chloride, nonsteroidal antiinflammatory drugs, antimetabolites
Radiation	Therapeutic, accidental
Idiopathic	Primary ulcer, Behçet syndrome

TABLE 36-2
Drug-Induced Small Bowel Disease

MECHANISM	DRUGS IMPLICATED
Erosive damage	Nonsteroidal antiinflammatory drugs, potassium chloride
Ischemic damage	
Hypotension	Antihypertensives, diuretics
Direct vasoconstriction	Norepinephrine, dopamine, vasopressin
Decreased splanchnic blood flow	Digoxin
Increased sympathetic stimulation	Cocaine
Vasospasm	Ergot compounds
Arterial/venous thrombosis	Oral contraceptives
Hematoma formation	Anticoagulants
Motility disorders	
Pseudoobstruction	Anticholinergics, phenothiazines, tricyclic antidepressants, opioids, verapamil, clonidine, cyclosporine
Neurotoxicity	Vincristine
Narcotic bowel syndrome	Narcotics
Malabsorption	
Interference with intralumenal digestion	Tetracycline, cholestyramine, mineral oil, aluminum and magnesium hydroxide
Increased intestinal transit	Prokinetic agents, cathartics
Mucosal injury	Colchicine, neomycin, methotrexate, methyldopa, allopurinol, mefenamic acid
Direct inhibition of absorption	Sodium aminosalicylate, thiazide diuretics
Inhibition of epithelial cell turnover	
Erosive enteritis	Methotrexate, 5-fluorouracil, actinomycin D, doxorubicin, cytosine arabinoside, bleomycin, vincristine, ara-C, interleukin-2

TABLE 36-3
Causes of Protein-losing Enteropathy

Increased interstitial pressure
    Congenital intestinal lymphangiectasia
    Mesenteric lymphatic obstruction
        Tuberculosis
        Sarcoidosis
        Lymphoma
        Retroperitoneal fibrosis
Increased central venous pressure
    Constrictive pericarditis
    Congestive heart failure
Ulcerative disease
    Erosive gastritis or enteritis
    Neoplasia—carcinoma or lymphoma
    Crohn's disease
    Pseudomembranous enterocolitis
    Acute graft-versus-host disease
Nonulcerative disease
    Giant hypertrophic gastropathy (Ménétrier disease)
    Hypertrophic hypersecretory gastropathy
    Viral enteritides
    Bacterial overgrowth
    Parasitic diseases (e.g., malaria, giardiasis, schistosomiasis)
    Whipple disease
    Allergic enteritis
    Eosinophilic gastroenteritis
    Gluten-sensitive enteropathy
    Tropical sprue
    Systemic lupus erythematosus

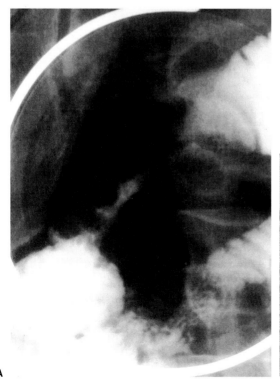

A

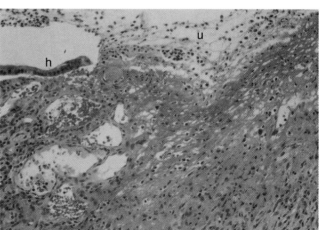

B

FIGURE 36-1. **A:** Small bowel follow-through image of a patient who sought treatment with clinical features obstruction of the small intestine shows intestinal spasm associated with ulceration and dilation of the proximal segment. The patient underwent exploratory laparotomy and resection of the affected bowel segment. (Courtesy of Dr. Dennis Balfe.) **B:** Histopathological section of the resected segment of small bowel shows ulceration (*u*) with epithelialization of the healing edge (*h*). A nifedipine capsule was found in the vicinity of the ulcer at operations, raising the possibility of a causative association. (Courtesy of Dr. Paul Swanson.)

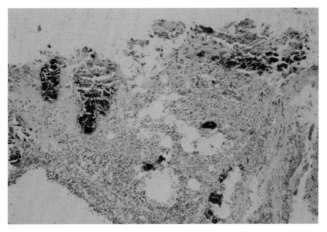

FIGURE 36-2. Prussian blue stain shows iron deposition in an ulcer of the terminal ileum. Iron tablets were thought to be the cause of small bowel ulceration and occult gastrointestinal bleeding in this patient. (Courtesy of Dr. Paul Swanson.)

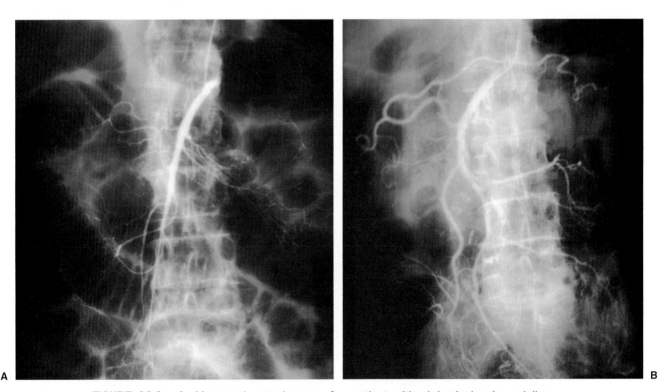

A   B

FIGURE 36-3. **A:** Mesenteric arteriogram of a patient with abdominal pain and ileus shows spasm of the superior mesenteric circulation. Prolonged spasm of the mesenteric vessels can lead to vascular insufficiency and intestinal ulceration. **B:** Repeat arteriography after intraarterial infusion of papaverine shows relief of the spasm and ileus and restoration of normal blood flow to the intestine. (Courtesy of Dr. Daniel Picus.)

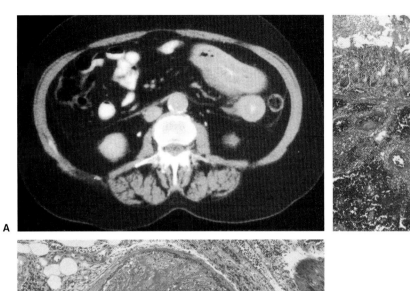

A

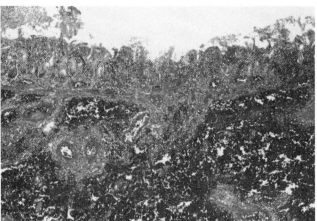

C

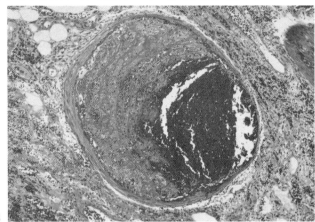

B

FIGURE 36-4. **A:** Computed tomographic scan of a patient with superior mesenteric venous thrombosis shows a thickened loop of small bowel. This can cause mucosal sloughing with ulceration and intestinal perforation that necessitates exploratory laparotomy and bowel resection. (Courtesy of Dr. Dennis Balfe.) **B:** Section through the superior mesenteric vein shows acute and organizing thrombus within the lumen. (Courtesy of Dr. Paul Swanson.) **C:** Section through surgically resected segment of bowel shows transmural hemorrhage and acute inflammation with focal epithelial necrosis. (Courtesy of Dr. Paul Swanson.)

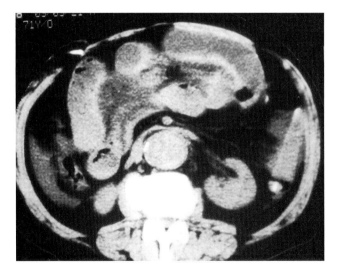

FIGURE 36-5. Abdominal computed tomographic scan of a patient who took an overdose of warfarin demonstrates bowel hemorrhage. The intestinal wall appears thickened because of the presence of intramural hematomas. Required therapeutic interventions included correction of coagulopathy and surgical resection of the affected bowel segments. (Courtesy of Dr. Dennis Balfe.)

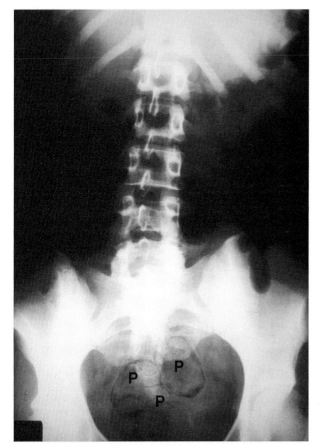

FIGURE 36-6. Plain radiograph of the abdomen of a drug smuggler shows multiple packets (*P*) of illicit drugs in the bowel lumen. Body-packer syndrome occurs when rupture of the drug-containing packets causes severe drug toxicity. (Courtesy of Dr. Dennis Balfe.)

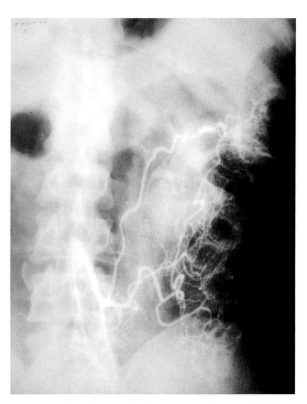

FIGURE 36-7. Mesenteric arteriogram of a patient with polyarteritis nodosa shows beaded appearance of the medium-sized arteries. Vasculitis of the arteries supplying the bowel can lead to intestinal ulceration. Angiography of other vessels, including the renal arteries, can show aneurysmal dilation. (Courtesy of Dr. Dennis Balfe.)

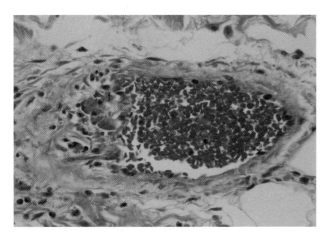

FIGURE 36-8. Section through a mesenteric artery shows evidence of vasculitis and fibrinoid necrosis (*f*) involving the arterial wall. This patient with Wegener granulomatosis had bowel ischemia, ulceration, and gastrointestinal bleeding that necessitated surgical resection of the affected bowel segment. (Courtesy of Dr. Paul Swanson.)

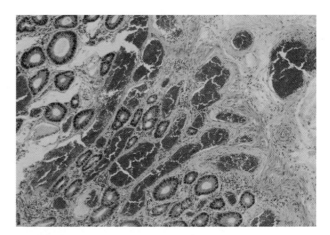

FIGURE 36-9. Section through angiodysplasia of the small intestine shows typical thickened and ectatic vasculature involving mucosa and submucosa (*red*). Rupture or erosion of the mucosa over areas of angiodysplasia can result in ulceration and gastrointestinal bleeding that can be difficult to localize. Intraoperative enteroscopy sometimes is necessary to identify the segment of bowel that needs surgical resection. (Courtesy of Dr. Paul Swanson.)

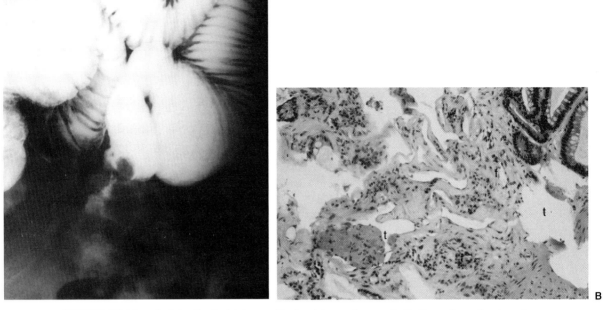

FIGURE 36-10. A: Intestinal stricture with food impaction and dilation of proximal segment in a patient who had received radiation therapy for lymphoma. This patient had clinical features of small bowel obstruction and underwent surgical resection of the affected segment. (Courtesy of Dennis Balfe.) **B:** Histopathological section of the surgically resected segment shows fibrosis of the lamina propria (*f*) with mucosal telangiectasis (*t*), a common finding with radiation-induced intestinal injury. (Courtesy of Dr. Paul Swanson.)

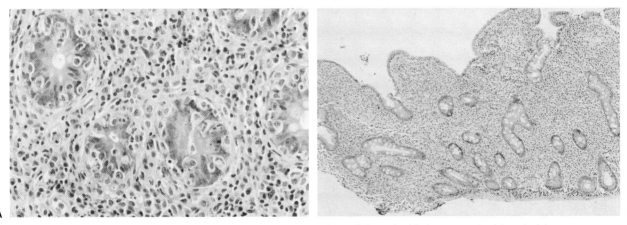

FIGURE 36-11. A: Infiltration of a segment of small bowel with large atypical lymphoid cells consistent with enteropathy-associated T-cell lymphoma in a patient with refractory celiac disease. This condition can present with malabsorption, ulceration of the intestine, and protein-losing enteropathy. **B:** Monotonous plasma cell infiltration of small-bowel mucosa in a patient with α–heavy-chain disease, which can also result in malabsorption and protein-losing enteropathy. (Courtesy of Dr. Paul Swanson.)

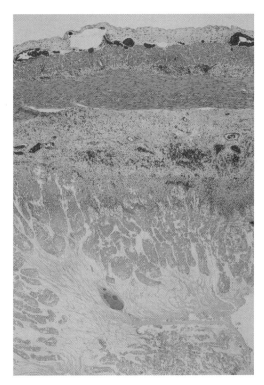

FIGURE 36-12. Section through a segment of bowel from a child with necrotizing enterocolitis shows submucosal hemorrhage, epithelial necrosis, and an acute inflammatory cell infiltrate. (Courtesy of Dr. Paul Swanson.)

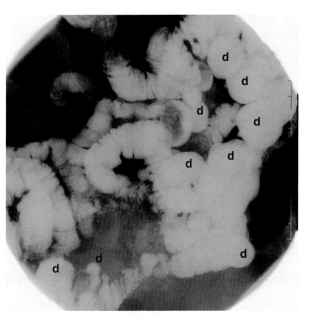

FIGURE 36-13. Images from small bowel follow-through series show multiple, large diverticula (*d*) of the small bowel. This patient had malabsorption caused by bacterial overgrowth. Treatment included long-term antibiotic therapy and correction of nutritional and vitamin deficiencies.

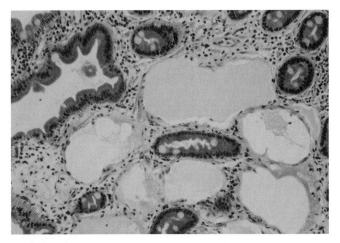

FIGURE 36-14. Intestinal lymphangiectasia can present as malabsorption and protein-losing enteropathy. Section shows lakes of ectatic lymphatic vessels within the lamina propria of the small intestine. (Courtesy of Dr. Paul Swanson.)

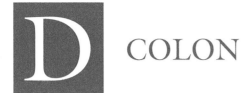

D COLON

COLON: Anatomy and Structural Anomalies

STEVEN M. COHN ■ ELISA H. BIRNBAUM

The gastroenterologist often encounters patients who have undergone previous surgical procedures involving the colon or rectum. An understanding of the postsurgical anatomy of the gastrointestinal tract often is crucial to effective treatment of these patients. Figures 37-1 and 37-2 illustrate the postsurgical anatomy that results from surgical procedures commonly performed on patients with inflammatory bowel disease or colorectal carcinoma.

Hirschsprung disease is rare among adults but must be considered in the evaluation of chronic constipation dating back to childhood. Hirschsprung disease can be a challenging diagnosis to establish for adult patients. It is a result of failure of neural crest cells (precursors of ganglion cells) to complete their caudal migration during normal colonic development. The aganglionic segment does not relax and causes functional obstruction. Anorectal manometry is often useful in the evaluation of suspected Hirschsprung disease. Figures 37-3 and 37-4 illustrate anorectal manometric findings for healthy adults and patients with Hirschsprung disease.

A normal sphincter profile (resting pressures 40–80 mm Hg and squeeze pressures 80–160 mm Hg) and an abnormal rectoanal inhibitory reflex typically occur among patients with Hirschsprung disease. The internal sphincter does not relax in response to rectal distention among patients with Hirschsprung disease, and an abnormal reflex during manometry aids in the diagnosis. However, the rectoanal inhibitory reflex may be normal among patients with short-segment Hirschsprung disease. These patients may have a short segment as the primary disease, or the short segment may be residual disease after surgical intervention. High anal resting pressures and impaired rectal emptying may occur.

Colonic volvulus is an infrequent cause of colonic obstruction. It may be difficult to diagnose without a high degree of suspicion. Volvulus is classified and managed according to its location in the colon. Figures 37-5 and 37-6 illustrate the radiographic findings for sigmoid volvulus and cecal volvulus. Sigmoid volvulus accounts for approximately 60% of all instances of volvulus in the United States. It usually occurs among elderly persons, patients in extended care facilities, or in patients with neuropsychiatric disorders. *Cecal volvulus* accounts for less than 20% of all cases of colonic volvulus and generally occurs among younger patients. It is believed to be caused by anomalous fixation of the right colon that leads to a freely mobile cecum. Other precipitating factors include adhesions from previous operations, pregnancy, and obstructing lesions of the left colon.

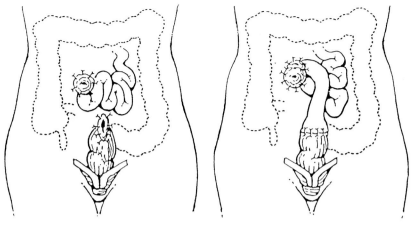

Abdominal colectomy and ileostomy
(rectum undisturbed)

Abdominal colectomy with
ileal-rectal anastomosis
(temporary ileostomy)

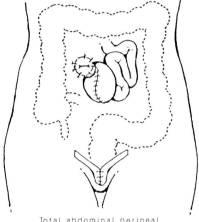

Total abdominal perineal
proctocolectomy with Koch
pouch (continent ileostomy)

JOHN A.CRAIG

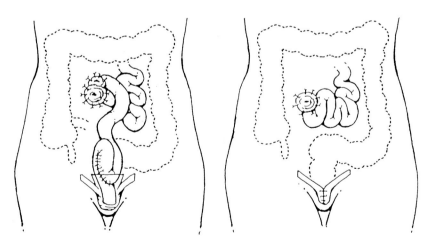

Total abdominal colectomy,
mucosal proctectomy, ileal
pouch anal anastomosis
(temporary ileostomy)

Total abdominal proctocolectomy

FIGURE 37-1. Surgical options for ulcerative colitis. Abdominal colectomy with ileostomy usually is performed as an emergency procedure when the diagnosis is unclear. The rectum is removed at a later operation. Total abdominal colectomy with ileal-rectal anastomosis is rarely performed for ulcerative colitis. It is a more common surgical approach for Crohn's colitis. Total abdominal perineal proctocolectomy with Koch pouch is a continent ileostomy performed for the rare patient who has undergone removal of the rectum. Ileostomy requires intubation for passage of fecal contents. It is never performed as a primary procedure. In total abdominal colectomy with ileal pouch anal anastomosis, a continent anal reservoir allows normal evacuation of stool. The ileostomy is closed once healing is complete. Total abdominal proctocolectomy with permanent end ileostomy is performed on patients with inadequate anal sphincters.

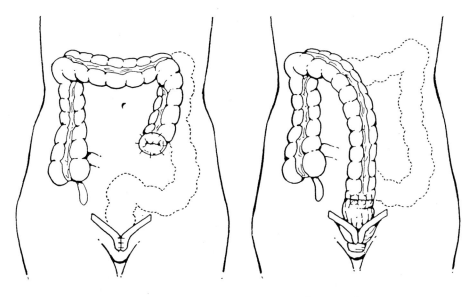

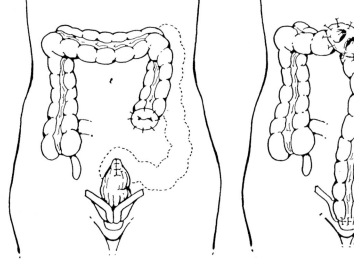

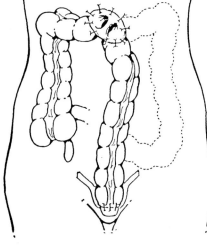

Abdominal perineal
proctosigmoidectomy with
permanent end colostomy

Low anterior resection
of rectosigmoid with
colorectal anastomosis

Hartmann resection

Low anterior resection
of rectosigmoid with
coloanal anastomosis
and protecting loop-
transverse colostomy

JOHN A. CRAIG—MD
©

FIGURE 37-2. Surgical options for rectal cancer. Abdominal perineal proctosigmoidectomy with permanent end colostomy is performed on patients with carcinoma in the lower third of the rectum. Low anterior resection of the rectosigmoid with colorectal anastomosis is performed for lesions in the upper and some lesions in the middle third of the rectum. Hartmann resection is performed as an emergency resection with an unprepared colon or inadequate anal sphincter to allow anastomosis without incontinence. Low anterior resection of the rectosigmoid with coloanal anastomosis and protecting loop-transverse colostomy is performed on patients with carcinoma in the lower third of the rectum who have a spared functional anal sphincter. The transverse colostomy is closed electively after healing of the coloanal anastomosis.

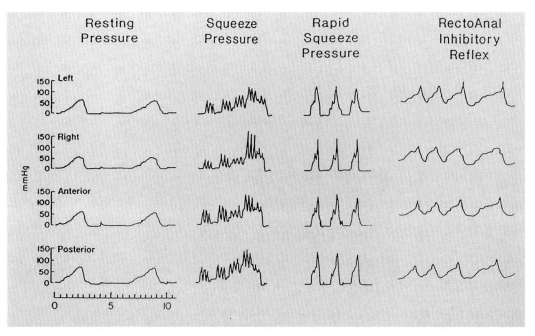

FIGURE 37-3. Normal anal manometric results with hydraulic capillary system. Resting pressures (normal 40–80 mm Hg) are obtained as the catheter is pulled through the anal sphincter with the patient at rest. Squeeze pressures (normal 80–160 mm Hg) are measured as the catheter is pulled through the anal sphincter in 0.5-cm increments with the patient squeezing. Rapid squeeze pressure (normal 80–160 mm Hg) is determined as the catheter is removed quickly while the patient is generating maximal squeeze effort. The rectoanal inhibitory reflex is measured with a catheter placed within the sphincter zone. The rectal balloon is distended in 10-cm increments. A normal rectoanal inhibitory reflex is manifested by an increase over baseline, followed by involuntary relaxation below baseline, followed by return to baseline.

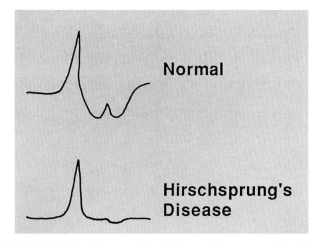

FIGURE 37-4. Rectoanal inhibitory reflex among healthy persons and those with Hirschsprung disease. Among healthy persons, sphincter presence increases over baseline, relaxes below baseline, and returns to baseline. Among persons with Hirschsprung disease, an increase over baseline occurs, but no relaxation of the internal anal sphincter is observed.

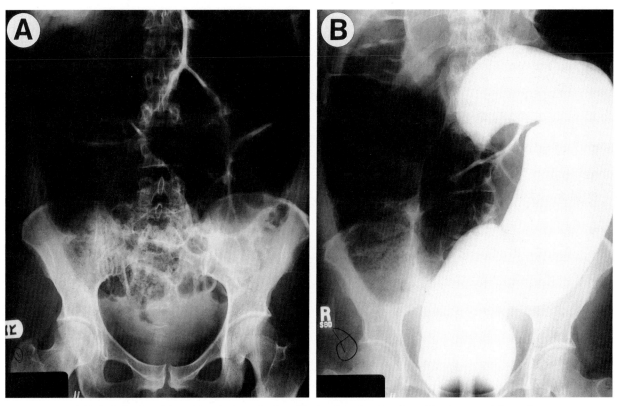

FIGURE 37-5. Sigmoid volvulus. **A:** Gas-filled, dilated colon is evident on a plain radiograph of the abdomen. There is a paucity of gas in the rectum. **B:** Hypaque enema image shows tapering of the column of contrast material at the site of torsion ("bird's beak sign") of the sigmoid colon.

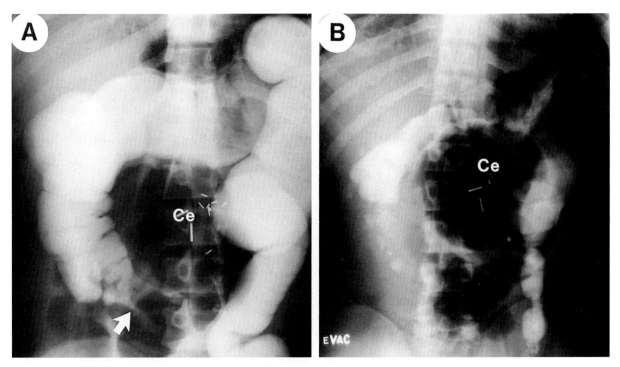

FIGURE 37-6. Cecal volvulus. **A:** Hypaque enema image shows tapering of the column of contrast material at the site of torsion (*arrow*) and displacement of the cecum toward the epigastrium. **B:** Postevacuation radiograph shows gas-filled, dilated cecum (*CE*) in the epigastrium. There is a paucity of gas in the normal location of the cecum in the right lower quadrant of the abdomen.

INFLAMMATORY BOWEL DISEASE

WILLIAM F. STENSON ■ **WILLIAM J. TREMAINE**

PATHOLOGY

Ulcerative Colitis

The gross appearance of ulcerative colitis may be uniform involvement throughout the colon or a sharp demarcation between abnormal mucosa distally and normal mucosa proximally (Fig. 38-1). The appearance also may be diffusely abnormal, with a gradation from mild edema in the cecum to submucosal hemorrhage in the transverse colon to frank ulceration in the rectum. Sometimes the ulcerations can be seen only in histological sections, but in other cases, large distinct ulcerations may be seen in the gross specimen.

At histological examination, the inflammatory infiltrate in ulcerative colitis usually extends down to the muscularis mucosae. The inflammatory infiltrate includes both neutrophils, a sign of acute inflammation, and macrophages and lymphocytes, signs of more chronic inflammation. Crypt abscess (Fig. 38-2), a collection of neutrophils in a colonic crypt, is characteristic of ulcerative colitis but also is seen in other diseases, including Crohn's colitis. Crypt branching (Fig. 38-3) occurs in many patients with ulcerative colitis and persists even when the disease is inactive and the mucosal inflammation has resolved. Crypt branching is uncommon in other disease processes. Inflammatory polyps in ulcerative colitis may be filiform (Fig. 38-4), or they may be broad based and sessile. Often they are covered with a whitish cap of exudate (Fig. 38-5).

It is possible to screen for carcinoma in ulcerative colitis by identifying areas of dysplasia (Fig. 38-6). Dysplastic mucosa can be villiform owing to the proliferation of epithelial cells. At low-power microscopic examination, low-grade dysplasia is marked by enlarged goblet cells and atypical hyperchromatic nuclei, whereas high-grade dysplasia is characterized by more marked nuclear pleomorphism and pseudostratification of the nuclei. Under higher-power magnification, low-grade dysplasia shows hyperchromatic cells with preservation of nuclear polarity, whereas high-grade dysplasia shows complete loss of nuclear polarity. Biopsy screening for dysplasia may reveal carcinoma in situ. Adenocarcinoma of the colon occurs with increased frequency in ulcerative colitis (Fig. 38-7) and Crohn's colitis. Adenocarcinoma of the small intestine occurs with increased frequency in Crohn's disease of the small intestine (Fig. 38-8).

The earliest pathological lesion in Crohn's disease is an aphthous ulcer. These small, sharply demarcated ulcers often occur over submucosal lymphoid aggregates.

As the disease progresses, aphthoid ulcers can grow to form transverse or round ulcers (Fig. 38-9). Gross specimens in Crohn's disease may show intersecting longitudinal and transverse ulcerations resulting in a "cobblestone" appearance (Fig. 38-10). In ulcerative colitis, involvement of the colon is continuous, whereas in Crohn's disease of either the intestine or colon, involvement may be discontinuous, with areas of involvement interspersed with grossly normal areas (Fig. 38-11).

The inflammatory process in Crohn's disease often is transmural. In transmural inflammation, there are areas of clustering of inflammatory cells in all layers of the intestinal wall. Frequently, this transmural inflammation includes granulomas and lymphoid aggregates with germinal centers (Fig. 38-12). In some sections, granulomas are seen in both the submucosa and the serosa. Narrowing of the small intestine as a result of Crohn's disease can lead to obstruction (Fig. 38-13).

EXTRAINTESTINAL MANIFESTATIONS

A common dermal manifestation of both ulcerative colitis and Crohn's colitis is pyoderma gangrenosum (Figs. 38-14 and 38-15), marked by sharply defined areas of ulceration with serpiginous borders. Iritis is a potentially serious ophthalmologic complication of ulcerative colitis and Crohn's disease. Iritis is accompanied by conjunctival injection (Fig. 38-16). Aphthous ulcers, which occur in the intestine and colon in Crohn's disease, also can occur on the tongue, oral mucosa, or lips (Fig. 38-17).

Perianal Crohn's disease is marked by fistulae, bluish discoloration, edematous tags, and ulceration (Figs. 38-18 through 38-20).

RADIOLOGY

Ulcerative Colitis

Plain radiographs are helpful in establishing the diagnosis of toxic megacolon, which is characterized by dilation of a colonic segment, typically the transverse colon (Fig. 38-21). Double-contrast studies identify early changes in ulcerative colitis that would not be seen with full-column studies. Early changes in ulcerative colitis include mucosal edema, granularity, and loss of haustral markings (Fig. 38-22A). As the disease progresses, ulcerations develop with penetration of the mucosal layer (see Fig. 38-22B). Undermining of the mucosal layer gives the characteristic appearance of collar-button ulcers (Fig. 38-23).

Although ulcerative colitis tends to involve the left colon more than the right, the inflammatory process may affect the cecum and result in severe narrowing. The terminal ileum is affected among about 10% of patients with pancolitis. Involvement of the terminal ileum is manifested radiographically with thickening of the mucosal folds, spasm, and irritability. The ileocecal valve in ulcerative colitis tends to be gaping, as opposed to its position in Crohn's disease, in which it tends to be narrowed.

Crohn's Disease

Crohn's disease can cause narrowing and obstruction of the duodenum (Fig. 38-24). Although isolated Crohn's disease in the duodenum can occur, disease usually is present elsewhere in the intestine as well.

One early radiographic finding in Crohn's disease is the presence of aphthous ulcers (Fig. 38-25). Another early radiographic finding in Crohn's disease is diffuse mucosal granularity. In the small bowel, this pattern is caused by widening and blunting of the villi with inflammatory infiltrate. As the inflammation progresses, there is thickening and distortion of the valvulae conniventes. Progression of the inflammatory process results in both transverse and longitudinal ulcers. These ulcers frequently cross each other in a grid pattern. The remaining islands of mucosa become thickened and have a cobblestone pattern on barium studies. Ulcers seen in cross section have a collar-button appearance (Fig. 38-26).

Infiltration and thickening of the bowel wall produce the radiographic appearance of separation of loops of small bowel (Fig. 38-27). The loops of barium-filled intestine are pushed apart by a thickened edematous mesentery and matted mesenteric nodes. Narrowing of the intestinal lumen makes the loops appear farther apart. Severe inflammation results in a rigid segment of bowel with a narrowed lumen and total loss of mucosal detail. This constellation results in the "string sign" (Fig. 38-28) and is most commonly seen in the terminal ileum.

Terminal ileal involvement includes stricture (Figs. 38-29 and 38-30), ulcers (see Fig. 38-30), and fissures (see Fig. 38-29). The standard surgical approach to Crohn's disease of the terminal ileum is resection of the affected segment with construction of an ileocolic anastomosis. Disease activity typically recurs on the ileal side of the anastomosis (Fig. 38-31). The terminal ileum or an ileocolic anastomosis can be depicted with oral barium examination (see Fig. 38-30), by means of enteroclysis (see Fig. 38-29), or by means of pneumocolon (oral administration of barium and insufflation of air into the colon).

Double tracking, which shows the presence of longitudinal extralumenal collections of barium paralleling the lumen, can be seen in diverticulitis as well as Crohn's disease. In Crohn's disease, this radiographic pattern reflects penetration of mucosa by ulcers and the development of a long intramural fistula.

Perianal Crohn's disease has a distinctive radiographic pattern of ulcers and deep lateral fissures. Extension of the ulcers results in branching sinus tracts and fistulae reaching to the skin.

ENDOSCOPY

Ulcerative Colitis

In quiescent ulcerative colitis, there is distortion of vascular markings without edema or erythema (Fig. 38-32). In mildly and moderately active disease, there is edema and erythema granularity and distortion of vascular markings (Figs. 38-33 and 38-34).

In severe ulcerative colitis, the mucosa is friable, erythematous, and edematous with ulceration (Fig. 38-35). Although the severity of inflammation seen endoscopically may lessen as one moves proximally in the colon in ulcerative colitis, the degree of inflammation at a given level is uniform through the entire circumference of the colon. Thus, ulceration in ulcerative colitis always occurs in areas of diffuse edema and erythema. The mucosa surrounding ulcerations may become so edematous that the result is a coarsely nodular deformity (Fig. 38-36). The more proximally one moves, the less severe the endoscopic changes are likely to be. Sometimes there is sharp demarcation between normal and inflamed tissue (Fig. 38-37).

Pseudopolyps can occur in ulcerative colitis of any degree of activity (Figs. 38-38 through 38-40; see Fig. 38-33).

Figure 38-41 shows sequential endoscopic studies of a patient with severe pancolitis. At the first colonoscopy (see Fig. 38-41*A*), there was almost universal ulceration with only a few islands of remaining mucosa. In Fig. 38-41*B*, the mucosa is beginning to heal, and less ulcer and more epithelium are seen. In Fig. 38-41*C*, there is further regression of ulcers with pseudopolyp formation. Full restoration of the epithelium with persistence of pseudopolyps is shown in Fig. 38-41*D*.

Dysplasia is most often found either when carcinoma is present in the colon or when the patient is at high risk for carcinoma. Dysplastic mucosa usually appears normal through an endoscope. When dysplasia is associated with a polypoid mass or other endoscopic abnormality, the lesion is called a *dysplasia-associated lesion or mass* (DALM) (Fig. 38-42). Identification of a DALM is an indication for resection because of the very high probability of an associated malignant tumor.

Ulcerative colitis can be treated surgically with total proctocolectomy and construction of an ileal pouch with an ileoanal anastomosis. Pouchitis (inflammation of the ileal pouch) occurs among some patients after this procedure. The endoscopic features of pouchitis include erythema, edema, mucous exudate, and superficial ulceration (Fig. 38-43).

Crohn's Disease

Aphthous ulcers are the earliest endoscopic lesions in Crohn's disease (Figs. 38-44 and 38-45). They are surrounded by erythematous rings (Fig. 38-46). The mucosa between aphthous ulcers is endoscopically normal. As Crohn's disease progresses, small aphthoid ulcers grow to form deep excavated ulcers with distinct margins (Fig. 38-47). These ulcers may be rounded (Fig. 38-48) or linear (Fig. 38-49). "Cobblestoning" is an endoscopic feature seen most often in Crohn's disease (Fig. 38-50). Cobblestoning is caused by the intersection of longitudinal and transverse ulcers in a grid pattern, with thickened erythematous mucosal bumps appearing between the ulcers. Severe Crohn's colitis can demonstrate diffuse ulceration in one portion of the colon (Fig. 38-51) and deep longitudinal ulcers in another portion (Fig. 38-52).

In some patients with involvement of the terminal ileum there is marked stenosis, and the colonoscope cannot be inserted into the ileum (Fig. 38-53). If the ileum can be entered, endoscopic examination reveals patterns similar to those in the involved part of the colon with longitudinal ulcers and cobblestoning (Fig. 38-54). This is differentiated from the endoscopic appearance of "backwash ileitis" in ulcerative colitis, in which there may be edema but no ulcers.

Crohn's disease of the cecum and terminal ileum often is managed with surgical resection of the affected segment and construction of an ileocolic anastomosis. Crohn's disease typically recurs on the ileal side of the anastomosis (Fig. 38-55). The endoscopic features of recurrent Crohn's disease are much the same as those of the initial presentation: ulcers, edema, erythema, and granularity.

Fistula formation is a common complication of Crohn's disease. Fistulae form between the affected segment of intestine and the skin, urinary bladder, vagina, or other segments of the intestine. Fistulae usually are easier to define with a barium enema or small bowel follow-through examination than with endoscopy. In some instances, however, fistulae can be easily appreciated with endoscopy (Fig. 38-56).

Successful medical therapy for active Crohn's disease results in healing of ulcers and loss of friability. In some cases, the endoscopic features revert to normal. In other cases, however, some superficial scarring, mucous exudate, and loss of vascular markings remain (Fig. 38-57).

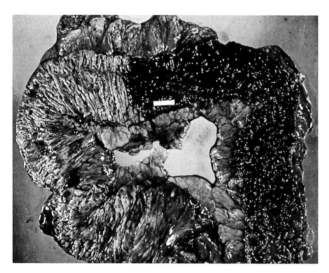

FIGURE 38-1. Colectomy specimen from a patient with ulcerative colitis demonstrates sharp demarcation in the midtransverse colon between involved and uninvolved mucosa. (Courtesy of Dr. Ira Kodner.)

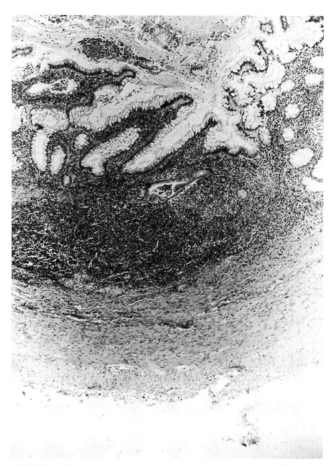

FIGURE 38-2. Ulcerative colitis in the appendix with mucosal inflammation and crypt abscesses. There is no inflammation in the muscularis propria. (Courtesy of Dr. David Lacey.)

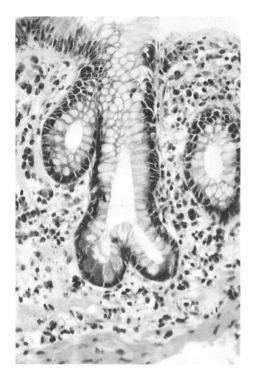

FIGURE 38-3. Crypt branching, Paneth cell metaplasia, increased neuroendocrine cells, and a prominence of eosinophils in the lamina propria all are features seen individually with increased frequency in ulcerative colitis. Their juxtaposition here makes this field diagnostic for quiescent ulcerative colitis (original magnification ×100).

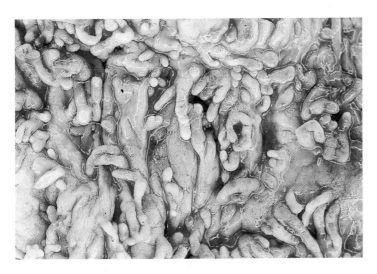

FIGURE 38-4. When inflammatory polyps assume the filiform appearance seen here, they are readily recognizable grossly; when smaller in numbers and rounded, they can be confused with adenomas or hyperplastic polyps.

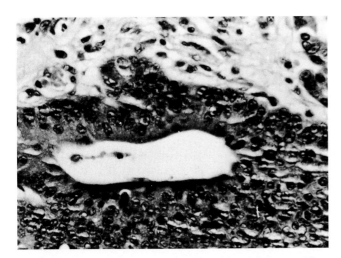

FIGURE 38-5. Multiple pseudopolyps in ulcerative colitis. Their surface is smooth and glistening. Detailed view of exudate creating whitish caps.

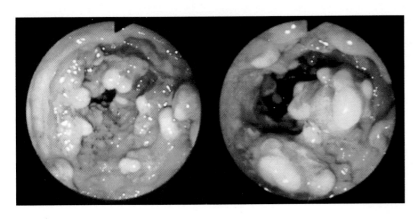

FIGURE 38-6. High-grade dysplasia with nuclear stratification, nuclear and cellular pleomorphism, and loss of nuclear polarity. Compare with Fig. 38-12, in which nuclear polarity is largely preserved, despite the presence of inflammation. (Courtesy of Dr. David Lacey.)

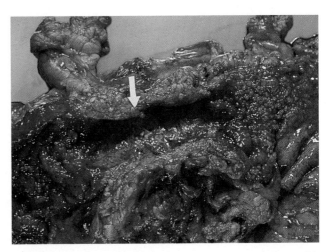

FIGURE 38-7. Adenocarcinoma (*arrow*) in a patient with ulcerative colitis. (Courtesy of Dr. Ira Kodner.)

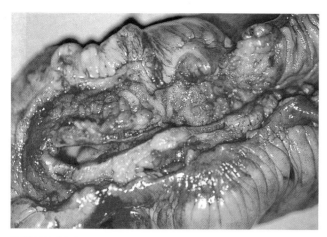

FIGURE 38-8. Gross specimen of Crohn's disease of the small intestine with adenocarcinoma. (Courtesy of Dr. Ira Kodner.)

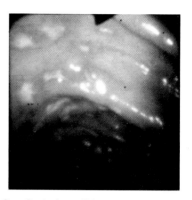

FIGURE 38-9. Crohn's colitis with discrete small, round ulcers separated by normal mucosa.

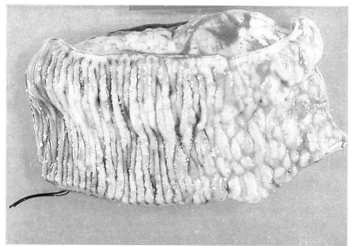

A

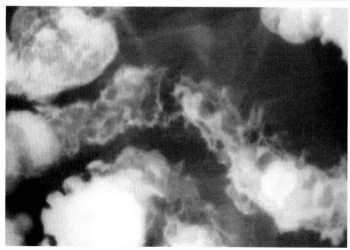

B

FIGURE 38-10. A: One end of this ileal segment shows prominent cobblestoning, believed to result from the combined effect of multiple, small, longitudinal and transverse linear ulcers isolating areas of edematous mucosa. The mucosa is nearly normal at the other end, although variably severe and patchy involvement is present as pale areas of mucosal swelling and distortion. **B:** Cobblestoning also can be detected radiographically, as in this case of Crohn's disease.

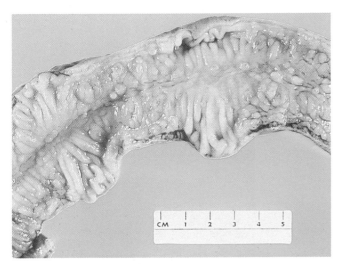

FIGURE 38-11. Skip areas in Crohn's disease of the jejunum are segments of involvement alternating with relatively normal segments. (Courtesy of Dr. Ira Kodner.)

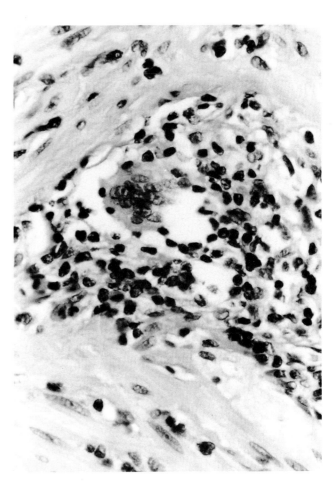

FIGURE 38-12. Surgical specimen shows granuloma in Crohn's disease. (Courtesy of Dr. David Lacey.)

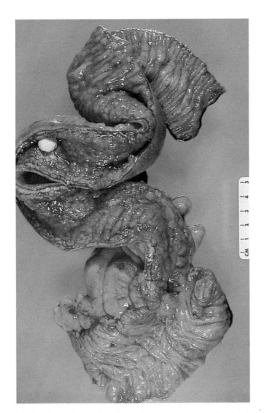

FIGURE 38-13. Ileal stricture in a patient with Crohn's disease. A pill is impacted in the lumen above a strictured area in the terminal ileum. An area of relatively normal cecum is at the **bottom**. (Courtesy of Dr. Ira Kodner.)

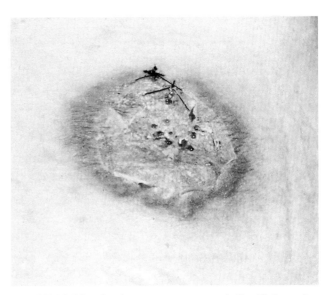

FIGURE 38-14. Pyoderma gangrenosum (with stitches after biopsy). (Courtesy of Dr. Ira Kodner.)

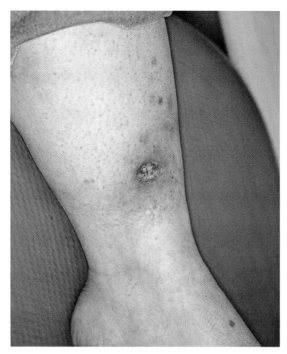

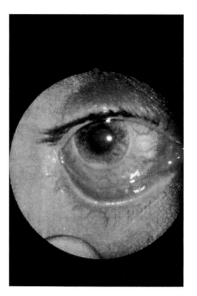

FIGURE 38-15.   Pyoderma gangrenosum. (Courtesy of Dr. Ira Kodner.)

FIGURE 38-16.   Marked conjunctival injection. A hypopyon also is present.

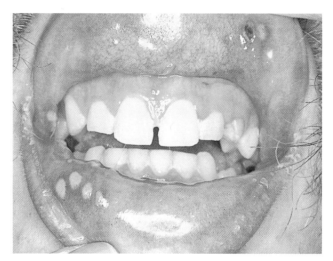

FIGURE 38-17.   Aphthous ulcers. (Courtesy of Dr. Ira Kodner.)

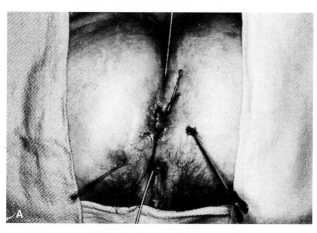
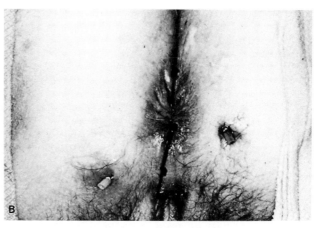

FIGURE 38-18. Perianal Crohn's disease with fistulae. Probes are placed intraoperatively to define fistulae (**A**). Use of mushroom catheters and setons allows adequate drainage (**B**). (Courtesy of Dr. Ira Kodner.)

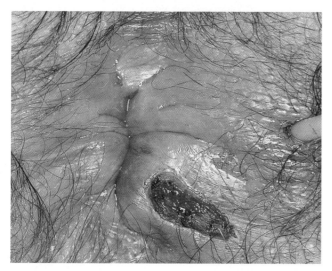

FIGURE 38-19. Perianal Crohn's disease with ulcer and catheter in a fistula. (Courtesy of Dr. Ira Kodner.)

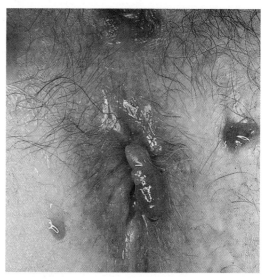

FIGURE 38-20. Perianal Crohn's disease with fistulae and an edematous tag. (Courtesy of Dr. Ira Kodner.)

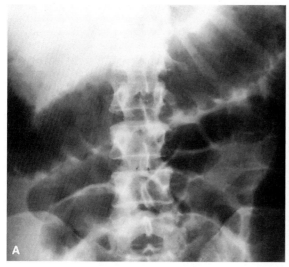
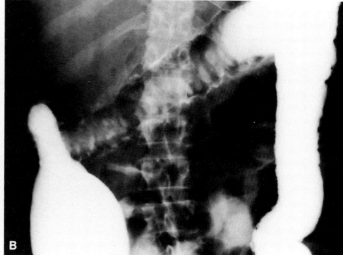

FIGURE 38-21. Toxic megacolon. **A:** Plain radiograph shows colonic dilation. **B:** Contrast radiograph reveals large ulceration. (Courtesy of Dr. Dennis Balfe.)

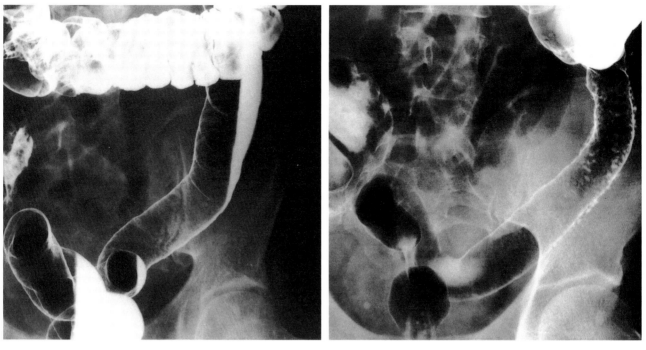

A   B

FIGURE 38-22. Progression of ulcerative colitis in the sigmoid and descending colon. **A:** Colon of a patient with mild ulcerative colitis. There is mucosal edema, granularity, and loss of haustral markings. **B:** Two years later, there is shortening of the colon and mucosal ulcers. Numerous collar-button ulcers are present in the descending colon. (Courtesy of Dr. Dennis Balfe.)

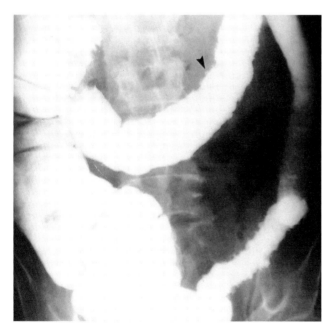

FIGURE 38-23. Ulcerative colitis extending to midtransverse colon with collar-button ulcerations in profile (*arrow*). (Courtesy of Dr. Dennis Balfe.)

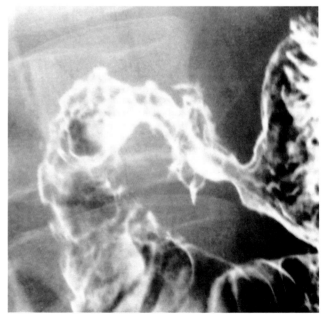

FIGURE 38-24. Crohn's disease involving the antrum and duodenum. (Courtesy of Dr. Dennis Balfe.)

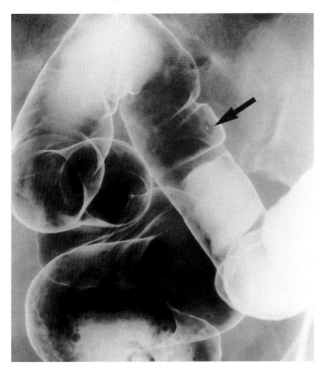

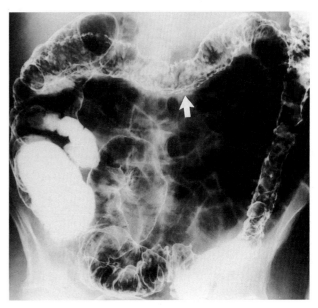

FIGURE 38-25. Early Crohn's colitis with a single aphthous ulcer in the sigmoid (*arrow*). (Courtesy of Dr. Dennis Balfe.)

FIGURE 38-26. Severe Crohn's colitis involving the sigmoid, descending, transverse, and ascending colon. Numerous collar-button ulcerations are present (*arrow*). (Courtesy of Dr. Dennis Balfe.)

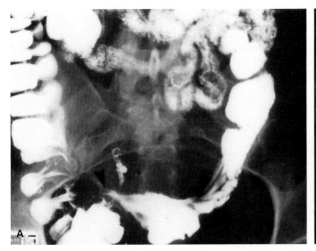

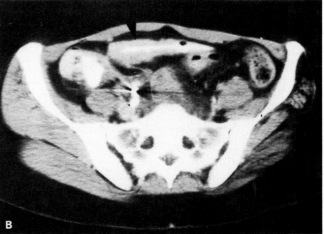

FIGURE 38-27. Crohn's disease of the terminal ileum (*arrows*) on small bowel follow-through image (**A**) and computed tomographic (CT) scan (**B**) of the same patient. Thickening of the intestinal wall is easily appreciated on the CT scan. On the small bowel follow-through image, wall thickening is indicated by the separation of the columns of barium. (Courtesy of Dr. Dennis Balfe.)

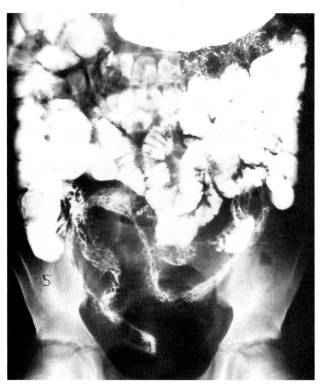

FIGURE 38-28. Crohn's ileitis with a long segment of involved ileum. The barium columns are widely separated because of wall thickening. (Courtesy of Dr. Dennis Balfe.)

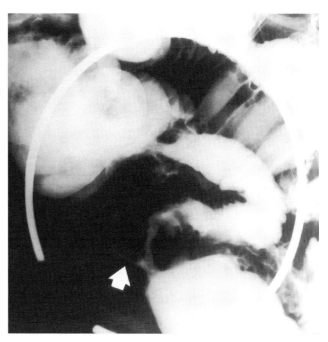

FIGURE 38-29. Crohn's disease of the terminal ileum. There is narrowing and ulceration of the terminal ileum with prestenotic dilation. There is also contrast material in a fissure (*arrow*). (Courtesy of Dr. Dennis Balfe.)

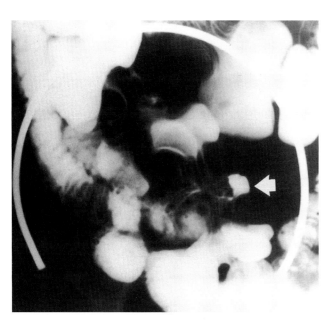

FIGURE 38-30. Crohn's disease of the terminal ileum with stricture and ulcer. (Courtesy of Dr. Dennis Balfe.)

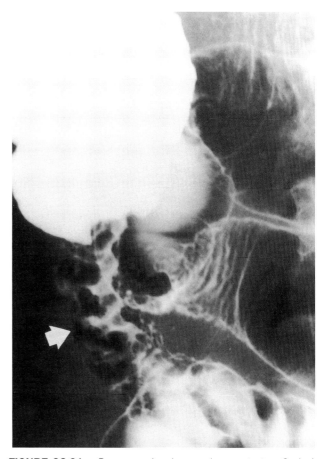

FIGURE 38-31. Pneumocolon image demonstrates Crohn's disease in a patient with an ileocolic anastomosis. There is active Crohn's disease with ulceration on the ileal side of the anastomosis (*arrow*). In a pneumocolon examination, barium is administered by mouth, and air is insufflated into the rectum. (Courtesy of Dr. Dennis Balfe.)

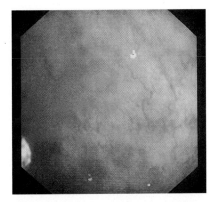

FIGURE 38-32. Quiescent (inactive) ulcerative colitis in a 39-year-old woman with ulcerative pancolitis for 11 years, now asymptomatic. There is distortion of the vascular markings but no granularity, edema, friability, mucus exudate, or ulcerations.

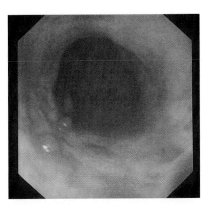

FIGURE 38-33. Mildly active ulcerative colitis with pseudopolyps. Same patient as in Fig. 38-32, 1 year after the endoscopic examination in Fig. 38-32, with a mild flare in symptoms. The disease now is responding to prednisone 20 mg daily and mesalamine 4 g daily. There are two small pseudopolyps; the mucosa is mildly granular and erythematous; and the vascular markings are distorted.

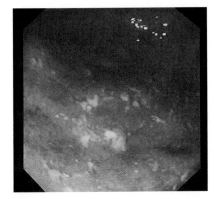

FIGURE 38-34. Moderately active ulcerative colitis in a 19-year-old woman with ulcerative pancolitis for 2 years. The patient has continuing symptoms despite oral mesalamine 4 g daily and prednisone 40 mg daily. Moderate granularity, edema, and mucus exudate is demonstrated.

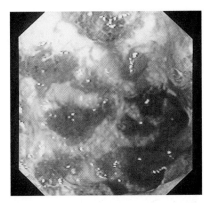

FIGURE 38-35. Severely active ulcerative colitis in a 54-year-old woman with left-sided ulcerative colitis for 7 years. There is marked ulceration. At least half of the surface area depicted is denuded by ulcers, and there are intervening areas of edematous granular mucosa.

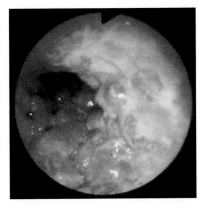

FIGURE 38-36. Coarsely nodular deformity of mucosal contour in ulcerative colitis. Mucosa is intensely erythematous and friable.

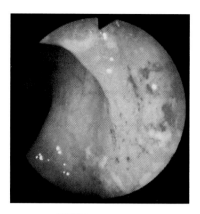

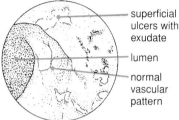

FIGURE 38-37. Sharp transition from normal to inflamed bowel is discernible at the rectosigmoid junction. Erythema and superficial ulceration of diseased mucosa contrast to the normal vascular pattern.

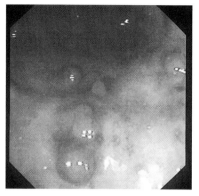

FIGURE 38-38. Mildly active ulcerative colitis with multiple pseudopolyps. This 54-year-old woman (same patient as in Fig. 38-35) about 1 year later after a course of topical 5-ASA (mesalamine) and prednisone 60 mg daily tapered and discontinued 9 months previously. There is mild granularity and erythema; the vascular markings are distorted, and multiple small pseudopolyps are present.

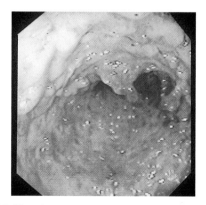

FIGURE 38-39. Long-standing ulcerative colitis with scarring and pseudopolyps. A 25-year-old man had a 9-year history of ulcerative colitis. The patient is now asymptomatic with azathioprine 150 mg daily and mesalamine 2.4 g daily. There is scarring and loss of the normal vascular markings. Two small pseudopolyps are present.

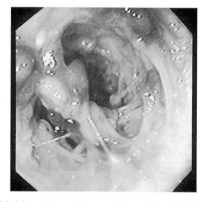

FIGURE 38-40. Ulcerative colitis with bridging pseudopolyps. A 25-year-old man has had ulcerative colitis for 9 years (same patient as in Fig. 38-39) and the disease is asymptomatic with azathioprine 150 mg daily and mesalamine 2.4 g daily. Endoscopic picture shows bridging pseudopolyps in the transverse colon.

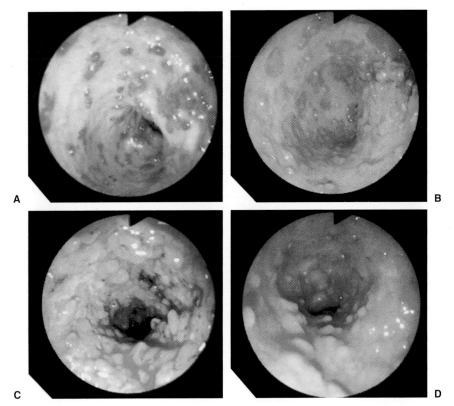

FIGURE 38-41.   Sequential study of severe pancolitis. Massive ulceration of the colon was studied at intervals of 4 to 6 weeks after institution of medical therapy. **A:** View of the proximal sigmoid shows extensive ulceration before therapy. Some islands of remaining mucosa are visible. **B:** Regression of inflammation and early reepithelialization. **C:** Ulcers are regressing with pseudopolypoid elevation of nonulcerated mucosal islands. **D:** Full re-epithelialization and pseudopolypoid transformation characterize healing.

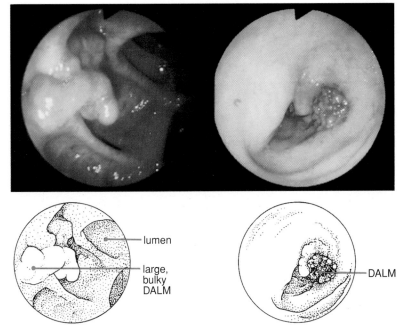

FIGURE 38-42.   Examples of dysplasia-associated lesions or masses in long-standing, inactive ulcerative colitis.

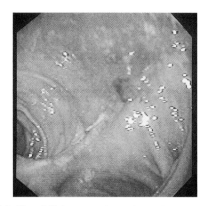

FIGURE 38-43. Mild to moderately active pouchitis. This 36-year-old woman has a history of ulcerative colitis for which she underwent colectomy with ileal J pouch–anal anastomosis 2 years previously. She had recurrent liquid stools and cramping discomfort relieved with bowel movements. Endoscopic image of the pouch, with views of the afferent limb of the neoterminal ileum in the **left** portion of the field and the blind end of the J pouch in the **inferior aspect** of the field, shows mucus exudate, superficial ulceration, and friability of the pouch mucosa but not of the mucosa in the neoterminal ileum.

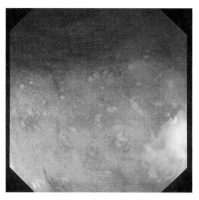

FIGURE 38-45. Crohn's disease involving the transverse colon with multiple aphthous ulcers. A 26-year-old woman with Crohn's disease for 2 years has persistent symptoms despite prednisone 25 mg daily and sulfasalazine 3 g daily. Endoscopic image shows multiple aphthous ulcers; edematous and erythematous mucosa with a loss of normal vascular markings; and mucous exudate.

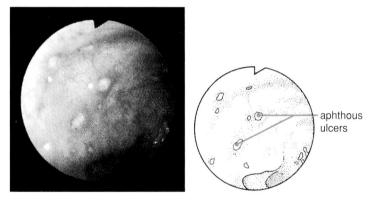

FIGURE 38-44. Colonoscopic appearance of aphthous ulceration.

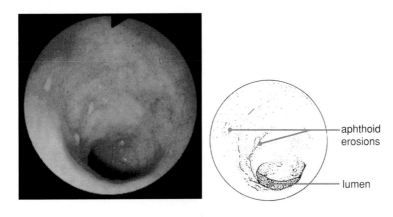

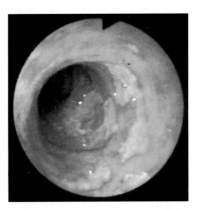

FIGURE 38-46. Characteristic superficial aphthoid erosions in Crohn's disease have erythematous rings.

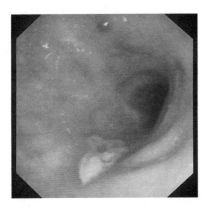

FIGURE 38-47. Crohn's disease of the colon with focal ulcer. A 24-year-old man with Crohn's disease for 2 years currently has minimal symptoms while taking metronidazole 250 mg three times daily and mesalamine 2.4 g daily. There is a focal ulcer in the distal sigmoid colon, mild inflammatory changes of the surrounding mucosa, distortion of the vascular markings, mild granularity, and erythema.

FIGURE 38-48. Multiple large, deep, excavated ulcers in severe ulcerating Crohn's disease show distinct margins. This patient has concomitant sclerosing cholangitis.

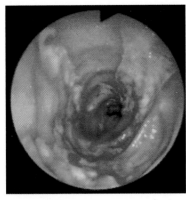

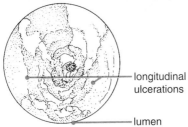

FIGURE 38-49. Longitudinal alignment of ulceration causes a railroad-track appearance in Crohn's disease.

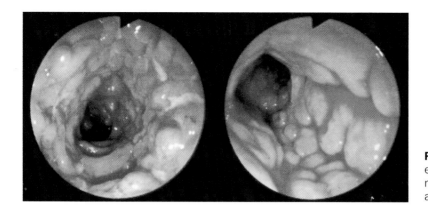

FIGURE 38-50. Active phase of Crohn's diseases shows cobblestoning caused by interconnecting ulcerations (**left**). Area of cobblestoning after therapy (**right**).

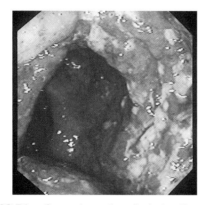

FIGURE 38-51. Severely active Crohn's disease of the colon. A 22-year-old man with a 1-year history of Crohn's disease has severe diarrhea, a 19-pound weight loss, and continuing symptoms despite prednisone 60 mg daily. Colonoscopic image shows severe ulceration in the transverse colon with markedly edematous, granular, and friable mucosa.

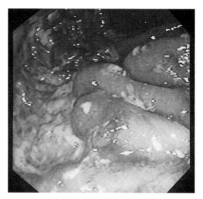

FIGURE 38-52. Severely active Crohn's disease of the colon (same patient as in Fig. 38-51). Deep rake ulcer in mid-descending colon with surrounding mucosal edema, granularity, and friability.

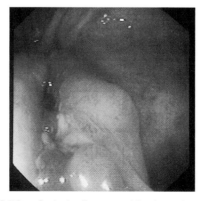

FIGURE 38-53. Crohn's disease with ulceration at the ileocecal valve. A 26-year-old woman with a history of Crohn's disease for 4 years has involvement of the terminal ileum. The disease was previously controlled with mesalamine 4 g daily, with worsening cramping abdominal pain in recent weeks. Colonoscopy revealed ulceration at the ileocecal valve with stenosis of the valve, which could not be intubated with a colonoscope. The colon otherwise appeared normal.

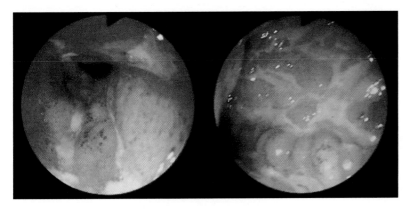

FIGURE 38-54. Diffuse, concentric involvement of the distal terminal ileum in Crohn's disease presents itself as swelling, erythema, punctiform bleeding, and ulceration (**left**). Circumferential involvement of the distal terminal ileum with longitudinal ulcers and cobblestoning (**right**).

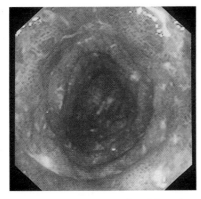

FIGURE 38-55. Crohn's disease involving the neoterminal ileum with multiple superficial ulcers. A 29-year-old woman with a history of Crohn's disease for 6 years had undergone resection of the terminal ileum and cecum with ileal–ascending colonic anastomosis. Symptoms of recurrent Crohn's disease (cramping abdominal pain and malaise) developed 4 months after resection. Colonoscopic image with visualization of the neoterminal ileum shows multiple focal superficial ulcers with edema, erythema, and granularity of the intervening mucosa.

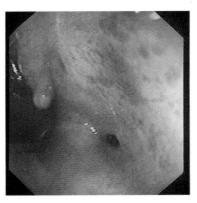

FIGURE 38-56. Crohn's disease—view of the rectum with rectovaginal fistula and prominent anal papilla. A 40-year-old woman has a 10-year history of Crohn's disease involving the colon. A symptomatic rectovaginal fistula developed with gas and stool passed per vagina. Retroflexed view of the rectum shows a central fistulous opening communicating with the vagina. The endoscope is in the **left** field of the photo, and a prominent anal papilla is present. The mucosa is granular, edematous, and friable.

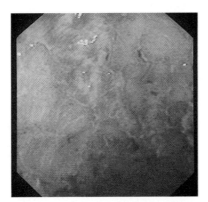

FIGURE 38-57. Mildly active Crohn's disease of the sigmoid colon in a 51-year-old man with a 4-year history of Crohn's colitis, now controlled with azathioprine 175 mg daily and metronidazole 250 mg twice daily. The mucosa shows superficial scarring, loss of normal vascular markings, and slight mucous exudate.

MISCELLANEOUS INFLAMMATORY AND STRUCTURAL DISORDERS OF THE COLON

DAVID H. ALPERS ■ DAVID H.B. CORT

A variety of structural and inflammatory conditions, apart from Crohn's disease and chronic ulcerative colitis involve the colon. They have been divided into inflammatory conditions associated with motor disorders (including solitary rectal ulcer and colitis cystica profunda), inflammatory conditions associated with therapeutic interventions (including radiation-induced, drug-induced, and cathartic-induced inflammation as well as diversion colitis), and other disorders (including microscopic and collagenous colitis, nonspecific ulcers of the colon, endometriosis, and pneumatosis cystoides intestinalis). Figure 39-1 shows the endoscopic appearance of solitary rectal ulcer. Figure 39-2 demonstrates the characteristic histological finding of fibromuscular hyperplasia in the lamina propria. These ulcers are believed to recur from repeated prolapse associated with the failure of the levator ani muscles to relax during defecation. More specific ulcers in the ascending colon can look quite similar, although their cause is probably different (Fig. 39-3). Colitis cystica profunda is possibly related to the solitary rectal ulcer syndrome. Polypoid masses can occur in the presence (Fig. 39-4) and absence (Fig. 39-5) of surface ulceration. The characteristic histological features of submucosal mucin-filled cysts are shown in Fig. 39-6. Inflammatory types of colitis other than idiopathic inflammatory bowel disease include Behçet disease (Fig. 39-7), radiation colitis (Figs. 39-8 through 39-10), and diversion colitis (Fig. 39-11). Pneumatosis cystoides intestinalis is a benign condition with submucosal gas cysts (Figs. 39-12 and 39-13).

414

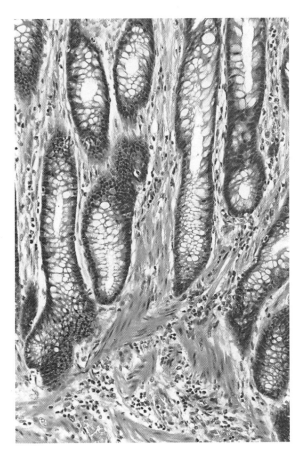

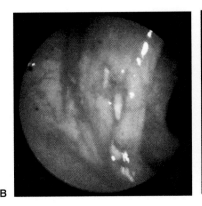

FIGURE 39-1. Solitary rectal ulcer. Well-demarcated margins and clean ulcer base with mild adjacent inflammatory change are depicted.

FIGURE 39-2. Solitary rectal ulcer syndrome. Biopsy specimen shows the characteristic appearance of fibroblasts (toward the 12 o'clock position) and muscle fibers (at the 6 o'clock position) within the lamina propria encircling crypts.

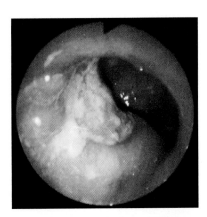

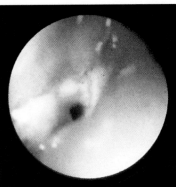

A, B

FIGURE 39-3. **A:** Nonspecific colonic ulcers in the ascending colon. Three discrete ulcers were found in an 80-year-old man with a history of hematochezia. The cause of these ulcers is unknown. **B:** Nonspecific colonic ulcer of the sigmoid with stricture. Deep ulceration in a patient with alcoholic pancreatitis and a pseudocyst was associated with stricture formation. There was no communication between the pancreatic pseudocyst and the stricture at operation, nor did the resected specimen show evidence of either inflammatory bowel disease or a malignant tumor. This was therefore considered to be nonspecific colonic ulceration.

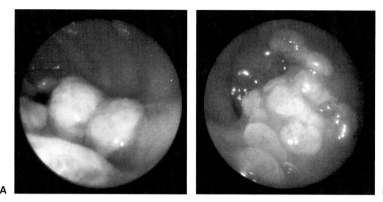

FIGURE 39-4. Solitary rectal ulcer syndrome. **A:** Ulcer stage with inflammatory polyps. Multiple 5- to 15-mm polypoid masses with ulcerated surfaces (composed of granulation tissue) are present rather than a discrete ulcer. **B:** Ulcer stage with polypoid masses. Rather than multiple discrete inflammatory polyps (**A**), these appear together as one large (1.5 × 2.5 cm), relatively discrete mass with nodules, the surfaces of which are composed of granulation tissue. In this case, large-particle biopsy showed superficial ulceration and fibromuscular hyperplasia of the lamina propria and muscularis mucosae. No submucosal mucin-containing cysts were found, although the endoscopic appearance and the location (rectosigmoid) cannot be differentiated from those of colitis cystica profunda.

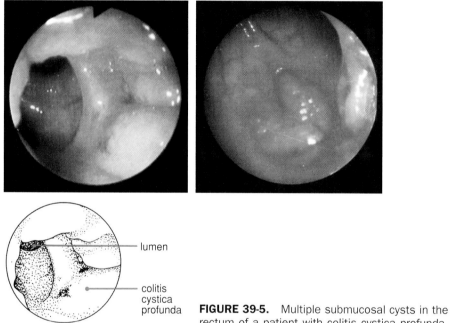

FIGURE 39-5. Multiple submucosal cysts in the rectum of a patient with colitis cystica profunda.

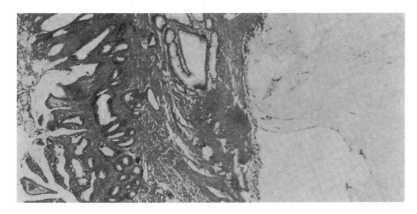

FIGURE 39-6. Submucosal mucin-filled cysts characteristic of colitis cystica profunda (hematoxylin and eosin).

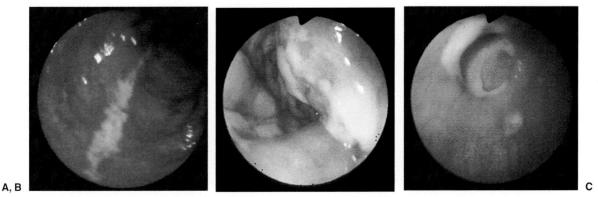

A, B   C

FIGURE 39-7. Behçet disease involving the colon. **A:** A discrete, long, linear ulceration set in a background of nonspecific erythema. This was observed in a patient with oral and vaginal ulcerations and iritis—the clinical constellation of Behçet disease. **B:** Discrete, deep ulceration of the sigmoid in a patient with clinical features favoring Behçet disease. The endoscopic appearance, however, does not allow differentiation from Crohn's disease, although colonic biopsies with evidence of vasculitis (lacking in this case) would have strongly favored Behçet disease. **C:** Discrete deep punched-out ulcerations are typical of colonic involvement in Behçet disease, not unlike those found in Crohn's colitis.

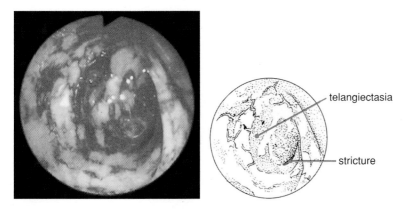

telangiectasia

stricture

FIGURE 39-8. Chronic radiation-induced telangiectasia and stricture of the rectosigmoid colon.

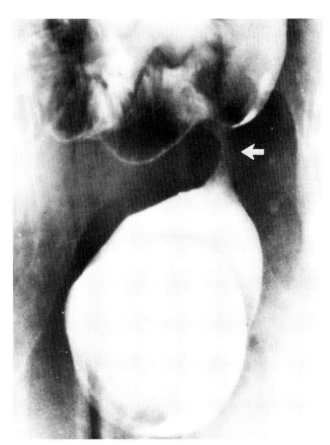

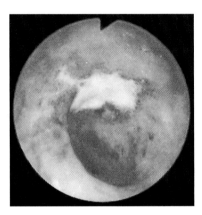

FIGURE 39-9. Chronic radiation-induced ulcer of the anterior wall of the rectum.

FIGURE 39-10. Barium enema image demonstrating chronic radiation-induced stricture of the rectosigmoid.

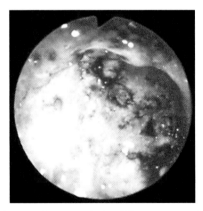

FIGURE 39-11. Characteristic diffuse mucosal inflammatory changes of diversion colitis. These findings are clinically indistinguishable from those of chronic idiopathic inflammatory bowel disease.

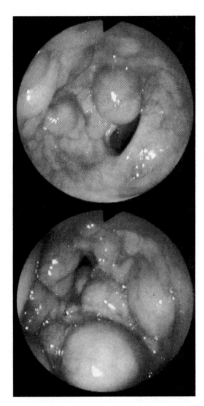

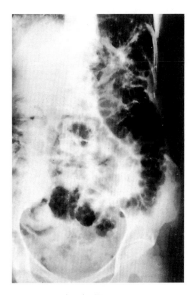

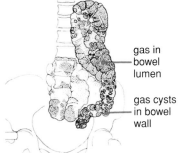

gas in
bowel
lumen

gas cysts
in bowel
wall

FIGURE 39-12. Multiple submucosal gas-filled cysts in pneumatosis coli. There is partial lumenal obstruction by the cysts.

FIGURE 39-13. Plain abdominal radiograph demonstrating gas-filled cysts in wall of sigmoid colon.

DIVERTICULAR DISEASE OF THE COLON

TONIA M. YOUNG-FADOK ■ MICHAEL G. SARR

Diverticular disease of the colon is an acquired condition. Diverticulosis, or the presence of diverticula, affects more than 50% of persons older than 80 years who live in industrialized countries. The etiology of diverticular disease appears to be multifactorial. Most important are age-related changes in the structure of the colon wall with decreased tensile strength and chronic exposure to excessive intralumenal pressures (Fig. 40-1). Insufficient dietary fiber in the western diet may be a leading contributing factor in the formation of diverticula, because African subjects with high-fiber diets rarely develop diverticula.

Diverticulosis involves primarily the sigmoid colon; in contrast, diverticula of the rectum are exceedingly uncommon. Diverticula are usually found in clusters, with sizes ranging from several millimeters to 1 to 2 cm. Diverticula are extralumenal structures composed of mucosa, submucosa, and serosa, but specifically lack the muscularis. They are, therefore, pseudodiverticula, characteristic of the pulsion, acquired type (Fig. 40-2).

The colon affected by diverticulosis undergoes changes that are signaled by muscular thickening (myochosis), which leads to shortening of the bowel and decreased lumenal diameter. These changes lead to a "concertina-like" or "picket fence" appearance radiographically (Fig. 40-3).

Most patients with diverticulosis have no symptoms. A small fraction of patients, approximately 15% to 25%, have intermittent abdominal pain and irregular bowel habits. Such symptomatic, uncomplicated disease may have an as yet undefined relationship to irritable bowel syndrome (IBS). Like IBS, uncomplicated diverticular disease is generally managed with increased dietary fiber. A high-fiber diet may ameliorate abdominal symptoms and may offer protection from the development and progression of diverticular disease.

Approximately 30% of patients with diverticulosis develop inflammation (diverticulitis) or bleeding, but rarely both. Diverticulitis is an inflammatory, peridiverticular process that begins with microperforation of a diverticulum typically filled with inspissated stool. Diverticulitis manifests classically with lower abdominal pain, frequently left-sided, tenderness, fever, and leukocytosis. The diagnosis of acute diverticulitis is frequently made on the basis of clinical presentation. Additional evaluation beyond plain abdominal radiography (to rule out free air) should proceed if there is diagnostic doubt or if a secondary complication is suspected (i.e., perforation, fistula, abscess, stricture, or obstruction). Further evaluation is also indicated in the patient whose disease is severe enough to merit hospitalization, because documentation of the diagnosis is a necessary part of subsequent surgical decision making. The use of a barium enema examination to diagnose acute diverticulitis is contraindicated because of the risks associated with extralumenal spillage of barium. The most widely used investigation is computed tomography (CT) (Figs. 40-4 and 40-5), which allows both confirmation of the diagnosis and also stages the extent of extralumenal inflammation. In the absence of ready access to CT facilities, water-soluble contrast enema may be useful (Fig. 40-6). CT colonography or "virtual colonoscopy" has the ability to image diverticula, but its role in the management of acute disease is not yet defined (Fig. 40-7A, B, C).

Management of acute diverticulitis includes bowel rest, correction of fluid and electrolyte abnormalities, and broad-spectrum intravenous antibiotics effective against aerobic and anaerobic organisms. Most patients respond to this medical management. After resolution of symptoms, a high-fiber diet may protect this subset of patients from recurrent attacks.

Elective operative intervention is reserved for patients with complicated diverticulitis (fistula [Fig. 40-8], abscess, and stricture), those with recurrent attacks, and when evaluation cannot exclude the possibility of an underlying carcinoma (Fig. 40-9). Elective surgical intervention is also indicated in the immunocompromised patient after just a single episode of diverticulitis. The management of young patients is more controversial; traditionally, operation has been offered after a single episode of diverticulitis, but with improved diagnostic modalities, it may be reasonable to base the need for operation on the severity of the disease rather than the age of the patient. Emergent operation is indicated for patients with free perforation or acute diverticulitis, which does not respond promptly to medical therapy.

For patients with a contained abscess (usually within the body of the colonic mesentery itself), CT-guided drainage (Fig. 40-10) may allow for postponement of surgical intervention until sepsis is controlled, the inflammatory process has subsided, and the bowel can be mechanically prepared for a one-stage resection of the affected colon with a primary colorectostomy. More urgent operations on an unprepared colon usually require a two-stage procedure with resection of the sigmoid colon and a diverting descending colostomy (Hartmann procedure). Formal resection of the diseased colonic segment rather than proximal colonic diversion via colostomy and drainage should be the aim of surgical management for perforated diverticulitis, because the affected bowel is a source of continuing sepsis that can lead to increased morbidity and mortality. Recurrent diverticulitis after appropriate resection of the entire sigmoid colon is uncommon.

A minimal access or laparoscopic approach increasingly is being used for surgical intervention. Most experience has been gained with elective sigmoid resection and with closure of colostomy after a Hartmann procedure. Laparoscopic techniques in the acute setting may be appropriate in skilled hands for Hinchey stages I and II, but not for stages III and IV. When resection with anastomosis is performed, an intracorporeal anastomosis is necessary (Fig. 40-11A, B) because the distal margin of resection should be in the proximal rectum to minimize the risk of recurrence.

Diverticular bleeding occurs much less frequently than acute diverticulitis. The true cause of erosion of the vasa recta at the neck of a diverticulum is unknown. The typical presentation involves an elderly patient with massive, painless bleeding that stops and starts abruptly and spontaneously. After initiating resuscitation, the site and source of bleeding should be sought. The timing and order of the diagnostic tests, including mesenteric angiography, red blood cell–tagged bleeding scintigraphy, and colonoscopy, depend on the clinical situation and the available facilities at the physician's institution. Mesenteric angiography is highly sensitive if performed when the rate of bleeding is greater than 0.5 mL/min (Fig. 40-12A,

B). Extravasation of intravenous contrast into a diverticulum is pathognomonic of diverticular bleeding. The radiographic pattern is different from that of bleeding angiectasis. Angiography has the additional benefit of allowing therapeutic infusion of vasopressin in an attempt to halt the bleeding. Red blood cell–tagged scintiscans (Fig. 40-13) may be helpful to determine whether bleeding is ongoing, but are often unreliable for localizing the precise site of bleeding, particularly in patients with chronic bleeding.

When significant bleeding persists, operative intervention is indicated. When the site of bleeding is known, segmental colonic resection is possible and is associated with low morbidity, mortality, and recurrence rates. When the site is unknown, intraoperative colonoscopy may be helpful. If the site cannot be identified, abdominal colectomy is usually indicated to deal effectively with the problem. This approach, however, is associated with increased morbidity among older patients, emphasizing the need to identify a site whenever possible to allow for the directed segmental resection.

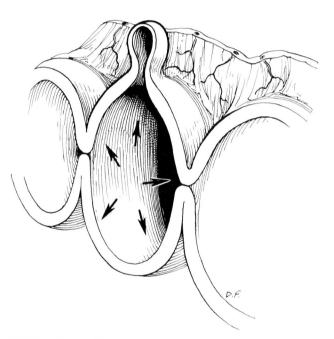

FIGURE 40-1. The concept of Painter and Burkitt of segmentation causing formation of pulsion diverticula.

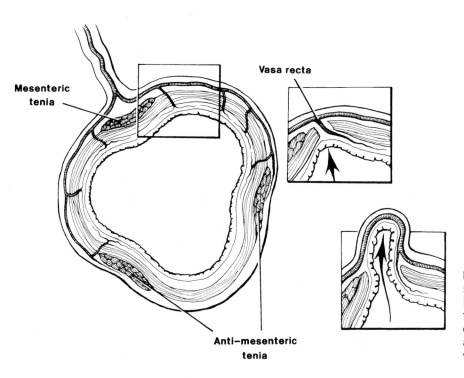

FIGURE 40-2. Cross section of the sigmoid colon. The main illustration indicates the points of penetration of the vasa recti around the bowel circumference. **Inset:** The development of a diverticulum at one such point of weakness.

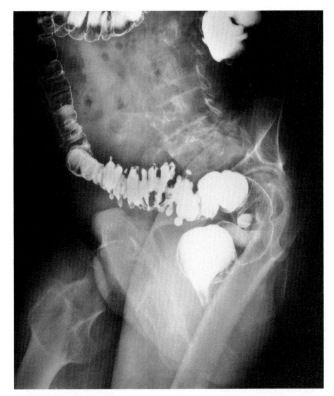

FIGURE 40-3. Contrast enema revealing picket fence appearance of the sigmoid colon, associated with symptoms of obstruction.

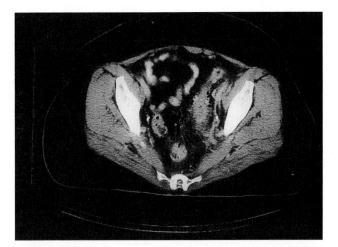

FIGURE 40-4. Computed tomography with oral and intravenous contrast in a 59-year-old woman with increasing abdominal pain for 3 weeks. Mild changes of diverticulitis are seen with narrowing of the colonic lumen, bowel wall thickening in the midsigmoid, tissue stranding in pericolic pelvic fat, and diverticula. There is no pericolic fluid collection.

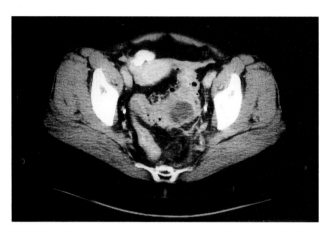

FIGURE 40-5. Computed tomography with oral and intravenous contrast in a 60-year-old woman with a 2-week history of crampy lower abdominal pain, fever, and chills showing a low-density mass adjacent to the sigmoid in the left pelvis. The central, low-density region within the mass, the pockets of surrounding gas, and inflammatory changes in pericolic tissues are consistent with diverticular disease.

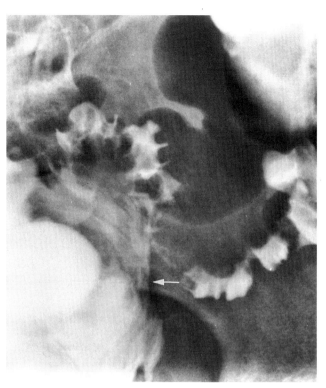

FIGURE 40-6. Hypaque enema in a 79-year-old woman shows nonanatomic distribution of contrast (*arrow*) around the rectum, demonstrating perforation.

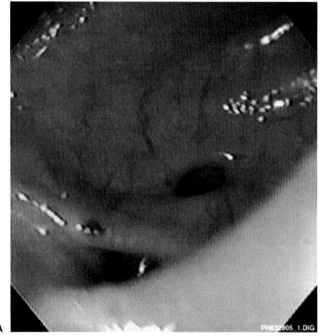

A

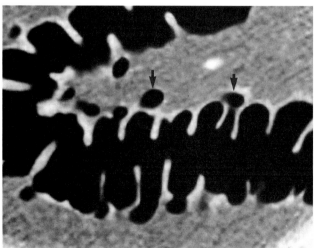

B

FIGURE 40-7. Virtual colonoscopy. **A:** View of diverticula as seen on routine colonoscopy. **B:** Two-dimensional image of diverticula (*arrows*) obtained by spiral computed tomography scan. *(Continued)*

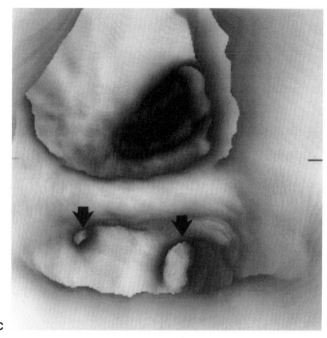

C

FIGURE 40-7.   C: Three-dimensional reconstruction (virtual colonoscopy) illustrating diverticula (*arrows*).

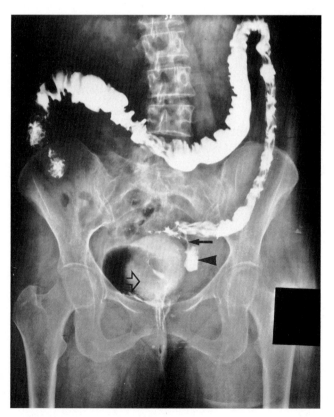

FIGURE 40-8. Barium enema in a 54-year-old woman with pneumaturia and left lower quadrant pain. A fistulous tract (*closed arrow*) arises in the midsigmoid passing into an abscess cavity (*arrowhead*) and then into bladder, where contrast is also seen (*open arrow*).

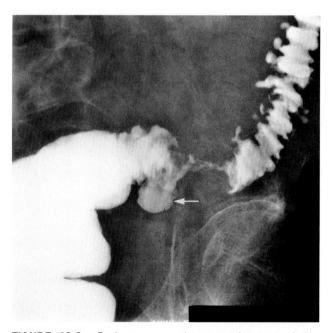

FIGURE 40-9. Barium enema demonstrating constricting lesion in sigmoid colon in a region of diverticulosis. There is also a 3-cm localized collection of barium (*arrow*) off the lateral colonic wall consistent with an abscess cavity. The most likely radiologic diagnosis is diverticulitis but carcinoma cannot be excluded.

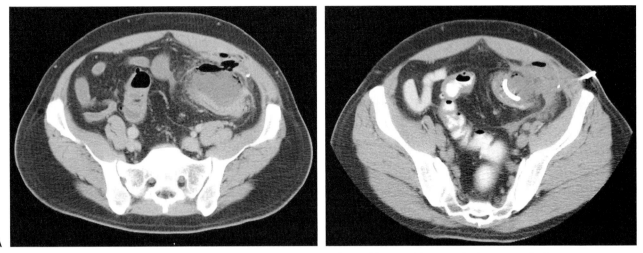

A   B

FIGURE 40-10. Computed tomographic scan in a 43-year-old man. **A:** Large pericolic abscess. **B:** Following placement of a pigtail catheter to drain the abscess.

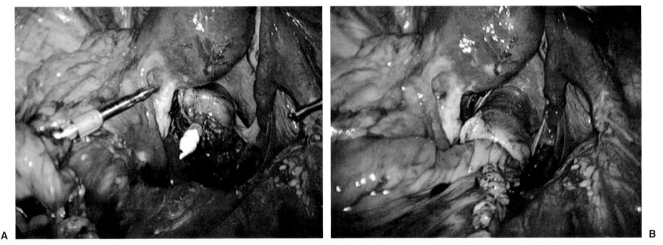

A   B

FIGURE 40-11. A 53-year-old woman undergoing elective laparoscopic sigmoid resection. **A:** The distal resection margin is in the proximal rectum, just below the sacral promontory. **B:** The completed anastomosis employing the circular stapler.

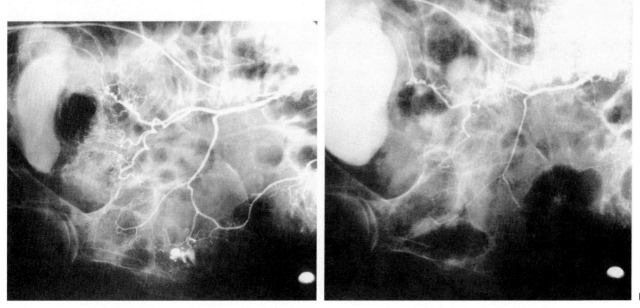

A

B

FIGURE 40-12. Arteriogram of the inferior mesenteric artery in a patient with diverticular bleeding. **A:** Extravasation of contrast medium into the lumen of the descending colon. **B:** Arteriogram of the same patient after infusion of vasopressin. Note the markedly reduced flow in the left colonic and sigmoidal branches.

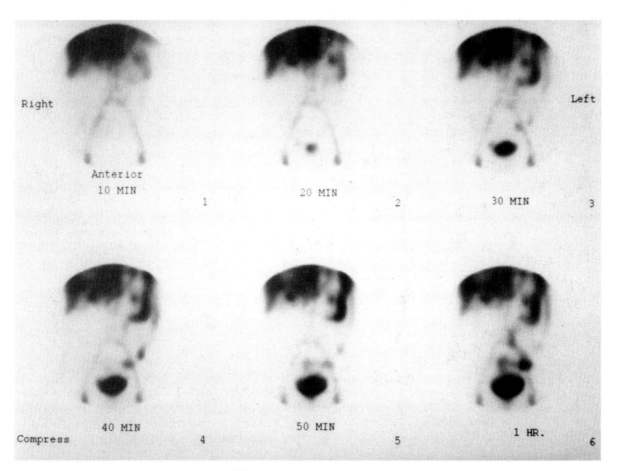

Right

Left

Anterior
10 MIN   20 MIN   30 MIN
1   2   3

40 MIN   50 MIN   1 HR.
Compress   4   5   6

FIGURE 40-13. Technetium (^{99m}Tc)-labeled red blood cell scan for evaluation of lower gastrointestinal bleeding in a 63-year-old woman with a 24-hour history of bright red blood per rectum. Increased activity in the distal transverse colon near the splenic flexure progresses toward the descending colon and sigmoid colon by termination of the examination at 1 hour. Findings are consistent with a bleeding source in the distal transverse colon near the splenic flexure.

BACTERIAL INFECTIONS OF THE COLON

GAIL HECHT ■ JERROLD R. TURNER

The spectrum of organisms that can infect and cause disease in the human colon includes bacteria, viruses, and protozoa. This chapter reviews the bacterial and viral pathogens of the large intestine. Although the symptoms associated with infection by enteric bacterial pathogens are essentially indistinguishable, including abdominal pain, diarrhea, and fever, the range of pathological appearances are somewhat more varied. For example, colonic biopsies of *Campylobacter* colitis have features similar to those seen in inflammatory bowel disease, including crypt abscesses (Fig. 41-1), but lack changes associated with chronicity. Infection with enterohemorrhagic *E coli* (EHEC) typically induces changes consistent with ischemic colitis (Fig. 41-2). Transmission of this pathogen to humans (Fig. 41-3) is most often from beef-derived food products, but may also be associated with ingestion of contaminated crops or water. Instances of secondary transmission from other infected humans or farm animals have also been reported. The histological features of colitis associated with enteroinvasive colitis and *Shigella* are typically identical (Fig. 41-4). This stems from the fact that the genes conferring the invasive phenotype are identical for these two pathogens. Despite these highlighted differences, colonic histology is usually not specific enough to conclusively determine the causative agent. The one exception to this statement is *C difficile*–associated pseudomembranous colitis. *C difficile* is the number one cause of healthcare-associated diarrhea because hospitals and long-term care facilities serve as reservoirs and establishment of infection in the colon by this spore-forming pathogen is dependent on disruption of the resident colonic microflora by antibiotics (Fig. 41-5). Although the diagnosis of *C difficile*–associated colitis is usually determined by assays that identify the presence of toxin A and/or B in the stool, the gross appearance of pseudomembranes seen at sigmoidoscopy (Fig. 41-6) and the characteristic histological volcano lesion (Fig. 41-7) are virtually pathognomonic for this infection. If a barium enema examination is performed (which is not recommended), the presence of pseudomembranes may be demonstrated (Fig. 41-8).

Infections of the anus and rectum are most commonly seen in homosexual men and heterosexual women who engage in anoreceptive intercourse. Primary anorectal syphilis appears as a chancre of the squamous epithelial lining of the anal canal or rectum (Fig. 41-9). Condyloma lata represents the secondary phase of syphilis (Fig. 41-10). Biopsy of anorectal lesions from patients infected with *Treponema pallidum* may reveal spirochetal organisms (Fig. 41-11) but nonpathogenic spirochetes can also reside in the rectum, thus reducing the significance of this finding.

More commonly seen are condyloma acuminata, or anal warts, caused by infection with human papilloma virus. These verrucous lesions are generally easy to differentiate from the flat, fleshy lesions of condyloma lata but histological examination easily distinguishes between the two and is recommended to confirm the diagnosis (Fig. 41-12).

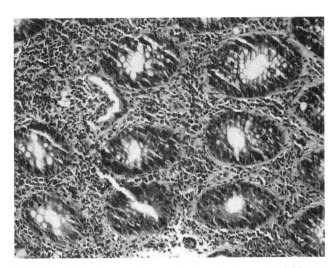

FIGURE 41-1. Photomicrograph of colonic mucosal biopsy from a patient with *C jejuni* colitis. Note the presence of crypt abscesses, crypt destruction, and lamina propria infiltrates of neutrophils, eosinophils, and lymphocytes. These features can overlap with those present in inflammatory bowel disease. However, the uniform spacing and shape of the crypts (i.e., a lack of architectural distortion) is unusual in inflammatory bowel disease and suggests that an alternative diagnosis, such as an infectious process, should be considered. (Case courtesy Dr. Neal S. Goldstein, William Beaumont Hospital, Royal Oak, MI.)

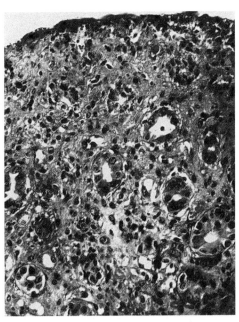

FIGURE 41-2. This colonic mucosal biopsy from a patient with *E coli* 0157:H7 colitis demonstrates superficial epithelial atrophy with crypt cell hyperplasia. These features are similar to those that can be present in ischemic colitis. In other cases the pathology associated with *E coli* 0157:H7 infection can be more severe, with the development of pseudomembranes. (Case courtesy Dr. Neal S. Goldstein, William Beaumont Hospital, Royal Oak, MI.)

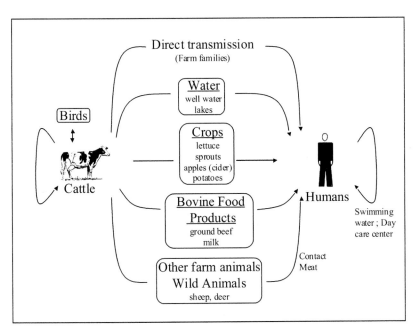

FIGURE 41-3. Schematic of modes of transmission of enterohemorrhagic *E coli* (EHEC) to humans. Cattle are the main reservoir of EHEC; therefore, the ingestion of contaminated bovine food products is most commonly associated with human infection. Crops and sources of water can also be contaminated by bovine feces through the use of manure for fertilizer or proximity to water sources. EHEC 0157:H7 has also been identified in birds, as well as other animals including deer and sheep, suggesting that they may also represent reservoirs of EHEC infection. Secondary infection between humans, especially between children in day-care centers, has also been reported.

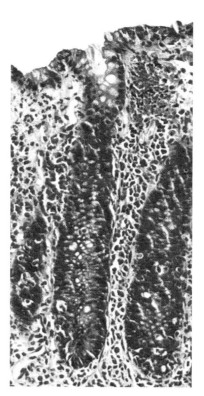

FIGURE 41-4. This colonic mucosal biopsy from a patient with enteroinvasive *E coli* colitis demonstrates pronounced infiltration of surface and crypt epithelium by neutrophils. The lamina propria also contains numerous neutrophils with admixed eosinophils and fewer lymphocytes and plasma cells. Some apoptotic epithelial cells can also be seen and can be present in even greater numbers in more severe cases. The clinical and pathological features can be indistinguishable from *Shigella* infection. The uniform spacing and shape of the crypts helps to exclude inflammatory bowel disease. (Case courtesy Dr. Neal S. Goldstein, William Beaumont Hospital, Royal Oak, MI.)

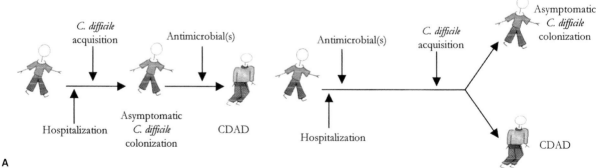

FIGURE 41-5. Hypothesized mode by which hospitalized patients acquire *C difficile* and the associated diarrhea. **A:** Depiction of the initial hypothesis that hospitalized patients become colonized with *C difficile* and upon exposure to antimicrobial agents develop the symptoms that typify this infection. More recently, a revised hypothesis has been put forth and is shown in **B**. In this case, the hospitalized patient may be exposed to *C difficile* throughout the course of stay, but is not susceptible to colonization until antibiotics are introduced. At that point, true acquisition of the organism occurs and host factors, such as the level of antibody production to the organism and/or its toxins, determines which patients will become colonized but remain asymptomatic, and which will manifest the associated symptom of diarrhea.

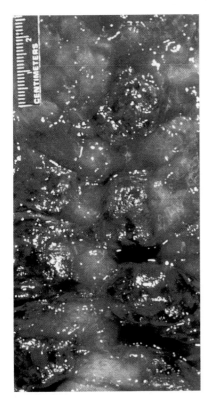

FIGURE 41-6. Gross appearance of *C difficile* pseudomembranous colitis. This photo shows the severe, nearly confluent, pale pseudomembranes that are typical of severe *C difficile* pseudomembranous colitis. The pseudomembranes are composed of purulent debris and contrast sharply against the surrounding dark edematous mucosa.

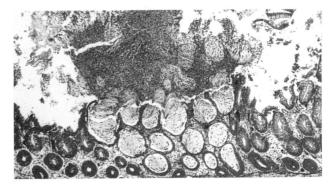

FIGURE 41-7. Histological appearance of *C difficile* pseudomembranous colitis. This photomicrograph shows a classical type II volcano-like eruption with a mushroom-shaped cloud of adherent inflammatory exudate.

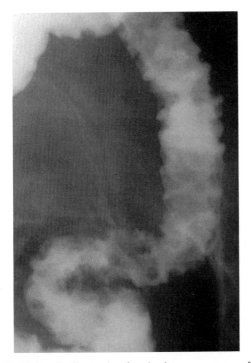

FIGURE 41-8. Radiograph of a barium enema performed on a patient with *C difficile*–induced pseudomembranous colitis. Note the presence of multiple filling defects within the colonic mucosa, which represent pseudomembranes and mucosal edema.

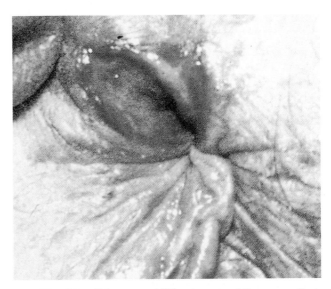

FIGURE 41-9. Primary syphilitic chancre of the anus. Such lesions occur in homosexual men and heterosexual women who engage in anoreceptive intercourse. Anorectal syphilitic chancres may be asymptomatic or painful, usually upon defecation.

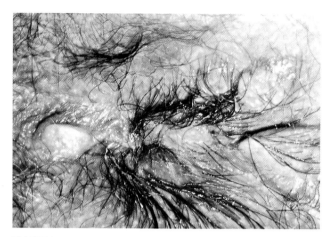

FIGURE 41-10. Condyloma lata of the anorectal area, shown here, represent the secondary stage of syphilis. Condyloma lata appear as smooth, moist, fleshy lesions, which can secrete a discharge that is highly infectious. Condyloma lata are distinguishable from the verrucous anal warts or condyloma acuminata caused by infection with human papilloma virus.

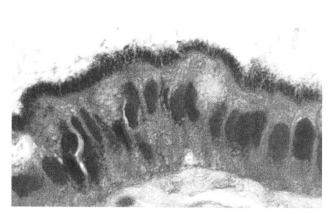

FIGURE 41-11. High-power photomicrograph of rectal spirochetosis showing the typical apical layer of spirochetes that stain dark blue on standard hematoxylin and eosin stain. The organisms are oriented parallel to the microvilli and, by electron microscopy, can be seen to interdigitate between the microvilli. Rectal spirochetes may represent *Treponema pallidum* or nonpathogenic organisms, diminishing the significance of such a finding.

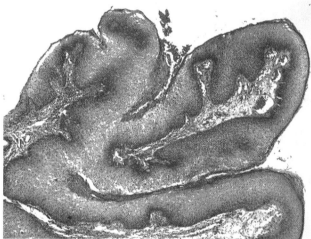

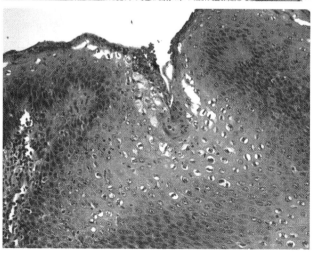

FIGURE 41-12. Condyloma acuminatum of the anal region. The low-power view (**upper panel**) shows the typical papillomatous growth pattern of this lesion. The higher-magnification photomicrograph (**lower panel**) demonstrates the typical vacuolization of koilocytotic human papilloma virus-infected squamous cells.

42

COLORECTAL POLYPS: Benign and Premalignant

FINLAY A. MACRAE ■ **GRAEME P. YOUNG** ■ **ANTHONY C. THOMAS**

Colorectal polyps may be classified in various ways. On the basis of location, they may be mucosal (such as an adenoma) or submucosal (such as a lipoma). Mucosal lesions are by far the most common and are further subdivided into neoplastic and nonneoplastic lesions. Neoplastic polyps are of greatest clinical significance because of their premalignant nature and their potential to progress to carcinoma. Nonneoplastic polyps have minimal or no premalignant potential. Submucosal lesions are rare, and their clinical significance depends on the underlying cause. A series of figures (photomicrographs, endoscopic and macroscopic photographs, radiologic studies) are presented in Figs. 42-1 through 42-85 as examples of the different types of polyps. In addition, some figures depict endoscopic therapy.

Polyps are generally asymptomatic and are usually detected in the context of screening or serendipitous diagnostic investigation. If the possibility of polyps is high, the definitive diagnostic procedure is colonoscopy, often coupled with polypectomy and histological examination to ascertain the true nature of the tissue. Endoscopic polypectomy is adequate management of most adenomatous polyps unless they are very large. Many sessile polyps can now be removed by a submucosal injection of saline (a "saline lift") followed by snare polypectomy. However, some malignant polyps may necessitate surgical resection if removal is incomplete, clearance is not certain, and histology is poorly differentiated. Because polyps are most often seen at endoscopy, many of the figures presented herein are taken at endoscopy. Selected radiographs are also presented because polyps are occasionally diagnosed in this way.

The potential for malignancy now or in the future depends on the size of an adenomatous polyp, the number of polyps, histological features such as degree of dysplasia, and architectural type such as degree of villous change. Polyps larger than 2 cm in diameter, those with a large villous architectural component, or those with severe dysplasia, carry a higher risk for malignancy. The natural history of the progression of adenomatous polyps is deduced from observational studies and remains largely speculative. It appears that most adenomas take 2 to 10 years to progress to frank malignant tumors. Exceptions include adenomas in hereditary nonpolyposis colorectal cancer (HNPCC) and perhaps some flat adenomas outside of this setting.

Because histopathological examination is the crucial issue for any polyp, examples of the histopathological features of the various types of polyps are provided. Figures are grouped and generally follow the following sequence: adenomas (Figs. 42-1 through 42-8), tubular adenomas (Figs. 42-9 through 42-15), villous adenomas (Figs. 42-18 through 42-22), serrated adenomas (Figs. 42-23 through 42-25),

433

examples of polypectomy (Figs. 42-26 through 42-39), malignant polyps (Figs. 42-16, 42-17, and 42-40 through 42-43), familial adenomatous polyposis (Figs. 42-44 through 42-50), other polyposis syndromes (Figs. 42-51 through 42-55), lymphoid accumulations (Figs. 42-56 through 42-59), hyperplastic polyps (Figs. 42-60 through 42-63), inflammatory polyps (Figs. 42-64 through 42-66), submucosal lesions (Figs. 42-67 through 42-77), and oddities and artifacts (Figs. 42-78 through 42-85).

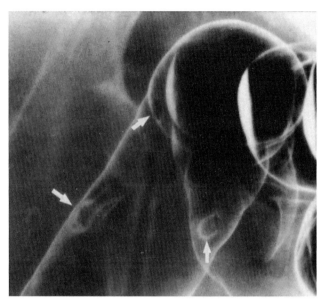

FIGURE 42-1. Double-contrast radiographic appearance of three small sessile polyps (*arrows*) ranging in size from 0.5 to 0.8 cm that were subsequently found to be tubular adenomas. The distinction between adenomas, which have malignant potential, and mucosal or hyperplastic polyps, which have no malignant potential, cannot be made at radiography or endoscopy. Biopsy (or polypectomy) and histological examination must be performed. Whenever possible, all polyps shown on this radiograph should be removed and retrieved for examination because they will not all be the same.

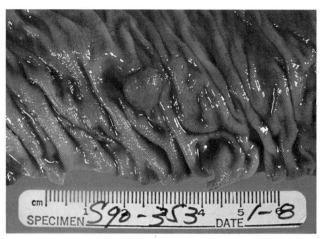

FIGURE 42-2. Typical macroscopic appearance of a 1-cm pedunculated tubular adenoma. Dark red coloration and fine granular surface are depicted. The surfaces of tubular adenomas are typically fine and granular, as shown here, or lobulated. However, a definitive diagnosis can be made only by means of histopathological study.

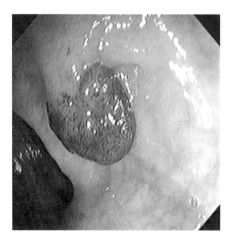

FIGURE 42-3. Colonoscopic photograph of an 8-mm tubular adenoma on a moderate sized stalk.

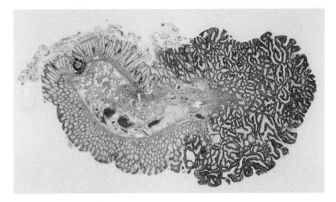

FIGURE 42-4. Low-power photomicrograph of a section of a small tubular adenoma with a long stalk (H&E stain). The adenoma comprises closely packed glands imparting a tubular appearance, and shows few goblet cells. There is no complexity of glandular architecture, and at higher power, the columnar cells had basal nuclei and a moderate amount of cytoplasm. These findings are characteristic of low-grade (mild) dysplasia. The diathermy burn is at the base of the stalk, well clear of the adenoma.

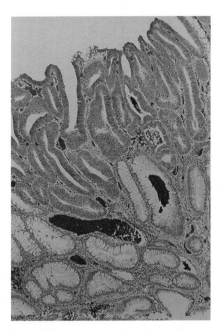

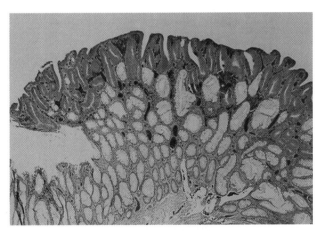

FIGURE 42-5. Histological appearance of a small tubular adenoma with mild dysplasia.

FIGURE 42-6. Higher-power view of another part of the specimen in Fig. 42-5 shows closely packed epithelial tubules, pseudostratification, scant cytoplasm, and enlarged and elongated hyperchromatic nuclei in the dysplastic area.

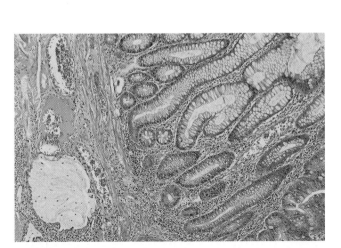

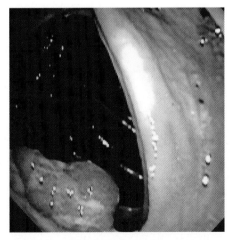

FIGURE 42-7. Medium-power photomicrograph of a section of part of a tubular adenoma (**lower right**) with "misplaced" mucin (**lower left**) within the submucosa deep to the muscularis mucosae (H&E stain). These appearances can be misinterpreted as invasive carcinoma, but note the absence of epithelium and the presence of lamina propria around the mucin pool indicating that this is not true invasion. Similarly, "misplaced" glands surrounded by lamina propria should not be interpreted as invasive carcinoma. Nonneoplastic mucosa is seen adjacent to the adenoma (**top right**).

FIGURE 42-8. Colonoscopic photograph of a large adenoma in the ascending colon of a patient with hereditary nonpolyposis colorectal cancer.

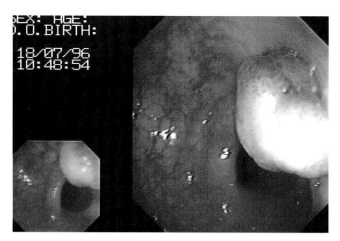

FIGURE 42-9. Endoscopic photograph showing semisessile sigmoid 1.5 cm tubulovillous adenoma partly obscured by a sigmoid fold in a patient without symptoms but at risk for hereditary nonpolyposis colorectal cancer.

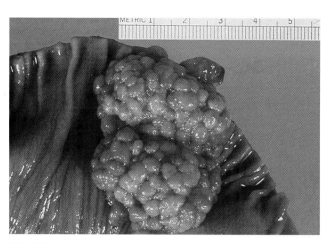

FIGURE 42-10. Macroscopic appearance of a tubulovillous adenoma.

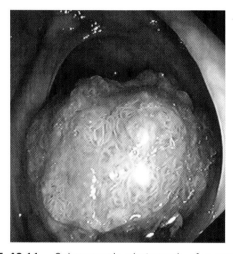

FIGURE 42-11. Colonoscopic photograph of a moderately large tubulovillous adenomatous polyp. (Courtesy of Dr. Michael Bourke.)

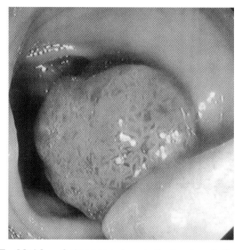

FIGURE 42-12. Colonoscopic photograph of the same polyp as in Fig. 42-11 from a different perspective and showing its thick stalk.

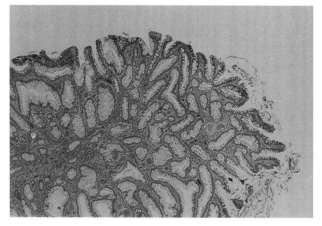

FIGURE 42-13. Histological appearance of a mixed tubulovillous adenoma. Image shows predominant epithelial tubules, villous projections at the surface, and the eosinophilic core of the polyp (**lower left corner**).

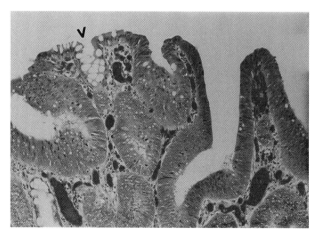

FIGURE 42-14. Histopathological appearance of a tubulovillous adenoma with high-grade dysplasia. There is marked variation in the cellular appearance of the dysplastic superficial cells with loss of basal polarity of nuclei and an increased nuclear-to-cytoplasmic ratio. Focal persistence of normal mucosa is present (*arrowhead*).

436

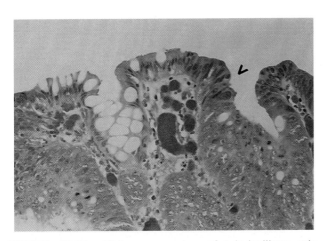

FIGURE 42-15. Higher-power view of tubulovillous adenoma in Fig. 42-14 shows marked variation in nuclear and cytoplasmic appearance (*arrowhead*), pleomorphic hyperchromatic nuclei, crowding of the glands, and frequent mitotic figures.

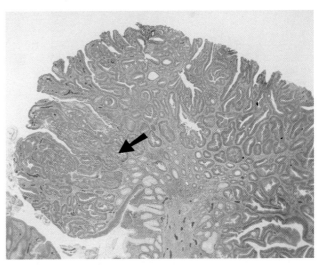

FIGURE 42-16. Low- to medium-power photomicrograph of a section of a portion of a 20-mm sigmoid polyp showing a tubulovillous adenoma with focal intramucosal carcinoma (*arrow*) (H&E stain). Note the complex glandular architecture with back-to-back arrangement and budding of glands. There is no submucosal invasion and the diathermy margin passed through normal epithelium (not apparent in this section).

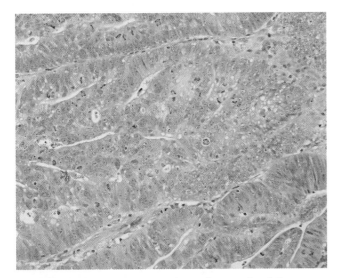

FIGURE 42-17. High-power photomicrograph of the same area of intramucosal carcinoma depicted in Fig. 42-16 showing more clearly the complex glandular architecture with crowding and distortion of crypts. In addition, there is high-grade cytological atypia with high nuclear-to-cytoplasmic ratio, prominent nucleoli, some stratification, and conspicuous mitotic figures. Despite the lack of an obvious desmoplastic response, the constellation of these features is often regarded as intramucosal carcinoma rather than merely high-grade dysplasia. Because the resection margin was well clear of neoplasia and there was no invasion of vessels in the stalk, polypectomy alone was considered adequate in this case.

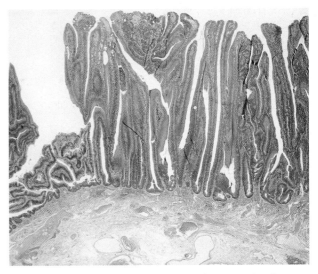

FIGURE 42-18. Medium-power photomicrograph of a section of a villous adenoma (H&E stain). Note the frond-like projections and relative lack of glandular architecture when compared with tubular adenomas.

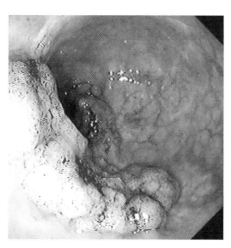

FIGURE 42-19. Colonoscopic photograph of an extensive, almost circumferential villous adenoma in the rectum that extended for 8 cm. This patient was not an ideal candidate for surgery and agreed to undergo attempted endoscopic removal.

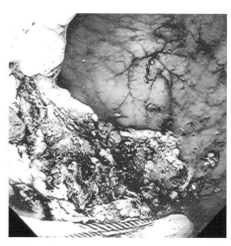

FIGURE 42-20. Colonoscopic photograph of the same villous adenoma as in Fig. 42-19 after submucosal saline injection to lift the adenoma followed by polypectomy. The submucosal injection elevates the base and makes polypectomy a little easier and more likely to remove the base of the adenoma.

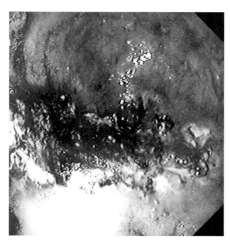

FIGURE 42-21. Colonoscopic photograph of the same villous adenoma as in Fig. 42-20 after polypectomy followed by destruction of residual adenoma at the margins by argon plasma coagulation. Close follow-up is required to check for recurrence because total destruction cannot be guaranteed.

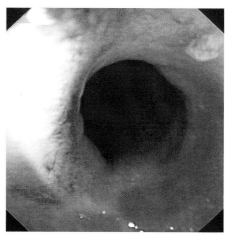

FIGURE 42-22. Colonoscopic photograph of the rectum of the same patient as in Fig. 42-21, 14 months later. There is scarring but no residual tumor on biopsy of the pale area. The yellow patch is fecal material.

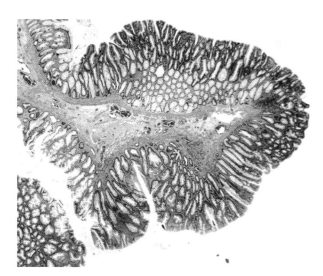

FIGURE 42-23. Low-power photomicrograph of a section of a typical serrated adenoma (H&E stain). Note the intermingling of the dysplastic component (imparting an appearance similar to that of a tubular adenoma) with the hyperplastic component characterized by the typical surface serrations. Some use the term "combined" or "mixed" when the adenomatous component lies adjacent to the hyperplastic component, reserving the term "serrated adenoma" when the two components are intimately intermingled, as in this case.

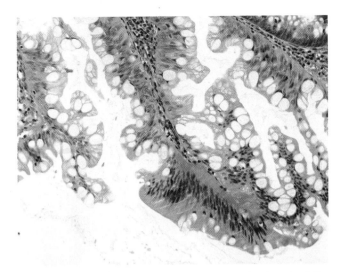

FIGURE 42-24. High-power photomicrograph of part of the same lesion depicted in Fig. 42-23 showing more clearly the intermingling of the two components. The serrated surface typical of a hyperplastic polyp can be clearly seen, but the surface epithelium is also hyperchromatic and stratified with, in some foci, a high nuclear-to-cytoplasmic ratio indicative of dysplasia.

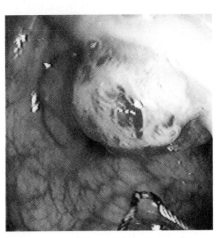

FIGURE 42-25. Colonoscopic photograph of a large serrated adenoma about to be removed from a patient with hyperplastic polyposis.

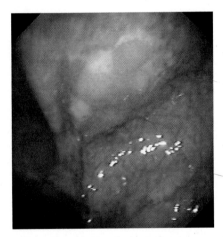

FIGURE 42-26. Endoscopic photograph shows a 1-cm flat, multilobulated polyp adjacent to the cecal sling fold. The polyp is pale pink, whereas the surrounding mucosa is brown because of melanosis. Adenomas do not take up melanin and stand out in melanosis coli.

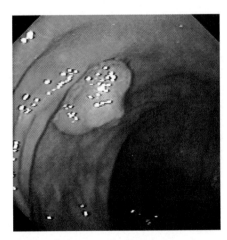

FIGURE 42-27. Colonoscopic photo shows a semisessile, 1.4-cm polyp in proximal rectum. Some irregularity of the surface and possible ulceration are evident by scalloping of the surface on the upper aspect.

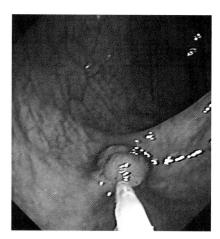

FIGURE 42-28. Polyp depicted in Fig. 42-27 grasped with colonoscopic snare before electrocauterization. Colonoscope has been rotated to allow better apposition of the snare to the polyp base to optimize clearance. Better clearance and safety could be facilitated by submucosal injection of up to 10 mL of saline (not shown).

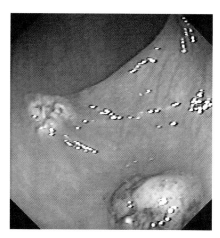

FIGURE 42-29. Clean polypectomy base interpreted by endoscopist as complete polypectomy of polyp depicted in Fig. 42-27. Separated free-lying polyp is present in the foreground.

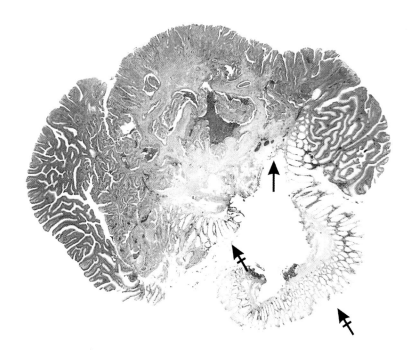

FIGURE 42-30. Histopathological examination of polyp depicted in Fig. 42-27 shows centrally placed, invasive, moderately differentiated adenocarcinoma arising in a sessile, moderately dysplastic tubulovillous adenoma. The malignant glands and surrounding desmoplastic stroma are approximately 600 μm from the closest point of the diathermized deep margin (*arrow*). Because of the closeness, this represents a relative indication to proceed to surgical resection. *Crossed arrows* point to the cuff of normal rectal mucosa included in the polypectomy specimen. The subsequent low anterior resection specimen did not contain any residual malignant tissue or lymph node metastases.

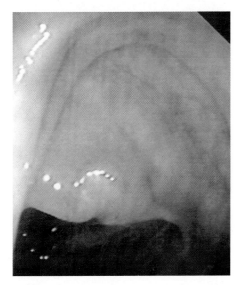

FIGURE 42-31. Colonoscopic photograph of a flat adenoma with slight central depression on the edge of a fold in sigmoid colon. These are likely to show high-grade dysplasia. Flat adenomas are recognized more commonly in Japan, and a recent study has shown that they may be as common in western countries such as the United Kingdom. (Courtesy of Dr. Michael Bourke.)

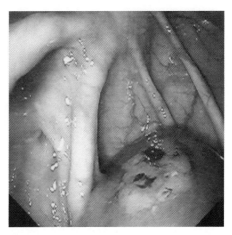

FIGURE 42-32. Colonoscopic photograph of a flat adenoma in the cecum which has been lifted by a submucosal injection of indigo carmine to facilitate colonoscopic removal. The wall of the cecum is thin and presents a higher risk of perforation than elsewhere in the colon. (Courtesy of Dr. Michael Bourke.)

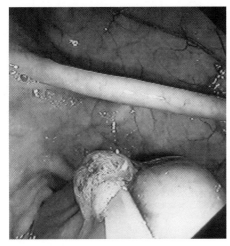

FIGURE 42-33. Colonoscopic photograph of the same lesion as in Fig. 42-32 after application of the snare for polypectomy. (Courtesy of Dr. Michael Bourke.)

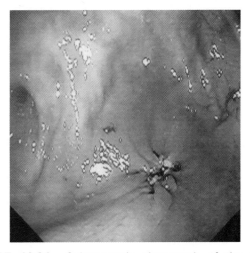

FIGURE 42-34. Colonoscopic photograph of the same lesion as in Fig. 42-33 after snare polypectomy. Note the clean base and how the saline-indigo carmine lift helps ensure complete removal with less chance of perforation. (Courtesy of Dr. Michael Bourke.)

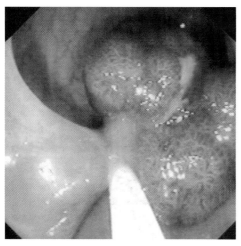

FIGURE 42-35. Colonoscopic photograph of a large, multilobulated tubulovillous adenoma showing the diathermy loop secured to the stalk a good distance below the adenoma tissue. Histopathology confirmed total removal with a 4-mm margin. Such polyps have a chance of containing a focus of carcinoma and complete removal at the first attempt is desirable. (Courtesy of Dr. Michael Bourke.)

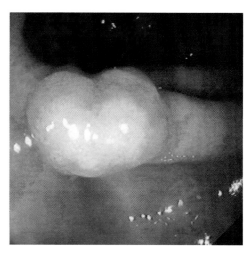

FIGURE 42-36. Colonoscopic photograph of a sessile polyp on a fold. Saline injection prior to polypectomy is desirable to aid complete removal and lessen the chance of perforation. (Courtesy of Dr. Michael Bourke.)

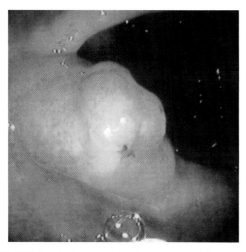

FIGURE 42-37. Colonoscopic photograph of the same sessile polyp as in Fig. 42-36 after saline injection. (Courtesy of Dr. Michael Bourke.)

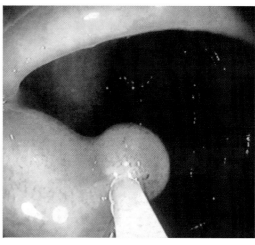

FIGURE 42-38. Colonoscopic photograph of the same sessile polyp as in Fig. 42-37 after saline injection and subsequent snaring. In this situation, it may be difficult to ensure that all the adenoma is included because there is no discrete stalk; histopathological examination and possible early follow-up examination within 1 year are required to ensure the adequacy of removal. (Courtesy of Dr. Michael Bourke.)

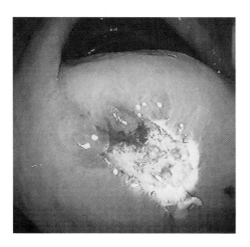

FIGURE 42-39. Colonoscopic photograph of the same sessile polyp as in Fig. 42-38 after polypectomy. There is no obvious residual material. Note the bulge on the fold remaining from the saline injection into the submucosa. (Courtesy of Dr. Michael Bourke.)

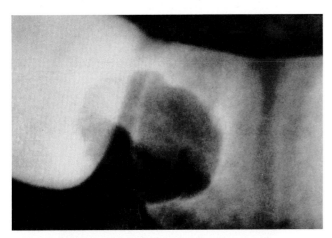

FIGURE 42-40. Radiographic appearance of a 2-cm sessile polyp with a somewhat lobulated surface. This was subsequently found to be tubulovillous adenoma with early invasive carcinoma. The carcinomatous invasion cannot be determined with radiography alone, or with endoscopy or biopsy. Large polyps must be removed in toto so the degree of carcinomatous invasion, if any, can be determined. The drawing in of a haustral fold suggests malignant tethering.

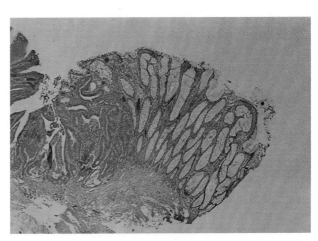

FIGURE 42-41. Histological appearance of a tubulovillous adenoma with severe dysplasia and invasion into and through the muscularis mucosae typical of a malignant polyp. There is marked cell crowding with hyperchromatic, elongated nuclei, marked loss of basal polarity, increased nucleus-to-cytoplasm ratio, and architectural distortion in the malignant focus. A lesion such as this highlights the inadequacy of biopsying such lesions because the carcinoma could easily be missed. All large polyps should be removed in toto and subjected to careful histological study.

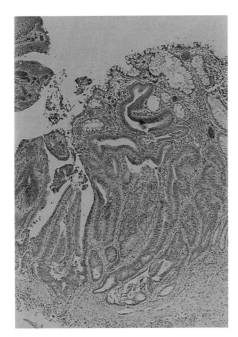

FIGURE 42-42. Higher-power view of the malignant focus of the adenoma in Fig. 42-41 showing cytologic detail with invasion into the muscularis mucosae.

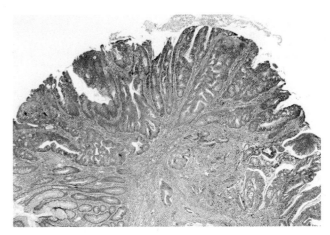

FIGURE 42-43. Medium-power photomicrograph of a section of an adenomatous polyp with a focus of invasive carcinoma in the submucosa of the stalk (H&E stain). In contrast to "misplaced" glands, note the lack of surrounding lamina propria and early desmoplastic response indicating true invasion.

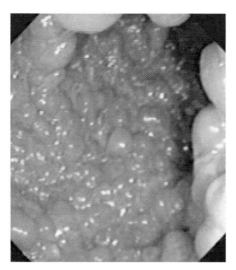

FIGURE 42-44. Colonoscopic photograph of the rectum of a teenage boy undergoing his first sigmoidoscopic surveillance for familial adenomatous polyposis. Many adenomas are apparent up to 10 mm in size. These extended well into the transverse colon and became sparse in the cecum. Residual fecal material accentuates the polyps.

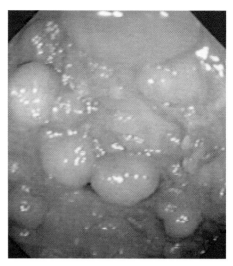

FIGURE 42-45. A close-up colonoscopic view of the same polyps from the patient shown in Fig. 42-44.

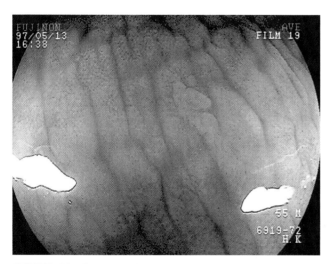

FIGURE 42-46. Magnifying colonoscopic view of a cluster of aberrant crypts with histopathological features of dysplasia. These are the earliest stage of adenoma formation. *APC* or *Ras* mutations (or both) may already be established in these lesions.

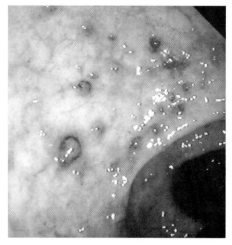

FIGURE 42-47. Colonoscopic photograph of scattered small polyps in the rectum of a patient with familial adenomatous polyposis who has undergone colectomy and ileorectal anastomosis.

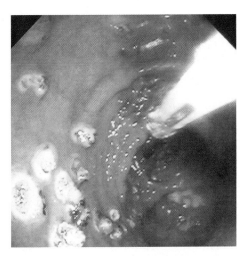

FIGURE 42-48. Colonoscopic photograph of the same patient shown in Fig. 42-47 after destruction of the polyps by argon plasma coagulation.

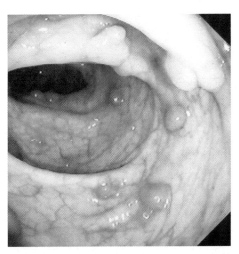

FIGURE 42-49. Colonoscopic photograph of sparse rectal polyps found at the first sigmoidoscopic examination of a patient in a family with attenuated (also termed "atypical") familial adenomatous polyposis. Compare the dramatic difference in density of the polyps with that shown in Fig. 42-44.

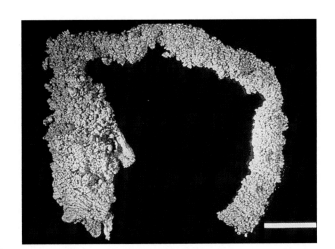

FIGURE 42-50. Colon resection specimen from a patient with familial adenomatous polyposis. The normal mucosa seems almost completely replaced by adenomas.

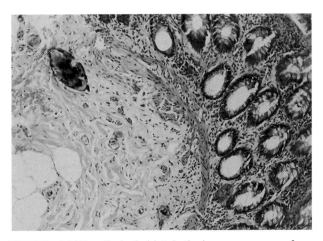

FIGURE 42-51. Typical histological appearance of an inflammatory polyp. The colonic glands are preserved and there is an increase of inflammatory cells in the lamina propria. This specimen was a result of schistosomiasis. A *Schistosoma haematobium* ovum, partially calcified, is lodged in the submucosa. Other inflammatory polyps, such as those found in inflammatory bowel disease, show similar histological features.

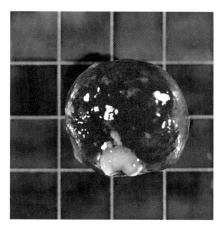

FIGURE 42-52. Macroscopic appearance of a juvenile polyp with a cherry-red, smooth, congested surface and a short, shiny mucosal stalk.

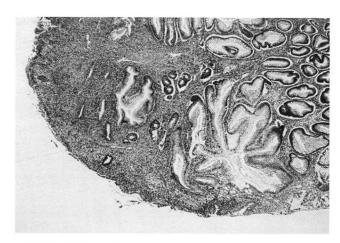

FIGURE 42-53. Histological features of the juvenile polyp from Fig. 42-52 include cystically dilated glands without mucosal hyperplasia and an edematous, mildly inflamed lamina propria. The surface erosion is common with inflammatory exudate. The cystic dilation seen here is not as marked, as is usually the case.

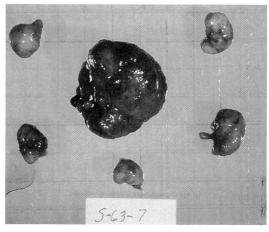

FIGURE 42-54. Macroscopic appearance of Peutz-Jeghers polyps: five small (0.3–0.8 cm) polyps and a 2.5-cm lobulated polyp. The polyps had a short stalk.

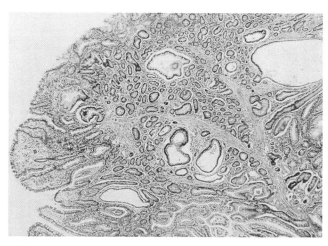

FIGURE 42-55. Histological features of Peutz-Jeghers polyps include atypical branching of the muscularis separating and surrounding islands of variably sized glands lined by normal colonic epithelium.

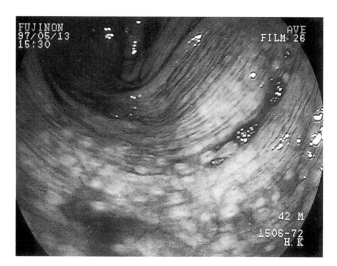

FIGURE 42-56. Colonoscopic photograph of lymphoid follicles highlighted by methylene blue dye. The methylene blue dye acts as a background against which the small follicles are raised above it like islands.

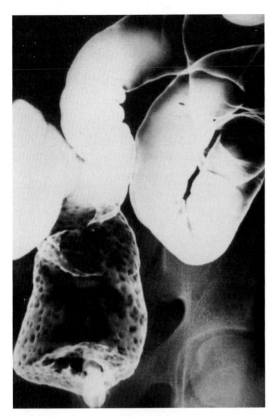

FIGURE 42-57. Large lymphoid polyps in the rectum typical of nodular lymphoid hyperplasia. Biopsy must be performed to differentiate this condition from multiple adenomas and lymphomas.

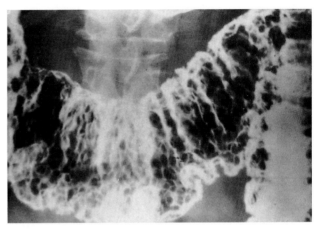

FIGURE 42-58. Radiological appearance of nodular lymphoma. Differentiation from lymphoid hyperplasia is difficult at radiology and biopsy is essential.

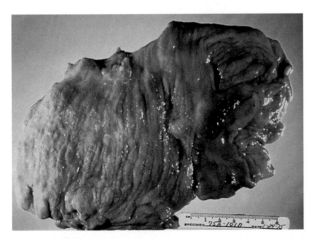

FIGURE 42-59. Macroscopic appearance of lymphosarcoma that appeared as multiple minute polyps, which suggest diffuse nodular lymphoid hyperplasia (which is benign).

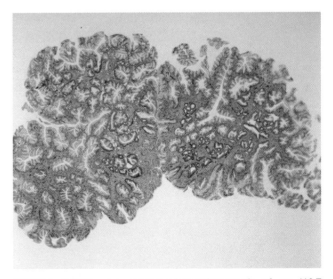

FIGURE 42-60. Low-power photomicrograph of an H&E stained section of a hyperplastic polyp showing the typical serrated appearance of the surface epithelium, and foci of hyperchromatic glandular epithelium within the crypts deeper in the lamina propria.

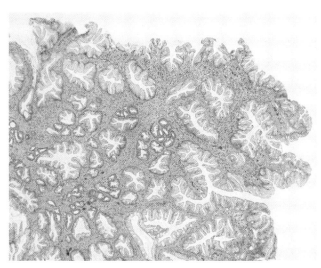

FIGURE 42-61. Medium-power photomicrograph of a section of a hyperplastic polyp showing the typical serrated appearance of the surface epithelium, and the hyperchromatic glandular epithelium of the crypts deeper in the lamina propria (H&E stain).

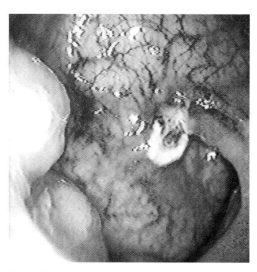

FIGURE 42-62. Colonoscopic photograph of hyperplastic polyps in the left colon of a patient with hyperplastic polyposis. These polyps are not distinguishable from adenomas without histological examination, preferably performed after polypectomy.

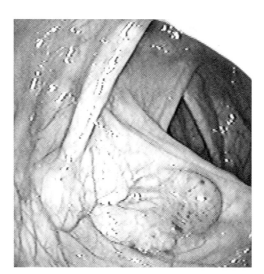

FIGURE 42-63. Colonoscopic photograph of sparse small polyps from the right side of the colon in the same patient as in Fig. 42-62 with hyperplastic polyposis.

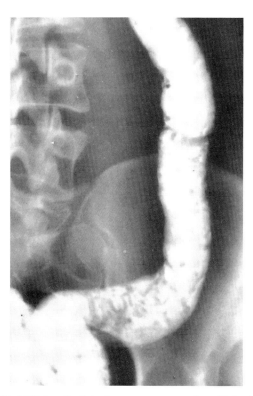

FIGURE 42-64. Radiologic appearance of multiple inflammatory polyps ("pseudopolyps") in the descending colon of a patient with ulcerative colitis. Colonoscopy and biopsy are necessary for proper characterization of the lesions. During colonoscopy, the endoscopist should perform a biopsy on atypical polyps and suspicious plaque-like areas, because these may show dysplasia. Dysplastic lesions, and not the inflammatory pseudopolyps, are the premalignant lesions.

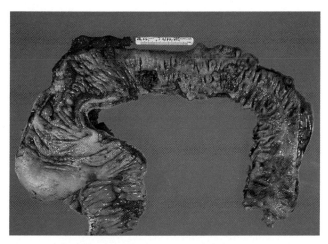

FIGURE 42-65. Total colon resection specimen from a 49-year-old man with a 20-year history of ulcerative colitis. In addition to the diffuse inflammatory mucosal changes and multiple inflammatory (pseudo) polyps, at least three distinct tumors, located 8, 15, and 25 cm distal to the ileocecal valve, are present.

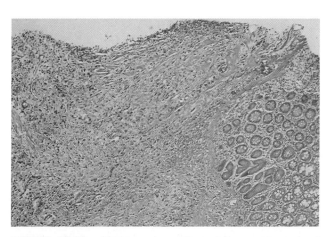

FIGURE 42-66. Microscopic section of the most proximal tumor from Fig. 42-65 shows the abrupt change from fairly normal lining mucosa to invasive pleomorphic, poorly differentiated carcinoma typical of ulcerative colitis.

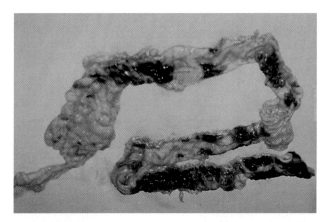

FIGURE 42-67. Colon resection specimen of pneumatosis cystoides intestinalis. Extensive pneumatosis and necrosis are depicted. The glistening, translucent, air-filled blebs vary in size. This case was caused by necrotizing enterocolitis, hence the poor state of the colon. Most cases of pneumatosis are idiopathic and asymptomatic.

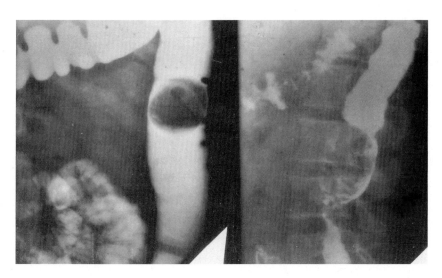

FIGURE 42-68. Characteristic radiographic appearance of a lipoma. The submucosal nature is suggested on the postevacuation radiograph (the image on the **right**) by the round, smooth, radiolucent appearance.

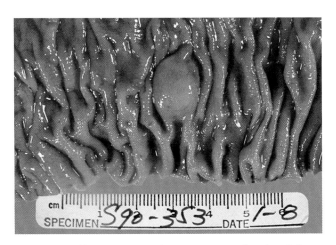

FIGURE 42-69. Macroscopic appearance of a 1 × 1.3 cm lipoma shows a normal smooth mucosal surface over the submucosal lipoma with a translucent yellowish color.

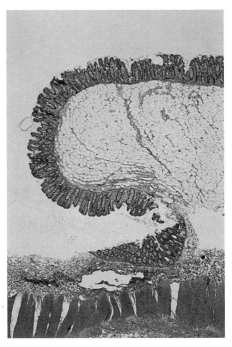

FIGURE 42-70. Histological section of the lipoma from Fig. 42-69 shows well-defined areas of mature, well-vascularized adipose tissue expanding the submucosal space and forming a sessile polyp covered by normal mucosa.

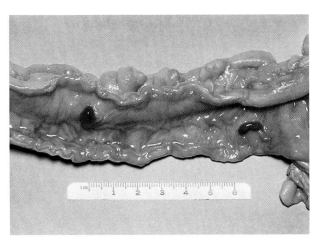

FIGURE 42-71. Macroscopic appearance of hemangiomas (blue rubber bleb syndrome). Two hemangiomas, one 0.5 × 0.5 cm, the other 1.0 × 0.3 cm, are depicted. The hemangiomas are cherry-red, vascular-appearing polypoid lesions. Biopsy of these and other vascular-appearing lesions may be hazardous.

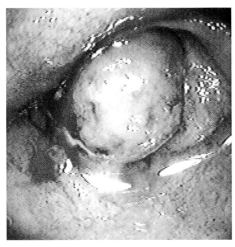

FIGURE 42-72. Colonoscopic photograph of an asymptomatic ileal carcinoid tumor (1.5 cm) found at surveillance colonoscopy for hereditary nonpolyposis colon cancer.

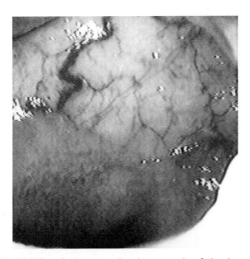

FIGURE 42-73. Colonoscopic photograph of the base adjacent to the carcinoid tumor shown in Fig. 42-72 depicting the "feeding" vessel characteristic of larger carcinoids.

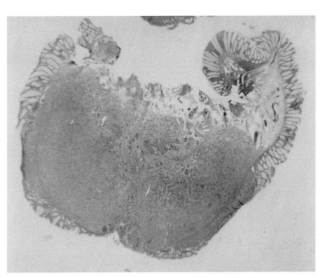

FIGURE 42-74. Low-power photomicrograph of a section from a biopsy of a 13-mm rectal polyp removed by loop diathermy and found to be a carcinoid (H&E stain). Note that although there is mucosal involvement and focal ulceration, the bulk of the lesion lies within the submucosa. Higher-power views showed the typical nests of small uniform cells having a stippled nuclear chromatin pattern characteristic of a carcinoid tumor. The tumor extends to the cauterized margin and complete removal cannot be guaranteed.

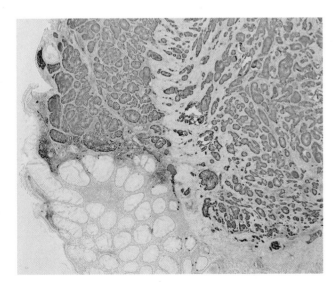

FIGURE 42-75. Medium-power photomicrograph of an immunoperoxidase-stained section of the same lesion shown in Fig. 42-74 using antibodies to the neuroendocrine marker chromogranin, with diaminobenzidine as the chromogen (brown reaction). Note the small rosettes and solid nests typical of a carcinoid tumor involving the mucosa and underlying submucosa. Adjacent mucosa shows only an occasional positively staining cell in keeping with the more normal distribution of neuroendocrine cells within the mucosa.

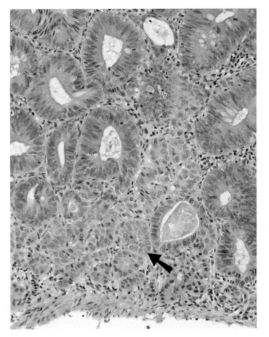

FIGURE 42-76. High-power photomicrograph of a section from a biopsy of a most unusual cecal polyp (H&E stain). This polyp was sessile and had an atypical appearance on endoscopy; hence, polypectomy was not attempted. Microscopic examination revealed the typical features of a tubular adenoma with low-grade dysplasia (**upper half of photograph**), but showed small rosettes of rounded, uniform cells with eosinophilic cytoplasm adjacent to the muscularis mucosae and suggestive of a neuroendocrine tumor (*arrow*).

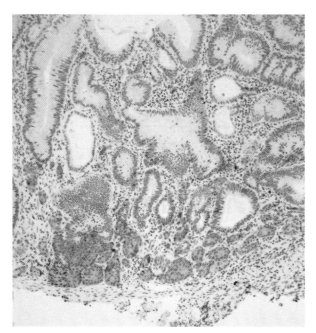

FIGURE 42-77. High-power photomicrograph of an immunoperoxidase-stained section of the same lesion shown in Fig. 42-76 using antibodies to the neuroendocrine marker chromogranin, with diaminobenzidine as the chromogen (brown reaction). In comparison to the tubular adenoma component, the small rosettes of cells noted in the section stain intensely brown (H&E stain), confirming that this is a composite tubular adenoma-carcinoid tumor. Co-occurrence of these two pathologies is rare. Provided excision is complete, and there is nothing to suggest more extensive infiltration by the carcinoid, polypectomy alone should be adequate because small benign carcinoids are not uncommon in the cecum.

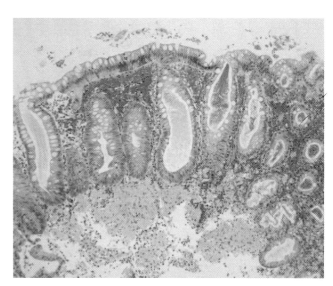

FIGURE 42-78. Medium-power photomicrograph of a section from a biopsy from an unusual rectal polypoid lesion caused by amyloidosis in a patient presenting with rectal bleeding (H&E stain). Note the pale-staining eosinophilic amyloid deposition, particularly at the base of the crypts, in contrast to the extravasation of red cells in the more superficial lamina propria.

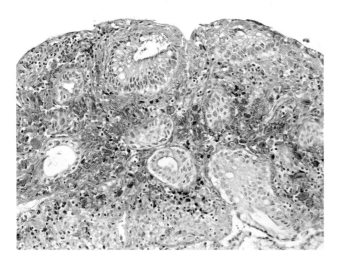

FIGURE 42-79. Corresponding photomicrograph of an immunoperoxidase-stained section of the biopsy shown in Fig. 42-78 using antibodies to amyloid P protein, with diaminobenzidine as the chromogen (brown reaction). Note the widespread deposition of amyloid throughout the lamina propria, which was previously masked in the section by the red cell extravasation (H&E stain).

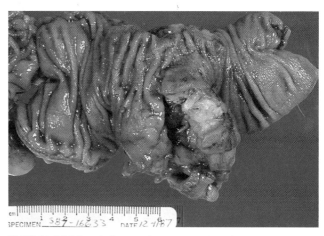

FIGURE 42-80. A firm, submucosal, ill-defined mass in the wall of the cecum of a 44-year-old woman with endometriosis appearing as a polypoid lesion at colonoscopy. The mass has been cut open for frozen-section studies.

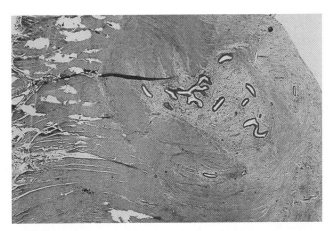

FIGURE 42-81. Histological section of the endometriosis depicted in Fig. 42-80 shows islands of endometrial tissue (glands lined by benign columnar epithelium and surrounded by spindle cell stroma) in the submucosa and muscularis of the colonic wall.

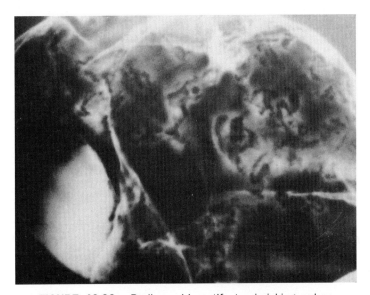

FIGURE 42-82. Radiographic artifact mimicking polyps caused by mucoid fecal material. Thorough colonic cleansing is important for radiographic and endoscopic studies.

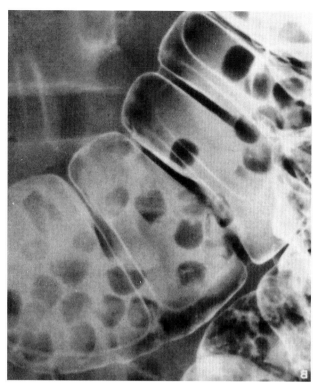

FIGURE 42-83. Radiographic artifact mimicking polyps caused by undigested kernels of corn. Undigested food remnants, especially corn and peas, often produce this artifact.

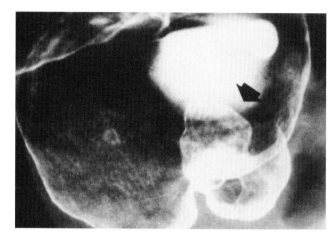

FIGURE 42-84. The appendiceal stump often mimics a polyp at radiologic and endoscopic examinations. A history of appendectomy within several years should alert the clinician to this artifact.

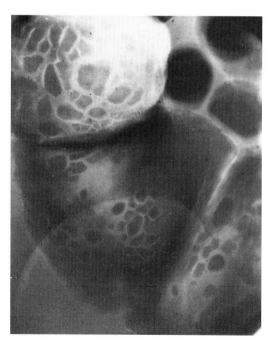

FIGURE 42-85. Radiographic appearance of cecal urticaria. The papular appearance of the urticarial lesions is depicted. These lesions often respond to antihistamine or corticosteroid therapy. They can be misdiagnosed as multiple polyps.

POLYPOSIS SYNDROMES

RANDALL W. BURT ■ RUSSELL F. JACOBY

The gastrointestinal polyposis syndromes are a set of uncommon diseases considered together because they each express multiple polypoid lesions of the gut. A number of separate syndromes can be defined in terms of pathological and clinical characteristics. Recent genetic advances have allowed an even more precise definition and categorization of these conditions. The syndromes are important because they each exhibit benign and malignant complications. They are sufficiently common that all gastroenterologists and gastrointestinal surgeons will deal with these conditions. Furthermore, because intestinal issues are central to the diagnosis and management of patients with polyposis, gastroenterologists are often the primary care physician of polyposis patients and families. The conditions are summarized in Tables 43-1 and 43-2.

(figures begin on page 458)

TABLE 43-1

Distinguishing Features of FAP and the Hamartomatous Polyposis Syndromes

SYNDROME	GENE (FREQUENCY MUTATION FOUND)	CRC RISK (AGE OF DIAGNOSIS)	POLYP HISTOLOGY	POLYP DISTRIBUTION	AGE OF GI SYMPTOM ONSET	MOST PROMINENT EXTRAINTESTINAL FEATURES	
						Benign	Malignant
FAP	APC (>90%)	100% (39 y) AFAP 80% (50 y)	Adenomatous, except stomach: fundic gland polyps	Stomach 23%–100%, duodenum 50%–90%, jejunum 50%, ileum 20%, colon 100%	33 y	Desmoid tumors, epidermoid cysts, fibromas, osteomas, CHRPE, dental abnormalities	Duodenal or periampullary: 3%–5%, rare pancreatic, thyroid, gastric, CNS, hepatoblastoma
Peutz-Jeghers syndrome (PJS)	STK11 (LKB1) (50%–60%)	39% (46 y)	Peutz-Jeghers	Stomach 24%, small bowel 96%, colon 27%, rectum 24%	22–26 y	Orocutaneous melanin pigment spots	Pancreatic 36%, gastric 29%, small bowel 13%, breast 54%, ovarian 21%, uterine 9%, lung 15%
Juvenile polyposis (JP)	SMAD4 (DPC4), BMPRA1 (53%)	9% to 68% (34 y)	Juvenile	Stomach, may occur; small bowel, may occur; colon, usually	18.5 y	Macrocephaly, hypertelorism, 20% congenital abnormalities in sporadic type	Stomach and duodenum combined up to 21%
Cowden syndrome* (CS)	PTEN (80%–90%)	Little, if any	Juvenile, lipomas, inflammatory, ganglioneuromas, lymphoid hyperplasia	Esophagus 66%, stomach 75%, duodenum 37%, colon 66%	Not determined	Facial trichilemmomas, oral papillomas, multinodular goiter, fibrocystic breast disease	Thyroid 3%–10%, breast 25%–50%, uterine 2%–5%
Hereditary mixed polyposis syndrome	Locus on chromosome 6	Increased, but uncertain (47 y)	Atypical juvenile, adenomatous, hyperplastic	Primarily colon	40 y	None known	None known
Gorlin syndrome	PTCH	Not known	Hamartoma	Only gastric reported	Not determined	Mandibular bone cysts, pits of palms and soles, macrocephaly	Basal cell carcinoma

*Includes Bannayan-Riley-Ruvalcaba syndrome and Lhermitte-Duclos disease.

AFAP, attenuated familial adenomatous polyposis; CHRPE, congenital hypertrophy of the retinal pigment epithelium; CNS, central nervous system; CRC, colorectal carcinoma; FAP, familial adenomatous polyposis (includes Gardner syndrome, two thirds of Turcot syndrome cases, and AFAP); GI, gastrointestinal.

TABLE 43-2
Additional Conditions That Exhibit Gastrointestinal Polyposis

CATEGORY	CONDITION	CAUSE	HISTOLOGY OF POLYPS	GI AREAS AFFECTED	OTHER DISEASE MANIFESTATIONS	
					Benign	*Malignant*
Syndromes in which polyps contain neural elements	Neurofibromatosis type I (NFI)	Mutations of *NF1* gene, autosomal dominantly inherited	Neurofibromas and ganglioneuromas	Small bowel > stomach > colon	Café au lait spots Cutaneous neurofibromas	Rare neurofibrosarcoma
	Multiple endocrine neoplasia type IIB (MEN2B)	Mutation at codon 918 of RET protooncogene, autosomal dominantly inherited	Ganglioneuromas	Lips to anus, but most common in colon and rectum	Pheochromocytoma parathyroid adenoma	Medullary thyroid carcinoma
Syndromes of uncertain etiology	Cronkhite-Canada syndrome	Possibly infectious	Juvenile polyps	Stomach to anus	Skin hyperpigmentation, hair loss, nail atrophy, hypogeusia	12%–15% colon cancer
	Hyperplastic polyposis	Possibly inherited	Hyperplastic	Colon	None known	Colon cancer risk probably increased
Conditions with inflammatory polyps	Inflammatory bowel disease	Crohn's disease and ulcerative colitis	Pseudopolyps	Colon	As in inflammatory bowel disease	
	Devon polyposis	Inherited	Fibroid polyps	Ileum, stomach	None	None
	Cap polyposis	Unknown, possibly internal prolapse	Similar to solitary rectal ulcer	Rectosigmoid	Rectal bleeding	None
Polyposis conditions arising from lymphoid tissue	Nodular lymphoid hyperplasia	Isolated > immuno-deficiency > lymphoma	Hyperplasia of lymphoid nodules	Small bowel, stomach, colon	Related to underlying disease	
	Multiple lymphomatous polyposis	A type of mantle cell lymphoma	Multiple malignant lymphomatous polyps	Small bowel and colon > stomach	None known	
	Immunoproliferative small intestinal disease	Not known, but acquired, end stage of α-heavy chain disease	Plasma cell proliferation	Small bowel	Malabsorption	
Miscellaneous noninherited polyposis conditions	Leiomyomatosis	Not known	Leiomyoma	Colon, other	None known	
	Lipomatous polyposis	Not known	Lipoma	Colon, other	None known	
	Multiple lymphangiomas	Not known	Lymphhiangoma	Colon	None known	
	Pneumatosis cystoides intestinalis	Not known	Inflammatory and air spaces	Colon and other GI locations	None known	

GI, gastrointestinal.

457

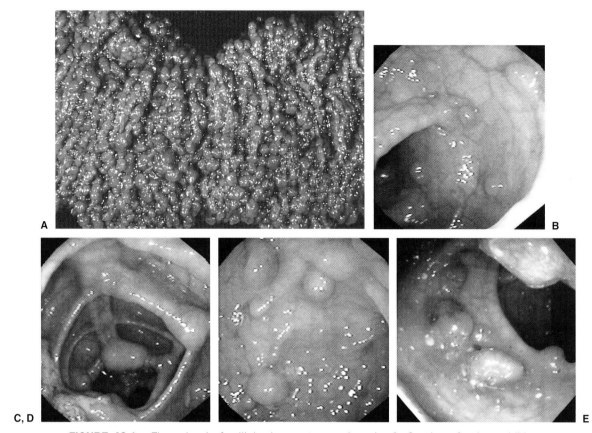

FIGURE 43-1. The colon in familial adenomatous polyposis. **A:** Section of colon exhibiting fully developed familial adenomatous polyposis. (Courtesy of Robert Flinner, M.D., Salt Lake City, UT.) **B–E:** Colonoscopic views of patients with familial adenomatous polyposis. (**B–D,** courtesy of Dr. Robert Kiyomura; **E,** courtesy of Dr. Robert J. Pagano.)

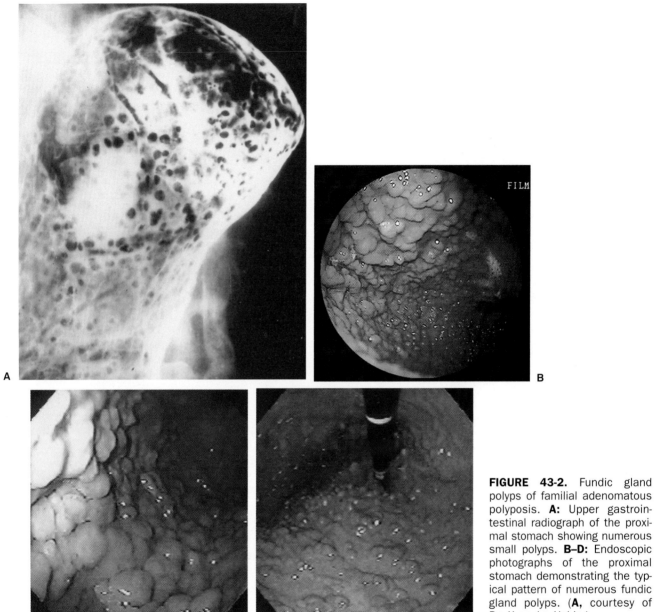

A

B

C, D

FIGURE 43-2. Fundic gland polyps of familial adenomatous polyposis. **A:** Upper gastrointestinal radiograph of the proximal stomach showing numerous small polyps. **B–D:** Endoscopic photographs of the proximal stomach demonstrating the typical pattern of numerous fundic gland polyps. (**A,** courtesy of Dr. Kyosuke Ushio.)

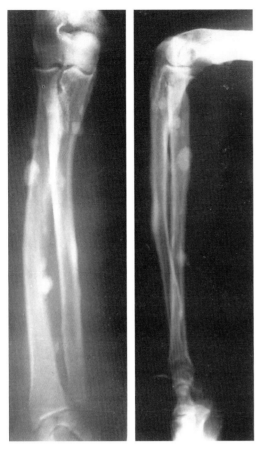

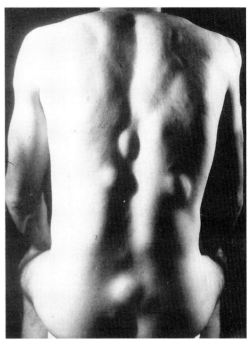

FIGURE 43-3. Osteomas of Gardner syndrome. Osteomas may form on any bone of the body in this syndrome. They occur most commonly at the angle of the mandible and elsewhere on the skull, but they may also be observed on long bones, as seen on the forearm and leg in these radiographs.

FIGURE 43-4. Epidermoid cysts on a patient with Gardner syndrome. These may occur anywhere on the cutaneous surface. They often occur before puberty and may grow to several centimeters in diameter.

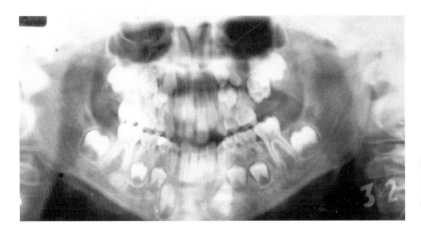

FIGURE 43-5. Dental abnormalities in a patient with Gardner syndrome. Opacities of the mandible as well as supernumerary teeth are evident in this panoramic radiograph of the maxilla and mandible.

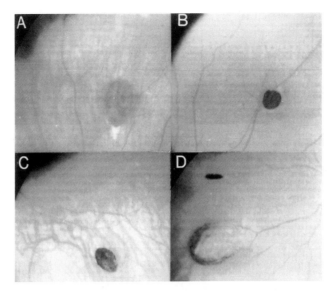

FIGURE 43-6. Congenital hypertrophy of the retinal pigment epithelium. **A–D:** Several sizes and hues of the retinal pigment are observed in pedigrees with adenomatous polyposis who exhibit *APC* mutations distal to exon 9. Although such lesions are common, the presence of bilateral or more than four retinal lesions is specific for familial adenomatous polyposis.

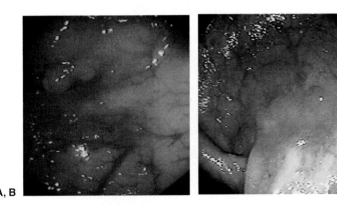

A, B

FIGURE 43-7. A, B: Small, more subtle colonic adenomas of attenuated adenomatous polyposis coli. (Courtesy of Dr. James DiSario.)

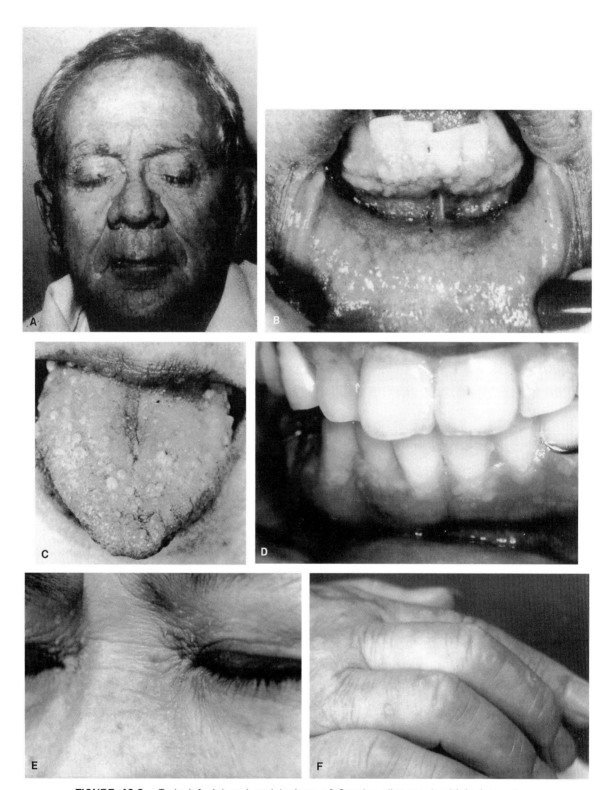

FIGURE 43-8. Typical facial and oral lesions of Cowden disease (multiple hamartoma syndrome). **A:** Face of a patient with Cowden disease demonstrating central papules. **B:** Labial mucosa and gingiva showing cobblestone papules. **C:** Tongue with typical papules. A second patient with Cowden disease had typical cutaneous features and gastrointestinal polyps. **D:** Gingiva. **E:** Face. **F:** Digits. *(Continued)*

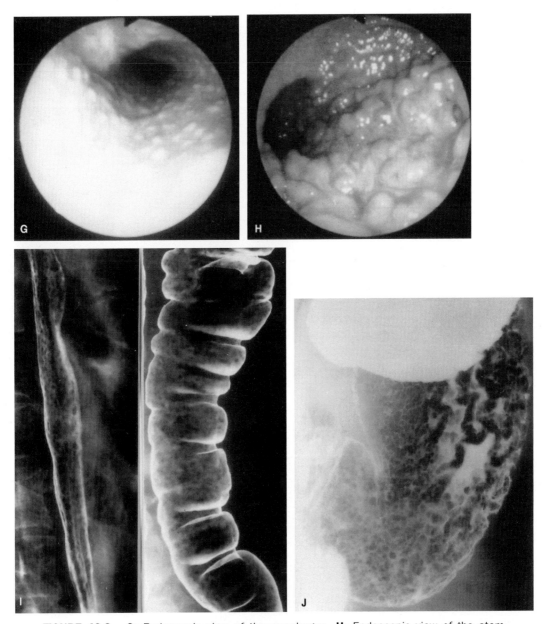

FIGURE 43-8. **G:** Endoscopic view of the esophagus. **H:** Endoscopic view of the stomach. **I:** Barium radiograph studies of the esophagus and colon. **J:** Barium radiograph of the stomach. (Courtesy of Dr. Kyosuke Ushio.)

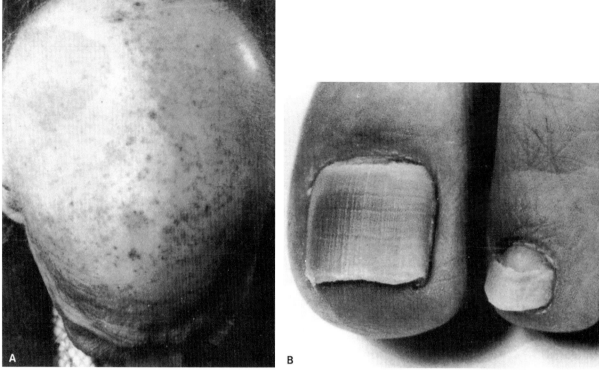

FIGURE 43-9. Cronkhite-Canada syndrome. **A:** Scalp showing almost total alopecia. **B:** Onychodystrophy of toenails with lines of separation from the normal nail.

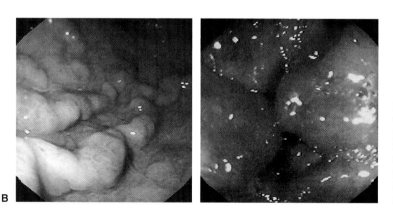

FIGURE 43-10. Endoscopic views of a patient with Cronkhite-Canada syndrome. The patient presented with dysgeusia, alopecia, onychodystrophy, and diarrhea. **A:** Stomach. **B:** Colon: the largest polyp is a pedunculated adenomatous polyp; all other polyps shown exhibited histology typical of Cronkhite-Canada lesions. (Courtesy of Dr. Edward L. Krawitt.)

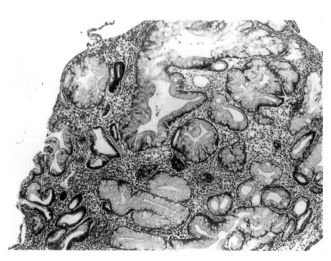

FIGURE 43-11. Polyp from a patient with Cronkhite-Canada syndrome. The polyp demonstrates cystically dilated glands with abundant generous, edematous, and inflamed lamina propria. The polyps of Cronkhite-Canada are very similar to those of juvenile polyposis. Intervening mucosa in Cronkhite-Canada syndrome, however, is abnormal, with edema and inflammation of the lamina propria.

44

MALIGNANT TUMORS OF THE COLON

DAVID H. ALPERS ■ C. RICHARD BOLAND

Cancer of the colon is very common in the western world, and its early detection has become a goal for gastroenterologists. Adenocarcinoma of the colon and rectum always begins in the mucosa and typically begins as a polypoid lesion that protrudes into the lumen. Flat, infiltrative lesions occasionally occur, particularly in the setting of ulcerative colitis. The bulk of the tumor in the lumen has no effect on survival. The Dukes classification and modifications of it have been developed to provide prognostic information to clinicians. This is of increased importance because of the development of effective adjuvant chemotherapy for Dukes class C tumors.

Illustrations of epidemiologic features of colon cancer are shown in Figs. 44-1 through 44-3 and Table 44-1. A model of genetic events in production of colon cancer is illustrated in Fig. 44-4.

The value of fecal occult blood for colorectal cancer screening has been demonstrated in many studies. Results from some of the major studies are documented in Tables 44-2 through 44-7, and in Figs. 44-5 and 44-6. An algorithm for screening of colon cancer is shown in Fig. 44-7. Family history is of importance in deciding who is at increased risk for colorectal cancer, and thus who should be screened. The data in Fig. 44-8 are the most comprehensive data available.

The importance of the natural history of colorectal cancer is emphasized by the fact that many patients present with disease that has spread beyond the mucosa, as shown in Table 44-8 and in Fig. 44-9. Distribution of another colon tumor (carcinoid) at time of presentation is shown in Table 44-9.

Illustrations of the pathological features of colon cancer are provided in Figs. 44-10 through 44-32. Most lesions are moderately differentiated or well-differentiated adenocarcinoma. Relatively few pathological features are effective predictors of the invasive and metastatic potential of a colon cancer. However, less well-differentiated and poorly differentiated tumors typically are associated with an adverse prognostic outcome.

A full spectrum of cellular atypia or architectural dysplasia may occur within adenomatous polyps. The cells within a small adenoma may look nearly normal, but one tends to see progressive degrees of cellular atypia as the polyps become larger. Foci of high-grade dysplasia may be found in adenomas, which is the equivalent of carcinoma in situ. The pathologist's report may not refer to this as "carcinoma in situ" when the high-grade dysplasia is entirely confined to the mucosa and does not penetrate the muscularis, because these lesions do not metastasize. Foci of carcinoma may be entirely confined to the polyp itself (see Fig. 44-16) and can be cured by means of polypectomy. A well-differentiated variant of colon cancer that is often associated with a poor clinical outcome is mucin-producing colon cancer (see Fig. 44-17). The production of large amounts of mucin is associated with enhanced ability to metastasize in animal models of the disease.

Figures 44-18 and 44-19 are instructive clinical cases. In the case in Fig. 44-18, a man without symptoms had occult fecal bleeding that was detected with a guaiac test. A barium enema examination appeared to be negative; however, a large mass ultimately was detected in the sigmoid by means of colonoscopy. In the second case (see Fig. 44-19), a man with several episodes of hematochezia was observed for a year; eventually a barium enema examination and rigid sigmoidoscopy were performed and showed no lesions. Cancer of the sigmoid colon was found soon thereafter at colonoscopy, although the lesion had metastasized by this time. This case illustrates the need to pursue suspicious symptoms to the point of diagnosis and highlights the limitations of a single-contrast barium enema study (see Fig. 44-20) and rigid sigmoidoscopic examination.

Adenocarcinoma is usually diagnosed at endoscopy and confirmed by means of mucosal biopsy. The lesions may appear plaque-like (see Fig. 44-21) or as lesions that occlude the lumen (see Figs. 44-22 and 44-23). The tumor can appear as a stricture with normal overlying mucus (see Fig. 44-22*A*), with exophytic growth (see Fig. 44-22*B*), or as an annular mass (see Fig. 44-22*C*). Often synchronous lesions are found (see Fig. 44-23). Malignant strictures in the colon occasionally result from metastases that arise from adjacent tissues such as the cervix (see Fig. 44-24). Malignant lymphoma occurs as either polypoid or ulcerating lesions (see Fig. 44-25) but does not usually occlude the lumen.

Strictures from adenocarcinoma can arise in areas of diverticular disease, and the malignant nature of the stricture may not be suspected without biopsy (see Fig. 44-26). If the carcinoma perforates and produces a localized inflammatory response, it may present itself in the same manner as diverticulitis (see Fig. 44-27).

Management of adenocarcinoma requires surgical resection. The portion of the colon involved should be removed with all of its draining lymphatic vessels (see Fig. 44-28). Restoration of lumenal continuity has been simplified with the use of the gastrointestinal anastomosis and triangulation anastomosis staplers (see Figs. 44-29 through 44-31). When cancer involves the rectum, the location of the tumor determines whether a rectal sparing operation can be performed. The location is usually reported as centimeters from the anal verge, but the surgical anal canal length is highly variable and may range from 2 to 7 cm depending on gender and body habitus (see Fig. 44-32). Thus, a tumor with its lower margin 8 cm from the anal verge may fall within the middle third of the surgical anal canal in a thin woman, but in the lower third of a heavily muscled man. These differences should be appreciated by endoscopists looking for rectal adenocarcinoma.

(figures begin on page 470)

TABLE 44-1
Age-Specific Incidence Rates per 10^5 Population for Cancers of the Colon and Rectum

AGE (y)	MEN	WOMEN
0–4	0.0	0.0
5–9	0.0	0.0
10–14	0.0	0.0
15–19	0.2	0.1
20–24	0.4	0.4
25–29	1.2	1.1
30–34	2.5	2.4
35–39	5.9	5.9
40–44	12.3	11.9
45–49	27.7	24.6
50–54	57.2	46.3
55–59	102.6	76.7
60–64	164.9	105.7
65–69	243.9	155.5
70–74	320.5	226.9
75–79	411.3	293.6
80–84	463.5	365.5
85+	497.6	391.5

From Eddy DM. Screening for colorectal cancer. Ann Intern Med 1990;113:373.

TABLE 44-2
Bleeding from Colorectal Cancers

LOCATION OF CANCER	MEAN BLOOD LOSS (^{51}Cr-LABELED ERYTHROCYTES)	POSITIVE HEMOCCULT II TESTS* Nonrehydrated	Rehydrated
Cecum, ascending colon ($n = 10$)	9.3 mL/d	83%	96%
Transverse and descending colon ($n = 5$)	1.5 mL/d	54%	54%
Sigmoid colon ($n = 13$)	1.9 mL/d	64%	97%
Rectum ($n = 18$)	1.8 mL/d	69%	93%
Total sample		69%	91%

*Hemoccult II tests performed with and without rehydration; Hemoccult II test considered positive if any of six tests are positive in a 3-day test period.

From Macrae FA, St. John DJB. Relationship between patterns of bleeding and Hemoccult sensitivity in patients with colorectal cancers or adenomas. Gastroenterology 1982;82:891.

TABLE 44-3
False-Negative Hemoccult II Tests Correlated with Duration of Testing in Patients with Known Colorectal Carcinoma

TEST RESULT	DURATION OF TESTING (d) 1	2	3	4	5	6	7	8	9	10
Hemoccult false-negative rate	181/359 (50%)	117/313 (37%)	84/267 (31%)	56/222 (25%)	41/177 (23%)	28/136 (21%)	18/100 (18%)	10/68 (15%)	5/39 (13%)	2/15 (13%)
Rehydrated Hemoccult false-negative rate	80/359 (22%)	39/313 (12%)	23/267 (9%)	15/222 (7%)	9/177 (5%)	7/136 (5%)	5/100 (5%)	3/68 (4%)	2/39 (5%)	1/15 (7%)

Note: Proportion and percentage of tests in which patients with known colorectal cancers had falsely negative Hemoccult II tests.

This demonstrates that 50% of cancers are missed by performing a single (unrehydrated) test; the false-negative rate decreases to 31% after 3 days of testing and is reduced to 13% with 10 days of testing. When the rehydrated test is used, the false-negative rate is only 9% with 3 days of testing, but the prohibitive rate of false-positives produced makes rehydration a maneuver of questionable value.

From Macrae FA, St. John DJB. Relationship between patterns of bleeding and Hemoccult sensitivity in patients with colorectal cancers or adenomas. Gastroenterology 1982;82:891.

TABLE 44-4

Relation Between Fecal Hemoglobin Concentration and Hemoccult II Tests in Patients with Colorectal Cancers

STOOL HEMOGLOBIN CONCENTRATION (mg Hb/g stool)	PROPORTION OF POSITIVE TESTS	
	HO	HO(R)
0–2	86/766 (11%)	212/758 (28%)
2–6	127/314 (40%)	213/304 (70%)
6–10	50/80 (63%)	75/80 (94%)
10–15	50/64 (78%)	60/64 (94%)
15–20	11/18 (61%)	14/18 (78%)
>20	30/58 (52%)	56/58 (97%)

HO, Hemoccult II developed without rehydration; HO(R), Hemoccult II developed with preliminary rehydration.

From Macrae FA, St. John DJB. Relationship between patterns of bleeding and Hemoccult sensitivity in patients with colorectal cancers or adenomas. Gastroenterology 1982;82:891.

TABLE 44-5

A Combination Strategy for Fecal Occult Blood Screening

TEST	POSITIVE TESTS*	TRUE-POSITIVE TESTS[†]	FALSE-POSITIVE TESTS[‡]	TRUE-NEGATIVE TESTS[‖]	FALSE-NEGATIVE TESTS[¶]	SENSITIVITY	SPECIFICITY	POSITIVE PREDICTIVE VALUE
Hemoccult II	2.5% (n = 198)	0.6% (n = 46)	1.9%	96.4%	1.2% (n = 96)	32.4%	98.1%	23.2%
Hemoccult SENSA	13.6% (n = 1073)	1.3% (n = 99)	12.3%	85.9%	0.5% (n = 40)	71.2%	87.5%	9.2%
HemeSelect	5.9% (n = 440)	1.2% (n = 90)	4.7%	93.5%	0.6%	67.2%	95.2%	20.5%
Sequential Strategy[#]	3.0% (n = 23)	0.92% (n = 72)	2.1%	96.2%	0.8% (n = 62)	53.7%	97.9%	30.9%

Note: Approximately 8000 patients were screened, although not all with every fecal occult blood test. Patients with positive tests were evaluated by colonoscopy, and followed further in a health maintenance organization, with chart follow-up of the screened population.

*Percent of asymptomatic, screened patients with positive test.

[†]Percent of all screened patients with a cancer or polyp ≥1 cm, *and* a positive test.

[†]Percent of all screened patients with a positive test, *but no* cancer or polyp ≥1 cm.

[‖]Percent of all screened patients with a negative test and no cancer or polyp ≥1 cm.

[¶]Percent of all screened patients with a cancer or polyp ≥1 cm who had a negative test.

[#]Stool screened first with Hemoccult SENSA, only positive stools rescreened with HemeSelect; positive test indicates both tests positive.

From Boland CR. Malignant tumors of the colon. In: Yamada T, Alpers DH, Owyang C, eds. Textbook of gastroenterology, 2nd ed. Philadelphia: Lippincott Williams & Wilkins, 1999.

TABLE 44-6

Development of Colorectal Neoplasms in 20,000 Patients During First Year After Screening

PATIENT GROUP	CARCINOMAS		ADENOMAS	
	Number	Rate per 1000	Number	Rate per 1000
Positive screening Hemoccult test (n = 77/3613)	13	3.6	42*	7.9
Negative screening Hemoccult test (n = 3536/3613)	1	0.3		
Offered Hemoccult test (refused or no response) (n = 6143)	8	1.3	3	0.5
Control group (not screened) (n = 10,272)	10	1.0	5	0.5

*In 29 patients.

From Hardcastle JD, Farrands PA, Balfour TW. Controlled trial of faecal occult blood testing in the detection of colorectal cancer. Lancet 1983;2:1.

TABLE 44-7
Pathological Stage of Cancers in 20,525 Patients Followed for 2 Years After Randomization to Screening or No Screening

	TEST GROUP			
STAGE	Responders* (3613)	Nonresponders† (6640)	Overall (10,253)	CONTROL GROUP (10,272)
A	12 (60%)	2 (14%)	14 (43%)	0
B	4 (20%)	7 (50%)	11 (33%)	8 (47%)
C	2 (10%)	1 (7%)	3 (9%)	6 (35%)
D	2 (10%)	4 (29%)	6 (15%)	3 (18%)
Total	20	14	34	17

*Responders: patients who completed the Hemoccult II fecal screening test.

†Nonresponders: patients randomized to be screened but who did not respond to request.

From Hardcastle JD, Farrands DA, Balfour TW. Controlled trial of faecal occult blood testing in the detection of colorectal cancer. Lancet 1983;2:1.

TABLE 44-8
Distribution of Colorectal Cancer Patients by Pathological Stage

STAGE*	ESTIMATED DISTRIBUTION†	DETECTION BY SCREENING‡
A	10%	60%
B	50% (±10%)	20%
B1	15%	
B2	35%	
C	25%	10%
C1	13%	
C2	13%	
D	15%	10%

*Pathological stage varies by the investigator.

†These are estimates drawn from several reported studies that used differing methods to recruit and exclude patients.

‡From Boland CR. Diagnosis and management of primary and metastatic colorectal cancers. Semin Gastrointest Dis 1992;3:33; in several large studies, 65%–90% of cancers were stage A or B when detected by screening.

TABLE 44-9
Distribution of 3000 Gastrointestinal Carcinoid Tumors

ORGAN	PERCENTAGE OF TOTAL	PERCENTAGE WITH METASTASIS
Stomach	3%	18%
Duodenum	1%	16%
Jejunum	2%	35%
Ileum	28%	35%
Appendix	47%	3%
Colon	2%	60%
Rectum	17%	12%

Adapted from Orloff MJ. Carcinoid tumors of the rectum. Cancer 1971;28:175.

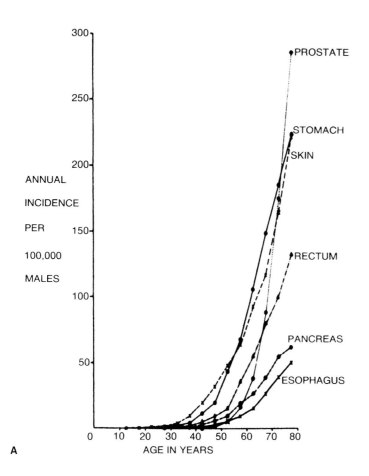

TOTAL	<15	15–24	25–34	35–44	45–54	55–64	65–74
306.7	12.4	36.3	118.9	200.9	407.9	789.6	1,344.0

B

FIGURE 44-1. The relation between cancer incidence and age. **A:** Site-specific increases in cancer incidence with advancing age. **B:** Crude age-specific total cancer incidence per 100,000 population for all sites.

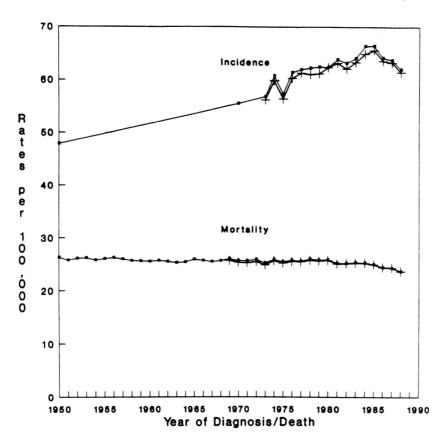

FIGURE 44-2. Incidence of colorectal cancer from five geographic regions of the United States from 1950 to 1988 (**top**) and mortality rates for the entire United States during that time (**bottom**). Both curves are age-adjusted to a 1970 standard population.

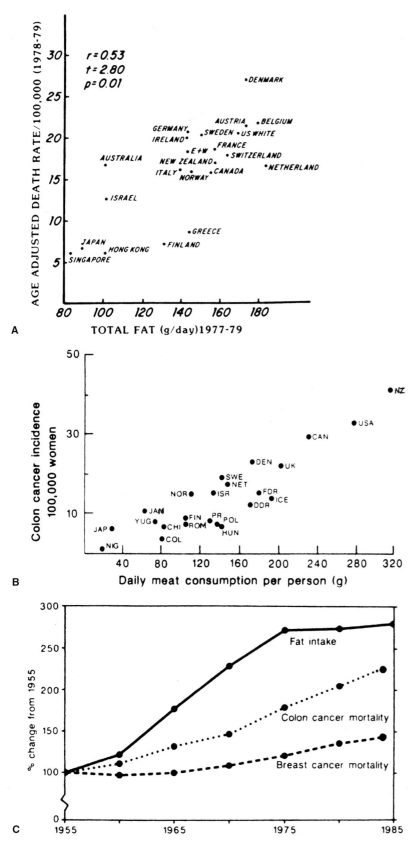

FIGURE 44-3. Influence of meat and fat intake on colorectal cancer incidence. **A:** Correlation between incidence of colon cancer and per capita fat consumption. **B:** Correlation between per capita meat consumption and colon cancer. **C:** Correlation between changing fat intake and age-adjusted mortality from cancer of the colon and breast from 1955 to 1985 in Japan, during which time an increase in fat intake of 180% occurred.

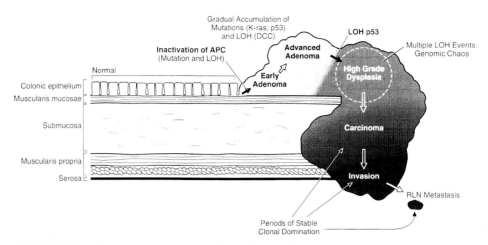

FIGURE 44-4. This is a proposed model of the genetic events by which normal colorectal epithelium first enters into a neoplastic growth pathway (i.e., by inactivation of the *APC* gene), undergoes additional growth in a variety of directions depending on the accumulated genetic events that might include k-ras mutations, *p53* mutations, or loss of heterozygosity (LOH) at tumor suppressor gene loci, and the adenoma-to-carcinoma transition that occurs upon the inactivation of the *p53* gene (which will involve processes that inhibit the expression of both *p53* alleles).

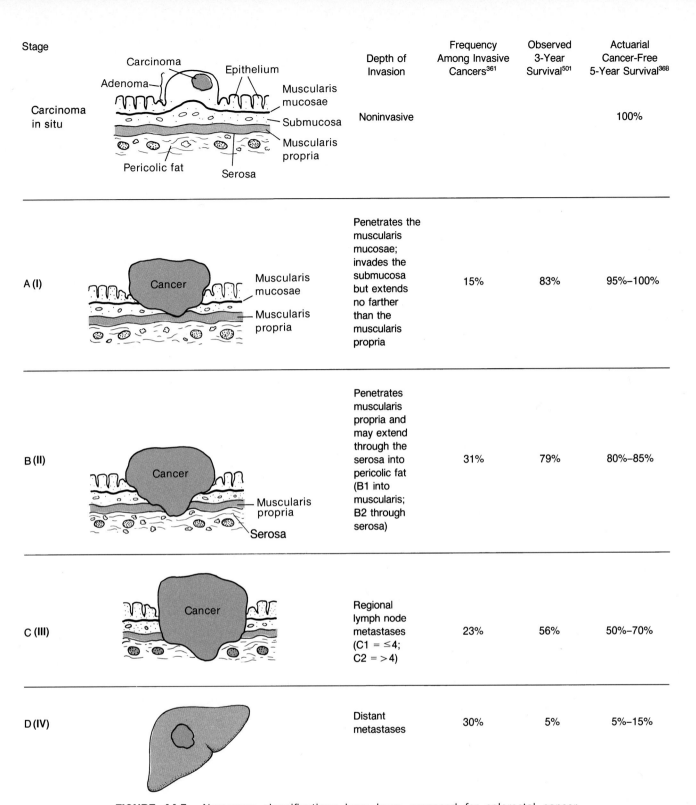

Stage		Depth of Invasion	Frequency Among Invasive Cancers[361]	Observed 3-Year Survival[501]	Actuarial Cancer-Free 5-Year Survival[368]
Carcinoma in situ		Noninvasive			100%
A (I)		Penetrates the muscularis mucosae; invades the submucosa but extends no farther than the muscularis propria	15%	83%	95%–100%
B (II)		Penetrates muscularis propria and may extend through the serosa into pericolic fat (B1 into muscularis; B2 through serosa)	31%	79%	80%–85%
C (III)		Regional lymph node metastases (C1 = ≤4; C2 = >4)	23%	56%	50%–70%
D (IV)		Distant metastases	30%	5%	5%–15%

FIGURE 44-5. Numerous classifications have been proposed for colorectal cancer. Demonstrated here is the Dukes-Turnbull classification A through D (accompanied by the tumor node metastasis [TNM] stage in parentheses), but it is not the only classification currently in use. Of potential importance are subclassifications in classes B and C. Subclass B1 has been proposed to include invasion to the muscularis propria but not through the serosa. Subclass B2 includes tumors that penetrate the serosa to the pericolic fat but do not have regional lymph node or distant metastases. Patients with B1 lesions have a better prognosis and 5-year survival rate than patients with subtype B2 lesions. Class C lesions have been subdivided into C1, with four or fewer involved regional lymph node metastases, and C2, with more than four involved regional lymph nodes. Patients with subtype C1 lesions have a better outcome than patients with C2 lesions. The observed 3-year survival and actuarial cancer-free 5-year survivals are estimated for each stage. The actuarial survival estimates reflect excessive disease-related mortality from the cancer, and the crude survival rates are considerably lower because of comorbidity.

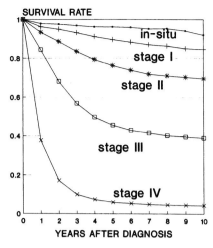

FIGURE 44-6. Relative rates of survival for patients with colon cancer, by stage of disease from a database of more than 110,000 patients using the tumor node metastasis (*TNM*) staging system. ($n = 4841$ stage 0; $n = 19,623$ stage I; $n = 33,798$ stage II; $n = 29,615$ stage III; $n = 23,233$ stage IV.)

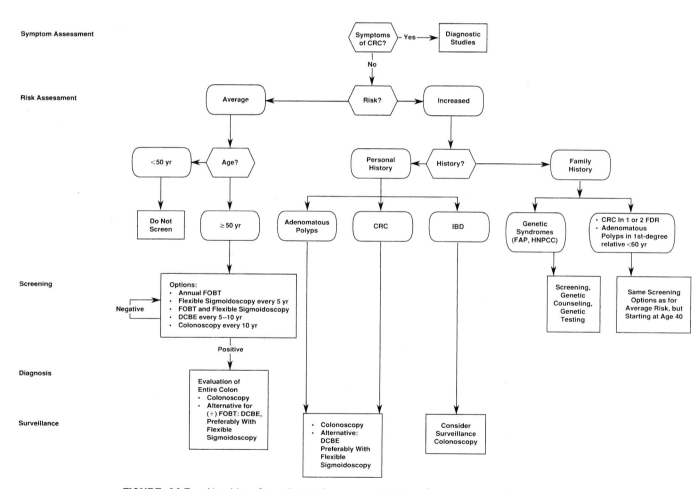

FIGURE 44-7. Algorithm for colorectal cancer screening for average and above-average risk groups.

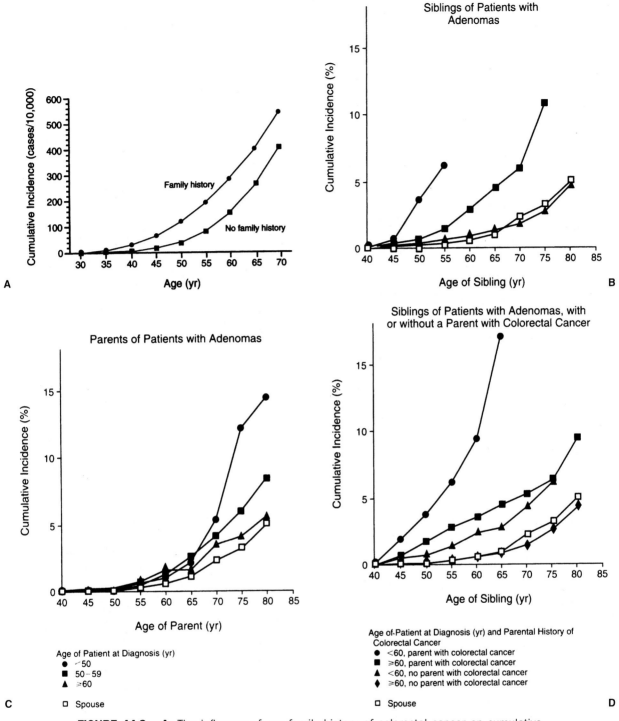

FIGURE 44-8. **A:** The influence of any family history of colorectal cancer on cumulative incidence of the disease. **B:** The influence of a history of colorectal cancer in siblings and the age at diagnosis on the cumulative incidence of colorectal adenomas. **C:** The influence of a history of colorectal cancer in parents and the age at diagnosis. **D:** The influence of the combined history of colorectal cancer in a parent and sibling and the age at diagnosis on the cumulative incidence of colorectal adenomas.

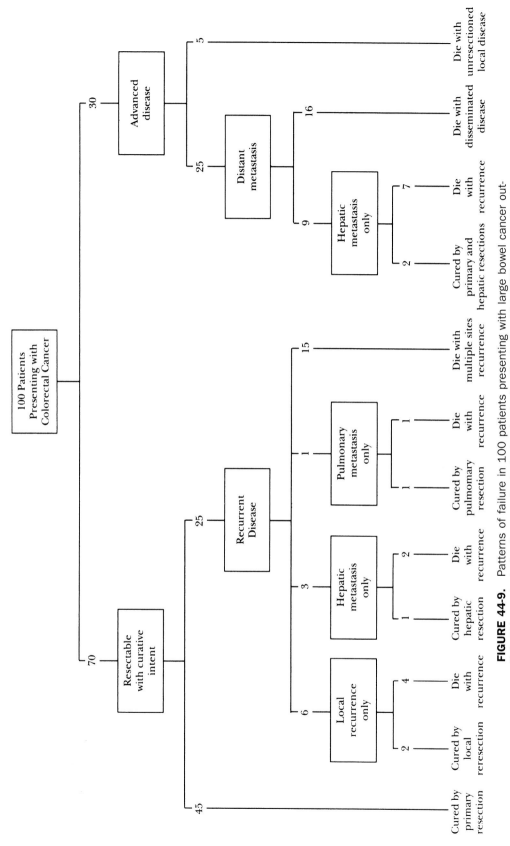

FIGURE 44-9. Patterns of failure in 100 patients presenting with large bowel cancer outlining the projected outcome of a typical cohort of patients in which 70% appeared to be resectable for cure; 64% of that group was cured by primary resection, but the other 36% experienced recurrent disease. A total of 55% either presented with advanced disease (30%) or developed postoperative recurrence (25%); about 11% of that group may be cured by additional surgery.

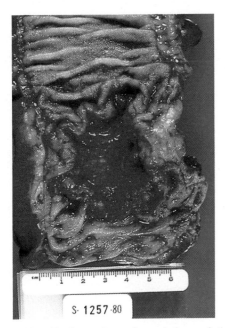

FIGURE 44-10. En face view of carcinoma of the colon. The features include heaped-up edges and the ulcerated center of the lesion.

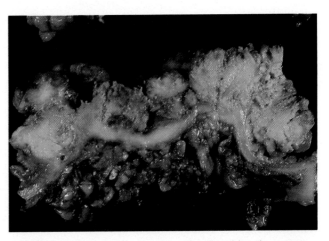

FIGURE 44-11. Cross section of polypoid colon cancer. Lesion is in Dukes class A because the neoplasm does not invade the muscularis propria. Although this lesion is a bulky intralumenal tumor, the prognosis after resection is excellent because of the minimal invasive capability.

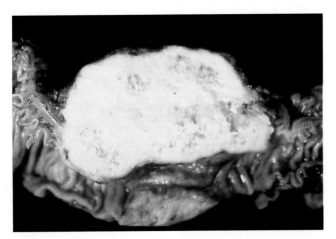

FIGURE 44-12. Cross section of a bulky tumor from the ascending colon that invades the serosa to the subserosal pericolonic fat layer, making it a Dukes class B2 lesion.

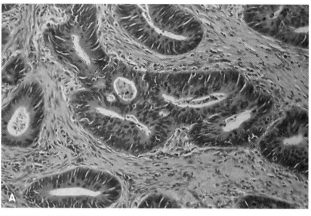

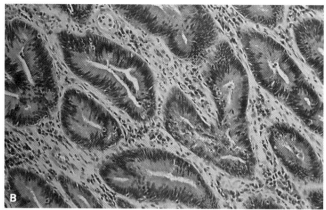

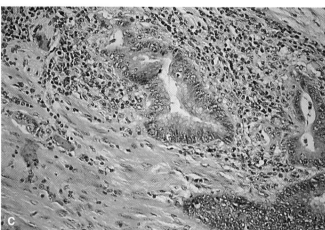

FIGURE 44-13. Histopathological features of well-differentiated carcinoma. **A:** High-power microscopic view of a well-differentiated carcinoma of the colon shows typical, darkly stained glands within a poorly stained stroma. The nuclear-to-cytoplasmic ratio is high, and the nuclei palisade away from the basal lamina. **B:** Microscopic field from a benign adenomatous polyp demonstrates the similarities it shares with a malignant neoplasm; however, the smaller nuclei with their basal orientation are more characteristic of a benign lesion. These glands are incapable of invading beyond the muscularis mucosae. **C:** Well-differentiated adenocarcinoma invading into the muscularis propria.

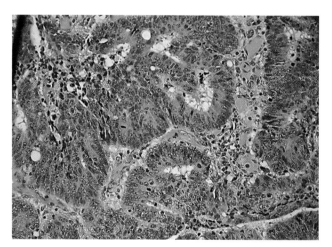

FIGURE 44-14. Less well-differentiated adenocarcinoma in which formation of the characteristic glands is less evident, and the nuclei are larger and more irregular. A poorly differentiated adenocarcinoma may consist of sheets of such bizarre cells and confers a poorer prognosis.

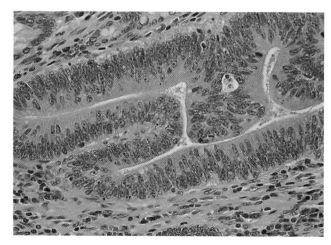

FIGURE 44-15. High-grade dysplasia in an adenomatous polyp. The nuclei are large with poorly condensed chromatin, and the nuclei palisade up from the basal lamina. This lesion, when it occurs in the confines of an adenomatous polyp, is the equivalent of carcinoma in situ but is not capable of invasion or metastasis.

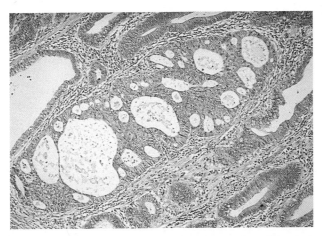

FIGURE 44-16. Histological appearance of carcinoma in situ in a polyp.

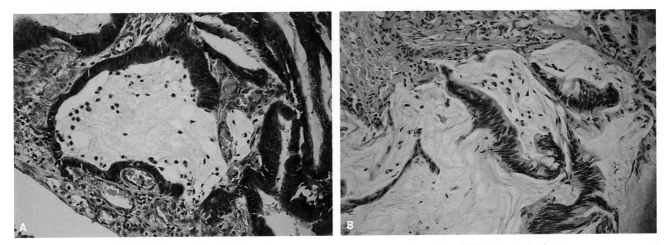

FIGURE 44-17. Mucinous colon cancer. **A:** Some tumors have the ability to secrete large amounts of mucus into a malignant gland. Darkly stained cancer cells are present, and the nuclei are suspended in the central pool of mucin. **B:** Liver metastasis of mucinous cancer. Nests of cells secrete large pools of mucin.

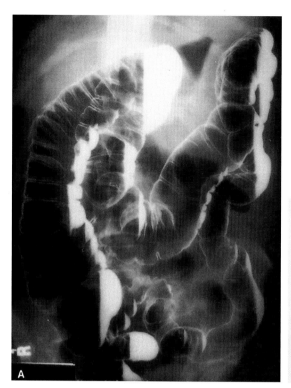

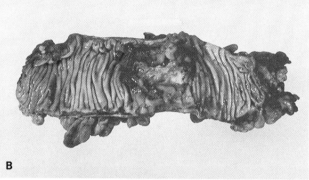

FIGURE 44-18. Large, but occult, colon cancer resectable for cure. A 42-year-old man had occult fecal bleeding detected at a routine examination (positive guaiac test) but had no symptoms of intestinal obstruction or overt bleeding. **A:** Air contrast barium enema study that was believed to be normal. On review, a constricting lesion was found in the midsigmoid colon. **B:** A 4.5 × 6 cm ulcerated mass in the sigmoid colon proved to be mucin-producing adenocarcinoma. The patient had no involved lymph nodes and was free of disease 3 years after his operation.

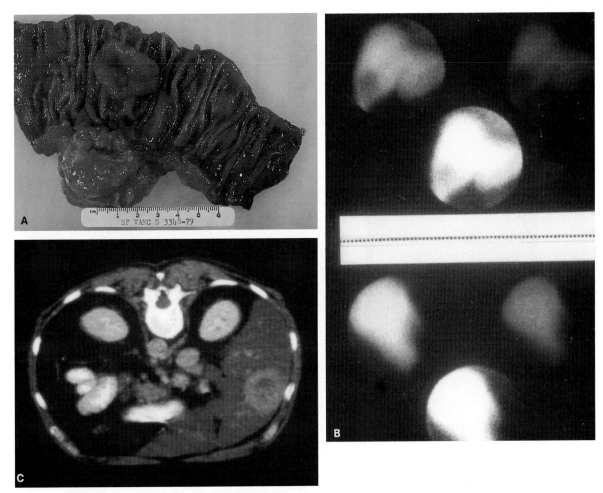

FIGURE 44-19. Metastatic colon cancer not detected with multiple diagnostic tests. A 55-year-old man had hematochezia and a 1-year history of guaiac-positive stools attributed to alcohol abuse and salicylate use. A single-contrast barium enema study was read as normal, and no lesions were seen at rigid sigmoidoscopy. **A:** A 3 × 4 cm elevated cancer in the sigmoid colon. The lesion was recognized on later review of the barium enema radiographs. **B:** Area of diminished uptake in the right lobe of the liver on a radionuclide scan. **C:** Metastatic lesion in the liver on a computed tomogram. The patient died of metastatic disease within 6 months. Although the primary lesion was smaller than that described in Fig. 44-17, this was an aggressive, Dukes class D lesion.

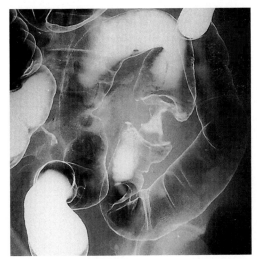

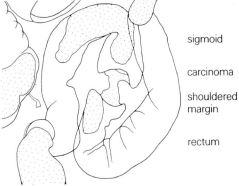

sigmoid

carcinoma

shouldered margin

rectum

FIGURE 44-20. Barium enema radiograph of annular colon carcinoma.

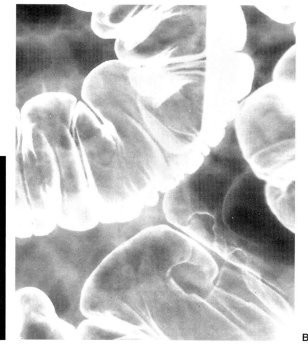

A

B

FIGURE 44-21. **A:** Adenocarcinoma, plaque-like mass. The lesion located proximal to the cecum (on the posterior wall at the 3 o'clock position) appears as a slightly raised, discrete mass with central depressions. **B:** Radiographic appearance of plaque-like adenocarcinoma. The lesion (**left lower quadrant**) has raised margins around a central depression, giving the appearance of a saddle.

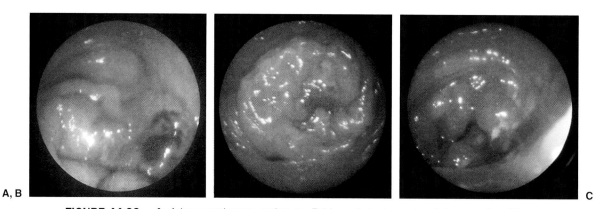

A, B

C

FIGURE 44-22. **A:** Adenocarcinoma, stricture. Folds radiate to a pinpoint narrowing. The intact overlying mucosa suggests an infiltrating rather than an exophytic growth pattern. Biopsies of the mouth of the stricture had normal results, but brush cytologic findings were abnormal, emphasizing the usefulness of this examination with this type of appearance. **B:** Adenocarcinoma, stricture. A mass effect is apparent, suggesting that this lesion may have an exophytic growth pattern. For the most part, the mucosa is intact, as in **A,** except for a small rim at the mouth of the stricture. **C:** Adenocarcinoma, annular mass. In this case, the stricture is entirely the result of this tumor, which has broken through at the point of lumenal narrowing.

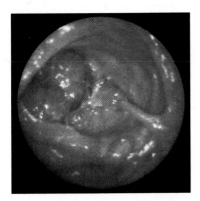

FIGURE 44-23. Adenocarcinoma, sigmoid with synchronous (sentinel) adenoma. A cancer with an ulcerated mass appearance was found at the splenic flexure (in the distance at the 3 o'clock position). Just distal to this in the proximal descending colon, a pedunculated polyp is present as a sentinel neoplasm. The possibility that other adenomas or even cancers are present in this colon suggests the need to perform colonoscopy 6 to 12 months after curative resection for this malignant growth.

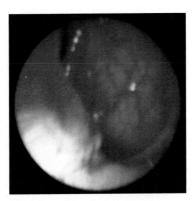

FIGURE 44-24. Metastatic carcinoma to the colon from a cervical primary lesion. Local spread produced a mass and cervical narrowing at the rectosigmoid junction. Biopsies showed squamous carcinoma similar to that found in the original cervical carcinoma.

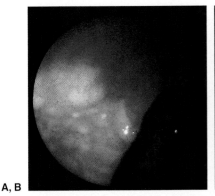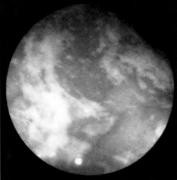

A, B

FIGURE 44-25. A: Lymphoma. Multiple polyps of the cecum of a patient with abdominal lymphoma always suggest involvement of this segment, even when the patient has no symptoms. **B:** Lymphoma simulating ulcerative colitis. Ulcerations and friability in this patient with watery diarrhea caused this appearance, which was initially mistaken for inflammatory bowel disease. Biopsies, however, showed poorly differentiated lymphoma.

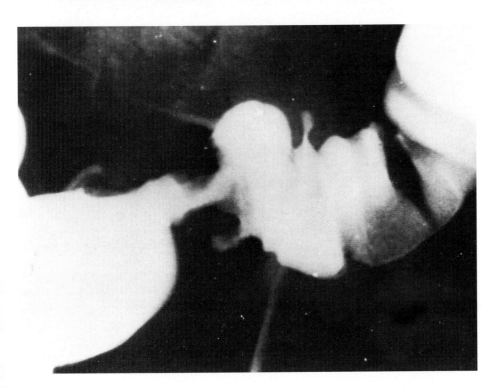

FIGURE 44-26. Carcinoma of the sigmoid with diverticular disease. Because of the relative frequency of both conditions, this is not an uncommon picture.

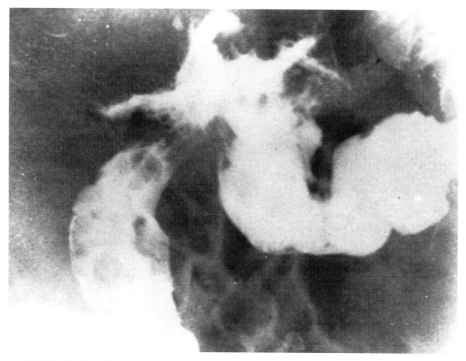

FIGURE 44-27. Perforated carcinoma may be indistinguishable from diverticulitis.

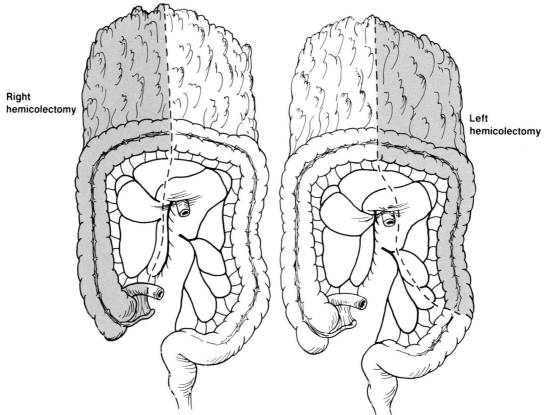

A   **B**

FIGURE 44-28. **A–E:** Oncologic colon resections. *(Continued)*

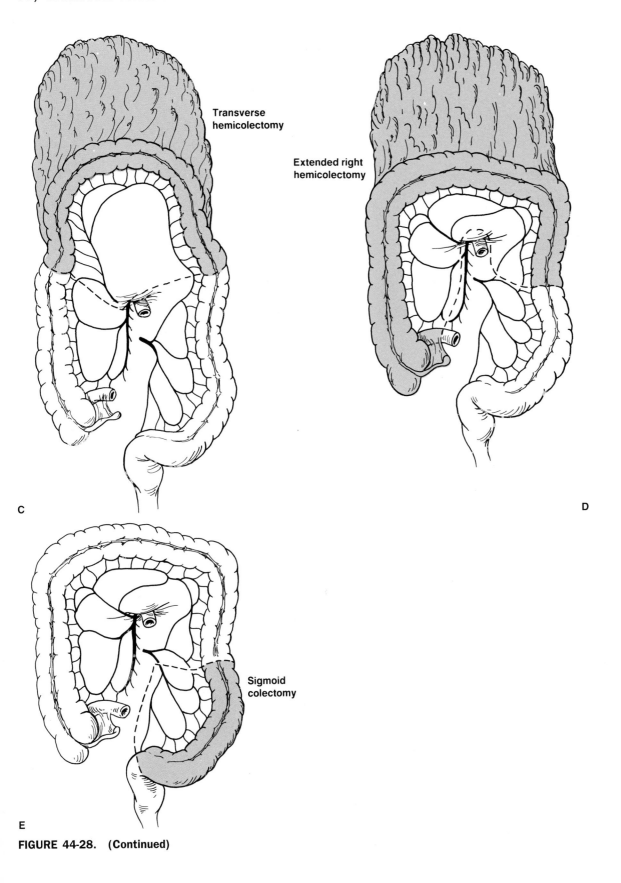

Transverse
hemicolectomy

Extended right
hemicolectomy

Sigmoid
colectomy

C

D

E

FIGURE 44-28. (Continued)

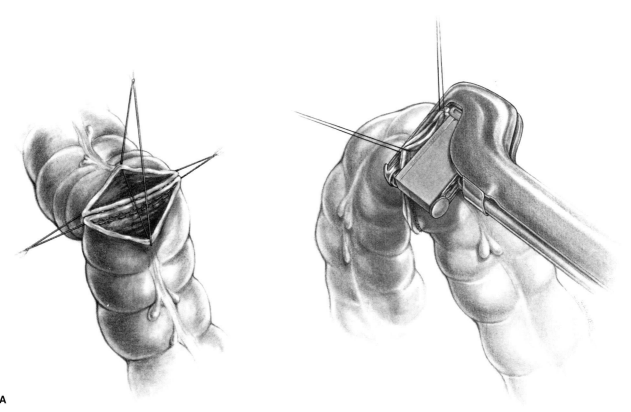

A   B

FIGURE 44-29. Triangulation anastomosis by means of inversion of the posterior (mesenteric) wall (**A**) and eversion of the anterior walls (**B**).

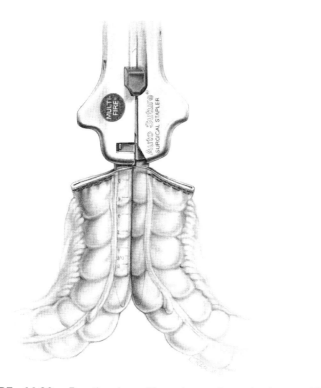

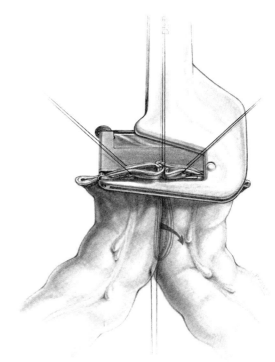

FIGURE 44-30. Functional end-to-end anastomosis by means of the closed technique after construction of two enterotomies for insertion of the separate limbs of the gastrointestinal anastomosis stapler.

FIGURE 44-31. Closure of the enterotomies with a triangulation anastomosis stapler.

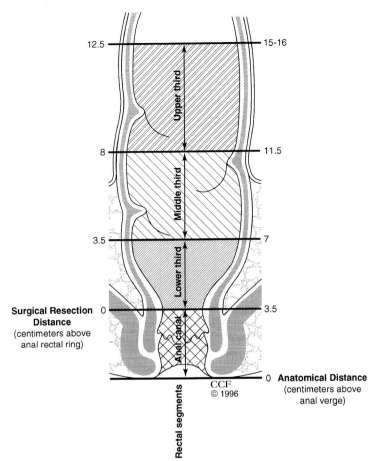

FIGURE 44-32. Surgical and purely anatomic regions of the rectum as they relate to the anal sphincters and pelvic floor.

45

ANORECTAL DISEASES

JEFFREY L. BARNETT

This chapter provides a visual introduction to some of the typical anal lesions encountered in clinical practice. We begin by showing some of the common instruments used by gastroenterologists and surgeons for anorectal examinations (Fig. 45-1). Typical anal retractors and anorectal examination instruments that require an external light source are shown in Fig. 45-1. Many of these instruments would more likely be used by a colorectal surgeon than a gastroenterologist, but I believe that it is important for the gastroenterologist to be familiar with this type of instrumentation. The equipment used for rigid proctosigmoidoscopy is shown in Fig. 45-1*A*. Because symptomatic internal hemorrhoids are one of the most common lesions seen by the practicing gastroenterologist, we have elected to show a photograph of the simplest, most widely used instrument for management of internal hemorrhoids, the Barron-type rubber band ligator with its ancillary equipment (see Fig. 45-1*C*).

Hemorrhoids are the most common anal lesions seen in practice; therefore, pictures of external and different degrees of internal hemorrhoids are critical to any atlas on anal disorders (Figs. 45-2 through 45-7). Hemorrhoids may be treated using a variety of nonsurgical techniques. One modality is banding using a ligator device attached to the tip of an endoscope (Fig. 45-8). Examples of a chronic anal fissure, anorectal abscess, anorectal fistula, and rectal prolapse are shown in Figs. 45-9 through 45-12. These important lesions are all best diagnosed by means of simple inspection. Finally, we show examples of carcinoma of the anus (Figs. 45-13 through 45-15). One fairly subtle lesion is Bowen disease (cutaneous squamous cell carcinoma in situ), which may be confused with the anal lesions of dermatitis and psoriasis.

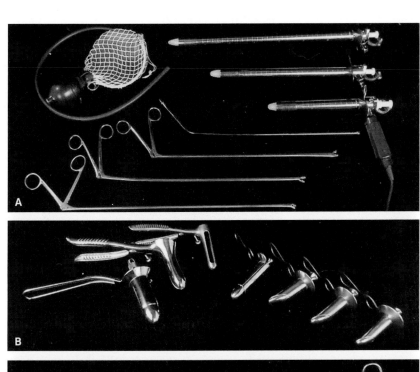

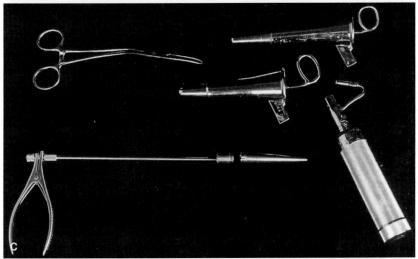

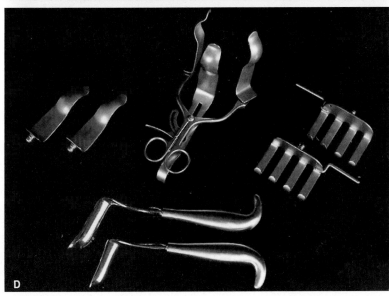

FIGURE 45-1. Instruments for anorectal examinations. **A:** Equipment necessary for performance of rigid proctosigmoidoscopy—air insufflator, interchangeable proctoscopes with light source, suction wand, and assorted biopsy forceps. **B:** Instruments for anorectal examination that require an external light source. **Left to right:** Fansler proctoscope, Pratt rectal speculum, Sims rectal speculum, Buie-Hirschman anoscope, and Hirschman anoscopes (small, medium, and large). Disposable anoscopes are also commonly used (not shown). **C:** Instruments for rubber-band ligation of internal hemorrhoids. Barron-type ligator with grasping forceps and device for loading bands (**left**). Welch-Allyn self-illuminated anoscope with large and small specula (**right**). **D:** Anal retractors. **Top to bottom:** Parks' anal retractor with interchangeable blades, Ferguson-Moon anal retractor, and Hill-Ferguson anal retractor.

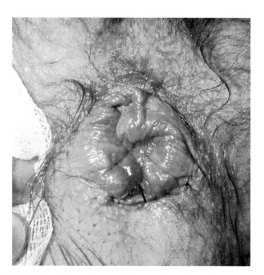

FIGURE 45-2. First-degree (nonprolapsing) internal hemorrhoid (*arrow*) and external hemorrhoids.

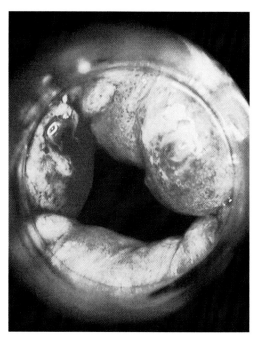

FIGURE 45-3. Anoscopic appearance of first-degree internal hemorrhoids.

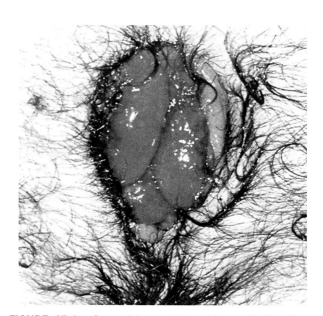

FIGURE 45-4. Second-degree internal hemorrhoids. These hemorrhoids prolapse but are spontaneously reducible.

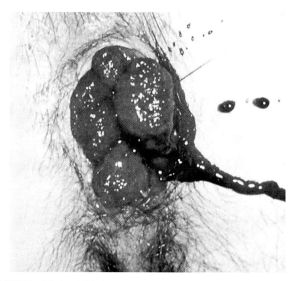

FIGURE 45-5. Third-degree internal hemorrhoids. These hemorrhoids prolapse and require manual reduction. Spontaneous bleeding is apparent.

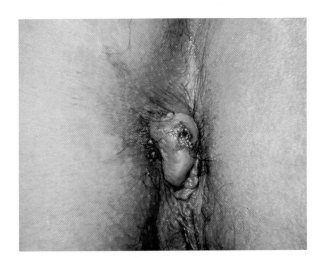

FIGURE 45-6. Thrombosed external hemorrhoid with cutaneous ulceration and superficial necrosis.

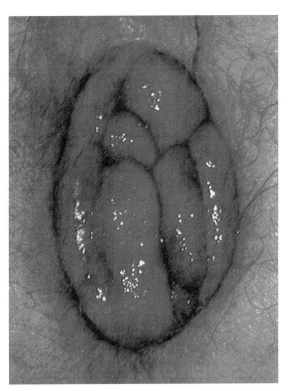

FIGURE 45-7. Fourth-degree (nonreducible) internal hemorrhoids.

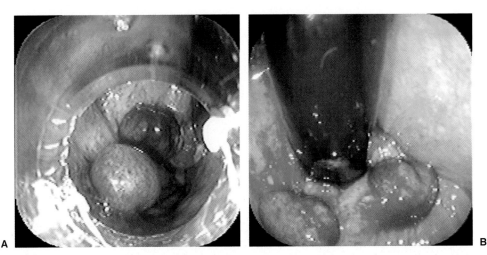

FIGURE 45-8. **A:** A view through the endoscope after placing bands on two separate internal hemorrhoids using a multibanding ligator device attached to the instrument tip. **B:** A retroflexed endoscopic view of banded internal hemorrhoids.

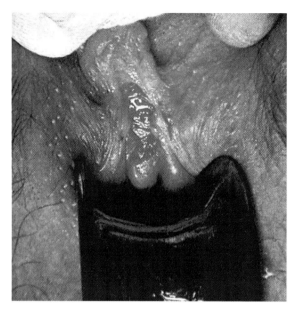

FIGURE 45-9. Typical appearance of a chronic anal fissure triad consisting of a sentinel pile (**top**), the fissure itself, and a hypertrophic papilla.

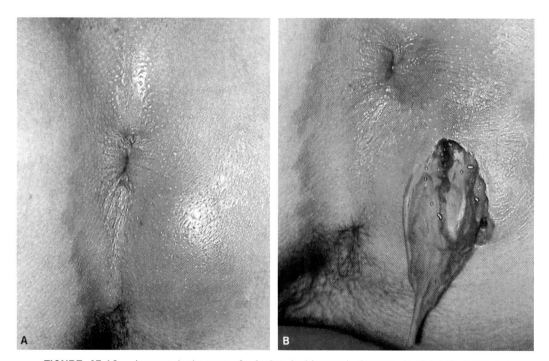

FIGURE 45-10. Anorectal abscess. **A:** A ripe ischiorectal abscess in the left posterior quadrant. **B:** The same abscess expressing pus immediately after incision.

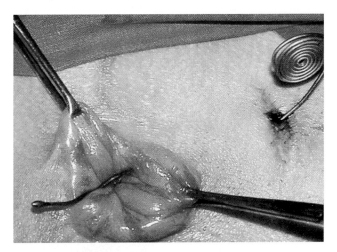

FIGURE 45-11. Anorectal fistula.

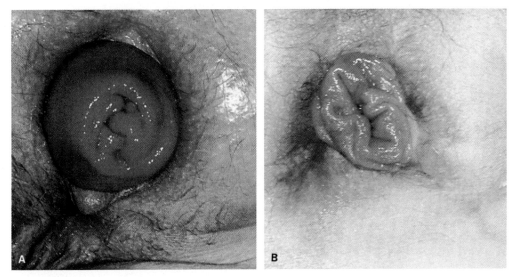

FIGURE 45-12. Rectal prolapse. **A:** Complete rectal prolapse. **B:** Incomplete rectal prolapse.

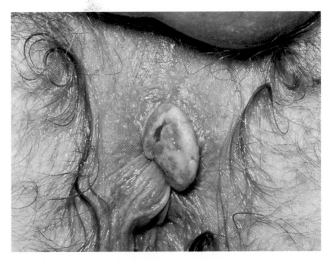

FIGURE 45-13. Squamous cell carcinoma of the anus. (Courtesy of Dr. Karen Guice.)

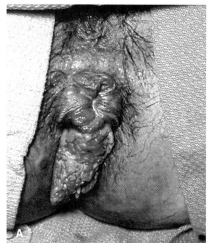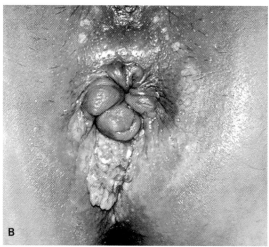

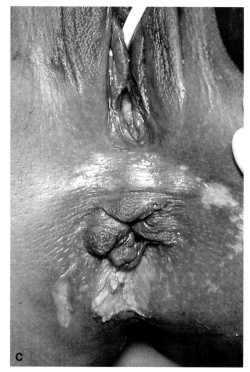

FIGURE 45-14. Large perianal squamous cell carcinoma just posterior to the anus. **A:** Bulky tumor at the time of initial diagnosis. **B:** The same tumor 3 weeks later, after partial treatment with radiation therapy and chemotherapy. **C:** Complete disappearance of tumor 3 months after diagnosis and a full course of radiation therapy and chemotherapy. (Courtesy of Dr. Karen Guice.)

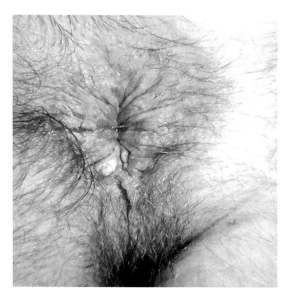

FIGURE 45-15. Bowen disease (cutaneous squamous cell carcinoma in situ) of the anus. The lesion has a scaly, plaque-like appearance. (Courtesy of Dr. Richard Burney.)

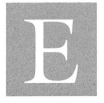

E PANCREAS

46

PANCREAS: Anatomy and Structural Anomalies

MICHAEL W. MULHOLLAND ■ DIANE M. SIMEONE

Knowledge of the anatomic and structural relations of the pancreas has become increasingly important with the advent of cross-sectional imaging, innovations in endoscopy, and the introduction of methods for percutaneous biopsy of the gland. The central location of the gland in the upper retroperitoneum complicates the medical and surgical management of pancreatic disease.

Pancreatic development begins during the fourth week of gestation from two primordial anlagen associated with the duodenum (Fig. 46-1). The dorsal pancreatic bud, destined to form a portion of the pancreatic head and all of the body and tail of the pancreas, enlarges more rapidly and extends into the dorsal mesentery. The ventral pancreatic bud, the source of the uncinate process and a portion of the pancreatic head, develops in association with the hepatic rudiment and biliary ductal structures. Rotation of the ventral pancreatic bud to the left of the duodenum brings it below the dorsal bud. Fusion occurs in the seventh week of gestation. In most instances, fusion of the ventral duct with the dorsal duct results in formation of a single pancreatic duct that empties through the ventral ductal segment (Fig. 46-2). Failure of ductal fusion results in formation of the congenital anomaly pancreas divisum (Figs. 46-3 and 46-4).

The pancreas is an elongated organ, 12 to 20 cm in length in adults, which lies transversely in the upper retroperitoneum. The gland may be divided arbitrarily into head, uncinate process, neck, body, and tail (Fig. 46-5). The head of the pancreas lies on the right in the concavity of the duodenal sweep. The head of the gland also is related to the gastroepiploic foramen, the right kidney, the inferior vena cava, and the right portion of the transverse mesocolon (Figs. 46-6 and 46-7). The distal common bile duct traverses the head of the pancreas before entering the duodenum.

The neck of the pancreas is bordered inferiorly by the transverse mesocolon and the root of the mesentery of the small intestine. Posteriorly, the neck of the pancreas is associated with the confluence of the superior mesenteric and splenic veins, which together form the portal vein (Fig. 46-8). The body and tail of the pancreas are related, along the superior border, to the splenic artery and vein (Fig. 46-9). The transverse mesocolon is attached to the inferior border of the tail of the gland; the stomach contacts the anterior surface. The tail of the pancreas extends to the left in the leaves of the splenorenal ligament to the hilum of the spleen. Some of these anatomic relations, as seen with cross-sectional imaging, are shown in Fig. 46-10. The arterial blood supply of the pancreas is derived from both the celiac axis and the superior mesenteric artery. Venous drainage is entirely portal.

The pancreas is a mixed endocrine and exocrine gland. The exocrine pancreas is organized in lobular units composed of ductules and acini. Acinar cells are pyramidal and have a highly basophilic cytoplasm. Numerous zymogen granules are visualized by means of electron microscopic examination of the cellular apex. Centroacinar cells and ductular cells are more columnar. The acini rest on a thin basal lamina penetrated by numerous blood vessels and nerve fibers.

The endocrine pancreas is composed of approximately 1 million islets of Langerhans. The islets contain endocrine cells that stain positively for insulin (75% to 80%), glucagon (10% to 20%), and somatostatin (5%). Pancreatic polypeptide and several other enteric peptides have been identified in the pancreatic islets.

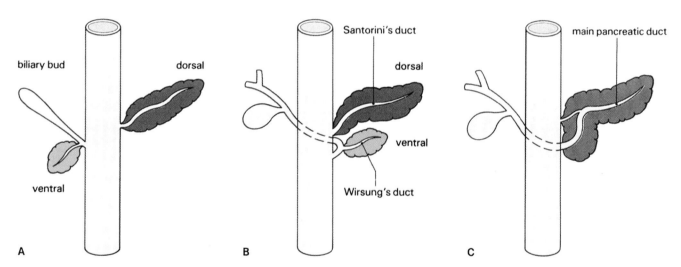

FIGURE 46-1. **A–C:** Developmental anatomy of the pancreas.

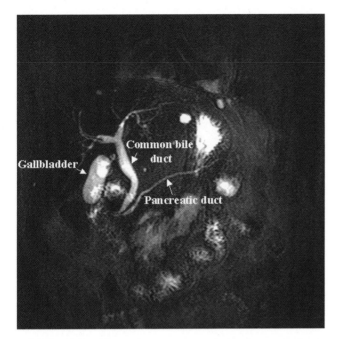

FIGURE 46-2. Magnetic resonance cholangiopancreatography demonstrates standard pancreatic ductal anatomy, with a single main pancreatic duct emptying through the ventral segment.

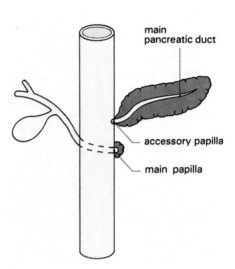

FIGURE 46-3. Failure of fusion of ventral and dorsal pancreatic buds results in pancreas divisum.

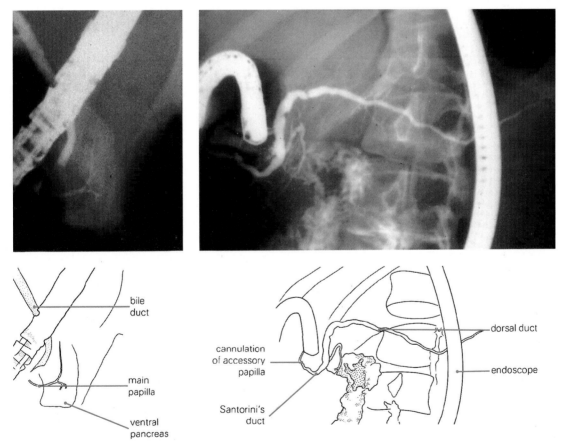

FIGURE 46-4. Endoscopic retrograde pancreatogram illustrates the congenital anomaly pancreas divisum. The ventral pancreatic duct (**right**) fills through the major papilla. The dorsal pancreatic duct is filled through the accessory pancreatic duct (**left**). The two ductal systems do not communicate.

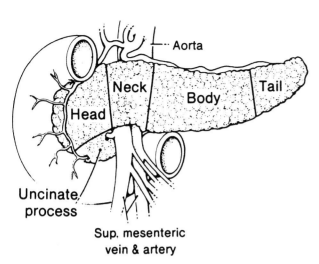

FIGURE 46-5. Anatomic regions of the pancreas.

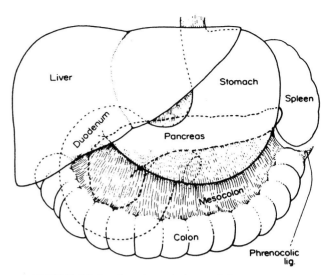

FIGURE 46-6. Anterior relations of the pancreas.

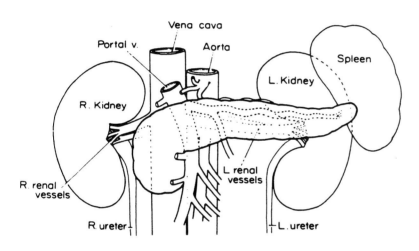

FIGURE 46-7. Anatomic relations posterior to the pancreas.

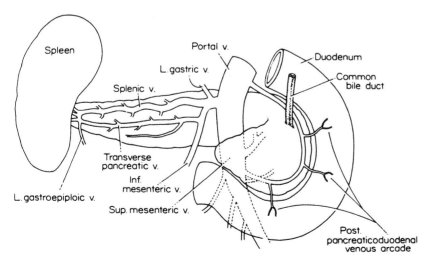

FIGURE 46-8. Posterior view of the pancreas demonstrates relations to portal venous tributaries.

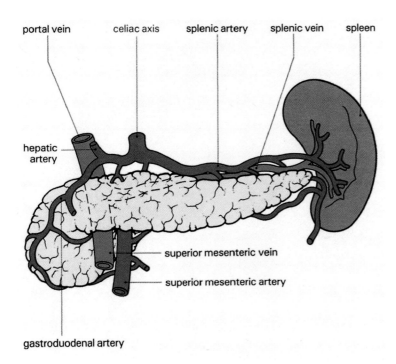

portal vein   celiac axis   splenic artery   splenic vein   spleen

hepatic
artery

superior mesenteric vein

superior mesenteric artery

gastroduodenal artery

FIGURE 46-9. Arterial supply to the pancreas.

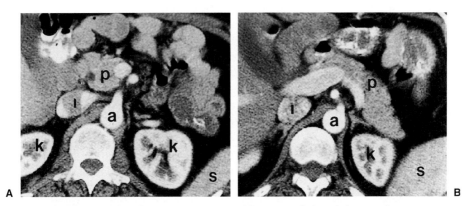

A   B

FIGURE 46-10. Computed tomographic scan of the abdomen demonstrates the relation of the head (**A**) and body and tail (**B**) of the pancreas
to surrounding structures. *a*, aorta; *l*, inferior vena cava; *k*, kidney; *p*,
pancreas; *s*, spleen.

47

ACUTE PANCREATITIS

ANIL NAGAR ■ FRED S. GORELICK

Acute pancreatitis is an acute inflammatory process of the pancreas. This inflammation may be mild with minimal abnormalities on imaging studies or severe with necrosis of the pancreas and accompanied multiorgan system failure. According to the Marseilles classification (1984), the acute inflammation should occur in an otherwise morphologically and functionally normal pancreas, thereby allowing for full functional recovery after treatment of precipitating factors and resolution of the acute attack. The two most common etiologies together accounting for 60% to 80% of acute pancreatitis are ethanol and gallstones (Table 47-1). Two histological forms of acute pancreatitis are recognized: acute interstitial and acute hemorrhagic. Macroscopic changes described in acute hemorrhagic pancreatitis (from autopsy and surgical specimens) include edema and necrosis of the pancreas with the surface showing areas of white chalky fat necrosis and hemorrhages. Fat necrosis of the omentum, mesentery, and retroperitoneum with turbid or hemorrhagic peritoneal fluid can also be observed. Hematomas may be present in the retroperitoneum. Rarely the gland may be transformed into a hemorrhagic mass. Microscopically, necrosis mainly involves the interlobular fatty tissue, and tends to spare the glandular elements. Arterial and venous thrombosis with acute granulocytic infiltration is usually present. In the life-threatening complication of infected necrosis, Gram stains can usually demonstrate the infectious pathogens.

Acute pancreatitis presents as severe midabdominal pain (which may radiate to the back), nausea, vomiting, and fever, and elevated amylase and lipase levels. A small percentage of patients do not complain of pain and the diagnosis of acute pancreatitis can be missed on presentation. These patients may present with acute respiratory changes or changes in mental status. Depending on the severity of disease and presence of distal organ failure, patients may develop tachycardia, hypotension, confusion, reduced urine output, and hypoxemia. In addition to tenderness, examination of the abdomen of patients with severe pancreatitis may demonstrate ileus, ascites, and rarely flank ecchymosis (Grey Turner sign) or periumbilical ecchymosis (Cullen sign). Periumbilical ecchymosis has been described in other causes of hemoperitoneum. Severe pancreatic necrosis may be accompanied by subcutaneous fat necrosis, which results in panniculitis.

In patients with acute and severe abdominal pain, plain films of the abdomen and chest should be taken to exclude intestinal perforation. Chest radiographic findings include pleural effusions (most commonly on the left, occasionally bilateral, and rarely right sided), atelectasis, and adult respiratory distress syndrome. The inflammatory exudates in acute pancreatitis can spread anteriorly and inferiorly to involve the transverse mesocolon, resulting in spasm of the transverse colon, which is observed as the colon cut-off sign. This finding is not specific for acute pancreatitis and may be seen in ischemic colitis or mechanical obstruction. Other findings on abdominal plain films include localized dilation of small bowel (sentinel loop) or generalized ileus.

Imaging studies establish the diagnosis of acute pancreatitis, provide prognostic information, document the presence or absence of biliary obstruction, and assess possible complications. Abdominal ultrasound examination is helpful in documenting cholelithiasis (>95% sensitive for gallbladder stones) and biliary obstruction. It is less sensitive for biliary sludge (microlithiasis) and choledocholithiasis. The inflamed pancreas is often not well-visualized secondary to overlying bowel gas. Ultrasound findings of acute inflammation include enlargement of the gland, loss of normal internal echoes, and hypoechogenicity secondary to increased water in the parenchyma.

Although the diagnosis of acute pancreatitis is made on the basis of elevated serum amylase and lipase levels, the level of elevation does not predict severity. Multiple biological markers and scoring systems have been proposed to predict severity, but the contrast-enhanced dynamic computed tomographic (CT) scan remains the most widely used diagnostic technique (Table 47-2). CT scanning is helpful in establishing the diagnosis of acute pancreatitis (edema and inflammatory stranding around the gland), predicting degree of necrosis (lack of contrast enhancement of >30% of the pancreas), and imaging of pancreatic and peripancreatic fluid collections. The severity of changes by dynamic CT scan correlates with morbidity and mortality in acute pancreatitis (Table 47-3). CT and other imaging procedures are useful in management and follow-up of local complications of acute pancreatitis (Table 47-4). Unlike ultrasonography, overlying bowel gas does not interfere with CT images. CT scanning is useful in follow-up examinations of peripancreatic and fluid collections and pseudocysts. CT scanning cannot differentiate sterile from infected necrosis; this requires percutaneous aspiration for Gram stain and culture of the necrotic area under CT or ultrasound guidance. The presence of air within a fluid collection suggests infection. Magnetic resonance imaging (MRI) may be used in acute pancreatitis. MRI changes in acute pancreatitis include edema, enlargement of the organ, and lack of tissue enhancement with intravenous gadolinium in the presence of necrosis. MRI is attractive as an alternative to CT scanning because it does not require iodine-containing intravenous contrast and can provide a magnetic resonance cholangiopancreatography (MRCP) image at the same setting. MRCP is a sensitive test to detect choledocholithiasis and is especially useful when there is a need to avoid endoscopic retrograde cholangiopancreatography (ERCP). MRI has not gained widespread use because of its lack of availability and relatively high cost. It is also a cumbersome test and results are difficult to obtain quickly. Endoscopic ultrasound (EUS) has a limited role in acute pancreatitis and may be helpful in detecting biliary sludge and choledocholithiasis not seen on abdominal ultrasound imaging. EUS can also aid in the diagnosis of pancreatic divisum and endoscopic drainage of pancreatic pseudocysts. This test is also limited by its availability.

Gallstones are among the most common causes of acute pancreatitis. Patients are usually treated conservatively. Emergent ERCP with biliary sphincterotomy and bile duct stone extraction is reserved for patients with persistent biliary obstruction or cholangitis. Occasionally, an impacted stone is seen at the ampulla and can usually be dislodged by a cannula. If sphincterotomy is difficult or contraindicated [e.g., in disseminated intravascular coagulation (DIC)], a temporary plastic biliary stent or nasobiliary drain can be placed to secure immediate bile duct drainage. ERCP is also a recognized cause of acute pancreatitis, with a reported incidence of 2% to 8%. The risk of ERCP-induced pancreatitis is associated with multiple pancreatic duct injections, acinarization (visualization of the pancreatic parenchyma with injected contrast), pancreatic sphincterotomy, and sphincter of Oddi manometry.

Pancreatic divisum results from congenital partial or absent fusion between the duct of Wirsung and the duct of Santorini, resulting in the dorsal duct draining most of the pancreas through the minor papilla. Some patients with pancreas divisum experience recurrent attacks of acute pancreatitis secondary to obstruction to the flow of pancreatic secretions at the duct of Santorini or at a diminutive orifice of the minor papilla. Diagnosis of pancreas divisum can be made by ERCP, MRCP, or EUS. In complete pancreas divisum, injection of the major ampulla demonstrates a short duct of Wirsung that terminates in the pancreatic head. To demonstrate filling of the pancreatic duct in the body and tail, the minor ampulla must be cannulated and injected with contrast. Careful examination of the ERCP images is required to distinguish pancreas divisum from duct obstruction caused by benign or malignant disease involving the main pancreatic duct. Treatment of pancreas divisum can consist of careful sphincterotomy of the intraduodenal portion of the minor papilla with short-term stenting to prevent obstruction to the minor ampulla caused by edema. Pancreatic duct disruption secondary to trauma is a common cause of acute pancreatitis in children. The midpancreatic duct, as it crosses the vertebral column, is particularly susceptible to blunt trauma. In suspected patients, ERCP or CT scan can demonstrate duct disruption. Pancreatic duct disruption can also be seen in acute pancreatitis not associated with abdominal trauma.

After an episode of acute pancreatitis, there is usually complete recovery of pancreatic morphology and function.

TABLE 47-1
Etiology of Acute Pancreatitis

Biliary tract disease
Alcohol
Tumors
Structural abnormality or obstruction of PD (pancreatic divisum, sphincter of Oddi
  dysfunction, helminths, foreign body)
Metabolic (hyperlipidemia, hypercalcemia)
Medications
Toxins (mushroom poisoning, scorpion bite)
Trauma
ERCP
Infection
Hereditary acute pancreatitis
Cystic fibrosis
Other (IBD, coronary bypass, peritoneal dialysis, peptic ulcer)
Idiopathic

ERCP, endoscopic retrograde cholangiopancreatography; IBD, inflammatory bowel disease; PD, pancreatic duct.

TABLE 47-2
CT Grading of Acute Pancreatitis

STAGING	SCORE
A. Normal	0
B. Focal or diffuse enlargement of gland	1
C. As for B plus involvement of peripancreatic fat	2
D. Single, ill-defined fluid collection	3
E. ≥2 ill-defined fluid collections and/or intrapancreatic gas	4

DEGREE OF NECROSIS (%) (NONENHANCEMENT WITH IV CONTRAST)

0	
<33 of pancreas	2
33–<50 of pancreas	4
≥50 of pancreas	6

Note: Add CT score + necrosis score = CT severity index.

CT, computed tomography; IV, intravenous.

From Balthazar EJ, Robinson DL, Megibow AJ, et al. Acute pancreatitis: value of CT in establishing prognosis. Radiology 1990;174:331.

TABLE 47-3
Computed Tomography Severity Index (CTSI) Correlates with Mortality in Acute Pancreatitis

CTSI	MORBIDITY	MORTALITY
0–3	8%	3%
4–6	35%	6%
7–10	92%	17%

From Balthazar EJ, Robinson DL, Megibow AJ, et al. Acute pancreatitis: value of CT in establishing prognosis. Radiology 1990;174:331.

TABLE 47-4
Selected Local Complications of Acute Pancreatitis

COMPLICATION	IMAGING	MANAGEMENT
Fluid collection	CT scan	Conservative management
Pancreatic abscess	CT scan with aspiration	Surgery
Pancreatic necrosis	Contrast CT scan, with needle aspiration for infection	Surgery for infected necrosis
Pseudocyst	CT scan or ultrasound	Conservative management; endoscopic or surgical for complications
Pancreatic fistula	ERCP, CT scan, MRCP	PD stenting, somatostatin, surgery
Splenic vein thrombosis	Contrast CT, MRA	Splenectomy for bleeding gastric or esophageal varices
Pseudoaneurysm formation	Contrast CT, angiography, MRA	Angiographic embolization of feeding artery

ERCP, endoscopic retrograde cholangiopancreatography; CT, computed tomography; MRA, magnetic resonance angiography; MRCP, magnetic resonance cholangiopancreatography; PD, pancreatic duct.

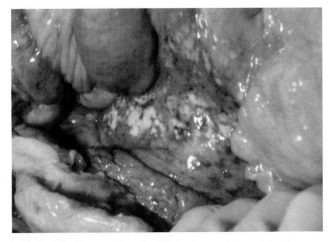

FIGURE 47-1. Gross specimen of acute hemorrhagic pancreatitis. White chalky fat necrosis and hemorrhage of the pancreas surface is seen. (Courtesy of Robert Homer, M.D., Yale University.)

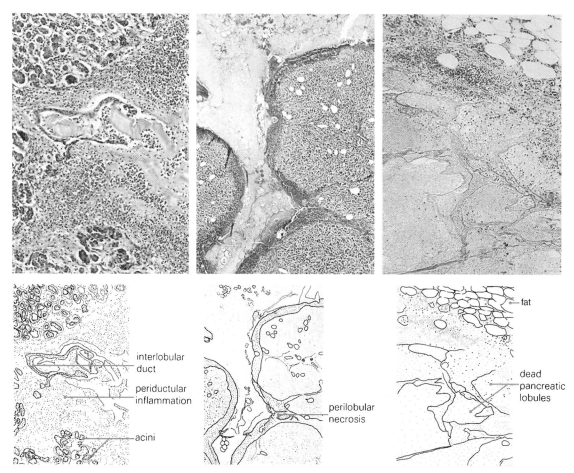

FIGURE 47-2.   Histology of acute pancreatitis.

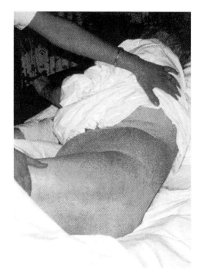

FIGURE 47-3.   Grey Turner sign.

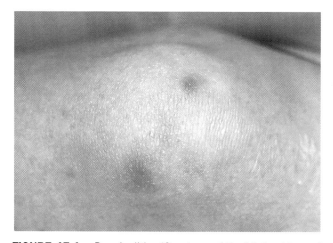

FIGURE 47-4.   Panniculitis. (Courtesy of Dr. Michael Lucey.)

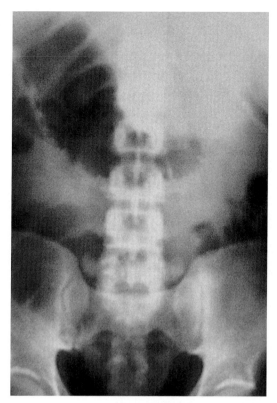

FIGURE 47-5.   Colon cut-off sign. (© Copyright 1990, The American Gastroenterological Association, 1990.)

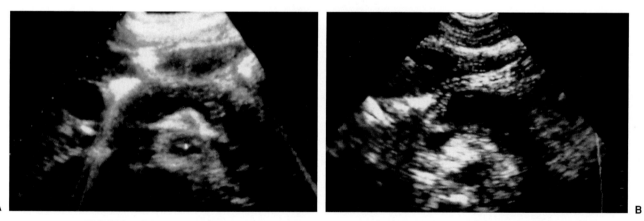

A   B

FIGURE 47-6.   Ultrasound image of pancreas. (© Copyright 1990, The American Gastroenterological Association, 1990.)

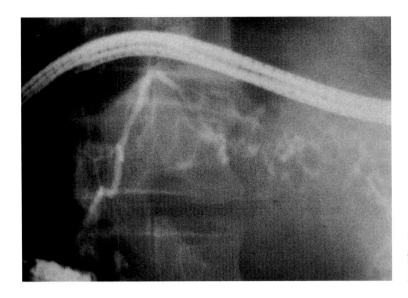

FIGURE 47-7. Endoscopic retrograde cholangiopancreatography of pancreatic duct trauma. (© Copyright 1990, The American Gastroenterological Association, 1990.)

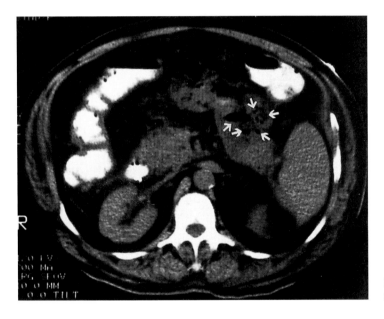

FIGURE 47-8. Computed tomographic scan of pancreatic abscess.

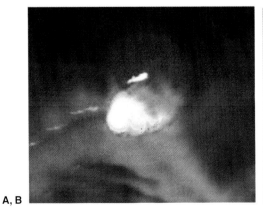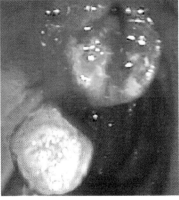

A, B

FIGURE 47-9. Endoscopic view of **A,** a bulging papilla caused by an impacted stone, which was revealed following biliary sphincterotomy and extraction **B.** (Courtesy of Mark Topazian, M.D.)

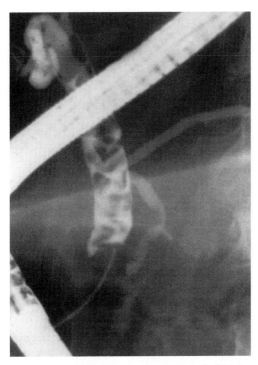

FIGURE 47-10. Endoscopic retrograde cholangiopancreatography with contrast injection into a dilated common bile duct in a patient with gallstone pancreatitis. Multiple stones appear as filling defects. Note the faceted edges of the stone. Normal filling of the pancreatic duct is observed.

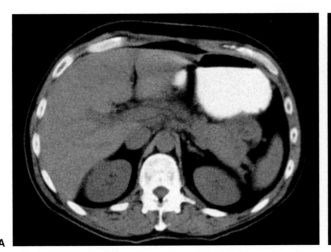
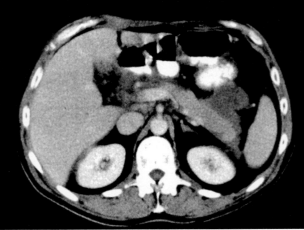

A　　　　　　　　　　　　　　　　　　　　　　　　　　　　　B

FIGURE 47-11. Computed tomographic (CT) scan of pancreas in pancreatitis. **A:** Without contrast. **B:** With intravenous contrast. The absence of contrast enhancement within the pancreas parenchyma is indicative of necrosis. Noncontrast CT scan cannot differentiate inflammation from necrosis.

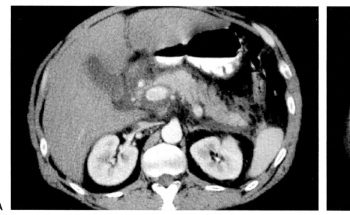
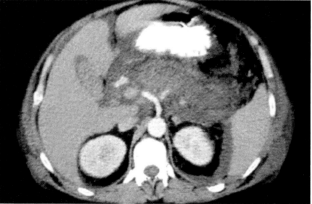

A   B

FIGURE 47-12. Contrast-enhanced computed tomographic scans of the pancreas. **A:** Day 1. Most of the pancreas demonstrates enhancement. **B:** Forty-eight hours later, there is absence of contrast enhancement, which suggests complete necrosis of the pancreas. The presence of necrosis is often inconspicuous at the onset of acute pancreatitis and is better detected 48 to 96 hours after the initial presentation. (Courtesy of Harold Schwartz, M.D.)

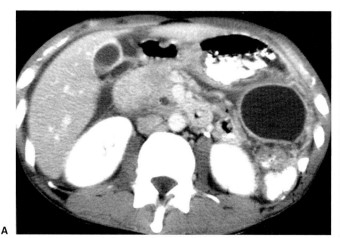
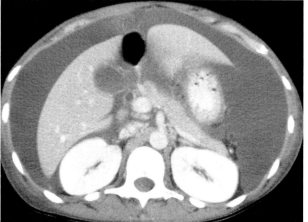

A   B

FIGURE 47-13. Contrast computed tomographic scan of pancreas. **A:** Pseudocyst is seen near the tail of pancreas. **B:** Ascites is observed with resolution of the pseudocyst following a rare complication of pseudocyst rupture. (Courtesy of Caroline Taylor, M.D.)

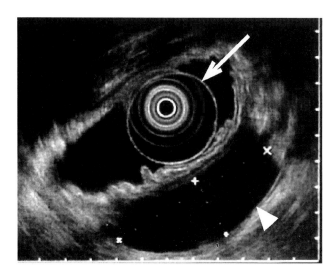

FIGURE 47-14. Endoscopic ultrasound (EUS) of a pseudocyst. The ultrasound probe (*arrow*) is seen in the water-filled stomach. A large pseudocyst (*arrowhead*) is noted adjacent to the stomach. EUS is helpful before endoscopic drainage of a pseudocyst to measure the distance between bowel wall and pseudocyst and to identify large blood vessels at the drainage site. (Courtesy of Mark Topazian, M.D.)

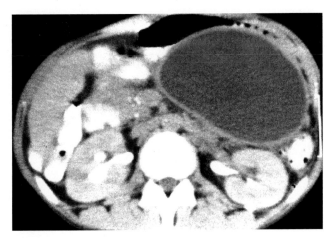

FIGURE 47-15. Contrast computed tomographic scan of pancreas, which demonstrates a large pseudocyst with thick walls.

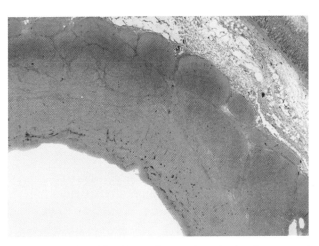

FIGURE 47-16. Histology of pseudocyst showing nonepithelial lining. The cyst is enclosed in a fibrous connective tissue from the inflammatory reaction.

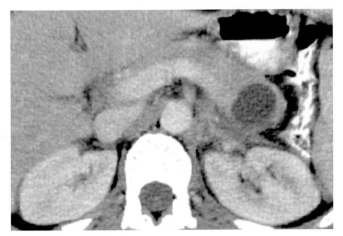

FIGURE 47-17. Contrast computed tomographic (CT) scan of pancreas showing a cystic lesion in the tail. CT scan may not differentiate a pseudocyst from a cystic neoplasm. (Courtesy of Howard Taubin, M.D.)

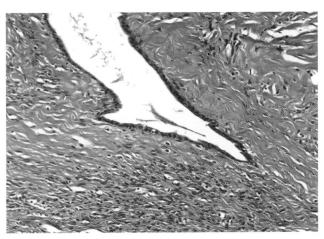

FIGURE 47-18. Histology of this cystic lesion demonstrated the columnar epithelial lining of a cystadenoma.

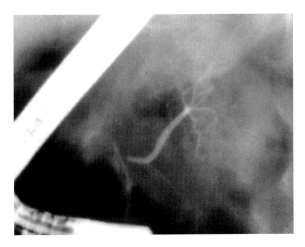

FIGURE 47-19. Endoscopic retrograde cholangiopancreatographic image in pancreas divisum. Injection of the major ampulla results in filing of the duct of Wirsung, which terminates in the pancreas head with arborization and does not fill the dorsal pancreatic duct. Injection of the minor ampulla would have filled the dorsal pancreatic duct in the body and tail.

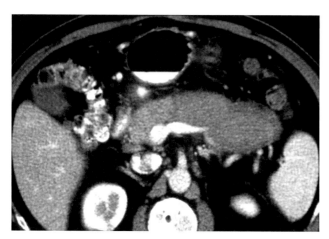

FIGURE 47-20. Contrast computed tomographic image of pancreas in a patient with autoimmune pancreatitis. The large smooth nodules are typical of this disease and are seen throughout the pancreas. These changes can be confused with neoplasms. (Courtesy of Jeff Lee, M.D. and David Carr-Locke, M.D.)

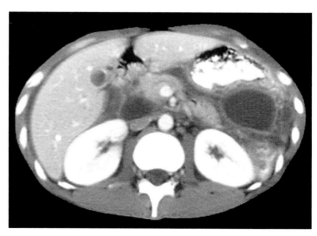

FIGURE 47-21. Contrast computed tomographic scan demonstrating multiple fluid collections complicating acute pancreatitis. These may resolve spontaneously, organize into pseudocysts, or rarely become infected.

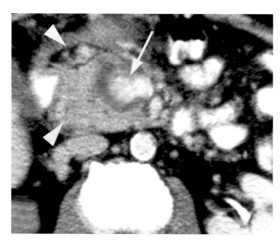

FIGURE 47-22. Contrast computed tomographic scan demonstrating acute bleeding observed as extravasation of intravenous contrast (*arrow*) into a pseudoaneurysm (*arrowheads*) of the splenic artery. The patient was successfully treated by angiographic embolization of the feeding vessel. (Courtesy of Caroline Taylor, M.D.)

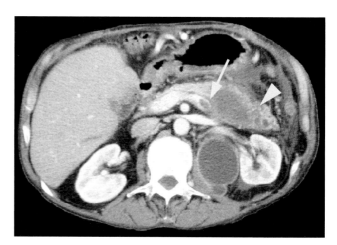

FIGURE 47-23. Contrast computed tomographic scan of abdomen demonstrating splenic vein thrombosis, which appears as a filling defect (*arrow*) within the splenic vein. Note the adjacent inflammation involving the pancreatic tail (*arrowhead*). (Courtesy of Caroline Taylor, M.D.)

48

CHRONIC PANCREATITIS

CHUNG OWYANG ■ POONPUTT CHOTIPRASIDHI

Chronic pancreatitis is defined as an inflammatory disease of the pancreas characterized by persistent and often progressive lesions resulting in functional impairment and structural alterations. Alcohol use in western societies (70% to 80%) and malnutrition worldwide represent the leading causes of chronic pancreatitis. Metabolic and mechanical disturbances and hereditary disposition also have been implicated (Fig. 48-1).

Pain is the most important symptom of chronic pancreatitis. Possible causes include inflammation of the pancreas, increased intrapancreatic pressure, neural inflammation, and extrapancreatic causes such as common bile duct stenosis and duodenal stenosis. Clinical and experimental evidence suggests that pain may be related to increased intraductal pressure caused by continued pancreatic secretion in the face of ductal obstruction caused by strictures, intraductal stones (Fig. 48-2), or destruction of pancreatic ducts (Fig. 48-3). Intrapancreatic neural inflammation is another factor that may play an important role in the genesis of pain in chronic pancreatitis. Morphologic studies indicate that there is an alteration in the perineurial sheath that ordinarily shields nerves from surrounding connective tissue (Fig. 48-4). The damaged perineurium allows penetration of biologically active materials from the surrounding extracellular matrix, and pain may result from continual stimulation of the sensory nerves by noxious substances. Malabsorption is a serious problem in chronic pancreatitis. Malabsorption, however, occurs only after the capacity for enzyme secretion is reduced by more than 90% (Fig. 48-5). In chronic pancreatitis caused by alcoholism, it usually takes 10 to 20 years for severe pancreatic insufficiency and steatorrhea to develop.

The multiple tests available for the diagnosis of chronic pancreatitis can be separated into chemical measurements of pancreatic function and radiologic procedures that provide information on pancreatic structure. Among the pancreatic function tests, the direct stimulatory tests with secretin or cholecystokinin are most sensitive and specific for evaluation of pancreatic function.

Pancreatic structural changes such as calcification, masses, ductal irregularities, enlargements, and cysts may be detected with various radiologic and ultrasonic techniques. The demonstration of diffuse, speckled calcification of the pancreas on a plain radiograph of the abdomen is diagnostic of chronic pancreatitis (Fig. 48-6). Although the sensitivity of this finding is limited (30% to 40%), plain radiography of the abdomen should be the first diagnostic test used to establish the diagnosis of chronic pancreatitis, because a positive finding obviates the need for additional testing.

The development during the last 15 years of ultrasound, computed tomographic (CT) scanning, and endoscopic retrograde cholangiopancreatography (ERCP) has made it possible to assess routinely the gross structure of the pancreas. These tests all have excellent specificity and reasonably good sensitivity. Ultrasound is the simplest and least expensive of the three imaging techniques. Characteristic findings include calcification, dilation of the pancreatic duct, and pancreatic enlargement (Fig. 48-7). The reported sensitivity of ultrasound scanning for chronic pancreatitis is on the order of 70% and the specificity is 90%. CT scanning is 10% to 20% more sensitive than ultrasound scanning in the diagnosis of chronic pancreatitis. The most helpful diagnostic findings on CT scans include ductal dilation, calcification (Fig. 48-8), and cystic lesions. Less helpful diagnostic findings include enlargement or atrophy of the pancreas and heterogeneous density of the parenchyma. ERCP is considered to be the most sensitive and specific test for the diagnosis of chronic pancreatitis. In minimal pancreatitis, the changes are limited to the branches and fine ducts, which show dilation and irregularity (Fig. 48-9). Moderate pancreatitis is characterized by the additional finding of minor irregularity of the main pancreatic duct. Advanced pancreatitis has the additional findings of cystic dilation of the main pancreatic duct and pancreatic atrophy (Fig. 48-10).

Endoscopic ultrasound (EUS) has emerged as a means of obtaining detailed images of the pancreas (Figs. 48-11 and 48-12). Several reports suggest that this technique is equivalent to ERCP; both tests exhibit sensitivities and specificities of greater than 80% in moderate and severe chronic pancreatitis. However, the role of EUS in the diagnosis of mild chronic pancreatitis remains to be determined. The diagnosis of chronic pancreatitis by EUS is based on abnormalities in the pancreatic duct and/or parenchyma. Most reports used nine features, of which a minimum of three must be present. Parenchymal abnormalities include hyperechoic foci, hyperechoic strands, glandular lobularity, and cysts. Ductal findings may include duct dilation, irregularity, hyperechoic ductal margins, dilated side branches, and stones. Unlike ERCP, EUS has no risk for inducing pancreatitis. EUS-guided fine-needle aspiration can differentiate chronic pancreatitis from malignancy. ERCP and EUS are costly, invasive procedures that should be used only when less invasive procedures fail to substantiate the diagnosis of chronic pancreatitis.

Pancreatic pseudocyst is the most common complication of chronic pancreatitis; it occurs in as many as 25% of cases in some series. It represents a collection of pancreatic juice outside the normal boundaries of the ductal system, which is enclosed by a fibrous tissue membrane (Fig. 48-13). Abdominal ultrasound is most frequently used in the diagnosis and management of pseudocyst (Fig. 48-14). CT scanning has emerged as the single most accurate method of diagnosing pancreatic pseudocyst (Fig. 48-15). In addition to having a high accuracy rate, CT scanning provides structural details, such as size of the common duct or pancreatic duct, that have important bearing on the choice of operative approach. ERCP may demonstrate the anatomic relation between a pseudocyst and the main pancreatic duct (Fig. 48-16). However, not all gastroenterologists and surgeons have found routine preoperative ERCP desirable because of the risk of secondary infection.

Splenic venous thrombosis occurs among at least 20% of patients with chronic pancreatitis. It is usually caused by compression and fibrosis resulting from pancreatitis. Splenic venous thrombosis may cause gastric varices (Fig. 48-17) and at times either esophageal or colonic varices. The most important symptom of splenic venous thrombosis is bleeding from varices. The diagnosis can be made by means of CT scanning with bolus injection, which demonstrates varices around the stomach and in proximity to the spleen (Fig. 48-18). The treatment of choice is splenectomy, which decreases venous outflow through the varices, thereby reducing pressure.

Medical treatment of chronic pancreatitis is aimed mainly at the control of pain and correction of malabsorption with adequate pancreatic enzyme replacement. Control of pain includes avoidance of alcohol, use of analgesics, and treatment with celiac plexus block. Celiac plexus block can be performed percutaneously (Figs. 48-19 and 48-20) and should be considered only for patients with refractory pain that does not respond to medical therapy. The outcome of celiac block, however, is not as good in pancreatitis as in pancreatic cancer. This may reflect the fact that pain from chronic pancreatitis usually has a "central" component, which means that specialized nociceptive impulses are not needed to experience pain, and thus a nerve block is not expected to have a significant beneficial effect.

Increase in intrapancreatic pressure is believed to play an important role in the pathogenesis of pain in chronic pancreatitis. Hence, strategies to reduce intrapancreatic pressure have been designed to combat pain in chronic pancreatitis. These include endoscopic stenting in patients with isolated stricture of the main pancreatic duct (Figs. 48-21 and 48-22), pancreatic enzyme replacement, and surgical decompression. A number of studies show that oral pancreatic enzymes may reduce pain in some patients with chronic pancreatitis.

The mechanism appears to involve a process termed "negative feedback inhibition"; that is, intraduodenal administration of trypsin or chymotrypsin is capable of inhibiting the release of cholecystokinin (CCK) and pancreatic enzyme secretion. It is conceivable that in patients with chronic pancreatitis, decreased enzyme secretion may result in hyperstimulation of the pancreas and produce pain. Effective enzyme replacement therapy might reduce pancreas stimulation, decrease intraductal pressure, and diminish pain.

After all medical measures have failed to relieve pain, surgery should be considered. The type of surgery is selected according to the perceived pain mechanism for the pain. Patients who have ductal dilation have a 60% to 70% chance of obtaining pain relief with either a partial resection with pancreaticojejunostomy or lateral pancreaticojejunostomy (modified Puestow) (Fig. 48-23). The modified Puestow pancreaticojejunostomy is particularly suitable for patients who have ductal obstruction and dilation. It is a safe and effective operation with less than 5% morbidity, less than 2% mortality, and approximately 60% effective pain relief. On the other hand, for patients with moderate to severe parenchymal disease and no ductal dilation, partial pancreatic resection should be considered. For patients with diffuse parenchymal disease, 95% distal resection is recommended, whereas local resection of the major site of involvement may be sufficient for those with regional parenchymal disease. Overall, 50% of these patients have had satisfactory results.

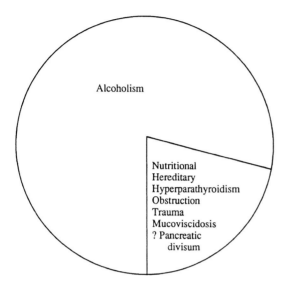

FIGURE 48-1. Etiologic factors in chronic pancreatitis. Factors associated with or known to cause chronic pancreatitis are shown. Alcoholism accounts for 70% to 80% of cases in western societies.

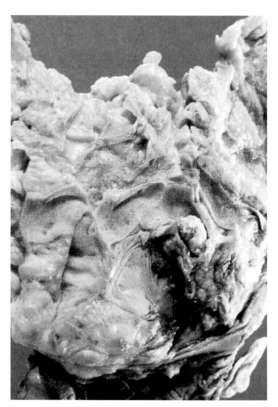

FIGURE 48-2. Surgical specimen of pancreas of a patient with advanced chronic pancreatitis. A pancreatic stone in the main pancreatic duct is causing obstruction.

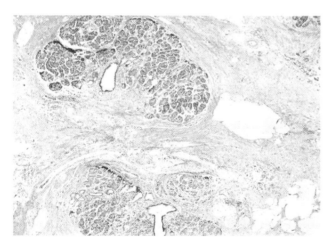

FIGURE 48-3. Histological appearance of chronic pancreatitis. Bands of fibrous tissue have replaced the acini, and the ducts have been destroyed (H&E stain). (Courtesy of Dr. Henry Appelman.)

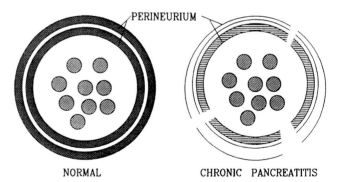

FIGURE 48-4. Diagram of damage to the perineurium that occurs in chronic pancreatitis. Intact perineurium normally provides a barrier, whereas damaged perineurium allows penetration of biologically active materials from the surrounding extracellular matrix.

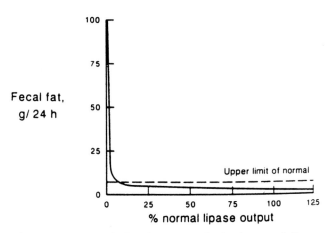

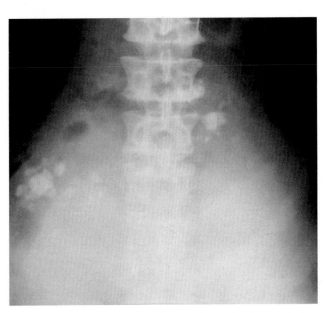

FIGURE 48-5. Relation between steatorrhea and lipase output. Steatorrhea does not occur until lipase output is reduced to less than 10% of normal.

FIGURE 48-6. Plain abdominal radiograph demonstrates extensive calcification in the duct system of a patient with chronic calcific pancreatitis caused by alcoholism.

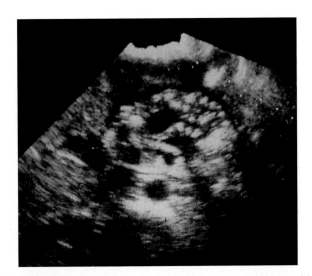

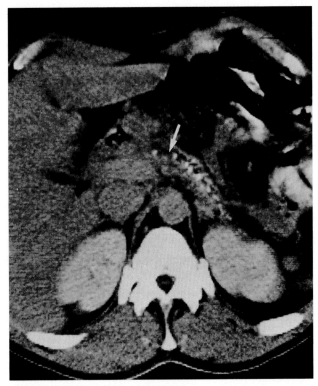

FIGURE 48-7. Transverse sonogram of a patient with chronic pancreatitis demonstrates a pancreas that is densely echogenic because of a combination of multiple calculi within the ducts and pancreatic fibrosis.

FIGURE 48-8. Chronic pancreatitis. Computed tomography scan shows pancreatic atrophy along with multiple intraductal calculi and dilation of the pancreatic duct (*arrow*).

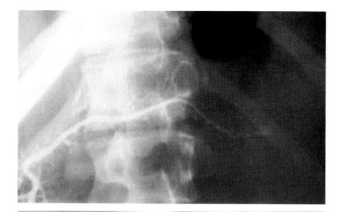

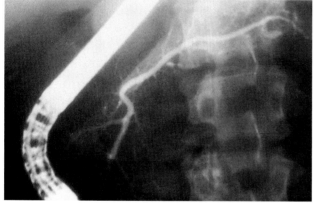

FIGURE 48-9. Endoscopic retrograde cholangiopancreatogram shows mild chronic pancreatitis. The main duct is of normal caliber, but the side branches are irregular. (Courtesy of Dr. Jeffrey L. Barnett.)

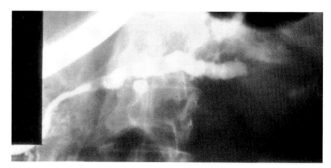

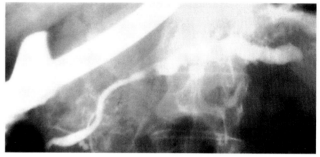

FIGURE 48-10. Endoscopic retrograde cholangiopancreatogram shows severe chronic pancreatitis (gross irregularity of side branches and irregular dilation of pancreatic duct). (Courtesy of Dr. Jeffrey L. Barnett.)

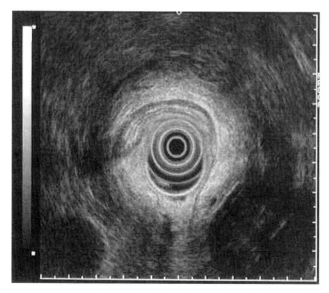

FIGURE 48-11. Endoscopic ultrasound showing mild chronic pancreatitis. Characteristic features include hyperechoic pancreatic duct margins and irregular contour of the pancreatic duct.

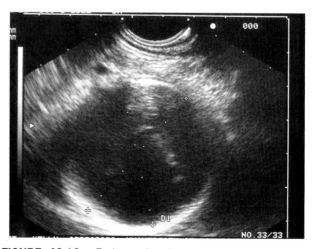

FIGURE 48-12. Endoscopic ultrasound showing a large pseudocyst (4.4 × 4.6 cm) with a calcified rim from a patient with chronic pancreatitis.

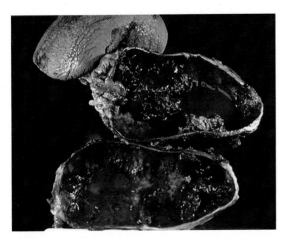

FIGURE 48-13. Pseudocyst in the tail of the pancreas. (Courtesy of Dr. Henry Appelman.)

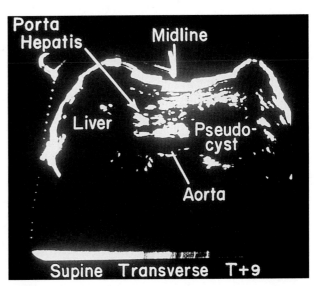

FIGURE 48-14. Transverse sonogram of a patient with chronic pancreatitis shows a large pseudocyst in the body and tail of the pancreas.

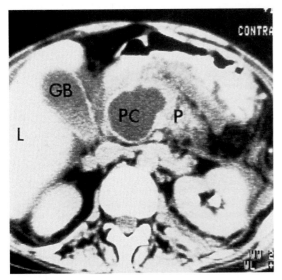

FIGURE 48-15. Computed tomographic scan of a patient with chronic pancreatitis demonstrates a pseudocyst (*PC*) in the head of the pancreas and diffuse enlargement of the pancreas (*P*). *GB,* gallbladder; *L,* liver.

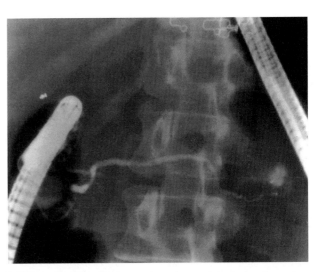

FIGURE 48-16. Endoscopic retrograde cholangiopancreatogram demonstrates extravasation of contrast material from the pancreatic duct into a pseudocyst.

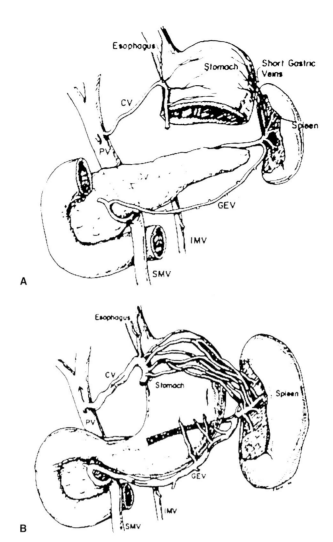

FIGURE 48-17. A: Normal venous anatomy. The splenic vein (*SV*) is posterior to the pancreas. **B:** Splenic venous thrombosis. Reversed direction of flow is shown (*arrow*). Left-sided portal hypertension leads to gastric varices and dilation of the short gastric veins, gastroepiploic vein (*GEV*), and coronary vein (*CV*). The portal vein (*PV*) is patent. *IMV,* inferior mesenteric vein; *SMV,* superior mesenteric vein.

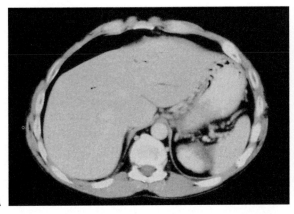

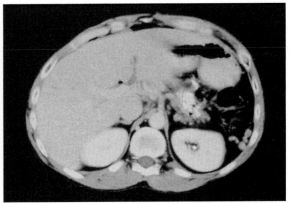

FIGURE 48-18. Computed tomographic scan shows splenic venous thrombosis. **A:** Varices of short gastric veins next to the enlarged spleen. Varices also are present next to the lesser curve of the stomach. **B:** Calcifications in the pancreas and varices (**lower right corner**).

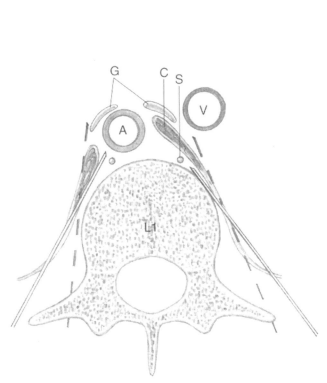

FIGURE 48-19. Diagram (transverse section) of needle position using classic and transcrural approaches to the celiac plexus. *A,* aorta; *C,* right diaphragmatic crus; *G,* celiac ganglia; *L1,* vertebral body of first lumbar vertebra (upper part); *S,* splanchnic nerve(s); *V,* vena cava.

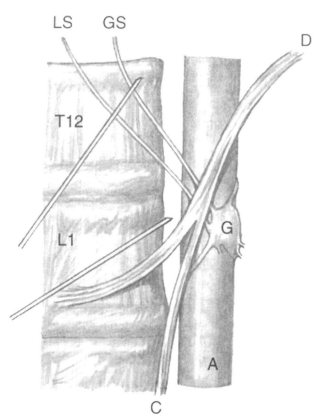

FIGURE 48-20. Diagram of needle position for classical (**lower needle**) celiac plexus block and for splanchnic (**upper needle**) nerve block. *A,* aorta; *C,* right crus; *D,* diaphragma; *G,* celiac ganglia; *GS,* greater splanchnic nerve; *L1,* vertebral body of first lumbar vertebra: *LS,* lesser splanchnic nerve; *T12,* vertebral body of twelfth thoracic vertebra.

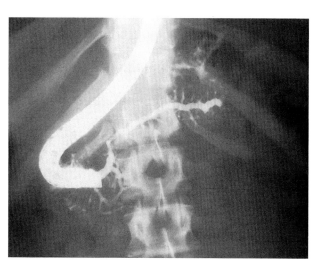

FIGURE 48-21. Endoscopic retrograde cholangiogram of a patient with chronic pancreatitis shows a stricture in the proximal pancreatic duct.

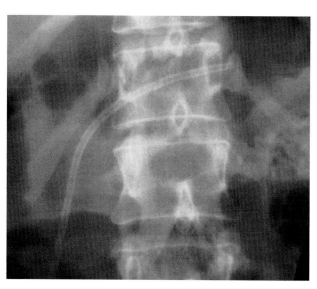

FIGURE 48-22. Endoscopic stent placement in the main pancreatic duct to facilitate pancreatic drainage.

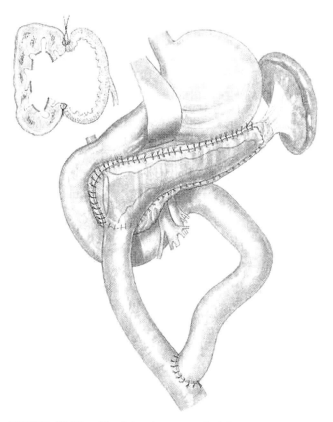

FIGURE 48-23. The lateral pancreaticojejunostomy is performed by anastomosing the jejunum to the anterior capsule of the pancreas. Nonabsorbable suture material is used to make this anastomosis. The procedure can be performed in a continuous or interrupted manner. The jejunojejunostomy is made approximately 40 cm distal to the pancreatico-jejunostomy.

49

NONENDOCRINE TUMORS OF THE PANCREAS

JOHN P. DUFFY ■ HOWARD A. REBER

Nonendocrine tumors of the pancreas include multiple pathological entities such as ductal adenocarcinoma, cystadenoma and cystadenocarcinoma of mucinous and serous varieties, intraductal papillary mucinous neoplasia (IPMN), solid and papillary epithelial neoplasms of the pancreas (SPENP), giant cell tumors, and acinar cell tumors. By far the most important of these, and the main focus of this chapter, is adenocarcinoma of the pancreas.

ADENOCARCINOMA OF THE PANCREAS

Adenocarcinoma of the pancreas is the fourth leading cause of cancer death in the United States, with approximately 29,000 new cases diagnosed each year. At diagnosis, the majority of patients have advanced disease, and only 15% to 20% of patients are candidates for potentially curative surgical resection. The overall 5-year survival rate for pancreatic adenocarcinoma remains dismal at 3%. However, recent series demonstrate operative mortality rates less than 2% and 5-year survival rates after resection of 17% to 20%. Patients whose tumors are resected with clean surgical margins and without microscopic nodal metastases have 5-year survival rates as high as 25%, and those with well-differentiated tumors may have a 5-year survival rate as high as 50%. These figures underscore the important role of surgical resection as the only therapy with the potential to cure this aggressive disease.

Ductal adenocarcinoma makes up more than 90% of all malignant exocrine pancreatic tumors. Most of these neoplasms (67%) occur in the head of the gland, where they often obstruct the intrapancreatic portion of the common bile duct as well as the pancreatic duct. More advanced tumors may invade or compress the duodenum, causing bleeding or duodenal obstruction. Tumors of the head of the pancreas are usually at least 2 cm in diameter when they are first diagnosed, and most tumors that are resected have a median diameter of 2.5 to 3.5 cm. The rest occur in the body or tail, or diffusely throughout the pancreas. Because they are anatomically distant from the common bile duct, tumors of the body and tail produce fewer early symptoms and commonly are larger (5–7 cm) and more advanced when discovered. Advanced body and tail tumors may produce abdominal or back pain as a result of malignant infiltration of retroperitoneal structures and nerves. Although nearly all body and tail pancreatic adenocarcinomas are unresectable by the time of diagnosis, resectable body tumors have a similar prognosis to resectable head tumors.

Several notable pathological characteristics of pancreatic ductal adenocarcinomas deserve mention. These tumors are usually associated with an intense desmoplastic reaction, producing a rock-hard mass capable of compressing nearby structures. These tumors also demonstrate a unique tendency to aggressively infiltrate lymphatic and perineural spaces. Seventy percent to 80% of adenocarcinomas of the head of the pancreas have metastasized to regional lymph nodes by the time they are discovered, which worsens the prognosis but does not preclude cure. Although distant metastases (e.g., to the lung) may occur, pancreatic cancer typically infiltrates locally into the adjacent structures such as the stomach, duodenum, colon, transverse mesocolon, portal and superior mesenteric veins, or celiac or superior mesenteric arteries. The liver is the most common site of intra-abdominal metastasis, and peritoneal seeding of the tumor can also occur. In patients without distant spread, vascular invasion by tumor is the most common reason for unresectability.

Patients with pancreatic cancer usually present with complaints such as weight loss, abdominal pain, back pain, and jaundice. The classical presentation of "painless" jaundice is actually uncommon. Pancreatic cancer can also manifest clinically as new-onset diabetes mellitus or, if pancreatic duct obstruction is present, as pancreatic exocrine insufficiency with malabsorption and steatorrhea. Light-colored acholic stools are associated with biliary obstruction and are accompanied by jaundice and biliuria. Hepatomegaly, a palpable abdominal mass, or ascites usually reflect advanced unresectable disease. The classical Courvoisier gallbladder is actually palpable in only one half of jaundiced patients with pancreatic cancer. Dermal lichenification or excoriation can be seen in those patients with intense pruritus associated with obstructive jaundice.

When the patient's history and physical examination suggest the diagnosis of pancreatic cancer, the workup should strive to achieve two main goals: to establish the diagnosis with a high degree of certainty (usually without a tissue diagnosis), and to determine if the patient is an appropriate candidate for surgical resection. The evaluation should be as cost and time efficient as possible to formulate an appropriate treatment plan. Transcutaneous ultrasound (US) can show large tumors and associated common bile or pancreatic duct dilation (Fig. 49-1), but usually provides limited information about resectability. The best overall test for the diagnosis and staging of pancreatic cancer is the dynamic helical contrast-enhanced computed tomographic (CT) scan of the abdomen. It provides extraordinary detail about the nature of the primary tumor, the adjacent vascular anatomy, and the presence of metastases (e.g., liver) (Fig. 49-2). Helical CT scan is better than conventional CT scan at both tumor detection and identification of metastatic disease (Fig. 49-3). Pancreatic adenocarcinomas are seen on CT as hypodense, nonenhancing areas of the pancreas because they are less well perfused with blood compared to the surrounding normal parenchyma. An experienced gastrointestinal radiologist can accurately predict resectability from a helical CT scan in 80% of patients. However, the study has its greatest sensitivity in the assessment of masses at least 2 cm in diameter. For smaller lesions, or in patients with a negative or equivocal CT scan, endoscopic ultrasound (EUS) may be indicated. EUS can demonstrate tumors as small as 1 centimeter. Its sensitivity for tumor detection may be as high as 99%, and it is also an accurate technique for local staging (70%). Other findings visible on EUS include a dilated common bile duct or a distended main pancreatic duct or side branch duct (Fig. 49-4). EUS may be particularly useful for evaluating vascular involvement, which manifests as abnormal vessel contour, loss of normal tumor-parenchymal interface, visible tumor within the vessel lumen, or nearby dilated peripancreatic venous collaterals. When tissue for diagnosis is desired, EUS allows for sampling of the tumor or nearby lymph nodes via fine-needle aspiration (EUS-FNA) with minimal morbidity (1%–2%) (Fig. 49-5). It is important to emphasize, however, that a negative FNA result never rules out the presence of malignancy.

With advances in other imaging techniques (e.g., CT, magnetic resonance imaging [MRI], EUS), endoscopic retrograde cholangiopancreatography (ERCP) is used less commonly for the diagnosis of pancreatic cancer. However, it does demonstrate certain typical abnormalities. The classical double duct sign can be seen on ERCP when pancreatic cancer obstructs and dilates both the common bile and pancreatic ducts in the head of the pancreas (Fig. 49-6). In tumors of the body or tail of the gland, the pancreatic duct may be narrowed or obstructed (Fig. 49-7). ERCP also allows for the collection of cytology brushings from pancreatic or common bile ductal strictures, which prove the diagnosis of malignancy in 40% to 60% of cases. ERCP has its greatest value as a therapeutic modality. Intraductal stents can be placed to relieve biliary obstruction preoperatively, or as palliation in those patients who are not surgical candidates. For patients whose clinical presentation suggests pancreatic cancer (e.g., pain, jaundice, weight loss) and with a CT scan that demonstrates a mass in the head of the pancreas, ERCP is unnecessary. If CT scan does not show a mass or raises questions about the diagnosis, ERCP or EUS examination should be performed, depending on the expertise available.

Additional techniques for diagnosis and staging of pancreatic cancer include MRI with angiography (MRA) or cholangiopancreatography (MRCP), percutaneous transhepatic cholangiography (PTC), CT-guided FNA (Fig. 49-8), and angiography. MRA and MRCP can provide excellent detail about vascular and biliary anatomy. PTC is most useful in the patient with proximal common bile duct obstruction (e.g., Klatskin tumor), whereas ERCP is preferred for those with evidence of periampullary disease. Angiography has been largely replaced by helical CT scan and MRA, which provide high resolution vascular detail.

The only potentially curative therapy for pancreatic adenocarcinoma is surgical resection in patients with disease localized to the pancreas and adjacent lymph nodes, and without distant metastases or involvement of nearby vascular structures. Neither advanced age nor large tumor size are contraindications to resection. At specialized high-volume pancreatic surgery centers, perioperative mortality rates for pancreaticoduodenectomy (Figs. 49-9 and 49-10) have been lowered from around 20% two decades ago to the current level of less than 2%. For tumors of the head of the pancreas, Whipple resection with pylorus preservation provides adequate tumor extirpation, and it has become the standard operation in most centers. Tumors of the body and tail of the pancreas require distal pancreatectomy and splenectomy.

Surgical resection begins with meticulous examination of the peritoneal cavity and its contents. Areas suspicious for metastatic disease are biopsied and sent for frozen-section analysis. In the absence of distant metastases, resectability usually depends on whether the tumor has invaded any major blood vessels. Assessment of vascular involvement requires mobilization of the tumor from surrounding structures. Involvement of the superior mesenteric, celiac, or hepatic arteries precludes resection. In most cases, so too does invasion of the superior mesenteric or portal vein. If the vessels appear to be free of tumor, the resection proceeds. It is unusual for vascular involvement to be found at the time of operation if it was not already suspected on the basis of helical CT scan or EUS examination performed preoperatively. It is more common (10%–15% of cases) to find small hepatic or peritoneal metastases, which were not evident from the preoperative studies.

For this reason, some surgeons prefer to begin with operative laparoscopy, which permits examination of the liver and peritoneal surfaces and biopsy of any suspicious lesions. If metastatic tumor is found, laparotomy may be avoided. In some cases, palliative gastric and biliary bypasses may even be completed laparoscopically. Laparoscopy may also be appropriate for patients with a high likelihood of unresectability unconfirmed by preoperative studies, for patients with body or tail masses (all have a lower chance of having resectable disease), and for patients with pancreatic masses and ascites (likely the result of unrecognized peritoneal tumor implants). The major drawbacks of laparoscopy are the additional time and expense required for the procedure and the inability to determine the presence of vascular invasion. The latter often requires more extensive dissection and the tactile sensation only afforded by laparotomy.

Despite being undertaken only in those patients with apparently curable disease, resection of pancreatic cancer is not curative in the majority of cases, and postoperative 5-year survival is 17% to 20%. There is evidence that survival is improved with the addition of adjuvant chemotherapy, however [European Study Group for Pancreatic Cancer (ESPAC)-1 Trial]. Other factors that favorably affect prognosis include absence of lymph node involvement, clear surgical resection margins, small tumor size, and well-differentiated tumor grade. The prognosis for patients with unresectable disease remains poor, with median survival only 6 months following diagnosis. For these patients, palliation is the main goal, and it can be achieved through surgical or non-surgical means. Biliary bypass via choledochojejunostomy or cholecystojejunostomy effectively relieves jaundice (Fig. 49-11), as do endoscopically placed bile duct stents. Duodenal obstruction occurs in the minority of patients, often as a near-terminal event. Surgical bypass (gastrojejunostomy) is the preferred therapy (Fig. 49-12), but endoscopically placed duodenal stents represent an alternative that may work well in some patients. Cholecystojejunostomy and gastrojejunostomy also can be performed laparoscopically, which minimizes postoperative morbidity. If a patient develops pancreatic exocrine insufficiency, enzyme replacement is useful to palliate steatorrhea and malabsorption. Palliative chemotherapy is also an option, and gemcitabine, in particular, has been associated with decreased pain and improved quality of life in some patients. The most effective treatment of these patients requires carefully orchestrated efforts from a multidisciplinary team of surgeons, gastroenterologists, and oncologists.

LESS COMMON PANCREATIC NEOPLASMS

Mucinous cystic neoplasms are large (often >5 cm), bulky, unilobular or multilobulated cysts containing mucin that comprise 1% to 2% of exocrine pancreatic tumors (Fig. 49-13). These tumors exhibit a marked female predominance (female-to-male ratio of 6:1) and have a peak age of occurrence in the fifth to seventh decades. The cysts are lined with a mucinous columnar epithelium that forms papillary projections, which may contain foci of dysplastic cells or invasive carcinoma. Radiographic studies reveal calcification within the cysts in about 10% of cases; calcification almost never occurs in pseudocysts. Mucinous cystadenomas are premalignant and should be resected. These tumors have a better prognosis than pancreatic adenocarcinoma; the 5-year survival after a curative resection of a mucinous cystadenocarcinoma is at least 50%.

Serous cystic neoplasms are typically large, encapsulated, multiloculated cystic tumors filled with watery fluid. They usually have a characteristic honeycomb appearance, and the individual cysts are usually smaller than the individual cysts in mucinous cystic neoplasms (Fig. 49-14). They account for about 1% of neoplastic pancreatic lesions and usually occur in elderly females in the sixth and seventh decades of life. These microcystic adenomas are usually asymptomatic and are often discovered incidentally on ultrasound examination or CT scan performed for another reason. Although uncommon, malignant transformation of serous lesions does occur, and these tumors should be resected if it can be accomplished safely. These fluid-filled neoplasms, as well as the mucinous cystic tumors just discussed, should not be confused with pseudocysts, which can be treated with internal or external drainage procedures.

SPENPs are rare neoplasms that are most common in adolescent girls and young women, usually occur in the pancreatic body or tail, can become large enough to produce vague abdominal discomfort, and have a characteristic appearance on CT scan (Fig. 49-15). SPENPs have a favorable prognosis, and most patients are cured by resection. Nevertheless, some may recur locally, and liver metastasis has been reported.

IPMN is an increasingly recognized disease often associated with repeated episodes of pancreatic inflammation. Intraductal tumor growth or secretion of mucus from these lesions can cause obstruction of the pancreatic duct and obstructive chronic pancreatitis. CT scans reveal a dilated pancreatic duct (Fig. 49-16), and EUS can demonstrate dilated main and side branch pancreatic ducts (see Fig. 49-4). ERCP can confirm the ductal dilation as well as intraductal tumor and mucus, which appear as filling defects. A glob of mucus emanating from the gaping orifice of the papilla of Vater is characteristically seen at the time of ERCP. Approximately half the lesions show papillary malignant changes, but even these tumors have a better prognosis than the usual ductal adenocarcinoma. Surgical resection is required to remove any premalignant or malignant disease that may be present and also to relieve the episodes of pancreatitis. This may require total pancreatectomy because the entire pancreatic duct may be affected.

Other less common nonendocrine tumors of the pancreas include giant cell tumors, which are rare tumors characterized by bizarre giant and sarcomatoid cells supported by minimal fibrous tissue. Giant cell tumors have a poor prognosis, even worse than ductal adenocarcinoma. Acinar cell carcinomas are uncommon and characterized by acinar arrangement of cells with little surrounding fibrous stroma. Zymogen granules are present and may be identified by electron microscopy. These tumors are most commonly seen in the elderly, and they can be associated with elevated serum lipase levels, nonsuppurative panniculitis of the extremities and bone marrow, subcutaneous nodules, and polyarthritis.

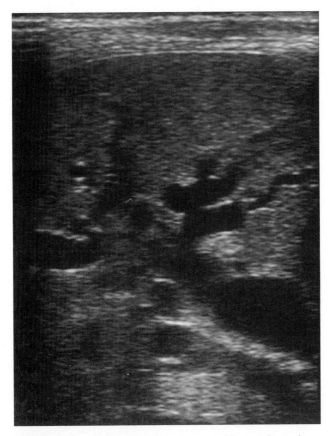

FIGURE 49-1. Transcutaneous ultrasound in a patient whose common bile duct is obstructed by a tumor in the head of the pancreas. The intra- and extrahepatic bile ducts are dilated.

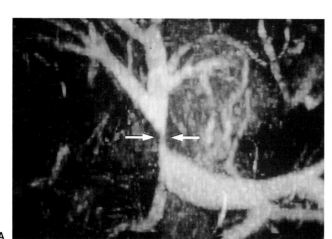
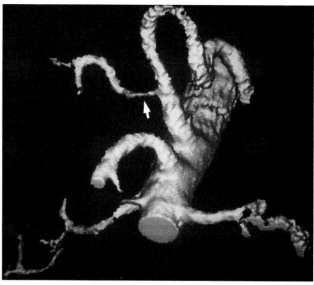

A

B

FIGURE 49-2. A: In this patient with unresectable pancreatic cancer, the helical computed tomographic (CT) scan shows that the tumor has compressed the portal vein (*arrows*). **B:** In another similar patient, the tumor is compressing the hepatic artery at its origin from the celiac axis (*arrow*), which indicates that the tumor is unresectable. In this case, computer reconstruction of the CT images was performed to demonstrate the detailed anatomy of the aorta and its branches. (Courtesy of David Lu, M.D., UCLA Department of Radiology, Los Angeles, CA.)

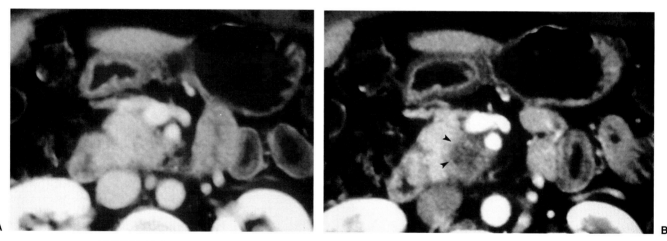

A

B

FIGURE 49-3. A: On a conventional computed tomographic (CT) scan, the primary tumor in the uncinate process of the pancreas is not seen. **B:** The helical (spiral) CT scan performed 4 days later reveals the tumor (*arrowheads*). *(Continued)*

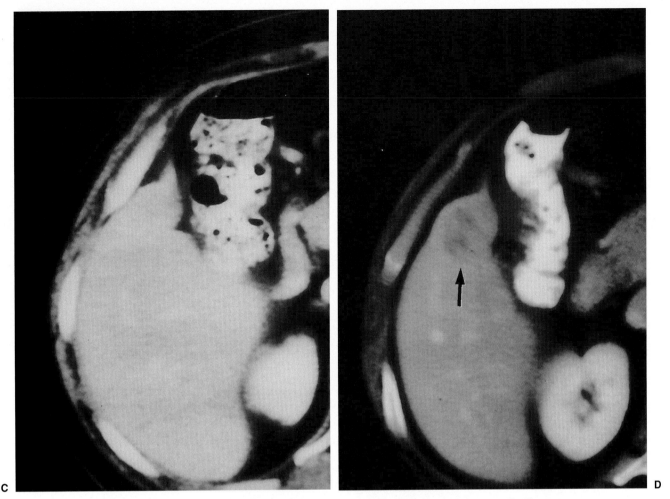

FIGURE 49-3. **C:** On a conventional CT scan, no liver metastases are seen. **D:** The helical CT performed 11 days later reveals an obvious metastatic lesion (*arrow*). (Courtesy of David Lu, M.D., UCLA Department of Radiology, Los Angeles, CA.)

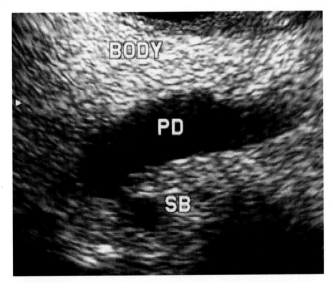

FIGURE 49-4. Linear array endoscopic ultrasound image of pancreatic body showing dilated main pancreatic duct (*PD*) and dilated pancreatic side branch duct (*SB*). Surgical resection confirmed main duct and side-branch intraductal papillary mucinous neoplasia. (Courtesy of James J. Farrell, M.D., Department of Gastroenterology, UCLA School of Medicine, Los Angeles, CA.)

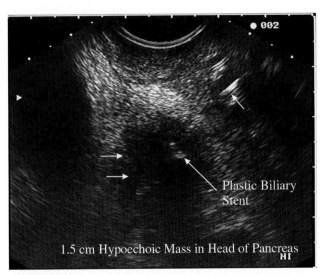

FIGURE 49-5. Endoscopic ultrasound and fine needle aspiration (FNA) of a 1.5-cm localized hypoechoic mass in the head of the pancreas. The FNA needle is seen in the top right-hand corner (*arrow*). A biliary stent is seen in the middle of the mass, which was not visualized on helical computed tomographic scan of the pancreas. Cytologic analysis of the FNA revealed adenocarcinoma. (Courtesy of James J. Farrell, M.D., Department of Gastroenterology, UCLA School of Medicine, Los Angeles, CA.)

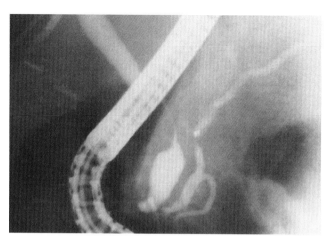

FIGURE 49-6. Endoscopic retrograde cholangiopancreatography of a patient with cancer of the head of the pancreas shows that both the pancreatic and bile ducts are compressed by the tumor. This produces the double duct sign.

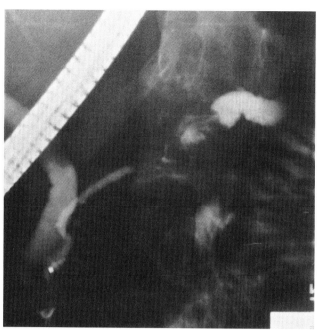

FIGURE 49-7. In this patient with cancer of the body of the pancreas, the duct is compressed in the body of the gland, and the obstructed ductal segment proximal to that point is dilated.

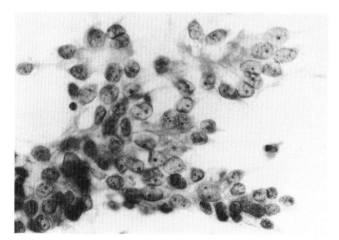

FIGURE 49-8. Fine-needle aspiration of a mass in the body of the pancreas shows cells characteristic of ductal adenocarcinoma of the pancreas. The tumor invaded the retroperitoneal structures and was unresectable.

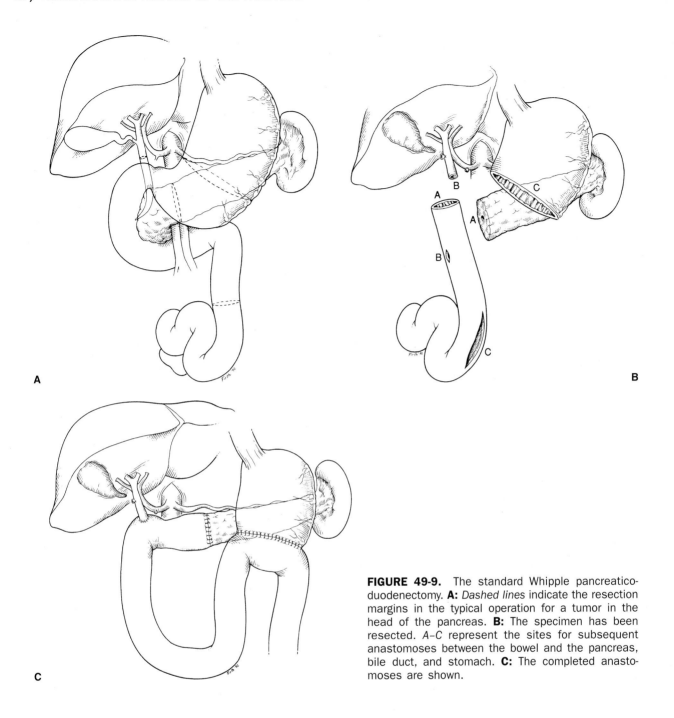

A

B

C

FIGURE 49-9. The standard Whipple pancreatico-duodenectomy. **A:** *Dashed lines* indicate the resection margins in the typical operation for a tumor in the head of the pancreas. **B:** The specimen has been resected. *A–C* represent the sites for subsequent anastomoses between the bowel and the pancreas, bile duct, and stomach. **C:** The completed anastomoses are shown.

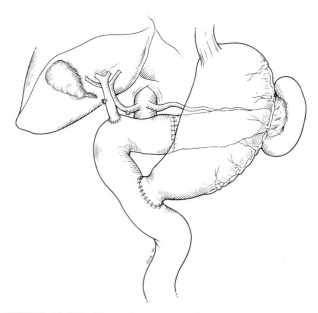

FIGURE 49-10. The pylorus-preserving modification of the standard Whipple pancreaticoduodenectomy is shown. The entire stomach, the pylorus, and several centimeters of duodenum are retained.

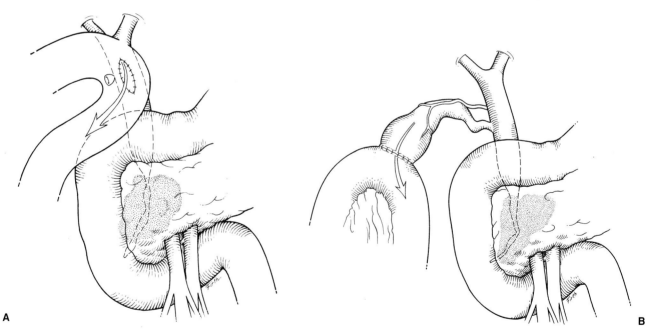

A   B

FIGURE 49-11. **A:** Choledochojejunostomy. **B:** Cholecystojejunostomy. Each of these operations effectively relieves biliary obstruction by diverting the bile into the small intestine proximal to the tumor.

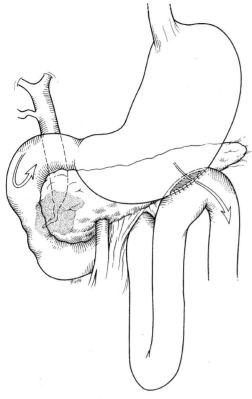

FIGURE 49-12. Gastrojejunostomy. The stomach can now empty into the small intestine directly when the tumor obstructs the duodenum.

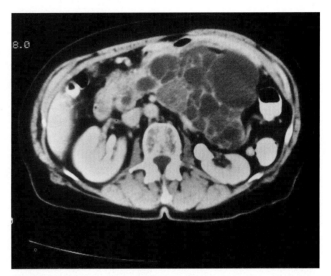

FIGURE 49-13. Computed tomographic scan of a patient with a malignant mucinous cystic neoplasm, which was resected. Note the large cystic structure with internal septations creating multiple large cysts.

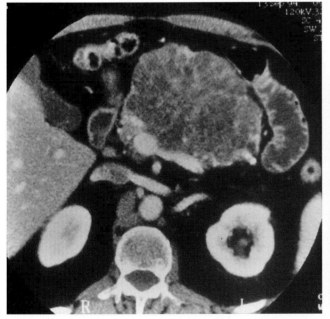

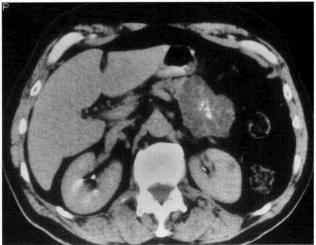

A

B

FIGURE 49-14. Computed tomographic scans of patients with benign serous cystadenomas, both of which were resected with a distal pancreatectomy. **A:** A large lesion suggests the honeycombed appearance of this tumor, which typically contains many very small cystic structures. It can be contrasted with the large cysts seen in Fig. 49-13. **B:** A smaller lesion demonstrates the central calcification, which is sometimes seen.

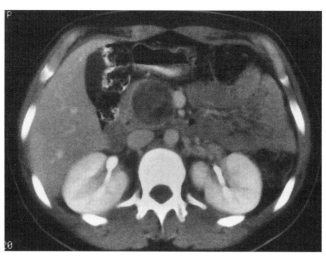

FIGURE 49-15. Computed tomographic scan of a solid and papillary neoplasm in a 21-year-old woman who underwent a Whipple resection. The tumor was removed completely.

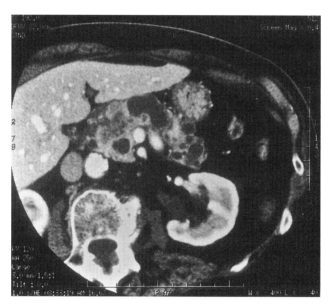

FIGURE 49-16. Computed tomographic scan of a patient with intraductal papillary mucinous neoplasia of the pancreas. In addition to multiple cystic lesions throughout the gland, there is a hypodense mass in the head of the pancreas consistent with a malignant neoplasm. The patient was 89 years old. Because a total pancreatectomy would have been required, surgery was not performed in this woman, who had multiple medical problems.

50

ENDOCRINE NEOPLASMS OF THE PANCREAS

ROBERT T. JENSEN ■ JEFFREY A. NORTON

Endocrine tumors of the pancreas are classified according to the type of clinical syndrome they cause. The seven generally accepted pancreatic endocrine tumor (PET) syndromes include gastrinoma that causes Zollinger-Ellison syndrome, insulinoma, glucagonoma, vasoactive intestinal peptide–secreting tumor (VIPoma) that causes the Verner-Morrison syndrome (also called pancreatic cholera or the watery diarrhea, hypokalemia, and achlorhydria syndrome [WDHA]), somatostatinoma, growth hormone releasing-factor–secreting tumor (GRFoma), and nonfunctional tumors. Other syndromes that should be included in this category are adrenocorticotropic hormone–secreting tumors (ACTHomas), PET-secreting factors that cause hypercalcemia (such as parathyroid hormone-related peptide [PTHrP]), PETs causing the carcinoid syndrome, and PETs secreting renin (one case). These latter syndromes are much more uncommon and not as well characterized as the seven well-established PETs. Some have proposed that pancreatic endocrine tumors (PETs) secreting neurotensin (neurotensinomas), PETs secreting calcitonin, and PETs secreting ghrelin, a 28 amino acid growth hormone secretogogue, also be included. There is no general agreement that these are distinct clinical syndromes and, therefore, are not included as a specific PET syndrome. In all cases except nonfunctional tumors, the ectopic hormone release is associated with a distinct clinical syndrome. With nonfunctional tumors, the clinical symptoms and signs are entirely due to the presence of the tumor itself (e.g., hepatomegaly, weight loss, abdominal mass) and not to the ectopically released peptides. Not all nonfunctional tumors are truly nonfunctional in that many release pancreatic polypeptide (PPomas), some release neurotensin, and almost all release chromogranin A; however, none of these secreted peptides is associated with specific clinical symptoms. All of these PETs share a number of common features, including various aspects of their natural history, pathology, medical treatment options, approaches to tumor localization, surgical options, and treatment options when the tumor is metastatic.

Even though these tumors are generally slow growing, recent studies show a subset that demonstrates aggressive growth. Therefore, effective therapy requires both treatment of the effects of the ectopic hormone overproduction and treatment directed at the tumor itself. With each of these tumors, surgical resection is the treatment of choice. However, except for insulinomas and gastrinomas, with the majority of the other tumors at the time of diagnosis, liver metastases are already present. Similar to carcinoids, almost all PETs except insulinoma possess high densities of somatostatin receptors. Their presence is used for novel localization methods using radiolabeled somatostatin analogs (discussed below) and for treatment with somatostatin analogs. With each of the symptomatic PETs except for insulinomas, the long-acting somatostatin analogs such as octreotide or lanreotide are frequently used to control medically the clinical syndrome caused by the ectopic hormone release and for their antigrowth effects. With this increased ability to control the symptoms caused by hormone overproduction, in the future the prognosis will be increasingly determined by the natural history of the tumor itself.

CLINICAL MANIFESTATIONS, PATHOGENESIS, DIFFERENTIAL DIAGNOSIS, AND DIAGNOSIS

Because these PET syndromes are uncommon, the proper diagnosis requires a continual awareness of the presenting manifestations of these tumor syndromes as well as an awareness that these syndromes can initially present with symptoms that are similar to other much more common conditions. In each instance, except with nonfunctional tumors, the early symptoms are caused by the actions of the ectopically released hormone, whereas late in the course of the disease symptoms caused by metastatic spread of the tumor per se (pain, bleeding, cachexia) may become increasingly important. The general approach to the diagnosis and treatment of all PET syndromes except insulinomas is shown diagrammatically in Fig. 50-1. In general, for these syndromes both inappropriate hormonal hyperfunction (such as increased stool output, acid output, effects on blood glucose) need to be demonstrated at the same time as an inappropriately elevated plasma hormone concentration is shown. After diagnosis, it is important to establish whether the PET is occurring alone (sporadic tumor) or is part of an inherited disorder. The most common inherited disorder associated with PETs is multiple endocrine neoplasia type 1 (MEN1) (nonfunctional > gastrinomas > insulinomas > GRFomas, VIPomas, and glucagonomas), but PETs can also occur with Von Recklinghausen disease (duodenal somatostatinomas), von Hippel-Lindau syndrome (nonfunctional), and tuberous sclerosis. It is important to establish if an inherited syndrome is present because it frequently affects the treatment approach and may determine the need for family studies. This should be followed by imaging studies both to localize the primary tumor and to assess the tumor extent (see Fig. 50-1). All of these investigations should be done preferably by a group with considerable experience with PETs because interpretation of these tests requires considerable expertise, and procedures such as sampling for hormone gradients and intraoperative ultrasound are very specialized techniques that may not be generally available (see Fig. 50-1).

The approach and treatment of a patient with possible insulinoma is summarized in Fig. 50-2. The essential point in the diagnosis is to demonstrate hypoglycemia in the presence of an inappropriately elevated insulin level. Important tests used to differentiate a patient with hypoglycemia due to an insulinoma from a patient with hypoglycemia due to the surreptitious use of either insulin or sulfonylureas are shown in Table 50-1. With the availability of human insulin and its low antigenicity, the traditional method of demonstrating anti-insulin antibodies for the diagnosis of surreptitious use of insulin will not generally be useful, thus compounding the difficulty of this diagnostic problem. At the time such a patient is hypoglycemic, if suppressed plasma C-peptide levels can be established this will add diagnostic verification (see Table 50-1). It is also important to note that free C-peptide should be measured because proinsulin bound to anti-insulin antibodies may cause false elevations of the C-peptide level. After diagnosis, tumor localization (Fig. 50-2) is essential and is discussed below.

Figure 50-3 outlines the approach to a patient suspected of having a VIPoma. Both patients with Zollinger-Ellison syndrome and VIPoma can present with secretory diarrhea. These two syndromes can be differentiated by measuring plasma VIP levels, which are normal in patients with gastrinomas and elevated in patients with VIPomas; measuring gastrin, which is elevated in Zollinger-Ellison syndrome and normal to minimally elevated in patients with VIPomas; measuring gastric acid secretion, which is elevated in Zollinger-Ellison syndrome and normal to low in patients with VIPomas; or measuring stool output during nasogastric aspiration or omeprazole treatment because increased stool output persists only in patients with VIPomas. In most series more than 50% of all patients with VIPomas have metastatic, unresectable disease at the time of diagnosis, and thus prolonged symptomatic treatment of the secretory diarrhea with a long-acting somatostatin analog such as octreotide or lanreotide is required. If tumor progression occurs, then treatment with chemotherapy as outlined in Fig. 50-13 may be required.

TUMOR LOCALIZATION

As indicated in Figs. 50-1 through 50-3, all patients with PET syndromes require imaging studies to assess both the extent of tumor and the possible location of the primary tumor. The best initial screening imaging test is somatostatin receptor scintigraphy (SRS) using ^{111}In-labeled octreotide (see Figs. 50-1 through 50-3). Except in patients with insulinomas, the ability of SRS to localize these tumors is based on the fact that all PETs except insulinomas have a high density of somatostatin receptors. For all PETs except insulinomas, SRS has higher sensitivity than conventional imaging studies (computed tomography [CT] scan, magnetic resonance imaging [MRI], angiography, ultrasound) for detecting metastatic disease to the liver and for detecting distant metastases. SRS also allows screening of all body regions with one study and detects the primary tumor with greater sensitivity than other imaging methods.

Because insulinomas frequently possess a low density of somatostatin receptors subtype 2 and 5, which are needed to bind radiolabeled octreotide with high affinity when SRS is performed, either CT or MRI scanning is recommended to detect liver metastases in the 5% to 15% with malignant disease (see Fig. 50-2). Endoscopic ultrasound is recommended as the initial study to localize insulinomas because insulinomas almost invariably are intrapancreatic in location and are small (<1 cm). If endoscopic ultrasound is negative, selective intraarterial injection of calcium with hepatic venous sampling for insulin gradients is particularly helpful for regional localization of the tumor (see Fig. 50-2). A typical result is shown in Fig. 50-4. In this patient, a marked increase in insulin release occurs with injection of calcium into the gastroduodenal artery, supplying the head of the pancreas. Subsequently, an insulinoma was found in the pancreatic head.

In other PETs except insulinomas, for SRS to have maximal sensitivity it is essential that single photon emission computed tomography (SPECT) imaging be used to analyze the results. If extensive metastatic disease to the liver is present, the diagnosis should be confirmed by biopsy. If metastatic disease is not present on SRS and no primary tumor is seen, additional imaging studies should be undertaken (see Fig. 50-1). SRS detects only 50% to 80% of primary PETs, primarily depending on their size. If SRS is negative, endoscopic ultrasound and angiography with determination of hormonal gradients after calcium (VIPoma, glucagonoma) or secretin (gastrinoma) should be performed to further localize the tumor. The ability of endoscopic ultrasound to localize a PET in a patient with the MEN1 syndrome is shown in Fig. 50-5. In this patient, a 3.5-cm tumor was localized in the pancreatic body with two adjacent lymph nodes, each of which were subsequently removed at surgery. At surgery all patients should have intraoperative ultrasound performed because small lesions missed by palpation can be detected (see Figs. 50-1 through 50-3).

Metastatic glucagonoma to the liver as well as metastatic disease with other PETs is frequently localized by CT scanning, especially if combined with intravenous contrast medium (Fig. 50-6). A number of recent studies show that PETs can also be detected by MRI, and results from a patient with primary VIPoma in the pancreatic tail are shown in Figs. 50-7 and 50-8; metastatic glucagonoma to the liver is shown in Fig. 50-9. With MRIs, variations of the magnetic field and imaging sequence allow the same tumor to appear dark on one scan (T1-weighted) and bright (T2-weighted) on another scan sequence (see Figs. 50-7 through 50-9). MRI scans have the additional advantage that no ionizing radiation is involved. Glucagonomas are hypervascular tumors, as are other PETs, and are seen clearly on angiography, as is demonstrated in Fig. 50-10 for a patient with metastatic glucagonoma to the liver. In some cases, small metastases in the liver and small primary tumors can be seen on angiography when SRS is negative; therefore, it is recommended that angiography be performed on a patient with a PET and a negative SRS, prior to surgery (Fig. 50-13; see Figs. 50-1 through 50-3).

SRS is particularly sensitive for detecting hepatic metastases, and in one recent comparative study it was equal in sensitivity to all conventional imaging studies combined (ultrasound, CT scan, MRI, and selective angiography). Figure 50-11 demonstrates this greater sensitivity compared to MRI in a patient with a metastatic PET to the liver with a serum chromogranin A level of 5200 ng/mL (normal <50). An additional left-lobe liver metastasis is seen on the SRS that is not seen on the MRI. Bone metastases are being diagnosed late in the disease course in patients with malignant PETs, and their detection is essential for determining appropriate therapy. SRS is superior to bone scanning for detection of bone metastases and has the advantage over MRI that distant metastases to ribs and nonspinous areas can easily be detected; SRS is therefore the recommended method. Figure 50-12 shows results of these three methods and the greater sensitivity of SRS for detecting bone metastases in a patient with a malignant PET releasing ACTH and causing Cushing syndrome.

Figure 50-13 outlines the approach to a patient with a metastatic PET syndrome. Whereas in patients with insulinoma only 5% to 15% of the tumors are found to be malignant, in older studies more than 50% of patients with the other PETs had metastatic disease at the time of diagnosis. In a small percentage of cases (<5% to 20%), it may be possible to resect the tumor either because it is localized to regional lymph nodes or to only one lobe of the liver. It has been recommended that surgical resection be considered in these cases (see Fig. 50-13). However, in the majority of cases the tumor is not resectable, and in these cases if the tumor is functional, a long-acting somatostatin analog such as lanreotide or octreotide should be used to control the symptoms (see Fig. 50-13). Progressive disease occurs in greater than 60% of patients with liver metastases. Among patients with symptomatic tumors, chemotherapy with dacarbazine should be considered to treat patients with malignant glucagonoma; therapy with streptozotocin and doxorubicin should be considered in patients with other PETs. Studies show that treatment with long-acting somatostatin analogs, either alone or in combination with α-interferon, may control the hormone excess state and decrease tumor growth rate. Because of its low incidence of side effects and ease of administration [monthly injection of octreotide long-acting release (LAR)], octreotide is the recommended initial antitumor treatment in patients with progressive disease. Chemoembolization of a symptomatic tumor may also help control symptoms (see Fig. 50-13). More than 80% of patients with nonfunctional tumors at presentation have metastatic disease to the liver. If progression occurs or symptoms develop because of the tumor itself, first treatment with somatostatin analogs (plus α-interferon) is recommended. If this treatment fails, then chemotherapy with streptozotocin and doxorubicin is recommended.

TABLE 50-1
Results of Laboratory Tests Used to Distinguish Factitious Hypoglycemia from Hypoglycemia Caused by Insulinoma

LABORATORY TEST	SURREPTITIOUS USE OF:		INSULINOMA
	Insulin	*Sulfonylureas*	
Plasma insulin	Normal or elevated	Normal or elevated	Normal or elevated
Plasma proinsulin	Normal or decreased	Normal	Increased in >85%
Plasma C-peptide	Decreased	Normal or elevated	Normal or elevated
Plasma antibodies to insulin	Present	Not present	Not present
Plasma or urine sulfonylureas detected	Not present	Present	Not present

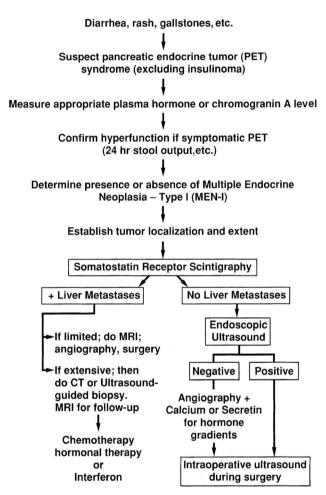

FIGURE 50-1. Schematic diagram of the general approach to diagnosis and treatment of all pancreatic endocrine tumor (PET) syndromes except insulinomas. Insulinomas are considered separately because they differ from all of the other PETs in frequency of not being imaged (30% to 50%) with somatostatin receptor scintigraphy (SRS) and being primarily nonmalignant (more than 90% are benign). SRS is shown to be the initial localization study because it is the most sensitive and allows imaging of the entire body. Other imaging studies detect few patients with liver metastases if the SRS is negative; however, endoscopic ultrasound or angiography with venous sampling for hormonal gradients can detect primary tumors in greater than 20% of patients who have normal finding at SRS.

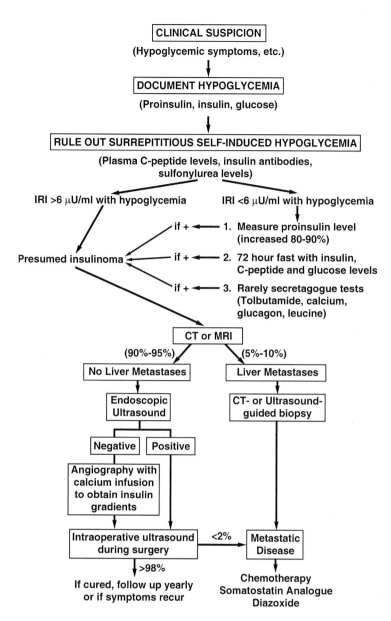

FIGURE 50-2. Algorithm for the diagnosis and treatment of a patient with insulinoma. After documentation of the hypoglycemia, it is important to rule out self-induced hypoglycemia caused by surreptitious use of insulin or sulfonylureas. If plasma insulin-like immunoreactivity (IRI) exceeds 6 μU/mL and hypoglycemia is present, then a presumed diagnosis of insulinoma can be made and one can proceed to tumor localization studies. In the small percentage of cases in which hypoglycemia is present but the IRI is less than 6 μU/mL, an additional evaluation is needed. The 72-hour fast is the most commonly used test to monitor plasma insulin, glucose, and C-peptide levels. Secretagogue provocative tests (tolbutamide, calcium, glucagon, or leucine) rarely are needed. Insulinomas are usually benign (90% to 95% of cases). The malignant cases can be detected with a computed tomographic scan or magnetic resonance imaging for liver metastases. Endoscopic ultrasound is more sensitive than other imaging studies for detection of insulinomas in 80% to 95% of cases. If endoscopic ultrasound does not localize the insulinoma, selective intraarterial injection of calcium with sampling of hepatic veins for insulin concentrations should be performed to localize the insulinoma to the appropriate pancreatic area. Intraoperative ultrasound should be used routinely.

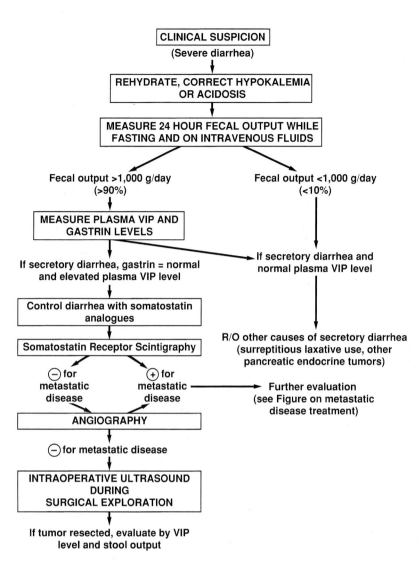

FIGURE 50-3. Algorithm summarizing approach and treatment of a patient with a suspected vasoactive intestinal polypeptide-secreting tumor (VIPoma) syndrome. It is important to measure 24-hour fecal output while the patient is completely fasting and is rehydrated after correction of electrolyte or acid-base imbalance by intravenous fluids. Greater than 80% of patients with VIPomas have more than 3000 g/day of stool output. It has been reported that no patients with VIPoma have daily stool output less than 700 g/day. Angiography is recommended if somatostatin receptor scintigraphy (SRS) is negative prior to surgery because it can detect small liver metastases not imaged by SRS. Intraoperative ultrasound should be used because recent studies with other pancreatic endocrine tumors demonstrate that some small tumors are only localized with this procedure. If metastatic disease is present and unresectable or if no tumor is found, postoperative treatment with long-acting somatostatin analogs (octreotide, lanreotide) should be continued. The dosage should be adjusted to control symptoms. If metastatic disease is present and there is progressive disease or symptoms are not controlled with octreotide, chemotherapy should be considered (see Fig. 50-13).

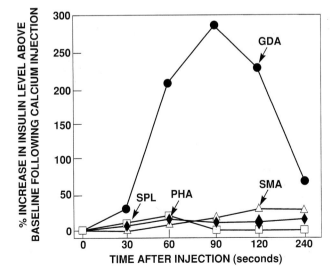

FIGURE 50-4. Localization of an insulinoma by selective intra-arterial injection of calcium with hepatic venous insulin sampling. Calcium (0.025 mEq Ca/Kg normally or 0.01 mEq Ca/Kg in obese patients) was injected selectively into the gastroduodenal artery (*GDA*), superior mesenteric artery (*SMA*), splenic artery (*SPL*), or proper hepatic artery (*PHA*), and hepatic venous blood was sampled for insulin concentration before and 30, 60, 90, 120, and 210 seconds after injection. A 275% increase over the preinjection value occurred with the gastroduodenal artery injection, which is consistent with a 0.9-cm insulinoma located in the pancreatic head area at operation.

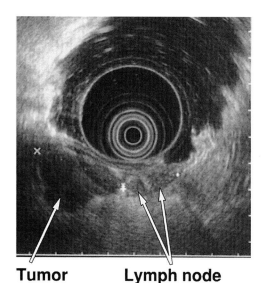

Tumor   **Lymph node**

FIGURE 50-5. Endoscopic ultrasound image in a patient with multiple endocrine neoplasia type 1. A 3-cm tumor was found in the pancreatic body (*labeled tumor*) and two adjacent enlarged lymph nodes. At operation, a 3.5-cm pancreatic endocrine tumor with two lymph nodes containing metastases were found.

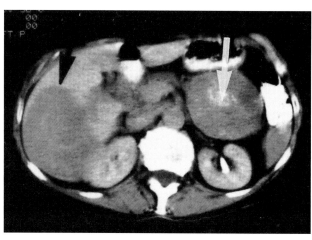

FIGURE 50-6. Computed tomographic scan in a patient with metastatic glucagonoma obtained with both intravenous and oral contrast media. This patient had a 7-cm glucagonoma in the pancreatic tail (*white arrow*) and a large 10-cm metastatic deposit in the right lobe of the liver (*black arrow*).

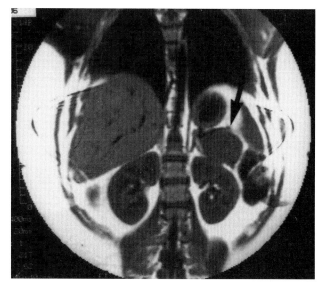

FIGURE 50-7. Magnetic resonance imaging scan of a patient with a large 5-cm vasoactive intestinal polypeptide–secreting tumor located in the tail of the pancreas (*arrow*). This scan represents a sagittal view of a T1-weighted sequence. The tumor is posterior to the stomach, medial to the spleen, and anterior to the kidney. The tumor appears dark on a T1-weighted sequence.

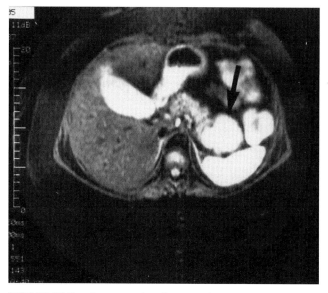

FIGURE 50-8. Cross-sectional magnetic resonance image of a patient with a vasoactive intestinal polypeptide–secreting tumor (VIPoma). This is the same patient as in Fig. 50-7. The tumor is a large VIPoma (*arrow*) located in the tail of the pancreas. The tumor appears bright (*white*) on this T2-weighted short time inversion recovery (STIR) sequence and is easier to see than on the T1-weighted STIR image (Fig. 50-7). The gallbladder, stomach, spleen, and colon also appear bright.

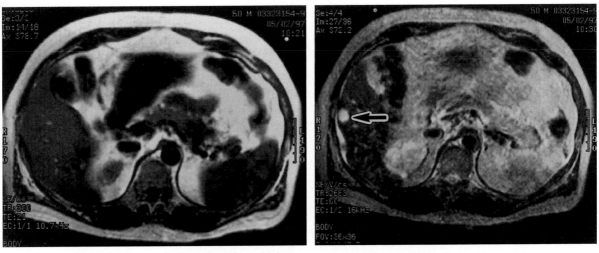

FIGURE 50-9.   Magnetic resonance imaging scan of a patient with metastatic glucagonoma to the liver. **A:** A T1-weighted image. **B:** A T2-weighted image. The metastasis is shown by the *arrow*. This case demonstrates that pancreatic endocrine tumor liver metastases are much better seen on the T2-weighted image.

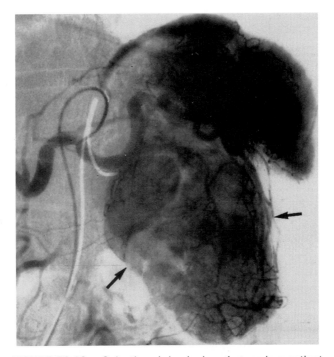

FIGURE 50-10.   Selective abdominal angiogram in a patient with metastatic glucagonoma demonstrates the primary glucagonoma. The splenic artery injection demonstrates a large 8-cm hypervascular primary tumor in the tail of the pancreas (*arrows*) next to the spleen. This is the same patient as in Fig. 50-6.

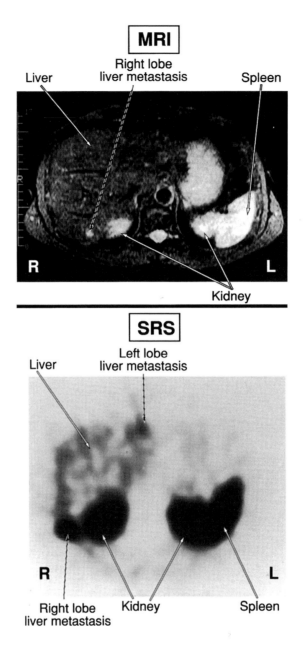

FIGURE 50-11. An example of the greater sensitivity of somatostatin receptor scintigraphy (*SRS*) than magnetic resonance imaging (*MRI*) for identifying bilateral liver metastases in a patient with a malignant pancreatic endocrine tumor metastatic to the liver. The **top panel** is an MRI image showing one metastasis in the right lobe of the liver. No left-lobe metastases were observed. The **bottom panel** is a single photon emission computed tomographic (SPECT) image of the SRS showing a left-lobe liver metastasis and a right-lobe liver metastasis.

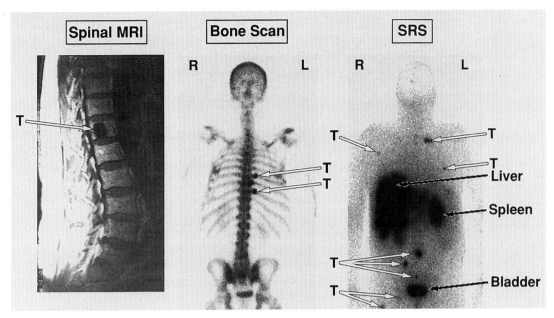

FIGURE 50-12. Detection of bone metastases in a patient with a malignant pancreatic endocrine tumor secreting adrenocorticotropic hormone and with liver metastases. The magnetic resonance image (**left**) shows a single metastasis (*T*) in a thoracic vertebral body. The bone scan (**middle**, posterior view) shows two new left rib metastases, whereas the somatostatin receptor scintigraphy (SRS) (**right**) shows new metastases to the left and right ribs, left scapula, thoracic and lumbar spine, right sacroiliac joint, and right femoral head. Extensive liver metastases are also observed on the SRS. Recent studies demonstrate that the SRS is the best overall method to detect bone metastases in malignant pancreatic endocrine tumors.

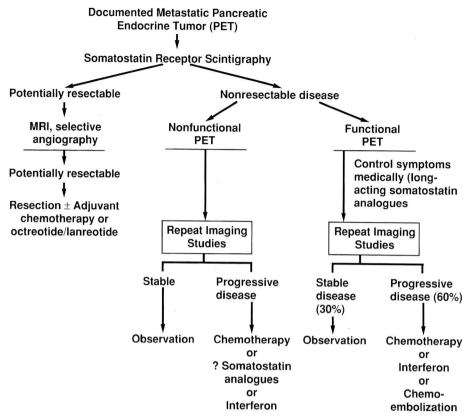

FIGURE 50-13. Algorithm of the treatment of a patient with a metastatic pancreatic endocrine tumor (PET). For all PETs except metastatic insulinoma, recent studies demonstrate that somatostatin receptor scintigraphy (SRS) should be the initial tumor localization method because of its greater sensitivity and ability to give a complete body scan. If surgical resection is feasible without a high morbidity, it should be considered by a surgeon experienced in the surgical treatment of such tumors. Additional imaging with magnetic resonance imaging and selective angiography are helpful for defining the location of the liver metastases and detecting possible small lesions not imaged on the SRS. If the tumor is not resectable in a patient with a functioning pancreatic endocrine tumor, symptoms should be controlled with a long-acting somatostatin analog (octreotide or lanreotide). If symptoms are not controlled or there is progressive disease, chemotherapy, interferon, or chemoembolization should be considered. Dacarbazine is recommended for such patients with metastatic glucagonomas, and streptozotocin or chlorozotocin with fluorouracil is advised for patients with the other functional PET syndromes or with nonfunctional tumors.

HEREDITARY DISEASE OF THE PANCREAS

ASIF KHALID ■ DAVID C. WHITCOMB

Recent developments in the field of molecular genetics have led to new insights encompassing all aspects of pancreatic structure, function, and disease. Specific genetic defects associated with developmental and hereditary diseases such as cystic fibrosis (CF) and hereditary pancreatitis (HP) have made significant contributions to our general understanding of pancreatic physiology and pathophysiology. The following section describes clinical findings in patients with genetic or developmental disorders of the pancreas.

DEVELOPMENTAL ABNORMALITIES

A variety of congenital abnormalities of the pancreas have been observed that reflect defective embryogenesis (see Chapter 46). The clinical features range from agenesis with complete pancreatic exocrine and endocrine insufficiency, to recurrent attacks of acute and chronic pancreatitis, to a variety of incidental findings.

Pancreas divisum is the most common disease-associated congenital abnormality of the pancreas and may be found in up to 7% of autopsy series. Anatomically, the two ductal systems do not unite or communicate and therefore separately drain via the two duodenal papillae; the dominant dorsal system drains through the minor papilla and the smaller ventral system drains through the major papilla (Fig. 51-1). A correlation between pancreas divisum and acute recurrent pancreatitis (ARP), chronic pancreatitis (CP), and abdominal pain syndromes has been noted. However, the majority of individuals with pancreas divisum never develop symptoms. Because the majority of exocrine flow is routed through the minor papilla, it is hypothesized that an increased resistance to flow across this small orifice may result in dorsal duct hypertension and clinical symptoms or an increased predisposition to injury from alcohol and drugs. Endoscopic retrograde cholangiopancreatography (ERCP) has been the diagnostic tool of choice, but the role of magnetic resonance cholangiopancreatography (MRCP) with or without secretin is increasing (Figs. 51-2 and 51-3). Endoscopic therapy aimed at the minor papilla is generally reserved for patients with ARP or CP on the basis of studies that demonstrate positive response rates of 80% and 50%, respectively.

Pancreatic agenesis is extremely rare, and can be caused by mutations in both alleles of the developmental and regulatory *PDX1* gene, rendering it nonfunctional.

The clinical features include intrauterine growth retardation, insulin-dependent diabetes, and pancreatic exocrine insufficiency. Serum C-peptide and glucagon are undetectable, and the pancreas is absent on imaging studies. Survival into childhood is possible with proper diagnosis and insulin and enzymatic supplementation. Pancreatic hypoplasia is thought to be a variant of pancreatic agenesis, and isolated agenesis of the dorsal or ventral pancreas has also been observed.

Annular pancreas is a rare congenital abnormality seen alone, in association with Down syndrome, or with other congenital abnormalities of the gastrointestinal tract. The clinical features, including abdominal pain and vomiting caused by duodenal stenosis, are related to a band of pancreatic tissue encircling the second portion of the duodenum (Fig. 51-4). The diagnosis should be suspected in a vomiting infant with the double bubble sign on an abdominal x-ray, caused by high-grade duodenal stenosis and air in the stomach and first portion of the (dilated) duodenum (Fig. 51-5). Traditionally, ERCP has been the most useful diagnostic test. With improved imaging techniques, computed tomography (CT) (Fig. 51-6), magnetic resonance imaging, or MRCP may replace ERCP as the test of choice, especially in children. The primary treatment for symptomatic annular pancreas is surgical.

Heterotopic-aberrant pancreas or pancreatic rest is a commonly observed developmental abnormality, but rarely is of clinical significance. Heterotopic pancreatic tissue usually appears as discrete, firm, yellow submucosal nodules from 2 mm to 4 cm in diameter and is typically seen in the stomach (60%–70%) (Fig. 51-7), and duodenum and jejunum (38%–45%). Foci of pancreatic tissue have also been reported in Meckel diverticulum, the appendix, omentum, and other locations. Most pancreatic rests contain pancreatic excretory ducts and exocrine glands. Islets of Langerhans are present in 33% to 84% of specimens. The heterotopic pancreatic tissue can occasionally present with biliary obstruction, mucosal ulceration with hemorrhage, intussusception, or intestinal obstruction, and very rarely pancreatic cancer. For symptomatic or suspicious lesions, the treatment remains surgical.

CONGENITAL SYNDROMES

CF is the most common lethal genetic defect of Caucasian populations. CF is caused by severe mutations in the *CFTR* gene located on chromosome 7q32 and is inherited as an autosomal recessive disorder. Patients with CF cannot adequately hydrate mucus and other macromolecules, which leads to accumulation of viscid material in ducts and inspissated glands and results in progressive organ destruction. In CF the pancreas is destroyed early in life, whereas pulmonary pathology develops later. CF is usually recognized and diagnosed before 5 years of age because of meconium ileus, maldigestion, and malabsorption, with frequent foul stools, failure to thrive, or rectal prolapse.

In patients with typical CF, the pancreas becomes shrunken, cystic, fibrotic, and fatty (Fig. 51-8). The histological appearance resembles other forms of chronic pancreatitis except for the inspissated secretions in the pancreatic ducts (Fig. 51-9*D*). Acinal cell atrophy, ductular hyperplasia, mild inflammatory changes, and progressive fibrosis gradually replace the pancreatic lobules.

The radiographic appearance of the pancreas in CF can vary between normal, incomplete or complete lipomatosis, cystic or macrocystic pancreas, or as an atrophic pancreas (Fig. 51-8).

HP is an autosomal dominant disorder with 80% disease penetrance. The clinical features encompass the spectrum of pancreatic inflammatory diseases. HP usually presents as recurrent acute pancreatitis in childhood, progresses to chronic pancreatitis by young adulthood, and is associated with an approximately 40% risk of pancreatic cancer by age 70 years. This risk is doubled if the patient smokes. The gene for HP was mapped to chromosome 7q35 and identified as the cationic trypsinogen gene (*PRSS1*) in 1996. Two point mutations N29I and R122H occurring in exon 2 and exon 3 respectively of cationic trypsinogen, account for the majority of cases. The R122H mutant cationic trypsin is thought to be resistant to autolysis. Trypsin is maintained in the inactive trypsinogen form within the pancreas, but is changed into a proteolytic enzyme in the duodenum, which in turn activates the majority of pancreatic digestive enzymes within the intestinal lumen (Fig. 51-10). When small amounts of trypsinogen are prematurely activated within the pancreas, the effect of activating other enzymes is inhibited by pancreatic secretory trypsin inhibitor (unigene symbol *SPINK1*) (see Fig. 51-10). However, *SPINK1* has the capacity to inhibit only approximately 20% of potential trypsin activity. During conditions that cause excessive trypsinogen activation, the *SPINK1* inhibitory capacity is overwhelmed and trypsin is inactivated by autolysis. With the R122H mutation that eliminates the autolysis site in HP, this second "fail-safe" mechanism is lost, trypsin activates the other digestive proenzymes, pancreatic autolysis ensues, and pancreatitis develops (see Fig. 51-10).

Shwachman-Diamond syndrome (SDS) remains the second most frequently recognized cause of pancreatic insufficiency in children. Rather than being a pancreas-destroying disease like CF and HP, the pancreas in patients with SDS appears to have fatty replacement of acinar cells. SDS is an autosomal recessive disorder with a disease gene at the centromere of chromosome 7. SDS is characterized by exocrine pancreatic insufficiency, normal sweat electrolytes (which distinguish SDS from CF), and hematologic abnormalities including cyclic neutropenias. Skeletal defects, short stature (Fig. 51-11), myelodysplastic syndromes, and acute leukemias are common. von Hippel-Lindau disease (VHL) is an autosomal dominant tumor predisposition syndrome, characterized by the presence of benign and malignant tumors. VHL is due to a germline mutation affecting a tumor suppressor gene mapped to chromosome 3. Hallmark lesions include retinal angiomas, cerebellar and spinal cord hemangioblastomas, and renal cell carcinomas. Pancreatic lesions are common in VHL and are most often limited to cysts. The cysts are often multiple and are present throughout the body of the pancreas (Fig. 51-12). They are frequently asymptomatic, but complications can occur because of space-occupying effects. Pancreatic islet cell tumors can occur in VHL, apparently independent of the pancreatic cyst formation. These are vascular tumors of neural origin. Most grow slowly and are asymptomatic, although they can be malignant. Once VHL is diagnosed in a patient, lifelong and close follow-up for multiple and recurrent tumors is necessary, as is screening of family members.

Autosomal dominant polycystic kidney disease is one of the most common hereditary disorders, and is 15 times more common than CF. The *ADPKD1* gene located on the short arm of chromosome 16 appears to be the causative gene in 90% or more of families in the Caucasian population. The extrarenal manifestations of autosomal dominant polycystic kidney disease occasionally involve cysts occurring in the pancreas.

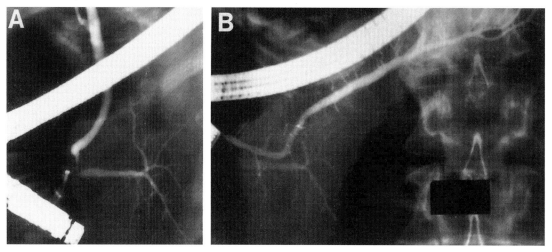

FIGURE 51-1.   A, B: Pancreas divisum. (Courtesy of Dr. Peter B. Cotton and Dr. David Gulliver.)

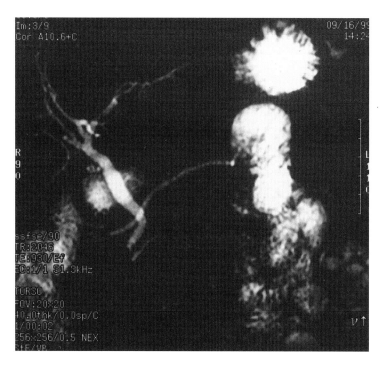

FIGURE 51-2. Pancreas divisum. Magnetic resonance cholangiopancreatography showing the biliary tree and the unconnected dorsal (dominant) and ventral pancreatic ducts in pancreas divisum.

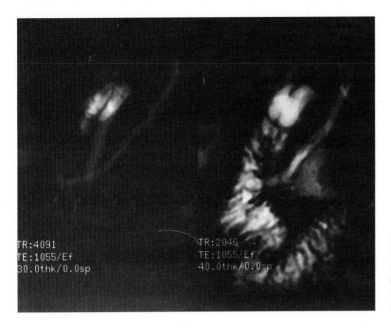

FIGURE 51-3. Pancreas divisum. Pre- (**left**) and post-secretin (**right**)–stimulated magnetic images of the dorsal pancreatic duct in pancreas divisum. Note the dilation of the dorsal duct and the bulging minor papilla (santorinicele) in the duodenum after secretin stimulation.

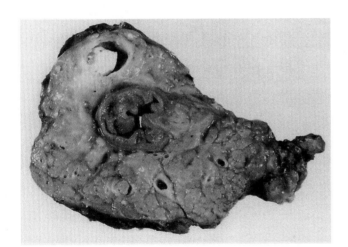

FIGURE 51-4. Annular pancreas. (Courtesy of Dr. J. Rode.)

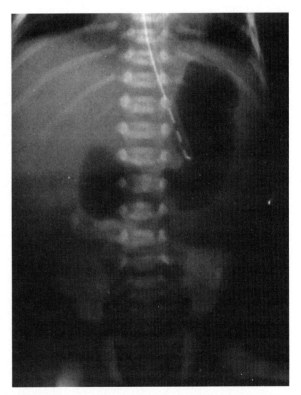

FIGURE 51-5. Annular pancreas. Abdominal film in an infant with annular pancreas. The nasogastric tube lies in the stomach. Note the dilated bulb of the duodenum and preantral gastric dilation giving the classical appearance of the double bubble.

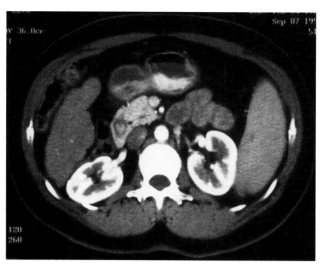

FIGURE 51-6. Annular pancreas. Contrast enhanced computed tomographic scan of the abdomen in a patient with annular pancreas. Note that the bowel is entirely encircled by pancreatic parenchyma. Part of the pancreatic duct is visualized medial to the annulus.

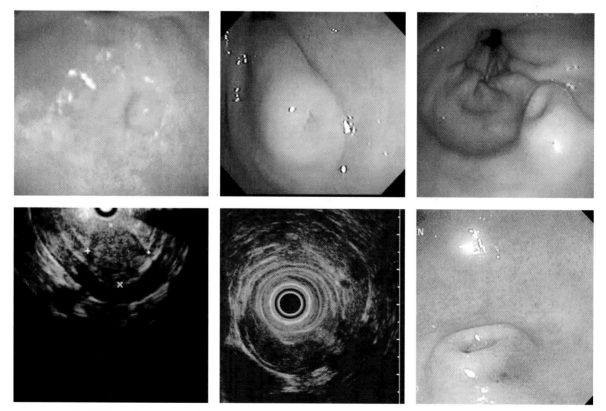

FIGURE 51-7. Pancreatic rests. Endoscopic images of pancreatic rests in the stomach. Two images with corresponding endosonographic visualization beneath revealing submucosally contained hypoechoic mass.

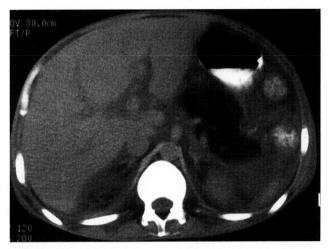

FIGURE 51-8. Cystic fibrosis (CF). Noncontrast computed tomographic scan of the abdomen revealing fatty replacement (*dark*) of the pancreas, one of a variety of radiologic findings seen in CF.

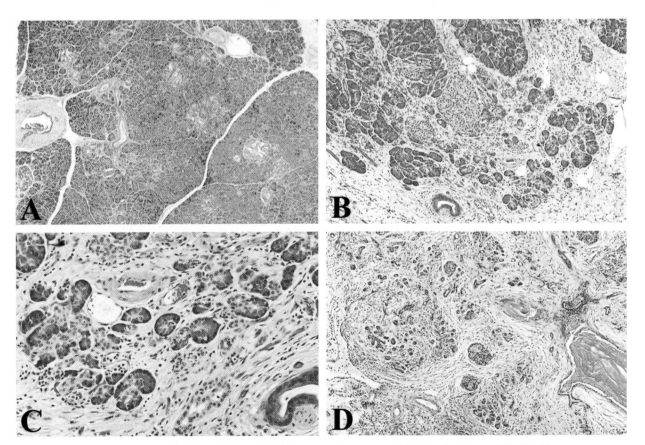

FIGURE 51-9. Pancreatic histology in a normal pancreas (**A**), chronic pancreatitis (**B, C**), and cystic fibrosis (CF) (**D**). Features of CF-related pancreatic histology include the inspissated secretions in the pancreatic duct.

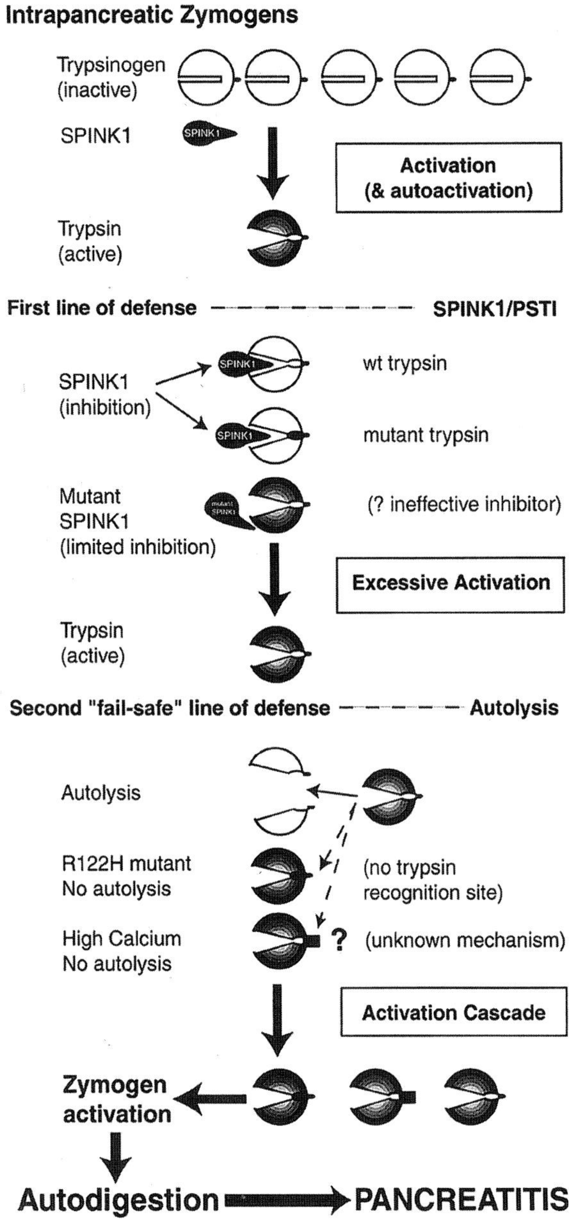

Intrapancreatic Zymogens

Trypsinogen (inactive)

SPINK1

Activation (& autoactivation)

Trypsin (active)

First line of defense — — — — — — **SPINK1/PSTI**

SPINK1 (inhibition)

wt trypsin

mutant trypsin

Mutant SPINK1 (limited inhibition)

(? ineffective inhibitor)

Excessive Activation

Trypsin (active)

Second "fail-safe" line of defense — — — — — **Autolysis**

Autolysis

R122H mutant No autolysis

(no trypsin recognition site)

High Calcium No autolysis

? (unknown mechanism)

Activation Cascade

Zymogen activation

Autodigestion ⟹ PANCREATITIS

FIGURE 51-10. Hereditary pancreatitis (HP). Postulated mechanism of pancreatitis in HP.

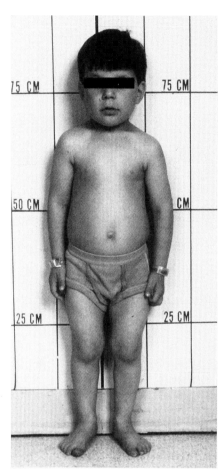

FIGURE 51-11. Shwachman-Diamond syndrome. Note the short stature and no overt signs of malnutrition. (Courtesy of Dr. Peter Durie.)

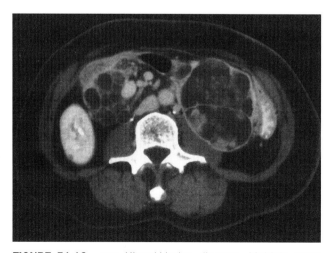

FIGURE 51-12. von Hippel-Lindau disease. Multiple cysts are seen throughout the pancreas.

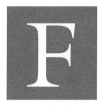

F GALLBLADDER AND BILIARY TRACT

52

GALLBLADDER AND BILIARY TRACT:
Anatomy and Structural Anomalies

DIANE M. SIMEONE

ANATOMY

The gallbladder lies in a depression along the inferior surface of the liver in a plane dividing the liver into its anatomic right and left lobes. The gallbladder is intimately attached to the liver by loose connective tissue that contains small veins and lymphatic vessels. The rest of the gallbladder, which is not in direct contact with the liver, is covered with peritoneum reflected from the liver and is in contact with the duodenum and hepatic flexure of the colon (Fig. 52-1). The gallbladder is divided into four anatomic areas: fundus, body, infundibulum, and neck. The neck tapers into the cystic duct, which joins the common hepatic duct to become the common bile duct. Although the cystic duct typically joins the common hepatic duct directly, it may join the extrahepatic biliary tract anywhere from the right hepatic duct down to the level of the ampulla (Figs. 52-2 and 52-3). The blood supply to the gallbladder and cystic duct is usually from a single artery arising from the right hepatic artery, although variations in this configuration are common (Fig. 52-4). The gallbladder is innervated by branches of both the sympathetic and parasympathetic nervous systems (Fig. 52-5), which play a role in modulating gallbladder contractility. The gallbladder has five layers: epithelium, lamina propria, muscularis, perimuscular connective tissue, and serosa. The gallbladder mucosa is lined with columnar epithelial cells that are covered with abundant microvilli and joined by tight junctions.

Bile drains from the liver into the right and left hepatic ducts, which join outside the liver to form the common hepatic duct. The cystic duct then joins the common hepatic duct to become the common bile duct. The common bile duct lies anterior to the portal vein and to the right of the hepatic artery. The common bile duct is divided into four segments: supraduodenal, retroduodenal, pancreatic, and intraduodenal. The intraduodenal common bile duct joins the main pancreatic duct to form the ampulla of Vater, which empties into the lumen of the duodenum. The intraduodenal common bile duct and ampulla of Vater are surrounded by a sheath of smooth muscle fibers referred to as the sphincter of Oddi (Fig. 52-6). Regulation of bile flow is controlled primarily by the sphincter of Oddi.

EMBRYOLOGY

The biliary tract is first apparent during the fifth week of gestation and develops as a ventral sacculation in the distal foregut (Fig. 52-7). This sacculation grows into the ventral mesentery, which divides into two buds: the cranial bud develops into the liver and intrahepatic bile ducts, and the caudal bud develops into the gallbladder and cystic duct (Fig. 52-8). Another small bud arises from the inferior aspect of the caudal bud and ultimately develops into the ventral pancreas (Fig. 52-9). The ventral pancreatic bud rotates 180° from right to left, fusing with the dorsal pancreatic bud to form the complete pancreas. Because the lower end of the common bile duct is attached to the ventral pancreatic bud, it also rotates and fuses with the duodenum along its posteromedial wall (Fig. 52-10). Variations in this developmental process give rise to structural anomalies in the biliary tract (Figs. 52-11 through 52-13).

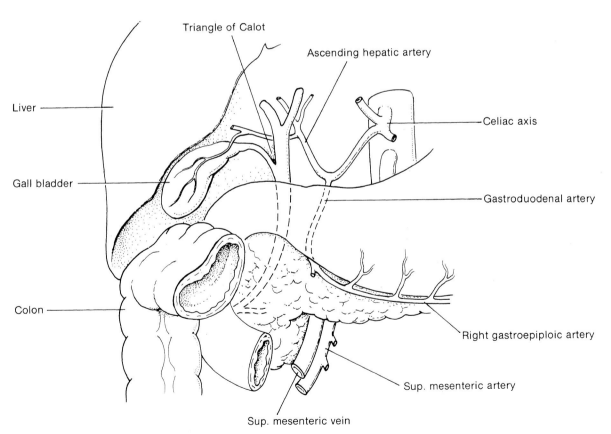

FIGURE 52-1. Relation of the gallbladder and extrahepatic biliary tract to the liver, duodenum, colon, and pancreas.

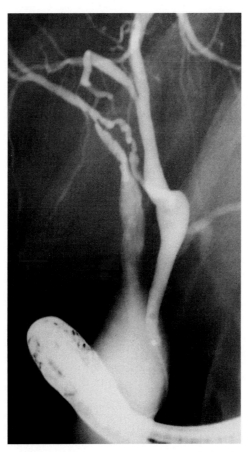

FIGURE 52-2. Endoscopic retrograde cholangiopancreatogram demonstrates an anomalous junction of the cystic
duct with an accessory right hepatic duct.

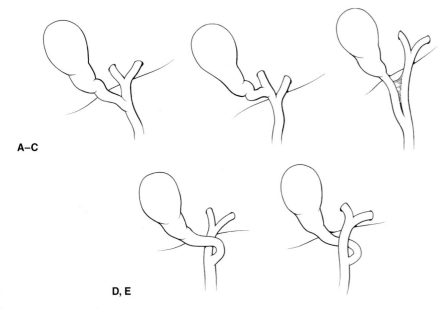

A–C

D, E

FIGURE 52-3. Variations in cystic duct
anatomy. **A:** Cystic duct joins common
hepatic duct directly (most common). **B:**
Cystic duct joins the right hepatic duct. **C:**
Low junction of cystic duct with common
hepatic duct. **D:** Anterior spiral of cystic duct
before joining common hepatic duct. **E:** Posterior spiral of cystic duct before joining
common hepatic duct.

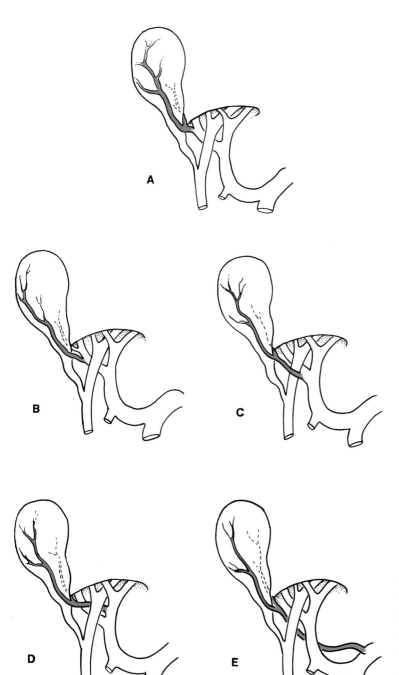

FIGURE 52-4. Common variations in the origin of the cystic artery. It originates most commonly from the right hepatic artery, traverses the triangle of Calot, and on reaching the gallbladder divides into two main branches (**A**). Occasionally, the two branches come off the right hepatic artery independently (**B**). The cystic artery may cross the hepatic duct anteriorly (**C**), come off the left hepatic artery (**D**), or more rarely, come directly from the celiac axis (**E**).

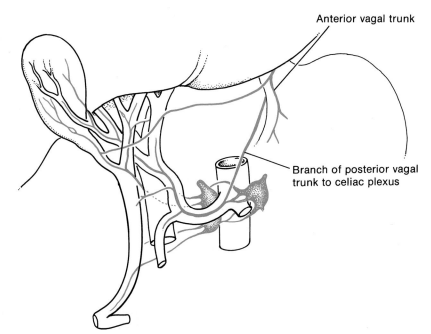

FIGURE 52-5. Schematic of the innervation of the gallbladder and extrahepatic biliary tract. The nerves originate from both vagi and from the celiac axis. They reach the biliary tract traveling along the walls of the hepatic artery, except for direct branches of the anterior vagus that cross through the gastrohepatic ligament.

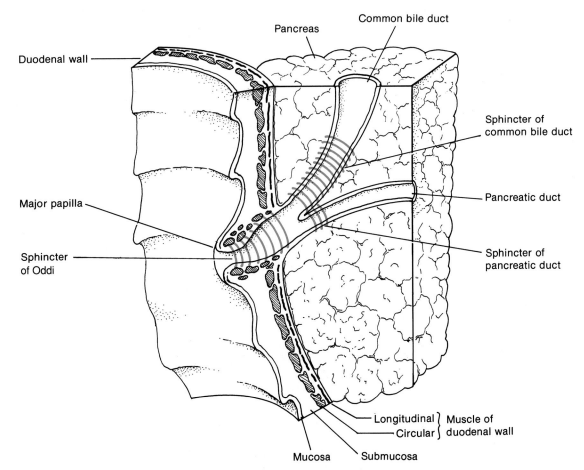

FIGURE 52-6. Muscular apparatus at the terminal end of the common bile duct. The bile duct is closely associated with the pancreatic duct, and they both enter the medial wall of the duodenum tangentially. Each duct has its own sphincter, which is poorly developed in the pancreatic duct.

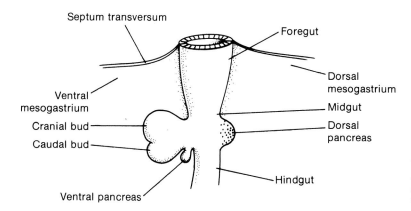

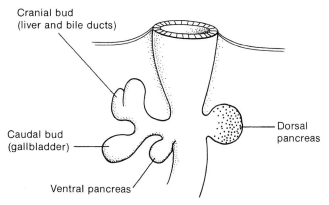

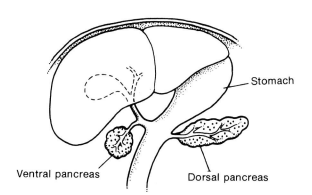

FIGURE 52-7. At the 3-mm stage of the embryo, the ventral bud enters the mesogastrium and soon divides into a cranial and a caudal bud. A smaller caudal bud represents the origin of the ventral pancreas.

FIGURE 52-8. As the embryo reaches 5 mm, the cranial bud (which will form the liver and intrahepatic biliary tract) moves toward the septum transversum, pulling the caudal bud (gallbladder and extrahepatic bile ducts).

FIGURE 52-9. When the embryo reaches 7 mm, the right and left lobes of the liver occupy the position under the septum transversum. The ventral pancreas and the extrahepatic biliary tract are visible. As the ventral pancreas rotates to reach the dorsal pancreas, it pulls the lower end of the common bile duct with it.

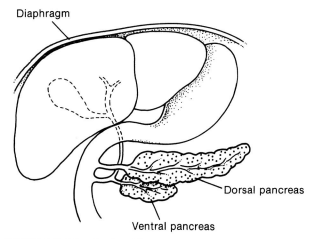

FIGURE 52-10. At the 12-mm stage, the ventral pancreas has rotated and the normal anatomic relations of the bile ducts and gastrointestinal tract have taken place.

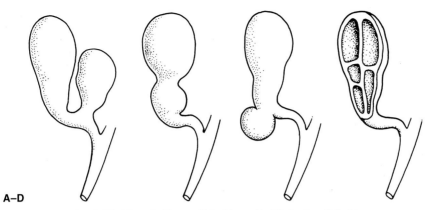

FIGURE 52-11. **A:** Two gallbladders. **B:** Bilobed gallbladder. **C:** Diverticulum at the neck. **D:** Septated gallbladder. All are anatomic variations that relate to the embryologic development of the biliary tract.

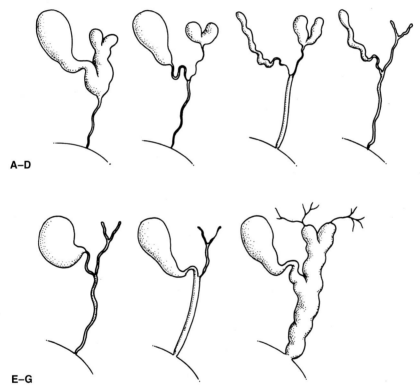

FIGURE 52-12. **A–G:** Different forms of biliary atresia. Biliary atresia may be partial, affecting the intrahepatic or extrahepatic portions of the biliary tract, or may be a complete process.

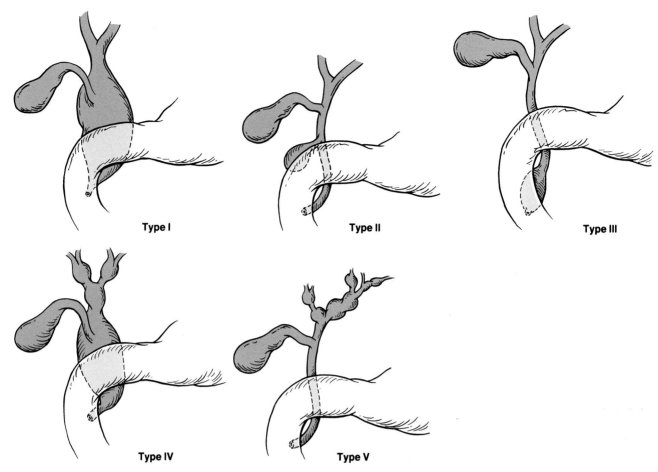

FIGURE 52-13. Classification of choledochal cysts.

53

GALLSTONES

SUM P. LEE ■ CYNTHIA W. KO

Cholelithiasis and its complications are the most prevalent diseases of the biliary tree. The incidence of gallstones varies greatly among ethnic and national groups. In the United States, more than 20 million persons harbor gallstones. Cholesterol stones predominate in western societies. During the last two decades, important advances have been made in understanding the pathogenesis and treatment of gallstones.

CLASSIFICATION OF GALLSTONES ACCORDING TO CHEMICAL COMPOSITION

Gallstones are classified by content as cholesterol or pigment stones. In western countries, about 80% of stones are cholesterol stones. About 5% of cholesterol gallstones are composed of pure cholesterol and often occur singly (*cholesterol solitaire*) (Fig. 53-1*A*). The highly pure cholesterol monohydrate crystalline structure is well appreciated in the fractured surface (Fig. 53-1*B*). This subgroup of cholesterol gallstones is characterized by an excellent response to oral bile acid therapy or lithotripsy. The long-term recurrence rate of these single cholesterol stones after medical treatment is surprisingly low—about 10% over 15 years.

More commonly, cholesterol gallstones contain other constituents, including proteins and calcium salts of bilirubin or carbonate. Although sometimes called mixed stones, they are still classified as cholesterol stones, because cholesterol is the predominant component (more than 70%) by weight. These stones are typically multiple and faceted (Fig. 53-2). The fractured surface shows a pigmented center and concentric "growth" rings, suggesting that the chemical composition of bile may have varied during the development of these stones. Sometimes smaller stones aggregate to form a larger concretion. Figure 53-3 shows a large cholesterol gallstone, the surface of which has a mulberry appearance composed of small subunits. In contrast, pigment gallstones are either dark brown or black, small, and amorphous (Fig. 53-4).

PATHOGENESIS OF CHOLESTEROL GALLSTONES

Applying the principles of physical chemistry has significantly advanced the basic scientific and clinical understanding of gallstone pathogenesis. Cholesterol is insoluble in water and bile. Cholesterol may be either secreted in its free form or metabolized to bile acids in the liver (Fig. 53-5). Cholesterol is initially secreted with phospholipids as unilamellar vesicles measuring 40 to 75 nm. If bile salt concentrations are low, the cholesterol in bile is predominantly carried in the vesicular form. With the addition of bile salts, mixed micelles form. Mixed micelles contain bile salts, lecithin, and cholesterol. In these mixed micelles, cholesterol is solubilized by the bile salts and phospholipids. Mixed micelles are high in buoyant density (>1.15 g/mL) and measure about 25 Å. This gives rise to the concept of "supersaturated" or "lithogenic" bile, which implies that the cholesterol content in bile has exceeded the cholesterol-carrying capacity of biliary mixed micelles. Implicit within this lithogenic bile hypothesis are two principles. First, the initial abnormality in gallstone formation comes from the liver, which secretes abnormal bile. Second, cholesterol supersaturation is a prerequisite factor for gallstone formation and differentiates persons who form gallstones from those who do not. Cholesterol solubility and biliary cholesterol saturation with various lipid concentrations can be defined using previously developed phase equilibrium diagrams.

A crucial step in cholesterol gallstone formation is nucleation, which is the formation of solid cholesterol crystals from lithogenic bile. The propensity of a bile sample to nucleate is a much better predictor of gallstone-forming risk than the degree of supersaturation. Figure 53-6 is a schematic summary of the physical and chemical events of biliary lipids in nucleation. It is believed that aggregation and fusion of vesicles precede nucleation. Fused vesicles can be seen at transmission electron microscopic examination as large lipid aggregates (Fig. 53-7) or at polarizing microscopic examination as lipid crystals. When cholesterol monohydrate crystals form, they are derived almost exclusively from vesicular cholesterol. Factors in addition to cholesterol supersaturation are important in nucleation. Biliary proteins may have a crucial role in promoting or inhibiting nucleation.

DIAGNOSIS OF GALLSTONES

Examination of bile with a polarizing microscope is a useful way of diagnosing gallstone disease. Macroscopic concretions greater than 2 mm often are not found in the gallbladder. Smaller cholesterol crystals may be found, and their presence in bile is referred to as biliary sludge, microcrystalline disease, or microlithiasis. Biliary sludge may be a precursor to gallstones in certain situations. Like patients with gallstones, most patients with sludge have no symptoms. However, patients may have typical biliary pain or complications such as pancreatitis. Biliary sludge may be detected by means of ultrasound scanning. On scans it appears as low-level echoes that layer in the dependent portion of the gallbladder without acoustic shadowing (Fig. 53-8). Sludge is composed of cholesterol monohydrate crystals, calcium bilirubinate, and calcium carbonate granules in bile high in mucus content (Figs. 53-9 through 53-12).

Gallstones are usually diagnosed with ultrasonography, at which they appear as high-amplitude, mobile echoes with postacoustic shadowing (Fig. 53-13). If choledocholithiasis is suspected, percutaneous transhepatic, endoscopic retrograde, or magnetic resonance cholangiography may be used (Figs. 53-14 and 53-15). Oral cholecystography is used infrequently (Fig. 53-16). Acute cholecystitis with obstruction of the cystic duct by stone or inflammatory edema can be diagnosed using hepatobiliary scintigraphy with high sensitivity (Figs. 53-17 and 53-18). Ultrasonographic features suggestive of cholecystitis include thickening of the gallbladder wall, the presence of pericholecystic fluid, and air in the gallbladder wall (Fig. 53-19).

Worldwide, a common biliary tract problem is recurrent pyogenic cholangitis (also known as Oriental cholangiohepatitis). This syndrome is characterized by intrahepatic stone formation with recurrent abdominal pain, fever, and jaundice. This syndrome often preferentially involves the left intrahepatic ducts (Fig. 53-20). Management of these patients is difficult, and often involves a combination of surgical and radiological techniques.

MANAGEMENT OF GALLSTONES

It is estimated that 60% to 80% of all gallstones are asymptomatic at a given time. When gallstones do form, the risk factors for developing symptoms are unknown. However, the rate at which stones to give rise to symptoms and complications is relatively small. More than 90% of complications, such as cholecystitis, cholangitis, and pancreatitis, are preceded by attacks of pain. Therefore, for most people with asymptomatic gallstones, watchful waiting is appropriate (Fig. 53-21). Once symptoms or complications develop, treatment should be considered. Because biliary sludge can cause symptoms or complications, treatment of sludge should be considered in situations similar to those for gallstones.

Surgery is the definitive curative method for treatment of gallstones. The advent of laparoscopic cholecystectomy and its widespread acceptance has revolutionized surgical treatment of gallstones. Laparoscopic cholecystectomy is now regarded as the treatment of choice for symptomatic gallstones. For patients unable or unwilling to undergo surgery, nonsurgical methods such as oral bile acid therapy are available (Table 53-1).

(figures begin on page 564)

TABLE 53-1
Therapeutic Options for Symptomatic Gallbladder Stones

THERAPY	CANDIDATES	STONE CLEARANCE (%)	MORTALITY (%)	DISADVANTAGES
Laparoscopic cholecystectomy	No prior abdominal surgery, normal gallbladder wall	100	<1	Invasive, requires general anesthesia, possible bile duct injury
Oral bile acids	Patent cystic duct, functioning gallbladder, floating radiolucent stones, <5 mm in diameter	80–90 (well selected)	0	Delayed stone clearance, possible stone recurrence
ESWL with oral bile acids	Patent cystic duct, functioning gallbladder, solitary radiolucent stones up to 20 mm in diameter	70–90	<0.1	Post-ESWL biliary pain and acute pancreatitis (3%–5%); delayed stone clearance, possible stone recurrence
Contact dissolution with MTBE	Radiolucent stones, GB attached to liver, patent cystic duct	50–90	Limited experience	Invasive, bile leakage (5%); leakage of MTBE (erosive duodenitis, hemolysis, pathologic somnolence); stone recurrence

ESWL, extracorporeal shock wave lithotripsy; GB, gallbladder; MTBE, methyl-tert-butyl ether.

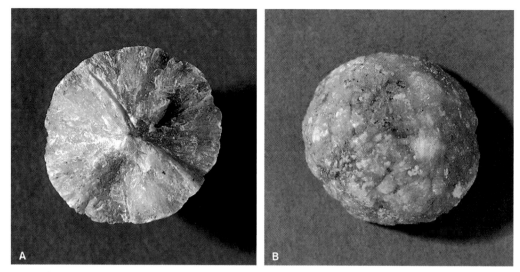

FIGURE 53-1. **A:** Pure, usually solitary, cholesterol gallstone (cholesterol solitaire). **B:** Almost 99% of this stone is cholesterol monohydrate. The crystalline structure arrangement can be seen in the fractured surface.

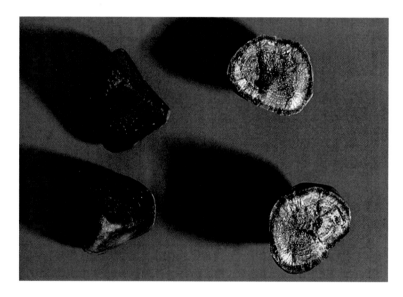

FIGURE 53-2. Mixed cholesterol gallstones. Usually multiple and faceted, the fractured surface shows a pigment center and concentric "growth" rings. These stones are at least 70% cholesterol by weight and thus are classified as a form of cholesterol gallstones. When multiple stones are present in the gallbladder, they usually are identical in chemical composition.

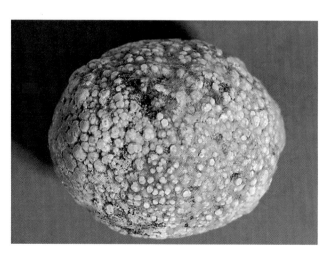

FIGURE 53-3. A large cholesterol gallstone, the surface of which has a mulberry appearance with multiple small subunits.

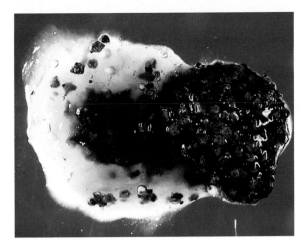

FIGURE 53-4. Pigment stones are either dark brown or black, small, and multiple. These pigment stones are embedded in a mucus gel.

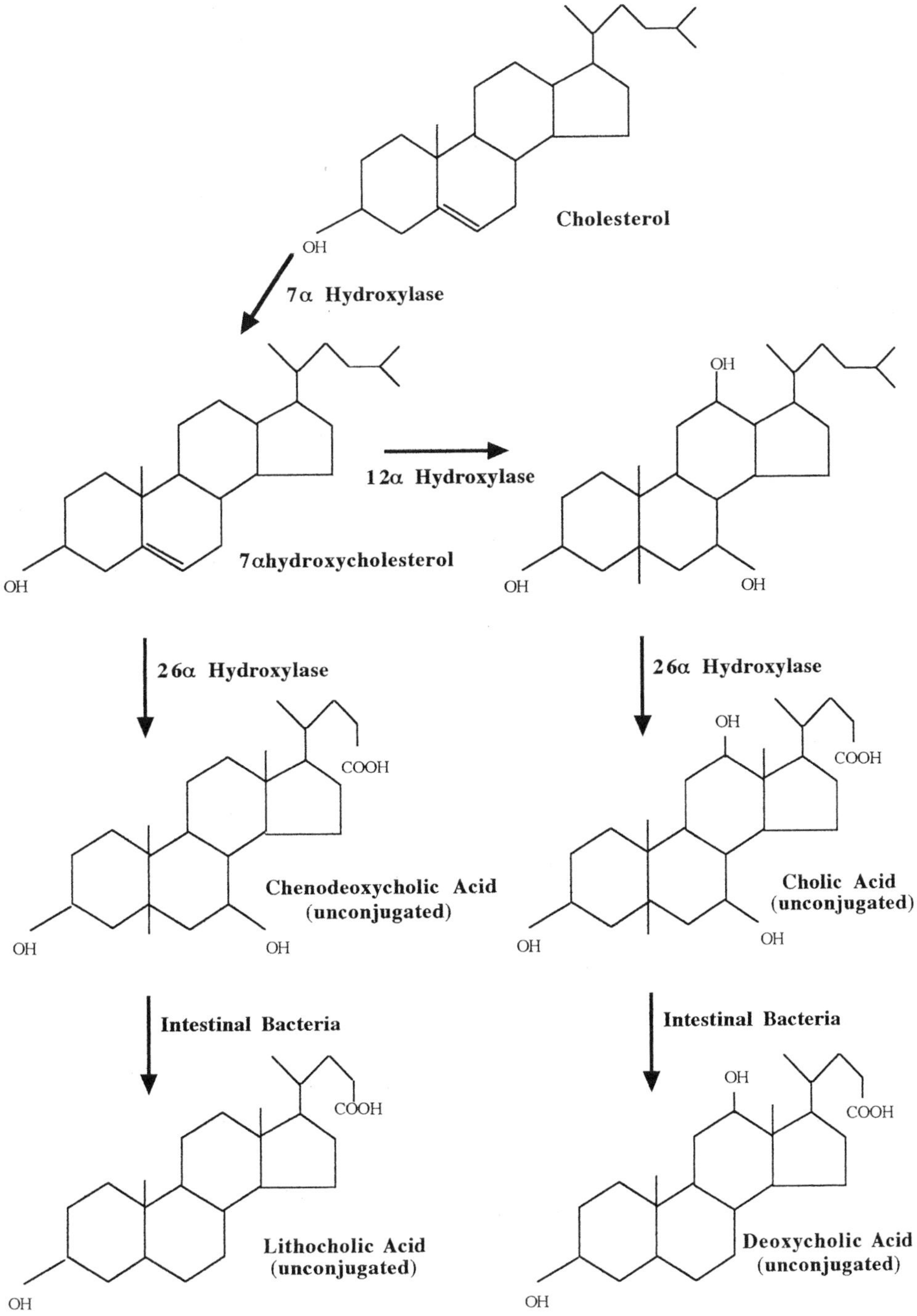

Cholesterol

OH

↓ **7α Hydroxylase**

7αhydroxycholesterol

OH

→ **12α Hydroxylase**

OH

OH   OH

↓ **26α Hydroxylase**

COOH

**Chenodeoxycholic Acid
(unconjugated)**

OH   OH

↓ **Intestinal Bacteria**

COOH

**Lithocholic Acid
(unconjugated)**

OH

↓ **26α Hydroxylase**

OH

COOH

**Cholic Acid
(unconjugated)**

OH   OH

↓ **Intestinal Bacteria**

OH

COOH

**Deoxycholic Acid
(unconjugated)**

OH

FIGURE 53-5. Schematic of bile acid synthesis and metabolism. The initial step in bile acid synthesis is hydroxylation of cholesterol by the enzyme 7α-hydroxylase. Further conversion of this metabolite by 12α-hydroxylase and 26α-hydroxylase results in synthesis of the primary bile acids cholic acid and chenodeoxycholic acid. After conjugation with glycine or taurine, secretion, and transport to the intestine, bacteria metabolize the primary bile acids to the secondary bile acids lithocholic acid and deoxycholic acid.

SOLUBLE FORMS   TRANSITIONAL FORMS   CRYSTALLINE FORMS

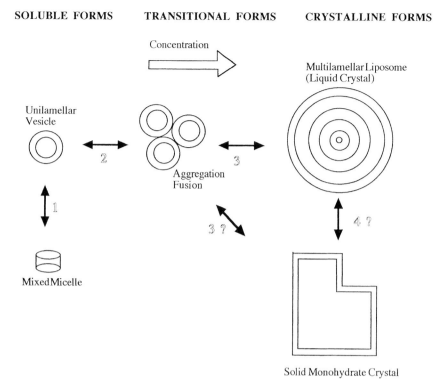

FIGURE 53-6. Schematic of cholesterol nucleation. In bile, cholesterol exists in two soluble forms: vesicles and mixed micelles. They are in dynamic equilibrium (*1*), depending on total bile salt concentration and total biliary lipid density. With concentration, the vesicles may be depleted with phospholipid and enriched with cholesterol, resulting in a tendency for the vesicles to aggregate and fuse (*2*). Pronucleators may aid vesicular fusion. The fused vesicles are transitional forms and lead to formation of multilamellar liposomes or liquid crystals (*3*). Cholesterol separates from the liquid to solid crystalline forms during nucleation (*4*). It is unclear whether fused vesicles can nucleate into solid cholesterol crystals.

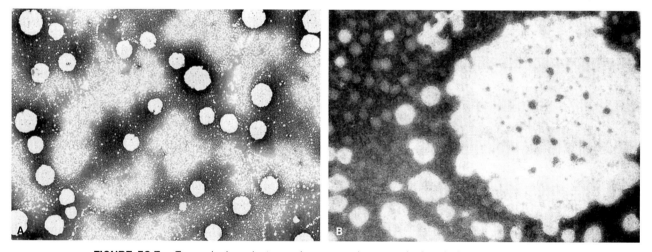

FIGURE 53-7. Transmission electron microscopy shows vesicular cholesterol and vesicular fusion. **A:** Monodispersed cholesterol-lecithin vesicles of approximately 600 Å in mean hydrodynamic radius. **B:** Vesicular fusion into large lipid aggregates, also known as multilamellar vesicles. At polarized microscopic examination, they appear as liquid crystals.

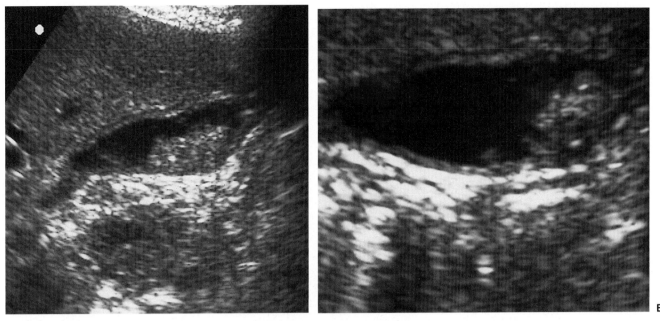

A   B

FIGURE 53-8. Ultrasound scan of gallbladder sludge. **A:** The particulate matter within the gallbladder generates low-amplitude echoes without postacoustic shadowing. **B:** With positioning changes, the material forms progressive layers in the most dependent part of the gallbladder. The high-amplitude echoes contained within the sludge may represent small, early gallstones.

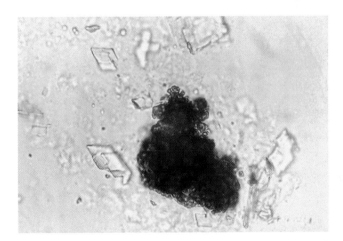

FIGURE 53-9. Phase-contrast photomicrograph of gallbladder sludge. A central, dark calcium bilirubin granule is surrounded by cholesterol monohydrate crystals. The crystals are typically rhomboidal with a notch. All are embedded within amorphous strands of mucus.

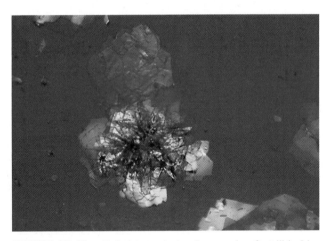

FIGURE 53-10. Polarizing photomicrograph of gallbladder sludge. A clump of cholesterol monohydrate crystals surrounds a pigmented center of calcium bilirubinate. These crystal aggregates have been referred to as biliary sludge.

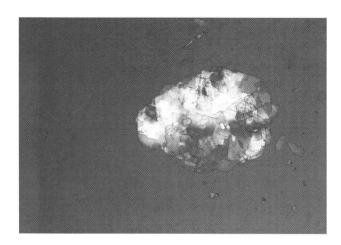

FIGURE 53-11. Polarizing photomicrograph of gallbladder sludge. Adherent cholesterol monohydrate crystals form a small oval structure. This is probably a cholesterol gallstone in its embryonic stage. This miniature gallstone will grow with further precipitation of cholesterol.

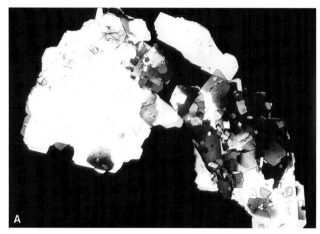
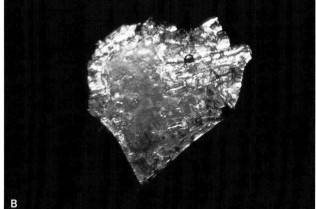

FIGURE 53-12.   A, B: Polarizing photomicrograph of gallbladder sludge. Crystals can be present in different shapes and sizes. In contrast to smooth, rounded cholesterol gallstones, crystals in sludge often have sharp, irregular edges. It is conceivable that such crystals can damage the mucosa of the bile ducts or the sphincter of Oddi, causing inflammation and symptoms.

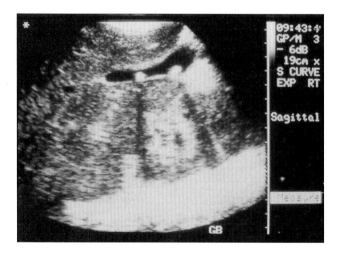

FIGURE 53-13. Ultrasound scan of gallstones. The stones generate high-amplitude echoes and are large and dense enough to constitute substantial acoustic impedance in the path of the ultrasound beam. This produces a void behind the stone, which is known as the postacoustic shadow.

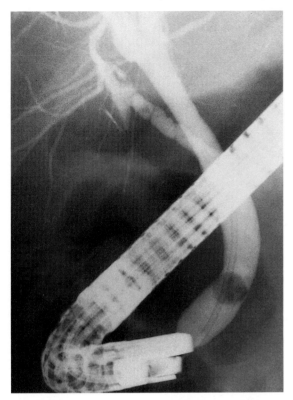

FIGURE 53-14. Endoscopic retrograde cholangiogram shows a stone within the common bile duct. There is also a small stone or debris within the cystic duct. (Courtesy of Dr. Scott Schulte.)

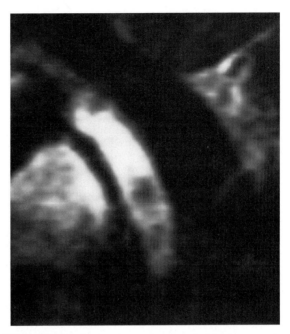

FIGURE 53-15. Magnetic resonance cholangiogram shows two stones within the common bile duct. The gallbladder is adjacent to the common bile duct. (Courtesy of Dr. Scott Schulte.)

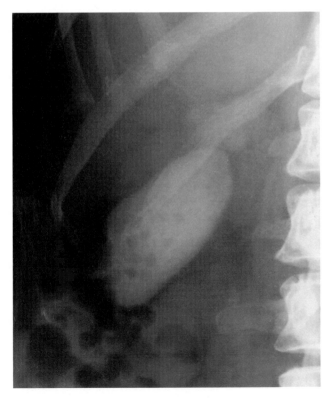

FIGURE 53-16. Oral cholecystogram shows several small stones within an opacified gallbladder.

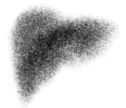
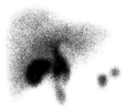

A   B

FIGURE 53-17. Technetium 99m iminodiacetic acid scintigraphy, normal study. **A:** Homogeneous hepatic uptake occurs within 5 minutes. **B:** Fifteen minutes after radionuclide administration, the gallbladder, common bile duct, and a portion of small bowel are visible. (Courtesy of Dr. Arnold Jacobson.)

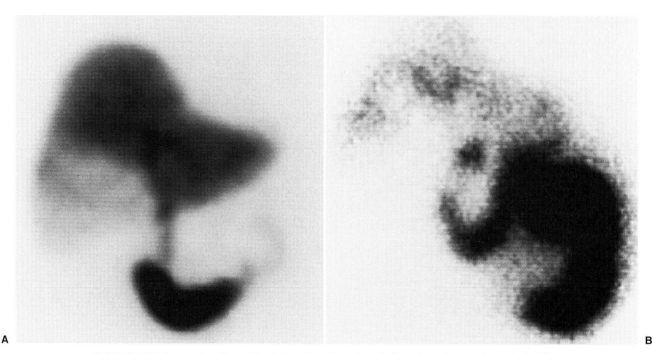

A   B

FIGURE 53-18. Technetium 99m iminodiacetic acid scintigraphy, abnormal study. **A:** The 5-minute scan demonstrates normal liver uptake. **B:** Morphine 0.04 mg/kg intravenously has been given to enhance gallbladder filling. Inability to visualize the gallbladder by 90 minutes after radionuclide administration if adequate images of the liver, common duct, and small bowel have been obtained is consistent with the diagnosis of acute cholecystitis. A rim sign, a region of increased activity in the liver adjacent to the gallbladder fossa, is present and represents transmural inflammation of the gallbladder. (Courtesy of Dr. Arnold Jacobson.)

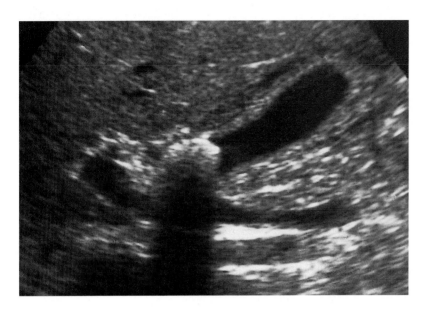

FIGURE 53-19. Ultrasound scan shows acute cholecystitis. A large gallstone is impacted within the neck of the gallbladder. Other findings that suggest acute cholecystitis include a thickened gallbladder wall and a small amount of pericholecystic fluid.

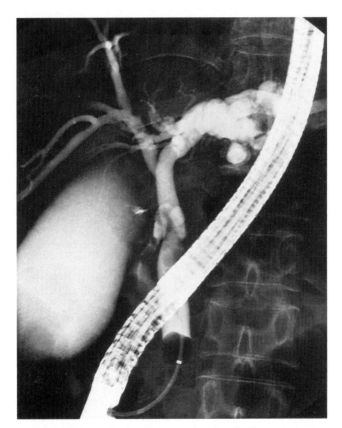

FIGURE 53-20. Cholangiogram showing findings characteristic of recurrent pyogenic cholangitis. The left intrahepatic duct is preferentially involved, with dilation and intraductal filling defects characteristic of intrahepatic stones. The right intrahepatic ducts show characteristic changes of pruning and decreased arborization. A balloon catheter is used to obtain the occlusion cholangiogram. (Courtesy of Dr. Charles Rohrmann.)

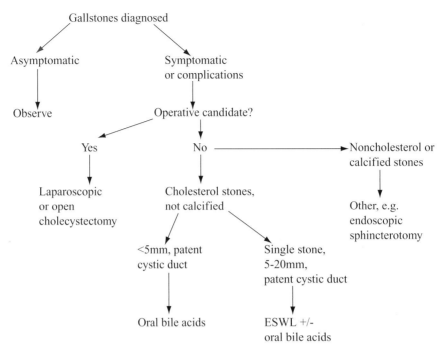

FIGURE 53-21. Algorithm for management of biliary sludge and gallstones.

54

PRIMARY SCLEROSING CHOLANGITIS AND OTHER CHOLANGIOPATHIES

JAYANT A. TALWALKAR ■ RUSSELL H. WIESNER

Primary sclerosing cholangitis (PSC) is a chronic cholestatic liver disease characterized by inflammation and fibrosis of the intra- and extrahepatic bile ducts. Disease progression often results in biliary cirrhosis and hepatic failure. Understanding the natural history of PSC has become important because of the success of liver transplantation as an effective therapeutic modality.

Fifty percent to 70% of patients with PSC are male with an average age of 40 years at diagnosis. A close association between PSC and inflammatory bowel disease (IBD) is also well established. Between 70% and 80% of PSC patients have chronic ulcerative colitis (UC). Conversely, about 2% to 4% of patients with UC have PSC.

Immunologic and genetic alterations have been cited as factors in the pathogenesis of PSC. Cellular abnormalities have focused primarily on T lymphocyte differentiation and function. Humoral serum markers including immunoglobulins G and M are seen in low but detectable titers. Elevated levels of circulating immune complexes are observed in 80% of cases. Human leukocyte antigen alleles A1, B8, and DR3 have been described in association with PSC. Non–immune-mediated etiologies associated with the development of PSC include infectious agents (bacterial, viral), immunodeficiency syndromes, and bile acid metabolites.

The clinical presentation of PSC ranges between asymptomatic to complaints of fatigue and pruritus at diagnosis. Jaundice (60%) and weight loss (40%) are uncommon and raise the suspicion of advanced disease. Serum hepatic biochemical parameters usually reflect a cholestatic profile with elevated alkaline phosphatase values in 95% of cases. Total bilirubin levels may be elevated and often fluctuate. Serum autoantibodies including antinuclear antibody, smooth muscle antibody, and perinuclear antineutrophil cytoplasmic antibody are variably detected but without known pathogenicity. Extrahepatic autoimmune disorders may also be associated with PSC. Primary conditions include UC (70%–80%), Crohn's disease (5%–8%), pancreatitis (10%–25%), diabetes mellitus (5%–15%), and autoimmune thyroid disease (3%–5%).

The diagnosis of PSC is made by cholangiography (Fig. 54-1). Intrahepatic duct involvement is nearly universal, with extrahepatic duct sparing in 20% of cases. Segmental bile duct fibrosis with subsequent saccular dilation of normal intervening areas results in the characteristic "beads on a string" appearance seen in

PSC. The use of abdominal computerized tomography or magnetic resonance cholangiopancreatography for accurate detection of suspected PSC has been increasingly useful (Fig. 54-2). Liver biopsy is required for staging disease severity in PSC. Periductal fibrosis with inflammation, bile duct proliferation, and ductopenia constitute the main histological findings (Fig. 54-3). Fibro-obliterative cholangiopathy (Fig. 54-4), considered the most diagnostic finding on liver biopsy, is present in only 10% of instances. Explant findings often reveal extreme fibrotic reactions surrounding large bile ducts (Fig. 54-5).

The recognition of elevated serum hepatic biochemistries consistent with cholestasis in a male patient with concurrent IBD is strongly suggestive of PSC. Inflammatory bowel disease occurs in 70% to 80% of patients with primary sclerosing cholangitis. In those PSC patients who undergo proctocolectomy, the formation of peristomal varices with severe bleeding can be a major complication and cause significant morbidity (Fig. 54-6). The differential diagnosis, however, also includes biliary obstruction from choledocholithiasis, stricture, or malignancy; primary biliary cirrhosis; autoimmune hepatitis; recurrent pyogenic cholangitis; fungal cholangitis; acquired immunodeficiency syndrome cholangiopathy; choledochal cysts; cystic fibrosis; cirrhosis; intrahepatic hepatocellular carcinoma; cholangitis glandularis proliferans; and eosinophilic cholangitis.

Several disease-related complications are recognized with PSC. The frequency of reported fatigue and pruritus in PSC is between 40% and 70%, respectively. Symptom severity appears to be independent of histological stage. Although no effective treatment has been identified for improving fatigue, a number of therapies for pruritus, including antihistamines, cholestyramine, phenobarbital, rifampin, ursodeoxycholic acid, naltrexone, activated charcoal hemoperfusion, and plasmapheresis, have been used with variable success. For intractable pruritus refractory to medical therapy, liver transplantation (LT) is the only existing therapeutic option. Metabolic bone disease is related to osteopenia rather than osteomalacia in PSC (Fig. 54-7). Approximately 50% of patients have osteopenia, whereas osteoporosis develops in 10% of cases. Initial treatment with calcium and weight-bearing activity is mandatory. Oral replacement therapy with vitamin D is indicated if measured serum levels are reduced. When present, steatorrhea may be caused by impaired small intestine bile acid delivery, celiac disease, or exocrine pancreatic insufficiency. Malabsorption of fat-soluble vitamins (A, D, E, K) is common with advanced PSC and usually responds to oral replacement therapy.

Cholelithiasis is common in PSC and often requires cholecystectomy for symptomatic disease in patients with nonadvanced hepatic disease. Choledocholithiasis occurs in 5% to 15% of cases in association with biliary strictures. Symptomatic disease has been successfully treated by endoscopic or percutaneous methods. Bacterial cholangitis is most commonly associated with a previous history of biliary tract surgery, bile duct calculi, or dominant stricture. Therapy includes empiric broad-spectrum intravenous antibiotics and biliary decompression when needed. Dominant strictures occur in 15% to 20% of PSC patients (Fig. 54-8). Clinical manifestations include a sudden asymptomatic increase in serum hepatic biochemistries, progressive jaundice, and bacterial cholangitis. Diagnosis and therapy with endoscopic or radiologic approaches often provide significant clinical improvement.

The most feared complication of PSC is cholangiocarcinoma. Primary anatomic sites of involvement include the hilum (75% of cases), intrahepatic ducts (16%), and gallbladder (8%). Risk factors include advanced age, long duration of IBD, advanced hepatic disease, cigarette smoking, and colorectal dysplasia or carcinoma. Confirming the diagnosis of cholangiocarcinoma in PSC is difficult. The distinction between benign and malignant biliary strictures with cross-sectional imaging and cholangiography is often unclear (Fig. 54-9). Serum tumor markers, including carbohydrate antigen 19-9 and carcinoembryonic antigen, remain insensitive for detecting early or advanced disease. Rarely, bile duct dysplasia or carcinoma can be diagnosed on liver biopsy (Fig. 54-10). Therapeutic options for cholangiocarcinoma in PSC are limited and include surgery, radiation therapy, chemotherapy, or a combination of therapies. Carefully selected patients with localized distal disease, however, may derive benefits from surgical resection. Although curative attempts with LT have traditionally resulted in poor outcomes, initial results with preoperative chemoradiation therapy may be associated with long-term survival.

Because of the variable nature of disease progression, there is no recognized effective medical therapy for PSC. Studies examining antifibrotic (D-penicillamine, colchicine) and immunosuppressive (corticosteroids, azathioprine, cyclosporine, methotrexate) agents have not been associated with improved survival in the absence of liver transplantation. Three randomized, placebo-controlled trials with ursodeoxycholic acid (UDCA) did not show significant improvements in histology or survival. Recent investigations of high-dose UDCA (25–30 mg/kg/day) have noted improved biochemical, cholangiographic, and histological parameters; these results await confirmation in placebo-controlled studies.

Endoscopic therapy in PSC has been successful in alleviating cholestasis aggravated by mechanical biliary obstruction. The current use of endoscopic dilation with sphincterotomy and/or stenting is associated with clinical response rates from 70% to 90%. Nasobiliary tube drainage provides no advantage compared to other techniques. Although short-term biliary stent placement appears effective for refractory strictures, its overall advantage compared to balloon dilation alone remains unknown. A recent investigation advocating the use of aggressive stricture dilation and/or stenting combined with UDCA therapy in PSC to improve survival was based on results in an uncontrolled trial setting. Among precirrhotic individuals with refractory extrahepatic biliary strictures, intraoperative resection has been successfully performed. A history of prior surgery, however, has been associated with increased risks for biliary complications after LT.

PSC is the fourth most common indication for LT in the United States, accounting for nearly 10% of all procedures. Recurrent cholangitis despite medical therapy, severe extrahepatic biliary obstruction precluding operative repair, and uncontrolled peristomal variceal bleeding may also benefit from LT. Patient survival rates between 90% and 97% (1 year) and 83% and 88% (5 years) are reported. Long-term graft survival is affected by a higher incidence of rejection and hepatic artery thrombosis. An increasing body of evidence suggests that PSC is a recurrent disease after LT (Fig. 54-11). If strict criteria are used, the recurrence rate is between 10% and 20%.

Despite a median survival of 9 to 12 years in PSC, a number of affected individuals will not experience progressive disease. Because of this significant variation in natural history, the use of mathematical prognostic models has allowed for improvements in estimating survival. The application of existing prognostic models for defining the optimal timing of LT requires further refinement.

Variant PSC syndromes have also been recognized. Small duct PSC occurs in patients with typical features of PSC, normal cholangiography, and compatible histological changes on liver biopsy. Eventual recognition of large duct PSC occurs in 40% of cases. Although it is uncommon, the progression to end-stage liver disease requiring hepatic transplantation has been associated with small duct PSC. Coexisting features reminiscent of autoimmune hepatitis in select PSC patients is called "overlap syndrome." The presence of typical cholangiographic features of PSC is often accompanied by histological changes in autoimmune hepatitis. Idiopathic adulthood ductopenia is a syndrome described by histological evidence of ductopenia and no evidence for PSC and IBD.

AIDS cholangiopathy describes a syndrome that resembles sclerosing cholangitis associated with papillary stenosis (Fig. 54-12). Among responsible pathogens, *Cryptosporidium* is the most commonly identified. However, up to 50% of patients have no identifiable opportunistic infection. The most common presentation is abdominal pain (64%–88%) with fever (20%–65%). Serum liver biochemistries are noted for elevations in alkaline phosphatase in more than 75% of cases. Ultrasonography or computed tomographic imaging can detect biliary duct dilation in most instances. The most common features on cholangiography include papillary stenosis with intrahepatic sclerosing cholangitis. Among individuals with severe pain and associated cholangitis, the identification of papillary stenosis is nearly universal. Treatment is directed at identified pathogens as well as biliary tract abnormalities. For patients with papillary stenosis alone, endoscopic sphincterotomy has been associated with improvement in abdominal symptoms.

Cholangiopathies may also develop after bone marrow transplantation. Acute graft versus host disease (GVHD) presents clinically with skin rash, gastrointestinal dysfunction, and elevated serum hepatic enzymes. Immunosuppressive agents are recommended for the prevention and treatment of acute GVHD. Cholangitis lenta is associated with fever and mild hyperbilirubinemia in the early posttransplant phase. Treatment of the underlying infection often improves cholestasis. Drug-induced cholestasis can occur by idiosyncratic or dose-dependent mechanisms. Discontinuation of potential offending agents is the initial step in treatment. Chronic hepatic GVHD is associated with the rapid or subacute onset of bile duct destruction and intrahepatic cholestasis. It may occur de novo or result from prior acute GVHD. Prednisone and cyclosporine are required for treatment; salvage therapy options include tacrolimus, thalidomide, or sirolimus. The development of jaundice, hepatomegaly, and weight gain over 5% of ideal body weight is consistent with the diagnosis of venoocclusive disease (VOD). Mild to moderate cases resolve with supportive measures. For severe cases, the use of thrombolytic therapy may improve hyperbilirubinemia but is associated with increased mortality. Transjugular intrahepatic portosystemic shunt (TIPS) placement has been associated with increased mortality in patients with severe VOD.

Cholangiopathies associated with LT can involve either intrahepatic or extrahepatic bile ducts. The overall incidence of biliary complications ranges from 9% to 15% and usually develops 2 to 6 months after LT. Anastomotic strictures occur in 3% to 7% of cases and may be early or late. Hilar strictures are associated with local ischemia or hepatic artery thrombosis. Bile leaks occur in up to 25% of recipients. Clinical manifestations of all biliary complications include elevations in serum alkaline phosphatase or total bilirubin. Exclusion of hepatic artery thrombosis by Doppler ultrasonography is mandatory. Cholangiography is required for diagnostic and therapeutic purposes. Allograft liver biopsy is warranted if cholangiography is unremarkable. Ensuring adequate immunosuppression in the presence of chronic ductopenic rejection is mandatory. Advances in endoscopic and radiologic techniques have demonstrated satisfactory results from balloon dilation and/or stenting. Refractory cases may then be considered candidates for biliary anastomosis reconstruction. Expandable metal stents are used in subjects with ischemic-type biliary strictures who are poor candidates for retransplantation.

Operative bile duct injury is most commonly associated with open and laparoscopic cholecystectomy. Risk factors include limited operative experience, acute or chronic biliary tract inflammation, and aberrant anatomy. Fever, abdominal pain, and/or wound drainage can be observed. Late complications include biloma formation and biliary stricture. Hepatobiliary scintigraphy can document the existence of bile leakage in 90% to 95% of cases. Endoscopic or percutaneous therapy has been employed with success. Injuries noted at laparoscopic surgery require conversion to an open procedure with immediate repair.

Biliary strictures associated with acute pancreatitis are usually transient. Operative therapy for chronic pancreatitis is associated with stricture formation in 60% to 70% of cases. Elevations in alkaline phosphatase without similar degrees of hyperbilirubinemia can occur. Complications may include cholangitis, choledocholithiasis, and secondary biliary cirrhosis. Surgical decompression is employed for high-grade obstruction complicated by jaundice, cholangitis, and/or progressive biliary fibrosis refractory to nonoperative approaches.

Spontaneous enteric biliary fistulae occur in 0.5% to 5% of cases after biliary tract operations. Cholecystoduodenal (75%), cholecystocolonic (15%), and cholecystogastric (6%) fistulae are the most frequent sites. Complications include ascending cholangitis, weight loss, bleeding, and bowel obstruction. Gallstone ileus can present with acute small bowel obstruction. The ileocecal area (75%) and jejunum (20%) are most common sites of obstruction. The treatment of choice is operative, when possible.

Operative biliary fistulae are most commonly observed with bile duct injury after cholecystectomy. Hepatobiliary scintigraphy and/or cholangiography can detect bile leaks and fistulae with greater than 90% accuracy. Endoscopic therapy has been successful; treatment failures require surgical intervention. Bronchobiliary fistulae occur in 4% to 10% of patients. Etiologies include hepatic and subphrenic abscess formation, blunt abdominal trauma, bile duct stenosis, choledocholithiasis, and congenital causes. Clinical manifestations include biliptysis, jaundice, and cholangitis. The diagnosis is made by cholangiography. The treatment of choice is surgical.

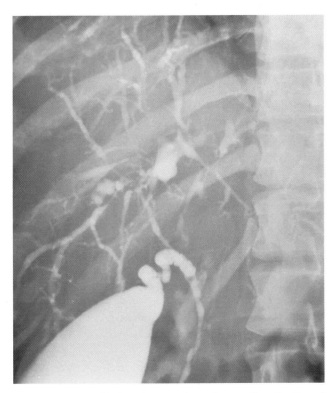

FIGURE 54-1. Cholangiogram that shows "beading" and irregularity of both the intra- and extrahepatic biliary tract typical of primary sclerosing cholangitis.

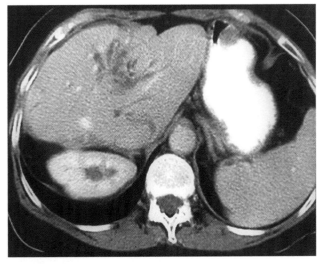

FIGURE 54-2. Computed tomographic scan of focal intrahepatic bile duct dilation in a patient with primary sclerosing cholangitis.

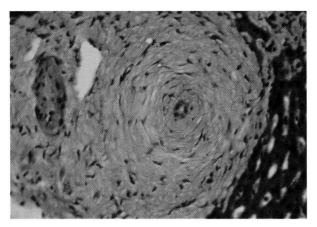

FIGURE 54-3. Liver biopsy that shows fibrotic duct lesion seen in primary sclerosing cholangitis.

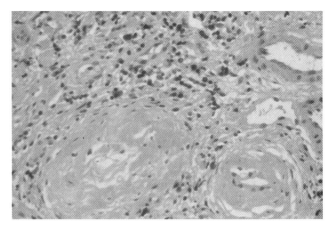

FIGURE 54-4. Liver biopsy that shows obliterative duct lesion seen in primary sclerosing cholangitis.

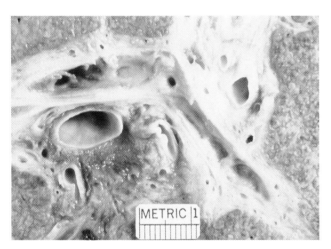

FIGURE 54-5. Explant liver with intense fibrosis surrounding the biliary tract, which is typical of primary sclerosing cholangitis.

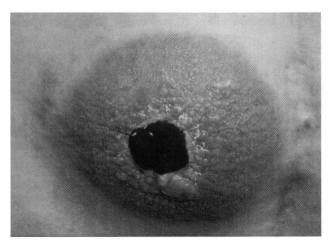

FIGURE 54-6. An abdominal photo of severe abdominal peristomal varices in a patient with primary sclerosing cholangitis with a history of chronic ulcerative colitis who underwent total proctocolectomy and ileostomy.

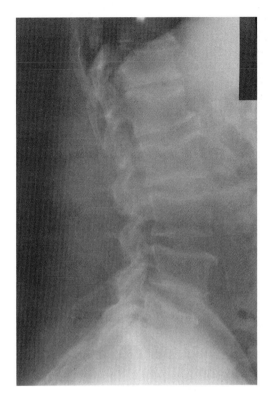

FIGURE 54-7. Spine x-ray of a patient with severe osteoporosis, a finding seen in 20% to 25% of patients with primary sclerosing cholangitis who undergo liver transplantation.

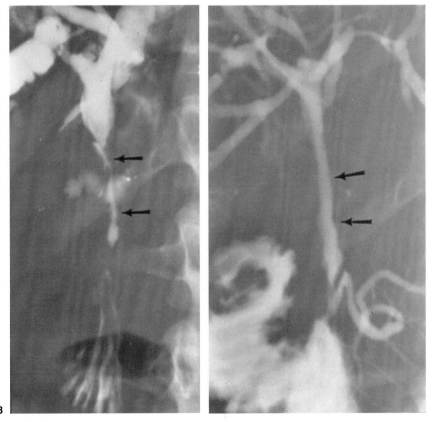

A, B

FIGURE 54-8. Cholangiogram of a dominant stricture of the common bile duct (**A**) before and (**B**) after balloon dilation.

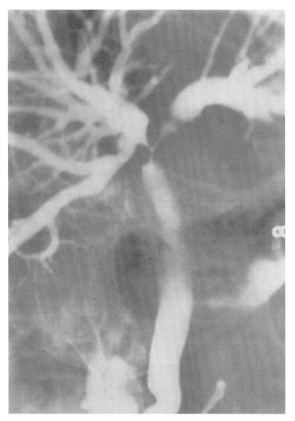

FIGURE 54-9. Cholangiogram of a hilar lesion typical of cholangiocarcinoma in a patient with long-standing chronic ulcerative colitis.

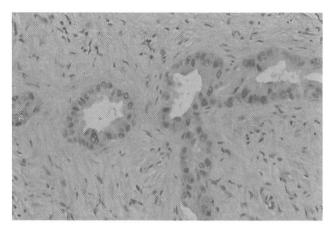

FIGURE 54-10. Liver biopsy that shows bile duct dysplasia and cholangiocarcinoma in a patient with long-standing primary sclerosing cholangitis and chronic ulcerative colitis.

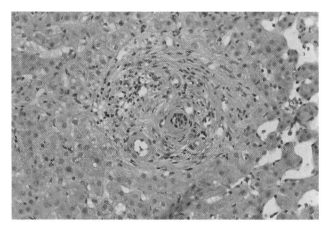

FIGURE 54-11. Liver biopsy that shows early recurrence of primary sclerosing cholangitis (PSC) in a patient who underwent liver transplantation for PSC 5 years ago. An early fibrosis obliterative duct lesion is present.

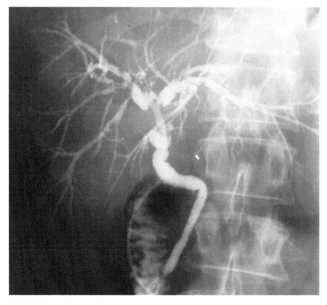

FIGURE 54-12. A patient with acquired immunodeficiency syndrome cholangiopathy who had a positive culture for cytomegalovirus and *Cryptosporidium:* the findings are indistinguishable from cholangiographic findings in primary sclerosing cholangitis.

55

CYSTIC DISEASES OF THE BILIARY TRACT

SHELLY C. LU ■ KHALDOUN A. DEBIAN

Biliary cysts are cystic dilations that can occur throughout the biliary system. They mainly afflict children and young adults; 83% to 90% of reported cases are diagnosed in patients younger than 30 years of age. Most biliary cysts are congenital but acquired forms occur. Todani and colleagues proposed the most useful classification of biliary cysts. Type I cysts are common bile duct (CBD) cysts or choledochal cysts, which encompass 75% to 85% of all cases of biliary cysts. Type II cysts are diverticulum cysts found anywhere in the extrahepatic ducts and make up 2% to 3% of reported cases. Type III cysts are choledochocele cysts, are rare, and represent 1.4% to 5.6% of reported cases. Type IV cysts are multiple cysts in the intrahepatic and extrahepatic ducts, and account for 18% to 20% of reported cases. Type V cysts are intrahepatic bile duct cysts (single or multiple), are also rare, and probably represent Caroli disease as originally described. Isolated cystic duct dilations are classified by some as type VI cysts. These are rarely found, and only three cases are described in the literature.

Clinical presentation of biliary cysts depends on the patient's age. In infancy, jaundice with or without acholic stools is the most common finding, occurring in as many as 80% of patients. Pain may or may not be a factor, but vomiting and failure to thrive have been reported in as many as 50% of patients. Hepatomegaly is often found, and 30% to 60% of patients have a palpable abdominal mass. The classic clinical triad of pain, jaundice, and a palpable abdominal mass has been found only in 11% to 63% of large series.

Chronic and intermittent pain appears to be the most common presenting symptom in patients older than 2 years of age, and has been reported in 50% to 96% of patients. Intermittent jaundice and recurrent cholangitis are also common, and have been reported in 34% to 55% of patients. Abdominal mass is much less common; it occurs in about 10% to 20% of cases. The classical triad of pain, jaundice, and a palpable mass has been reported in 3% to 13% of patients. Cirrhosis and portal hypertension are encountered less often than the infantile form. Recurrent pancreatitis has been reported only in the noninfantile form, although whether there is actual pancreatic inflammation is debatable. Sometimes the patient may present with carcinoma of the biliary tract, which is the most feared complication of biliary cysts.

Diagnosis of biliary cysts requires a high index of suspicion. Percutaneous transhepatic cholangiography (PTC) and endoscopic retrograde cholangiopancreatography

(ERCP) provide the most detailed examinations (Figs. 55-1, 55-2*A*, 55-4, 55-5*A*, and 55-6*A*). In infants, ultrasonography and hepatobiliary scintigraphy provide a sound basis for diagnosis (Figs. 55-2*B* and 55-3). Ultrasonography is an excellent screening tool but provides little anatomical or functional information. Hepatobiliary scintigraphy provides information about excretory patterns (see Fig. 55-2*B*) and is excellent for postoperative patient follow-up. Computed tomography is superior to ultrasonography in older patients (Figs. 55-2*C* and 55-6*B*). Recent advances in magnetic resonance imaging (MRI) have made magnetic resonance cholangiopancreatography (MRCP) an attractive alternative to ERCP or PTC (Fig. 55-7). Several studies have shown MRCP to be just as effective as conventional cholangiopancreatography, such as ERCP, in evaluating biliary cysts.

An anomalous pancreaticobiliary ductal anatomy occurs commonly in choledochal cysts (see Fig. 55-4*A, B*). In many patients with choledochal cysts, the CBD enters the pancreatic duct at a right angle, abnormally far from the ampulla of Vater. This abnormal anatomy impairs normal sphincteric function at the pancreaticobiliary junction, which may lead to reflux of pancreatic juice into the bile duct, destruction of the bile duct by pancreatic enzymes, and cystic malformation.

Cholangiography best diagnoses choledochoceles (see Fig. 55-5*A*). Typically, the distal CBD appears "clubbed." Emptying of contrast material is often delayed. Choledochoceles are easily distinguished from duodenal diverticula and duodenal duplication cysts because they fill during cholangiography but not during upper gastrointestinal contrast studies (see Fig. 55-5*B*). Duodenal diverticula fill on upper gastrointestinal series but not on cholangiography. Duplication cysts will not fill with either diagnostic method. Sarris and Tsang proposed an additional anatomic classification of choledochoceles (Fig. 55-8). In type A, the ampulla opens into the choledochocele, which communicates with the duodenum through another small opening. Type A choledochoceles can be further subclassified into A1, in which the pancreatic and CBD share a common opening into the cyst (33% of cases); A2, in which the openings are distinct (4% of cases); and A3, in which the choledochocele is small and entirely intramural (25% of cases). In type B, the ampulla opens directly into the duodenum, and the choledochocele communicates only with the distal CBD (21% of cases). This scheme is useful because of important therapeutic implications.

Type IV cysts are multiple cysts in the intrahepatic and extrahepatic ducts. They are further subclassified into type IVA and IVB. Type IVA cysts are multiple cysts in the intrahepatic and extrahepatic ducts, which account for 18% to 20% of reported cases. Type IVB multiple cysts occur only in the extrahepatic duct and are much less common.

Type V intrahepatic bile duct cyst represent Caroli disease as originally described (see Fig. 55-6). After the original description, Caroli soon realized that there is a simple type and a perifibrosis type. The periportal fibrosis type is also known as Caroli syndrome. In addition to intrahepatic cystic dilation, congenital hepatic fibrosis, cirrhosis, portal hypertension, and esophageal varices are frequently seen. It is often associated with the renal abnormalities of autosomal recessive polycystic kidney disease.

Congenital hepatic fibrosis refers to a unique congenital liver histology characterized by bland portal fibrosis, hyperproliferation of interlobular bile ducts within the portal areas with variable shapes and sizes of bile ducts, and preservation of normal lobular architecture (Fig. 55-9). Congenital hepatic fibrosis is often associated with biliary cysts and appears to be caused by phosphomannose isomerase deficiency, a genetic defect that results in impaired protein *N*-glycosylation, in some cases. This finding means that congenital hepatic fibrosis is potentially treatable in some patients. It also highlights the importance of normal protein glycosylation in ductal plate formation.

The treatment of choice in patients with biliary cysts is total cyst excision for choledochal cysts and diverticulum cysts. The malignant potential of choledochoceles is low, but is dependent on the type of epithelium that lines the cysts. Carcinoma has only been reported in choledochoceles that were lined by biliary or undifferentiated epithelium internally (up to 20% in some reports). Thus, some investigators advocate complete excision of the choledochocele by separation and reinsertion of the CBD and pancreatic duct into the duodenal wall if the choledochocele is lined by biliary or undifferentiated epithelium, whereas sphincteroplasty should be reserved only for those lined by duodenal epithelium.

Intrahepatic cyst (i.e., types IVA and V) treatment depends on the degree of involvement. When segmental cystic disease is confined to one lobe (more often the left lobe), then lobectomy is usually curative. If both lobes are involved, some have advocated establishing a permanent-access hepaticojejunostomy after partial hepatectomy to allow easy biliary tract access when necessary. Chronic antibiotic therapy in multilobar Caroli disease may have some benefit. Ultimately, if attacks of cholangitis are frequent and quality of life is poor, hepatic transplantation may be a therapeutic option. Cholecystectomy should be performed at the time of cyst excision because the gallbladder has shown clinical and histological evidence of cholecystitis in patients that required secondary operations. The gallbladder appears to be predisposed to malignant change in patients with biliary cysts. If definitive surgical procedure is successful, the prognosis is generally excellent. Reversal of cirrhosis has even been reported.

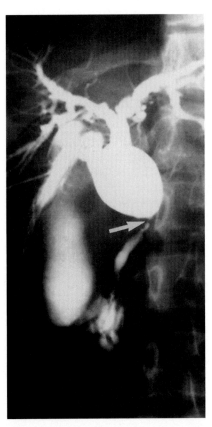

FIGURE 55-1. Choledochal cyst: type IA. Mild stenosis (*arrow*) of the common bile duct immediately distal to the cyst contributes to the slight intrahepatic ductal distention.

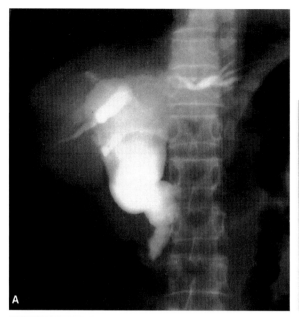

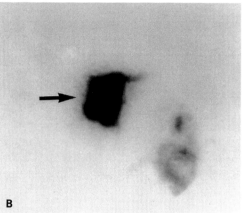

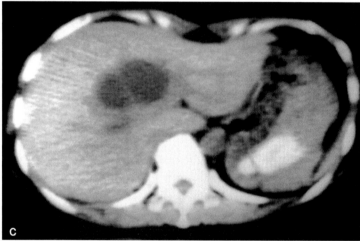

FIGURE 55-2. Choledochal cyst: type IC. **A:** Diffuse enlargement of the common bile duct with distal tapering. **B:** Radionuclide scan with activity predominantly in the cyst (*arrow*) and left hepatic duct. Bowel activity indicates patency of the common bile duct. **C:** Computed tomographic scan at the level of the cephalic portion of the cyst shows slight extension of the dilation into both right and left hepatic ducts.

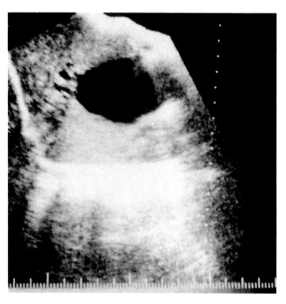

FIGURE 55-3. Choledochal cyst: sonographic findings. The anechoic mass with enhanced through-transmission is characteristic of a cystic structure. Note one and possibly two ducts entering the cephalic aspect of the cyst. Absence of dilation of the bile ducts proximal to the cystic mass is typical for most type I cysts.

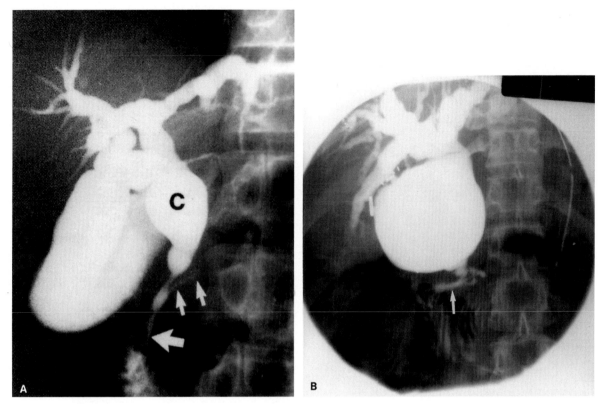

FIGURE 55-4. Choledochal cyst: anomalous ductal relationship. **A:** Cystic enlargement of the common bile duct (C) with associated dilation of the common hepatic and intrahepatic ducts. The abnormal junction of pancreatic (*small arrows*) and common bile duct and long common channel (*large arrow*) are displayed. **B:** A large cyst involves the common hepatic and common bile duct accompanied by intrahepatic ductal dilation. A long common channel (*arrow*) results from the abnormally high junction with the pancreatic duct.

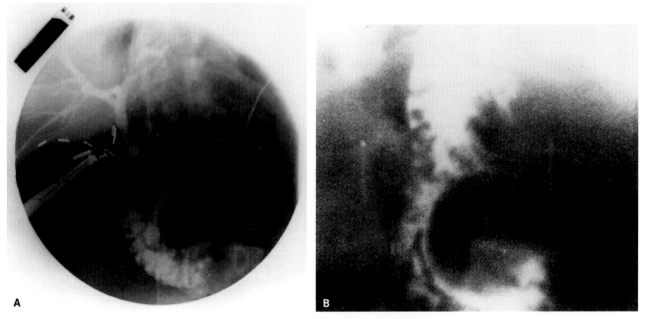

FIGURE 55-5. Choledochocele: type III cyst. **A:** Cholangiography reveals a club-shaped enlargement of the distal common bile duct bulging into the duodenum. **B:** Upper gastrointestinal series reveals a smoothly rounded filling defect in the second portion of the duodenum.

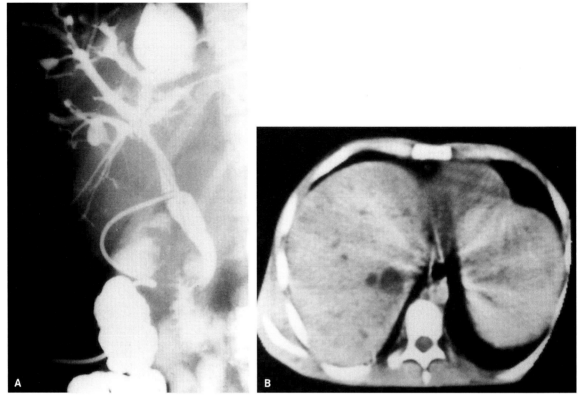

FIGURE 55-6. Caroli disease: type V cyst. **A:** T-tube cholangiography demonstrates cystic dilation of multiple intrahepatic bile ducts representing type V biliary cyst. **B:** Computed tomographic scan of the same patient showing several of the intrahepatic cysts.

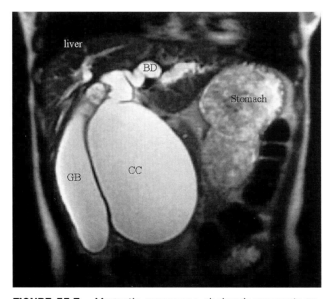

FIGURE 55-7. Magnetic resonance cholangiopancreatography (MRCP) of choledochal cyst. A coronal FSE T2 MRCP performed on a 16-year-old female patient presenting with right upper quadrant pain, jaundice, and amylasemia shows a very dilated segment of the common bile duct compatible with choledochal cyst distal to the origin of the cystic duct. The intrahepatic ducts are normal in size and shape. (Courtesy of Dr. Fergus Coakley, Department of Radiology, UCSF.)

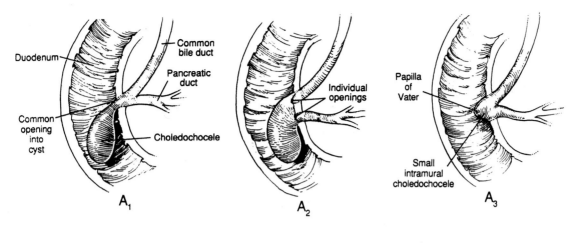

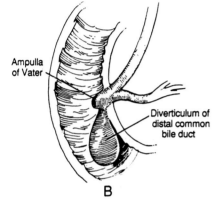

FIGURE 55-8. Proposed subclassification of choledochoceles (type III biliary cyst). Type A: The ampulla opens into the choledochocele, which in turn communicates with the duodenum via another small opening. Type A is subclassified into A1, in which the pancreatic and common bile duct share a common opening into the cyst (33% of cases); A2, in which the openings are distinct (4% of cases); and A3, in which the choledochocele is small and entirely intramural (25% of cases). Type B: The ampulla opens directly into the duodenum with the choledochocele communicating with the distal common bile duct (21% of cases).

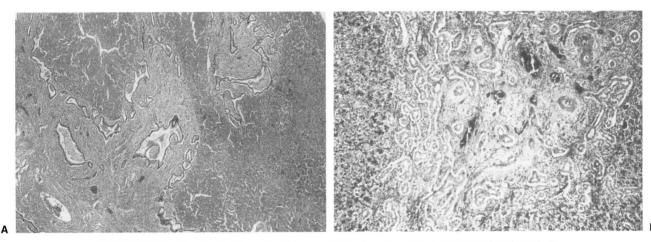

FIGURE 55-9. Congenital hepatic fibrosis. A 27-year-old woman presented with periodic right upper quadrant discomfort and persistent mildly elevated alkaline phosphatase levels. A liver biopsy showed (**A**) the liver parenchyma is normal but the portal areas show prominent portal fibrosis without inflammation. The interlobular bile ducts are numerous, dilated, and some contain inspissated bile (H&E stain; low power) and (**B**) marked portal fibrosis as demonstrated by trichrome staining. Note the sharp demarcation of the fibrotic area from the parenchyma (trichrome stain; high power). (Courtesy of Dr. Gary Kanel, Department of Pathology, Rancho Los Amigos Medical Center.)

TUMORS OF THE BILIARY TRACT

JOSEPH J.Y. SUNG

TUMOR OF THE BILE DUCTS

Bile duct cancer, or cholangiocarcinoma, is rare in the western world but is relatively common in Asia. The cause of cholangiocarcinoma is unclear, but chronic inflammation and bile stasis are considered to be important in the development of the disease. Risk factors include chronic infestation by liver flukes; chronic suppurative cholangitis (recurrent pyogenic cholangitis); inflammatory bowel disease associated with sclerosing cholangitis; congenital bile duct disorders (choledochal cyst and Caroli disease); and use of Thorotrast, a radiologic contrast medium, in the 1930s and 1940s. Evidence of old or current infestation by clonorchis (*Clonorchis sinensis*) and opisthorchis (*Opisthorchis viverrini*) has been associated with cholangiocarcinoma in China and Southeast Asia. The leaf-shaped adult worms live and proliferate in the intrahepatic biliary tract and cause chronic inflammation, ductal proliferation, and mucin secretion of the biliary epithelium (Fig. 56-1). Cholangiocarcinoma also is associated with hepatolithiasis and strictures of the bile duct (Fig. 56-2). The chemical composition of primary bile duct stones, mostly calcium bilirubinate with less than 25% cholesterol content, is very different from that of stones in gallbladders. Because bacteria form an integral part of these pigment stones, patients usually have recurrent attacks of suppurative cholangitis. Patients with sclerosing cholangitis and choledochal cyst may have bile duct cancer in the fourth decade of life, 20 to 30 years younger than the mean age of other patients with cholangiocarcinoma. Reflux of pancreatic juice into the bile duct because of an anomalous pancreatic-biliary junction has been suggested as the cause of cancer.

At macroscopic examination, cholangiocarcinoma is a solid, grayish-white tumor with a nodular, sclerosing, or diffuse infiltrative appearance. The distribution of extrahepatic bile duct cancer is 49% in the upper third, 25% in the middle third, 19% in the lower third, and diffuse among 7% of patients, according to Tompkins and colleagues. Cholangiocarcinoma originating from the hilum of the liver is called Klatskin tumor. These tumors usually are small and can be missed even during an operation and remain localized at the confluence of the right and left hepatic ducts. Bismuth and colleagues classified these tumors according to extent of involvement and communication between the right and left ductal system as follows:

Type I: Unobstructed primary confluence (tumor in the main hepatic duct).
Type II: Obstruction limited to primary confluence (tumor at the confluence).

Type III: Obstruction of the primary confluence with extension to either the right (IIIa) or left (IIIb) secondary confluence.

Type IV: Tumor growth along both hepatic ducts causing multiple segmental obstructions.

Most Klatskin tumors present themselves in type II or type III distribution. This classification reflects increasing difficulty in treatment options as the tumor grows into segmental bile ducts.

At microscopic examination most bile duct cancers are adenocarcinoma. They usually are differentiated tubular adenocarcinoma with abundant fibrous stroma and variable mucin-secreting ability (Fig. 56-3). The tumor penetrates lymphatic vessels and regional lymph nodes, portal vessels, and adjacent neural tissues. Despite advances in biliary imaging, the treatment results of cholangiocarcinoma have not improved substantially. Only 25% of patients have tumors that are resectable at the time of diagnosis. Most patients die within 6 to 12 months of diagnosis, usually as a result of local invasion and biliary obstruction that lead to cholangitis and liver failure. The prognosis is worst for lesions affecting the confluence of bile ducts and is best for tumors involving the distal common bile duct.

Benign tumors of the biliary tract, such as papillomas, adenomas, and granular cell myoblastoma, are extremely rare. Inflammatory reactions in recurrent cholangitis that cause strictures, dilation, and fibrosis of the bile duct can be difficult to differentiate from malignant growths in the biliary tract.

TUMOR OF THE GALLBLADDER

Tumor of the gallbladder is the most common biliary tract cancer in the western world. Gallbladder cancer occurs more frequently among women. Gallbladder stones, found among 75% of patients, are considered an important risk factor for gallbladder cancer. The causal relation to gallstones was supported by results of a prospective cohort study in Rochester, Minnesota. It is hypothesized that gallstones cause chronic trauma to and inflammation of the gallbladder mucosa, which induce dysplastic changes and carcinogenesis. Duration of the presence of gallstones appears to be a crucial factor in the development of cancer. Porcelain gallbladder also is associated with high risk for infiltrative carcinoma of the gallbladder; some experts advocate prophylactic cholecystectomy for such patients. There appears to be a high incidence of an anomalous junction between the cystic duct and common bile duct among patients with gallbladder cancer. The malignant potential of benign lesions such as adenoma (gallbladder polyp) and adenomyoma is unconfirmed. No clear adenoma-to-carcinoma sequence has been demonstrated as it has with colonic cancer.

At macroscopic examination the tumor is seen to produce diffuse thickening of the gallbladder wall. Fungating growth in the gallbladder lumen and infiltration of surrounding structures are commonly found. Most gallbladder cancers are mucin-secreting adenocarcinoma. Squamous cell carcinoma and undifferentiated carcinoma constitute only 10% of cases. Gallbladder cancer spreads by means of direct local invasion of the liver, duodenum, and colon. The common hepatic duct often is invaded by cancer that arises from the neck of the gallbladder or the Hartmann pouch and mimics cholangiocarcinoma in clinical presentation. The diagnosis often is made at laparotomy for a presumptive diagnosis of chronic cholecystitis. Only about 20% of patients with gallbladder cancer have a correct preoperative diagnosis. Eighty percent of tumors are considered unresectable at surgical exploration. The overall 5-year survival rate remains less than 5%. Benign tumors of the gallbladder are not uncommon. They are often detected incidentally during ultrasound examination of the abdomen for other reasons. In general, follow-up ultrasonography in

3 to 6 months is recommended for gallbladder polyps. If no enlargement is detected, cholecystectomy is unnecessary.

PERIAMPULLARY TUMORS

Tumors of the papilla and ampulla of Vater are grouped together as periampullary tumors. The cause of periampullary cancer is unclear. The tumors appear as papillary growth at the periampullary region, which makes identification of the opening of the ampulla difficult (Fig. 56-4). Like other biliary tract cancers, periampullary cancers are adenocarcinoma. Periampullary tumor is considered a separate entity from carcinoma of the pancreas. It has a different clinical presentation, and the prognosis is much better than that of pancreatic cancer. It is the most rare type of malignant tumor among the biliary tract cancers. Because of the early presentation, most periampullary tumors are resectable, and the postoperative survival rate is very high. Adenoma of the ampulla is extremely rare.

CLINICAL FEATURES

Patients with biliary tract cancers usually have vague symptoms such as anorexia, malaise, weight loss, and pain. Cholangiocarcinoma and gallbladder cancer cause jaundice when the confluence of the common hepatic duct or the common bile duct is obstructed. On the other hand, intermittent jaundice is an early sign of periampullary cancer. In complete biliary obstruction, urine turns dark and stool turns pale. Unlike choledocholithiasis or benign biliary strictures, cholangitis is an uncommon presenting feature of cholangiocarcinoma. Sepsis of the biliary tract usually occurs only after endoscopic or radiologic intervention. Cholangitis is distinctly more common with periampullary cancer. Periampullary cancer occasionally ulcerates and causes frank gastrointestinal bleeding or iron deficiency anemia. A mass can be palpated in the right upper quadrant in some cases of gallbladder cancer.

DIAGNOSIS

An initial ultrasound or computed tomographic (CT) scan provides valuable information about the level of obstruction and invasion of adjacent structures. In cholangiocarcinoma, dilated intrahepatic ducts proximal to the tumor and normal or collapsed gallbladder usually are seen (Figs. 56-5 and 56-6). It is uncommon to see a mass with bile duct cancers. Segmental or lobar atrophy of the liver resulting from portal vein or bile duct occlusion is an important finding on CT scans, because it might affect decisions about surgical resection and biliary drainage. A complex mass shadow in the region of the gallbladder or intralumenal mass with thickened wall is highly suggestive of gallbladder cancer (Fig. 56-7). A low-density area of the liver adjacent to the tumor may imply local invasion. Periampullary cancers are usually too small to be detected with ultrasonography or CT scanning. Dilation of the common bile duct that extends to the most distal end and distention of the gallbladder suggest periampullary tumor.

Cholangiography is the most accurate method for delineating the extent of tumor involvement and defining segmental ducts. The choice of cholangiography lies between percutaneous transhepatic cholangiography (PTC) and endoscopic retrograde cholangiopancreatography (ERCP). For tumors involving the proximal biliary tract, PTC is preferred because it is better for delineating the proximal involvement of the malignant growth. For tumors at the distal biliary tract, ERCP is often the choice. A cholangiogram that shows dilated intrahepatic ducts with a normal common bile duct suggests cholangiocarcinoma (Figs. 56-8 and 56-9). Gallbladder cancer may cause extrinsic compression or direct invasion into the common bile duct (see Fig. 56-7). Patients with periampullary tumors have a distended gallbladder and dilated ductal system up to the level of the distal common bile duct (see Fig. 56-4).

A definitive diagnosis of biliary cancer rests on histologic or cytologic proof of malignant growth. Fine-needle aspiration cytologic examination guided by ultrasound or CT scanning often confirms the diagnosis of gallbladder cancer. Unfortunately, a mass is seldom detected in bile duct cancer, making direct aspiration difficult. Brush cytologic specimens can be obtained at ERCP or PTC (Fig. 56-10). The sensitivity of brush cytologic examination ranges from 35% to 70%, depending on the type and location of tumor, method of brushing, and experience of the cytologist. On the other hand, endoscopic biopsy of the ampulla provides good tissue samples for histological diagnosis. Biopsy after endoscopic sphincterotomy may further improve the diagnostic yield.

Angiography is important in assessing the resectability of a tumor. It shows a nonvascular mass in the biliary tract that is nonspecific for the diagnosis. The main purpose of angiography is to exclude invasion of the blood vessels and major arterial anatomic variants.

TREATMENT

The two objectives in the treatment of patients with biliary tract cancer are to cure the patient of the tumor or to relieve bile duct obstruction by means of establishing biliary-enteric drainage. The only curative therapy available for bile duct cancer is radical surgical resection. The criteria for unresectability according to Blumgart and Benjamin are as follows:

- bilateral intrahepatic duct spread of tumor
- involvement of main trunk of portal vein
- bilateral involvement of hepatic artery or portal venous branches
- a combination of vascular involvement with cholangiographic evidence of extensive contralateral ductal spread.

Resection of the proximal bile duct (with or without hepatic resection) and reconstruction by means of hepaticojejunostomy is the standard procedure for the management of cholangiocarcinoma. Patients with complete resection of tumor and histologically verified tumor-free margins have a satisfactory chance of survival. Cholangiocarcinoma is not considered suitable for transplantation at most centers. Most cases of resectable gallbladder cancer are found incidentally at cholecystectomy. In confirmed cases, cholecystectomy with resection of the liver and dissection of lymph nodes and hepatoduodenal ligament is recommended for gallbladder cancer. In these cases, survival is good. Whipple procedure is widely accepted as therapy for periampullary cancer, although some surgeons claim local resection is sufficient. The outcome among these patients is the best among all tumors of the biliary tract.

Initial attempts to relieve biliary obstruction before an operation are aimed at optimizing hepatic and renal function. Unfortunately, preoperative biliary drainage has not shown to be beneficial. Neither surgical morbidity and mortality nor the nutritional status of the patients is significantly improved. Introduction of a foreign body into the biliary tract increases risk for infection.

Palliative treatment is aimed at relieving the obstruction of bile flow to preserve liver function and metabolism. It can be achieved with endoscopic-radiologic drainage of the bile ducts or surgical biliary-enteric bypass. Successful endoscopic insertion of a biliary endoprosthesis can be achieved in 80% to 90% of cases (Fig. 56-11) and results in normalization of bilirubin levels in the blood. Several randomized trials have compared endoscopic stenting with surgical bypass in the treatment of patients with distal malignant biliary obstruction. Endoscopic stenting results in lower immediate mortality and morbidity rates and shorter hospital stays, and thus is less expensive. However, the long-term results of surgical bypass are better than those of endoscopic drainage. The latter is associated with recurrent cholangitis in subsequent months. For proximal bile duct obstruction, the success of endoscopic stenting is reduced, and higher procedural complication rates and lower rates of resolution of jaundice occur. Percutaneous drainage would be a better option. The plastic stents in current use tend to clog as result of bacterial colonization and sludge formation on the stent. Patients experience recurrent jaundice, fever, and cholangitis. The median patency interval for a 10F stent is about 4 to 5 months.

Self-expanding metallic stents have been developed to avoid early clogging of endoprostheses. The Wallstent endoprosthesis (Schneider, Minneapolis, MN), which opens to a much larger diameter in the bile duct than a plastic stent, allows good drainage of bile (Fig. 56-12). The metal mesh of this stent also facilitates drainage of segmental bile ducts in proximal cholangiocarcinoma. Tumor ingrowth may still cause obstruction to bile flow in a period of 6 to 9 months (Fig. 56-13). The obstruction can be relieved with insertion of a plastic stent into the metal stent to resume bile drainage. A "removable," self-expanding stent made of a coil spring of nickel-titanium alloy, the Endocoil prosthesis (Instent, Eden Prairie, MN), is more suitable for drainage of distal biliary obstruction (Fig. 56-14). There is little evidence to support the use of radiation therapy and chemotherapy in the palliation of biliary tract cancers.

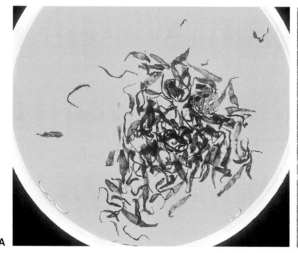
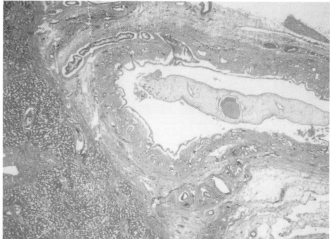

FIGURE 56-1. *Clonorchis sinensis* infestation. **A:** Liver fluke extracted from the bile of a patient with cholangiocarcinoma. **B:** Liver fluke in the bile duct causing chronic inflammation and ductal injury.

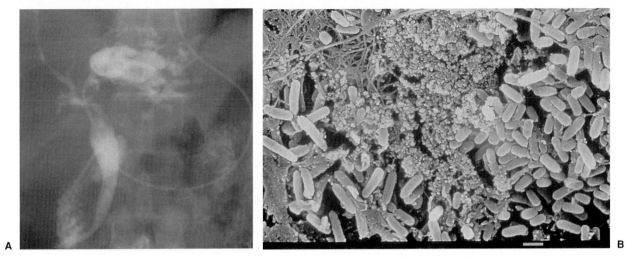

FIGURE 56-2. Intrahepatic pigment stones. **A:** Intrahepatic ductal dilation and stone impaction in the left hepatic duct of a patient with bile duct cancer. **B:** Bacteria inside the pigment stones.

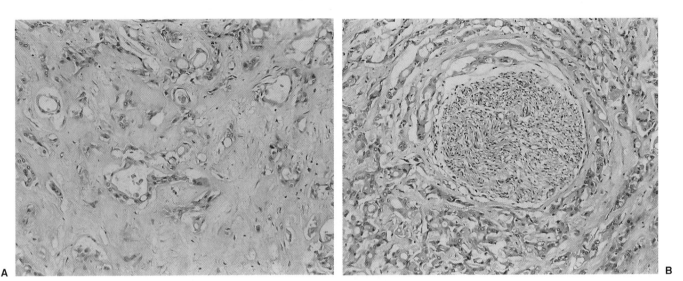

FIGURE 56-3. Cholangiocarcinoma. **A:** Cholangiocarcinoma is adenocarcinoma with abundant fibrosis. **B:** Perineural infiltration by cholangiocarcinoma.

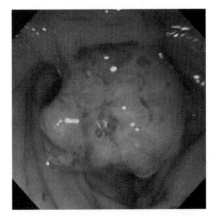

FIGURE 56-4. Periampullary cancer. Papillary growth of periampullary cancer obscures the opening of the ampulla.

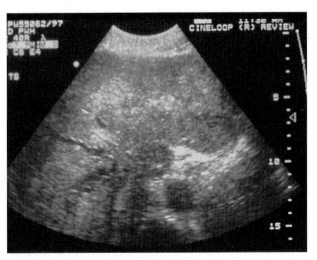

FIGURE 56-5. Ultrasound scan demonstrates intrahepatic ductal dilation in cholangiocarcinoma.

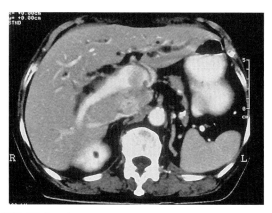

FIGURE 56-6. Computed tomographic scan demonstrates intrahepatic ductal dilation with tumor invasion in the portal vein.

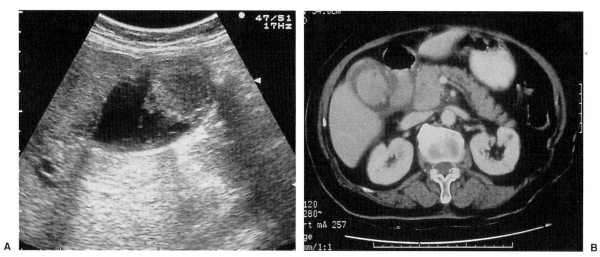

FIGURE 56-7. Cancer of gallbladder. **A:** Ultrasound scan shows a complex mass in the gallbladder. **B:** Computed tomographic scan shows tumor filling the lumen of the gallbladder.

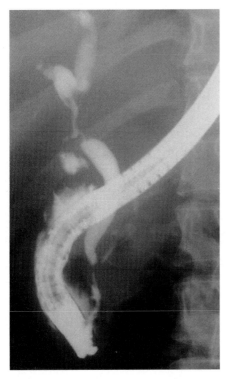

FIGURE 56-8. Endoscopic retrograde cholangiopancreatogram shows a stricture at the common hepatic duct and a normal-sized common bile duct.

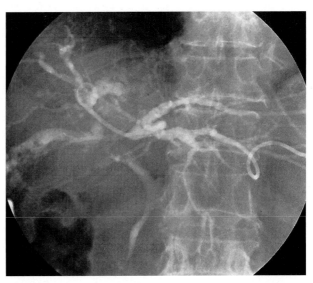

FIGURE 56-9. Percutaneous transhepatic cholangiogram shows a bile duct cancer at the confluence causing proximal ductal obstruction. A pigtail catheter is inserted for drainage.

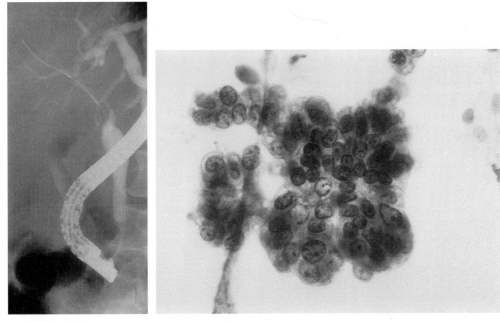

A   B

FIGURE 56-10. Brush cytologic examination. **A:** Cytologic brush is inserted through the endoscope into the proximal biliary tract. **B:** The presence of malignant cells confirms the diagnosis of bile duct cancer.

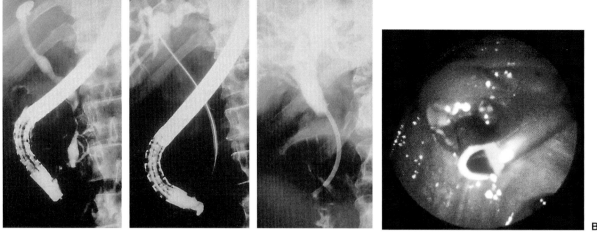

FIGURE 56-11. Endoscopic stenting. **A:** Endoscopic insertion of a polyethylene stent to manage distal bile duct cancer. **B:** Good drainage of bile after stenting.

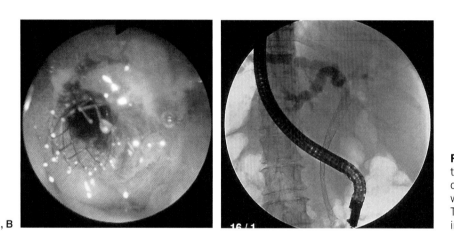

FIGURE 56-12. Wallstent endoprosthesis for drainage of bile duct cancer. **A:** Endoscopic view shows mesh wire extending into the duodenum. **B:** The metallic stent opens the lumen in instances of biliary stricture.

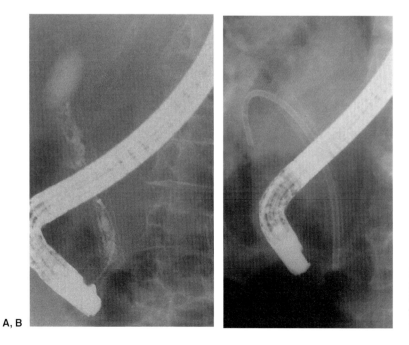

FIGURE 56-13. Blockage of Wallstent endoprosthesis. **A:** Tumor ingrowth in a Wallstent causing recurrent biliary obstruction. **B:** A plastic stent is inserted inside the Wallstent to resume the drainage of bile.

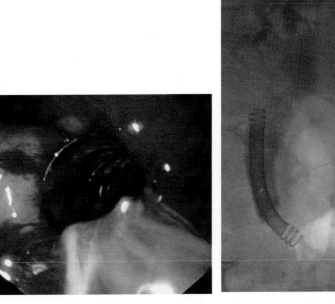

FIGURE 56-14. Endocoil prosthesis for drainage of periampullary cancer. **A:** Endoscopic view of Endocoil prosthesis inserted for a case of ampullary cancer with purulent bile drainage. **B:** The metal stent opens a wide lumen in the common bile duct.

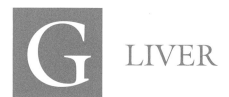

G LIVER

57

ANATOMY, MICROSCOPIC STRUCTURE, AND CELL TYPES OF THE LIVER

GARY C. KANEL

EMBRYOLOGY

The hepatic primordium anlage first appears toward the end of the third week of gestation, and is seen as a hollow midline outgrowth stalk (hepatic diverticulum); by the fourth week the diverticulum enlarges by proliferation of the endodermal cell strands (hepatoblasts), and projects cranially into the mesoderm of the septum transversum, eventually giving rise to the hepatic parenchyma and intrahepatic duct structures.

The mesoderm of the septum transversum initially surrounds the liver and is in continuity with the lesser curvature of the stomach, duodenum, and the ventral body wall. The mesoderm is the main focus for the development of hematopoiesis (Fig. 57-1), which begins at approximately 6 weeks and becomes most active during the sixth and seventh months, then rapidly regresses because of developing bone marrow activity.

The vascular network is originally derived from the development of both the vitelline and umbilical veins. The hepatic cords and vessels anastomose, forming the hepatic sinusoids. The sinusoidal plexus initially receives blood via the vitelline vein and is drained into the sinus venosus, but by the fifth week the right and left umbilical veins also supply blood to the sinusoidal plexus. By week 5, most of the major vessels are identified, and include the right and left umbilical vein, the transverse portal sinus, and the ductus venosus. The portal vein develops from the vitelline vein, and then subdivides into the right and left branches.

The biliary apparatus develops from membranous infolding occurring between the junctional complexes of adjacent hepatoblasts and appears initially as intercellular spaces with no distinct wall. The biliary canaliculi are first seen at week 6, with bile synthesis occurring by week 9, and bile secretion by week 12. A ductal plate develops from the hepatoblasts immediately adjacent to the portal mesenchyme, eventually forming an anastomosing network of portal duct structures (Fig. 57-2).

The individual cell functions become apparent at different but early times in the embryological development. The α-fetoprotein (Fig. 57-3), which is in high quantities at birth, initially is present by 1 month gestation. Glycogen may be seen by 2 months, with glycogen synthesis becoming most apparent by 3 months. Fatty change within the hepatocyte also parallels that of glycogenesis.

GROSS ANATOMY

The liver takes up the majority of the right upper abdominal cavity, and extends from the right lateral aspect of the abdomen 15 to 20 cm transversely toward the xiphoid (Figs. 57-4 and 57-5). The weight of the adult liver varies from 1200 to 1800 g, dependent on the overall body size, and consumes approximately from 1.8% to 3.1% of the total body weight. The liver anatomically has four lobes: right, left, caudate, and quadrate. The right lobe accounts for one half to two thirds of the total liver volume; however, functionally the right and left lobes are of approximately equal size, and are divided by a line extending from the inferior vena cava superiorly to the middle of the gallbladder fossa inferiorly. A total of eight functional segments are present, each demarcated by the vascular and biliary drainage (Fig. 57-6).

Figure 57-7 demonstrates the intrahepatic branching of the portal vein, hepatic artery, and bile duct. The portal vein is the main route of vascular drainage of the gastrointestinal tract, and is formed through the merger of the superior mesenteric and splenic veins. The hepatic vein is composed of three major tributaries (right, middle, and left), each having intrahepatic branches. The hepatic artery is a branch of the celiac artery, and ascends along the hepatoduodenal ligament and eventually divides into the right and left main branches.

The biliary system originally arises from the bile canaliculi, and can grossly be demonstrated in the larger interlobular branches. The biliary drainage of the right lobe is derived from anterior and posterior segmental branches that merge to form the right hepatic duct. Lateral and medial segmental branches merge to form the left hepatic duct that drains the left lobe. The caudate lobe is drained from three duct branches directly into the right and left hepatic ducts.

MICROANATOMY

The portal tract (Fig. 57-8) is often referred to as a portal triad; this term is misleading because more than three components are present. One to two interlobular bile ducts occur per portal structure. The ducts are usually seen immediately adjacent to the hepatic arterioles, which are responsible for their blood supply. The portal venule is a single vascular structure. The fibrous tissue, which supports the major portal components, varies in amount dependent on the distance of the portal tract from the hepatic hilum. The infiltrating cellular inflammatory components within the fibrous tissue consist of scattered lymphocytes, which are scanty, but often present to some degree even in normal livers.

In the adult, the hepatic lobules (Fig. 57-9) comprise approximately 80% of the total hepatic volume, and are composed predominantly of liver cell cords one cell thick containing polyhedral hepatocytes. The adjacent sinusoids are lined by both endothelial and Kupffer cells. The perisinusoidal space is located between the endothelial cells and hepatocytes. Stellate cells and collagen fibers are also present along the perisinusoidal space.

The hepatocyte comprises approximately two thirds of the total number of cells within the liver and approximately four fifths of the total liver volume. The cells average from 25 to 40 μm in diameter, dependent on their zonal location and the patient's age, and are polyhedral and multifaceted. The cells in the adult are arranged in cords that are one cell thick and have three distinct cell boundaries: sinusoidal, lateral (intercellular), and canalicular membranes. The liver cell nucleus is centrally located within the hepatocytes, measures approximately 10 μm in diameter, and contains clumped chromatin and nucleoli.

The liver cell cytoplasm comprises approximately 90% of the volume of the hepatocytes, and contains numerous functionally important organelles (Fig. 57-10). The cytoplasm and intracellular components vary in size, ultrastructure, and function dependent on the zonal location of the hepatocytes. The superstructure is maintained by the cytoskeleton of the hepatocyte. These include three major subdivisions: the microfilaments, microtubules, and intermediate filaments. The mitochondria are one of the most prominent intracellular organelles, averaging up to 2200 per hepatocyte. Mitochondria have numerous critical functions that include oxidative phosphorylation and fatty acid oxidation, and contain components essential for the urea and citric acid cycles. The endoplasmic reticulum (ER) is composed of a convoluted network of cisternae, saccules, tubules, and vesicles that are distributed throughout the liver cell cytoplasm, and is divided into two components, the rough ER and smooth ER. The Golgi apparatus is composed of highly polarized parallel flattened dilated saccules or vesicles, are approximately 1 μm in diameter, and are most often present adjacent to the liver cell nucleus and biliary canaliculi. Lysosomes appear as electron-dense pleomorphic single membrane-bound vesicles containing various enzymes such as acid phosphatase, esterases, proteases, and lipases, and are most frequently identified adjacent to the canalicular membrane.

The Kupffer cells are sinusoidal lining cells that function as tissue macrophages, represent more than 75% of fixed macrophages throughout the body, and take up approximately one third of the hepatic sinusoidal cell volume. The endothelial cells are flattened elongated sinusoidal cells ranging in size from 50 to 80 nm, and represent almost one half of the sinusoidal cell volume. Numerous cytoplasmic projections and clustered fenestrae or gaps that range in size from 0.1 to 0.2 μm are present. The stellate cells, also termed "fat-storing (Ito) cells," are located within the perisinusoidal liver cell recesses along the space of Disse, and comprise approximately one fifth of the sinusoidal cell volume. The cytoplasm often contains variably sized lipid droplets, which carry a high concentration of vitamin A (retinol palmitate). The space of Disse lies between the hepatocyte and the endothelial cells, measures from 0.2 to 1.0 μm wide, and forms a space usually not appreciated on routine light microscopy of biopsy material.

The stroma component comprises approximately 10% of the liver volume, and overall supports the basic hepatic architectural arrangement, produces intercellular cohesion and communication, and effects cellular differentiation. Five basic types of collagen are seen; types I and III represent more than 95% of the total collagen. Type I represents mature collagen strands, whereas type III represents new collagen (reticulin fibers).

The main function of the biliary tract is to transport bile synthesized in the hepatocyte into the gastrointestinal tract by way of the extrahepatic biliary network. It can be divided into its structural components, the smallest of which are the biliary canaliculi (Fig. 57-11). These are located along the intercellular spaces between hepatocytes, range in size from 0.5 to 1.0 μm in diameter, and are lined by microvilli. The canaliculi that enter the portal tracts are labeled the terminal ductules, periportal cholangioles, or ducts of Hering. These duct structures are derived from hepatocytes located at the limiting plate, and communicate with the interlobular bile ducts. The interlobular bile ducts range in size from 15 to 20 μm in diameter within the smaller portal structures, and are lined by a single layer of cuboidal cells with discrete round nuclei, usually inconspicuous nucleoli, and scanty eosinophilic cytoplasm. The larger interlobar and septal ducts measure more than 100 μm in diameter, have a fibrous wall, and are lined by a single layer of cuboidal to columnar epithelium with nuclei located toward the basement membrane. These lead into the segmental ducts that measure up to 800 μm in diameter, which eventually form the major hilar ducts that measure up to 1.5 mm in diameter. The hilar ducts ultimately branch into the main right and left hepatic ducts.

The major blood vessels that supply the liver are the portal vein and hepatic artery. The portal vein sequentially develops interlobar, segmental, interlobular veins and preterminal branches. The terminal portal venules measure approximately 20 to 30 μm in diameter and are seen in the smaller triangular portal tracts. The hepatic artery branches accompany the portal vein, and divide within the smaller portal tracts into two segments: the periportal plexus, which branches around the portal vein itself and drains into the sinusoids, and the peribiliary plexus, which provides blood supply to the accompanying interlobular bile ducts through small capillaries that are layered around the ducts.

The hepatic acinus can be divided into three segments: simple, complex, and acinar agglomerate. The simple acinus is the smallest functional parenchymal unit, and centers on a portal tract (smaller preterminal portal venule, hepatic arteriole, and terminal bile ductule). The acinus is divided into three zones (zones of Rappaport): periportal (zone 1), which includes the limiting plate; midzone (zone 2); and perivenular (zone 3) with the terminal hepatic venule at its outer lateral margin (Fig. 57-12). The complex acinus is derived from three adjacent simple acini fed by a preterminal portal vein and arterial branches. The acinar agglomerate is composed of approximately four complex acini and is fed by a portal venous branch measuring from 300 to 1200 μm in diameter.

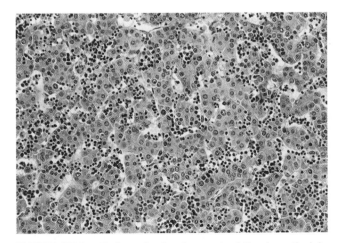

FIGURE 57-1. Embryonic development of the hepatic lobule. Extramedullary hematopoiesis is prominent in the hepatic lobules, begins at approximately 6 weeks, and is most active during the sixth and seventh months of gestation.

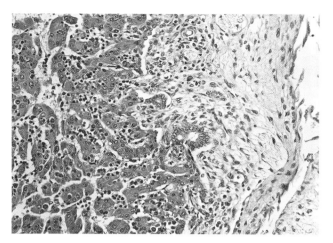

FIGURE 57-2. Embryonic development of the duct plate. Duct plates form by invasion of hepatoblasts into the portal mesenchyme.

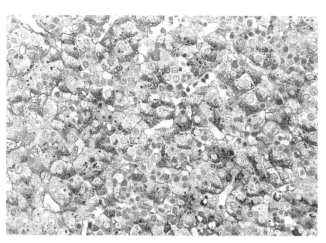

FIGURE 57-3. α-Fetoprotein during embryonic development. This protein, which is in high concentration at birth, is initially identified in the liver at 1 month gestation.

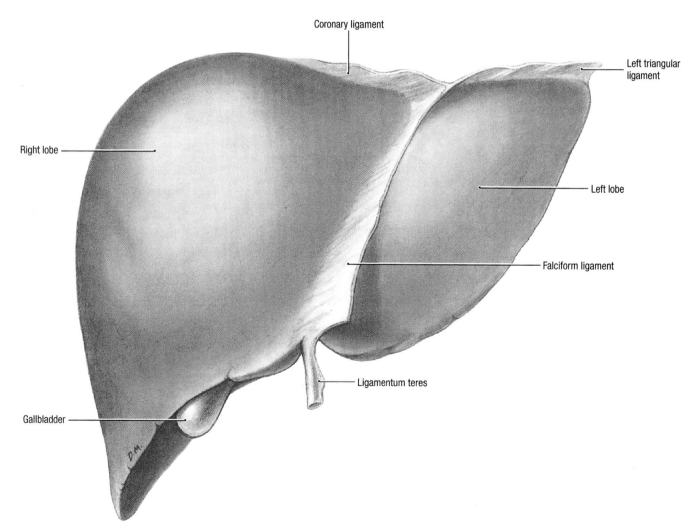

FIGURE 57-4. Anterior surface of the liver. The right and left lobes are divided by the falciform ligament, with the ligamentum teres lying along its free edge.

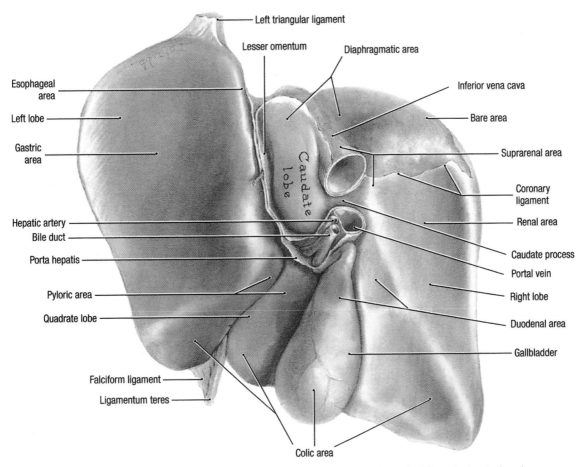

FIGURE 57-5. Inferior and posterior hepatic surfaces. The hepatic hilum is best visualized from this angle.

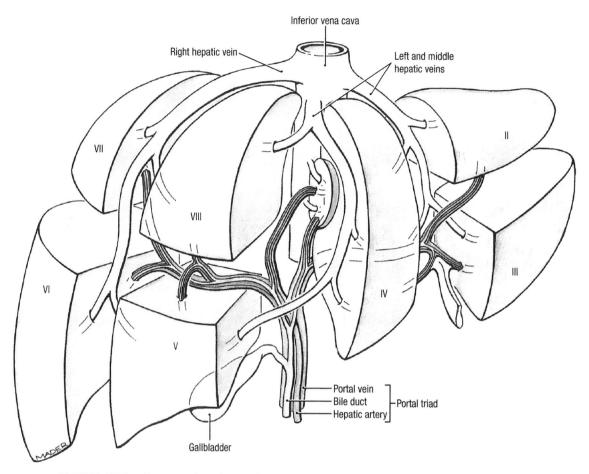

FIGURE 57-6. Segmental and vascular hepatic components. The eight functional components are demarcated by their vascular supply and biliary drainage.

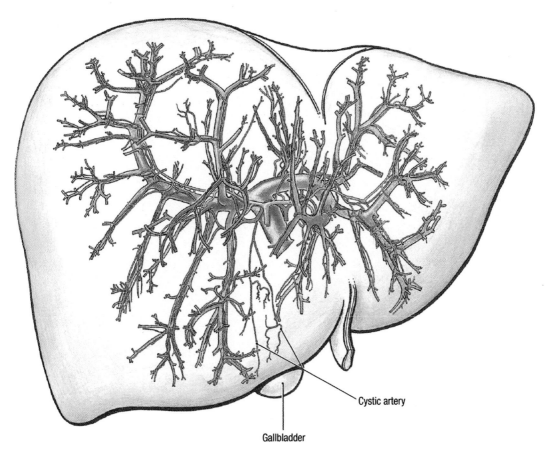

Cystic artery

Gallbladder

FIGURE 57-7. Intrahepatic network of the portal vein, hepatic artery, and bile duct. The branching patterns follow along a segmental distribution.

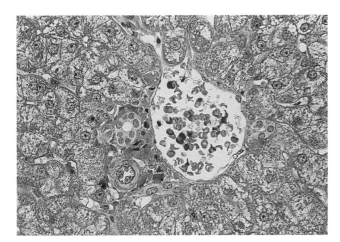

FIGURE 57-8. Portal tract (Masson trichrome). The major components include the hepatic arteriole, portal venule (large vessel), and bile ductule (cuboidal epithelium). There is a normal amount of collagen seen in this portal tract.

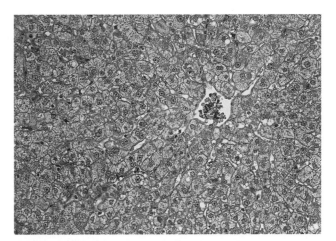

FIGURE 57-9. Parenchyma (Masson trichrome). The liver cell plates are one cell thick, and are divided by sinusoids lined by Kupffer and endothelial cells, with vascular outflow via the terminal hepatic venule. No sinusoidal collagen deposition is appreciated on light microscopy in the normal liver.

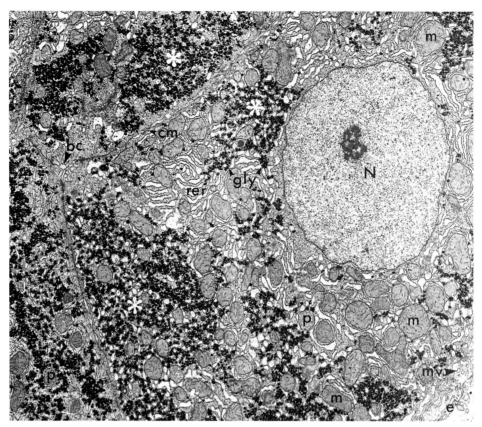

FIGURE 57-10. Hepatocyte (electron microscopic image). The hepatocyte is composed of a single nucleus (*N*); the cytoplasm demonstrates many mitochondria (*m*), rough (*rer*) and smooth (*) endoplasmic reticulum, glycogen (*gly*), peroxisomes (*p*), bile canaliculus (*bc*), cell membrane (*cm*), endothelium (*e*), and microvilli (*mv*).

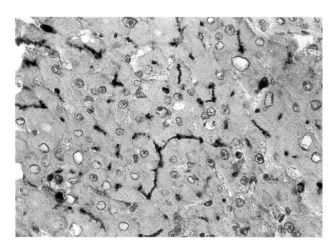

FIGURE 57-11. Biliary canaliculi (immunoperoxidase stain). Polyclonal carcinoembryonic antigen stains biliary glycoprotein, and is useful in demonstrating the biliary canalicular network.

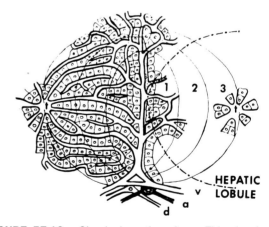

FIGURE 57-12. Simple hepatic acinus. This drawing of a simple acinus demonstrates its relationship with the preterminal portal venule (*v*), small hepatic arteriole (*a*), and ductule (*d*), and is divided into three zones (zones of Rappaport) with the terminal hepatic venule (*t*) located along its outer margins.

58

ACUTE VIRAL HEPATITIS

T. JAKE LIANG

Primary infection of the liver by viruses that cause injury to hepatocytes results in the condition called acute viral hepatitis characterized by a constellation of clinical, biochemical, and pathological features. Five hepatotropic viruses (A, B, C, D, and E) account for more than 90% of cases. The hepatotropic viruses are found worldwide (Figs. 58-1 through 58-5); the prevalence varies greatly from region to region and their individual distribution is partly dependent on their mode of transmission. Hepatitis A virus (HAV) and hepatitis E virus (HEV) are transmitted enterically, whereas hepatitis B, C, and D (HBV, HCV, and HDV, respectively) are transmitted via the percutaneous-permucosal routes. The liver is the primary site of infection and replication of hepatotropic viruses. Four viruses (HAV, HCV, HDV, and HEV) are single-stranded RNA viruses and HBV is a partially double-stranded DNA virus.

The genomic organization of HAV is shown in Fig. 58-6. The replication process of HAV has been inferred from studies of other picornaviruses. Entry of the virus into the host is mediated by a cell surface receptor, which has been recently proposed to be a mucin-like class 1 integral membrane glycoprotein. Viral entry is followed by uncoating and initiation of viral protein synthesis. Viral RNA synthesis proceeds from negative to positive strand and occurs in the cytoplasm. Viral assembly follows a sequence similar to that of picornaviruses in a cellular membrane compartment.

The infectious HBV virion (Dane particle) has a 42-nm spherical, double-shelled structure, consisting of a lipid envelope containing hepatitis B surface antigen (HBsAg), which surrounds an inner nucleocapsid. The hepatitis B core antigen (HBcAg) complexes with viral-encoded polymerase and viral DNA genome to form the nucleocapsid. The genome of HBV is a partially double-stranded circular DNA of approximately 3.2 kbp. The viral genome encodes four overlapping open reading frames (ORFs) from which four mRNA transcripts are derived and code for seven viral proteins (see Fig. 58-7 for details). HBV replicates through an RNA intermediate and this process is summarized in Fig. 58-8.

The HCV has a positive sense, single-strand RNA genome of approximately 9.6 kb in length with a single large ORF and highly conserved untranslated regions (UTRs) at the 5′ and 3′ ends. The genomic organization is summarized in Fig. 58-9. HCV replicates in the cytoplasm, presumably in a membrane-associated compartment. The replication process is illustrated in Fig. 58-10.

HDV requires coinfection with HBV for replication. Delta antigen is the inner ribonucleoprotein component of a subviral particle that is enveloped by the HBV surface antigen. The ribonucleoprotein complex consists of small (SHDAg) and large (LHDAg) delta antigens and a single-stranded circular RNA genome of 1.7 kb in length which has extensive self-complementation to form a rodlike structure (Fig. 58-11). The antigenome is synthesized from the genomic RNA and is the template for HDV mRNA encoding the delta antigens. The antigenome also serves as the template for genome synthesis. The HDV genome uses host RNA polymerase II to carry out RNA-directed RNA synthesis that is dependent on the SHDAg. Both genomic and antigenomic RNAs possess ribozyme activities that catalyze RNA self-cleavage and self-ligation. Transcription and replication are integrated into a single process using a double rolling circle mechanism. After entry into cells, HDV genome serves as a template for replication, resulting in the production of multimeric antigenomes. Nascent antigenomes, through their intrinsic ribozyme activities, form circular monomeric RNAs, which, in turn, serve as templates for the production of HDV genomes. Alternatively, the elongating product can be cleaved and released as polyadenylated mRNAs, which then direct delta antigen synthesis. HDV assembly begins with the association of the delta antigens with the newly synthesized genome to yield a ribonucleoprotein complex (RNP). The RNP is transported from nucleus to cytoplasm, and is presumably mediated by the nucleocytoplasmic shuttling function of delta antigens. The LHDAg of the RNP interacts with HBsAg to facilitate assembly. LHDAg is required for particle assembly, whereas SHDAg is copackaged but not required for particle formation.

The HEV genome is a single-strand, positive-sense RNA of approximately 7.5 kb. The genome is organized into three overlapping ORFs flanked by noncoding regions (Fig. 58-12). Replication of HEV has not been characterized. The mechanisms of viral attachment, entry, and uncoating are unknown.

During primary infection, the initial pathway of antiviral immune response is largely unknown. Initial viral infection is associated with activation of innate immunity in the liver. Recognition of infected hepatocytes by resident natural killer (NK) or natural killer T (NK-T) cells leads to activation of these cells and induction of antiviral cytokines including interferons. This phase of innate immunity leads to the initial control of viral replication. Because this antiviral response is likely associated with a noncytopathic mechanism, little or no hepatocellular injury is evident. The innate immunity also plays a critical role in the activation of the adaptive immunity, including humoral and cellular responses. Induction of a humoral immune response with production of neutralizing antibodies prevents viral spread and leads to subsequent elimination of circulating viruses. For HBV, the antibody response to the envelope proteins is a T-cell–dependent process.

The other limb of the immune response, the cell-mediated immunity (CMI) is critical for the long-term control of viral infections, including the hepatitis viruses. In acute HBV infection, individuals can mount a vigorous, multispecific, and polyclonal cellular immune response to HBV. In contrast, chronically infected patients have a weak or barely detectable anti-HBV response. This is true for both CD4 and CD8 responses. During acute HBV infection, a vigorous human leucocyte antigen (HLA) class II-restricted, CD4+, helper T-cell response to multiple epitopes of HBc/eAg predominates in virtually all patients. By helping B cells produce neutralizing antienvelope antibodies and activating HBV-specific cytotoxic T lymphocytes (CTLs), this CD4+ T helper population may direct the initial antiviral response.

In most viral infections, the activation of virus-specific CD8+ cytotoxic T lymphocytes is critical for viral clearance. Patients acutely infected with HBV develop a strong, polyclonal, HLA class I-restricted CTL response that is directed against multiple epitopes in all viral proteins. This response appears to persist for many years after recovery from acute HBV infection.

Knowledge of the molecular and cellular mechanisms of viral clearance and hepatocellular injury has been elucidated for HBV infection (Fig. 58-14). CD8+, class I-restricted HBsAg-specific CTLs target the liver through interaction between the HBV-specific T-cell receptors and the antigen-presenting HLA class I molecules on the hepatocytes and cause scattered apoptosis of hepatocytes. By secreting cytokines including interferons, the CTLs recruit a variety of antigen-nonspecific inflammatory cells into the liver, resulting in more extensive necroinflammatory injury of the liver. The predominant infiltrating effector cells are the macrophages, which probably mediate the majority of hepatocellular injury. The CTLs, although not primarily responsible for the majority of hepatocellular injury, initiate the cascade of immunological events leading to hepatitis. They also play a role in elimination of infected hepatocytes through noncytolytic inhibition of HBV gene expression and viral replication. The detection of virus-specific CD4 and CD8 cells in the peripheral blood and liver of chronically infected individuals suggests a pathogenic relationship between the indolent cellular immune response and necroinflammatory liver disease associated with chronic hepatitis. Therefore, the CMI is a double-edged sword: vigorous response leads to viral clearance, whereas ineffective response results in chronic hepatocellular injury.

Following infection, the hepatotropic viruses give rise to similar clinical, biochemical, and pathological features. Serologic testing is the only reliable way to determine the infecting agent (see Figs. 58-14 through 58-19). The incubation period differs for each virus, and ranges from 2 weeks to 6 months. The clinical course ranges from an asymptomatic illness to fulminant hepatitis and is typified by three phases (prodromal, symptomatic, and convalescent), lasting from 6 weeks to 6 months. Approximately 20% of cases present with jaundice. The primary biochemical abnormality is an acute increase in serum alanine and aspartate aminotransferases, which are markers of hepatocellular necrosis, to greater than 2.5 times the upper limit of normal—more commonly to greater than 10 times the upper limit of normal. The basic pathological lesion is an acute inflammation of the entire liver. The severity can range from mild, involving a few hepatocytes, to moderate, or massive necrosis involving almost all hepatocytes (Figs. 58-20 through 58-22). The classic pathological features of acute viral hepatitis are swollen hepatocytes, apoptotic hepatocytes (acidophil bodies) and the presence of inflammatory cells within the hepatic lobule, predominantly lymphocytes and macrophages, which result in distortion of the normal liver architecture.

HAV and HEV do not lead to chronic infection, and development of antibody protects against reinfection for HAV. HBV, HCV, and HDV have the propensity to cause chronic infection and are associated with an increased risk of hepatocellular carcinoma. Effective and safe vaccines exist for the prevention of infection with HAV and HBV, and are recommended in the pre- and postexposure setting and for persons with non-A, non-B hepatitis–related chronic liver disease. Institution of risk behavior modifications is the only effective way to prevent HDV superinfection in persons with chronic HBV. No vaccine exists for HCV and strategies for preventing infection include screening of blood donors and risk behavior modification. Improving hygiene and providing safe drinking water should lower the risk of HEV infection.

Treatment is supportive, with the aim of maintaining adequate nutrition and hydration, and monitoring for the development of fulminant hepatitis. Antiviral therapy is rarely indicated, especially for HAV and HEV, for which the course is benign and recovery is the rule. Most adults with acute HBV infection recover spontaneously, and given the low response rate of current regimens, specific antiviral treatment is not currently advised. Household contacts with known exposure and sexual contacts of an acute case of HBV should receive HBV immunoglobulin and HBV vaccine. On the basis of recent data indicating a high response rate to interferon therapy, it may be reasonable to treat patients with acute hepatitis C.

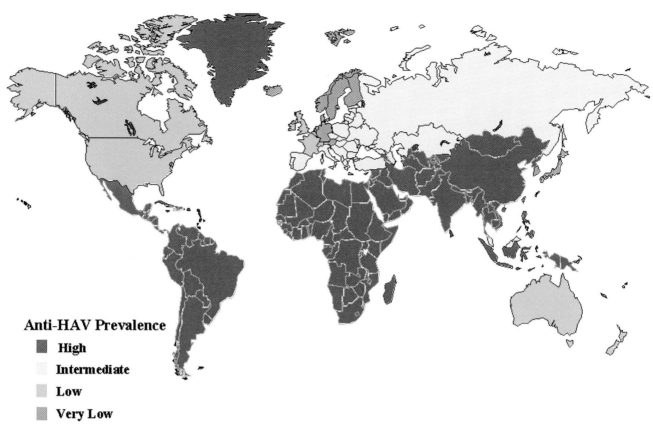

Anti-HAV Prevalence

■ High

□ Intermediate

■ Low

■ Very Low

FIGURE 58-1. Worldwide prevalence of hepatitis A virus infection.

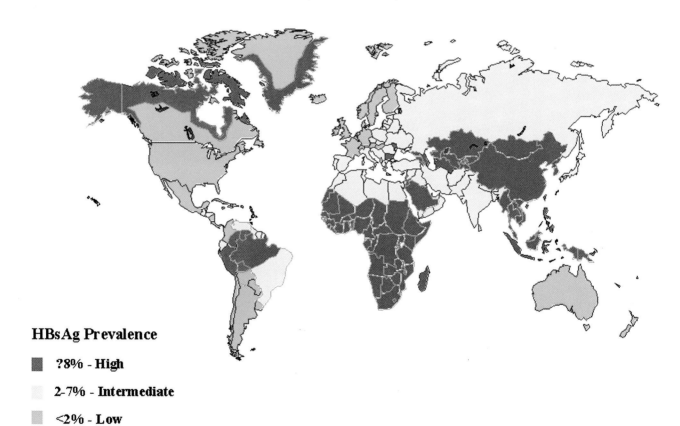

HBsAg Prevalence

■ ?8% - High

□ 2-7% - Intermediate

■ <2% - Low

FIGURE 58-2. Worldwide prevalence of hepatitis B infection (HBV). Almost 50% of the world's population lives in regions with the highest prevalence of HBV infection, where 8% to 20% of the population is hepatitis B surface antigen (HBsAg) positive. Another 40% of global population lives in areas with intermediate prevalence, where 1% to 5% of the population is positive for HBsAg.

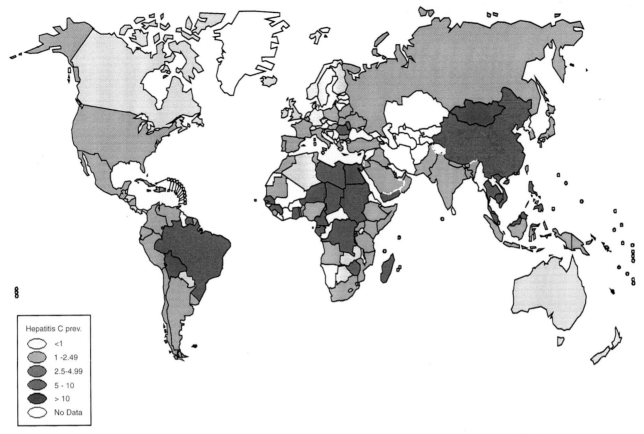

FIGURE 58-3. Worldwide prevalence of hepatitis C virus infection (HCV). Worldwide the prevalence of anti-HCV is fairly consistent, and ranges from 0.5% to 2%. Note areas of high prevalence in Egypt and Japan compared to the low prevalence in Northern Europe. Based on published data updated June 1999.

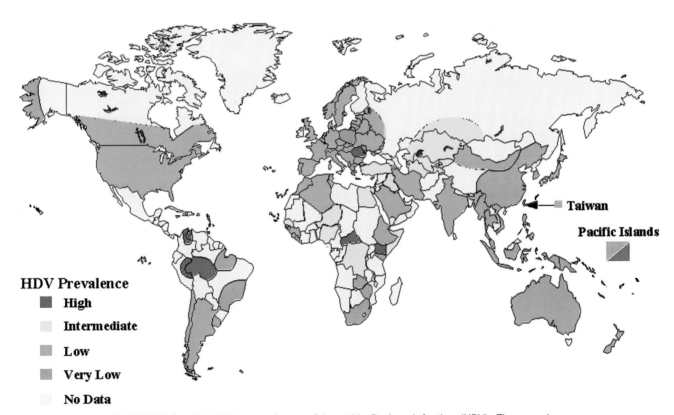

FIGURE 58-4. Worldwide prevalence of hepatitis D virus infection (HDV). The prevalence of HDV mimics that of hepatitis B virus (HBV) because of its dependency on HBV for its life cycle. However, areas of discordance exist, such as China, where the rate of HDV infection is low but the rate of HBV infection is high. The reasons for this finding are not known.

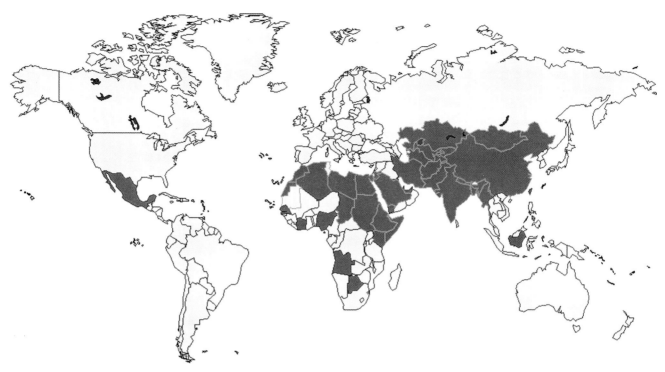

FIGURE 58-5. Worldwide prevalence of hepatitis E virus infection (HEV). Prevalence of anti-HEV in the darkly highlighted areas is estimated to be greater than 2.5% to 25%. In lightly shaded areas, prevalence of anti-HEV is estimated to range from 0% to 2.5%.

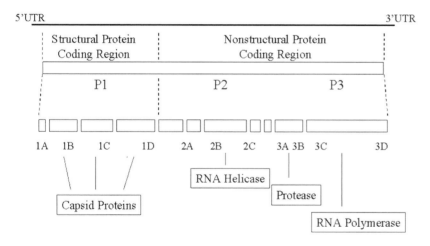

FIGURE 58-6. Structure of the hepatitis A virus (HAV) and genetic organization. The **top line** represents the hepatitis A virus RNA genome. The HAV has a linear, positive-sense, single-stranded RNA genome of approximately 7.5 kb. Translation of the genome yields a single polyprotein, divided into three main functional domains (P1, P2, and P3) from which the individual viral proteins are cleaved. P1 encodes the viral capsid proteins, whereas P2 and P3 encode the nonstructural proteins. The **lower diagram** illustrates the three regions of the polyprotein and the individual protein products. Four capsid proteins designated 1A to 1D are encoded in P1, and the P2 and P3 regions encode proteins 2A to 2C and 3A to 3D, respectively.

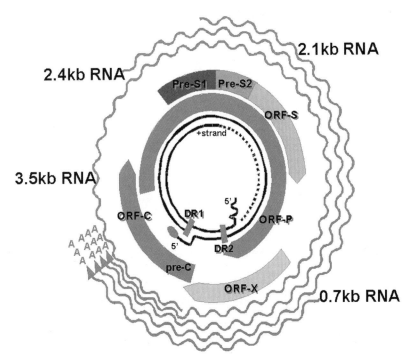

FIGURE 58-7. Genome structure and organization of hepatitis B virus (HBV). The HBV open reading frames: precore (*preC*) and core proteins; polymerase protein (*P*); L, M, and S surface envelope proteins (*PreS1, PreS2,* and *S*); and X protein (*X*) are shown. The viral genome structure is composed of the full-length (−)-DNA strand and variable length (+)-DNA strand (*solid followed by dashed line*). The polymerase protein is covalently attached to the 5′ of the (−) strand and a capped oligoribonucleotide (*angulated line*) to the (+) strand. Direct repeats 1 and 2 (*small rectangular boxes*) are shown on the genome. The *outer lines* represent the four transcripts, all terminating at a common polyadenylation site. The S open reading frame (*ORF*) encodes the viral surface envelope proteins, the hepatitis B surface antigen (HBsAg), and comprises the pre-S1, pre-S2, and S regions. The core gene consists of precore and core regions; separate initiation codons give rise to the hepatitis B early antigen and the viral nucleocapsid (HBcAg). The polymerase ORF encodes the polymerase protein, which is involved in encapsidation and initiation of negative strand synthesis, possesses reverse transcriptase activity, and catalyzes genome synthesis and RNAse H activity, which degrades pregenomic RNA and facilitates replication. The HBX protein is translated off the X transcript and is a viral protein with pleotrophic functions that plays an integral role in the viral life cycle.

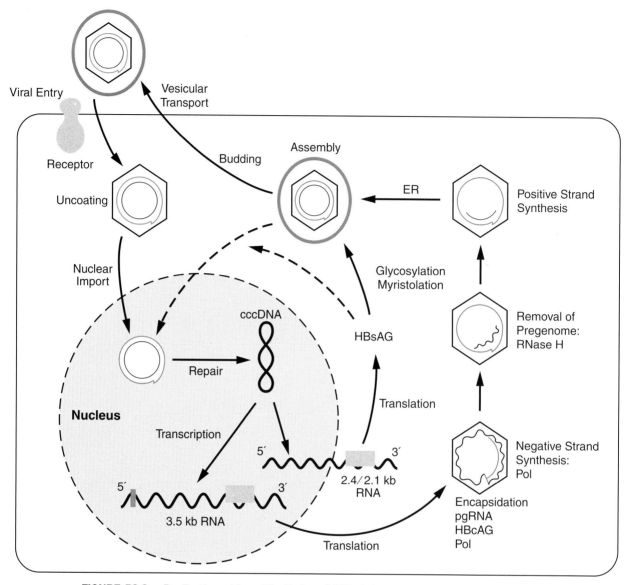

FIGURE 58-8.   Replication of hepatitis B virus (HBV). Infectious virions probably attach to hepatocytes via the pre-S1 domain of the L protein. Upon entering, the nucleocapsid is delivered to the nucleus and the viral genome is repaired to the covalently closed circular form (cccDNA). Viral transcripts are translated in the cytoplasm, and the core and polymerase proteins interact with the genomic length RNA to form the nucleocapsids. Reverse transcription occurs, and the mature virions are assembled in the endoplasmic reticulum, where they acquire the surface proteins. The virion is then secreted via vesicular transport. The encapsidation signal and posttranscriptional regulatory element on the HBV transcripts are shown as *rectangular boxes.*

FIGURE 58-10.   Replication of hepatitis C virus (HCV). The virion attaches and enters the susceptible cell via pathways that ▶ are not yet completely defined. The viral genome is then directed to a membranous component in the perinuclear endoplasmic reticulum region and serves as template for HCV protein synthesis. The nonstructural proteins form a replication complex with the genomic RNA and direct RNA replication (to negative and then positive strands). The structural proteins, which are retained in the endoplasmic reticulum, interact with the progeny genomes and assemble into virions. The virions are then secreted via an unknown exocytotic pathway, and probably do not pass through the Golgi compartment.

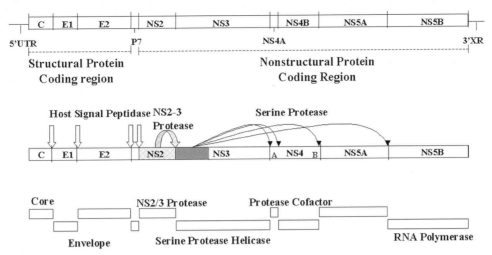

FIGURE 58-9. Genome organization of hepatitis C virus (HCV). The 5′ and 3′ untranslated regions (*UTR*) flanking a polyprotein open reading frame are shown at the **top**. Numbering refers to nucleotide positions of genes, which are based on the sequence of a HCV genotype 1a infectious clone. The HCV polyprotein of approximately 3000 amino acids is processed co- and posttranslationally by cellular and viral proteases to produce the individual gene products. Cellular proteases in the endoplasmic reticulum catalyze the cleavage of the structural proteins, whereas viral encoded proteases cleave the nonstructural proteins. The **middle panel** shows HCV polyprotein processing with cleavage sites of host signal peptidase (*open arrows*), NS2-3 protease (*gray arrow*), and NS3 serine protease (*thin arrows*). Numbering denotes amino acid position upstream of cleavage sites. The processed HCV proteins are shown at the **bottom**. The highly conserved core protein is the putative viral nucleocapsid and encompasses the first 191 amino acids of the polyprotein. The E1 and E2 are envelope glycoproteins with C-terminal hydrophobic transmembrane domains. The NS2 region encodes a metalloproteinase. The NS2-3 protease mediates autocatalytic cleavage between the NS2 and NS3. The NS3 region encodes a multifunctional protein with a N-terminal serine protease and a C-terminal RNA helicase and nucleotide triphosphatase (NTPase). The NS3 protease, distinct from the NS2-3 protease activity, is involved in processing the downstream polyprotein. The NS4A interacts with and acts as a cofactor for the NS3 protease. The function of NS4B is unknown. The NS5A may play a role in sensitivity to interferon. The NS5B is the RNA-dependent RNA polymerase that mediates viral replication.

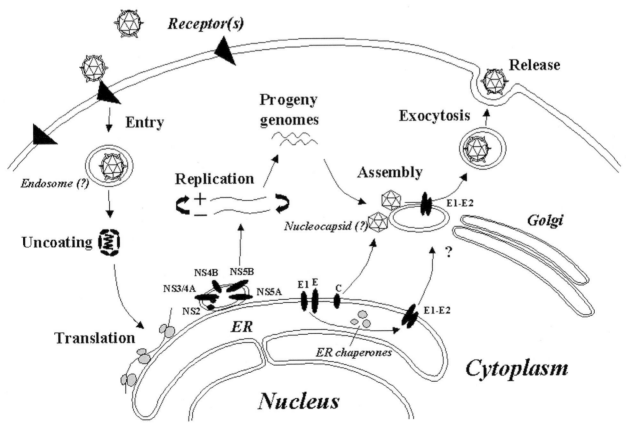

FIGURE 58-10.

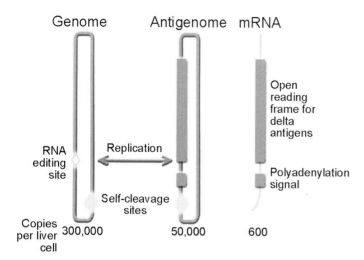

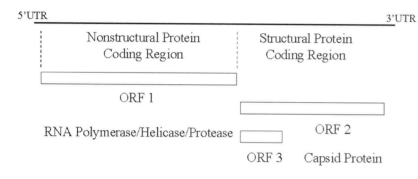

FIGURE 58-11. Genomic organization of hepatitis D virus (HDV). The RNA genome has a rodlike structure and contains an RNA editing and a self-cleavage site (*circle*). The antigenome is synthesized from the genomic RNA and is the template for HDV mRNA encoding the delta antigens. The antigenome also serves as the template for genome synthesis. The estimated copy numbers of the RNA species in the infected liver are shown at the bottom of the figure.

FIGURE 58-12. Genomic organization of hepatitis E virus. The genome is organized into three overlapping open reading frames (ORFs) flanked by 5' and 3' noncoding regions and a 3' polyadenylation. The ORF 1 appears to encode the nonstructural gene products: methyl transferase (*MT*), unknown functions (*X* and *Y*), protease (*Pro*), helicase (*Hel*), proline-rich hinge region (*H*), RNA-dependent RNA polymerase (*Pol*). ORF 2 codes for the capsid and ORF 3 codes for a protein with possible nucleocapsid function.

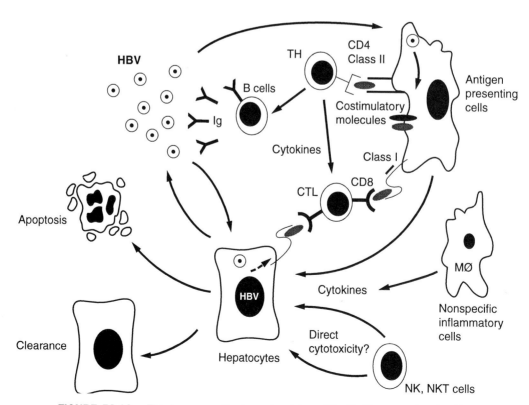

FIGURE 58-13. The immunopathogenesis of hepatitis B. (See text for details.)

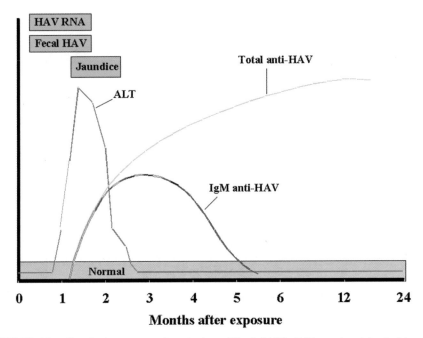

FIGURE 58-14. Serologic course of acute hepatitis A (HAV). HAV can be detected in stool before the onset of clinical symptoms by electron microscopy and polymerase chain reaction. Persons are therefore infectious during the incubation period. Levels of virus decrease and become almost undetectable with the onset of symptoms and the peak of the alanine aminotransferase level. Antibody to HAV (anti-HAV) first becomes detectable during this period. The initial antibody response is immunoglobulin M (IgM) anti-HAV; levels usually peak at 3 months following acute exposure and rapidly decline to undetectable by month 5 or 6. Occasionally, IgM anti-HAV may remain detectable for up to 1 year or longer. IgG anti-HAV is also present at low levels during acute infection, but levels increase as IgM anti-HAV begin to decrease. IgG anti-HAV persists for life and confers protection against reinfection. Thus, diagnosis of acute HAV rests on the demonstration of IgM anti-HAV in serum. IgG anti-HAV is a marker of past infection. One caveat is that commercial assays for total anti-HAV measure both IgM and IgG and therefore are not helpful in diagnosing acute infection.

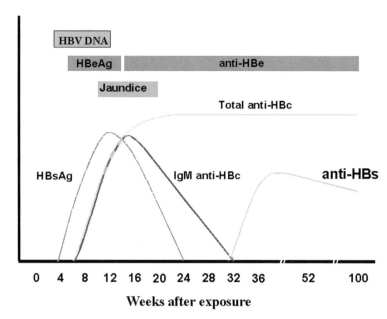

FIGURE 58-15. Serologic course of acute hepatitis B (HBV). Diagnostic tests are available for most of the HBV antigens and corresponding antibodies. The presence or absence of each of these antigens and antibodies serologically defines the stage of illness as acute, chronic, or recovered. Detection of hepatitis B surface antigen (HBsAg) in serum is the serologic hallmark of HBV infection. It usually appears in serum 1 to 10 weeks after acute exposure and 2 to 6 weeks before the onset of symptoms. It is detectable in both acute and chronic sera. Hepatitis B early antigen (HBeAg) is the next viral antigen to appear in serum soon after HBsAg. Its presence correlates with other markers of viral replication such as HBV DNA, and it is a useful marker of infectivity. Hepatitis B core antigen (HBcAg) is not detectable in serum but can be demonstrated in liver tissue. With the onset of symptoms, HBeAg and HBV DNA levels may become undetectable and the level of HBsAg also begins to decline. HBsAg may persist in the convalescent phase but should disappear by 6 months. Antibody against HBc, anti-HBc, appears before the onset of symptoms. Immunoglobulin M (IgM) anti-HBc is usually the first to appear and the titer peaks with the onset of symptoms but declines to undetectable levels within 6 months. IgG anti-HBc is also present during acute infection but unlike IgM anti-HBc, remains elevated lifelong and is a marker of past infection. Thus, diagnosis of acute HBV infection is made by the demonstration of HBsAg and IgM anti-HBc in serum. During the convalescent phase, HBsAg disappears and antibodies to HBsAg, anti-HBs, appear. Therefore, loss of HBsAg, HBeAg, and development of anti-HBs indicates recovery from acute infection and immunity against reinfection. Rarely are all markers of HBV infection, HBsAg, HBeAg, and HBV DNA, cleared from serum before the development of anti-HBs. If testing is performed during this period, IgM anti-HBc may be the only marker to indicate HBV infection, and this "serologically silent" period is referred to as the window period.

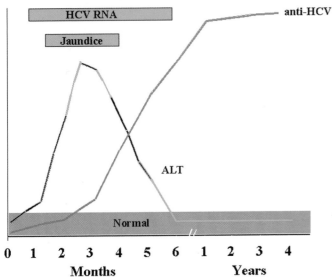

FIGURE 58-16. Serologic course of acute hepatitis C virus (HCV) infection. Following exposure to HCV, the virus can be detected within 2 weeks in serum and liver using sensitive polymerase chain reaction assays. An antibody response can be demonstrated as early as week 4, but more commonly by week 12, coinciding with the onset of clinical symptoms. Anti-HCV usually persists for life but may disappear in up to 25% of persons who recover spontaneously. Anti-HCV does not confer immunity against reinfection.

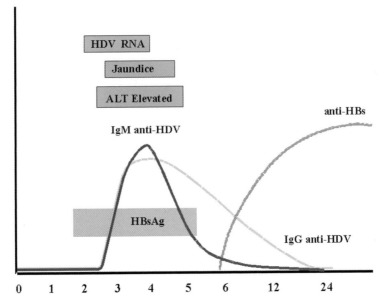

FIGURE 58-17. Serologic course of hepatitis D virus (HDV) coinfection. Acute HDV occurs in two settings: simultaneously with acute hepatitis B virus (HBV) infection-coinfection or following exposure in a patient with chronic HBV infection-superinfection. The serologic course is different in each instance. In acute coinfection, markers of HBV are usually evident before HDV is detected. HDV antigen and HDV RNA can be detected in serum before the peak in alanine aminotransferase level; however, these are research tests and not commercially available. Immunoglobulin M anti-HDV can be detected by week 4 following exposure but is often weak and may disappear before the development of IgG anti-HDV. IgG anti-HDV is usually delayed for several weeks following exposure, and in some cases is only present transiently during convalescence. Therefore, both acute and convalescent sera should be tested for anti-HDV. Following recovery, levels of anti-HDV may decline to undetectable and no serologic markers of HDV may remain. Thus, some cases may be diagnosed as acute HBV infection alone. The presence of IgM anti-hepatitis B core (HBc), which is associated with acute HBV infection, is an important marker for distinguishing HDV coinfection from superinfection. Thus, the diagnosis of HDV coinfection is determined by the presence of IgM anti-HDV, hepatitis B surface antigen, and IgM anti-HBc.

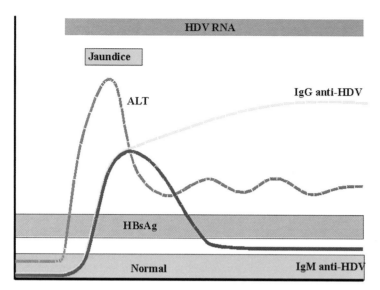

FIGURE 58-18. Serologic course of hepatitis D virus (HDV) superinfection. The incubation period of HDV superinfection is usually shorter than for coinfection. HDV RNA and hepatitis D virus antigen (HDVAg) are present during the incubation period and symptomatic phase. The titer of hepatitis B surface antigen (HBsAg) usually decreases when HDVAg appears in serum. Most cases of HDV superinfection result in chronic infection and HDV RNA and HDVAg persist in serum. In contrast to HDV coinfection, immunoglobulin M (IgM) and IgG anti-HDV are both present during the symptomatic phase of infection and persist indefinitely. IgM anti-hepatitis B core (HBc) is usually absent or present in low titer. Thus, diagnosis of acute HDV superinfection rests on the detection of anti-HDV and HBsAg and the absence of IgM anti-HBc.

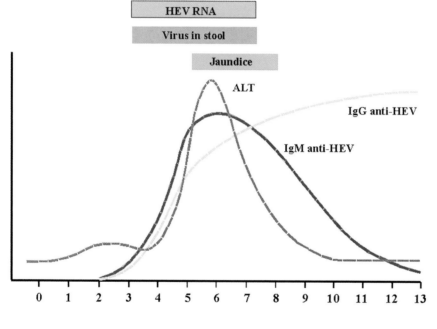

Weeks after Exposure

FIGURE 58-19. Serologic course of hepatitis E virus (HEV) infection. Following acute exposure to the virus, viral excretion is detectable within 2 weeks in serum and stool. Similar to HAV infection, virus levels are highest during the incubation phase and begin to decline with the onset of symptoms. Both immunoglobulin M (IgM) and IgG antibody are elicited during acute infection. IgM anti-HEV is detectable within 2 weeks of exposure and peaks with the onset of symptoms and alanine aminotransferase levels. It disappears rapidly over 4 to 5 months. IgG anti-HEV is present during the acute illness and remains elevated for several years and then levels begin to decline. Current assays for anti-HEV vary widely in their sensitivity and false-negative results can cause diagnostic error.

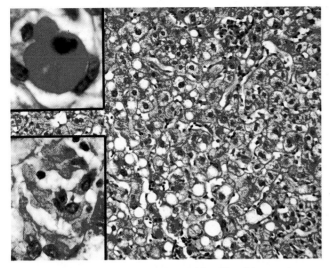

FIGURE 58-20. Acute viral hepatitis. The biopsy demonstrates typical features of acute viral hepatitis with a mild inflammatory infiltrate, ballooning degeneration, scattered acidophil bodies, and mild lobular disarray. **Upper left insert** shows a high-power view of an acidophil body with densely eosinophilic, irregularly shaped cytoplasm and pyknotic nucleus. **Lower left insert** shows a high-power view of the inflammatory infiltrate. There are lymphocytes, pigmented macrophages, and occasional plasma cells. Mild steatosis is present. (H&E stain; low-power magnification.)

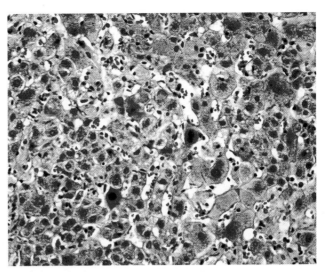

FIGURE 58-21. Acute viral hepatitis, moderate severity. Note ballooned hepatocytes together with scattered acidophil bodies (toward the center of biopsy). There is a moderate inflammatory infiltrate. (H&E stain, low-power magnification.)

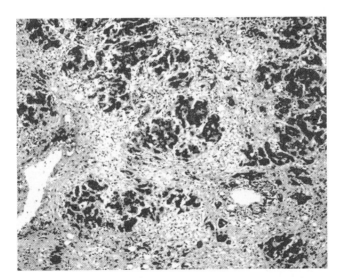

FIGURE 58-22. Acute viral hepatitis with submassive necrosis. There is almost complete involvement of the acini with extensive loss of parenchyma. Islands of hepatocytes are seen, separated by reticulin and inflammatory cells that form bridges. (H&E stain; low-power magnification.)

59

CHRONIC HEPATITIS B VIRAL INFECTION

ROBERT G. GISH ■ **RICHARD GARCIA-KENNEDY**

Hepatitis B viral infection (HBV) remains one of the most common chronic infections in the world. HBV accounts for one of the most devastating and common cancers in the world: hepatocellular carcinoma. The lifetime risk of death caused by HBV is approximately 30% in individuals who are chronically infected. Unfortunately, most patients remain undiagnosed because of the lack of population screening. If a diagnosis of chronic HBV infections is made, often little intervention takes place because of the lack of symptoms in most patients and a lack of knowledge of the rapidly evolving therapies available for HBV. It is important for all practitioners to understand that HBV infection is curable and in many patients, viral suppression can markedly improve long-term outcomes. Understanding all aspects of HBV disease is essential to the management of this complex problem. The physician managing HBV infection must be a virologist, radiologist, clinician, pathologist, and oncologist combined. Each physician must understand the natural history of the various forms of chronic HBV infection and recognize the multiple ways in which a patient may present. Each patient group with chronic HBV is quite heterogeneous in the initial presentation and clinical course. Each patient needs to be monitored for changes in liver enzymes, liver function tests, and serum tests of viral replication at least every 6 months. This monitoring process allows intervention to take place for those patients who have progressive liver disease. Ultrasound testing every 6 months for patients with cirrhosis or for those who have carried HBV infection for more than 40 to 50 years will identify many patients who develop hepatocellular carcinoma. Liver biopsy should be considered in all patients with elevated liver enzymes. Understanding the scoring system for liver fibrosis and inflammation, and applying this system to the liver biopsy for each patient is important. This information can be used to counsel patients about the chances of developing cirrhosis, the presence or absence of cirrhosis, the risk of liver cancer, and the possibility of identifying additional diagnoses.

A 26-year-old man who had a history of more than 50 sexual partners presented with elevated liver enzymes that normalized after 1 month of follow-up. The serum liver enzyme levels were markedly elevated again 3 months later. The patient underwent a liver biopsy and had active liver disease with positive core and surface antigen immunoperoxidase stain as well as grade 3 inflammation and stage 3 fibrosis (Figs. 59-1 and 59-2A, B, C). The patient was treated with interferon therapy, but could not tolerate the severe fatigue associated with the treatment. Treatment was discontinued. The patient's liver tests normalized for 4 months and serum levels of HBV DNA were below 2 pg/mL. After this 4-month interval, there was a sudden increase in liver enzymes and the serum level of HBV DNA increased to more than 400 pg/mL. Lamivudine (100 mg orally per day) was initiated. There was a subsequent rapid decrease in liver enzyme levels and the serum HBV DNA became unmeasurable after 2 months of therapy. The patient's serum became negative for hepatitis B early antigen (HBeAg) and positive for anti-HBe. The serum levels of liver enzymes were normal 1 year after lamivudine therapy was stopped. Figure 59-3*A, B, C* outlines the suggested patient groups for observation or treatment with interferon or lamivudine.

A 35-year-old Romanian woman who was infected with HBV and hepatitis D virus (HDV) presented with jaundice, ascites, and encephalopathy. She rapidly developed coma within the ensuing 6 weeks and underwent a liver transplant. A liver biopsy was performed 6 months before her clinical presentation with rapidly progressive liver disease. The patient died of recurrent HDV infection and liver failure after liver transplant despite hepatitis B immunoglobulin therapy and adequate serum levels of immunoglobulin. Liver tissue photomicrographs are shown in Fig. 59-4*A, B, C*, and demonstrate hematoxylin and eosin, trichrome, and delta antigen staining, respectively.

A 23-year-old woman with chronic HBV infection after a liver transplant developed a rapidly progressive liver disease, jaundice, and liver dysfunction, and liver biopsy indicated fibrosing cholestatic hepatitis (Fig. 59-5*A, B*) and positive in situ DNA stain throughout the liver tissue. The clinical course in this patient was modified by the addition of nucleoside analogs (Fig. 59-6). Her jaundice, ascites, and abnormal coagulation tests corrected to normal within 3 months of initiating antiviral therapy. She remains well 8 years later and a liver biopsy shows early cirrhosis but no evidence of progression by physical exam or by liver synthetic abnormalities.

A 45-year-old man presented with chronic HBV infection and cirrhosis, and waited 2 years before undergoing a liver transplant. The patient had a known single hepatoma at the time of transplant that was single and less than 5 cm without evidence of vascular invasion by computed tomography. After the liver transplant, the explant and tumor (Fig. 59-7*A*) were examined microscopically in detail by the pathologist and were found to have vascular invasion (Fig. 59-7*B*). The patient died 1 year later of brain metastasis. The finding of vascular invasion often portends a poor prognosis and signifies that the patient may have stage 4 disease (disseminated).

Fortunately, the incidence of acute HBV infection (Fig. 59-8) has been decreasing in the United States during the last two decades. With the introduction of neonatal vaccination and screening of pregnant mothers throughout the world, there is a clear expectation that not only will early deaths due to hepatocellular carcinoma decline, but that the incidence of end-stage liver disease caused by HBV will also decrease. The mandate for occupational safety, vaccination of adolescents, and education of individuals involved in high-risk activities are also very important public health policies.

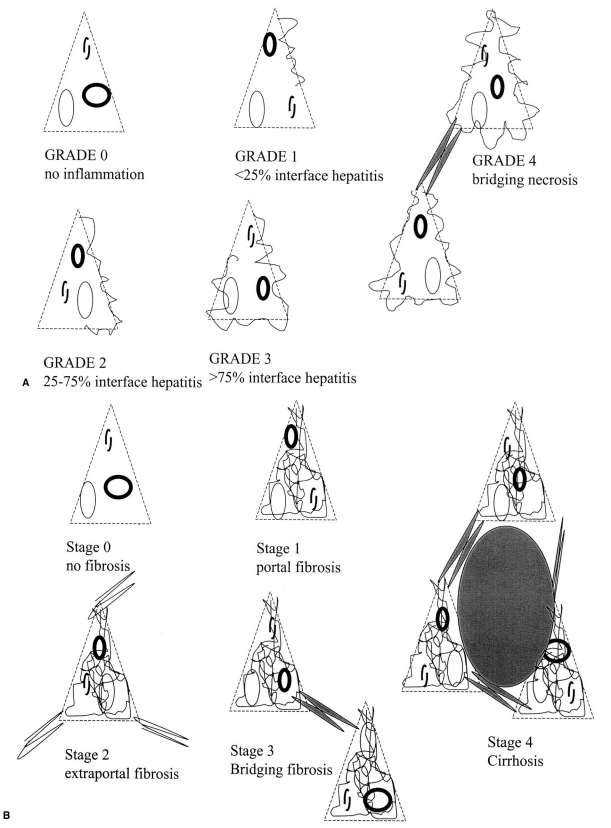

FIGURE 59-1. **A:** Grading of liver biopsy inflammation. **B:** Staging of liver biopsy fibrosis score.

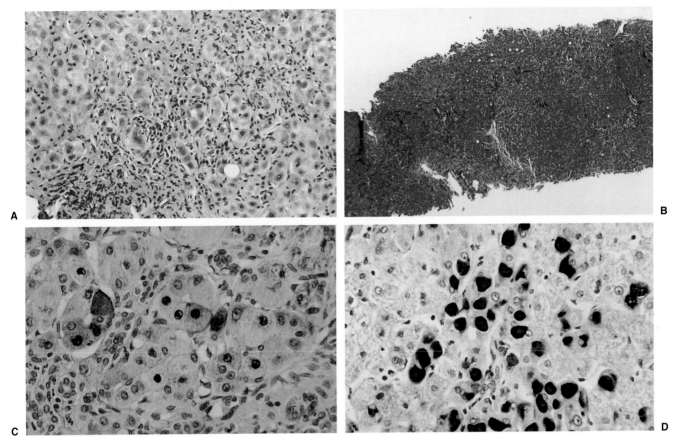

FIGURE 59-2. A: H&E stain of a liver biopsy from a patient with HBV infection demonstrating grade 3 inflammation. **B:** Trichrome staining demonstrating stage 3 fibrosis. **C:** Immunoperoxidase staining for hepatitis B core antigen. **D:** Immunoperoxidase staining for hepatitis B surface antigen.

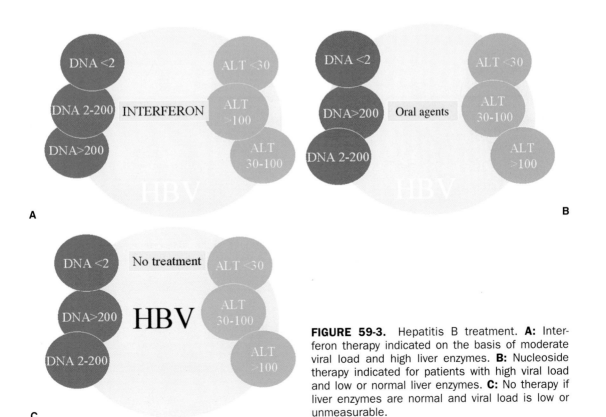

FIGURE 59-3. Hepatitis B treatment. **A:** Interferon therapy indicated on the basis of moderate viral load and high liver enzymes. **B:** Nucleoside therapy indicated for patients with high viral load and low or normal liver enzymes. **C:** No therapy if liver enzymes are normal and viral load is low or unmeasurable.

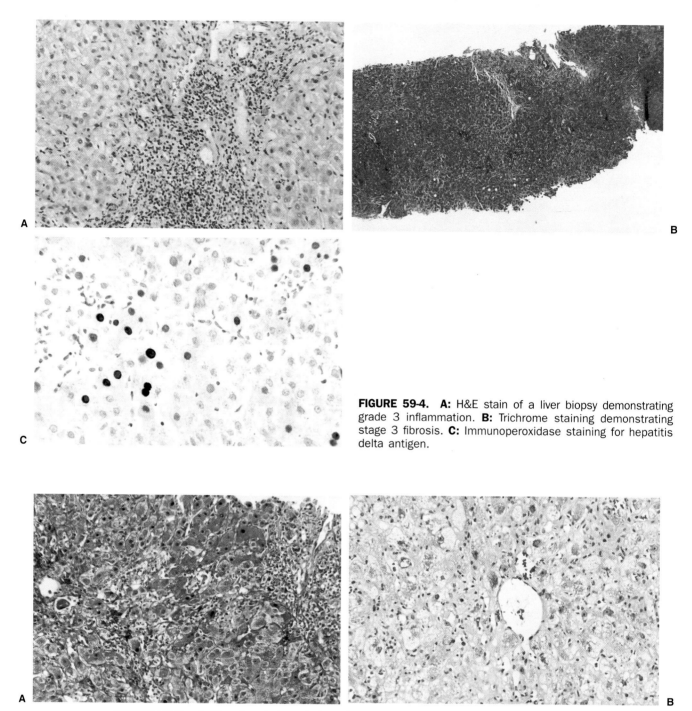

FIGURE 59-4.   **A:** H&E stain of a liver biopsy demonstrating grade 3 inflammation. **B:** Trichrome staining demonstrating stage 3 fibrosis. **C:** Immunoperoxidase staining for hepatitis delta antigen.

FIGURE 59-5.   **A:** Fibrosing cholestatic hepatitis (trichrome stain). **B:** Fibrosing cholestatic hepatitis (H&E stain).

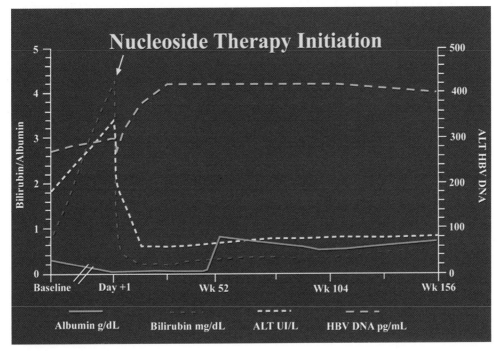

FIGURE 59-6. Graph of clinical course of liver enzymes and bilirubin after the initiation of antiviral therapy.

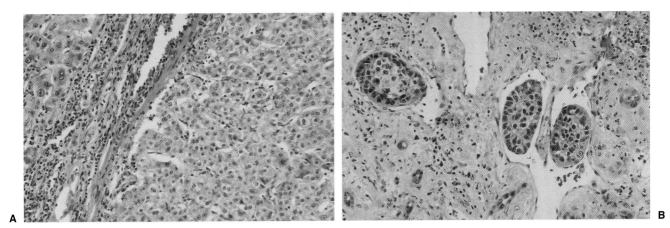

FIGURE 59-7. **A:** Liver cancer (hepatoma, hepatocellular carcinoma). **B:** Liver cancer invading a blood vessel.

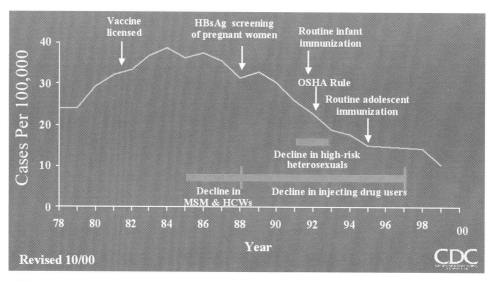

FIGURE 59-8.   The decline in the incidence of acute hepatitis B virus in the United States from 1978–1999.

HEPATITIS C VIRUS INFECTION

AIJAZ AHMED ■ EMMET B. KEEFFE

Chronic hepatitis C virus (HCV) infection is a major global public health problem, with an estimated 170 million individuals infected worldwide. Data from population-based studies demonstrates that chronic HCV infection accounts for 40% of chronic liver disease and results in an estimated 8000 to 10,000 deaths annually in the United States. Chronic HCV is the most common chronic blood-borne infectious disease in the United States, even though the annual incidence rate has declined from 180,000 to 30,000 cases during the last decade. The Third National Health and Nutrition Examination Survey (NHANES III), conducted from 1988 to 1994, provided data on the past incidence of acute HCV infection using national seroprevalence and age-specific incidence data from the sentinel counties' surveillance program. The overall national prevalence of antibody to HCV (anti-HCV) was 1.8%, which corresponds to an estimated 3.9 million individuals infected with HCV (Tables 60-1 through 60-3). Approximately two thirds of these individuals were between 30 and 49 years of age. Serum HCV RNA was detectable in 74% cases, which corresponds to an estimated 2.7 million actively infected individuals nationwide. Of these chronically infected individuals, 74% were infected with genotype 1, which is also the predominant genotype worldwide (Table 60-4).

New adult patients undergoing initial intake evaluation should be screened for a history of risk factors associated with HCV infection. During the history and physical examination, findings suggestive of chronic liver disease include encephalopathy, ascites, edema, spider angiomas, palmar erythema, a firm liver edge, and splenomegaly. The majority of patients with chronic HCV have constitutional symptoms, such as fatigue and decreased energy level, which are nonspecific and thus not diagnostically helpful in suggesting the presence of chronic HCV infection. A test for anti-HCV should be performed if an elevated alanine aminotransferase (ALT) level is found, if there is a positive history of risk factors for HCV infection, or if physical findings suggest the presence of chronic liver disease (see Table 60-2). A test for HCV RNA is warranted in patients who test positive for anti-HCV, particularly those with normal ALT levels or no HCV risk factors, to confirm HCV infection and rule out a false-positive test or recovery from past HCV infection (Table 60-5 and Fig. 60-1). Serologic testing for anti-HCV is the most practical screening test for HCV infection in hemodialysis patients, who often have normal ALT levels; however, serum HCV RNA is detectable in about 10% of HCV-seronegative patients, suggesting that patients in this high-risk population with negative anti-HCV testing should undergo a confirmatory HCV RNA test.

The primary goal of antiviral therapy in patients with chronic HCV infection is long-term viral eradication as determined by an undetectable HCV RNA in serum and liver. Secondary objectives of treatment include normalization of ALT levels and reduced inflammation and fibrosis on liver biopsy, which logically should decrease progression to cirrhosis, hepatocellular carcinoma, and premature death. The National Institutes of Health and European consensus conferences recommended that a liver biopsy be performed when considering treatment for chronic HCV infection to distinguish patients most likely to benefit from therapy (i.e., those with moderate histological disease) from those who may be less likely to benefit from therapy (i.e., those with mild disease and no or minimal fibrosis or those with advanced disease and cirrhosis). However, these recommendations were developed when only interferon monotherapy was available, and a decision to perform a liver biopsy may be influenced by many factors, such as patient preferences, cost effectiveness, presence of contraindications, and suspicion of coexistent liver diseases (Table 60-6). Liver biopsy is the most reliable method of establishing the severity of liver disease caused by chronic HCV infection by determination of the stage of fibrosis and grade of inflammation, but provides no superiority to overall clinical and laboratory assessment in ruling out other unsuspected coexisting liver diseases. In addition, percutaneous liver biopsy can cause pain in 30%, severe complications in 0.3%, and death in 0.03% of patients. On the basis of cost-effectiveness considerations, the most suitable strategy in the management of chronic HCV infection may be to initiate therapy in all patients without performing liver biopsy. Moreover, with recent advances in antiviral therapy resulting from the addition of ribavirin to interferon-based therapy, patients with genotypes 2 and 3 have sustained virologic response rates of about 65% with regular interferon plus ribavirin and 80% with peginterferon plus ribavirin. The role of liver biopsy thus might be thought of as selective rather than mandatory in identifying candidates for antiviral therapy; that is, patients with genotype 1 (sustained virologic response rates still less than 50%) may prefer to defer therapy if mild disease with no or minimal fibrosis is present.

The evolution of interferon-based therapy for chronic HCV, particularly combination therapy with ribavirin and pegylation of interferon, has resulted in incremental improvement in the sustained virologic response rates; that is, 10% to 15% with interferon monotherapy for 24 weeks, 15% to 25% when interferon monotherapy was extended to 48 or 72 weeks, 40% with interferon plus ribavirin, and 55% with peginterferon plus ribavirin. Factors that predict a favorable response to antiviral therapy are shown in Table 60-7. The combination of peginterferon with ribavirin is the most efficacious antiviral therapy of chronic HCV infection. Peginterferon alfa 2b at a weekly dose of 1.5 μg/kg plus ribavirin 800 mg per day showed a significantly higher response rate when compared to standard interferon plus ribavirin combination in a large pivotal trial. The sustained virologic response rate was 54% overall, 42% in patients with genotype 1, and 82% in patients with genotype 2 or 3 (Table 60-8). Secondary analysis of the data from the peginterferon alfa 2b plus ribavirin study suggested better efficacy with weight-based dosing. Results with peginterferon alfa 2a and ribavirin were similar to those with peginterferon alfa 2b and ribavirin. The use of peginterferon monotherapy is only appropriate if there are contraindications to ribavirin use or patients are not candidates for therapy (Table 60-9). On the basis of data from these trials, peginterferon and ribavirin combination therapy is the standard of care in treating patients with chronic HCV infection (Fig. 60-2). Consensus recommendations regarding antiviral therapy of HCV infection in special populations are displayed in Table 60-10.

Patients should be informed that, although the risk of transmitting HCV infection by sexual contact is low (3% to 5%), HCV is potentially transmissible. Patients should be careful about blood exposure of any type to partners and family contacts. Open wounds must be covered, and razors or toothbrushes should not be shared. Exposed persons should undergo postexposure baseline and follow-up testing

(Table 60-11). Although sexual or intrafamilial HCV transmission is rare, testing sexual partners or other family members if there is a concern regarding infection usually provides reassurance. Patients with chronic HCV infection should be counseled to avoid excessive consumption of alcohol, which can accelerate the progression of HCV when used in moderate or large amounts. It has been recommended that the less alcohol consumed the better, and that complete abstinence is ideal. In addition, acute hepatitis A or B may be more severe in patients with chronic HCV, and thus it is recommended that HCV patients without immunity to hepatitis A and B undergo vaccination (Table 60-12). Finally, a comprehensive strategy to prevent and control HCV infection, outlined in Table 60-13, is an important public health agenda during the next decade.

(figures begin on page 635)

TABLE 60-1
Viral Hepatitis in United States: Centers for Disease Control Data from 1984 to 1994

	HEPATITIS A	HEPATITIS B	HEPATITIS C
Acute hepatitis ($\times$1000/y)	125–200	140–320	35–180
Fulminant hepatitis (deaths/y)	100	150	7
Chronic hepatitis (prevalence)	0	1–1.25 million (0.3%)	3–4 million (1.8%)
Chronic liver disease (deaths/y)	0	4–5000	8–10,000

From *www.cdc.gov.*

Alter MJ, Kruszon-Moran D, Nainon OV, et al. The prevalence of hepatitis C virus infection in United States, 1998 through 1994. N Engl J Med 1999;341:556.

TABLE 60-2
Modes of Transmission: Risk Factors for HCV Infection

Illicit drug use
  Injection drug use
  Intranasal cocaine use
Sexual and vertical transmission
  High-risk sexual activity (homosexual contact, multiple partners)
  Children born to HCV-positive mothers
Health care-related transmission
  Transfusion of blood or blood products before July 1992
  Recipient of solid organ transplant before July 1992
  Chronic hemodialysis
  Health care and public safety workers with history of needle stick or mucosal exposure
    to HCV-positive blood
  Receipt of injections in a third-world country
Miscellaneous
  Body piercing or tattoos
  Patients with elevated ALT levels independent of other risk factors

ALT, alanine aminotransferase; HCV, hepatitis C virus.

From Wasley A, Alter MJ. Epidemiology of hepatitis C: geographic differences and temporal trends. Semin Liver Dis 2000;20:1.

Alter MJ, Kruszon-Moran D, Nainon OV, et al. The prevalence of hepatitis C virus infection in United States, 1998 through 1994. N Engl J Med 1999;341:556.

Alter MJ. The epidemiology of acute and chronic hepatitis C. Clin Liver Dis 1997;1:559.

TABLE 60-3
Modes of Transmission: Percentage Risk

Injection drug use	60%
Sexual	15%
Transfusion (before screening)	10%
Other (hemodialysis, health care worker, etc.)	5%
Unknown	10%

From Alter MJ, Kruszon-Moran D, Nainon OV, et al. The prevalence of hepatitis C virus infection in United States, 1998 through 1994. N Engl J Med 1999;341:556.

TABLE 60-4
Distribution of Hepatitis C Virus Genotypes

GENOTYPE	GEOGRAPHICAL PREDOMINANCE
1a	United States and developed western countries
1b	United States, Japan, and Europe
2	Developed countries
3	Developed countries
4	Middle East and North Africa
5	South Africa
6	Asia

Note: Prevalence in United States: 74% genotype 1, 26% genotype 2 and 3. Genotypes 1 and 4 are less responsive to antiviral therapy.

From Alter MJ, Kruszon-Moran D, Nainon OV, et al. The prevalence of hepatitis C virus infection in United States, 1998 through 1994. N Engl J Med 1999;341:556.

TABLE 60-5
Diagnostic Tests for Hepatitis C Infection

	ALT	EIA	RIBA	RT-PCR
Chronic hepatitis C	↑	+	+	+
HCV carrier	N	+	+	+
Recovered HCV infection	N	+	+	−
False positive anti-HCV	N	+	−	−

ALT, alanine aminotransferase; anti-HCV, antibody to HCV; EIA, enzyme immunoassay; HCV, hepatitis C virus; RIBA, recombinant immunoblot assay; RT-PCR, reverse transcriptase polymerase chain reaction; ↑, elevated levels; +, positive; −, negative.

TABLE 60-6
Role of Liver Biopsy in HCV: Selective Versus Routine

Arguments for routine liver biopsy
  Determine fibrosis stage and need for therapy, that is, treatment indicated for stages 2–4; treatment optional or not needed for stages 0–1 (particularly patients with genotype 1; may not apply for patients with genotypes 2 or 3)
  Exclude coexisting unsuspected secondary liver diseases, such as autoimmune hepatitis or nonalcoholic fatty liver disease (not commonly found on biopsy)
  Provide assistance in the management of side effects during antiviral therapy (use of adjunctive agents such as antidepressive drugs, epoetin, or G-CSF in patients with advanced stages of fibrosis)
Arguments for selective liver biopsy
  Improved efficacy of antiviral therapy, particularly in patients with genotypes 2 and 3
  Invasive procedure with risk of fatality
  Favorable cost-effectiveness analysis
  Patient preference

G-CSF, granulocyte colony-stimulating factor; HCV, hepatitis C virus.

TABLE 60-7

Favorable Response Determinants: Interferon and Ribavirin Therapy

Host determinants
  Female gender
  Caucasian or Asian versus African or Latino American
  Age younger than 40 y
  Absence of stage 3 or 4 fibrosis
  HIV-negative status
  Low hepatic iron levels
  Elevated ALT levels
Viral determinants
  Genotype 2 and 3*
  Low baseline serum HCV RNA level (<2–3×10^6 copies/mL)*
  Short duration of infection
  Small number of quasispecies
  Mutation at interferon sensitivity determining site (NS5A)
Drug determinants
  Prolonged duration of treatment
  Early response to therapy based on ALT and HCV RNA levels

*Most important determinants.

ALT, alanine aminotransferase; HCV, hepatitis C virus; HIV, human immunodeficiency syndrome.

TABLE 60-8

Peginterferon Plus Ribavirin Therapy for Chronic HCV Infection

	OVERALL	GENOTYPE 1	GENOTYPES 2, 3
Peginterferon alfa-2a plus ribavirin	56%	46%	76%
Peginterferon alfa-2b plus ribavirin	54%	42%	82%
Peginterferon alfa-2b plus ribavirin (weight-based dosing)	61%	48%	88%

HCV, hepatitis C virus.

From Manns MP, McHutchison JG, Gordon SC, et al. Peginterferon alfa-2b plus ribavirin compared to interferon alfa-2b plus ribavirin for initial treatment of chronic hepatitis C: a randomized trial. Lancet 2001;358:958.

Fried MW, Shiffman ML, Reddy RK, et al. Pegylated (40 kDA) interferon alfa-2a (Pegasys®) in combination with ribavirin: efficacy and safety results from a phase III, randomized, actively-controlled, multicenter study [Abstract]. Gastroenterology 2001;120:A55.

TABLE 60-9

Candidates for Peginterferon Monotherapy

Patients not eligible for ribavirin
  Severe anemia
  Coronary artery disease
  Renal failure (hemodialysis)
  Severe pulmonary disease
  Prior ribavirin toxicity
Patients receiving maintenance therapy

TABLE 60-10
Therapy for Special HCV Patient Populations

SPECIAL HCV POPULATION	THERAPY
Acute hepatitis C	Recommended
Children with HCV infection	Recommended
Histologically mild HCV infection	Recommended
Mixed cryoglobulinemia and glomerulonephritis	Recommended
Normal ALT levels	Not recommended
Autoimmune hepatitis	Not recommended
Immunocompromised status	Clinical trial
Compensated cirrhosis	Cautiously recommended
Decompensated cirrhosis	Clinical trial

ALT, alanine aminotransferase; HCV, hepatitis C virus.

TABLE 60-11
Postexposure Testing and Follow-up for HCV Infection

Source
  Baseline testing for anti-HCV
Person exposed to HCV-positive source
  Baseline anti-HCV and ALT activity
  Follow-up testing for anti-HCV and ALT at 4–6 mo. If earlier diagnosis of HCV infection
    is desired, testing for HCV RNA may be performed at 4–6 wk.
  All EIA-based positive anti-HCV must be confirmed by PCR testing for HCV RNA
  Prophylactic antiviral therapy not recommended

ALT, alanine aminotransferase; anti-HCV, antibody to HCV; EIA, enzyme immunoassay; HCV, hepatitis C virus; PCR, polymerase chain reaction.
From *www.cdc.gov.*

TABLE 60-12
Efficacy of Hepatitis A and B Vaccination in Chronic Hepatitis C

PATIENTS	SEROCONVERSION RATE	
	HAV Vaccine	*HBV Vaccine*
Chronic hepatitis C		
Mild	Good	Good
Moderate	Good	Fair to good
Advanced (OLT candidates)	+/−*	Poor†
OLT recipients	+/−*	Poor†

*Data limited.
†Consider accelerated, high-dose regimen.
HAV, hepatitis A virus; HBV, hepatitis B virus; OLT, orthotopic liver transplant.

TABLE 60-13

Comprehensive Strategy to Prevent and Control HCV Infection

Primary prevention
  Screening and testing of blood, plasma, organ, tissue, and semen donors
  Virus inactivation of plasma-derived products
  Risk-reduction counseling and services
  Implementation and maintenance of infection-control practices
Secondary prevention
  Identification, counseling, and testing of persons at risk
  Medical management of infected persons
Professional and public education
Surveillance to monitor disease pattern and efficacy of prevention measures

---

From *www.cdc.gov.*

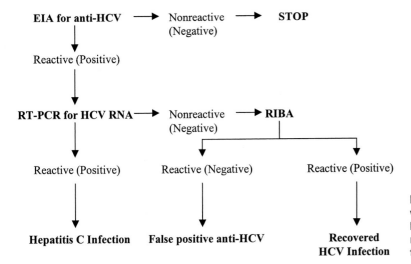

FIGURE 60-1. Diagnostic algorithm for patients with hepatitis C virus risk factors. *Anti-HCV,* antibody to HCV; *EIA,* enzyme immunoassay; *RIBA,* recombinant immunoblot assay; *RT-PCR,* reverse transcriptase polymerase chain reaction.

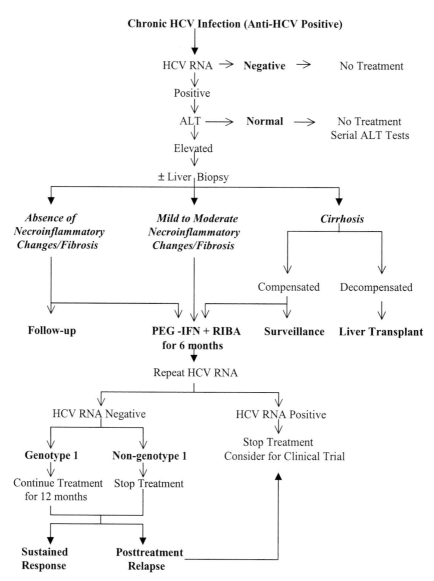

FIGURE 60-2. Treatment of chronic hepatitis C virus infection. *ALT*, alanine aminotransferase; PEG−IFN+RIBA, peginterferon plus ribavirin combination.

DRUG-INDUCED LIVER INJURY

FRANK V. SCHIØDT ■ WILLIAM M. LEE

Drugs can cause hepatotoxicity either in a dose-dependent or dose-independent (idiosyncratic) fashion. Both types of drug-induced liver injury are very frequent causes of acute liver failure with hepatic encephalopathy and coagulopathy (Fig. 61-1), even though the proportion of acute liver failure caused by drugs varies greatly worldwide (Table 61-1).

Idiosyncratic drug reactions occur rarely (in 1:10,000 to 1:100,000 people using the specific drug), and enzyme polymorphism in one of the cytochrome P450 (*CYP*) or other genes undoubtedly play a role in many susceptible patients, but the clinical role and value of pharmacogenetics are just beginning to emerge.

Acetaminophen is probably the best example of a dose-dependent hepatotoxic drug. Acetaminophen is extremely safe when taken within recommended doses (4 g/day), but doses of 8 to 10 g/day may cause severe liver necrosis. Figure 61-2 describes the metabolic pathways of acetaminophen. It is widely accepted that toxicity is ascribed to the highly reactive metabolite *N*-acetyl-*p*-benzoquinone imine (NAPQI). NAPQI can bind covalently to cellular proteins, and cause blebbing and later lysis of the hepatocyte. Acetaminophen-induced acute liver failure is a hyperacute disease in which liver failure may develop only days after ingestion of the overdose. Biochemical characteristics include very high aminotransferase levels (5000 to 25,000 IU/L) and often also elevated creatinine because of a direct nephrotoxic effect of acetaminophen. Frequently, liver transplantation is not performed for patients with acetaminophen-induced acute liver failure, because the disease progresses too rapidly, or medical or social contraindications preclude transplantation. In addition, the spontaneous (transplant free) survival is better (approximately 70%) than for other causes of acute liver failure (Fig. 61-1), and liver transplantation is not needed for most patients.

Idiosyncratic drug-induced hepatotoxicity has been described for a very large number of drugs, and Fig. 61-3 outlines implicated agents from a U.S. database. The majority of reactions are directed against hepatocytes, but biliary injury and combined hepatocyte-biliary injury or damage to specific organelles produce the different disease patterns observed. The proportion of drug-induced liver disease varies greatly among drug classes as evidence of class effect.

Idiosyncratic drug-induced liver injury differs from acetaminophen-induced acute liver failure in a number of ways, including a slower onset of symptoms and lower spontaneous (transplantation free) survival. Biochemical differences are apparent in lower aminotransferase and creatinine levels and higher bilirubin levels.

Figure 61-4 displays some of the different histological patterns of acute liver failure caused by drugs.

TABLE 61-1

The Presumed Etiology of Acute Liver Failure in Different Parts of the World

	ACM	HAV	HBV	DRUG	SHOCK	INDET.	OTHER
Argentina: 1996–2001 (n = 83)	0%	8%	22%	14%	0%	25%	31%
Denmark: 1973–1990 (n = 160)	19%	2%	31%	17%	3%	15%	13%
France: 1972–1990 (n = 502)	2%	4%	32%	17%	?	18%	27%
India: 1987–1993 (n = 423)	0%	2%	31%	5%	0%	0%	62%
Japan: 1992–1999 (n = 38)	0%	3%	18%	0%	0%	71%	8%
United Kingdom: 1993–1994 (n = 342)	73%	2%	2%	2%	3%	8%	9%
United States: 1994–1996 (n = 295)	20%	7%	10%	12%	3%	15%	33%
United States: 1998–2001 (n = 308)	39%	4%	7%	13%	6%	17%	15%

Note: All studies have cases of hepatitis A and hepatitis B, whereas acetaminophen-induced ALF is a feature of western countries. Idiosyncratic drug reactions typically constitute 12% to 17% of cases, but India, Japan, and the United Kingdom see fewer cases.

ACM, acetaminophen; ALF, acute liver failure; drug, idiosyncratic drug reactions; HAV, hepatitis A virus; HBV, hepatitis B virus; indet., indeterminate; shock, ischemic hepatitis.

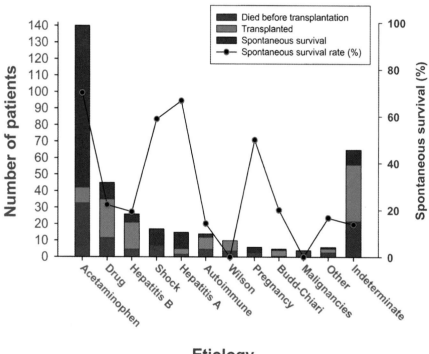

FIGURE 61-1. Breakdown of presumed etiologies and outcomes for 353 patients with acute liver failure, enrolled in the U.S. Acute Liver Failure Study Group between January 1998 and October 2001. Presumed etiologies were determined by the site investigators using standardized criteria. The most common cause was acetaminophen hepatotoxicity (40% of cases). Idiosyncratic drug reactions comprised 13% of cases; hepatitis B, 7%; shock liver, 5%; hepatitis A, 4%; and indeterminate etiology, 18%. *Stacked bars* reflect the number of patients who died, were transplanted, and survived spontaneously. The *line-dots* indicate short-term survival without transplantation rate (percent). Transplant-free survival rates greater than or equal to 50% were observed in acetaminophen, shock-liver, pregnancy, and hepatitis A cases, but were less than 25% for all other etiologies. Note that there are two different vertical axes.

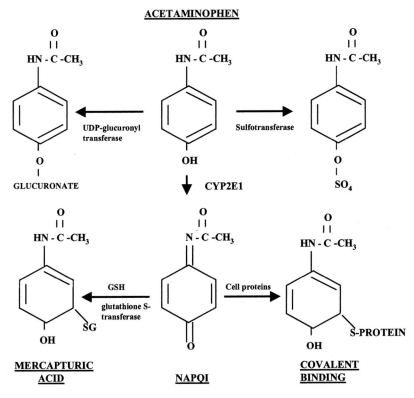

FIGURE 61-2. The metabolic pathway of acetaminophen. The major hepatic pathways of acetaminophen include glucuronidation or sulfation (**top**), yielding nontoxic conjugates excreted by the kidney. A second pathway involves the cytochrome P-450 (*CYP*) system, especially CYP2E1, by which acetaminophen is metabolized to the highly reactive metabolite *N*-acetyl-*p*-benzoquinone imine (*NAPQI*), that may bind covalently with hepatic proteins and cause cellular necrosis (**bottom**). The toxic effect of NAPQI is eliminated by the natural antidote glutathione (*GSH*), yielding mercapturic acid, which is excreted in the kidneys. Chronic alcoholism could increase acetaminophen toxicity either by short-lived induction of the CYP2E1 pathway or by decreasing the hepatic contents of the glutathione.

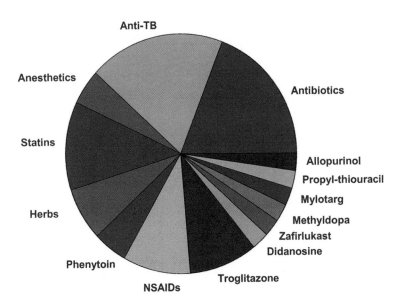

FIGURE 61-3. Presumed agents implicated in 44 cases of idiosyncratic drug reactions from the U.S. Acute Liver Failure Study Group, 1998 to 2001. Anti-tuberculosis agents included isoniazid (5 patients), pyrazinamide-rifampin (2 patients), rifampin (1 patient). Antibiotics included nitrofurantoin (2 patients), sulfadiazine (1 patient), amoxicillin (1 patient), trimethoprim-sulfamethoxazole (1 patient), clarithromycin (1 patient), itraconazole (1 patient), and terbinafine (1 patient), whereas all nonsteroidal antiinflammatory cases were due to bromfenac (which has been withdrawn from the market). Statins included cerivastatin (2 patients), simvastatin (1 patient), stavudine (1 patient), and pravastatin (1 patient). Troglitazone (4 patients) has also been withdrawn from the market.

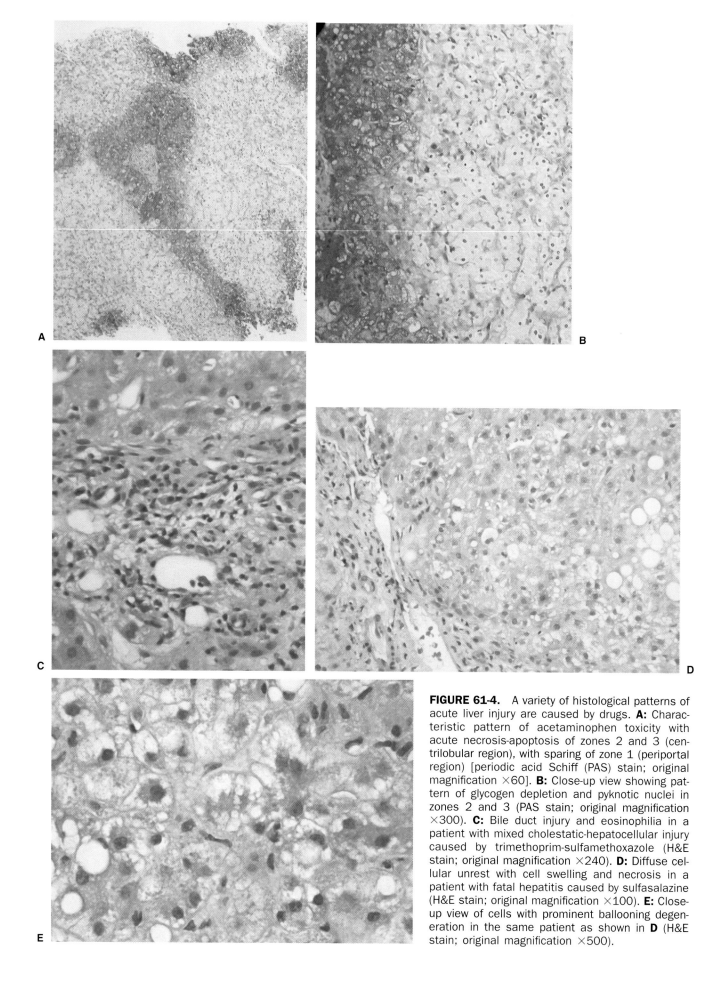

FIGURE 61-4. A variety of histological patterns of acute liver injury are caused by drugs. **A:** Characteristic pattern of acetaminophen toxicity with acute necrosis-apoptosis of zones 2 and 3 (centrilobular region), with sparing of zone 1 (periportal region) [periodic acid Schiff (PAS) stain; original magnification ×60]. **B:** Close-up view showing pattern of glycogen depletion and pyknotic nuclei in zones 2 and 3 (PAS stain; original magnification ×300). **C:** Bile duct injury and eosinophilia in a patient with mixed cholestatic-hepatocellular injury caused by trimethoprim-sulfamethoxazole (H&E stain; original magnification ×240). **D:** Diffuse cellular unrest with cell swelling and necrosis in a patient with fatal hepatitis caused by sulfasalazine (H&E stain; original magnification ×100). **E:** Close-up view of cells with prominent ballooning degeneration in the same patient as shown in **D** (H&E stain; original magnification ×500).

62

AUTOIMMUNE HEPATITIS

E. JENNY HEATHCOTE

When the disease entity autoimmune hepatitis (AIH) was first described, patients generally presented with decompensated cirrhosis. Now that liver enzymes are often checked at the time of a routine screen, it is apparent that AIH may be associated with a wide range of liver disease severity. Some individuals have no symptoms, but the majority have various nonspecific symptoms with or without evidence of liver failure. Rarely, AIH presents as an acute fulminant hepatitis, although liver biopsy at the time often shows that cirrhosis is already present. Both asymptomatic and symptomatic patients may have underlying cirrhosis when first diagnosed.

This disease typically affects women more so than men. All age groups and racial groups may be affected. When symptoms are present they are nonspecific and consist of fatigue, anorexia, arthralgia, and secondary amenorrhea, with or without signs of liver failure. Sometimes, other nonhepatic autoimmune diseases may be present or develop later, such as thyroid disease. Laboratory test abnormalities include a fairly marked elevation in serum aminotransferase levels (5- to 10-fold elevation) and a minimally elevated alkaline phosphatase (ALP), with or without hyperbilirubinemia, hypoalbuminemia, and/or prolonged coagulation. The serologic hallmarks of AIH are the non–organ-specific antibodies antinuclear antibody (ANA) and/or smooth muscle antibody (SMA) in those with type 1 AIH, or antiliver/kidney microsomal antibody (LKM-1) in those with type 2 AIH (Table 62-1). However, these first two autoantibodies may be detected in up to one third of individuals with a wide range of chronic liver diseases, so they are not sufficient to make a diagnosis of AIH on their own. Hypergammaglobulinemia is a prerequisite, and levels need to be elevated greater than 1.5 times normal; sometimes they are very high. In type 2 AIH, immunoglobulin levels are less elevated and serum IgA may even be low.

Any other hepatitis can mimic AIH, particularly drug-induced liver disease, chronic viral hepatitis B or C, and occasionally Wilson disease. Rarely alcoholic hepatitis and nonalcoholic fatty liver disease may resemble AIH. Hence, in addition to a thorough history, tests for hepatitis B and C and serum ceruloplasmin should be performed.

A liver biopsy is required to confirm the diagnosis and assess the severity of AIH. It is necessary that a well-trained hepatopathologist interpret the liver biopsy findings. Typically, there is a lymphoplasmacytic infiltration of both the portal tracts and the liver parenchyma, with variable degrees of fibrosis (Fig. 62-1). If a coagulopathy is present and cannot be corrected, the biopsy must be performed via the transjugular route rather than percutaneously. In children, it is not unusual for both

AIH and primary sclerosing cholangitis (PSC), to be present simultaneously. Up to 50% of children who present with typical AIH also have features of PSC, and thus it is recommended that all children thought to have AIH also undergo examination of the biliary tract. This overlap of AIH and PSC is much less common in adults, although it is described.

It is helpful to confirm the diagnosis of AIH by calculating the AIH score (Table 62-2). A score of 15 or more determines definite AIH. A score of 10 to 15 indicates probable AIH. It is best to assess this score prior to the institution of therapy. The score can be recalculated once the response to therapy is known.

NATURAL HISTORY

The majority of individuals recruited to the classical therapeutic trials initiated in the late 1960s had decompensated cirrhosis. In the 21st century, patients may be given a diagnosis of AIH when they have few or no symptoms. The natural history of asymptomatic AIH is poorly documented; some patients subsequently develop symptomatic disease. The natural history of untreated symptomatic AIH (gleaned from the placebo groups in the early therapeutic studies) indicates that survival without therapy is only 50% and 10% at 5 and 10 years.

Death generally is due to liver failure, often complicated by sepsis. With therapy the 10-year survival of patients with AIH with or without cirrhosis is close to 100% at 5 years and 80% at 20 years. Even when treatment is successful, cirrhosis may still develop in 40% of patients; that is, therapy markedly improves survival, but does not necessarily prevent the development of cirrhosis.

Whereas fertility may be reduced in the untreated patient with AIH, women with well-controlled AIH can become pregnant and their ongoing therapy should be continued during the pregnancy. Therapy has no adverse effects on the fetus. Flare-ups may occur, most often in the postpartum period.

TREATMENT

Three well-conducted studies published in the early 1970s indicated that corticosteroid therapy markedly improved the survival of patients with AIH. Successful treatment was obtained with prednisone, alone or in combination with azathioprine (Imuran), but the latter was ineffective as monotherapy. A dose of 30 mg prednisone is generally sufficient to initiate therapy. Azathioprine 1 to 2 mg/kg may be started simultaneously or a little later. Once the serum aminotransferase values decrease to less than 2-fold elevated, the dose of prednisone should be reduced slowly. It is often possible to stop the administration of prednisone altogether, and to maintain adequate disease suppression with azathioprine 50 to 100 mg/day (Table 62-3). Few patients fail to respond to treatment, but relapse off treatment is frequent (83%). The optimal duration of immunosuppressive therapy required to induce and sustain remission is unknown, although it is generally advised that treatment be maintained for at least 1 and perhaps 2 years after the ALT and immunoglobulin levels have returned to normal. Some clinicians advocate repeat liver biopsy before stopping therapy to ensure that there is no disease activity present. In those rare individuals who fail to respond to treatment, a higher dose of corticosteroid therapy may first be tried. Once doses greater than 40 mg/day are employed, there is a high side effect profile, and it is reasonable under these circumstances to attempt suppression of disease with other immunosuppressants, such as cyclosporin, mycophenolate mofetil, methotrexate, or cyclophosphamide. In individuals who present with fulminant hepatitis, a liver transplant may be needed before the individual has a chance to respond to standard immunosuppressive therapy. Liver transplantation may also be required in individuals with burned-out, decompensated cirrhosis in whom immunosuppressive therapy is inappropriate. AIH may return in the transplanted liver, but this is not a reason to deny a transplant. It is not known whether those with asymptomatic AIH should receive immuno-suppressive therapy, because their natural history is uncertain.

Immunosuppressive therapy frequently produces side effects. If there is time before the patient starts treatment with prednisone, baseline measurements of bone mineral density, blood glucose, and systemic blood pressure, and ophthalmologic examination for glaucoma and cataracts should be performed; subsequently moni-toring during therapy is recommended. Patients should be warned to treat any infection promptly, and advised appropriately about travel overseas. Because of the drug's effect on the bone marrow, patients taking azathioprine should have their white blood count checked frequently. Pancreatitis and even hepatitis are rare com-plications of azathioprine, but gastrointestinal side effects of azathioprine are com-mon, and when severe may render the patient intolerant to this treatment. It is safe for women to conceive while taking prednisone and/or azathioprine. In individu-als who are known to have cirrhosis and in all women who are pregnant, upper panendoscopy should be performed to check for the presence of large esophageal varices. Prophylactic beta-blocker therapy should be given to those with large varices.

(figure on page 645)

TABLE 62-1

Comparison of the Clinical and Immunological Features of Types 1 and 2 Autoimmune Chronic Active Hepatitis

	TYPE 1 (ANTIACTIN)	TYPE 2 (ANTI-LKM)	ANTI-SLA
Age at presentation	10–25 and 45–70 y	Less than 15 y	Mean age, 37 y
Associated disorders	10%	17%	58%
Immunoglobulins	37 ± 11	23 ± 8	Mean, 32.2
γ-globulins (g/L)			Range, 1.8–5.2
IgG	37 ± 16	25 ± 10.4	
IgA	3.7 ± 1.3	1.8 ± 0.9	
IgM	1.7 ± 1.1	2.4 ± 1.5	
Autoantibodies			
Anti-SMA (%)	100	0	74
ANA (%)	33	2	29
AMA (%)	2	0	14
Progression to cirrhosis after 3 y (%)	43	82	75

AMA, antimitochondrial antibody; ANA, antinuclear antibody; IgG, immunoglobulin G; LKM, antiliver/kidney microsome; SLA, soluble liver antigen.

From Johnson PJ, McFarlane IG, Eddleston ALWF. The natural course and heterogeneity of auto-immune type chronic active hepatitis. Semin Liver Dis 1991;11:189.

TABLE 62-2
Summary of Autoimmune Hepatitis Scoring Revised Sheet

PARAMETERS	SCORE
Gender: female	+2
Biochemistry	
(IU ALP:unl ALP):(IU AST:unl AST)	+2, 0, −2
<1.5, 1.5−3, >3	
Total globulin or IgG (fold elevation)	+3, +2, +1, 0
>2, 1.5−2, 1−1.5, <1	
Autoantibodies (ANA, SMA, LKM-1) titer	+3, +2, +1, 0
>1:80, 1:80, 1:40, <1:40 (IF)	
Antimitochondrial antibody	
AMA positive	−4
Viral hepatitis markers	
IgM HAVAb, HBsAg, IgM HBcAb,	Positive −3
anti-HCV, and HCV RNA, ?CMV/EBV Ab	Negative +3
Hepatotoxic drug history (current)	Positive −4
	Negative +1
Average alcohol intake (current)	
<25 g/d	+2
>60 g/d	−2
Liver histology	
Interface hepatitis	+3
Mostly lymphoplasmacytic infiltrate	+1
Rosetting of liver cells	+1
None of the above	−5
Biliary changes	−3
Other changes	−3
Other autoimmune diseases in patients or	+2
first-degree relatives	
Optional Additional Parameters	
Seropositivity of other defined autoantibodies	+2
(pANCA, anti-LC1, anti-SLA, anti-ASGPR,	
anti-LP, antisulfatide)	+2
HLA DR3 or DR4	+1
Response to therapy	
Complete	+2
Relapse	+3
No response (cholangiography required)	

ALP, alkaline phosphatase; AMA, antimitochondrial antibody; ANA, antinuclear antibody; ASGPR, asialoglycoprotein receptor Ab; AST, aspartate aminotransferase; CMV/EBV, cytomegalovirus or Epstein-Barr virus; HAVAb, hepatitis A virus antibody; HBcAb, hepatitis B virus core antibody; HBsAg, hepatitis B surface antigen; HCV, hepatitis C virus; HLA, human leukocyte antigen; IgG, immunoglobulin G; IU, international unit; LC1, liver cytosol antibody type 1; LKM-1, antiliver/kidney microsomal antibody 1; LP, liver pancreas; pANCA, perinuclear antineutrophilic cytoplasmic antibody; SLA, soluble liver antigen; unl, upper normal limit.

From Alvarez F, Berg PA, Blanchi FB, et al. International autoimmune hepatitis group report: review of criteria for diagnosis of autoimmune hepatitis. J Hepatol 1999;31:929.

TABLE 62-3
Suggested Therapeutic Regimen: AIH

Initial therapy: prednisone 30–60 mg/d monotherapy or prednisone 30 mg/d and
  azathioprine 50–100 mg/d combined therapy
Dose reduction: slowly reduce prednisone (2.5–5 mg every 1–3 mo) if ALT remains
  <1.5 uln
Maintenance: minimum dose prednisone and/or azathioprine to maintain ALT <1.5 uln
Stop therapy: if ALT <1.5 uln for 1–2 y +/−, liver biopsy indicates inactivity
Retreatment of relapse: reintroduce therapy as for initial treatment
Failure to respond: use either high-dose prednisone 40–60 mg/d or another
  immunosuppressant, or consider liver transplant if appropriate

AIH, autoimmune hepatitis; ALT, alanine aminotransferase; uln, upper limit normal; +/−, with/without.

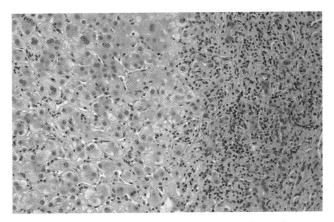

FIGURE 62-1. Typical histological picture of autoimmune hepatitis.

63

PRIMARY BILIARY CIRRHOSIS

MARLYN J. MAYO ■ M. HOSSEIN SABOORIAN ■ DWAIN L. THIELE

Primary biliary cirrhosis (PBC) is a chronic liver disease that is defined by its clinical presentation, histological features, and serological findings. The underlying abnormality in PBC is a slowly progressive, nonpurulent inflammatory destruction of the biliary epithelial cells lining the small- to medium-sized interlobular ducts. Autoantibodies are a characteristic feature of the disease; more than 90% of PBC patients have antimitochondrial antibodies (AMA) and about 30% have antinuclear antibodies (ANA). Loss of normal biliary drainage eventually leads to a clinical picture of chronic hepatic cholestasis and its potential complications.

HISTOLOGY

Several authors have developed histological staging systems that group the histological abnormalities of PBC into four distinct stages (Fig. 63-1). Stage I is characterized by lymphocytes infiltrating the portal tracts (Fig. 63-2). Stage II is characterized by a greater degree of inflammation, extending beyond the limiting plate, and the presence of bile ductular proliferation (Fig. 63-3). Stage III is defined by the presence of bridging fibrosis (Fig. 63-4), and the presence of cirrhosis represents stage IV (Fig. 63-5). The most specific (although not pathognomonic) histological finding is the "florid duct lesion," in which the bile duct is surrounded by an intense lymphocytic or granulomatous infiltrate, and the basal integrity of the bile duct has been breached by individual lymphocytes (Fig. 63-6). Bile staining and cholate stasis with feathery degeneration of hepatocytes (Fig. 63-7) is evident in some patients, and Mallory hyaline may be found in the affected hepatocytes (Fig. 63-8). As the disease advances, ductopenia becomes evident. Stains for copper and copper binding protein are often positive in PBC liver (Fig. 63-9). The degree of copper retention correlates with disease severity, and it may reach levels comparable to that seen in Wilson disease.

CLINICAL MANIFESTATIONS

The diagnosis of PBC is suspected when a patient presents with evidence of chronic cholestasis. In the early stages, this may be an asymptomatic elevation of serum alkaline phosphatase levels and/or γ-glutamyltransferase. Over time, fatigue or clinical signs of chronic cholestasis such as pruritus or hypercholesterolemia may develop. Jaundice occurs late in the disease process and is a poor prognostic sign.

Xanthomas and hyperpigmentation are the primary skin findings expressed in PBC patients. Xanthomas are most often seen around the eyes (xanthelasma), but may also develop over tendons and in palmar-digital creases (Fig. 63-10). Hyperpigmentation (Fig. 63-11) results from increased melanin deposition, and is most often found on the trunk and arms. Skin may also darken in areas that are repetitively scratched, which may result in a butterfly pattern of sparing in the middle of the back.

PBC is frequently accompanied by other extrahepatic conditions, many of which are also believed to be autoimmune in nature. The most common symptomatic co-morbid condition is Sjögren syndrome, which occurs in 30% to 58% of patients with PBC. Xerostomia and xerophthalmia of sicca syndrome are the usual manifestations. The calcinosis, Raynaud phenomenon, esophageal dysmotility, sclerodactyly, and telangiectasias (CREST) syndrome is present in about 5% of PBC patients. The most common features seen are Raynaud (Fig. 63-12) and telangiectasias (Fig. 63-13). Isolated Raynaud syndrome occurs in an additional 7% to 14% of patients.

CLINICAL COURSE AND THERAPY

PBC may exist for relatively long periods of time in an asymptomatic state. However, the majority of asymptomatic individuals eventually become symptomatic, and most individuals with established disease eventually progress to cirrhosis. Clinical progression is foretold by worsening of specific biochemical parameters, particularly serum bilirubin levels.

Therapy with ursodeoxycholic acid (ursodiol) at a dose of 13 to 15 mg/kg/day has become the mainstay of therapy for PBC. Five large, randomized, double-blind, controlled trials have demonstrated the beneficial effects of ursodeoxycholic acid therapy (Table 63-1). In all trials, improvement in serum liver tests was noted, usually within the first 1 to 2 months of therapy, with a maximal response by about 6 months. Effects on symptoms were unimpressive, and no effect on the development of cirrhosis or portal hypertension, or death or transplantation could be detected at 2 years in any of the individual trials. Subsequent combined analyses and metaanalyses have reached conflicting conclusions regarding the ability of ursodiol to improve survival. The difficulty in clearly demonstrating survival benefits of ursodiol is not surprising considering the slowly progressive course of PBC and the relatively short duration of the placebo phase in most randomized controlled trials. Nevertheless, because of its excellent safety profile, proven ability to improve markers of cholestasis, and suggestion of long-term benefits, ursodiol is currently recommended as treatment for all stages of PBC. Patients with complicated cirrhosis or poor estimated survival should be considered for transplant referral.

Treatment of the symptoms and complications of chronic cholestasis comprises a significant portion of the management of PBC patients (Fig. 63-14). Pruritus is a common and often vexing symptom of patients with PBC. Bile acid sequestrants, such as cholestyramine and colestipol, are the first line of medical treatment for cholestatic pruritus. Other medications that have been demonstrated to relieve cholestatic itching in small controlled trials include rifampin, phenobarbital, opioid receptor blockers, and ondansetron. Antihistamines, plasmapheresis, and phototherapy have also been anecdotally successful in ameliorating cholestatic pruritus. Some patients have intractable itching, which has been an independent indication for liver transplantation.

Accelerated osteoporosis can be a devastating complication of chronic cholestasis, and careful monitoring and preventative treatment are warranted. The severity of bone disease correlates with the severity of the liver disease, and therefore patients with stage IV disease should be screened with bone densitometry at regular intervals. Calcium supplementation is well tolerated and widely used. The majority of postmenopausal PBC patients can benefit from transdermal or low-dose oral estrogen replacement without experiencing a clinically significant increase in cholestasis.

The ability of bisphosphonates to increase bone density has been demonstrated in PBC patients, so these agents are indicated when bone density is already decreased.

Deficiencies in fat-soluble vitamins should be replaced. Because of potential toxicity from overdoses, levels of vitamin A and D should be monitored in patients receiving supplements.

Many PBC patients have sicca syndrome and are troubled by xerophthalmia and xerostomia. Liberal use of moisturizers and regular evaluation by a dental professional are recommended.

(figures begin on page 650)

TABLE 63-1

Summary of Double-Blind, Randomized, Placebo-Controlled, Trials of Ursodeoxycholic Acid (UDCA) for the Treatment of Primary Biliary Cirrhosis

	POUPON ET AL.[*,†]	HEATHCOTE ET AL.[‡]	LINDOR ET AL.[‖]	COMBES ET AL.[¶]	PARES ET AL.[#]
No. subjects	145	222	180	151	192
Histological stage					
I, II (%)	53	45	32	33	70
II, IV (%)	47	55	68	67	30
Follow-up period	2 y	2 y	Up to 50 mo (mean 2 y)	2 y	Median 3.4 y (range 0.3–6.1 y)
Dosing of UDCA	13–15 mg/kg/d in two doses	14 mg/kg with evening meal	13–15 mg/kg/d, in three doses with meals	10–12 mg/kg/qhs	14–16 mg/kg/d in three doses
Changes in symptoms in UDCA group	No effect on hyperpigmentation, xanthoma, arthritis, CREST	No effect on fatigue, pruritus, xanthelasma, ascites, or encephalopathy	No effect on fatigue, pruritus	No effect on fatigue, pruritus	Improved pruritus, fatigue, and xanthomas
Changes in laboratory tests in UDCA group	Improved bili, AP, GGT, AST, ALT, IgM, cholesterol; small improvement in IgG, and AMA titer; no effect on IgA, PT, alb	Improved bili, AP, AST, ALT, IgM, cholesterol; no effect on IgG or IgA	Improved bili, AP, AST	Improved bili, AP, GGT, AST, ALT, IgM; prevented alb decline	Improved AP, GGT, AST, ALT, IgM, IgG, cholesterol
Changes in histology in UDCA group	Improved hepatocyte necrosis, portal and lobular inflammation, cholestasis, ductopenia, and ductular proliferation; no effect on fibrosis	Prevented progression of hepatocyte necrosis and ductopenia; no effect on fibrosis, ductular proliferation, portal or lobular inflammation	No effect on stage	Prevented progression of hepatocyte necrosis and improved fibrosis in subgroups of patients without jaundice; no effect seen in patients with bili ≥2	Beneficial effect on histological stage, portal inflammation, hepatocyte necrosis, bile duct paucity
Development of portal hypertension (% in UDCA group/% in placebo group)	3% versus 7%	Not stated	Trend toward beneficial effect of ursodiol	No difference	No difference

(continued)

TABLE 63-1. *(Continued)*

	POUPON ET AL.[*,†]	HEATHCOTE ET AL.[†]	LINDOR ET AL.[‖]	COMBES ET AL.[¶]	PARES ET AL.[#]
Death or trx (% in UDCA group versus % in placebo group)	7% versus 7% (estimated from graph at 2 y, Fig. 63-2)	11% versus 17% (NS)	8% versus 13% (NS)	16% versus 15% (NS)	17% versus 12% (NS)
Time to death or trx	Not stated	No difference	No difference	Trend toward beneficial effect of ursodiol in patients with bili <2	No difference

[*]Poupon RE, Balkau B, Eschwege E, Poupon R, and the UDCA-PBC study group. A multicenter, controlled trial of ursodiol of the treatment of primary biliary cirrhosis. N Engl J Med 1991;324:1548.

[†]Poupon RE, Poupon R, Balkau B, and the UDCA-PBC study group. Ursodiol for the long-term treatment of primary biliary cirrhosis. N Engl J Med 1994;330:1342.

[‡]Heathcote EJ, Cauch-Dudek K, Walker V, et al. The Canadian multicenter double-blind randomized controlled trial of ursodeoxycholic acid in primary biliary cirrhosis. Hepatology 1994;19:1149.

[‖]Lindor KD, Dickson ER, Baldus WP, et al. Ursodeoxycholic acid in the treatment of primary biliary cirrhosis. Gastroenterology 1994;106:1284.

[¶]Combes B, Carithers RL, Maddrey WC, et al. A randomized double-blind, placebo-controlled trial of ursodeoxycholic acid in primary biliary cirrhosis. Hepatology 1995;22:759.

[#]Pares A, Caballeria L, Rodes J, et al. Long-term effects of ursodeoxycholic acid in primary biliary cirrhosis: results of a double-blind controlled multicentric trial. J Hepatology 2000;32:561.

alb, albumin; ALT, alanine aminotransferase; AST, aspartate aminotransferase; AMA, antimitochondrial antibody; AP, alkaline phosphatase; bili, bilirubin; CREST, calcinosis, Raynaud phenomenon, esophageal dysmotility, sclerodactyly, and telangiectasia; GGT, gamma glutaryl transferase; IgM, immunoglobulin M; NS, not significant; PT, prothrombin time; trx, treatment.

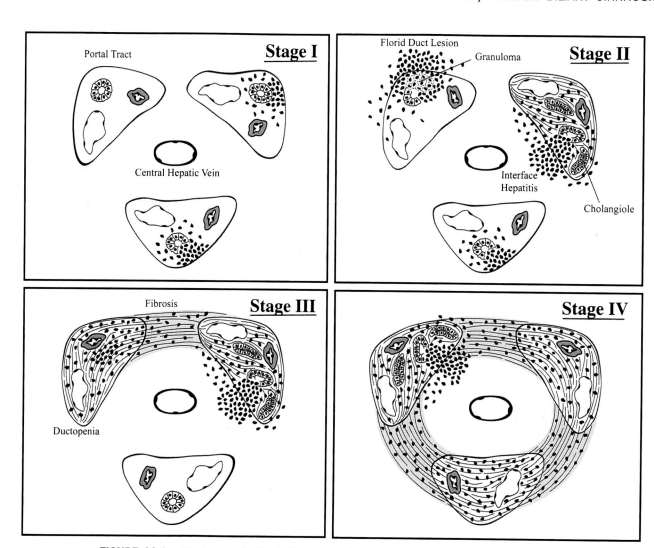

FIGURE 63-1. Diagrammatic illustration of the four stages of histological progression of primary biliary cirrhosis. Characteristic features of each stage are illustrated here, but the lesions are often patchy in nature. Stage I: mononuclear portal tract infiltrates, sometimes involving the bile duct. Stage II: intense mononuclear portal tract infiltrate with interface hepatitis, a florid duct lesion (granulomatous involvement of bile duct), and pseudoductular (cholangiolar) proliferation. Stage III: bridging fibrosis, mononuclear portal tract infiltrates with interface hepatitis, pseudoductular proliferation, and ductopenia. Stage IV: cirrhosis, mononuclear portal tract infiltrates with interface hepatitis, pseudoductular proliferation, and ductopenia.

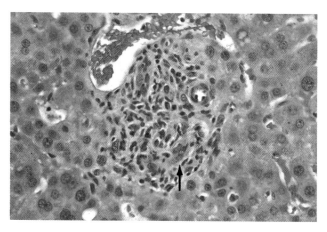

FIGURE 63-2. Primary biliary cirrhosis (PBC), stage I, is characterized by a mononuclear cell portal infiltrate that does not extend beyond the limiting plate. The inflammatory infiltrate consists predominantly of T lymphocytes, but it may also contain plasma cells and eosinophils. The arrow points to residual biliary epithelial cells of a native bile duct destroyed by the inflammatory process. Bile duct destruction suggests the diagnosis of PBC, but may not be evident in biopsy specimens during stage I disease.

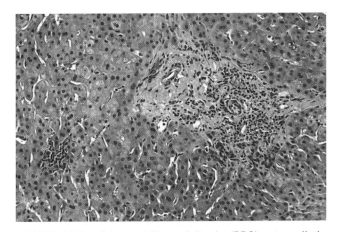

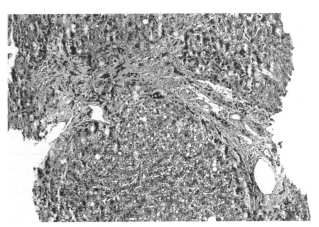

FIGURE 63-3. Primary biliary cirrhosis (PBC), stage II, is characterized by a mononuclear cell infiltrate (predominantly of T lymphocytes, also plasma cells and eosinophils) of the portal tract that extends beyond the limiting plate. Bile ductules are usually found at the periphery of the portal tract (as opposed to the native bile ducts, which tend to be located adjacent to the portal arteriole) and they frequently have poorly defined basement membranes and lumens. Proliferation of bile ductules (pseudoducts or cholangioles) that arise from hepatic cell plates or putative stem cells under conditions of chronic cholestasis are a common feature of stage II disease. Nonsuppurative cholangitis, portal granulomas, and granulomatous cholangitis (see Fig. 63-6) are present in about 50% of stage II PBC biopsies. Septal fibrosis or ductopenia (not shown in this figure) may also be present. Lobular hepatitis, as noted in the lower left corner of the photomicrograph, may also be seen in primary biliary cirrhosis.

FIGURE 63-4. Primary biliary cirrhosis (PBC), stage III, is defined by the presence of bridging fibrosis. All of the features seen in stage II PBC (see Fig. 63-2) may be present, but ductopenia is more common in later stages of the disease. The diagnosis of ductopenia is often difficult to make because of insufficient diagnostic material. A minimum sample of 4 portal tracts (with all 4 portal tracts containing arterioles but no ducts) or ideally 20 portal tracts (with at least 10 portal tracts containing arterioles but no ducts) are needed to make a diagnosis of ductopenia.

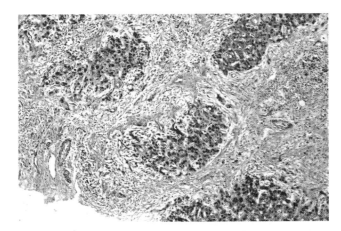

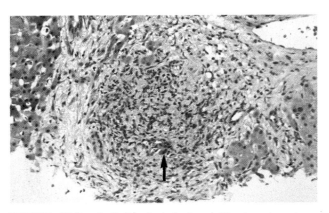

FIGURE 63-5. Primary biliary cirrhosis (PBC), stage IV, is defined by the presence of cirrhosis. Although any of the characteristic histological features of PBC (see Fig. 63-2) may be present, they may also be absent if much of the liver has been replaced by fibrous tissue. Ductopenia is usually evident in stage IV PBC.

FIGURE 63-6. A florid duct lesion with granulomatous involvement of the bile duct is the most specific histological finding suggestive of the diagnosis of primary biliary cirrhosis (PBC). The granulomas in primary biliary cirrhosis are often poorly defined. Portal granulomas without bile duct involvement are also seen in PBC, but lobular granulomas are much less common. In this photomicrograph, the *arrow* points to a damaged bile duct associated with portal granulomatous inflammation.

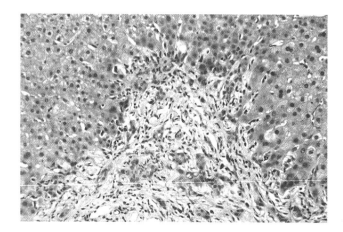

FIGURE 63-7. Biliary piecemeal necrosis in which there is death of periportal hepatocytes associated with an inflammatory infiltrate may also be evident in primary biliary cirrhosis. The injured hepatocytes appear swollen (feathery degeneration) as a result of cholate stasis.

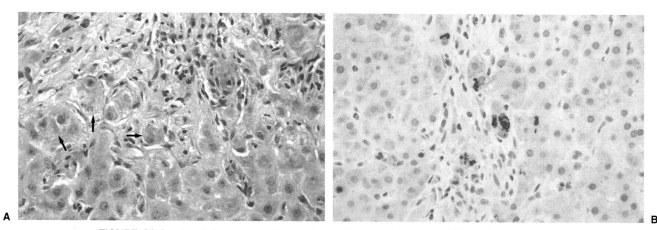

A   B

FIGURE 63-8. **A:** Mallory bodies (*arrows*) may be seen in primary biliary cirrhosis (PBC). They are typically located in the periportal hepatocytes, as opposed to localization in the hepatic lobule in steatohepatitis. **B:** Immunohistochemistry for ubiquitin (*red pigment*) highlights the presence of Mallory hyaline in PBC liver tissue.

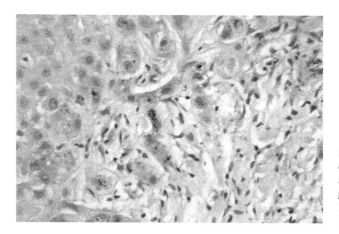

FIGURE 63-9. A rhodanine stain (*red pigment*) demonstrates copper granules in primary biliary cirrhosis liver tissue. Copper accumulates in the periportal hepatocytes as cholestasis progresses. It is frequently accompanied by Mallory hyaline (see Fig. 63-8) and is typically found in areas of cholate stasis (see Fig. 63-7).

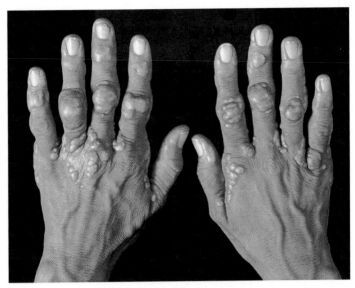

FIGURE 63-10. Hands of a primary biliary cirrhosis (PBC) patient with severe xanthomas. Xanthomas are most often seen around the eyes (xanthelasma), but may also develop over tendons and in palmar-digital creases. Xanthomas are more often seen in PBC patients with prolonged cholestasis but can also be seen before the onset of cirrhosis.

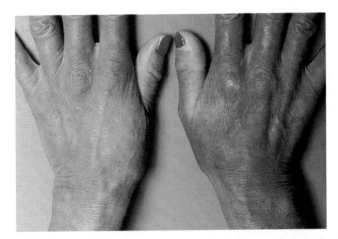

FIGURE 63-11. Hyperpigmentation, which results from increased melanin deposition, is usually seen in primary biliary cirrhosis (PBC) patients with prolonged cholestasis but can also be seen before the onset of cirrhosis. Pictured here is one PBC patient with asymmetric hyperpigmentation of the hands. Hyperpigmentation is most often found on the trunk and arms. Skin may also darken in areas that are repetitively scratched, which may result in a butterfly pattern of sparing in the middle of the back.

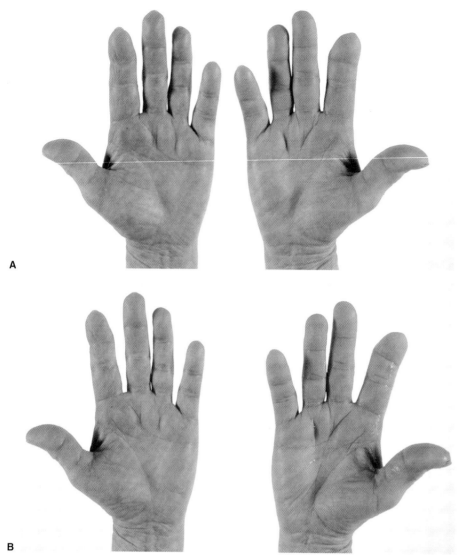

A

B

FIGURE 63-12. Raynaud phenomenon is present in about 15% of patients with primary biliary cirrhosis. It may be an isolated feature, or a part of the calcinosis, Raynaud phenomenon, esophageal dysmotility, sclerodactyly, telangiectasias (CREST) syndrome. **A:** The patient's fingertips are cyanotic at room temperature. **B:** After the patient has soaked her hands in warm water, the bluish color disappears.

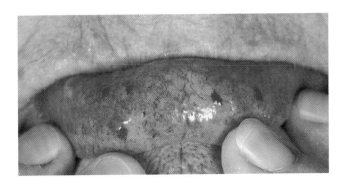

FIGURE 63-13. Telangectasias are seen as part of the calcinosis, Raynaud phenomenon, esophageal dysmotility, sclerodactyly, telangiectasias (CREST) syndrome in 5% to 7% of primary biliary cirrhosis patients. Telangiectasias are most commonly found on the lips (shown here) and the fingertips.

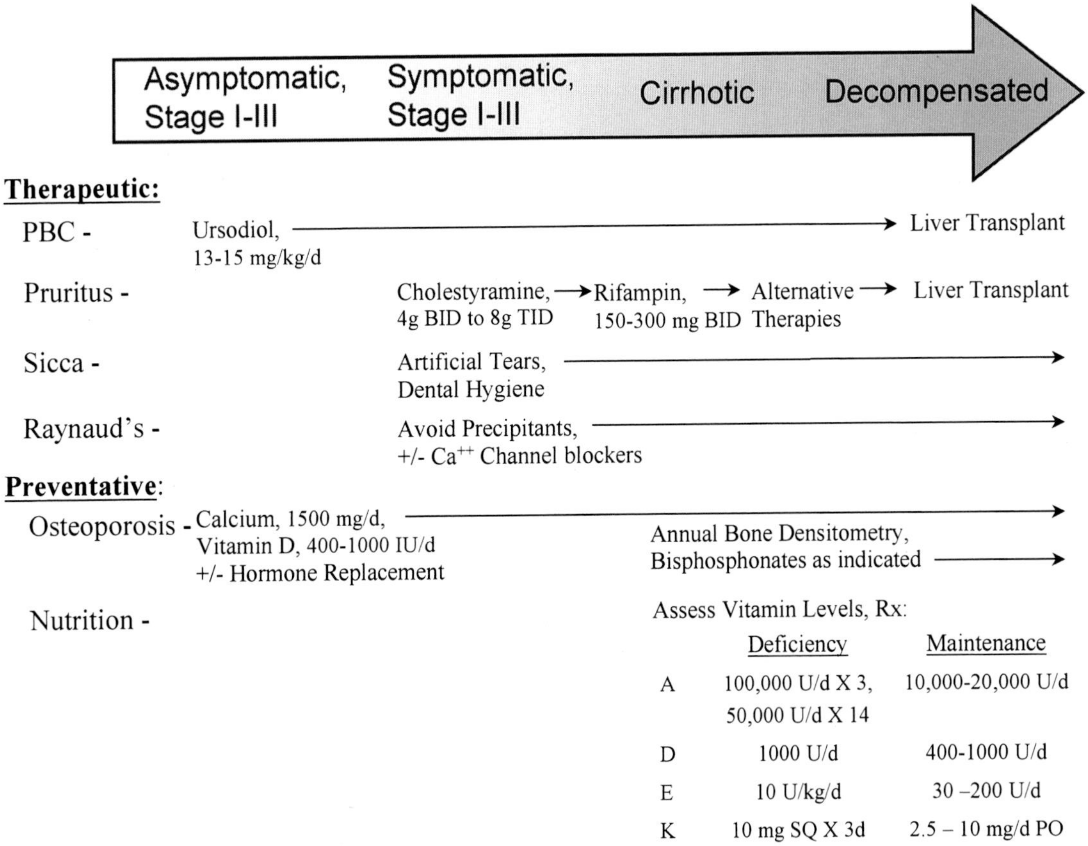

Asymptomatic, Stage I-III	Symptomatic, Stage I-III	Cirrhotic	Decompensated

Therapeutic:

PBC - Ursodiol, 13-15 mg/kg/d ——————————————→ Liver Transplant

Pruritus - Cholestyramine, →Rifampin, → Alternative → Liver Transplant
4g BID to 8g TID   150-300 mg BID Therapies

Sicca - Artificial Tears, ————————————————————→
Dental Hygiene

Raynaud's - Avoid Precipitants, ——————————————————→
+/- Ca++ Channel blockers

Preventative:

Osteoporosis - Calcium, 1500 mg/d, ——————————————————→
Vitamin D, 400-1000 IU/d
+/- Hormone Replacement
Annual Bone Densitometry,
Bisphosphonates as indicated ————————→

Nutrition - Assess Vitamin Levels, Rx:

	Deficiency	Maintenance
A	100,000 U/d X 3, 50,000 U/d X 14	10,000-20,000 U/d
D	1000 U/d	400-1000 U/d
E	10 U/kg/d	30 –200 U/d
K	10 mg SQ X 3d	2.5 – 10 mg/d PO

FIGURE 63-14. Overview of the management of primary biliary cirrhosis and associated conditions. Complications of portal hypertension (not shown) are managed in the same manner as in other forms of cirrhosis.

HEMOCHROMATOSIS

PAUL C. ADAMS

INTRODUCTION

Hemochromatosis is one of the most common genetic diseases and may lead to iron accumulation in the liver, heart, pancreas, and endocrine organs. Early diagnosis and treatment are essential to prevent organ damage.

GENETICS

Since the discovery of the gene for hemochromatosis (*HFE*) in 1996, a simple genetic blood test has been developed that can be performed on a blood sample or stored tissue.

The C282Y mutation on chromosome 6 of the *HFE* gene is present in 93% to 100% of homozygotes in pedigree studies. In less well-defined patients with iron overload, the prevalence ranges from 60% to 80%. A second mutation, H63D, is less common and its relationship to hemochromatosis is less well defined. There have been other iron overload diseases associated with mutations in other iron-related genes (transferrin receptor 2, *IREG1*).

USE OF THE C282Y GENETIC TEST FOR HEMOCHROMATOSIS

The genetic test is most useful in a patient who is suspected of having hemochromatosis clinically or who has an elevated transferrin saturation and/or serum ferritin. It is also useful when investigating siblings and other family members of a C282Y homozygote. It will replace human leucocyte antigen (HLA) typing in pedigree studies.

Several reported cases within hemochromatosis families are homozygous for the C282Y mutation without iron overload. This may represent incomplete penetrance, and the frequency of these phenomena in the general population has not been clearly established. However, population studies in North America, Europe, and Australia suggest that the gene is more common than the clinical disease. This may reflect a high degree of incomplete penetrance or underdiagnosis of the disease.

TREATMENT OF HEMOCHROMATOSIS

Patients are initially treated by the weekly removal of 500 mL of blood. Patients attend an ambulatory care facility and the venesection is performed by a nurse using a kit containing a 16-gauge straight needle and collection bag (Blood Pack MR6102, Baxter, Deerfield, IL). Blood is removed with the patient in the reclining position during 15 to 30 minutes. A hemoglobin level is assessed at the time of each venesection. If the hemoglobin decreases to less than 100 g/L, the venesection schedule is modified to 500 mL every other week. Serum ferritin is measured periodically (every 3 months in severe iron overload, monthly in mild iron overload) and weekly venesections are continued until the serum ferritin is approximately 50 μg/L. Transferrin saturation often remains elevated despite therapy. Patients may then begin maintenance venesections three to four times per year. Iron reaccumulation is an inconsistent observation and many patients will continue for years without treatment without an increase in serum ferritin. Chelation therapy is not used for the treatment of hemochromatosis.

TABLE 64-1
Phenotypic Diagnostic Tests for Hemochromatosis and Iron Overload

Transferrin saturation: is better than serum iron alone; is available and inexpensive; fasting is better than random. This test is elevated even in children with hemochromatosis. Thresholds for investigation vary from >45% to 62%.
Unsaturated iron binding capacity: is an old test that can be done for <$1 and has shown promise as a screening test.
Serum ferritin: is a good indirect measurement of body iron stores. Increases with age in hemochromatosis. Can be elevated in all liver diseases and chronic inflammation.
Liver biopsy: Since the development of genetic testing, liver biopsy has gone from a diagnostic test to a prognostic test. A biopsy should be considered in the hemochromatosis patient with liver dysfunction and in the patient with iron overload that does not have the typical genetic pattern. Hepatic iron concentration is useful and can be expressed as the hepatic iron concentration/age (hepatic iron index). This is particularly useful in the alcoholic patient. All types of end-stage liver disease can have mild to moderate iron overload.
Magnetic resonance imaging: The sensitivity of the technique continues to improve. It does not replace liver histology and liver iron concentration. It can be helpful in a patient with a contraindication to liver biopsy.

TABLE 64-2
Interpretation of Genetic Testing for Hemochromatosis

C282Y homozygote: This is the classical genetic pattern which is seen in >90% of typical cases. Expression of disease ranges from no evidence of iron overload to massive iron overload with organ dysfunction. Siblings have a 1 in 4 chance of being affected and should have genetic testing. For children to be affected, the other parent must be at least a heterozygote. If iron studies are normal, false-positive genetic testing or a nonexpressing homozygote should be considered.
C282Y/H63D—compound heterozygote: This patient carries one copy of the major mutation and one copy of the minor mutation. Most patients with this genetic pattern have normal iron studies. A small percentage of compound heterozygotes have been found to have mild to moderate iron overload. Severe iron overload is usually seen in the setting of another concomitant risk factor (alcoholism, viral hepatitis).
C282Y heterozygote: This patient carries one copy of the major mutation. This pattern is seen in about 10% of the Caucasian population and is usually associated with normal iron studies. In rare cases, the iron studies are high in the range expected in a homozygote rather than a heterozygote. These cases may carry an unknown hemochromatosis mutation, and liver biopsy is helpful to determine the need for venesection therapy.
H63D homozygote: This patient carries two copies of the minor mutation. Most patients with this genetic pattern have normal iron studies. A small percentage of these cases have been found to have mild to moderate iron overload. Severe iron overload is usually seen in the setting of another concomitant risk factor (alcoholism, viral hepatitis).
H63D heterozygote: This patient carries one copy of the minor mutation. This pattern is seen in about 20% of the Caucasian population and is usually associated with normal iron studies. This pattern is so common in the general population that the presence of iron overload may be related to another risk factor. Liver biopsy may be required to determine the cause of the iron overload and the need for treatment in these cases.
No *HFE* mutations: There are other iron overload diseases associated with mutations in other iron-related genes (transferrin receptor 2, *IREG1*). There will likely be other hemochromatosis mutations discovered in the future. If iron overload is present without any *HFE* mutations, a careful history for other risk factors must be reviewed and liver biopsy may be useful to determine the cause of the iron overload and the need for treatment. Most of these cases are isolated and nonfamilial. There have been cases of familial iron overload associated with other non-*HFE* mutations (*TfR2* mutation, *IREG1* mutation).

TABLE 64-3
Differential Diagnosis of Iron Overload

HFE-related hemochromatosis
    C282Y homozygotes (95%)
    C282Y/H63D compound heterozygotes (4%)
    H63D homozygotes (1%)
Non–*HFE*-related hemochromatosis
    Familial (rarely described in Italy)
    Transferrin receptor 2 mutation
    IREG1 mutation
    Nonfamilial (may be a heterogeneous collection of conditions resulting in iron overload)
    Juvenile hemochromatosis (young adults with cardiac and endocrine dysfunction)
    Neonatal hemochromatosis
Miscellaneous iron overload
    African-American iron overload
    African iron overload
    Polynesian iron overload
    Transfusional iron overload
    Insulin-resistance–related iron overload
    Aceruloplasminemia
    Alcoholic siderosis
    Iron overload secondary to end-stage cirrhosis
    Porphyria cutanea tarda
    Post-porta-caval shunt

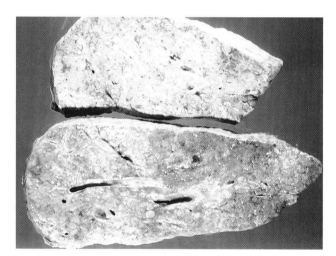

FIGURE 64-1. A cirrhotic liver from a patient with hemochromatosis. The **upper** specimen has been stained for iron, which appears blue and illustrates the diffuse iron distribution throughout the liver. (Courtesy of L.W. Powell.)

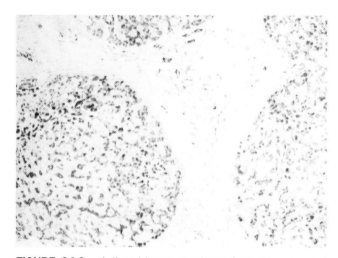

FIGURE 64-2. A liver biopsy specimen from an untreated C282Y homozygote with cirrhosis. The cirrhotic nodules are stained for iron (Prussian blue stain).

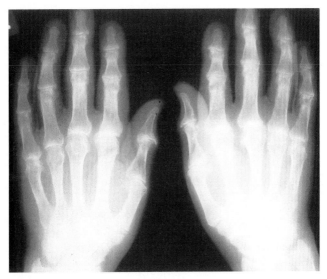

FIGURE 64-3. The arthropathy of the metacarpal phalangeal joints in hemochromatosis. In this case, a 55-year-old surgeon had to give up surgical practice because of severe disabling arthritis.

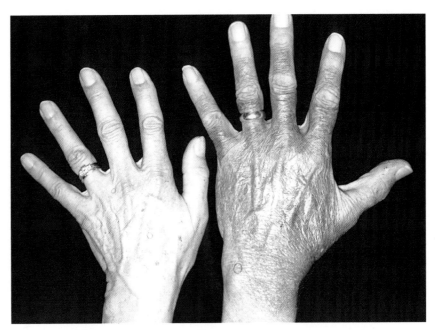

FIGURE 64-4. The skin pigmentation of hemochromatosis is illustrated in a hemochromatosis patient (**right**) compared to his wife (**left**).

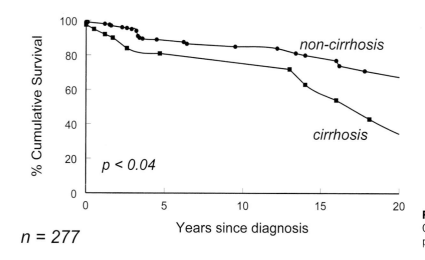

n = 277

FIGURE 64-5. Actuarial survival of treated C282Y homozygotes in cirrhotic and noncirrhotic patients.

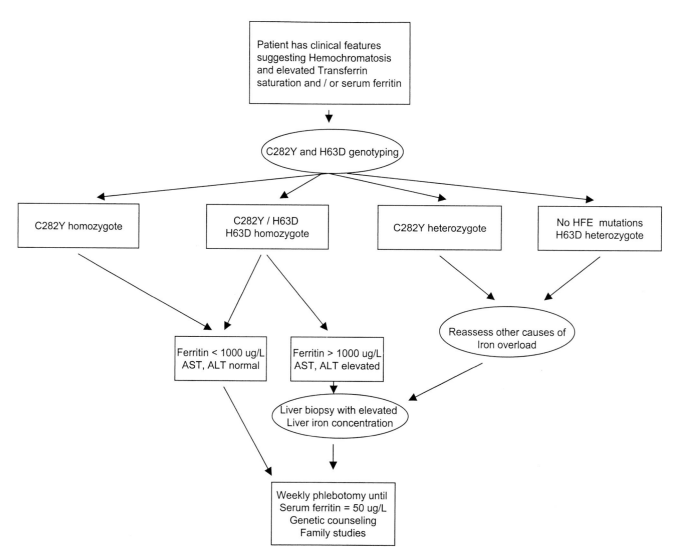

FIGURE 64-6. Algorithm for the diagnosis of hemochromatosis.

65

METABOLIC DISEASES OF THE LIVER

RONALD J. SOKOL ■ MARK A. LOVELL

Metabolic liver diseases comprise a diverse group of genetic disorders in which an enzyme or transport protein is deficient or dysfunctional. Most present during childhood with symptoms of neonatal cholestasis, chronic progressive hepatic fibrosis, or a metabolic syndrome (hypoglycemia, acidosis, encephalopathy, hyperammonemia). Identification of the precise etiology is important so that therapy can be initiated to prevent irreversible injury to the liver, brain, kidneys, or other organs. Several of the most common and important metabolic liver diseases are summarized and the histology of the liver is illustrated.

α_1-antitrypsin (AAT) deficiency is an autosomal recessive disorder in which the ZZ phenotype of AAT leads to liver involvement in 10% to 20% of affected individuals and emphysema in those exposed to cigarette smoke. The incidence of AAT deficiency varies with ethnic group, from 1 in 800 to 1 in 2000. Mutant AAT, which accumulates in the endoplasmic reticulum of the hepatocyte, can be detected as periodic acid-Schiff (PAS)–positive, diastase-resistant globules, and is thought to be responsible for initiating injury to the hepatocyte (Fig. 65-1). There is no effective treatment for this liver disease; liver transplant is required for end-stage liver disease and is curative of all manifestations of AAT deficiency because normal circulating levels are restored after transplantation.

Wilson disease is an autosomal recessive disorder of copper storage primarily involving the liver, brain, eye, and kidney, with a frequency of 1 in 30,000. It is caused by a mutation in the *ATP7B* gene, which codes for a P-type ATPase that is essential for copper transport out of the hepatocyte into bile and for incorporation of hepatic copper into ceruloplasmin, which is secreted into the systemic circulation. In Wilson disease, copper first accumulates in the liver, leading to acute or chronic hepatitis, fulminant liver failure, or cirrhosis. Copper then accumulates in the brain, causing psychiatric symptoms and dystonic or pseudoparkinsonian symptoms. The Kayser-Fleischer ring of the cornea is a hallmark. Liver lesions characteristically demonstrate steatohepatitis, glycogen-filled nuclei of periportal hepatocytes, varying degrees of portal tract inflammation, and periportal fibrosis advancing to cirrhosis (Fig. 65-2). Copper chelation and zinc therapies are effective; liver transplantation is required for acute fulminant cases and those with advanced cirrhosis unresponsive to medical therapy.

Several physical findings suggest Wilson disease. The Kayser-Fleischer ring (Fig. 65-6) is a greenish-brown ring in Descemet membrane at the periphery of the cornea on its posterior surface. It is best detected by slit-lamp examination by an experienced ophthalmologist, but can occasionally be seen by the naked eye, particularly in people with blue or green pigmentation of the iris. The ring, composed of granules rich in copper and sulfur, disappears during appropriate copper chelation therapy. Skin pigmentation may be increased, particularly on the anterior aspect of the lower leg, because of melanin deposition (Fig. 65-7). Blue lunulae of the fingernails may also occur, presumably from copper deposition (Fig. 65-8).

Glycogen storage diseases (GSDs) are a heterogeneous group of defects in degradation or synthesis of hepatic and muscle glycogen. Several GSDs primarily affect the liver. In GSD type I, glucose-6-phosphatase is defective, leading to massive hepatomegaly, profound fasting hypoglycemia, lactic acidosis, hyperlipidemia, hyperuricemia, and growth failure. Liver biopsies (Fig. 65-3) show swollen hepatocytes with clear cytoplasm (so-called "mosaic" appearance), macrovesicular and microvesicular steatosis, and a general lack of inflammation, cell death, or portal fibrosis. Treatment is aimed at maintaining normal blood sugar, and includes frequent high-starch meals, oral doses of uncooked cornstarch throughout the day, and nocturnal nasogastric tube or gastrostomy tube drip feedings of a formula high in carbohydrate or awakening every 3 to 4 hours at night to ingest cornstarch. GSD type IX is a generally benign disease manifested by hepatomegaly without the metabolic symptoms of type I. Liver biopsy (Fig. 65-4) shows swollen hepatocytes with clear cytoplasm and varying degrees of periportal fibrosis. Occasional patients progress to develop portal hypertension.

Reye syndrome, the prototypic mitochondrial hepatopathy, is called encephalopathy with fatty degeneration of the viscera. Its onset follows a viral infection (most often influenza or varicella) with the sudden onset of vomiting and lethargy in the absence of central nervous system infection; elevated aminotransferases, prothrombin time, and ammonia but normal bilirubin; and progression to coma. Most patients in the United States have been exposed to salicylates during the prodromal viral illness. Liver biopsy (Fig. 65-5) demonstrates diffuse, panlobular microvesicular steatosis characterized by swollen hepatocytes with central nuclei. Because the fat droplets may be so fine, the steatosis is frequently not appreciated unless special fat stains are used (see Fig. 65-5). There is no portal tract inflammation, although dead hepatocytes are occasionally observed. Special stains will demonstrate a marked decrease in mitochondrial enzyme activity (e.g., succinic acid dehydrogenase) with normal microsomal enzyme activity. Electron microscopy shows markedly swollen and pleomorphic mitochondria with hypodense matrix and loss of dense bodies. The hepatopathy is accompanied by cerebral edema, which becomes the primary clinical challenge in managing the patients, because the patient eventually fully recovers from liver injury. The diminished use of aspirin products in febrile children in the early 1980s after several government warnings about the association with Reye syndrome has been associated with a marked decline in the number of cases. Some of the cases, however, are probably now being correctly diagnosed as defects of mitochondrial fatty oxidation and related metabolic disorders, which were possibly triggered in the past by viral infections and the effect of salicylates on mitochondrial oxidative phosphorylation.

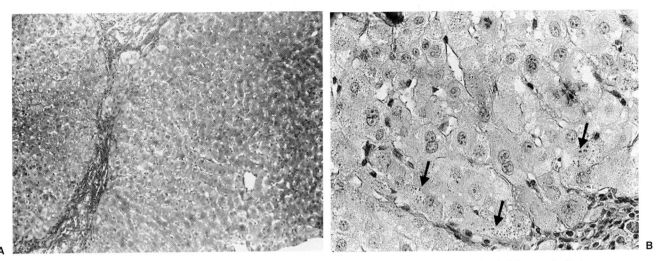

FIGURE 65-1. Liver biopsy of 8-year-old boy with PiZZ phenotype of α_1-antitrypsin deficiency. **A:** Note periportal bridging fibrosis with mild portal tract inflammation (trichrome stain; original magnification ×10). **B:** Periodic acid-Schiff–diastase staining reveals typical globules (*arrows*) of α_1-antitrypsin trapped within periportal hepatocytes (original magnification ×40).

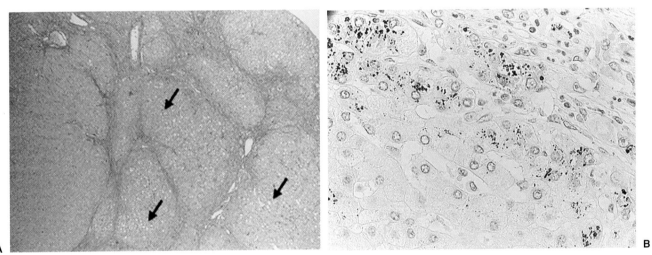

FIGURE 65-2. Liver removed at time of liver transplantation in 12-year-old girl with acute fulminant presentation of Wilson disease. **A:** Note established cirrhosis with regenerative nodules and mild macrovesicular steatosis (*arrows*) (H&E stain; original magnification ×4). **B:** Rhodanine staining reveals increased copper-associated proteins (*brownish pigment*) present in hepatocytes (original magnification ×40).

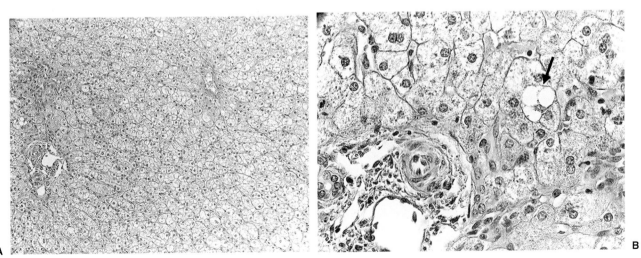

FIGURE 65-3. Liver biopsy from 2-month-old Hispanic girl with glycogen storage disease type Ib. **A:** Extensive hepatocyte ballooning with clear cytoplasm and lobular disarray are prominent; fibrosis and portal tract inflammation are absent (H&E stain; original magnification ×10). **B:** Macrovesicular steatosis (*arrow*) is also present (H&E stain; original magnification ×40).

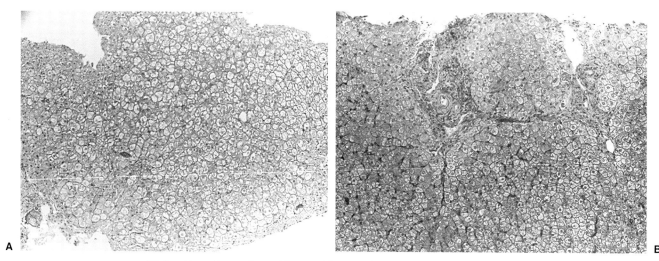

FIGURE 65-4. Liver biopsy from 19-year-old man with glycogen storage disease type IX. **A:** Note swollen pale hepatocytes with clear cytoplasm exhibiting "mosaic" appearance (H&E stain; original magnification ×10). **B:** Mild periportal and early bridging fibrosis is present, although there is no indication of chronic inflammation or hepatocellular death (trichrome stain; original magnification ×10).

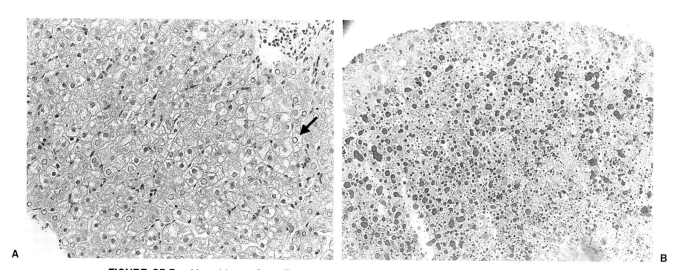

FIGURE 65-5. Liver biopsy from 5-year-old boy with Reye syndrome. **A:** Hepatocytes are swollen (*arrow*) with microvesicular steatosis that is difficult to discern on routine stains, absent portal tract inflammation and no hepatocyte death. Bile ducts are normal (H&E stain; original magnification ×20). **B:** Oil-red-O stain reveals extensive neutral lipid responsible for microvesicular steatosis (original magnification ×20).

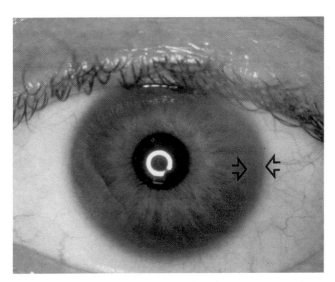

FIGURE 65-6. Kayser-Fleischer ring (*between arrows*) on cornea of 30-year-old man with Wilson disease.

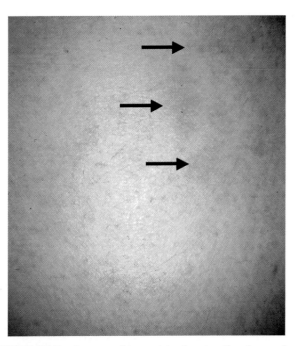

FIGURE 65-7. Increased brownish discoloration (*arrows*) of skin over tibia in a 10-year-old Cambodian boy with subfulminant Wilson disease.

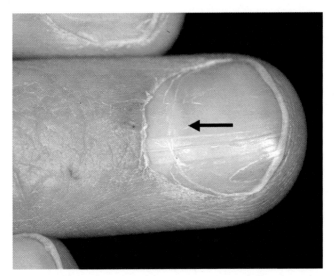

FIGURE 65-8. Blue lunula of fingernails in a 10-year-old boy presenting with acute fulminant Wilson disease.

Acknowledgment

This work is supported in part by grants from the National Institutes of Health (RO1 DK38446 and MO1 RR00069) and the Abbey Bennett Liver Research Fund.

66

ALCOHOLIC LIVER DISEASES

LAWRENCE LUMENG ■ DAVID CRABB

EPIDEMIOLOGY

Alcoholic liver disease (ALD) prevalence correlates with national per capita drinking. There appears to be a threshold level of daily alcohol consumption (20 g of ethanol for men and 10 g of ethanol for women) above which the risk of ALD increases. The peak age of onset of clinical ALD is 40 to 55 years in men and 10 years earlier in women. No more than 35% of heavy drinkers develop alcoholic hepatitis and 20% develop cirrhosis; thus, an alcoholic patient with liver disease cannot be assumed to have alcoholic liver injury, and they need careful evaluation to exclude other possible diagnoses; in particular, chronic viral hepatitis.

PATHOGENESIS

The pathogenesis of ALD is complex. The enzymes that metabolize alcohol, alcohol dehydrogenase and cytochrome P4502E1, generate potentially toxic substances (acetaldehyde and reactive oxygen species). The redox stress of alcohol oxidation contributes to the development of fatty liver, which may increase the sensitivity of the liver to endotoxin. Oxidative stress results in lipid peroxidation. Additional forms of toxicity include formation of protein adducts, dysfunction of the cytoskeleton, activation of Kupffer cells by endotoxin present in the portal blood, and ultimately activation of hepatic stellate cells, with fibrosis and cirrhosis. These processes are summarized in Figs. 66-1 and 66-2.

CLINICAL MANIFESTATIONS

ALD comprises three classical states: fatty liver, alcoholic hepatitis, and cirrhosis, which may coexist. Fatty liver can develop within 2 to 3 weeks of heavy drinking, and resolves in 4 weeks with abstinence. It may cause vague symptoms and mild abnormalities of liver tests, but is usually benign (Fig. 66-3). Alcoholic hepatitis is nearly always seen in the setting of moderate to severe malnutrition, with hepatomegaly, abnormal liver tests, jaundice, and signs of chronic liver disease. Prognosis correlates with the degree of jaundice, encephalopathy, and coagulopathy (Fig. 66-4). Cirrhosis from alcoholism is indistinguishable from cirrhosis from other causes, except that feminization is more common (Fig. 66-5). Other variants of ALD are seen less frequently (Table 66-1).

666

DIFFERENTIAL DIAGNOSIS

The differential diagnosis for ALD includes all other causes of liver disease. Alcoholic fatty liver needs to be differentiated from fatty liver that results from drug side effects, obesity, diabetes, and other conditions of insulin resistance, as well as numerous conditions that cause hepatomegaly. Alcoholic hepatitis may mimic other forms of chronic hepatitis, especially nonalcoholic steatohepatitis, and may resemble biliary tract disease when leukocytosis, fever, and abdominal pain are prominent. The differential diagnosis of cirrhosis is broad, but particular attention should be paid to the possibility of chronic hepatitis C (which commonly coexists with alcoholic liver disease) and hemochromatosis.

COURSE AND COMPLICATIONS

The course of fatty liver is typically prompt resolution of hepatomegaly and liver test abnormalities when the patient stops drinking. Alcoholic hepatitis may be mild, but often is life threatening. The development of infection, hepatic encephalopathy, or renal dysfunction is an ominous sign. Some patients progress to cirrhosis as they recover; continued drinking after an attack of alcoholic hepatitis carries a very high risk of development of cirrhosis and liver failure. The complications of alcoholic cirrhosis are common to other forms of cirrhosis, including a relatively high risk of hepatocellular carcinoma. All forms of alcoholic liver disease may be acutely worsened by concurrent acute hepatitis (especially hepatitis A) or acetaminophen overdose.

TREATMENT

Fundamental to the treatment of ALD is control of alcoholism. The current best therapy includes detoxification followed by behavioral or cognitive therapy to help the patient understand factors that precipitate relapse, ongoing involvement in Alcoholics Anonymous or other support programs, and in some patients, the use of medications to reduce the risk or severity of relapse. These medications include naltrexone; European experience with acamprosate is also promising. The long-term prognosis with treatment is better than many practitioners realize.

The treatment of alcoholic fatty liver is abstinence from alcohol and a nutritious diet. Alcoholic hepatitis requires treatment if the patient is sufficiently ill. The Maddrey discriminant function [bilirubin + (4.6 × prolongation of the prothrombin time)], if greater than 32, predicts a more than 50% mortality at 30 days, and has been used as an indicator of the need for therapy. Infections are common in these patients and should be sought and treated. Corticosteroids reduce mortality by about 25%, but also may worsen infection in these patients. Pentoxifylline has been shown to improve short-term survival, largely through reduction in the frequency of hepatorenal syndrome. Most patients with alcoholic hepatitis suffer from protein-calorie malnutrition, which must be addressed. Clinical trials of S-adenosylmethionine for cirrhosis suggest a survival benefit, although the drug is not approved for this indication in the United States. Preliminary reports of results of Veterans Administration cooperative studies of dilinoleoylphosphatidylcholine and of colchicine for hepatic fibrosis are discouraging. The other option for therapy for alcoholic cirrhosis is liver transplantation in carefully selected patients who have succeeded in abstaining from alcohol, typically for a minimum of 6 months.

It is important to recognize medical problems related to the underlying alcoholism as well as liver disease. Alcoholics are prone to fasting hypoglycemia, ketoacidosis, many kinds of infection, alterations in mental status that are not due to acute intoxication (meningitis, hepatic encephalopathy, electrolyte abnormalities, withdrawal syndromes, inadvertent poisoning with methanol or ethylene glycol, and Wernicke-Korsakoff syndrome), and to the toxicity of acetaminophen. They are subject to problems with numerous drug interactions because of the induction of hepatic microsomal enzymes as well as pharmacodynamic interactions of psychoactive drugs when the patients drink. Worsening liver disease in an alcoholic should prompt a search for common bile duct stones, drug toxicity, acute viral hepatitis, and hepatoma.

TABLE 66-1
Pathological Features and Variants of Alcoholic Liver Disease

Alcoholic fatty liver
Alcoholic hepatitis
Alcoholic cirrhosis
Less common variants of alcoholic liver disease
   Alcoholic fatty liver with perivenular fibrosis
   Alcoholic foamy degeneration (alcoholic microvesicular steatosis)
   Sclerosing hyaline necrosis
   Alcoholic cirrhosis with chronic hepatitis (often concomitant hepatitis B or C)
   Cholestasis
   Hepatic iron overload
   Lipogranuloma
   Massive hepatic necrosis (caused by acetaminophen ingestion)
   Focal fatty liver or focal fat sparing

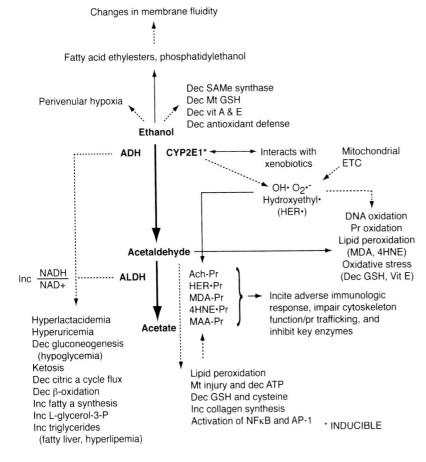

FIGURE 66-1. Pathway of alcohol metabolism and its effect on metabolism of hepatocytes. Alcohol is metabolized by alcohol dehydrogenase (*ADH*) or cytochrome P4502E1 (*CYP2E1*) to acetaldehyde. Acetaldehyde is then oxidized by aldehyde dehydrogenase (*ALDH*). The ADH and ALDH reactions generate the reduced form of nicotinamide adenine dinucleotide (*NADH*) more rapidly than it can be re-oxidized by the mitochondria. The increased NADH to the oxidized form of nicotinamide adenine dinucleotide$^+$ (NAD$^+$) ratio (*NADH:NAD$^+$*) modifies many intermediary metabolism pathways, indicated in the **lower left**, and contributes to formation of reactive O_2 species by the mitochondrial electron transfer chain (*ETC*). CYP2E1 also contributes to the formation of reactive O_2 species and hydroxyethyl radical (HER·), which promote oxidation and peroxidation of DNA, proteins and lipids. Acetaldehyde (*Ach*) and aldehyde products of lipid peroxidation (4-hydroxynonenal [*4HNE*] and malondialdehyde [*MDA*]) participate in the formation of various aldehyde-protein adducts (malondialdehyde-acetaldehyde protein [*Pr*] adducts [*MAA*]). Other effects include changes in membrane fluidity and depletion of antioxidants (including *S*-adenosyl-L-methionine [*SAMe*]). These effects are important mechanisms that lead to liver cell injury and cell death. Other abbreviations: AP-1, activator protein-1; *Dec*, decrease; *Fe*, iron; *GSH*, glutathione; *Inc*, increase; *Mt*, mitochondrial; *NF-κB*, nuclear factor-κB.

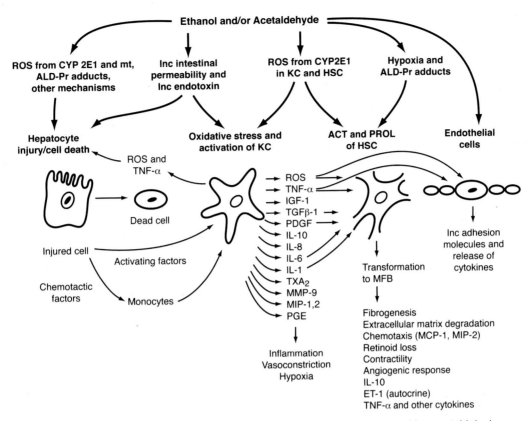

FIGURE 66-2. Effects of hepatocyte injury, endotoxin, and ethanol- and/or acetaldehyde-induced changes (including hypoxia and oxidative stress) on autocrine and paracrine pathways of activated Kupffer cells (*KCs*), hepatic stellate cells (*HSCs*), and endothelial cells. Although not shown, other cell types in liver, such as bile duct epithelium, lymphocytes, and platelets, are also involved. Fibrogenesis includes synthesis of matrix proteins (e.g., type 1 and 3 collagens, proteoglycans, hyaluronate, and several specialized glycoproteins including fibronectin), release of metalloproteinases, and secretion of tissue inhibitors of metalloproteinases. Abbreviations: *ALD-Pr*, aldehyde-protein; *ACT*, activation; *ET*, endothelin; *IGF-1*, insulin-like growth factor-1; *IL*, interleukin; *MCP*, monocyte chemotactic protein; *MFB*, myofibroblast; *Inc*, increase; *MIP*, macrophage inflammatory protein; *MMP*, matrix metalloproteinase; *PDGF*, platelet-derived growth factor; *PGE*, prostaglandin E; *PROL*, proliferation; *TGFβ-1*, transforming growth factor-β1; *TNFα*, tumor necrosis factor-α; *TXA$_2$*, thromboxane A$_2$; *ROS*, reactive oxygen species.

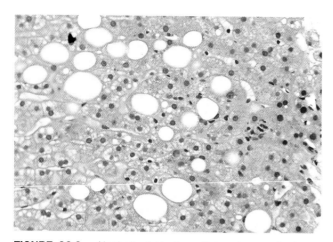

FIGURE 66-3. Alcoholic fatty liver. This micrograph shows the typical macrovesicular fat seen with heavy alcohol consumption. There is no evidence of inflammation or neutrophil infiltration, cell death, or fibrosis.

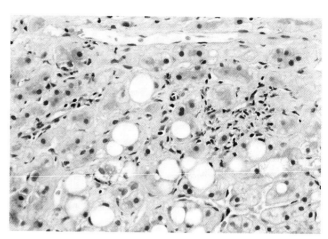

FIGURE 66-4. Alcoholic hepatitis. This biopsy specimen shows evidence of macrovesicular fat, infiltration of the liver with polymorphonuclear cells, and the presence of Mallory bodies in the **lower left** field.

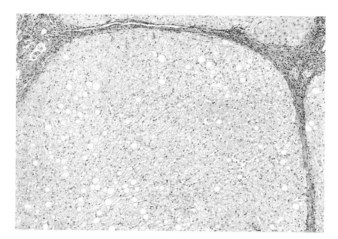

FIGURE 66-5. Alcoholic cirrhosis. The biopsy, at a lower magnification than in Figs. 66-3 and 66-4, shows persistent macrovesicular fat, as well as the formation of fibrous septae. Liver architecture is disrupted, hence this represents a cirrhotic nodule. There is little evidence of inflammation to suggest concurrent alcoholic hepatitis. This biopsy does not distinguish between alcoholic cirrhosis and cirrhosis secondary to a number of other liver diseases.

67

NONALCOHOLIC FATTY LIVER DISEASE

OLIVER F.W. JAMES

The term nonalcoholic steatohepatitis (NASH) was coined as recently as 1980 by Ludwig and colleagues. It referred to "the pathological and clinical features of non-alcoholic disease of the liver associated with the pathological features commonly seen in alcoholic liver disease itself." The term steatohepatitis excludes the appearance of fat alone in the liver, yet pure fatty liver (FL) is part of the spectrum of nonalcoholic fatty liver disease (NAFLD) that can be used to describe the entire spectrum from simple fat to steatohepatitis and fibrosis to cirrhosis. It is becoming clear that NAFLD is an important part of the insulin resistance, obesity, hyperlipidemia, hypertension constellation (the metabolic syndrome or syndrome X), and like the other features is becoming rapidly more common in western society. In the Third National Health and Nutrition Examination Survey study (NHANES III; United States), cryptogenic elevation in serum alanine aminotransferase (ALT) was seen in 2.6% of the population after other possible causes were excluded. This was independently associated with increased waist-to-hip ratio and indices of insulin resistance. Although researchers have limited additional data about the incidence and prevalence of NASH, it can be confidently stated that in office practice, this is one of the three (with hepatitis C virus [HCV] and possibly alcoholic liver disease [ALD]) most common liver diseases.

NATURAL HISTORY

The natural history of NAFLD is outlined in Fig. 67-1. Fatty deposition in the liver is the precursor of steatohepatitis, steatonecrosis, fibrosis, and ultimately cirrhosis. It is believed that a proportion of individuals, very probably the majority, who develop FL have an excellent prognosis. Almost all individuals who have simple fat alone on liver biopsy (without steatohepatitis, necrosis, or fibrosis) show little evidence of significant progression up to 10 years. Presumably, as with alcoholic FL and steatohepatitis, a proportion of individuals with FL also develop features of steatohepatitis and subsequently fibrosis at a relatively early stage (this is likely to be determined by several genes). A consensus is emerging from the increasing number of studies of natural history that age older than perhaps 45 years, presence of overt type 2 diabetes (T2DM), and greater degrees of obesity are all associated with increased likelihood of development of significant fibrosis and ultimately cirrhosis.

Although a number of algorithms have been described using a variety of laboratory, anthropometric, and clinical parameters with which to predict the likelihood that an individual patient will have or will develop more advanced disease, these algorithms are, as yet, imperfect. In addition to the factors described above, an ALT level greater than two times the upper limit of normal indicates increasing likelihood of disease progression.

Summarizing information from major clinical studies, the median age of patients with NASH but without cirrhosis is 45 to 50 years. There is a gap in our knowledge but it is increasingly clear that in a substantial proportion of patients with cryptogenic cirrhosis—perhaps 60%—the underlying cause is NASH. Physicians are beginning to realize that most of the 60- to 65-year-old patients they see with cryptogenic cirrhosis were obese 10 or 20 years ago and may have developed T2DM. We still do not understand how an obese 50-year-old patient with liver inflammation and possibly fibrosis, with a lot of fat in the liver, becomes a less obese but probably diabetic 60-year-old patient with histologically well-developed cirrhosis and little fat. Recent studies from France, Japan, and Italy have extended our knowledge to suggest that patients with (previous) NASH-related cryptogenic cirrhosis are at similar risk of developing hepatocellular cancer as individuals with other forms of cirrhosis—that caused by HCV, for example. Histological progression of pure FL, steatohepatitis, steatohepatitis with moderate fibrosis, and inactive cryptogenic cirrhosis (in a formerly obese patient with diabetes) is illustrated in Figs. 67-2 through 67-6.

PATHOGENESIS

The pathogenesis of NASH can be considered to be a "two-hit" process. In metabolic syndrome excess central fat and peripheral insulin resistance lead to increased delivery of free fatty acids (FFAs) to the liver, which leads to increasing hepatic steatosis and subsequent hepatic insulin resistance—the first hit (Fig. 67-7). Two mechanisms are then principally responsible for the second hit—necroinflammation and fibrosis—in the FL. The first of these is oxidative stress. FFAs are endogenous ligands for peroxisome proliferator activated receptor-α (PPARα). PPARα regulates the transcription of some CYP450 enzymes involved in long-chain FFA oxidation, including fatty acyl-CoA oxidase and CYP4A family members. This metabolism generates reactive oxygen species. Just as ethanol induces some CYP450 enzymes, so fatty acids are both substrates and inducers of enzyme activity. In marked central obesity, there is increased lipocyte production of tumor necrosis factor-α (TNF-α), and portal TNF-α leads to release of a proinflammatory cytokine cascade, which is also responsible for inflammation and fibrosis in parallel with oxidative stress. It has been demonstrated that TNF induces insulin resistance in both peripheral fat and the liver via inactivation of I Kappa B kinase (IKK), thus establishing a potential series of paracrine "vicious circles" of increased insulin resistance, consequent increased fatty acid oxidation, subsequent increased production of reactive oxygen species, increased IKK and TNF, and further insulin resistance.

Clearly, these metabolic pathways are susceptible to at least two sets of genes. These may be genes causing susceptibility to the metabolic syndrome, and genes governing FFA oxidation or TNF production and sensitivity together with the development of the proinflammatory cytokine cascade.

DIAGNOSIS

The diagnosis of the full spectrum of NAFLD and FL through steatohepatitis to cirrhosis is partly one of exclusion. Important points to be considered in the history of NAFLD are outlined in Table 67-1.

Laboratory Investigation

The laboratory investigation and definition of NASH/NAFLD can be considered in two parts: investigations of exclusion and investigations of assessment. These are listed in Table 67-2. Parameters used to distinguish between ALD and NASH/NAFLD are described in Table 67-3.

Imaging

Abdominal ultrasound examination or unenhanced computed tomography (CT) with assessment of the difference between liver and spleen attenuation values is the best (and simplest) method to assess the presence and severity of FL.

Liver Biopsy

Liver biopsy should be considered for making a diagnosis, staging the disease, and assessing treatment. It is also vital in aspects of clinical research—particularly in relation to clinical trials or treatment. If history, relevant laboratory investigations, and ultrasound are all suggestive of NAFLD/NASH, particularly in an overweight or obese individual, the overall diagnosis is not in doubt. Far more important is the question of staging the disease. Histology, particularly the distinction between simple FL and NASH, is very important for determining the likely natural history and prognosis in an individual patient. This distinction cannot be reliably made without liver biopsy, despite the clinical and laboratory parameters described above that are suggestive of more advanced disease. Furthermore, a physician cannot confidently distinguish between mild steatohepatitis or necrosis with or without a little fibrosis compared with more advanced fibrosis or early cirrhosis without biopsy (see Figs. 67-2 through 67-6).

ASSOCIATED FEATURES

NAFLD is almost always part of the metabolic syndrome. Other rare causes of a histological appearance of NASH are detailed in Table 67-4. Figure 67-4 shows steatohepatitis as a rare adverse effect of amiodarone treatment. In general, in evaluation and management of a patient with NAFLD, the features of the metabolic syndrome and some other possibly related conditions should be considered. These are summarized in Table 67-5.

TREATMENT

A wide variety of medical therapies for NASH are under consideration in clinical trials. There is no evidence from well-conducted, large-scale control trials to indicate a preferred treatment, so practical clinical management must rely on a pragmatic approach. Clinicians should bear in mind the key etiologic factors in NASH. Pragmatic management is described in Table 67-6.

(figures begin on page 676)

TABLE 67-1
History and Examination of NAFLD

Note known metabolic associations
Careful history of medications
Family history of NAFLD or cryptogenic cirrhosis or T2DM
Careful history and assessment of alcohol consumption (NAFLD may be excluded if
    consumption >14 units/wk)
Weight, height, and body mass index (BMI)—definitions of "obese" vary, so a pragmatic
    definition is overweight, BMI > 26; obese, BMI > 30
  Waist measurement
    Men: ideal < 37 in., obese > 40 in.
    Women: ideal < 32 in., obese > 35 in.
Blood pressure
General and abdominal examination as for other patients with liver disease

NAFLD, nonalcoholic fatty liver disease; T2DM, type 2 diabetes mellitus.

From Han TS, van Leer EM, Seidell JC, et al. Waist circumference action levels in the identification of
cardiovascular risk factors: prevalence study in a random sample. BMJ 1995;311:1401.

TABLE 67-2
NAFLD/NASH Investigations of Exclusions

EXCLUSION	ASSESSMENT
HBV markers	ALT
Anti-HCV	AST
HFE genotype	γ-GT
Autoantibodies[*]	Albumin
	Globulins
	Bilirubin
	Prothrombin time
	Alkaline phosphatase

[*]Low-titer anti–smooth muscle antibodies may be seen in NASH in the complete absence of any other
clinical, laboratory-based, or histological features to suggest autoimmune disease.

ALT, alanine aminotransferase; AST, aspartate aminotransferase; γ-GT, γ-glutamyl transpeptidase; HBV,
hepatitis B virus; HCV, hepatitis C virus; NAFLD, nonalcoholic fatty liver disease; NASH, nonalcoholic
steatohepatitis.

TABLE 67-3
**Laboratory Investigation: Distinction Between Alcoholic Liver Disease
and NAFLD/NASH**

TEST	ALCOHOLIC	NONALCOHOLIC
AST/ALT	Often >1	Often <1 (if mild)
Bilirubin	↑ or ↑↑	Normal
Alkaline phosphatase	Normal or ↑	Normal
Albumin	Normal or ↓	Normal (until late cirrhosis)
Prothrombin time	↑	Normal
Gamma glutamyl transpeptidase	↑	↑
Mean corpuscular volume	↑	Normal
Cholesterol	Often ↑	Often ↑
Blood ethanol	Present	Absent

ALT, alanine aminotransferase; AST, aspartate aminotransferase; NAFLD, nonalcoholic fatty liver disease;
NASH, nonalcoholic steatohepatitis.

TABLE 67-4
Rare Causes of NASH

Rapid weight cycling
Obesity related surgery—jejunoileal bypass has by far the strongest association
Total parenteral nutrition in adults
Other surgeries associated with massive weight loss
Jejunal diverticulosis and bacterial contamination of small bowel
Congenital syndromes of severe insulin resistance (the lipodystrophies)
Drug induced
    Amiodarone
    Perhexiline
    Possibly also calcium channel blockers or tamoxifen

NASH, nonalcoholic steatohepatitis.

TABLE 67-5
NAFLD Associations Checklist

Metabolic syndrome
    Obesity
    Type 2 diabetes or insulin resistance
    Hypertension
    Hyperlipidemia
Other possible associations[*]
    Celiac disease
    Sleep apnea syndrome
    Autoantibodies (SMA and ANA) without other manifestations of autoimmunity
    Heterozygote of *HFE C282Y* mutation

---

[*]None of these is well established. The association between iron overload and NASH is controversial. If patients have a liver biopsy, stainable iron should be sought, although it is rarely found. Some authors suggest that heterozygotes of the *HFE* gene, are more common in NASH patients and should be treated by venesection to reduce likelihood of iron-related lipid peroxidation.

ANA, antinuclear antibody; NAFLD, nonalcoholic fatty liver disease; NASH, nonalcoholic steatohepatitis; SMA, smooth muscle antibody.

TABLE 67-6
Practical Management of NAFLD

FEATURE	MANAGEMENT
Obesity	Weight-reducing diet; aim for American Heart Association dietary balance; ? ± orlistat (Zenical)
T2DM or insulin resistance	Metformin or a thiazolidinedione (↓ insulin resistance) Exercise (↓ insulin resistance) In overt T2DM manage or screen for complications of diabetes
Hyperlipidemia	Diet ± statin
Hypertension	Treat: follow WHO-ISH guidelines[*]; lipid-lowering diet
Alcohol consumption	Recommend reduction to zero or below 7 units/wk
Iron overload	If *C282Y* heterozygote or stainable iron on biopsy, then venesection

---

Note: Trials of antioxidants, ursodeoxycholic acid, other means of weight reduction, and lipid-lowering medications are currently being carried out.

[*]From Blood Pressure 1999;8:1.

NAFLD, nonalcoholic fatty liver disease; T2DM, type 2 diabetes mellitus; WHO-ISH, World Health Organization and International Society of Hypertension (J Hypertension 1996;9:342–360).

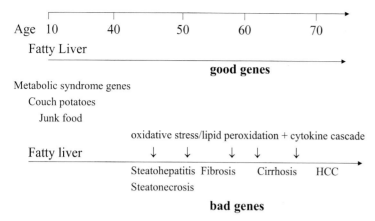

Age   10   40   50   60   70

Fatty Liver

good genes

Metabolic syndrome genes

Couch potatoes

Junk food

oxidative stress/lipid peroxidation + cytokine cascade

Fatty liver

Steatohepatitis Fibrosis   Cirrhosis   HCC

Steatonecrosis

bad genes

FIGURE 67-1. Natural history of nonalcoholic fatty liver disease. Individuals with simple fatty liver seldom progress. Individuals with fat and susceptibility (genes plus environment) may progress from fat and slight necroinflammation through more severe necroinflammation and fibrosis to cirrhosis. Ultimately, an unknown proportion (possibly 10% to 20%) will develop cryptogenic cirrhosis and some will progress to hepatocellular cancer.

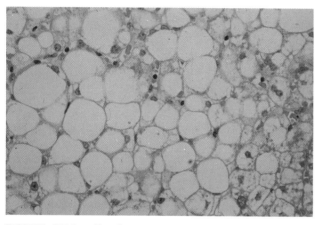

FIGURE 67-2. Simple macrovesicular hepatic steatosis (H&E stain).

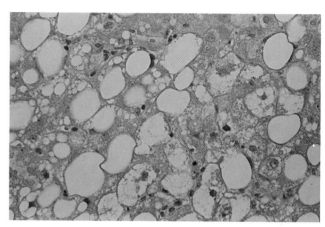

FIGURE 67-3. Steatohepatitis, ballooning degeneration, and Mallory bodies. Note that the marked presence of Mallory bodies may indicate likelihood of histological progression (H&E stain).

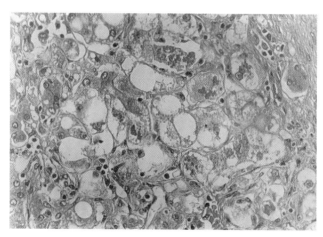

FIGURE 67-4. Steatohepatitis and abundant Mallory bodies with associated phospholipidosis (typically seen, as here, in amiodarone-induced steatohepatitis) (H&E stain).

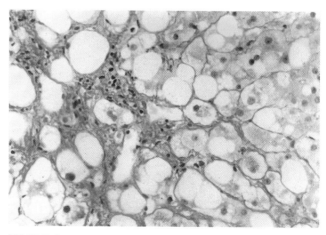

FIGURE 67-5. Marked perivenular and pericellular fibrosis associated with steatohepatitis (picro-Mallory stain).

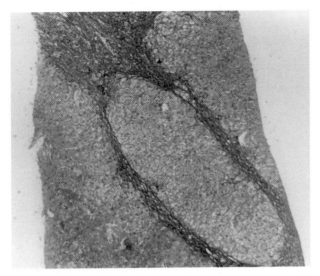

FIGURE 67-6. Cryptogenic cirrhosis; a small amount of fat remains (van Gieson stain).

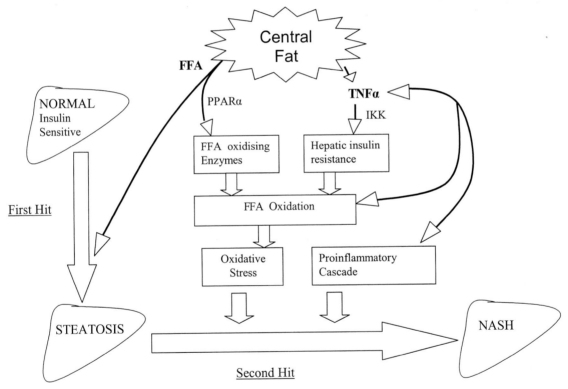

FIGURE 67-7. The two-hit pathogenesis of NASH.

CENTRAL NERVOUS SYSTEM AND PULMONARY COMPLICATIONS OF END-STAGE LIVER DISEASES

MICHEL H. MENDLER ■ **JOHN A. DONOVAN** ■ **ANDRES T. BLEI**

INTRODUCTION

Portal hypertension is usually the result of chronic liver disease and cirrhosis. Increased portal pressure is a cause of portal to systemic shunting of splanchnic blood. Shunting of portal blood to the systemic circulation results in an unusual translocation of humoral mediators not usually present in the systemic circulation. Portal blood not completely metabolized by the cirrhotic liver contributes further to a humoral imbalance. This imbalance of humoral mediators is implicated in the pathogenesis of diseases associated with cirrhosis and portal hypertension. Among these pathologies are hepatic encephalopathy (HE), hepatopulmonary syndrome (HPS), and portopulmonary hypertension (PPHTN). These complications of portal hypertension, and, as discussed elsewhere, variceal bleeding, ascites, and hepatorenal syndrome, represent the major manifestations of end-stage liver disease.

HE, HPS, and PPHTN can cause significant morbidity and a poor quality of life in patients with cirrhosis and portal hypertension. Medical therapies may often attenuate the severity of symptoms associated with each of these conditions but are not considered curative. Liver transplantation, if not otherwise contraindicated, may be indicated as the treatment of choice in the selected patient.

A suspected diagnosis of HE, HPS, or PPHTN is made during evaluation of the patient with suspected or confirmed portal hypertension. Existence of each condition is suggested by sometimes-subtle findings noted in the history of illness or by physical examination. Initial clinical suspicion is indication to pursue a diagnostic evaluation by screening and then more advanced diagnostic techniques.

HEPATIC ENCEPHALOPATHY

HE can be defined by the presence of a wide variety of neuropsychiatric disturbances secondary to either end-stage liver disease in a chronic setting (cirrhosis) or in an acute setting (fulminant hepatic failure), or in a patient with either intrahepatic or extrahepatic portosystemic shunting. The Working Party of experts on HE from the Organisation Mondiale de Gastroentérologie in 1998 elaborated the following multiaxial nomenclature. This novel nomenclature describes three HE types: A, B, and C. Type A HE refers to encephalopathy associated with acute liver failure. Type B HE refers to encephalopathy associated with portosystemic bypass and no intrinsic hepatocellular disease. Type C HE refers to encephalopathy associated with cirrhosis and portal hypertension or portosystemic shunts. Type C is characterized by three subcategories and other subdivisions: episodic HE, which may be precipitated, spontaneous, or recurrent; persistent HE, which may be mild, severe, or treatment-dependent; and minimal HE (MHE).

The signs and symptoms of HE may be overt or only detectable by neuropsychometric testing and referred to as MHE. Overt HE (OHE) can present with a wide variety of signs and symptoms. The most typical are changes in consciousness, intellectual function, behavior, and neuromuscular abnormalities. Onset is most often rapid unless in the setting of persistent HE. The clinical features can worsen or improve rapidly within hours or days and most often respond as rapidly to treatment. Figure 68-1 summarizes the many complex and progressive facets of OHE according to four clinical stages. In routine clinical practice, the West Haven criteria (I–IV) should be used for changes in consciousness, intellectual function, and behavior (Table 68-1); and the Glasgow coma scale can be used in addition for patients in stages III and IV (Table 68-2). The dynamics of OHE present differently in a patient with chronic liver disease compared to a patient with acute liver failure (Table 68-3). To diagnose MHE in routine clinical practice, the number connection tests (NCTs) A and B are the most widely used (Fig. 68-2). In the setting of OHE, routine blood biochemistry analysis will complete the clinical presentation of underlying liver disease in the form of suspected cirrhosis or hepatic failure. Venous or arterial ammonia levels cannot be reliably used in clinical practice to make the diagnosis of HE.

HE without underlying liver failure is observed in the setting of either spontaneous or iatrogenic extrahepatic portosystemic shunting (EPS). Etiologies of spontaneous EPS include congenital vascular malformations and the development of shunts secondary to partial occlusion of the portal system at the extrahepatic or intrahepatic level. As in side-to-side surgical shunts, transjugular intrahepatic portosystemic shunts (TIPS) are plagued by an increased rate of postprocedure HE, but improvements in techniques (smaller diameter stents) and a better understanding of predictive factors of post-TIPS mortality have decreased the rate of post-TIPS HE to approximately 30%.

In a patient with cirrhosis or portosystemic shunting, HE can develop spontaneously and even remain persistent without treatment. Spontaneous HE is typically observed in acute liver failure or in large-bore portosystemic shunts that may be either iatrogenic (surgical shunt and TIPS) or spontaneous (Fig. 68-3). However, in most instances symptoms of HE are precipitated by a number of factors that exacerbate latent or MHE (Table 68-4).

The pathophysiology of HE is complex and still not completely understood. The mechanisms involve neurochemical alterations and changes in the functional status of cerebral neurotransmitter systems. Permanent structural disorders of the brain are not believed to be involved. Clinical observations and research in animals suggest the role of at least four phenomena: gut-derived neurotoxins, altered neurotransmitters, modifications in cerebral energy metabolism, and the altered astrocytes. The principal toxin implicated is ammonia, derived by bacteria acting on ingested food. Ammonia is also produced from catabolism of dietary protein, metabolism of glutamine, and deamination and transamination pathways of amino acids (Fig. 68-4). Low levels of ammonia are constantly maintained by the production of urea (liver) and the production of glutamine from glutamate by glutamine synthetase (liver, muscle, and brain). In the brain, only astrocytes contain glutamine synthetase. In patients with cirrhosis or acute liver failure, reduction in hepatocellular function is believed to explain the observed elevations of blood ammonia levels. Portosystemic shunting increases ammonia levels by bypassing hepatic metabolism. The deleterious effect of ammonia is due to the facilitated passage of ammonia across the blood-brain barrier involving multiple mechanisms leading to the development of Alzheimer type II astrocytosis, regarded as the cardinal pathological central nervous system (CNS) change associated with HE (Fig. 68-5). At low levels, ammonia suppresses inhibitory postsynaptic potential formation and depolarizes neurons. At high concentrations, ammonia increases the resting membrane potential and inhibits axonal conductance and excitatory postsynaptic potential formation, thereby depressing CNS function. These abnormalities involve the inhibition of cellular chloride channels by ammonia. Other mechanisms whereby ammonia may play a role in HE include a reduction in brain glucose and oxygen consumption, an increase in neurotoxic glutamine, increase in serotonin by increased cerebral tryptophan uptake, and a reduction in glutamatergic neurotransmission (Table 68-5). The γ-aminobutyric acid (GABA) -ergic neurotransmission hypothesis is considered by many authorities to be the most important in the manifestation of HE. This hypothesis involves the interplay of GABA, so-called endogenous or "natural" benzodiazepines (BZs), and the diazepam binding receptor (Fig. 68-6). The phenomena of HE could be explained by an up-regulation and increase in number of $GABA_A$ receptors. More important, it is believed that natural BZ receptor agonists are elevated in HE and are responsible for the experimentally observed GABA-mediated responses. Despite compelling evidence for the natural BZ hypothesis in HE, many issues including the precise role of BZs remain unresolved (Table 68-6). Abnormalities in cerebral catecholamine transmitters may play a small role in HE. The "false neurotransmitter" hypothesis described by early authors is based on the observation that tyrosine hydroxylase is inhibited in HE. Certain amines (tyramine, octopamine, and β-phenylethanolamine) can be synthesized from tyrosine via alternative pathways. It was hypothesized that these amines acted as weak neurotransmitters, competing with standard catecholamines. None of the above hypotheses alone correlate adequately with symptoms of HE. Synergism between each individual pathway most likely occurs. Ammonia could directly potentiate inhibitory GABA-ergic neurotransmission and synergistically augment the actions of natural BZ receptor agonists (Fig. 68-7).

Finally, the presence of Alzheimer type II astrocytes in HE and their relation to hyperammonemia and glutamine metabolism and the observation of abnormalities in astrocyte osmolarity have prompted a recently developed hypothesis that disturbances in astrocyte cell volume homeostasis may be the initial event in chronic HE. The pathogenic model described in Fig. 68-8 describes a common astrocytic pathway explaining both the role of multiple factors triggering HE and the multiple abnormalities in neurotoxins and neurotransmitters. This model may be applicable to acute HE as well, except kinetics and degree of swelling may be different.

In a patient with known cirrhosis, with or without spontaneous or iatrogenic portocaval shunting, the onset of abnormal consciousness concomitant to a recognized precipitating factor of HE usually leaves little doubt about the positive diagnosis of HE. The many differential diagnoses of HE described in Table 68-7 should nevertheless be addressed, if the clinical setting is appropriate.

Treatment of HE must begin with rigorous search and elimination of a precipitating factor (Table 68-8). Meanwhile, supportive care and measures to decrease the nitrogenous load should be implemented, as outlined in Tables 68-8 and 68-9. Nutritional management should include careful limitation of animal proteins and supplementation of any vitamin or mineral deficiencies, especially zinc. The recommendations for protein restriction are no less than 1 to 1.5 g protein/kg/day mostly in the form of vegetables and dairy products. Reduction of gut-derived ammonia or other putative compounds of HE is the mainstay and first-line treatment of HE. The majority of ammonia involved in the pathogenesis of HE enters the circulation from the intestinal tract, and is derived from colonic bacteria and deamination of glutamine in the small intestine. The ammonia is absorbed via passive diffusion. Other putative substances are derived from the gut: BZ-like substances or precursors, toxic short-chain fatty acids, phenols, and mercaptans.

The therapeutic goal is to shorten bowel transit to eliminate ammonia-producing bacteria and to lower the available absorbable colonic ammonia. This can be achieved with nonabsorbable disaccharides. These agents promote the incorporation of lumenal ammonia into the bacterial protein wall, and promote catharsis by acidification of the colon as the result of the bacterial production of acetic and lactic acid by bacterial fermentation (Fig. 68-9). Despite controversies about the lack of ample randomized controlled trials, oral lactulose is the standard treatment, given orally and titrated from 15 to 45 mL every 8 to 12 hours to achieve two or three loose and acidic (pH < 6) stools daily. The inconveniences are flatulence, abdominal cramping, diarrhea, and excessively sweet taste. Comatose or fasting patients can be given lactulose enemas (300 mL in 1 L of tepid water) every 4 to 8 hours as needed to achieve resolution of HE. The use of oral antibiotics to eliminate the urease-producing bacteria should be a second-line treatment. Despite their comparable efficacy to nonabsorbable disaccharides, certain undesirable effects limit their use. Neomycin is the most widely used antibiotic for this indication, at the oral dose of 6 g daily. Despite its limited intestinal absorption (3%), long-term use can expose patients to nephrotoxicity and ototoxicity, especially in instances of renal failure. The most frequent complication is malabsorption and bacterial superinfection. For these reasons, neomycin should be tapered rapidly after 2 to 3 days of treatment for a total of 1 week of treatment. The effectiveness of a combination of nonabsorbable disaccharides and antibiotics is debated. The consensus is to start antibiotics only after failure of lactulose alone, and to stop lactulose if stool pH increases above 6.

The use of L-ornithine-L-aspartate has been proposed in Europe for the treatment of HE with the hypothesis that this molecule decreases ammonia by recycling through the urea cycle and by increasing glutamine. Studies on treatments targeting false neurotransmitters such as branched-chain amino acids, levodopa, and bromocriptine have not shown significant beneficial results to warrant formal recommendations on their use. Flumazenil (1 mg intravenous bolus) may be beneficial in selected patients with severe HE, but no oral preparation is available for long-term treatment. This drug can also be considered when BZ use is suspected.

HEPATOPULMONARY SYNDROME AND PORTOPULMONARY HYPERTENSION

HPS and PPHTN are two pulmonary syndromes that can complicate portal hypertension. The shunting of blood from the hypertensive portal circulation to the systemic circulation is common to the pathophysiology of both conditions (Fig. 68-10). Both can cause significant morbidity in the patient with cirrhotic or, less frequently, noncirrhotic portal hypertension.

HPS and PPHTN should be considered when the patient with a diagnosis of portal hypertension presents with respiratory symptoms. A suspected diagnosis of HPS or PPHTN is established by initial screening tests and confirmatory diagnostics.

HPS is most often manifested by exertional hypoxia. Arterial blood gas analysis indicated a resting, room air, hypoxia ($PaO_2 < 70$ mm Hg) and an increase A-a gradient (>15–20 mm Hg) not responsive to 100% O_2 supplementation. Contrast echocardiography ("bubble study") that demonstrates the early appearance of bubbles in the left atrium further supports a diagnosis of HPS. Radionucleotide lung scanning is employed as a more specific and confirmatory test of the HPS diagnosis. Pulmonary angiography is not usually required (Table 68-10).

Portopulmonary syndrome is also a cause of respiratory symptoms in patients with portal hypertension. Dyspnea on exertion, when present, is the most common symptom. Unsuspected PPHTN in the asymptomatic patient with cirrhosis and other complications of portal hypertension may be detected. During 2D echocardiography, an indirect measurement of an elevated pulmonary artery pressure can further suggest the diagnosis of PPHTN. Confirmation of PPHTN requires right heart catheterization (Table 68-11).

The classification of PPHTN as mild, moderate, or severe is dependent on the pulmonary artery pressure measured by a confirmatory Swan-Ganz catheterization required to establish the diagnosis of PPHTN. In addition, the definition of PPHTN requires that the wedged pulmonary capillary pressure does not exceed 15 mm Hg (Table 68-12).

Treatment of the patient with HPS usually includes O_2 administration. The patient with PPHTN should be considered a candidate for long-term vasodilator therapy (usually epoprostenol) if a therapeutic response to short-term treatment is established. Patients with cirrhosis complicated by HPS or PPHTN, who are otherwise appropriate candidates, should be considered for potentially curative liver transplantation (see Tables 68-11 and 68-12).

(figures begin on page 689)

TABLE 68-1

The West Haven Criteria for Altered Mental State in Hepatic Encephalopathy

Stage 0: Lack of detectable changes in personality or behavior; asterixis absent

Stage 1: Trivial lack of awareness; shortened span; impaired addition or subtraction; hypersomnia, insomnia, or inversion of sleep pattern; euphoria or depression; asterixis can be detected

Stage 2: Lethargy or apathy; disorientation; inappropriate behavior; slurred speech; obvious asterixis

Stage 3: Gross disorientation; bizarre behavior; semistupor to stupor; asterixis generally absent

Stage 4: Coma

From Atterbury CE, Maddrey WC, Conn HO. Neomycin-sorbitol and lactulose in the treatment of acute portal-systemic encephalopathy. A controlled, double-blind clinical trial. Am J Dig Dis 1978;23:398.

TABLE 68-2

The Glasgow Coma Scale

EYES OPEN		BEST MOTOR RESPONSE		BEST VERBAL RESPONSE	
Spontaneously	4	Obeys verbal orders	6	Oriented, conversant	5
To command	3	Localizes painful stimuli	5	Disoriented, conversant	4
To pain	2	Painful stimulus, flexion	3	Inappropriate words	3
No response	1	Painful stimulus, extension	2	Inappropriate sounds	2
		No response	1	No response	1

Note: The best ocular, verbal, and motor responses are summed. The best score is 15; the worst is 3. Severe hepatic encephalopathy is defined by a score less than 12.

From Teasdale G, Jennett B. Assessment and prognosis of coma after head injury. Acta Neurochir 1976;34:45.

TABLE 68-3

Differences Between ALFA HE (Acute Liver Failure Associated HE) and HE in Chronic Liver Dysfunction

	ALFA HE	HEPATIC ENCEPHALOPATHY IN CHRONIC LIVER DISEASE
Hepatic disorder	Acute (<8 wk)	Chronic (>6 mo)
Animal model	Galactosamine rabbit and rat	Portocaval shunted rat
Pathology	Acute hepatocellular necrosis and hepatic insufficiency	Hepatocellular insufficiency and circulatory bypass of liver
Clinical profile		
Onset	Acute	Variable: insidious to acute
Precipitating factors	Uncommon	Common
Documented prior hepatic disease	No	Yes
Liver size	Reduced—serial evaluation may show nonpercussible liver	Shrunken, firm left lobe of liver (±)
Cerebral edema	Common	Very rare
Nutritional state	Normal	Cachexia may be present
Ascites	Often clinically absent	Present
Treatment	Acute hepatic support	Acute followed by long-term support
Collateral veins	Very rare	Usual
Survival	Low (without transplant)	High
Persistent neuropsychiatric sequelae	No	Not uncommon (chronic HE)
Follow-up hepatic function	Excellent	Deranged

HE, hepatic encephalopathy.

From Mullen KD, Dasarathy S. Hepatic encephalopathy. In: Schiff ER, Dorrell MF, Maddrey WC. Schiff's diseases of the liver, 8th ed. Philadelphia: Lippincott Williams & Wilkins, 1999.

TABLE 68-4

Precipitating Factors for HE

PRECIPITANT	POSSIBLE MECHANISM	ASSOCIATED COPRECIPITANT
GI bleeding	Nitrogen load, hepatic hypoperfusion, arterial hypoxemia	Infection, banked blood transfusion (ammonia), benzodiazepines (endoscopic procedure)
Sepsis	Protein catabolism	Azotemia, arterial hypotension, anemia
Hypokalemia (diarrhea, diuretics)	Ammonia generation	GI bleeding, alkalosis
Dehydration (diuretics, paracentesis, laxatives)	Hepatic hypoperfusion	Hypokalemia, azotemia
Azotemia	Increased ammonia production (urealysis)	GI bleeding, hypotension
Acute hepatitis	Hepatocellular dysfunction, impaired detoxication	Sepsis
Benzodiazepines, narcotics	Enhanced CNS sensitivity	—

CNS, central nervous system; GI, gastrointestinal; HE, hepatic encephalopathy.

From Mullen KD, Dasarathy S. Hepatic encephalopathy. In: Schiff ER, Sorrell MF, Maddrey WC. Schiff's diseases of the liver, 8th ed. Philadelphia: Lippincott Williams & Wilkins, 1999.

TABLE 68-5

Changes in Brain and Cerebrospinal Fluid (CSF) Metabolites in Ammonia-Precipitated Encephalopathy in Chronic Liver Disease

METABOLITES (LOCALIZATION)	AMMONIUM ACETATE TREATED	
	Precoma	*Coma*
Ammonia (brain)	↑	↑
Ammonia (CSF)	↑	↑
Energy metabolites		
Lactate (brain)	↑	↑
Lactate (CSF)	↑	↑
α-Ketoglutarate (brain)	NC	NC
ATP	NC	↓
ADP	NC	NC
ATP-to-ADP ratio	NC	↓
Amino acids		
Glutamine (brain)	NC	↑
Glutamine (CSF)	↑	↑
Glutamate (brain)	NC	↓
γ-Aminobutyric acid (brain)	NC	NC
Alanine (brain)	↑	↑
Alanine (CSF)	↑	↑
Monoamine transmitters and metabolites		
Homovanillic acid (brain)	↑	↑
Dopamine turnover (brain)	↑	↑
Serotonin (brain)	↓	↓
Serotonin (extracellular)	NC	↑
5-Hydroxyindoleacetic acid (brain)	↑	↑
Serotonin turnover (brain)	↑	↑

NC, no change.

Adapted from Buttterworth RF. Pathogenesis of acute hepatic encephalopathy. Digestion 1998;59[Suppl 2]:16.

TABLE 68-6

The Concept That Natural Benzodiazepines Contribute to Hepatic Encephalopathy

Evidence supporting the concept
  Studies in animal models
    BZ receptor antagonist (BZRA)-induced ameliorations of HE
    In HE, BZRAs induce excitation of CNS neurons in vitro
    In HE, BZ agonists occupy BZ receptors
    In HE, the BZ levels in CSF, blood, and brain tissue are increased
    Levels of BZs correlate with severity of HE
  Findings in humans
    BZRA-induced ameliorations of HE
    In HE, increased levels of BZs in CSF, blood, and postmortem brain tissue
    Levels of BZs correlate with severity of HE
Unresolved issues
  The source of the BZs is unknown
  The identity of many BZ receptor ligands in HE is unknown
  The properties of many BZ receptor ligands in HE are unknown
  Whether BZ levels in HE are sufficient to depress the CNS is unknown
  The precise role of BZs in the pathogenesis of HE is unclear
  Interactions between BZs and other putative toxins in HE is unexplored

BZ, benzodiazepine; CNS, central nervous system; CSF, cerebrospinal fluid; HE, hepatic encephalopathy.

Adapted from Mullen KD, Jones EA. Natural benzodiazepines and hepatic encephalopathy. Semin Liver Dis 1996;16:255.

TABLE 68-7

Chronic Liver Dysfunction with Change in Mental Status—Differential Diagnostic Investigations

	INVESTIGATIONS
Metabolic encephalopathies	
Hypoxia	Blood gas, clinical chemistry, pulmonary evaluation
Hypercapnia	Blood gas, clinical chemistry, pulmonary evaluation
Hypoglycemia	Blood chemistry
Hyponatremia	Blood chemistry, urinalysis; evaluate for chronic cardiac, renal, hepatic disease
Azotemia	Blood chemistry, urinalysis, renal imaging
Diabetic coma (ketoacidosis, hyperosmolar coma)	Blood chemistry, urinalysis, blood gases
Intracranial disorders	
Cerebrovascular disorders: intracerebral hemorrhage, thrombosis	Neurological imaging: CT scan, MRI
Subarachnoid hemorrhage	
Intracranial tumors	
Subdural hematoma	
Intracranial infections: meningitis, encephalitis, cerebral abscess	CT, MRI, lumbar puncture
Seizure disorders	CT, MRI, EEG
Toxins	
Alcohol	Urine and blood toxin screen, blood alcohol level, postchelation urinalysis
Drugs	
Hypnotics	
Tranquilizers	
Analgesics	
Heavy metals: lead, manganese, mercury	

CT, computed tomography; MRI, magnetic resonance imaging; EEG, electroencephalogram.

From Mullen KD, Dasarathy S. Hepatic encephalopathy. In: Schiff ER, Sorrell MF, Maddrey WC. Schiff's diseases of the liver, 8th ed. Philadelphia: Lippincott Williams & Wilkins, 1999.

TABLE 68-8
TABLE 68-8
Treatment Strategies for a Patient with Acute HE

Supportive measures
  General management of a patient with change in mental status
    Nutrition—amino acids, lipids, glucose, essential elements
    Fluid and electrolyte maintenance
    Bladder and bowel function—catheter care
    Intravenous catheters, central line
    Aspiration pneumonitis prevention
    Sepsis prevention
    Pressure sore prevention or treatment
  Management of problems associated with chronic liver dysfunction (ascites, variceal bleeding, hepatotropic
    viral infection)
    Hepatic support
      Hepatotropic agents
      Alcohol abstinence
Rule out other causes of encephalopathy
Identify and treat precipitating factors

PRECIPITATING FACTORS	POSSIBLE CAUSES	INTERVENTION
GI bleeding	Variceal; nonvariceal	Endoscopy: variceal ligations and sclerotherapy
Infection	Pneumonitis, urinary tract infection, bacterial peritonitis	Antibiotics
Hypokalemia, alkalosis	Diuretics, fluid and electrolyte management problems	Correct electrolyte abnormality, avoid diuretics, fluid restriction
Sedatives, tranquilizers	Narcotics, benzodiazepine	Flumazenil, naloxone challenge
Dietary proteins	Animal protein	Restrict protein, encourage vegetable protein
Azotemia	Drug (NSAID, others) induced dysfunction, catabolic states (sepsis), hepatorenal syndrome, GI bleed, hypovolemia	Control sepsis, avoid nephrotoxic agents, correct circulatory volume abnormalities, stress ulcer prophylaxis
Acute hepatic injury	Hepatotoxic drugs, reactivation and superinfection of hepatotropic virus, progressive hepatic dysfunction	Avoid hepatotoxic drugs, avoid antivirals, place on transplant list

Empiric measures
  Ammonia
    Decrease ammonia substrate
      Gut clearance: cathartics, enemas
      Decreased protein intake
    Decrease ammonia formation
      Gut bacterial suppression (antibiotics)
      Nonabsorbable disaccharides: lactulose, lactitol, lactose
      Enteric flora modification
    Biochemical neutralization of ammonia
      L-Glutamic acid
      Sodium benzoate
      L-Ornithine L-aspartate
      Keto analogs of amino acids
      Acidifying enemas
  False neurotransmitters (octopamine, phenylethanolamine)
    Suppress gut bacterial flora
    L-Dopa, bromocriptine
  Altered amino acid balance
    Branched-chain amino acid infusion
    Substitute vegetable protein for animal protein
  Endogenous benzodiazepines
    Flumazenil

GI, gastrointestinal; NSAID, nonsteroidal antiinflammatory drug.

From Mullen KD, Dasarathy S. Hepatic encephalopathy. In: Schiff ER, Sorrell MF, Maddrey WC. Schiff's diseases of the liver, 8th ed. Philadelphia: Lippincott Williams & Wilkins, 1999.

TABLE 68-9
Therapeutic Strategies for Chronic HE

Decrease ammonia content
   Substrate reduction
      Protein restriction
      Regular diet
      Vegetable proteins
      Oral BCAA
   Bowel movements—cathartics
   Colonic exclusion surgery
Decrease ammonia production
   Antibiotics
   Nonabsorbable disaccharides
   Bacterial replacement
Improve hepatic perfusion
   Shunt narrowing/obliteration
   TIPS narrowing
Convert ammonia to nontoxic products
   Sodium benzoate
   L-Ornithine L-aspartate
   Keto analogs of BCAA
Benzodiazepine antagonists
   Long-term flumazenil/alterations
Hepatic support
   Artificial liver
   Hepatocyte transplantation
   Liver transplantation

BCAA, branched-chain amino acids; HE, hepatic encephalopathy; TIPS, transjugular intrahepatic portosystemic shunt.

From Mullen KD, Dasarathy S. Hepatic encephalopathy. In: Schiff ER, Sorrell MF, Maddrey WC. Schiff's diseases of the liver, 8th ed. Philadelphia: Lippincott Williams & Wilkins, 1999.

TABLE 68-10
Hepatopulmonary Syndrome

Suspicion
   Portal hypertension
   Exertional dyspnea
   Platypnea

	EXAMINATION	RESULT
Screening	Arterial blood gas analysis	Hypoxia (PaO$_2$ < 70 mm Hg) A-a gradient > 15–20 mm Hg Orthodeoxia
Confirmatory testing	Contrast echocardiography bubble study	Bubbles in right atrium within 3–5 heart beats
	Radionucleotide lung perfusion scan	Brain uptake > 6%
	Pulmonary angiography	Usually not necessary
Treatments	Supplemental O$_2$	Variable
	Medication (i.e., somatostatin, garlic)	Inconclusive
	Transjugular portosystemic shunt	Unproven
	Liver transplantation	Usually curative

TABLE 68-11
Portopulmonary Hypertension

	EXAMINATION	RESULT

Suspicion
  Portal hypertension
  Exertional dyspnea		

Screening	Echocardiogram	Tricuspid regurgitation Increased tricuspid regurgitant jet velocity
Confirmatory testing	Right heart catheterization	Pulmonary vascular resistance: PVR > 120 dynes/sec/cm^{-5} Increased pulmonary artery pressure (PAP) PCWP < 15 mm Hg
Treatments	Epoprostenol infusion Liver transplantation	Variable Variable

TABLE 68-12
Classification of Portopulmonary Hypertension (PPHTN)

MPAP (mm Hg)	PPHTN
<25	Normal
25–35	Mild
35–50	Moderate
>50	Severe

MPAP, mean pulmonary artery pressure.

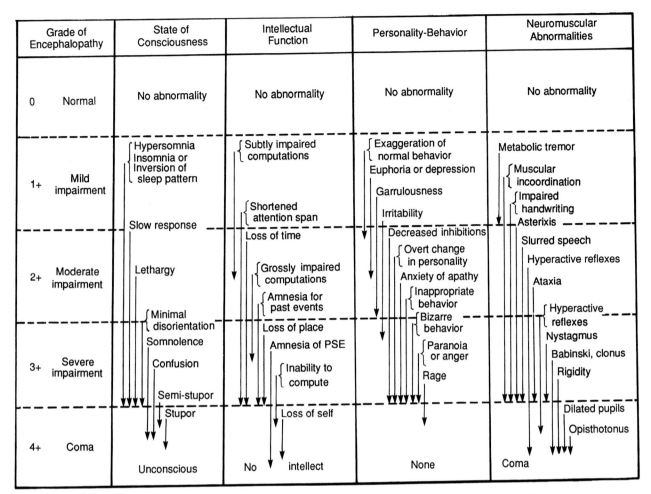

FIGURE 68-1. A detailed description of symptoms and signs of portal-systemic encephalopathy.

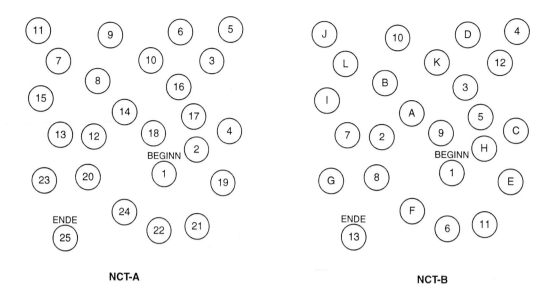

NCT-A   **NCT-B**

FIGURE 68-2. An example of number connection tests (NCTs) A and B used to assess minimal hepatic encephalopathy. In the NCT-A, the subject must connect in the correct order as quickly as possible the sequence of scattered circles numbered 1 through 25. The score is the time required for the subject to complete the trail, including time to correct errors. A low score indicates a good performance. The concept of the NCT-B is similar, except for an alternating sequence of scattered numbered and lettered circles, 1-A through 13-L. The subject must be given the opportunity to practice either test before doing a timed run, thereby decreasing training bias in follow-up testing. With a normal upper time limit of 30 seconds for NCT-A and 100 seconds for NCT-B, the sensitivity and specificity in detecting minimal hepatic encephalopathy is estimated to be respectively 56% and 100% for the NCT-A and 68% and 99.2% for the NCT-B.

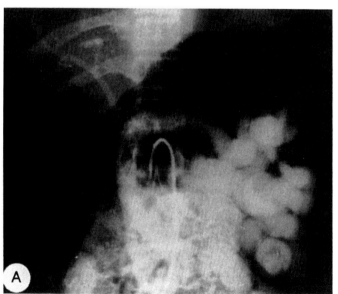

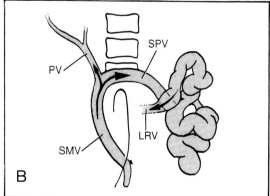

FIGURE 68-3. A, B: Large splenorenal collateral in a patient with cirrhosis and spontaneous hepatic encephalopathy. *PV,* portal vein; *SMV,* superior mesenteric vein; *SPV,* splenic vein; *LRV,* left renal vein. Radiographic contrast has been injected via a catheter in the superior mesenteric artery.

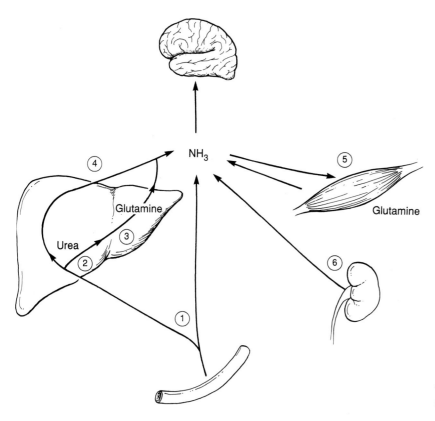

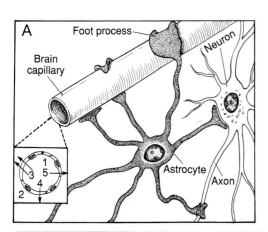

NH$_3$

Glutamine

Urea

Glutamine

FIGURE 68-4. Several factors combine to increase ammonia levels in liver disease. As the hepatic extraction of ammonia is high (>0.9), portal-systemic shunting (1) is a major factor. Hepatic metabolism of ammonia, via the formation of urea (periportal area [2]) or glutamine (perivenular hepatocyte [3]), may be impaired. Intrahepatic shunts (4) are present in cirrhosis. Metabolism of ammonia in muscle (5) becomes an important alternative pathway; loss of muscle mass may reduce the formation of glutamine. Renal vein ammonia levels (6) increase as a consequence of primary respiratory alkalosis.

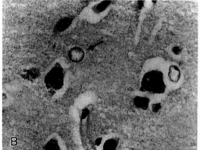

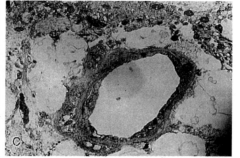

FIGURE 68-5. A: A scheme that depicts the relation of cortical astrocyte foot-processes with the brain capillary endothelial cell and neuronal elements. *Inset:* The anatomic substrate of the blood-brain barrier. The capillary endothelial cell with its tight junctions (1) and abundant mitochondria (2) possesses several carrier mechanisms (3–5) to transport solutes into the brain parenchyma. **B:** An Alzheimer type II astrocyte (*arrow*), with an enlarged pale nucleus, with chromatin displaced to the side. (Courtesy of Dr. Roger Butterworth, University of Montreal.) **C:** Marked swelling of astrocyte foot-processes surrounding a brain capillary in an edematous brain of a rat with fulminant ischemic liver failure.

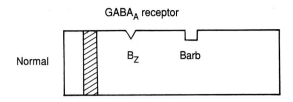

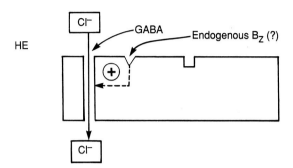

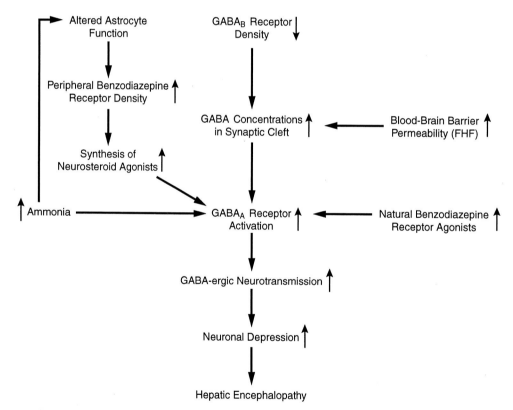

FIGURE 68-6. Current views of the γ-aminobutyric acid (GABA)$_A$ receptor have modeled a common site of action for *GABA*, benzodiazepines (*B$_z$*), and barbiturates (*Barb*). In the most recent hypothesis of the pathogenesis of hepatic encephalopathy (*HE*), GABA-ergic neurotransmission could be facilitated when binding of an endogenous benzodiazepine ligand allows the GABA-mediated opening of a chloride channel; entry of chloride results in cellular hyperpolarization with a decrease in excitability.

FIGURE 68-7. Postulated interrelationships between elevated brain concentrations of ammonia and increased γ-aminobutyric acid (GABA) -ergic neurotransmission in the pathogenesis of HE. The mechanisms depicted, alone or in combination, can account for a substantial increase in GABA-ergic neurotransmission, which is a major factor contributing to the manifestations of hepatic encephalitis.

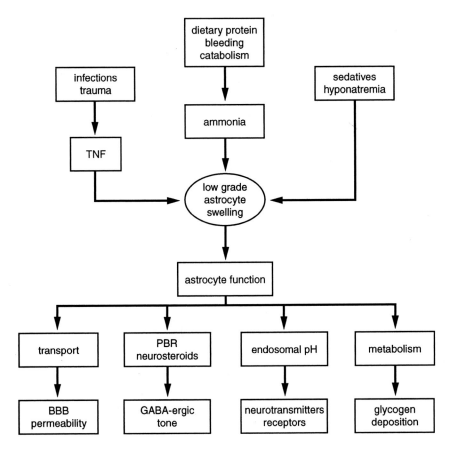

FIGURE 68-8. Proposed mechanism through which various precipitating factors can induce hepatic encephalopathy (HE). This model views a disturbance of astrocyte hydration (low-grade cerebral edema) as a key event and one (not the only) major mechanism leading to astrocyte dysfunction and the clinical picture of HE.

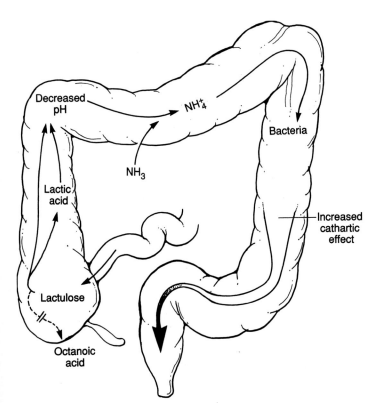

FIGURE 68-9. Mechanism of the beneficial effects of lactulose in hepatic encephalopathy. Bacterial fermentation results in an increased transformation to lactic acid and short-chain fatty acids, while decreasing the formation of medium-chain fatty acids such as octanoic acid and favoring catharsis. The resultant reduction in intestinal pH favors the passage of ammonia into the intestinal lumen, with conversion to ammonium ion. Bacteria incorporate NH_4^+ for their own metabolism.

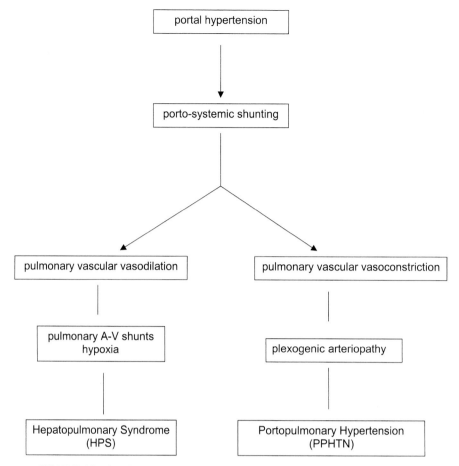

FIGURE 68-10. Pulmonary syndromes complicating portal hypertension.

69

LIVER TRANSPLANTATION

FRANCIS Y. YAO ■ NATHAN M. BASS

Liver transplantation is a highly successful treatment for patients with life-threatening, advanced liver disease and is performed in more than 120 centers in the United States. The success of this procedure in recent years is attributed to improved patient selection and pretransplant management, advances in surgical technique, improved organ preservation using the University of Wisconsin preservation fluid, new immunosuppressive agents, and effective prophylaxis against and management of infectious complications and recurrent disease. The conventional transplant procedure matches the recipient to a cadaveric donor of compatible ABO blood type and involves orthotopic transplantation of the donor organ (i.e., in the normal anatomic location). The bile duct is most commonly anastomosed in a direct duct-to-duct fashion or by a Roux-en-Y choledochojejunostomy. The latter is used mainly in patients with preexisting bile duct abnormalities (e.g., primary sclerosing cholangitis [PSC] and biliary atresia) or when technical difficulty is encountered with a conventional anastomosis.

The 1-year patient survival for all adult liver transplants in the United States is 87% (United Network for Organ Sharing [UNOS] data from 1998 to 2000) and many centers have achieved 1-year patient survival rates of about 90%, and 5-year survival rates of 70% to 80%. Liver transplantation improves the quality of life in patients with end-stage liver disease, and facilitates return to gainful employment in more than 50%. The applicability of liver transplantation as a therapy is, however, limited by donor organ shortage. As of June 2001, 17,983 patients in the United States were placed on the waiting list for liver transplantation, whereas only 4934 liver transplantation operations were performed in the year 2000 (Fig. 69-1). The rapid increase in the number of patients on the waiting list has led to increased length of waiting time and a greater number of deaths each year among patients on the list (see Fig. 69-1). In contrast, the rate of organ donation has remained relatively stagnant in recent years.

The critical shortage of donor livers has led to strategies that make use of high-risk donors, including hepatitis B core antibody–positive donors (for all recipients) and hepatitis C antibody–positive donors (for hepatitis C antibody–positive recipients). There has also been an increase in the use of segmental grafts, which includes splitting of cadaveric livers between two recipients, and the use of living donors. The latter has become almost routine in the case of pediatric liver recipients, in whom a left lateral segment is usually obtained from a blood-type–compatible parent. Living adult-to-adult donor procedures have been developed and increasingly used. This procedure usually involves removing the right lobe from the donor and transplanting it orthotopically into the recipient (Fig. 69-2). In both the donor and the recipient, there is rapid regeneration of the liver, with full size regained over 6 to 8 weeks. Living donor liver transplantation (LDLT) in adults carries inherent risks for the healthy donor, the full extent of which are not yet fully known. There have been at least two known donor deaths among close to 1000 adult-to-adult living donor liver transplants performed in the United States. Practice guidelines for LDLT have been established by the American Society of Transplant Surgeons.

Liver transplantation should be considered for patients with complications of cirrhosis (end-stage liver disease), fulminant hepatic failure, and certain metabolic disorders (Table 69-1). Patients with portal hypertensive bleeding or refractory ascites as the main complications of cirrhosis may undergo transjugular intrahepatic portosystemic shunt as a bridging procedure. Patients with end-stage liver disease who meet UNOS minimal listing criteria (i.e., a Child-Turcotte-Pugh [CTP] score of 7 or greater) are eligible for placement on the liver transplant waiting list. The Model for End-Stage Liver Disease prognostic score has recently been implemented by UNOS as a disease severity index to determine priority for organ allocation, replacing the previous system based on the CTP score and other clinical criteria (Table 69-2). Patients with fulminant liver failure, who are at greatest risk for short-term mortality, are classified in a separate category and listed at the highest priority (status 1).

The approach to the evaluation of patients for liver transplantation typically involves a multidisciplinary team including hepatologists, transplant surgeons, transplant nurse coordinators, social workers, and individuals with expertise in substance abuse issues (Fig. 69-3). Major items that are addressed during evaluation include the presence of appropriate indications and absence of contraindications (Table 69-3) for transplantation, cardiopulmonary fitness to undergo major surgery, abstinence from substance abuse and appropriate rehabilitation, and adequacy of social support.

The relative frequencies of disease indications for liver transplantation in the United States on the basis of recent UNOS data are presented in Fig. 69-4. Although the outcomes for liver transplantation have been excellent for most of the conditions shown in Fig. 69-4, recurrent disease is a limiting factor in long-term graft and patient survival and quality of life. The most significant problem in this respect is recurrent hepatitis C infection, which is almost universal following transplantation and for which currently available options for prophylaxis and treatment are limited and poorly effective. Treatment with interferon plus ribavirin is commonly used, but is poorly tolerated and results for the control of recurrent hepatitis C disease have been suboptimal. Severe recurrent liver disease occurs in up to 25% of patients transplanted for end-stage hepatitis C, with 10% to 20% progressing to cirrhosis within the first 5 years after liver transplantation. Long-term survival may be adversely impacted in these patients by the recurrent disease. Factors predictive of more severe recurrent disease and worse outcome after liver transplantation have not been clearly elucidated. Prevention and treatment of recurrent hepatitis B is currently achieved in most patients with a combination of currently available nucleoside analogs (i.e., lamivudine and adefovir dipivoxil) and high-dose intravenous hepatitis B immunoglobulin. Recurrence of autoimmune diseases (autoimmune hepatitis, primary biliary cirrhosis, and PSC) is usually mild, and an infrequent cause of graft loss. The results of transplantation for hepatocellular carcinoma have improved substantially with careful patient selection of those who have limited disease according to strict criteria that define acceptable tumor burden and absence of vascular invasion.

A major focus of management following transplantation is the prevention and treatment of rejection, which is commonly based on a triple-drug regimen of calcineurin inhibitors (cyclosporine or tacrolimus), a nucleoside analog (azathioprine and/or mycophenolate mofetil), and prednisone. Sirolimus is a nonnephrotoxic immunosuppressive that has been used in place of the calcineurin inhibitors in patients with impaired renal function. Most patients can be maintained on lower doses of immunosuppression with time and in the absence of acute rejection. Lower levels of maintenance immunosuppression are used, in general, for patients transplanted for chronic hepatitis B or C, whereas higher levels are often used in patients with autoimmune hepatitis, primary biliary cirrhosis, and possibly fulminant hepatic failure. Prednisone can be withdrawn with close monitoring in some patients at 6 months to 1 year after liver transplantation.

Acute cellular rejection occurs in 30% to 60% of all liver transplant recipients within the first year after transplantation, and most commonly within the first 6 weeks following surgery. Histologically, acute cellular rejection is characterized by the triad of portal mixed cellular inflammation with predominantly lymphocytes, bile ductular injury, and subendothelial inflammation of the portal or terminal hepatic venules (endotheliitis) (Fig. 69-5*A*). At least two of the three features are required for the diagnosis. Eosinophils are commonly present in the mixed cellular infiltrate, although this is a nonspecific feature (Fig. 69-5*B*). A single episode of mild acute rejection has not been shown to exert an overall detrimental impact on patient and graft survival, but patients with an episode of severe rejection are at increased risk for death or retransplantation. Initial treatment for acute cellular rejection is usually a high dose, and subsequently tapering corticosteroid regimen. Steroid-resistant rejection is treated with murine monoclonal antibody to the CD3 receptor on T lymphocytes (Muromonab-CD3, OK-T3). Chronic rejection is characterized by small bile duct loss (chronic ductopenic rejection) and is seen in about 10% of all liver transplant recipients. It usually occurs beyond 60 days after transplantation and is characterized by progressive loss of interlobular bile ducts and an obliterative arteriopathy. Chronic rejection may also result in diffuse bile duct stricturing in the allograft.

Graft dysfunction and loss following liver transplantation occurs mainly secondary to rejection, recurrent primary disease, vascular complications (mainly hepatic artery thrombosis), biliary complications (anastomotic and nonanastomotic strictures, bile leaks), and primary graft nonfunction. Liver retransplantation, especially for severe acute or chronic rejection and recurrent primary disease, is associated with worse survival compared to primary liver transplantation. There are significant medical risks associated with the use of immunosuppressive drugs in liver transplantation. These are listed in Table 69-4.

The most important short- and long-term complications of immunosuppression are infections (bacterial and opportunistic viral and fungal), malignancies (including posttransplant lymphoproliferative disease), as well as cardiovascular, renal, and metabolic disease. Cytomegalovirus (CMV) is one of the most important infectious complications after organ transplantation, and has been suggested to be an important cause of reduced survival and high resource utilization among liver transplant recipients. Histologically, the classical intranuclear inclusion bodies (Cowdry type A) (Fig. 69-6) are not always identified. A number of diagnostic assays for the early detection of CMV infection are now available, including the CMV antigenemia assay, the polymerase chain reaction, and the hybrid capture CMV DNA assay. Treatment of CMV disease with intravenous ganciclovir is effective in the majority of patients.

Hypertension, obesity, altered lipid profiles, and impaired glucose tolerance are all aggravated by immunosuppressive drugs, and contribute to an increased risk of ischemic heart disease and stroke in many patients after liver transplantation. Long-term follow-up data regarding the risks and incidence of cardiovascular events and mortality following liver transplantation are only beginning to emerge, and strategies to correct potentially reversible cardiovascular risk factors following liver transplantation will be an important challenge for the future.

(figures begin on page 700)

TABLE 69-1

Indications for Liver Transplantation

Complications of end-stage liver disease
    Failure of hepatic synthetic function
    Ascites
    Spontaneous bacterial peritonitis
    Hepatorenal syndrome
    Hepatic encephalopathy
    Hepatopulmonary syndrome
    Refractory portal hypertensive bleeding

Fulminant hepatic failure
    Drug-induced liver failure
    Viral hepatitis
    Wilson disease
    Idiopathic
    Acute fatty liver of pregnancy
    Primary liver graft nonfunction

Primary hepatic malignancy
    Hepatocellular carcinoma
    Hepatoblastoma
    Epithelioid hemangioendothelioma

Impaired quality of life secondary to liver disease
    Complications of cholestatic liver disease
        Intractable pruritus
        Symptomatic osteopenia
        Xanthomatous neuropathy
        Recurrent bacterial cholangitis
    Nutritional failure or failure to thrive

Extrahepatic complications of metabolic diseases
    Familial amyloid polyneuropathy
    Severe familial hypercholesterolemia
    Primary oxaluria
    Methylmalonic aciduria
    Crigler-Najjar syndrome

TABLE 69-2

The MELD Scoring System Determining Disease Severity and Priority for Organ Allocation

	3-MO MORTALITY ACCORDING TO THE MELD SCORE[†]				
MELD score	≤9	10–19	20–29	30–39	≥40
Hospitalized cirrhotic patients	4% (6/148)	27% (28/103)	76% (16/21)	83% (5/6)	100% (4/4)
Outpatient cirrhotics	2% (5/213)	6% (14/248)	50% (15/30)	—	—

Note: MELD risk score* = 10 × [0.957 × log e (creatinine mg/dL) + 0.378 × log e (bilirubin mg/dL) + 1.120 × log e (INR)] + 6.43.

Current calculation of a MELD score uses a minimum value for the creatinine of 1.0 mg/dL, bilirubin of 1.0 mg/dL, and INR of 1.0. A maximum value of 4.0 mg/dL applies to creatinine. The scores are rounded to the nearest whole number with a score range of 6 (minimum) to 40 (maximum).

*The MELD calculator is available via the Internet: *http://calc.med.edu/UNOS.htm.*

[†]Data from Wiesner RH, McDiarmid SV, Kamath PS, et al. MELD and PELD: application of survival models to liver allocation. Liver Transpl 2001;7:567–580.

INR, international normalized ratio; MELD, model for end-stage liver disease.

TABLE 69-3
Contraindications to Liver Transplantation

Absolute contraindications
   Severe, irreversible co-morbid medical illnesses that adversely impact short-term life expectancy
   Severe pulmonary hypertension (mean PAP $\geq$ 50 mm Hg)[*]
   Extrahepatic malignancy (excluding some skin cancers)
   Extensive hepatocellular carcinoma or with macrovascular or lymph node invasion[*]
   Cholangiocarcinoma[*]
   Uncontrolled systemic sepsis
   Extensive portal vein and mesenteric vein thrombosis
   Active alcohol and/or drug abuse
   Noncompliance
   Unacceptable risks for recidivism from drugs or alcohol
   Severe, uncontrolled psychiatric disease
   AIDS (HIV[*])
Relative contraindications
   Moderate pulmonary hypertension (mean PAP between 35 and 50 mm Hg)[*]
   Severe hepatopulmonary syndrome with PaO_2 of $\leq$50 mm Hg
   Severe obesity (body mass index $\geq$35)
   Poor social support
   Advanced age ($\geq$70 y)

[*]Liver transplantation has been performed in some centers under an experimental treatment protocol.

AIDS, acquired immunodeficiency syndrome; HIV, human immunodeficiency syndrome; PAP, pulmonary arterial pressure.

TABLE 69-4
Side Effects of Immunosuppressive Drugs

CORTICOSTEROIDS	AZATHIOPRINE	MYCOPHENOLATE MOFETIL	SIROLIMUS
Infection	Leukopenia	Leukopenia	Leukopenia
Poor wound healing	Thrombocytopenia	Thrombocytopenia	Thrombocytopenia
Osteonecrosis	Hepatotoxicity	Gastrointestinal	Hyperlipidemia
Cataracts	Gastrointestinal	Nausea/vomiting	Interstitial pneumonitis
Diabetes	Pancreatitis	Abdominal pain	
Cushingoid habitus	Cough	Ulceration/gastritis	
Peptic ulcer	Arthralgia	Pancreatitis	
Hypertension	Retinopathy	Arthralgia	
Obesity	Hypersensitivity		
CNS symptoms			
Growth retardation			

	CYCLOSPORINE	TACROLIMUS
Nephrotoxicity	++	++
CNS toxicity	++	++
Headaches		
Tremor		
Paresthesia		
Confusion		
Nightmares		
Seizure		
Hypertension	++	+
Glucose intolerance	++	++
Hyperkalemia	+	++
Hypomagnesemia	++	++
Hyperuricemia	+	+
Gastrointestinal	++	++
Diarrhea		
Nausea/vomiting		
Abdominal pain		
Anorexia		
Hirsutism	++	−
Alopecia	−	+
Gingival hyperplasia	+	−
Hyperlipidemia	++	+

CNS, central nervous system.

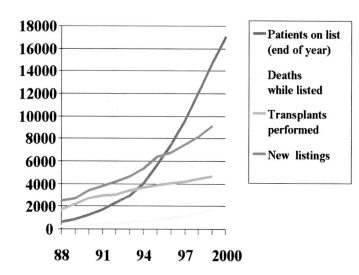

FIGURE 69-1. United Network for Organ Sharing (UNOS) data showing the trends in the liver waiting list, liver transplantation performed, and waiting list deaths during the last decade in the United States. Data for listed patients are for the end of each year up to and including 2000.

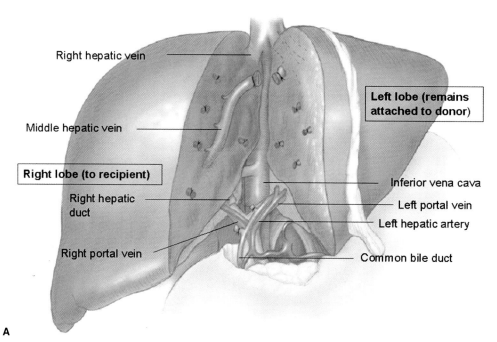

A

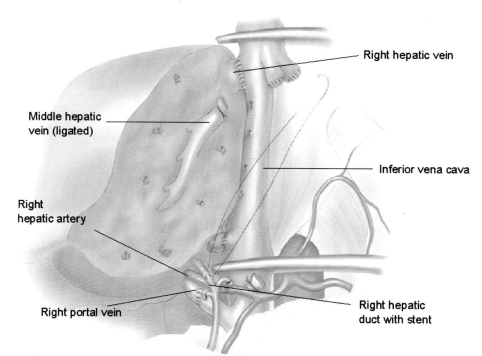

B

FIGURE 69-2. Illustration of the technique of living donor liver transplantation. **A:** Right donor hepatic lobectomy. **B:** Right lobe implantation into donor. (Courtesy of John P. Roberts, M.D., Department of Surgery, University of California, San Francisco.)

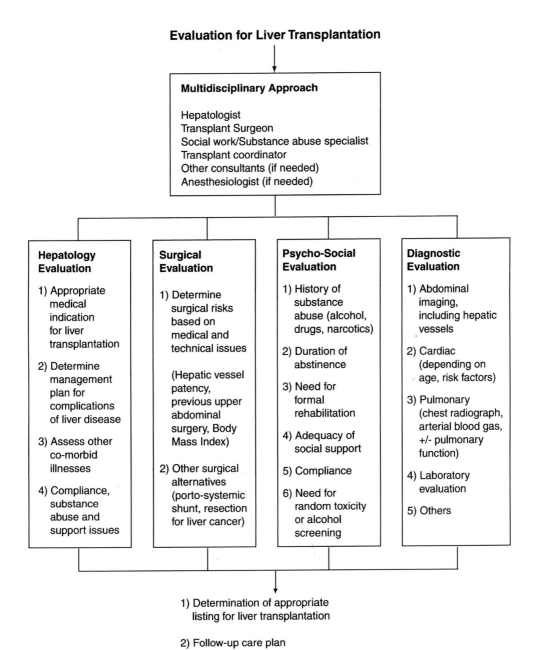

FIGURE 69-3. Principles in the evaluation of potential candidates for liver transplantation.

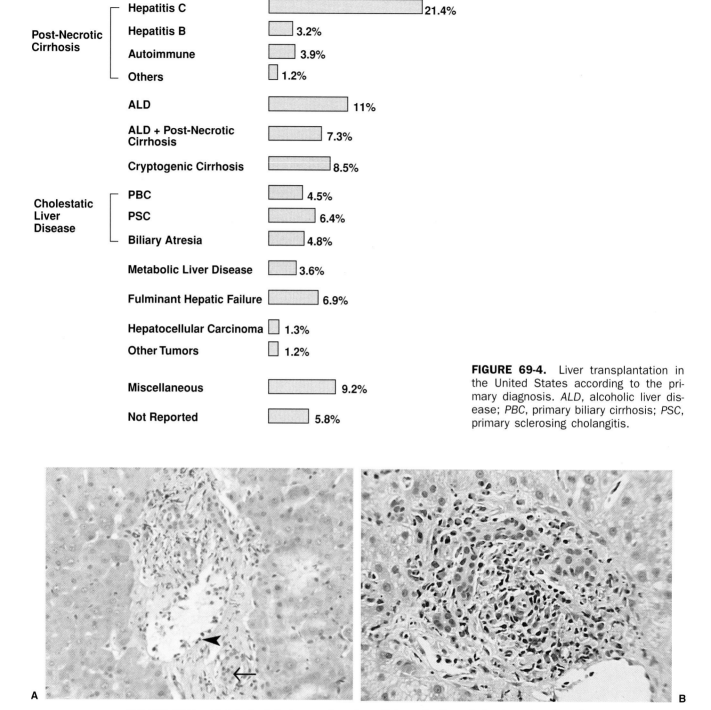

FIGURE 69-4. Liver transplantation in the United States according to the primary diagnosis. *ALD*, alcoholic liver disease; *PBC*, primary biliary cirrhosis; *PSC*, primary sclerosing cholangitis.

FIGURE 69-5. Histological features of acute cellular rejection of the hepatic allograft. **A:** The portal tract shows a mixed inflammatory infiltrate, bile ductular injury (*arrow*), and subendothelial inflammation involving a portal venule (endotheliitis) (*arrowhead*). **B:** A close-up view of the portal tract in another patient shows an inflammatory infiltrate with an abundance of eosinophils. Eosinophils are commonly seen in acute cellular rejection but are nonspecific for the diagnosis. (Courtesy Robert S. Brown, Jr., M.D., M.P.H., Department of Medicine, Columbia University College of Physicians and Surgeons, New York.)

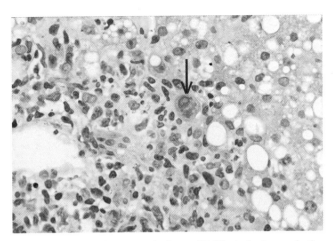

FIGURE 69-6. Cytomegalovirus (CMV) infection of the hepatic allograft. An intranuclear CMV inclusion body (Cowdry type A) is shown (*arrow*).

HEPATOCELLULAR CARCINOMA

LEWIS R. ROBERTS ■ GREGORY J. GORES

EPIDEMIOLOGY OF HEPATOCELLULAR CANCER

Hepatocellular cancer (HCC) is the fifth most common cancer and the third most common cause of death from cancer worldwide, with an estimated 560,000 new cases per year (Table 70-1). The incidence in the United States is 4/100,000 persons/year and has increased by 75% during the last 20 years. There are strong etiologic associations with cirrhosis caused by chronic hepatitis B virus (HBV), chronic hepatitis C virus (HCV), alcohol, hemochromatosis and other causes of chronic liver disease, and dietary aflatoxin exposure. Consequently, the worldwide geographic distribution of HCC cases parallels the distribution of chronic HBV infection, chronic HCV infection, and chronic dietary aflatoxin exposure. The regions with the highest incidence of HCC are in Asia and sub-Saharan Africa (Table 70-2, Fig. 70-1).

PATHOGENESIS OF HEPATOCELLULAR CARCINOMA

The pathogenesis of malignant primary liver tumors has been intensively explored. The hepatocellular injury and inflammation that characterize chronic HBV and HCV infection presumably result in cycles of liver cell death and regeneration, which lead to accelerated hepatocellular senescence, telomeric crisis, and chromosomal and genomic instability that contribute to carcinogenesis. Molecular pathways implicated in liver carcinogenesis include the p53/p21 pathway, the p16/*cyclin D1*/pRB pathway, and the Wnt/wingless signaling pathway. In addition, multiple growth factors (including tumor necrosis factor-α and transforming growth factor-β), oncogenes (particularly c-*myc*), and tumor suppressor genes (including *IGF2R, SMAD2, SMAD4, DLC1, HIC1*) have been implicated in hepatocarcinogenesis. The molecular mechanisms involved in hepatocarcinogenesis include promoter hypermethylation, deletions, and mutations. Mechanisms specific to HBV-induced HCC include HBV integration, which leads to the production of novel fusion transcripts, the interruption of genes, genomic instability with secondary insertion and deletion events, and transactivation of cellular genes by HBV proteins, particularly the X and pre-S gene products. HCV, which is an RNA virus, does not integrate into the host genome, however, the HCV core protein and nonstructural proteins NS4B and NS5A have been shown to have potentially tumorigenic effects. Chronic aflatoxin exposure predisposes to mutations in the *p53* gene; in particular, a G to T transversion at codon 249 of the *p53* gene has been shown to cause specific mutations in the *p53* gene. In populations exposed to aflatoxin approximately 50% of HCCs contain the G249T transversion.

Recently, quantitative and qualitative alterations of β-catenin, a member of the Wnt/wingless signal transduction pathway, have been reported in HCC. Mutations in exon 3 of the β-catenin gene disrupt the serine-threonine phosphorylation sites normally phosphorylated by glycogen synthetase kinase-3β (GSK-3β). This interferes with the proteosomal degradation of β-catenin, leading to its accumulation in cells. Aberrantly accumulated β-catenin translocates to the nucleus and binds to members of the T-cell factor/lymphoid enhancer factor protein family; the resulting complexes then activate target genes such as c-*myc* and *cyclin D1*, which regulate cellular growth and apoptosis. Because β-catenin gene mutations are only observed in a portion of the liver tumors with β-catenin accumulation, it is reasonable to expect that defects in other molecules that disrupt the normal β-catenin pathway may also be responsible for tumorigenesis in liver cancers. Recent studies have suggested that AXIN1, a scaffold protein for adenomatous polyposis coli (APC), GSK-3β, and β-catenin that mediates the phosphorylation of β-catenin by GSK-3β, could be another mutational target in HCC.

DIAGNOSIS, GROWTH PATTERNS, AND NATURE OF SPREAD OF HEPATOCELLULAR CARCINOMA

The prognosis of untreated hepatocellular carcinoma depends on the extent of disease at the time of diagnosis. Because current treatment of early HCC is effective, high-risk patients should be screened to allow for early diagnosis of the tumor. In the United States, many HCCs occur in patients without known risk factors, in whom the tumor is usually detected at a late stage because of a lack of symptoms or signs of early HCC. The high-risk population includes persons with chronic HBV (with or without cirrhosis), chronic HCV with cirrhosis, hereditary hemochromatosis with cirrhosis, alcoholic cirrhosis, primary biliary cirrhosis, α$_1$-antitrypsin deficiency, and cryptogenic cirrhosis. Histopathologic findings placing the patient with cirrhosis at high risk for HCC include dysplasia (Fig. 70-2), positive immunohistochemistry for proliferating cell nuclear antigen, and the presence of argyrophilic nucleolar organizer regions, macroregenerative nodules, and irregular regeneration. High-risk individuals have an incidence rate of HCC of 3% to 8% per year. Histological variants of HCC include trabecular, pseudoglandular (Fig. 70-3), scirrhous, and fibrolamellar types (Fig. 70-4). Macroscopically, HCCs usually present as an expansile mass with a fibrous capsule (Fig. 70-5). Often, a high-grade focus arises within a low-grade early stage tumor, leading to a nodule-in-nodule appearance (Figs. 70-6). Spread of HCCs usually occurs by invasion into blood vessels, most often the portal vein (Fig. 70-7).

Intrahepatic metastases are predominantly caused by tumor spread via portal vein branches.

Extrahepatic metastasis is most frequently to the lungs and regional lymph nodes. Periodic liver ultrasonography is the recommended screening tool for HCC (Fig. 70-8). Ultrasonography has been shown to be cost effective at incidence rates greater than or equal to 1.5%/year. Most centers perform liver ultrasonography in high-risk patients every 6 months. Positive ultrasounds are usually followed up with multiphasic spiral computed tomography (CT) or gadolinium contrast-enhanced magnetic resonance image (MRI) scanning (Fig. 70-9; see Fig. 70-8). If possible, most experienced centers avoid the use of biopsy for the diagnosis of HCC because of a 3% to 5% risk of needle track seeding. Radiographic and laboratory criteria for the diagnosis of HCC without biopsy include the presence of cirrhosis, a mass greater than or equal to 2 cm, identified by two imaging modalities, and either the presence of an arterial hypervascular lesion demonstrated by CT, MRI, or angiography, or the presence of a serum α-fetoprotein greater than 400 ng/mL. The serum α-fetoprotein level is often used in screening for HCC. It has an overall sensitivity of 39% to 64%, a specificity of 76% to 91%, and a positive predictive value of only 9% to 32%. Because α-fetoprotein is seldom elevated in small HCCs (<2 cm), its usefulness as a screening tool is limited. The serum α-fetoprotein level is most useful for identifying a high-risk group of patients that requires close follow-up.

TREATMENT OPTIONS FOR HEPATOCELLULAR CARCINOMA

The selection of an appropriate treatment strategy for patients with HCC depends on careful tumor staging and assessment of the underlying liver disease (Fig. 70-10). The best prognostic group includes patients with performance status 0 with no constitutional symptoms, Child's A cirrhosis, no vascular invasion, and no extrahepatic spread. All patients with localized HCC (involvement of one single lobe, no vascular invasion or extrahepatic disease) should be evaluated for the potentially curative therapy options of partial hepatectomy or orthotopic liver transplantation (OLT). Candidates for partial hepatectomy must have no liver disease or Child's A cirrhosis, normal portal pressure, and normal serum bilirubin. For patients not meeting these criteria, OLT should be considered if there is a solitary lesion less than 5 cm or fewer than three lesions less than 3 cm. Local ablative therapies such as percutaneous ethanol injection (PEI), radiofrequency ablation (RFA), and chemoembolization (CE) offer palliation for patients with contraindications to surgical approaches (Fig. 70-8). PEI and RFA are minimally invasive and can be used on an outpatient basis, usually for tumor nodules less than 3 cm. When used for small tumors, the survival rates can be similar to those achieved by partial hepatectomy. CE may be used as an interim treatment for patients waiting for OLT. Given the paucity of efficacy data, there are no proven systemic chemotherapy regimens, immunotherapy approaches, or hormonal therapies that can be recommended.

(figures begin on page 708)

TABLE 70-1
Estimated Worldwide Annual Mortality from Major Cancers

MEN				WOMEN				BOTH GENDERS			
Site		Number	Percentage	Site		Number	Percentage	Site		Number	Percentage
1.	Lung	810	25.6%	1.	Breast	373	15.9%	1.	Lung	1103	20.0%
2.	Stomach	405	12.8%	2.	Lung	293	12.5%	2.	Stomach	647	11.7%
3.	Liver	384	12.1%	3.	Stomach	241	10.3%	3.	Liver	549	10.0%
4.	Colon/rectum	255	8.1%	4.	Colon/rectum	238	10.1%	4.	Colon/rectum	492	8.9%
5.	Esophagus	227	7.2%	5.	Cervix uteri	233	9.9%	5.	Breast	373	6.8%
6.	Prostate	204	6.5%	6.	Liver	165	7.0%	6.	Esophagus	338	6.1%
7.	Pancreas	112	3.5%	7.	Ovary etc.	114	4.9%	7.	Cervix uteri	233	4.2%
8.	Leukemia	109	3.5%	8.	Esophagus	111	4.7%	8.	Pancreas	213	3.9%
9.	Bladder	99	3.1%	9.	Pancreas	101	4.3%	9.	Prostate	204	3.7%
10.	Non-Hodgkin's lymphoma	93	3.0%	10.	Leukemia	86	3.7%	10.	Leukemia	195	3.5%
11.	Oral cavity	81	2.6%	11.	Non-Hodgkin's lymphoma	68	2.9%	11.	Non-Hodgkin's lymphoma	161	2.9%
12.	Larynx	79	2.5%	12.	Brain/nervous system	56	2.4%	12.	Bladder	132	2.4%

TABLE 70-2

World Age-Standardized Incidence of Hepatocellular Carcinoma

	MALE	FEMALE	MALE-TO-FEMALE RATIO
World	14.97	5.51	2.72
Eastern Africa	14.44	6.02	2.40
Middle Africa	24.21	12.98	1.87
Northern Africa	4.95	2.68	1.85
Southern Africa	6.16	2.07	2.98
Western Africa	13.51	6.16	2.19
Caribbean	7.58	4.17	1.82
Central America	2.06	1.64	1.26
South America	4.8	3.68	1.30
Northern America	4.11	1.68	2.45
Eastern Asia	35.46	12.66	2.80
South-Eastern Asia	18.35	5.7	3.22
South Central Asia	2.77	1.45	1.91
Western Asia	5.6	2.06	2.72
Eastern Europe	5.8	2.55	2.27
Northern Europe	2.61	1.39	1.88
Southern Europe	9.84	3.45	2.85
Western Europe	5.85	1.61	3.63
Australia/New Zealand	3.6	1.19	3.03
Melanesia	20.19	10.24	1.97
Micronesia	8.94	5.02	1.78
Polynesia	9.83	3.89	2.53

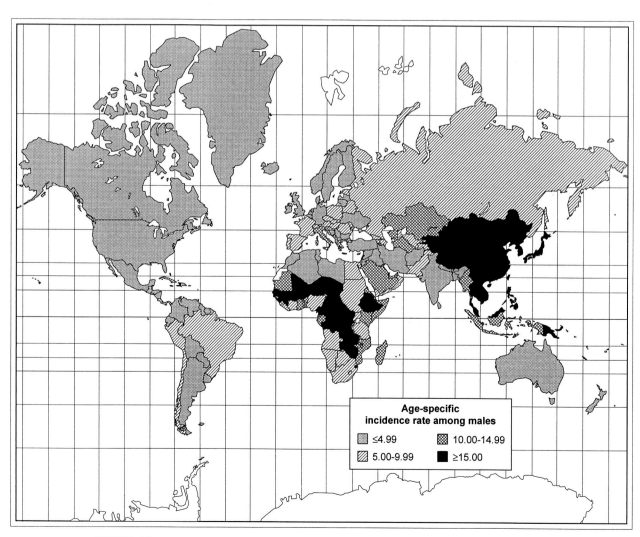

FIGURE 70-1. Worldwide age-specific incidence of hepatocellular carcinoma in males.

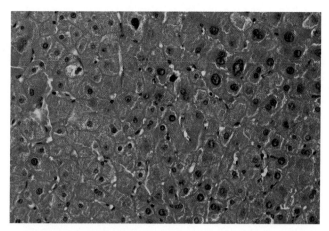

FIGURE 70-2. Liver cell dysplasia. This nodule from a patient with post-hepatitis cirrhosis shows a moderate increase in cell density, an irregular trabecular pattern, and increased cellular atypia.

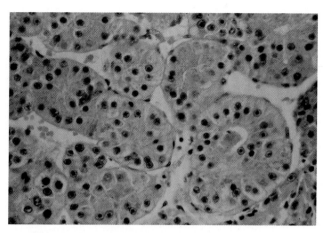

FIGURE 70-3. Hepatocellular carcinoma. The tumor has a mixed pseudoglandular and trabecular pattern with bile plugs. The sinusoid-like blood spaces show variable dilation.

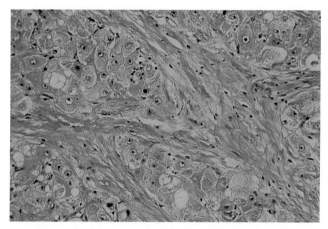

FIGURE 70-4. Fibrolamellar hepatocellular carcinoma is characterized by sheets of large polygonal tumor cells separated by hyalinized collagen bundles with a lamellar pattern. This variant of hepatocellular carcinoma usually affects adolescents or young adults who have no known risk factors for hepatocellular carcinoma.

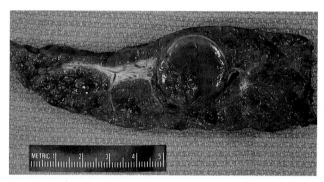

FIGURE 70-5. Nodular type of hepatocellular carcinoma. The tumor is expansile with a fibrous pseudocapsule. Prominent bile production gives the tumor its green color. The surrounding liver is cirrhotic, with multiple regenerative nodules.

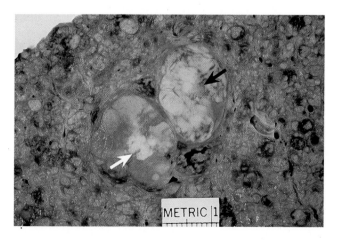

FIGURE 70-6. Nodule-in-nodule type of hepatocellular carcinoma. A lighter-colored, higher-grade focus of hepatocellular carcinoma (*black arrow*) has arisen within the upper right nodule and is compressing the original lower-grade tumor toward the pseudocapsule. There is a small, high-grade focus of hepatocellular carcinoma arising in the center of the lower left nodule (*white arrow*), surrounded by well-differentiated tumor.

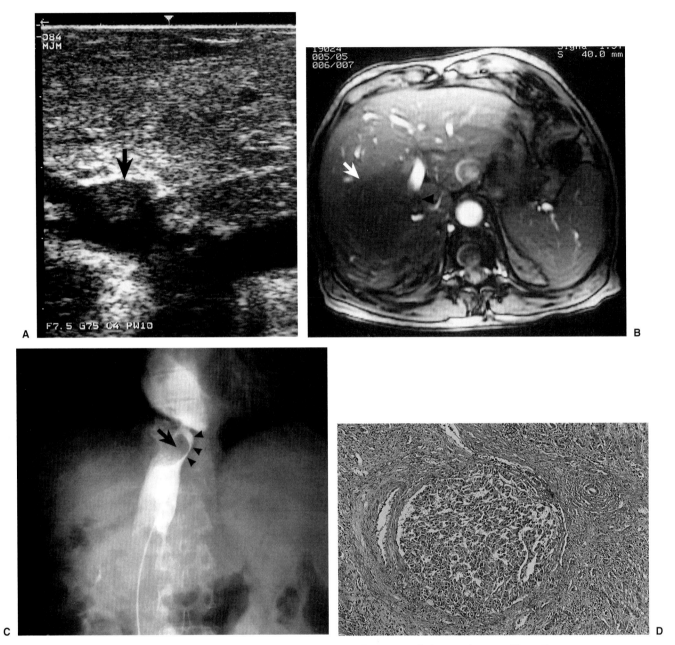

FIGURE 70-7. Vascular invasion is a hallmark of hepatocellular carcinoma. More than 70% of patients with advanced hepatocellular carcinoma develop tumor thrombi in the portal vein, which lead to intrahepatic dissemination of the tumor. **A:** Ultrasound image showing extension of hepatocellular carcinoma into the portal vein (*black arrow*). **B:** Magnetic resonance image scan demonstrating a tumor mass (*white arrow*) and an abrupt cutoff of the right portal vein (*arrowhead*). **C:** Angiogram showing near-occlusion of the inferior vena cava (*arrowheads*) by hepatocellular carcinoma within the lumen (*black arrow*). **D:** Histology of hepatocellular carcinoma invading a portal vein branch.

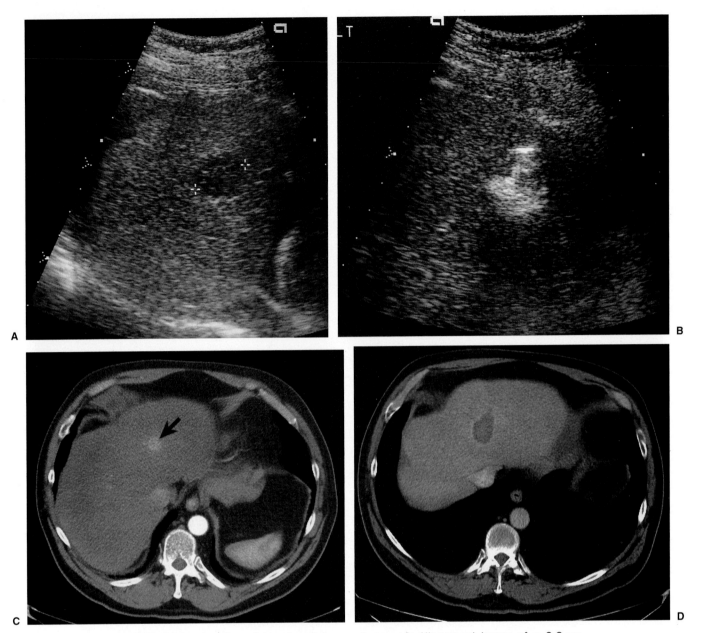

FIGURE 70-8. Imaging of hepatocellular carcinoma. **A:** Ultrasound image of a 2.2-cm small hepatocellular carcinoma (marked by *asterisks*). **B:** Ultrasound image immediately after percutaneous ethanol injection for treatment of the hepatocellular carcinoma in **A.** The tissue injury produced results in an enhanced echogenic signal. **C:** Computed tomography (CT) scan of a 1.8-cm small enhancing hepatocellular carcinoma (*arrow*). **D:** CT image after treatment of the hepatocellular carcinoma in panel **C** by radiofrequency ablation.

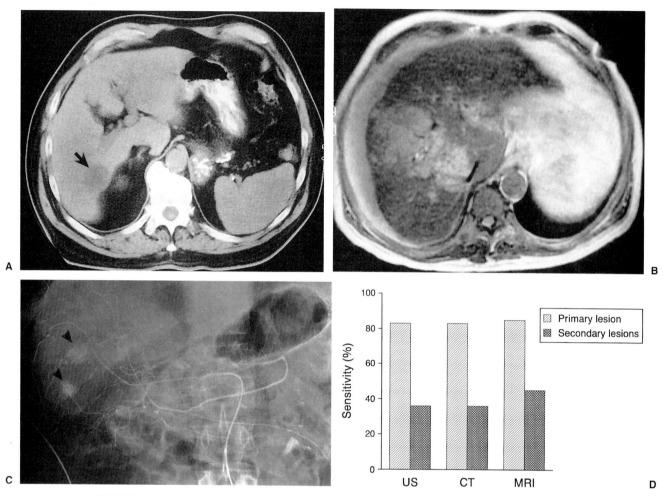

FIGURE 70-9. Imaging of hepatocellular carcinoma. **A:** Computed tomography (CT) image showing a hypodense hepatocellular cancer (HCC) with a visible capsular rim (*arrow*). **B:** Magnetic resonance image (MRI) showing a large HCC located centrally within the liver. **C:** Angiogram demonstrating two enhancing HCC lesions in the right lobe of the liver (*arrowheads*). **D:** Ultrasound, CT, and MRI each have a sensitivity of more than 80% for primary lesions and about 40% for secondary lesions.

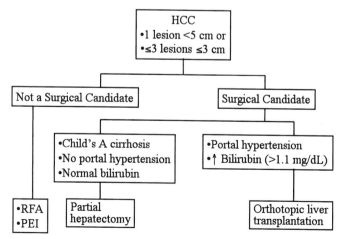

FIGURE 70-10. Treatment of hepatocellular carcinoma. Algorithm for the management of patients with hepatocellular carcinoma.

71

LIVER ABSCESS

DAVID S. RAIFORD

AMEBIC VERSUS PYOGENIC ABSCESS

Although there is considerable overlap in the clinical presentation and imaging characteristics of amebic and pyogenic abscesses, differences in epidemiology, associated conditions, treatment, and prognosis underscore the need for the physician to distinguish these entities. Effective management depends critically upon prompt and correct definition of the abscess type.

EPIDEMIOLOGY

Because intestinal amebiasis is a necessary prelude to hepatic amebic abscess, persons with amebic abscess typically have emigrated from or traveled to areas where intestinal amebiasis is prevalent. In contrast, the ethnicity and travel history of patients with pyogenic abscess does not differ from that of the general hospital population. Over the last few decades, biliary obstruction, both benign and malignant, has emerged as the most common etiology of pyogenic liver abscess, and accounts for 50% to 60% of cases.

SYMPTOMS

Fever and right upper quadrant pain are the principal symptoms of hepatic abscess, both amebic and pyogenic. Fever is evident in virtually all patients. Although spiking fever and chills favor pyogenic abscess, these may be seen with amebic abscess. Pain is reported by 75% to 90% of patients, is usually constant, is of variable intensity, and may exhibit pleuritic features with radiation to the right shoulder if diaphragmatic involvement is present. The majority of patients will have symptoms for less than 2 weeks before seeking medical care. Nonspecific symptoms such as weakness, anorexia, nausea, and weight loss are common. Approximately one third of persons with either type of liver abscess will report diarrhea and one fourth will have a nonproductive cough.

PHYSICAL FINDINGS

On physical examination, sequential measurements of body temperature should be made to detect fever. Hepatic enlargement and tenderness are typical, but not

713

invariably present. Jaundice is rare in amebic abscess and, when present, should suggest biliary tract obstruction with pyogenic infection and/or underlying chronic liver disease. Percussion dullness, diminished breath sounds, or other chest findings at the right lung base are evident in 20% to 30% of patients and suggest involvement of the superior portion of the right hepatic lobe. Occasionally, signs of weight loss, dehydration, and anemia will be evident.

IMAGING MODALITIES IN DIAGNOSIS

The clinical constellation of fever, right upper quadrant discomfort, and hepatic enlargement with tenderness should prompt an imaging study early in the diagnostic assessment. Depending on the age of the patient and level of clinical suspicion for cholelithiasis or biliary obstruction, either ultrasonography (US) or computerized tomography (CT) will be performed. These techniques facilitate discrimination of liver abscess from cholecystitis, bile duct obstruction, or pancreatitis. Radionuclide liver-spleen scanning after administration of ^{99m}Tc sulfur-colloid has been supplanted by US and CT because the latter two are more sensitive for small lesions (<3 cm in size) and offer better precision in localizing lesions that may require percutaneous aspiration or drainage. Of note, lesions near the dome of the right hepatic lobe may be difficult to visualize by US. Typically, on US an abscess appears as a rounded, hypoechoic mass, sometimes with internal echoes (Fig. 71-1). CT scanning with intravenous contrast will identify an abscess as a low-density lesion (Fig. 71-2), often with peripheral enhancement, and may provide better definition of extrahepatic pathology associated with pyogenic abscess (e.g., appendiceal or diverticular abscess). Although both modalities are sensitive for detecting abscesses and biliary obstruction, neither can distinguish reliably between amebic and pyogenic abscesses. Although less widely used, magnetic resonance imaging (MRI) also has high sensitivity for detection of hepatic abscess. Characteristically, liver abscesses are hypointense on T1-weighted and hyperintense on T2-weighted images and wall enhancement soon after gadolinium infusion is typical. Thus, MRI may provide complementary data if US and CT findings are ambiguous or when coronal images will help guide management of a lesion in the superior portion of a hepatic lobe (Fig. 71-3). The majority of abscesses, both amebic and pyogenic, occur in the right hepatic lobe. The presence of multiple abscesses strongly suggests pyogenic infection, as does identification of concomitant biliary tract obstruction. Chest radiographs in patients with an abscess adjacent to the diaphragm may show elevation of the right diaphragm, subpulmonic effusion, and right lower lobe atelectasis or infiltrate. Note that hepatic tumors may present with necrosis and secondary infection, mimicking a primary abscess.

NEEDLE ASPIRATION

Key to diagnosis and treatment of liver abscess is identification of the organism(s) in the abscess. Needle aspiration of an abscess is the best and most direct method to distinguish amebic from pyogenic abscess. Material from an amebic abscess will be brown-red in color and typically is not particularly malodorous (Fig. 71-4). A pyogenic abscess will yield material that is creamy, tan-green in color, and often putrid, reflecting anaerobic infection. Gram stains of amebic abscess contents will show neutrophils but no bacteria, unless secondary infection is present. Smears of pyogenic abscess contents will usually identify at least one bacterial form. Meticulous handling of aspirated material to avoid exposure to air enhances recovery and identification of anaerobic species. Reliable and complete identification of infectious agents ensures proper selection of an antibiotic treatment regimen.

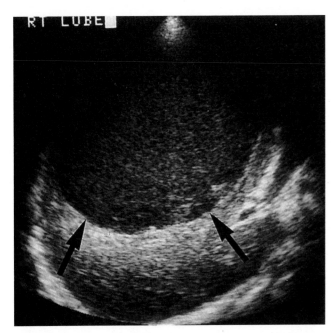

FIGURE 71-1. Transverse sonogram of the right hepatic lobe showing a large hypoechoic amebic abscess (*arrows*). This lesion is homogeneous, as is typical, although any sonographic pattern may occur. The image is from a 26-year-old man who had strongly positive amebic serology and recovered rapidly with metronidazole treatment.

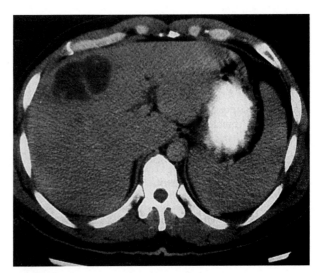

FIGURE 71-2. Computerized tomography showing a low-density lesion in the anterosuperior segment of the right hepatic lobe of a 34-year-old man. *Klebsiella pneumoniae* was cultured from the blood and from the abscess cavity. The patient recovered with antibiotic treatment and a single abscess aspiration.

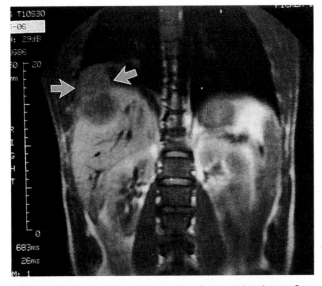

FIGURE 71-3. Magnetic resonance image showing a 6-cm lesion in the dome of the right hepatic lobe with apparent penetration into the thoracic cavity (*arrows*). The patient was a 35-year-old Hispanic man with 3 weeks of pleuritic, right-sided chest pain and fever. Red-brown material was aspirated from the right chest. Amebic serology was strongly positive. He recovered with metronidazole therapy.

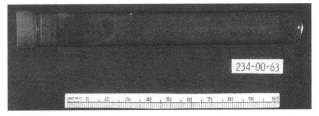

FIGURE 71-4. Material aspirated from a large right lobe amebic abscess in a 31-year-old man who had been ill for 2 weeks with fever and right upper quadrant pain. He recovered completely with chloroquine therapy.

VASCULAR DISEASES OF THE LIVER

LAURIE D. DELEVE ■ GARY C. KANEL

This chapter reviews images of Budd-Chiari syndrome, sinusoidal obstruction syndrome (hepatic venoocclusive disease), nodular regenerative hyperplasia, and peliosis hepatitis. These diseases are all thought to be primary circulatory problems that lead to secondary changes in the hepatic parenchyma.

In Budd-Chiari syndrome, severity of liver injury will depend on the extent of the involvement of the hepatic veins, the time course over which the obstruction of the hepatic veins develops, and the duration of untreated disease. Slower development of the obstruction or occlusion allows formation of collaterals to alleviate sinusoidal congestion as the obstruction progresses. These collaterals produce the characteristic spiderweb appearance shown in Fig. 72-1. In acute Budd-Chiari syndrome, there is perivenular and sometimes midzonal sinusoidal congestion, acute hemorrhage, and liver cell ischemia. Figure 72-2 demonstrates hemorrhage within the hepatic cords with red blood cells replacing the damaged hepatocytes. In chronic Budd-Chiari syndrome, chronic outflow obstruction may lead to bridging fibrosis between terminal hepatic venules with sparing of the portal tracts and fibrosis that obliterates the terminal hepatic venules, as demonstrated in Fig. 72-3.

Sinusoidal obstruction syndrome (SOS) is initiated by damage to sinusoidal endothelial cells. Figures 72-4 and 72-5 demonstrate the ultrastructural changes in the sinusoid that occur prior to "clinical" evidence of disease in the experimental model, notably formation of gaps in the sinusoidal endothelial cells and penetration of red blood cells through the gaps into the space of Disse. Figure 72-6 demonstrates the ultrastructural features of early SOS with denudation of the sinusoidal lining and loss of hepatocyte microvilli during early SOS. The histological features of early SOS shown in Fig. 72-7 include subendothelial and sinusoidal hemorrhage and perivenular necrosis. Occlusion of terminal hepatic venules is not present in all patients, but is seen more commonly in patients with more severe disease. Narrowing of terminal hepatic venules in early SOS is due to subendothelial accumulation of plasma and some formed elements or frank subendothelial hemorrhage. In late SOS, there is fibrosis within perizonal sinusoids and adventitial or subendothelial fibrosis with narrowing or occlusion of the terminal hepatic veins (Fig. 72-8). Unlike more subtle changes in the sinusoid, venular occlusion is easily recognized on histology and this led to the previous name, hepatic venoocclusive disease. With the recognition that the disease is initiated in the sinusoid and that venular involvement is not present in a sizable minority of patients, the disease was renamed sinusoidal obstruction syndrome.

Current thinking is that nodular regenerative hyperplasia is due to uneven perfusion of the liver. In areas of hypoperfusion, hepatocytes atrophy or undergo apoptosis, with reactive hyperplasia in areas in which perfusion is maintained. Impaired perfusion may occur at the level of the portal vein or the sinusoids. Hypoperfusion resulting from obstruction of the portal vein may occur in collagen vascular diseases or immune complex diseases when inflammation of the hepatic artery leads to inflammatory destruction of adjacent portal veins. Nodular regenerative hyperplasia may accompany portal vein thrombosis caused by prothrombotic disorders such as agnogenic myeloid metaplasia, polycythemia vera, or antiphospholipid syndrome. Perfusion deficits at the level of the sinusoid are seen with toxicity to sinusoidal endothelial cells, such as by long-term azathioprine therapy in renal or liver transplantation patients or after conditioning therapy for hematopoietic stem cell transplantation. Figures 72-9 and 72-10 demonstrate small regenerative nodules, which are composed of cytologically benign hepatocytes. The nodules displace portal structures and are surrounded by areas with atrophic hepatocytes.

Patients with chronic wasting illnesses or who have been exposed to androgenic anabolic steroids or long-term azathioprine therapy may develop one or multiple peliotic lesions in the liver or spleen (Figs. 72-11 and 72-12). The peliotic lesion consists of well-defined vascular cavities without a discrete endothelial lining (Fig. 72-13). In patients with acquired immunodeficiency syndrome, peliosis may occur because of infection with *Bartonella* species (Fig. 72-14). Although it had been suggested that sinusoidal endothelial cells were the initial target in peliosis, this concept has been most clearly supported by studies of peliosis caused by *Bartonella* species. *Bartonella* bacilli can be detected by electron microscopy in sinusoidal endothelial cells. This leads to disruption of the sinusoidal endothelial cell barrier, with initial sinusoidal dilation and subsequent formation of peliotic cavities.

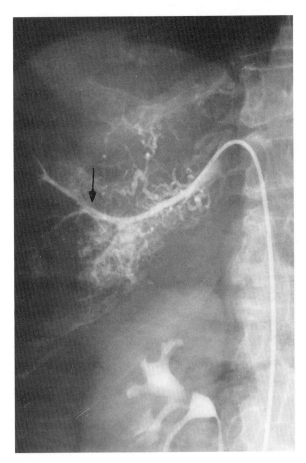

FIGURE 72–1. Budd-Chiari syndrome. The angiogram demonstrates the spiderweb pattern characteristic of Budd-Chiari syndrome. A residual, narrowed hepatic vein is indicated by the *arrow*. (Courtesy of Dr. Sue Ellen Hanks, University of Southern California.)

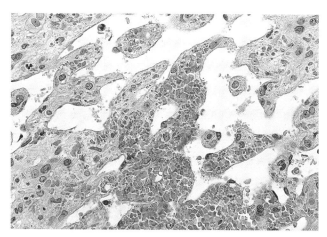

FIGURE 72-2. Budd-Chiari syndrome, acute. The sinusoids in the perivenular zone (zone 3 or Rappaport) show marked dilation and are virtually devoid of erythrocytes. The red blood cells are present within the hepatic cords, replacing the damaged hepatocytes.

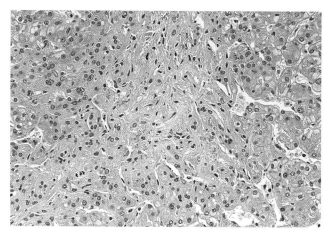

FIGURE 72–3. Budd-Chiari syndrome, chronic. The terminal hepatic venule has been replaced by intraluminal fibrosis, which has extended into the perivenular zone as well.

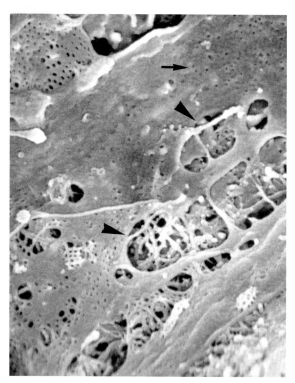

FIGURE 72–4. Sinusoidal obstruction syndrome (SOS), "pre-SOS." A scanning electron microscopic image (original magnification ×10,300) was taken from the rat model of SOS 1 day after administration of monocrotaline. This demonstrates changes that occur before clinical or light microscopy images are observed in this model: gaps in sinusoidal endothelial cells (*arrowheads*) that allow penetration of red blood cells into the space of Disse and loss of fenestrae organized as sieve plates (*arrow*). (Courtesy of Dr. Robert McCuskey, University of Arizona.)

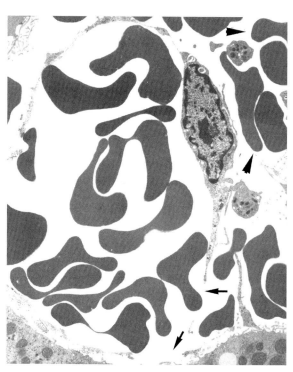

FIGURE 72–5. Sinusoidal obstruction syndrome (SOS), "pre-SOS." A transmission electron microscopy image, taken from the rat model of SOS, demonstrates gaps in the sinusoidal endothelial cell (*arrows*) and red blood cells in the space of Disse (*arrowheads*) (original magnification ×10,300). (Courtesy of Dr. Robert McCuskey, University of Arizona.)

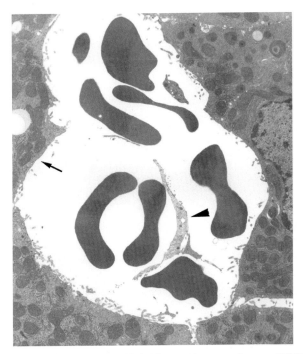

FIGURE 72-6. Sinusoidal obstruction syndrome (SOS), early. A transmission electron microscopy image, taken from the rat model of SOS during early SOS, demonstrates loss of sinusoidal lining and of microvilli on the hepatocyte (*arrow*) and a remnant of a sinusoidal endothelial cell in the lumen (*arrowhead*). (Courtesy of Dr. Robert McCuskey, University of Arizona.)

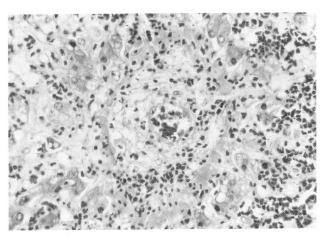

FIGURE 72-7. Sinusoidal obstruction syndrome (SOS), early. A photomicrograph demonstrates the changes of early SOS in a hematopoietic stem cell transplantation patient. Features demonstrated here are marked subendothelial and sinusoidal hemorrhage and perivenular necrosis. (Courtesy of Dr. Howard Shulman, Fred Hutchinson Cancer Research Center and the University of Washington.)

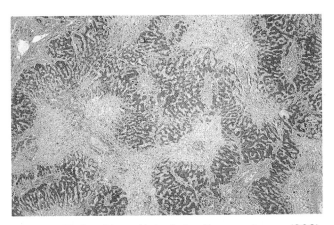

FIGURE 72-8. Sinusoidal obstruction syndrome (SOS), late. Marked sinusoidal and venular fibrosis is present in the perivenular zone in the liver of a patient 63 days after conditioning therapy for hematopoietic stem cell transplantation. (Courtesy of Dr. Howard Shulman, Fred Hutchinson Cancer Research Center and the University of Washington.)

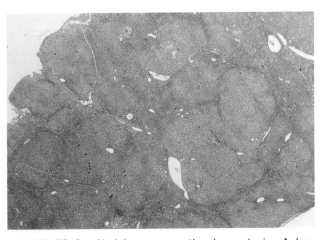

FIGURE 72-9. Nodular regenerative hyperplasia. A low-power photomicrograph shows small regenerative nodules ranging in size from 3 to 6 mm, displacing portal structures.

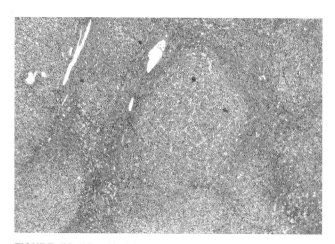

FIGURE 72–10. Nodular regenerative hyperplasia. A high-power photomicrograph shows that the nodule is composed of cytologically benign hepatocytes. The liver cells adjacent to these nodules are smaller with mild atrophy of the eosinophilic cytoplasm.

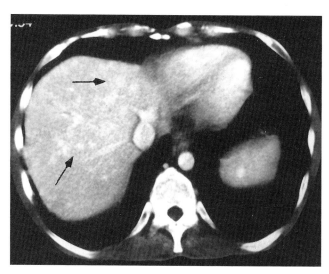

FIGURE 72–11. Peliosis hepatis. A computed tomography image demonstrates multiple peliotic lesions, two of which are indicated by *arrows*. (Courtesy of Dr. Randall Radin, University of Southern California.)

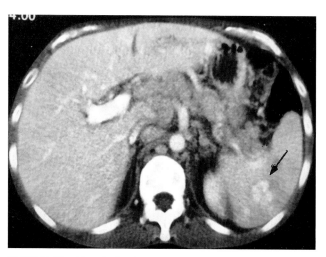

FIGURE 72–12. Peliosis. A computed tomography image demonstrates a large peliotic lesion in the spleen (*arrow*). (Courtesy of Dr. Randall Radin, University of Southern California.)

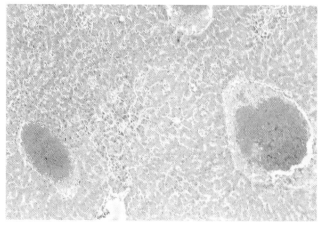

FIGURE 72–13. Peliosis hepatis. Scattered randomly within the hepatic parenchyma are well-defined vascular spaces filled with red blood cells. A closer inspection would show that the cysts have no discrete endothelial lining.

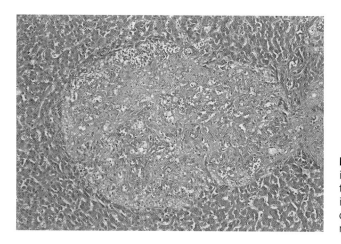

FIGURE 72–14. Peliosis hepatis. Peliosis hepatis may occur in immunocompromised patients because of organisms from the rickettsial *Bartonella (Rochalimaea)* species, which can be identified as gram-negative bacilli in the lesion. The well-circumscribed lesion is composed of numerous vascular channels within a loose fibroconnective stroma.

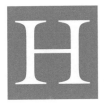

73

ABDOMINAL CAVITY: Anatomy, Structural Anomalies, and Hernias

SAREH PARANGI ■ **RICHARD A. HODIN**

This chapter introduces the reader to the anatomy of the abdominal cavity, as well as discusses structural anomalies and hernias. More common issues are discussed here, and significantly more detail is included in Chapter 121 of the *Textbook of Gastroenterology,* 4th edition.

EMBRYOLOGY OF THE ABDOMINAL CAVITY

The Abdominal Cavity

Understanding of the embryology of the abdominal contents is imperative to understanding the pathophysiology of the various congenital and structural anomalies of the abdominal cavity. The upper gastrointestinal tract develops from the foregut and includes the esophagus, stomach, duodenum, liver, gallbladder, and pancreas. The midgut develops into the small bowel, and the right and transverse colons. The hindgut development forms the left colon, sigmoid, rectum, and the upper part of the anal canal. The abdominal cavity in the adult is defined by the diaphragm superiorly, the abdominal walls laterally, and the pelvis inferiorly. The peritoneal covering is the endodermal investment of the surface of the organs of the abdominal cavity. The pancreas, parts of the duodenum, right and left colon, and the rectum, which are all retroperitoneal, are covered only anteriorly by peritoneum.

CONGENITAL ANOMALIES

In the embryo the abdominal cavity is too small to accommodate the intestines, and a physiological herniation occurs into the umbilical cord with return of the intestines to the abdominal cavity by the tenth week. An omphalocele (*Textbook of Gastroenterology*, 4th edition Chapter 121: Fig. 121-3*A*) is failure in the growth of the celomic walls with a large herniation of the abdominal viscera into the base of the umbilical cord. The herniated viscera are covered by a sac composed of amnion. Gastroschisis (*Textbook of Gastroenterology*, 4th edition Chapter 121: Fig. 121-3*B*) is a similar anomaly, but the defect in the abdominal wall is located lateral to the umbilicus, and is caused by failure of closure of the abdominal wall. No sac is present to cover the herniated intestines and the size of the defect is often smaller.

Congenital Diaphragmatic Hernias

The diaphragm appears in the third week of development as a septum transversum that separates the thorax from the abdomen. A diaphragmatic hernia is one of the more common malformations of the newborn and is most frequently caused by failure of the pleuroperitoneal membranes to completely separate the peritoneal and pleural cavities posteriorly.

Posterolateral hernia defects (hernia of Bochdalek) are usually large, and on the left side; the intestinal loops, stomach, spleen, and part of the liver may enter the thoracic cavity (Fig. 73-1*A*). The presence of abdominal viscera in the chest results in compression of the heart and hypoplasia of the lung (Fig. 73-1*B*). The neonate presents with acute respiratory distress; the heart, mediastinum, and lungs are displaced to the right and the abdomen may be scaphoid. Respiratory sounds are absent on the affected side and heart sounds may be audible in the right chest. The diagnosis is easily made with a chest radiograph showing one or more air-fluid levels in the left thorax, displacement of the mediastinum, and loss of the sharp diaphragmatic line separating the thorax and abdomen (*Textbook of Gastroenterology*, 4th edition Chapter 121: Fig. 121-4*B*). Lung hypoplasia results in acute respiratory distress and is the main cause of death in these patients. Mortality depends on the age of the patient, associated malformations, and most importantly the degree of lung hypoplasia.

Occasionally, a small part of the muscular fibers of the diaphragm fails to develop and a hernia may remain undiscovered until later in life. Such a defect is seen in the anterior portion of the diaphragm and is known as a parasternal hernia (hernia of Morgagni; *Textbook of Gastroenterology*, 4th edition Chapter 121: Fig. 121-4*A*). These hernias are usually small and can contain stomach, omentum, colon, or small intestine with a peritoneal covering.

HERNIAS OF THE ABDOMINAL CAVITY IN ADULTS

"Hernia is a protrusion of any viscus from its proper cavity" (Sir Astley Cooper, 1804). Hernias are composed of a herniated viscus, the hernia sac, and the opening of the hernia (the hernial ring) (*Textbook of Gastroenterology*, 4th edition Chapter 121: Figure 121-5). The hernial sac is the internal wall of the hernia lined by peritoneum. An external hernia is composed of a viscus abnormally located outside the abdomen; an internal hernia occurs when the viscus is abnormally located within the intra-abdominal space. Any viscus can become part of a hernia, but most commonly a segment of intestine is partially or completely herniated.

A reducible hernia occurs when the hernial sac contents return to the abdominal cavity spontaneously or with external manipulation. The major complications of hernias are incarceration, bowel obstruction, and bowel strangulation. A complication is more likely to occur if the hernial opening is small and in hernias where the bowel has access to the sac. Bowel incarceration greatly increases the chance that strangulation will occur. An incarcerated hernia occurs when the hernial contents cannot be dislodged from the sac. Incarceration occurs when there are adhesions from the hernial contents or around the opening of the hernia making reduction impossible, or when there is edema or contortion of the hernial contents such that hernial contents, once entered into the sac, cannot exit. A hernia, reducible or incarcerated, becomes a strangulated hernia when the blood supply to the herniated viscus is compromised.

Diagnostic Considerations

Most hernias are detected using a history and physical exam. The patient needs to be questioned about the presence of a bulge, conditions that make the bulge appear and disappear, and any associated pain or gastrointestinal symptoms. A complete physical examination of the abdomen and rectum should be done. All scars should be noted. Radiographic studies are rarely needed, but may be useful in cases where the abdominal wall fat layer prevents accurate diagnosis. Ultrasound is rarely helpful, but in some cases can delineate the abdominal wall musculature and note the presence of air or peristalsing bowel. Computed tomography (CT) is effective for detecting abdominal and pelvic defects; use of the Valsalva maneuver may sometimes be helpful during imaging. In some cases, attenuation of the abdominal fascia can be seen in the midline with no herniation; this is termed diastasis of the rectus muscle (Fig. 73-2).

Epigastric Hernias
Epigastric hernias occur in the midline of the abdominal wall between the umbilicus and the xiphoid in 5% of the population.

Umbilical Hernias
Umbilical hernias in adults often occur in obese, multiparous women and patients with ascites. The diagnosis is usually self-evident, with a protuberant mass at the umbilicus.

Ventral Hernias
Ventral hernias occur in the midline of the abdominal wall and can enlarge slowly. If history and physical examination do not provide an accurate diagnosis, a CT scan of the abdomen can be performed and will show a defect with herniated viscera (Fig. 73-3).

Groin Hernias
Hernias of the groin are the most common of all hernias. The inguinal canal contains the spermatic cord in males (vas deferens, spermatic artery and vein, and cremasteric muscle) and the round ligament in females, in addition to the ilioinguinal nerve. The inguinal ligament is the landmark between the abdomen and thigh. Inguinal hernias include direct and indirect forms found above the inguinal ligament, and femoral hernias found below the inguinal ligament in the femoral canal. The inferior epigastric artery serves as an important defining anatomic landmark. Indirect hernias originate lateral to this artery and protrude into the inguinal canal along the spermatic cord. Direct hernias are located medial to the inferior epigastric artery and come through a weakened inguinal floor composed of the transversalis aponeurosis and fascia (*Textbook of Gastroenterology,* 4th edition Chapter 121: Figs. 121-6*A, B*). An example of a giant inguinal hernia containing nearly all of the small intestine is shown in Fig. 73-4.

Without an operation it is difficult to determine if bowel loops are strangulated, therefore all painful tense hernias should be considered strangulated and repaired emergently. Surgical treatment is generally recommended for most inguinal and femoral hernias, because of the chance of strangulation. Suitable native tissue can be used for repair; however, polypropylene mesh repair is now widely used as standard repair for all direct and larger indirect hernias. Recurrence rates are thought to be somewhat lowered by the use of mesh, but a higher risk of infection must be taken into consideration. The laparoscopic approach to repair of hernias has recently been popularized.

Pelvic and Lumbar Hernias

The intestine can herniate through the pelvic floor (weakness, perhaps, from multiparity or previous trauma) in areas such as the obturator foramen, the greater or lesser sciatic foramina, or through the perineal muscle. The most common of these hernias is the obturator hernia. The obturator foramen is covered by a membrane except for one small area, and herniation occurs when the intestine (usually ileum) enters the foramen through this small defect and moves into the obturator region of the thigh (*Textbook of Gastroenterology*, 4th edition Chapter 121: Fig. 121-9). Most obturator herniations present with acute intestinal obstruction and no previous signs or symptoms. Sciatic hernias are extremely rare, and can present with a slowly enlarging mass in the gluteal fold area. In lumbar hernias, the posterior abdominal wall has two naturally weak areas. Lumbar hernias should be surgically repaired when first noted because they tend to enlarge, and larger hernias are more difficult to repair.

Spigelian Hernias

A spigelian hernia is rare, and occurs through the linea semilunaris, lateral to the rectus abdominis, with protrusion through the external oblique fascia (Fig. 73-5). Spigelian hernias occur in the elderly, are often small and difficult to diagnose, and always present below the arcuate line of Douglas. Symptoms include local pain or discomfort worsened by increased intra-abdominal pressure. Diagnosis can be made with ultrasound or CT scan if physical examination is difficult because of obesity or if differentiation is needed from abdominal wall tumor. Surgical repair is needed because of the risk of incarceration; the results are excellent.

Diaphragmatic Hernias

Acquired diaphragmatic hernias are the result of blunt or penetrating trauma. Most hernias occur on the left, and herniated viscera can include stomach, spleen, colon, or the left lobe of the liver.

Internal Hernias

An internal hernia is a protrusion of any intraperitoneal viscus into a compartment within the abdominal cavity. There is no hernia sac, and most often the herniated viscus is entering a known anatomical space or foramen; some hernias occur in surgically created or congenital defects.

Incisional Hernias

Incisions of the abdominal wall result in future herniation 2% to 5% of the time. Multiple factors are responsible for a postoperative incisional hernia, including defective suture material, undue tension on the sutured fascia, obesity, previous incisions, infections, seromas or hematomas, malnutrition, and smoking (Fig. 73-6). Different incisions have different rates of future herniation. Midline incisions have the highest rates; paramedian and transverse incisions have lower rates of herniation.

The diagnosis of incisional hernia is usually evident by history as well as physical exam. The hernial ring is often palpable with the edges of the muscle retracted laterally. Incisional hernias often incarcerate but tend not to strangulate. Operative repair should be undertaken in most patients. For many years, the repair of incisional hernia was associated with a high recurrence rate. Most recurrences are thought to be due to infection, insufficient dissection, and exposure of other defects, or closure under excess tension. Tension should be avoided at the time of repair and prosthetic mesh is often needed. In recent years, the introduction of synthetic prosthetic materials has provided the opportunity to perform a tension-free repair, thereby reducing the rate of recurrence. Note that recurrent herniation can occur even with mesh in place (Fig. 73-7).

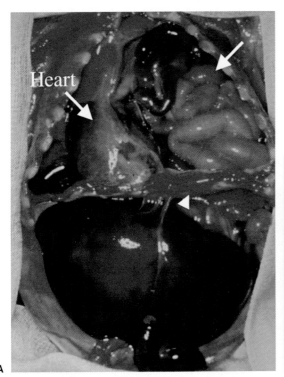

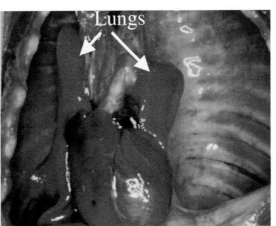

FIGURE 73-1. Congenital diaphragmatic hernia. **A:** A posterolateral diaphragmatic hernia (hernia of Bochdalek) is seen in autopsy pictures of a newborn baby. Note the intestinal loops (*arrow*) present in the left chest cavity. The diaphragmatic defect is marked with the *arrowhead*. The presence of abdominal viscera in the chest results in compression of the heart and hypoplasia of the lungs. **B:** The pulmonary hypoplasia associated with this condition. (Photographs courtesy of J. Wilson, M.D.)

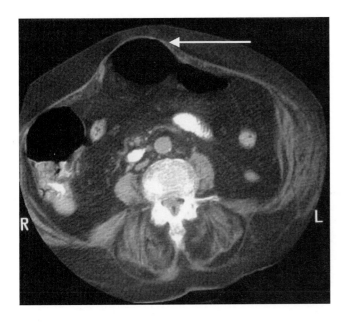

FIGURE 73-2. Diastasis recti (*arrow*). Computed tomography scan of the abdomen shows that the rectus muscle is attenuated in the midline, but there is no fascial defect; this is not a hernia. (Radiograph courtesy of J. Kruskal, M.D.)

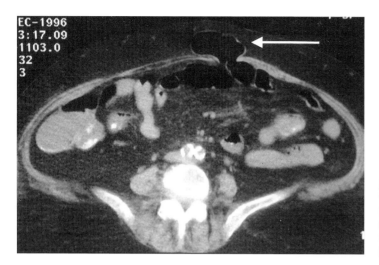

FIGURE 73-3. Ventral hernia seen on computed tomography scan of the abdomen. Note the gas-filled loop of intestine (*arrow*) going through the fascial defect and presenting in the subcutaneous tissue of the anterior abdominal wall. (Radiograph courtesy of J. Kruskal, M.D.)

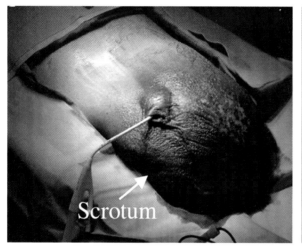

A

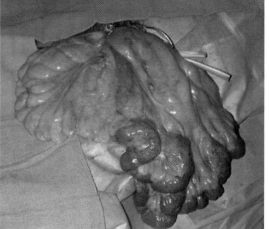

B

FIGURE 73-4. Giant inguinal hernia. **A:** Large bilateral inguinal hernia. **B:** At operation, most of the small and large intestinal contents were present in the hernia sac in the scrotum. Repair was performed with polypropylene mesh.

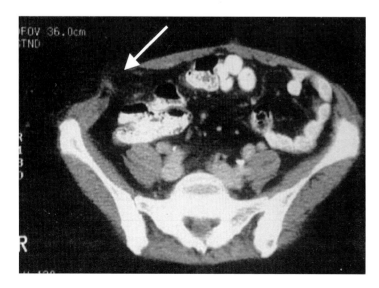

FIGURE 73-5. Spigelian hernia. Computed tomography scan of the abdomen demonstrating a spigelian hernia. These hernias are rare and occur through the linea semilunaris (*arrow*), lateral to the rectus abdominis, with protrusion through the external oblique fascia. (Radiograph courtesy of J. Kruskal, M.D.)

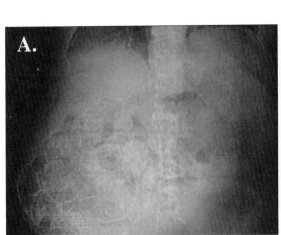

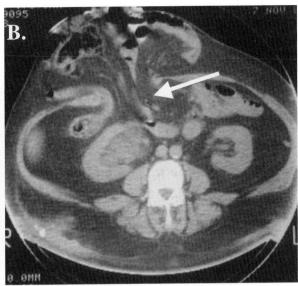

FIGURE 73-6. Large incisional hernia. Abdominal x-ray (**A**) and computed tomography scan of the abdomen (**B**) of a patient with a large incisional hernia. Note that the mesentery of the intestine is engorged and fat stranding is seen where the hernia traverses the fascia. Delay in surgical repair can result in intestinal ischemia. (Radiographs courtesy of J. Kruskal, M.D.)

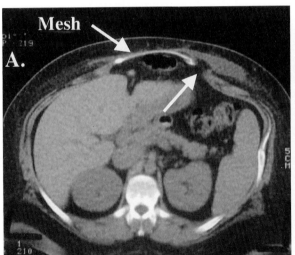

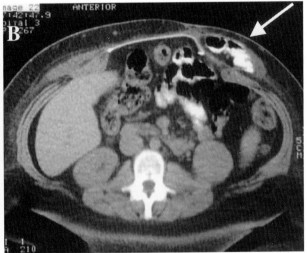

FIGURE 73-7. Recurrent ventral hernia after mesh repair. Computed tomography scan of the abdomen in a patient with a bulge 1 year after ventral hernia repair with polypropylene mesh. **A:** A fascial defect can be seen lateral to the mesh (*arrow*). **B:** A loop of intestine filled with contrast is seen in the subcutaneous tissue of the abdomen lateral to the mesh (*arrow*). (Radiographs courtesy of J. Kruskal, M.D.)

74

INTRA-ABDOMINAL ABSCESSES AND FISTULAE

FREDERIC E. ECKHAUSER ■ JAMES A. KNOL ■ MICHAEL W. MULHOLLAND
ALICIA M. TERANDO

INTRA-ABDOMINAL ABSCESSES

An intra-abdominal abscess is a well-defined collection of pus that is isolated from the rest of the peritoneal cavity by inflammatory adhesions, omentum, abdominal viscera, and loops of intestine. Abscesses may or may not contain viable bacteria, and they represent successful but incomplete attempts of normal host defense mechanisms to eradicate peritoneal infection. Intra-abdominal abscesses may occur within the peritoneal cavity or the retroperitoneum; they may be either within or adjacent to abdominal viscera. Visceral abscesses usually result from lymphatic or hematogenous spread of bacteria to the organ. Intraperitoneal, nonvisceral abscesses most commonly follow perforation of an abdominal viscus or are due to an anastomotic dehiscence. Retroperitoneal abscesses may occur as a result of perforation of the gastrointestinal tract or via lymphatic or hematogenous spread of bacteria to retroperitoneal organs. Pancreatic abscess is an example of the latter mechanism.

Intra-abdominal abscesses frequently arise in a postoperative context, with one half to three fourths occurring after an abdominal, particularly colonic, operation. Most postoperative abscesses result from an anastomotic leak. In decreasing order of frequency, diverticular disease, appendicitis, inflammatory bowel disease, and perforated visceral carcinomas account for primary, noniatrogenic intra-abdominal abscesses.

Computed tomography (CT) is the single most useful mode for investigating patients with suspected intra-abdominal abscesses. CT scanning is much less operator dependent than ultrasonography, the visual information is less abstract, and CT provides better anatomic resolution that is not affected by surgical incisions, bandages, body habitus, or the presence of bowel gas. Intralumenal fluid collections, interloop areas, and retroperitoneal structures all can be visualized. The presence of an abscess is suggested by a localized accumulation of fluid of low attenuation. CT provides information about the size and shape of cavity walls as well as the presence of loculations, gas, or debris.

728

GASTROINTESTINAL FISTULAE

A fistula is defined as an abnormal communication between the lumen of a hollow viscus and another hollow organ or the skin. Abdominal fistulae generally are classified by their sites of origin and termination, by the volume and composition of drainage, and by their etiology. The major clinical problems include fluid and electrolyte losses, skin excoriation, hypermetabolism, abscess formation, sepsis, and malnutrition. Operative or radiologic drainage of a postoperative abscess also may demonstrate an unsuspected fistula.

Fistula management is multifaceted. Adequate external drainage, control of infection, and intensive nutritional support are the keys to improved patient survival. Effective drainage of the fistula tract should be established to prevent pooling of contaminated secretions. A fistulogram should be obtained to identify the source organ and to establish optimal drainage.

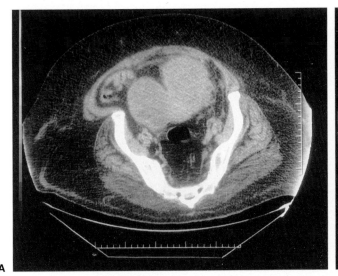
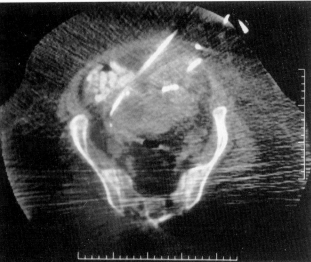

A

B

FIGURE 74-1. **A:** Computed tomographic scan of a patient with diverticular abscess as a complication of diverticular disease. **B:** The abscess was drained, allowing the diverticular disease to be treated by a one-stage sigmoid colon resection.

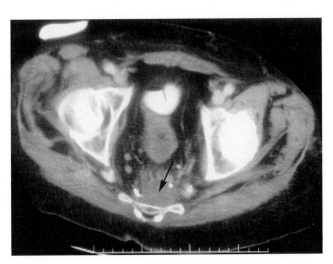

FIGURE 74-2. Computed tomographic scan of a patient with a presacral abscess (*arrow*) following abdominoperineal resection for ulcerative colitis. The abscess was suspected after purulent drainage exited the perineal wound.

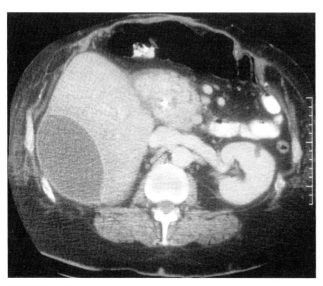

FIGURE 74-3. Computed tomogram of a patient with a hepatic abscess resulting after placement of a percutaneous transhepatic biliary drain. There are no features distinguishing this patient's fluid collection as infected, such as debris or the presence of gas bubbles.

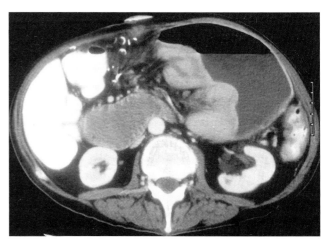

FIGURE 74-4. Computed tomogram of a patient with sepsis after a small bowel resection for Crohn's disease: The computed tomogram reveals a large abscess represented by the left anterior abdominal fluid collection containing gas (with an air-fluid level), with the medial wall bounded by small bowel.

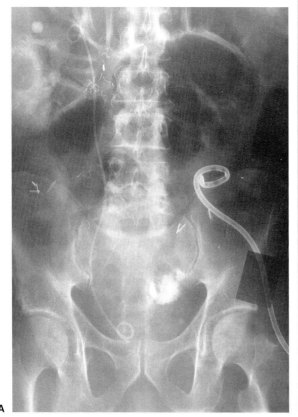
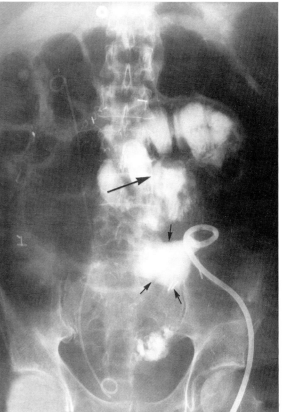

A   B

FIGURE 74-5. The sequence of radiographs demonstrates the presence of an intestinal fistula associated with a residual abscess cavity, which had been drained percutaneously. **A:** The scout film, preinjection of radiographic contrast. **B:** The coil of the all-purpose drain lies within the residual abscess cavity, which fills with contrast (*small arrows*) and then opacifies the small bowel (*large arrow*).

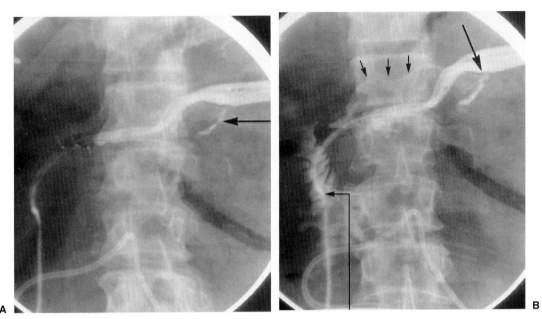

FIGURE 74-6. The sequence of radiographs demonstrates a pancreatic fistula. The patient had had Jackson-Pratt drains placed at operative debridement of infected para-pancreatic necrosis complicating acute pancreatitis. **A:** Initial contrast injection through the drain shows a linear retroperitoneal residual space (*arrow*). **B:** Additional contrast injection shows a pancreatic fistula—a connection to the pancreatic duct (*large arrow*) with contrast demonstrating the duct (*small arrows*), and emptying into the duodenum (*right-angle arrow*).

DISEASES OF THE PERITONEUM, RETROPERITONEUM, MESENTERY, AND OMENTUM

B. MARK EVERS

The peritoneum is the mesothelial lining of the peritoneal cavity that covers the walls (parietal peritoneum) and the combined viscera (visceral peritoneum) of the peritoneal cavity. Embryologically, the peritoneum is derived from the primitive coelom, which is formed by splitting of the lateral mesoderm into somatic and splanchnic layers. Diseases of the peritoneum include inflammation of the peritoneal lining (peritonitis), primary mesothelioma, and pseudomyxoma peritonei.

Peritonitis involves a local or generalized inflammatory condition of the parietal and visceral peritoneum. Although other classifications exist, a simplistic method of classifying peritonitis divides this condition into primary and secondary peritonitis. Primary peritonitis is less common and involves spontaneous infection of preexisting ascites. Different forms of secondary peritonitis can occur. Acute suppurative peritonitis is the most common. It results from spillage of intestinal contents into the peritoneal cavity as the result of an inflammatory process, perforation, or penetrating trauma. Common symptoms include abdominal pain, rebound tenderness, fever, and leukocytosis. Radiographic findings can include free air under the diaphragm if rupture of a viscus is the cause.

Management of peritonitis includes resuscitation with intravenous fluids, use of broad-spectrum antibiotics, and operative management to control the source of peritoneal contamination and irrigate the peritoneal cavity. If the source of infection is not completely eliminated with the initial operation, a planned reoperation with further debridement and irrigation is performed. In this situation, opening and closing of the abdominal cavity may be facilitated by placement of a large abdominal zipper (Fig. 75-1).

Granulomatous peritonitis, characterized by inflammation and granuloma formation, can be caused by diseases such as tuberculosis. Tuberculous peritonitis usually is associated with a primary focus elsewhere (most commonly the lung), with spread to the abdomen in approximately 1% of cases (Fig. 75-2).

Other conditions that may affect the peritoneum include the rare malignant process, primary mesothelioma, which is linked to asbestos exposure. Clinical manifestations are relatively nonspecific. The diagnosis may be obtained by means of ultrasound and computed tomographic (CT) studies (Fig. 75-3). Therapy for mesothelioma is quite disappointing because of the usually advanced stage of the disease at diagnosis and the local aggressiveness of the tumor.

Pseudomyxoma peritonei is another rare condition that can involve the peritoneal cavity and omentum. It is caused by mucinous neoplasms arising from either the appendix or the ovary. Most patients with this disease are women between the ages of 45 and 55 years. They seek treatment because of an increasing abdominal girth. Sonographic findings include multiple intraperitoneal multilocular cysts and ascitic septation. Characteristic CT findings of pseudomyxoma peritonei include scalloping of the hepatic and intestinal margins caused by extrinsic compression by ascitic spaces containing gelatinous material (Fig. 75-4). Management of pseudomyxoma peritonei is primarily surgical with aggressive debulking of all intraabdominal tumors and omentectomy. Reports suggest a survival advantage with early postoperative chemotherapy.

The retroperitoneum is the space behind the abdominal cavity that extends superiorly from the diaphragm and inferiorly to the levator muscles of the pelvis. Anteriorly, the retroperitoneal space is bounded by the posterior parietal peritoneum and the spaces between the leaves of the mesenteries of the small and large intestine. Contained within this space are the pancreas; duodenal loop; ascending and descending colon; the perinephric space with kidneys, ureters, and adrenal glands; and an extensive network of blood vessels, lymphatic vessels, and neural structures. Diseases of the retroperitoneum include retroperitoneal hemorrhage, inflammation, fibrosis, and neoplasia.

The most common cause of retroperitoneal bleeding is traumatic injury to the pelvis, vertebral column, or kidneys (Figs. 75-5 through 75-7). Other causes include anticoagulation therapy and rupture of abdominal aortic aneurysms. Signs of profuse retroperitoneal hemorrhage include those of hypovolemic shock. A CT scan often is useful, if the patient is in stable condition, to evaluate the possible cause and extent of hemorrhage. Treatment depends on the specific cause and may include fracture stabilization or arteriography for patients with a pelvic fracture, or emergency surgical intervention for ruptured abdominal aneurysm.

Retroperitoneal infections may be caused by diseases of the surrounding abdominal organs, the urinary tract, or the vertebral column (Figs. 75-8 and 75-9). Clinical manifestations include fever, chills, and nonspecific pain in the lower back and abdomen. CT scanning is the most useful diagnostic modality to establish the diagnosis. Depending on the cause, percutaneous drainage may be effective management of some of these conditions.

Retroperitoneal fibrosis is an uncommon disease characterized by progressive nonspecific inflammation and fibrosis of connective and adipose tissue in the retroperitoneal space. The main complications of this disease are compression and obstruction of the tubular structures, particularly the ureter, in the retroperitoneal space. A useful imaging study for establishing the diagnosis is intravenous pyelography, in which the triad of findings includes hydronephrosis, narrowing of the ureters, and medial displacement of the ureters (Fig. 75-10). CT scanning and magnetic resonance imaging (MRI) are useful in the diagnosis and follow-up management of this condition (Fig. 75-11). Surgical management is directed at ureterolysis for ureteral obstruction with intraperitoneal transposition of the ureters.

Tumors of the retroperitoneal space arise from mesodermal, neuroectodermal, or embryonic remnants (Fig. 75-12). Most of the rare primary neoplasms of the retroperitoneum are sarcomas, such as liposarcoma and leiomyosarcoma. Retroperitoneal tumors may grow to a large size before becoming symptomatic. The most common physical finding is the presence of a nontender abdominal mass. CT scanning is a useful imaging modality to identify the mass, determine the size and origin, and assess relations to and possible invasion of surrounding structures. MRI has become an increasingly important diagnostic tool in the management of retroperitoneal neoplasms. It allows a better degree of definition between the mass and surrounding muscle groups and vascular structures compared with CT scanning. Surgical excision offers the greatest prospect for cure and remains the best option for management of these retroperitoneal malignant tumors. Malignant tumors have a recurrence rate in the range of 30% to 50% over a 3-year period.

As the peritoneal cavity develops, the splanchnic mesoderm covers the developing gut. The ventral mesentery is mostly resorbed, except for the portion that forms the gastrohepatic omentum. The greater omentum develops from the dorsal mesogastrium. It extends from the greater curvature of the stomach caudally to fuse with the transverse colon and mesocolon. The mesentery or omentum may become involved in a variety of disease processes, most of which originate in adjacent visceral organs. These include inflammatory and vascular processes, mesenteric-omental cysts, and tumors (benign, malignant, and metastatic) (Table 75-1).

Mesenteric and omental cysts are uncommon lesions representing benign proliferation of ectopic lymphatics that lack communication with the normal lymphatic system. Some authors differentiate between mesenteric-omental cysts and cystic lymphangiomas. Lymphangiomas characteristically are found in children and are frequently large and almost always symptomatic. Ultrasonography, CT, and MRI may demonstrate the multilocular or unilocular nature of the cysts, which may have homogeneous or nonhomogeneous contents. Of the three imaging modalities, ultrasonography probably yields the most information for the least expense (Fig. 75-13).

Nonlymphangiomatous mesenteric cysts may have cuboidal or columnar lining cells or even an absent lining; however, they lack smooth muscle or lymphatic elements in their walls. The definitive diagnosis and treatment of these lesions are with surgical resection. Most types of mesenteric cysts simply can be excised (Fig. 75–14).

TABLE 75-1
Classification of Mesenteric and Omental Diseases

MESENTERIC DISEASES	OMENTAL DISEASES
Primary mesenteric inflammatory diseases	Mass lesions
Mesenteric panniculitis	Primary tumors and cysts
Retractile mesenteritis	Metastatic disease
Mesenteric cysts	Vascular lesions damaging blood supply
Embryonic and developmental cysts	Torsion
Traumatic or acquired cysts	Primary
Neoplastic cysts	Secondary: hernia, adhesion, tumor
Infective and degenerative cysts	Infarction
Mesenteric tumors	Primary
Benign tumors	Secondary: torsion, incarceration in hernia
Lipoma	
Hemangioma	
Leiomyoma	
Ganglioneuroma	
Malignant tumors	
Leiomyosarcoma	
Liposarcoma	
Rhabdomyosarcoma	
Metastatic disease	
Mesenteric fibromatosis	

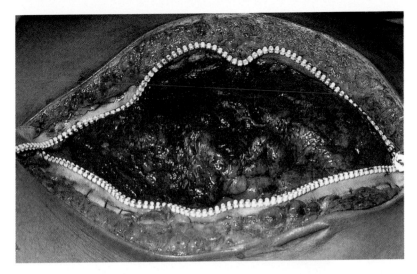

FIGURE 75-1. Patient with severe necrotizing pancreatitis with abscess requiring multiple reoperations for debridement, irrigation, and packing. An abdominal zipper was placed to facilitate abdominal opening and closing. It was removed at definitive fascial closure.

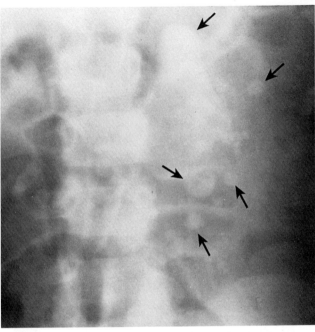

FIGURE 75-2. Abdominal radiograph of a patient with tuberculous peritonitis shows extensive calcification of the peritoneum, omentum, and lymph nodes (*arrows*). (Courtesy of Dr. Luis B. Morettin.)

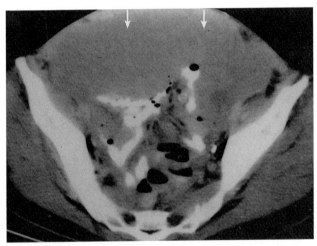

FIGURE 75-3. Computed tomographic scan of a patient with peritoneal mesothelioma demonstrates diffuse mesenteric and peritoneal involvement of a soft tissue mass (*arrows*) causing displacement of intra-abdominal organs. (Courtesy of Dr. Eric van Sonnenberg.)

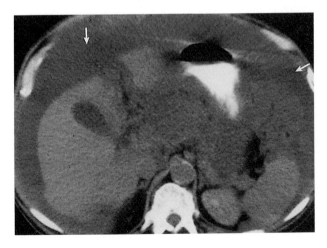

FIGURE 75-4. Computed tomographic scan of a patient with pseudomyxoma peritonei caused by adenocarcinoma of the appendix demonstrates a large amount of high-density gelatinous fluid (*arrows*) compressing the surrounding bowel. (Courtesy of Dr. Luis B. Morettin.)

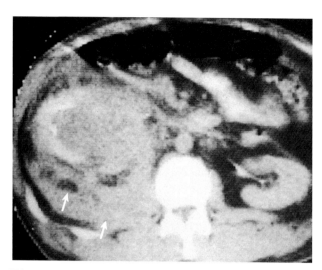

FIGURE 75-5. Computed tomographic scan demonstrates a large retroperitoneal hematoma (*arrows*) caused by hemorrhage from renal carcinoma. (Courtesy of Dr. Luis B. Morettin.)

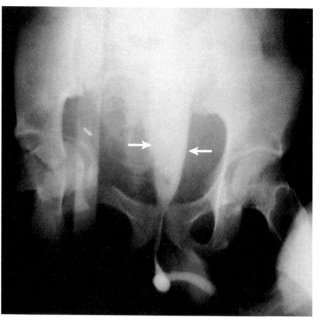

FIGURE 75-6. Cystogram of a trauma patient with a severe pelvic fracture and large retroperitoneal hematoma compressing the bladder (*arrows*).

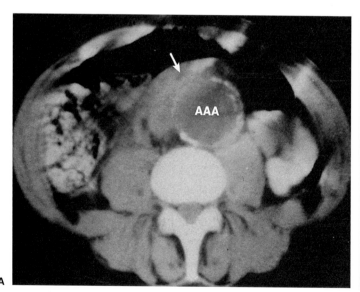

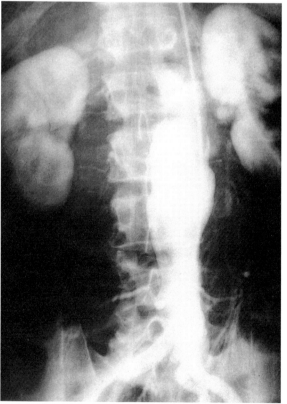

FIGURE 75-7. A: Computed tomographic scan demonstrates a large abdominal aortic aneurysm (*AAA*) with calcification in the wall of the aneurysm. A contained retroperitoneal hematoma is shown (*arrow*). **B:** Arteriogram demonstrates the abdominal aortic aneurysm shown in **A.** On arteriograms one often underestimates the size and extent of the aneurysm. (Courtesy of Dr. Luis B. Morettin.)

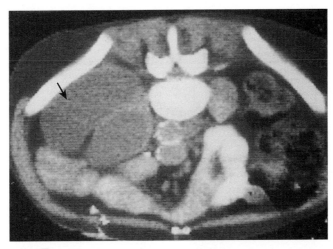

FIGURE 75-8. Computed tomographic scan shows a large retroperitoneal abscess (*arrow*) originating from an infection of a previously placed aortobifemoral graft. (Courtesy of Dr. Luis B. Morettin.)

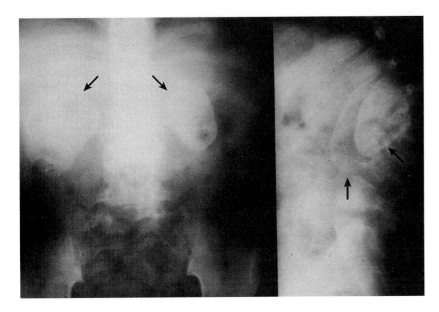

FIGURE 75-9. Abdominal radiographs (anteroposterior and lateral) demonstrate bilateral calcified psoas abscesses (*arrows*) caused by tuberculosis. (Courtesy of Dr. Luis B. Morettin.)

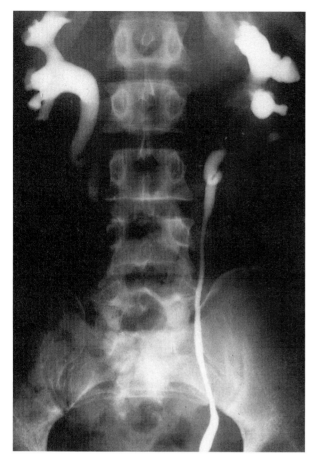

FIGURE 75-10. Intravenous pyelogram of a patient with retroperitoneal fibrosis demonstrates bilateral hydronephrosis, ureteral dilation, and narrowing without complete obstruction. (Courtesy of Dr. Luis B. Morettin.)

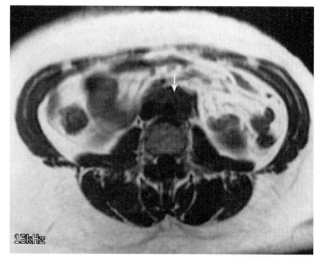

FIGURE 75-11. Axial T1-weighted magnetic resonance image of a patient with retroperitoneal fibrosis demonstrates a periaortic soft-tissue mass (*arrow*) that obliterates the fat plane. (Courtesy of Dr. Greg Chalchub.)

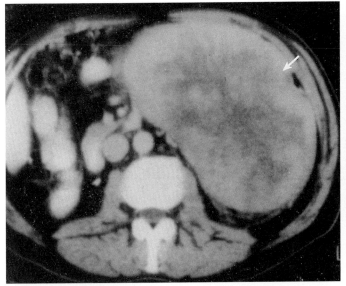

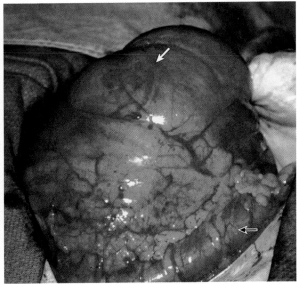

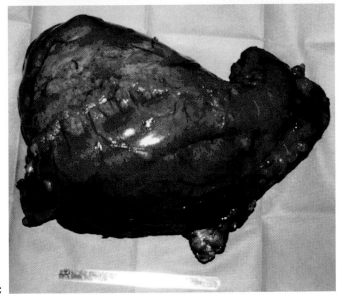

FIGURE 75-12. **A:** Computed tomographic scan demonstrates a large left retroperitoneal mass (*arrow*). **B:** Intraoperative view of the large retroperitoneal tumor shown in **A**. The tumor (*white arrow*) was contiguous with but does not invade the left kidney and descending colon (*black arrow*). **C:** Retroperitoneal tumor after resection. The kidney and descending colon were resected en bloc with the tumor, which was a hemangiopericytoma.

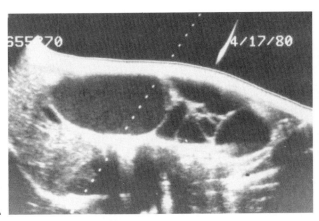

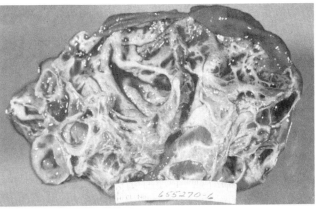

FIGURE 75-13. Sonographic appearance of a lymphangioma with gross specimen correlation. **A:** As in this sagittal section of the right abdomen, the loculi of a lymphangioma can be anechoic and contain echogenic debris and fluid-fluid levels. **B:** The corresponding gross specimen demonstrates the multilocular nature of a lymphangioma and the different kinds of fluid contained in the loculi, ranging from hemorrhagic to serous.

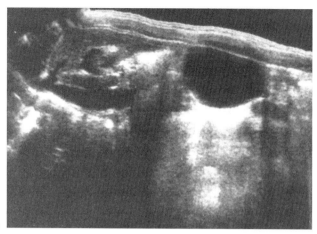

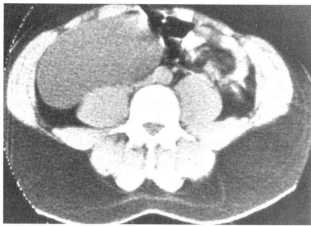

A

B

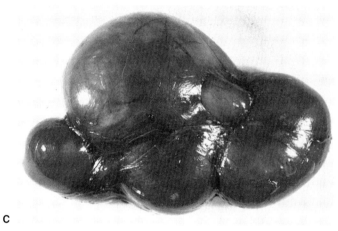

C

FIGURE 75-14. Sonographic and computed tomographic (CT) appearance of a mesothelial cyst with a pathologic correlation. **A:** A longitudinal abdominal sonogram (sagittal section, to the right of the midline) reveals an anechoic mass with acoustic enhancement. The anterior location suggests an omental location. **B:** A CT scan of another patient demonstrates a fluid-filled mass in the right lower abdomen. There is no discernible wall. **C:** Specimen corresponding to **B** shows an elongated, thin-walled cyst.

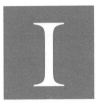

76

GASTROINTESTINAL COMPLICATIONS OF THE ACQUIRED IMMUNODEFICIENCY SYNDROME

PHILLIP D. SMITH ■ KLAUS E. MÖNKEMÜLLER ■ C. MEL WILCOX

The gastrointestinal and hepatic complications of the acquired immunodeficiency syndrome (AIDS) are caused predominantly by infection. Parasitic (mainly protozoal), viral, bacterial, and fungal pathogens cause a spectrum of mucosal disease, depending on the location and severity of the infection and the level of underlying immunosuppression. These pathogens are considered opportunistic agents in immunosuppressed persons with human immunodeficiency virus-1 (HIV-1) infection because they occur more frequently, cause more severe disease, are associated with more prolonged or recurrent infection, and more frequently develop resistance to antimicrobial drugs than the same pathogens in immunocompetent persons. Endoscopic and histological findings are key aspects of the diagnostic evaluation for these pathogens in persons with HIV-1 infection. This chapter focuses on the endoscopic and histological manifestations of representative protozoal, viral, and bacterial opportunistic pathogens of the gastrointestinal tract and recently appreciated hepatic complications in patients with AIDS (Figs. 76-1 through 76-13).

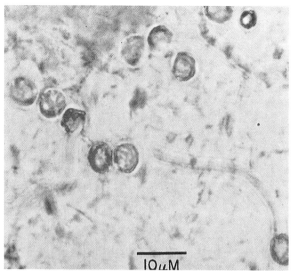

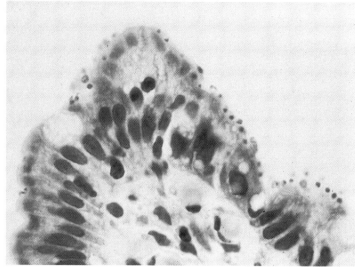

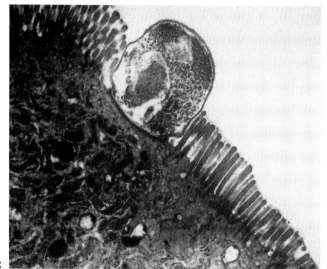

FIGURE 76-1. *Cryptosporidium* is a genus of parasitic protozoa that causes prolonged, often profuse, watery diarrhea among immunosuppressed persons with human immunodeficiency virus-1 infection, particularly in the developing world. **A:** Acid-fast–stained stool specimen shows round *Cryptosporidium* oocysts, which average 4 to 6 μm in diameter (modified Kinyoun stain; original magnification ×630). **B:** Light microscopic image shows *Cryptosporidium* protozoa lining the lumenal surface of the epithelium in an intestinal biopsy specimen from a patient with chronic diarrhea (H&E stain; original magnification ×400). **C:** Electron micrograph of an intestinal biopsy section shows a *Cryptosporidium* trophozoite that has displaced the microvilli to attach to the apical surface of an epithelial cell (original magnification ×12,500). (Courtesy of Dr. Edward N. Janoff.)

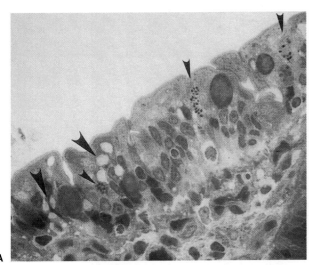

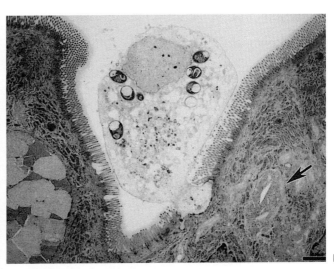

FIGURE 76-2. Microsporidan protozoa in the small intestine of persons with human immunodeficiency virus-1 infection are associated with a chronic diarrheal illness that clinically resembles cryptosporidiosis. **A:** The intensity of infection is greatest in the jejunum, where densely stained elliptic spores (*arrowheads*) are detected in epithelial cell cytoplasm by means of light microscopic examination (semithin plastic section, methylene blue-azure II, basic fuchsin stain, original magnification ×630). **B:** Electron micrograph shows a necrotic intestinal enterocyte in the final stage of being sloughed into the lumen; the enterocyte contains six microsporidian spores (*arrow*) (original magnification ×10,000). (Courtesy of Dr. Jan M. Orenstein.)

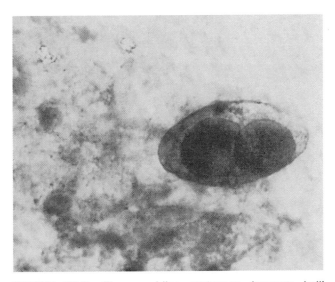

FIGURE 76-3. The coccidian protozoan *Isospora belli* causes a mild, self-limited diarrheal illness among immunocompetent persons but prolonged diarrhea among immunosuppressed persons. Infection with *I belli* is diagnosed by identification of large (20 to 30 μm × 10 to 19 μm), oval, acid-fast oocysts that contain two sporoblasts in a fresh stool specimen (modified Kinyoun stain, original magnification ×630).

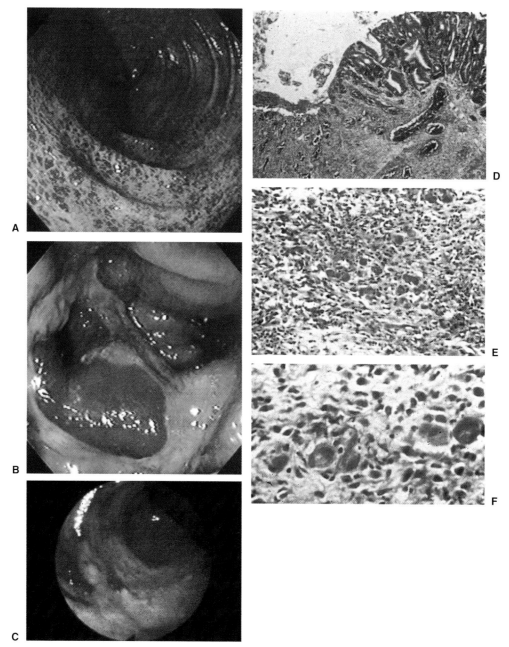

FIGURE 76-4. Cytomegalovirus infection is a common cause of inflammation and ulceration in virtually all organs of the gastrointestinal tract in persons with human immunodeficiency virus-1 infection, but colitis is the most common manifestation. **A:** Endoscopic view of diffuse colitis with prominent subepithelial hemorrhage in a patient with cytomegalovirus colitis. **B:** Endoscopic visualization of a large, well-circumscribed ulcer involving the ileocecal valve in a patient with cytomegalovirus colitis. **C:** Endoscopic view of mucosal inflammation, ulceration, and bleeding in a patient with cytomegalovirus colitis. **D:** Light microscopic examination of a colon biopsy specimen from the patient in **C** shows ulceration and hemorrhage, **(E)** infiltration by large numbers of inflammatory cells, and **(F)** numerous cytomegalic inclusion cells, which are pathognomonic of the infection. (**D, E, F,** H&E stain; **D,** original magnification ×30; **E,** original magnification ×62; **F,** original magnification ×125).

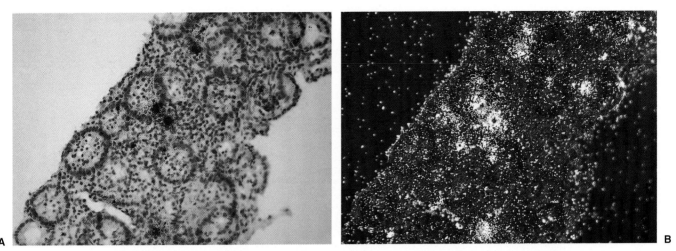

FIGURE 76-5. Cytomegalovirus infection of mononuclear inflammatory cells in the gastrointestinal tract mucosa may induce local production of certain cytokines, such as tumor necrosis factor-α (TNF-α), which mediates inflammation. **A:** Light-field and (**B**) dark-field illumination of cells expressing TNF-α mRNA in colonic tissue sections by means of in situ hybridization with a TNF-α RNA-specific (antisense) probe (original magnification ×125).

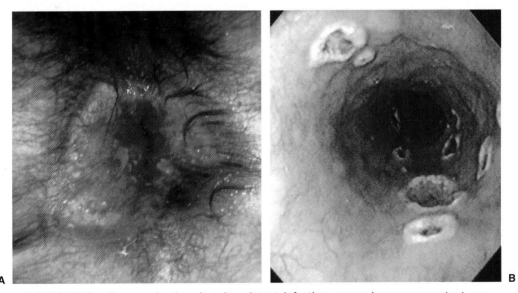

FIGURE 76-6. Herpes simplex virus is a latent infection among immunocompetent persons, but in persons infected with human immunodeficiency virus-1 (HIV-1), the virus can cause severe inflammation and ulceration of the anus and perianal region, rectum (proctitis), and esophagus (esophagitis). **A:** The perianal ulceration of this severely immunosuppressed patient with HIV-1 infection caused pain, tenesmus, and bleeding. A culture from the ulcer bed revealed herpes simplex virus. **B:** Multiple small, well-circumscribed shallow ulcers are typical of herpes simplex virus esophagitis.

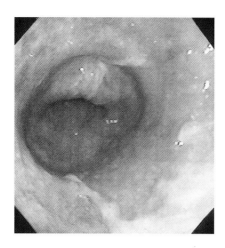

FIGURE 76-7. Bacterial infections with *Salmonella* species, *Shigella flexneri,* and *Campylobacter jejuni* cause a similar clinical illness in persons infected with human immunodeficiency virus-1 (HIV-1), characterized by recurrent or chronic diarrhea commonly associated with fever and abdominal cramps. Endoscopic visualization of the colon of a patient infected with HIV-1 shows superficial erosions, erythema, pus, and loss of the normal vascular pattern. A biopsy specimen of the area grew *C jejuni*.

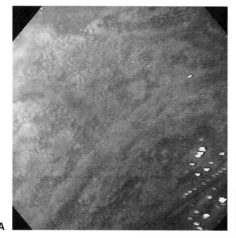

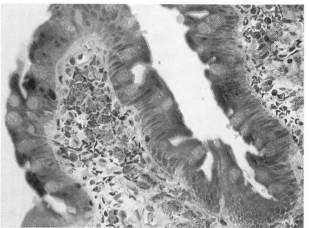

FIGURE 76-8. *Mycobacterium avium* complex is one of the most common bacterial pathogens identified in the gastrointestinal tract of immunosuppressed patients infected with human immunodeficiency virus-1. Gastrointestinal involvement usually indicates disseminated infection and is associated with diarrhea, weight loss, and fever. **A:** Endoscopic image of the duodenum in a patient with acquired immunodeficiency syndrome with disseminated *M avium* complex infection who had diarrhea, abdominal pain, weight loss, and fever shows multiple small yellow plaques, some of which have coalesced in the second portion of the duodenum. **B:** Light micrograph of a biopsy section from the duodenum shows numerous lamina propria macrophages engorged with mycobacteria (methylene blue-azure II, basic fuchsin stain; original magnification ×100).

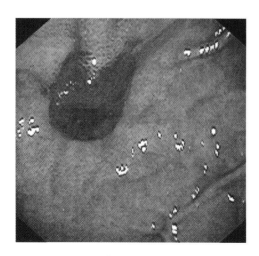

FIGURE 76-9. Kaposi sarcoma of the stomach in a patient with acquired immunodeficiency syndrome. Endoscopic view shows the typical nodularity and dark red color of such lesions. With the widespread use of highly active antiretroviral therapy, Kaposi sarcoma, a neoplasm associated with human herpes virus type 8 infection, has become an uncommon malignancy associated with immunosuppression in patients infected with human immunodeficiency virus-1.

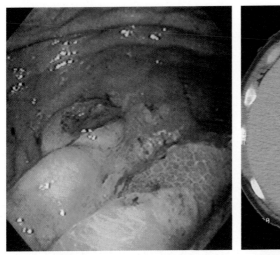
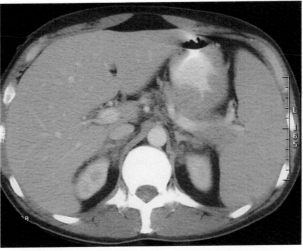

A   B

FIGURE 76-10. **A:** Endoscopic view of the stomach of a patient with acquired immunodeficiency syndrome (AIDS) and non-Hodgkin lymphoma of the stomach shows thickened gastric folds with superficial erosions and edema. **B:** Abdominal computed tomography scan with contrast from the same patient shows markedly thickened gastric mucosa; gastric distention is limited because of the hardened stomach walls that are infiltrated by tumor. Although the overall survival of AIDS patients with non-Hodgkin lymphoma has increased since the introduction of highly active antiretroviral therapy (HAART), the incidence of this tumor among AIDS patients has not decreased significantly.

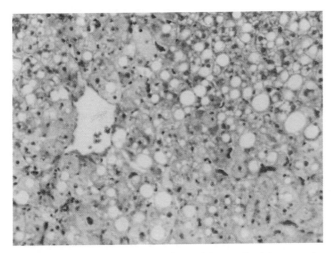

FIGURE 76-11. A female patient with acquired immunodeficiency syndrome (AIDS) taking stavudine presented with abdominal pain, nausea, vomiting, myalgias, hepatomegaly, elevated liver enzymes, and type B lactic acidosis. Liver biopsy shows macro- and microvesicular steatosis without cholestasis. Fatty infiltration is the most common hepatic complication in patients with AIDS, particularly those taking antiretroviral drugs, such as zidovudine, didanosine, and stavudine. In addition to hepatic steatosis, these agents have been associated with myopathy, type B lactic acidosis, and fulminant hepatic failure.

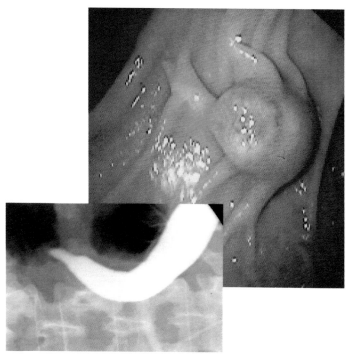

FIGURE 76-12. Endoscopic view of the ampulla of Vater in a patient with acquired immunodeficiency syndrome (AIDS) with abdominal pain and an elevated alkaline phosphatase shows a protuberant papilla that is edematous, erythematous, and partially covered by exudate. The **insert** shows an endoscopic retrograde cholangiogram of the patient's stenotic distal common bile duct. The bile duct wall shows an irregular "fuzzy" wall typical of human immunodeficiency virus (HIV) cholangiopathy. Biopsy of the ampulla of Vater revealed *Cryptosporidium*. AIDS cholangiopathy is defined as inflammation of the biliary tract in a patient infected with HIV-1, and is most commonly due *Cryptosporidium*, cytomegalovirus, and microsporidia.

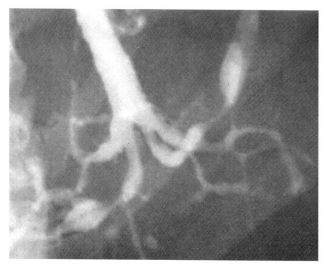

FIGURE 76-13. Endoscopic retrograde cholangiogram in a patient with acquired immunodeficiency syndrome with cholangiopathy shows an irregular and distorted biliary tract with multiple areas of dilation and stricture.

Acknowledgment

This work is supported in part by the National Institutes of Health (DK-47322 and HD-41361) and the Medical Research Service of the Department of Veterans Affairs.

77

PARASITIC DISEASES: Protozoa

ELLEN LI ■ SAMUEL L. STANLEY JR.

The intestinal parasitic protozoa are being increasingly recognized as important causes of diarrheal illness worldwide. Infestation with *Entamoeba histolytica*, the causative agent of amebic dysentery and amebic liver abscess, is primarily a disease of developing countries. Infestation with *Giardia lamblia*, *Cryptosporidium parvum*, and *Cyclospora cayetanensis*, however, poses serious threats to public health in the United States and the rest of the world. Large-scale outbreaks of cryptosporidiosis and cyclosporiasis in the United States have greatly increased physician and public awareness of these diseases. Physicians (gastroenterologists in particular) must consider these pathogens in the differential diagnosis of acute and chronic diarrhea and should be familiar with the optimal diagnostic (Table 77-1) and therapeutic approaches to these diseases.

AMEBIASIS

Improved sanitation conditions have greatly reduced the number of cases of amebiasis in the United States. Disease in the United States is probably most commonly detected among immigrants from countries where amebiasis is endemic. The diagnosis of amebiasis should be considered for all persons with dysentery and an appropriate travel or exposure history. *E histolytica* trophozoites can be seen in wet mounts of stool, ulcer scrapings, or intestinal aspirates obtained during endoscopy and in fixed specimens stained with trichrome (Fig. 77-1). Trophozoites are usually 10 to 20 μm in diameter but can be as large as 60 μm.

Important morphologic clues in the identification of an ameba as *E histolytica* are a pale, round nucleus with a small central karyosome and the presence of ingested erythrocytes (erythrophagocytosis). *E histolytica* trophozoites can be confused with other *Entamoeba* organisms and, not uncommonly, fecal leukocytes. Cysts are 9 to 25 μm in diameter and contain four nuclei. An important diagnostic problem is the fact that *E histolytica* is morphologically identical to the genetically distinct nonpathogenic *Entamoeba dispar* species. New antigen-detection enzyme-linked immunosorbent assays (ELISA) that specifically recognize *E histolytica* and not *E dispar* in stool may replace microscopic examination as the test of choice for the diagnosis of intestinal amebiasis.

E histolytica trophozoites invade the colonic mucosa and cause ulcer formation. The appearance of the colon in symptomatic amebic colitis can include discrete ulcers covered with yellowish-white exudate (Fig. 77-2*A*), multiple well-defined ulcers (Fig. 77-2C), diffuse erythema and ulceration (Fig. 77-2D), and rarely, heaped-up inflammatory and granulation tissue that forms an ameboma (Fig. 77-2B). Pseudomembrane formation can be seen.

The most frequent extraintestinal manifestation of *E histolytica* infestation is amebic liver abscess. Patients usually have the triad of fever, right upper quadrant pain and tenderness, and a space-occupying lesion in the liver. Amebic serologic tests almost always have positive results among patients with amebic liver abscess and should be performed when amebic liver abscess is suspected. Patients can seek treatment years after residing in an endemic area and with no history of diarrheal illness, so a complete travel and immigration history is important. Rupture of an amebic liver abscess into the pleural cavity is not uncommon. As illustrated in Fig. 77-3, an initial clue to the presence of amebic liver abscess may be an abnormal chest radiograph showing elevation of the right hemidiaphragm, right pleural effusion, and possibly a right basilar infiltrate. Amebic liver abscesses often are solitary, usually involve the right lobe, and often are visible on computed tomographic (CT) scans as large, generally homogenous, low-attenuation lesions (Fig. 77-4). However, multiple abscesses can develop.

BLASTOCYSTIS

Blastocystis hominis is one of the protozoan organisms frequently detected in stools. It inhabits the colon and is typically seen in stool as a spherical organism with nuclei and other organelles arranged around a large central vacuole (Fig. 77-5). The pathogenicity of this organism continues to be controversial. Symptomatic *Blastocystis* infestation (mild diarrhea, nausea, anorexia, and fatigue) should be considered a diagnosis of exclusion. If symptoms persist after therapy, there should be further investigation for other causes of intestinal disease. Optimum therapy has not been established, but metronidazole, iodoquinol, and furazolidone all have been reported to have some degree of efficacy in anecdotal reports.

GIARDIASIS

G lamblia has been the most common intestinal parasitic cause of diarrhea in the United States in recent years. Groups at high risk for giardiasis include children in day-care facilities and their adult contacts, travelers, and persons who consume contaminated water. *Giardia* can cause both an acute, self-limited, watery, nonbloody diarrheal syndrome and a chronic diarrhea syndrome with prominent signs of malabsorption and considerable weight loss. Chronic and severe infections are more likely to develop among persons with hypogammaglobulinemia, selective immunoglobulin A deficiency, and nodular hyperplasia. Abundant *Giardia* trophozoites may be seen in the biopsy samples from the small intestine of these persons (Fig. 77-6). The diagnosis of *G lamblia* infestation is based primarily on detection of trophozoites and cysts in the stool by means of microscopic analysis of stained stool specimens (Fig. 77-7). Many persons, however, appear to only intermittently excrete trophozoites and cysts, making diagnosis difficult. Antigen detection tests are available that permit detection of *G lamblia,* as well as *E histolytica* and *C parvum*. These tests may be valuable as initial screening tests for individuals with diarrhea. Another rapid screening test is an immunofluorescence assay (MeriFluor, Meridian Bioscience, Inc., Cincinnati, OH), which can be used to detect both *G lamblia* cysts and *C parvum* oocysts (Fig. 77-8).

DIENTAMOEBA FRAGILIS

Dientamoeba fragilis is a species of flagellated protozoa increasingly identified in stool samples. The organism is ameboid in shape and ranges in size from 5 to 15 μm; the flagella are not visible (Fig. 77-9). There is no known cyst form. Symptoms ascribed to this organism include mild diarrhea, abdominal pain, anorexia, and fatigue. Adults are treated with diiodohydroxyquin (650 mg three times a day for 3 weeks); tetracycline (500 mg four times a day for 1 week) is an alternative. For children, metronidazole is recommended; paromomycin is an alternative.

BALANTIDIASIS

Balantidium coli is a ciliate parasite that is a rare cause of intestinal disease among humans. It can invade the colonic mucosa (Fig. 77-10) and cause colonic ulceration. Diagnosis is made by observation of the large motile trophozoites in saline mounts of stool. Cysts are more rarely seen and are 50 to 75 μm in diameter with a large macronucleus. Optimum therapy is unclear, but tetracycline (500 mg four times a day for 10 days) or iodoquinol (650 mg three times a day for 3 weeks) is recommended.

COCCIDIA (*CRYPTOSPORIDIUM, ISOSPORA, AND CYCLOSPORA*)

Since the onset of the acquired immunodeficiency syndrome (AIDS) epidemic, coccidial organisms from the genera *Cryptosporidium, Cyclospora,* and *Isospora* have emerged not only as important gastrointestinal protozoan pathogens among immunocompromised hosts but also as causative agents of diarrhea among immunocompetent hosts. These organisms cause an acute self-limited diarrheal illness among immunocompetent hosts that can be somewhat prolonged, and they can cause severe, chronic diarrhea among patients with AIDS and other forms of immune dysfunction. *C parvum* is a common cause of diarrhea among patients with AIDS in the United States. It is one of the leading causative agents of water-borne disease outbreaks and has become a serious public health problem in the United States. *Cyclospora* and *Isospora* are seen less commonly in the United States but are prevalent in developing countries and should be suspected among travelers returning from endemic areas. Multiple outbreaks (encompassing nearly 1500 cases) of food-borne (associated with the consumption of contaminated raspberries) cyclosporiasis in the United States during the summer of 1996 increased public awareness of this disease.

These organisms are intracellular pathogens with similar life cycles (Fig. 77-11), which may account for their similar clinical manifestations. All these organisms undergo asexual replication within the enterocyte to produce a merozoite stage, which leads to autoinfection of other enterocytes and rapid spread of the infection within the epithelium. They also undergo a sexual stage that leads to generation of cysts or spores, which are sloughed into the gastrointestinal lumen and excreted in stool. Cryptosporidia can form infectious sporozoites within the host, leading to further autoinfection. Unlike the situation with *Cyclospora* and *Isospora,* maturation of infectious sporozoites must take place outside the host.

The diagnosis of these parasitic diseases generally is made by examination of the stool. The acid-fast stain may be the most useful stain for detecting these organisms (Figs. 77-12 and 77-13). Some laboratories may not routinely search for these organisms, and the physician may need to submit special requests to the laboratory. The organisms differ in size and shape (see Figs. 77-12 and 77-13; Table 77-1).

Cryptosporidium and *Cyclospora* organisms are particularly difficult to differentiate from each other, and measurements must be made to confirm the size difference. Smears and biopsies of small intestine aspirates may be useful for the diagnosis of infestation with these organisms (Figs. 77-14 through 77-16; see Table 77-1). Cryptosporidia can be easily detected at routine light microscopic examination as 4-μm basophilic dots on the apical surface of enterocytes and are typically located within crypt cells (see Fig. 77-14). The organism is intracellular but extracytoplasmic (see Fig. 77-15). Direct fluorescence assay allows screening by fluorescent microscopic examination, which can provide rapid and accurate results (see Fig. 77-8). *Isospora* organisms can be detected at light microscopic examination as 20-μm inclusions within the enterocyte and are typically located within villous enterocytes (see Fig. 77-16). With a heavy organism burden, *Cyclospora* organisms have been identified at light microscopic examination of duodenal biopsy specimens, but transmission electron microscopic examination may be a more sensitive approach.

Treatment with trimethoprim-sulfamethoxazole shortens the course of isosporiasis and cyclosporiasis in immunocompetent hosts and is required for cure among immunocompromised hosts. *Cryptosporidium* infestation is difficult to manage, although nitazoxanide appears to have some efficacy. Patients with AIDS need life-long suppressive therapy to prevent relapse.

(figures begin on page 754)

TABLE 77-1
Morphologic Features of Human Gastrointestinal Protozoan Parasites

TYPE OF PARASITE	STOOL	INTESTINAL BIOPSY
Extracellular ameboid		
Entamoeba histolytica	Trophozoite 10–20 μm Pale, round nucleus with small central karyosome Cyst 9–25 μm, four nuclei Morphologically indistinguishable from *Entamoeba dispar* ELISA: fecal antigen detection of trophozoite antigen can differentiate *E histolytica* from *E dispar*; serologic testing may be useful adjunct	Trophozoites but not cysts seen invading colonic mucosa causing colonic ulcerations
Blastocystis hominis (pathogenicity is controversial)	Organisms 6–40 μm, round with large central body or vacuole	
Flagellates		
Giardia lamblia	Trophozoite pear shaped, 10–20 μm long, characteristic face-like image because of two nuclei, each with prominent karyosome Cyst oval, 7–10 μm long Direct fluorescence antibody test available in many laboratories for detection of cysts ELISA for fecal antigen detection may be available in some laboratories	Trophozoites seen most commonly on duodenal mucosal surface, but also on jejunal and ileal biopsy specimens Histologic features usually normal, but villus atrophy seen in severe infections
Dientamoeba fragilis	Appears ameboid in shape, 10–15 μm, with flagella not visible, one or two nuclei No known cyst form	
Ciliate		
Balantidium coli (rare)	Trophozoite 50–200 μm in length, motile Cysts are rarely seen in stool and are 50–75 μm in diameter	Trophozoites can invade into colonic mucosa causing ulceration
Intracellular		
Coccidia		
Cryptosporidium parvum	*May need to submit special request to laboratory* Modified acid-fast stain: oocysts stain uniformly, are round, 4–6 μm, contains four sporozoites that may or may not be visible Direct fluorescence assay may be helpful in detecting cysts	Intracellular forms seen as 4–μm extracytoplasmic dots on the apical surface of enterocytes Distribution may be patchy
Isospora belli	May be observed on wet preparation *May need to submit special request to laboratory* Modified acid-fast stain: oocysts stain uniformly, appear oval, 20–30 μm, with two sporocysts, each containing four sporozoites	Intracellular forms seen as 20–μm intracytoplasmic inclusions within the enterocyte at light microscopic examination Distribution may be patchy
Cyclospora catayensis	May be observed on wet preparation *May need to submit special request to laboratory* Modified acid-fast stain: oocysts stain variably, resemble *Cryptosporidia* oocysts but are larger, 8–10 μm Contains two sporocysts each with two sporozoites Oocysts autofluoresce under ultraviolet light (365 nm)	Intracellular forms difficult to see at light microscopic examination Intracellular forms have been seen at electron microscopic examination as intracytoplasmic inclusions

ELISA, enzyme-linked immunosorbent assay.

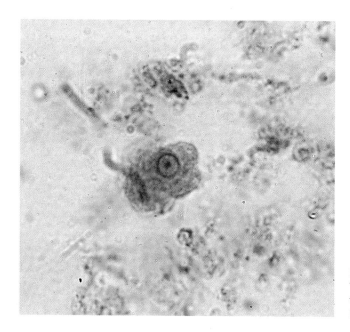

FIGURE 77-1. *Entamoeba histolytica* trophozoite in stool. This trophozoite is approximately 20 μm in diameter and has the characteristic round nucleus with a small, centrally placed karyosome. (Courtesy of Patrick Murray, Ph.D.)

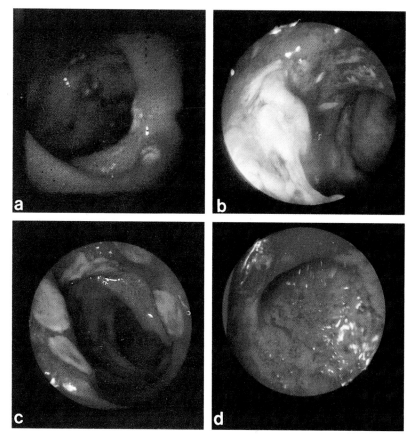

FIGURE 77-2. Rectosigmoidoscopic images show part of the pathological spectrum of intestinal amebiasis. **A:** Ulcers covered with yellowish-white secretion. **B:** Heaped-up granulation tissue forming an ameboma. **C:** Multiple well-defined ulcers. **D:** Diffuse erythema and ulceration.

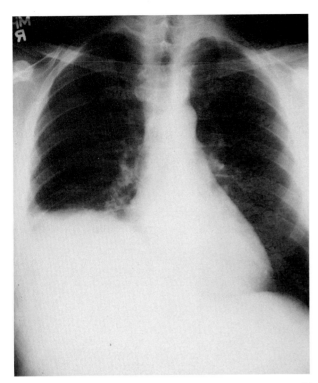

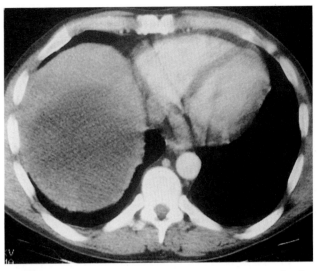

FIGURE 77-3. Chest radiograph of a patient with amebic liver abscess that has ruptured into the right pleural space. Elevated right hemidiaphragm, pleural effusion, and basilar infiltrate are depicted. This patient was initially thought to have bacterial pneumonia and empyema.

FIGURE 77-4. Computed tomographic scan of the abdomen demonstrates a large amebic liver abscess in the right lobe of the liver.

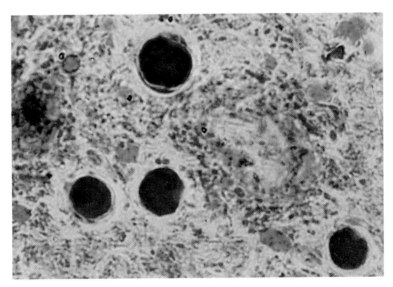

FIGURE 77-5. Trichrome stain of *Blastocystis hominis* organism.

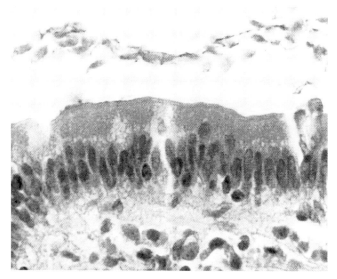

FIGURE 77-6. Multiple *Giardia lamblia* trophozoites that were lying on the surface of duodenal mucosa.

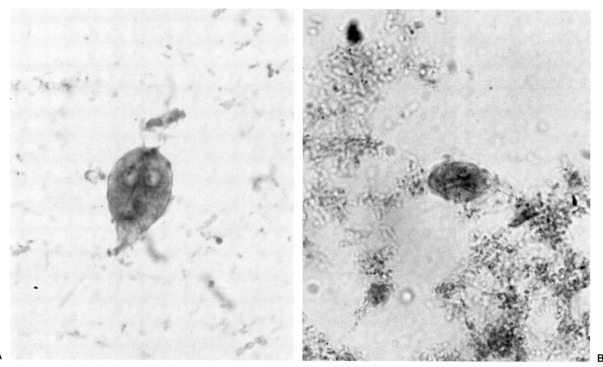

A

B

FIGURE 77-7. Trichrome stain of *Giardia lamblia* trophozoite (**A**) and cyst (**B**) in stool. (Courtesy of Patrick Murray, Ph.D.)

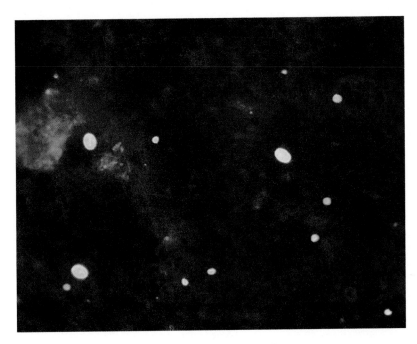

FIGURE 77-8. *Giardia lamblia* cysts (larger ellipsoid, with some internal detail present) and *Cryptosporidium parvum* oocysts (smaller, spherical) in a stool sample are revealed by direct fluorescence assay. (Courtesy of Meridian Diagnostics, Inc.)

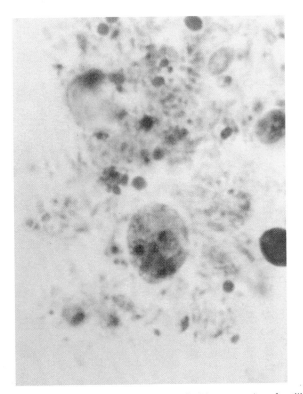

FIGURE 77-9. Trichrome stain of *Dientamoeba fragilis* organism. Although this organism is a flagellate, its appearance mimics that of amebas.

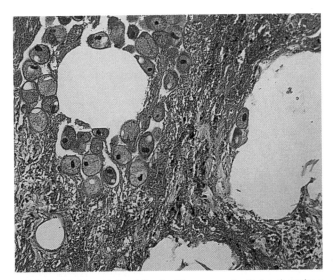

FIGURE 77-10. Balantidiasis. Numerous large trophozoites in the wall of the intestine in a patient with acquired immunodeficiency syndrome.

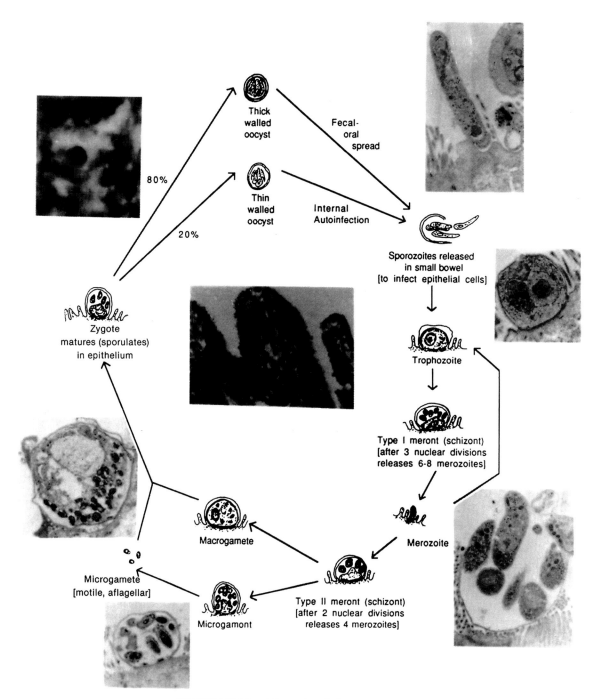

FIGURE 77-11. Life cycle of *Cryptosporidium*.

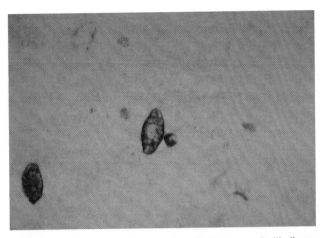

FIGURE 77-12. Acid-fast stain of *Isospora belli* (large oocyst) and *Cryptosporidium* oocyst (small oocyst) in a patient from Haiti. (Courtesy of Dr. Madeline Boncy and Dr. Rosemary Soave.)

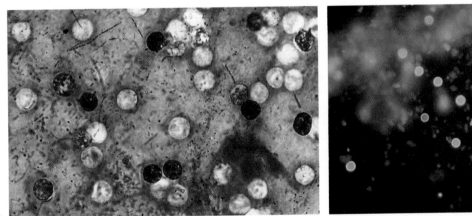
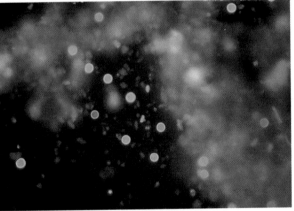

FIGURE 77-13. *Cyclospora catayensis.* **A:** Modified acid fast stain of *Cyclospora* oocysts shows multiple, well-stained, poorly stained, and unstained oocysts within the same field. **B:** Autofluorescence of *Cyclospora* oocysts. (Courtesy of Earl G. Long.)

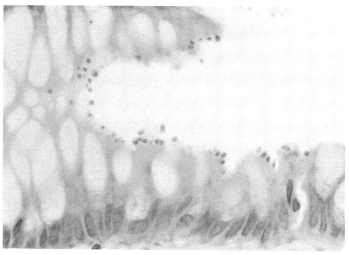

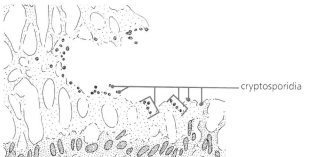

FIGURE 77-14. Cryptosporidia are seen as 4-μm dots on the apical surface of enterocytes.

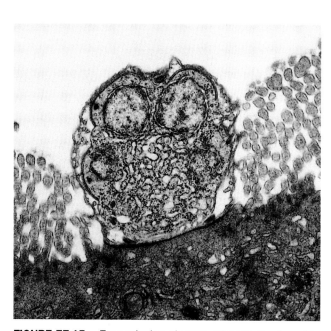

FIGURE 77-15. Transmission electron micrograph of a schizont stage of *Cryptosporidium parvum* attached to the intestinal epithelium. The organism is surrounded by the enterocyte plasma membrane but is separated from the cytoplasm by the membrane of a parasitophorous vacuole. (Courtesy of Dr. Paul Swanson.)

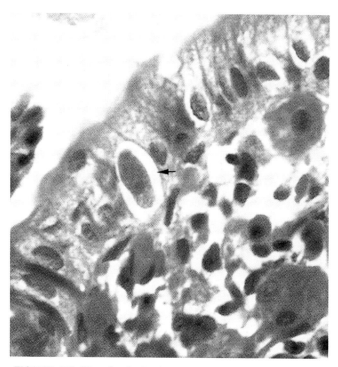

FIGURE 77-16. A single *Isospora belli* organism (*arrow*) appears as a 20-μm inclusion within an enterocyte.

78

PARASITIC DISEASES: Helminths

RICHARD D. PEARSON

The intestinal helminths are classified as nematodes (roundworms) or platyhelminths (flatworms), which are further divided into the cestodes (tapeworms) and trematodes (flukes). This classification is useful clinically because related helminths often have similar life cycles, metabolic pathways, and susceptibilities to chemotherapeutic agents.

INTESTINAL NEMATODES

Intestinal nematodes are among the most prevalent of the parasites that infect humans. They have complex and varied life cycles. Ova of some, such as *Trichuris trichiura*, are ingested in fecally contaminated food or water and release larvae that develop within the confines of the gastrointestinal tract. Adult female worms release characteristic ova in the stool (Fig. 78-1). *Enterobius vermicularis*, the pinworm, likewise develops in the gastrointestinal tract. Mature adult females migrate from the anus. Perianal or perineal pruritus results after ova are deposited on the skin by means of uterine contraction or death of the worm. On rare occasion, adult pinworms migrate into the genital tract of girls or women. Egg-induced granulomas have been identified in the vagina, uterus, salpinx, or peritoneal cavity (Fig. 78-2).

Ascaris lumbricoides is the most prevalent intestinal helminth in the world. Ova in fecally contaminated food or water are ingested and hatch in the intestine. Larvae traverse the intestinal wall, enter the circulation, travel to the lungs, break into the alveoli, and ascend the trachea. They are swallowed and complete their development in the gastrointestinal tract. *A lumbricoides* is the only intestinal nematode that has the length and size of an earthworm (Fig. 78-3). Adult *A lumbricoides* worms occasionally migrate into or obstruct the common bile duct. If large numbers are present, the worms form a bolus that obstructs the intestine. The diagnosis is usually made by means of identifying unembryonated (Fig. 78-4) or embryonated ova in the stool. Adult worms occasionally are seen in the feces or migrate from the oropharynx or nose.

Worldwide, the hookworms, *Necator americanus* and *Ancylostoma duodenale*, are important causes of iron deficiency anemia. Infectious filariform larvae in the soil enter the skin, pass through the lungs, are swallowed, and reach maturity in the gastrointestinal tract. Adult hookworms (Fig. 78-5) secrete an anticoagulant that keeps the blood flowing into their gastrointestinal tracts. Examination of unconcentrated stool is sufficient to identify clinically significant infestation. Ova (Fig. 78-6) of the two hookworm species are indistinguishable from one another.

Strongyloides stercoralis has a life cycle similar to that of the hookworms, but it is unique among the intestinal nematodes in its ability to autoinfect and cause disseminated hyperinfection among immunocompromised persons. Those concurrently infected with human T-lymphotropic virus-1 (HTLV-1) or taking corticosteroids are at greatest risk of hyperinfection. In such cases, large numbers of filariform larvae invade through the intestine. Mucosal damage may be severe; larvae can enter the lungs, central nervous system, and other organs. Death can result either because of the larvae or infection caused by enteric bacteria that accompany them. Identification of larvae confirms the diagnosis (Fig. 78-7).

Trichinella spiralis has a complex life cycle. Encysted larvae in the muscle of wild or domestic hogs, bears, or other infested animals are released in the human gastrointestinal tract when raw or inadequately cooked meat is eaten. Larvae develop to adulthood over a period of several days. Adult female worms subsequently produce larvae that invade the human intestine, disseminate throughout the body, and encyst in muscle (Fig. 78-8). Severe myalgia, periorbital edema, and eosinophilia are common among persons with trichinosis (Fig. 78-9).

On occasion, humans become infested with intestinal nematodes that are primarily pathogens of animals. For example, ingestion of animal ascarids such as *Toxocara canis* can result in visceral larva migrans. Penetration of the skin by *Ancylostoma braziliense,* an animal hookworm, can result in cutaneous larva migrans (Fig. 78-10), and another animal hookworm, *Ancylostoma caninum,* has been associated with eosinophilic enteritis among humans.

CESTODES

Cestodes, or tapeworms, live as adults in the gastrointestinal tract of their definitive hosts and as solid or bladder larvae in the tissues of their vertebrate or invertebrate intermediate hosts. *Diphyllobothrium latum,* which is acquired through ingestion of inadequately cooked fish, has broad, short proglottids (Fig. 78-11) and distinctive ova (Fig. 78-12), and competes with its human host for vitamin B_{12}.

Adult *Taenia saginata,* the beef tapeworm (Fig. 78-13), and *Taenia solium,* the pork tapeworm, have long, rectangular proglottids. Ova of these species (Fig. 78-14) are indistinguishable from one another. A species-specific diagnosis can be made by examining the proglottids (Fig. 78-15).

T solium can use humans as either a definitive or an intermediate host. In the latter instance, ova ingested in fecally contaminated food or water excyst in the intestine, releasing larvae that invade the mucosa, disseminate throughout the body, and form cysticerci (Fig. 78-16) in the brain, muscle, and other tissues. Cysticerci can be particularly troublesome in the central nervous system. They may damage critical structures as they enlarge, or they may cause no symptoms. There is usually little surrounding inflammatory response when a cysticercus is viable (Fig. 78-17), but parasite antigens that are released from dying cysticerci can elicit inflammatory responses. The diagnosis of neurocysticercosis is usually made by computed tomographic scanning or magnetic resonance imaging.

Humans also serve as an intermediate host for *Echinococcus granulosus* and *Echinococcus multilocularis.* The adult tapeworms of these species live in dogs or other canines. *E granulosus* is the most prevalent. It tends to cause large, multiloculated cysts, which are usually found in the liver (Fig. 78-18). The cysts contain "hydatid sand" composed of protoscolices (Fig. 78-19).

TREMATODES

Schistosoma species are the most prevalent of the flukes that infest humans. Adult female and male schistosomes live as pairs in venules in their human hosts (Fig. 78-20). *Schistosoma mansoni* lives primarily in the distribution of the superior mesenteric vein, whereas *S japonicum* usually is found in the distribution of the inferior mesenteric vein. Lytic enzymes allow ova to penetrate the walls of the venules and ultimately to reach the lumen of the intestine. Schistosomiasis is diagnosed by identification of ova (Figs. 78-21 and 78-22) in concentrated stool samples or in biopsy specimens of colonic mucosa. Ova that are carried to the liver through the portal circulation can elicit inflammatory responses, fibrosis, and hepatosplenic schistosomiasis that may ultimately be complicated by portal hypertension.

Other trematodes inhabit the biliary tract or intestine. *Clonorchis sinensis,* the Chinese liver fluke, and the closely related *Opisthorchis viverrini,* are acquired by eating inadequately cooked or raw contaminated freshwater fish. The adult flukes live in the biliary tract, and ova are excreted in the feces (Fig. 78-23). Although infestations with these flukes are often asymptomatic, they can persist for decades and have been associated with biliary tract pathology and the development of cholangiocarcinoma. The diagnosis of other liver and intestinal flukes is usually made by identifying their characteristic ova in the stool.

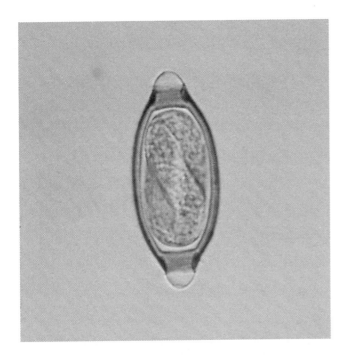

FIGURE 78-1. *Trichuris trichiura,* embryonated fertile ovum. The ovum has a characteristic bile-stained, thick, smooth-walled shell with prominent polar plugs at each end. Eggs are 50 to 54 by 23 μm. (From Smith JW, Ash LR, Thompson JH Jr, et al. Intestinal helminths. In: Atlas of diagnostic medical parasitology series. Chicago: American Society of Clinical Pathologists, 1984.)

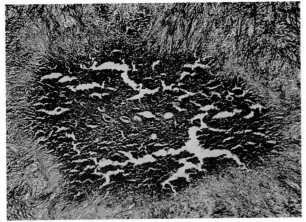

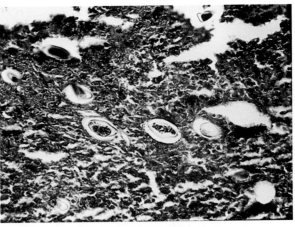

FIGURE 78-2. Adult female *Enterobius vermicularis,* on rare occasion, reach the pelvic peritoneum through the female genital tract. **A:** Ova can elicit a granulomatous response as in this biopsy specimen from a woman who underwent exploratory laparotomy for abdominal pain (Grocott modification of Gomori methenamine-silver stain). **B:** *Enterobius vermicularis* ova in the granuloma at high power. (JAMA. 1981;245:1340–1341. Copyrighted 1981, American Medical Association.)

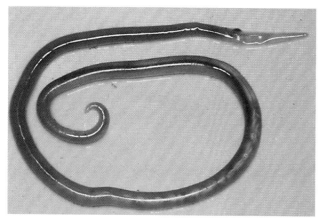

FIGURE 78-3. *Ascaris lumbricoides* adult. Adults are white or pink. Males range from 10 to 31 cm in length and females range from 22 to 35 cm. Adults occasionally migrate from the gastrointestinal tract and appear in the feces or oropharynx. *A lumbricoides* is the only helminth that infests humans that resembles an earthworm in size and shape.

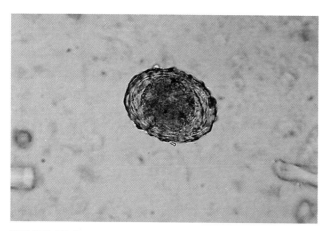

FIGURE 78-4. *Ascaris lumbricoides,* unembryonated fertile egg. This egg demonstrates the characteristic bile-stained, external, mammillated layer of the relatively thick shell. The egg is in the one-cell stage normally found in fresh feces. *Ascaris* eggs measure 45 to 70 by 35 to 50 μm. (From Smith JW, Ash LR, Thompson JH Jr, et al. Intestinal helminths. In: Atlas of diagnostic medical parasitology series. Chicago: American Society of Clinical Pathologists, 1984.)

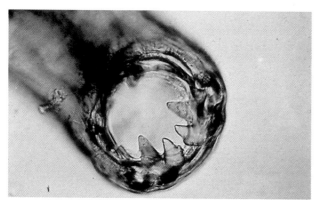

FIGURE 78-5. The characteristic buccal capsule of *Ancylostoma duodenale* has two teeth on each side of the capsule. (From Smith JW, Ash LR, Thompson JH Jr, et al. Intestinal helminths. In: Atlas of diagnostic medical parasitology series. Chicago: American Society of Clinical Pathologists, 1984.)

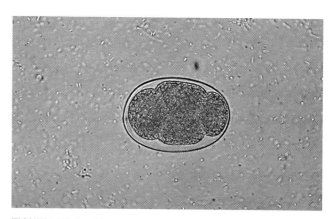

FIGURE 78-6. Hookworm, segmented egg. This is a typical, thin-shelled egg in the four-cell stage. Hookworm eggs are usually in the four- to eight-cell stage in fresh fecal specimens. Hookworm species that infest humans cannot be differentiated from one another on the basis of their eggs. Eggs measure 55 to 75 by 35 to 47 μm. (From Smith JW, Ash LR, Thompson JH Jr, et al. Intestinal helminths. In: Atlas of diagnostic medical parasitology series. Chicago: American Society of Clinical Pathologists, 1984.)

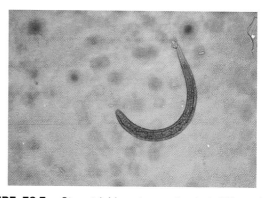

FIGURE 78-7. *Strongyloides stercoralis* rhabditiform larva, 225 by 16 mm, in the stool of a patient with epigastric pain and eosinophilia. (Courtesy of Richard L. Guerrant, M.D., Charlottesville, VA.)

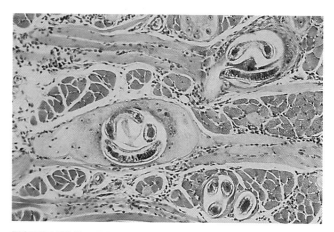

FIGURE 78-8. *Trichinella spiralis,* infective larvae, tongue, tissue section (H&E stain). Infective larvae, approximately 1 mm long, are encysted in striated muscle. (From Smith JW, Ash LR, Thompson JH Jr, et al. Intestinal helminths. In: Atlas of diagnostic medical parasitology series. Chicago: American Society of Clinical Pathologists, 1984.)

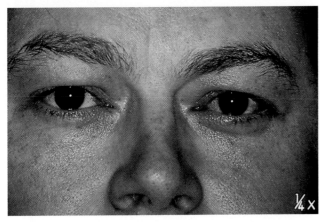

FIGURE 78-9. Periorbital edema and conjunctivitis in association with severe myalgia and eosinophilia are common manifestations of trichinosis. (Courtesy of William A. Petri Jr., M.D., Ph.D., Charlottesville, VA.)

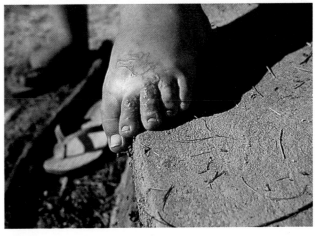

FIGURE 78-10. Cutaneous larva migrans. *Ancylostoma braziliense,* a hookworm of dogs and cats, is the most frequent but not the only cause of this syndrome. The lesions are characterized by pruritic, serpiginous tracts in which the infective-stage larvae have migrated. (From Smith JW, Ash LR, Thompson JH Jr, et al. Intestinal helminths. In: Atlas of diagnostic medical parasitology series. Chicago: American Society of Clinical Pathologists, 1984.)

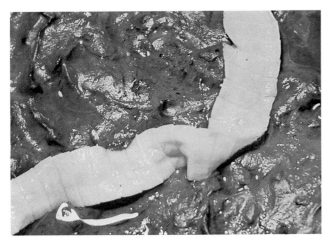

FIGURE 78-11. *Diphyllobothrium latum,* adult tapeworm. Adult *D latum* worms are characterized by broad proglottids with a central uterus. Intact proglottids are not ordinarily shed by this species, unlike the *Taenia* species, and eggs are the diagnostic stage usually found in feces. (From Smith JW, Ash LR, Thompson JH Jr, et al. Intestinal helminths. In: Atlas of diagnostic medical parasitology series. Chicago: American Society of Clinical Pathologists, 1984.)

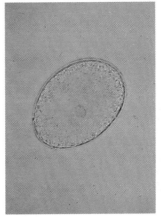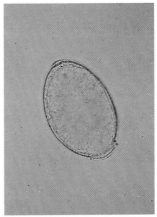

FIGURE 78-12. *Diphyllobothrium latum,* eggs. One egg (**left**) has an indistinct but visible operculum and does not show a knob on the abopercular end. Pressing on the coverslip of a wet mount bursts the operculum, as seen in the other egg (**right**), showing that the egg is operculate. The egg on the **right** shows the abopercular knob. Eggs measure 58 to 75 by 40 to 51 μm. (From Smith JW, Ash LR, Thompson JH Jr, et al. Intestinal helminths. In: Atlas of diagnostic medical parasitology series. Chicago: American Society of Clinical Pathologists, 1984.)

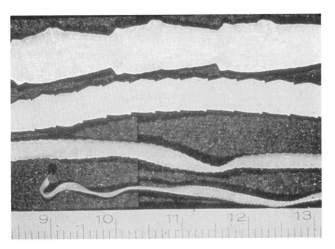

FIGURE 78-13. *Taenia saginata.* The scolex with its four suckers is seen (**lower left**). Mature proglottids are found at the distal end of the worm (**top**). (From Smith JW, Ash LR, Thompson JH Jr, et al. Intestinal helminths. In: Atlas of diagnostic medical parasitology series. Chicago: American Society of Clinical Pathologists, 1984.)

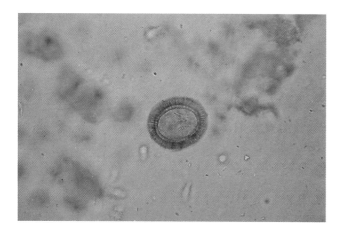

FIGURE 78-14. *Taenia* species, egg. This egg demonstrates a thick, bile-stained, radially striated shell enclosing a six-hooked embryo. The eggs of *Taenia solium* and *Taenia saginata* are indistinguishable from each other. The shell may stain so darkly with iodine that the egg resembles a pollen grain. To confirm the diagnosis, one should see the six hooks of the embryo. The eggs measure 31 to 43 μm in diameter. (From Smith JW, Ash LR, Thompson JH Jr, et al. Intestinal helminths. In: Atlas of diagnostic medical parasitology series. Chicago: American Society of Clinical Pathologists, 1984.)

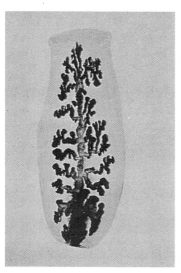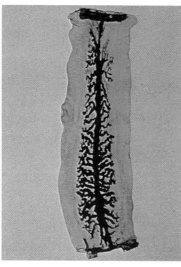

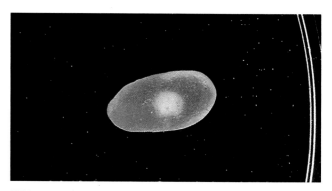

FIGURE 78-15. India ink-injected proglottids of *Taenia solium* (**left**) and *Taenia saginata* (**right**). Proglottids of *T saginata* have more lateral uterine branches than those of *T solium*. (From Smith JW, Ash LR, Thompson JH Jr, et al. Intestinal helminths. In: Atlas of diagnostic medical parasitology series. Chicago: American Society of Clinical Pathologists, 1984.)

FIGURE 78-16. *Taenia solium,* cysticercus. This larval cyst of *T solium,* also known as *Cysticercus cellulosae,* contains a single scolex that is inverted into a fluid-filled bladder. (From Smith JW, Ash LR, Thompson JH Jr, et al. Intestinal helminths. In: Atlas of diagnostic medical parasitology series. Chicago: American Society of Clinical Pathologists, 1984.)

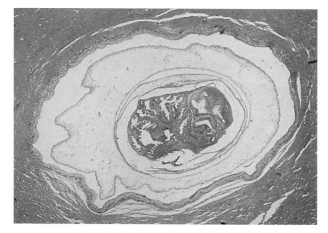

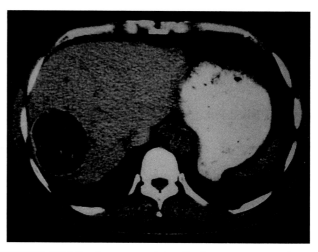

FIGURE 78-17. *Taenia solium,* cysticercosis. Tissue section (H&E stain) shows cysticercus in brain tissue. The scolex region of the cysticercus is in the center. Typical hooks are evident within the inverted scolex. (From Smith JW, Ash LR, Thompson JH Jr, et al. Intestinal helminths. In: Atlas of diagnostic medical parasitology series. Chicago: American Society of Clinical Pathologists, 1984.)

FIGURE 78-18. Large, septate *Echinococcus granulosus* cyst in the right lobe of the liver (computed tomographic scan without contrast medium). The patient was raised in Greece and emigrated to the United States. He sought treatment with intermittent right upper quadrant abdominal pain and two prior episodes of anaphylaxis.

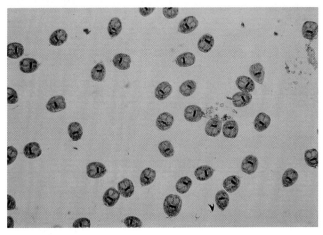

FIGURE 78-19. *Echinococcus granulosus.* Aspiration of fluid from a hydatid cyst may yield numerous protoscolices and hooklets that are referred to as hydatid sand. The protoscolices characteristically are invaginated, as in this photomicrograph. (From Smith JW, Ash LR, Thompson JH Jr, et al. Intestinal helminths. In: Atlas of diagnostic medical parasitology series. Chicago: American Society of Clinical Pathologists, 1984.)

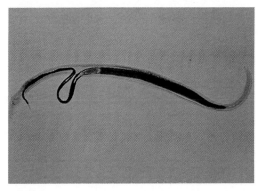

FIGURE 78-20. *Schistosoma mansoni,* adult worm pair. The long, slender female is protruding from the gynecophoral canal of the larger male. *S mansoni* pairs such as these usually reside in the mesenteric plexus in the distribution of the superior mesenteric vein (carmine stain). (From Smith JW, Ash LR, Thompson JH Jr, et al. Intestinal helminths. In: Atlas of diagnostic medical parasitology series. Chicago: American Society of Clinical Pathologists, 1984.)

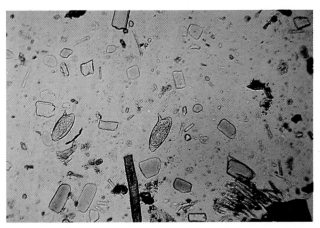

FIGURE 78-21. *Schistosoma mansoni,* egg (iodine stain). The egg has a relatively thin, yellowish, transparent shell with a prominent, sharply pointed lateral spine. A miracidium is within the egg. In wet mounts, tapping the coverslip to reorient eggs so that the lateral spine lies to the side may facilitate identification. Eggs measure 114 to 180 by 45 to 73 μm. (From Smith JW, Ash LR, Thompson JH Jr, et al. Intestinal helminths. In: Atlas of diagnostic medical parasitology series. Chicago: American Society of Clinical Pathologists, 1984.)

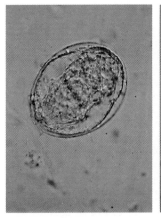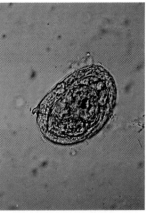

FIGURE 78-22. *Schistosoma japonicum,* egg. In this composite photomicrograph, one egg (**left**) is more typical in that the small spine is not visible; in the other egg (**right**) the spine is readily visible. The spine may be hooklike, as it is here, or more knoblike, but in most instances, it is difficult to see. These eggs are smaller and more rounded than eggs of either *Schistosoma mansoni* or *Schistosoma haematobium.* They contain a miracidium when found in feces and measure 70 to 100 by 45 to 80 μm. (From Smith JW, Ash LR, Thompson JH Jr, et al. Intestinal helminths. In: Atlas of diagnostic medical parasitology series. Chicago: American Society of Clinical Pathologists, 1984.)

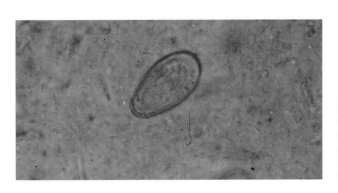

FIGURE 78-23. *Opisthorchis viverrini,* egg. Photomicrograph of an embryonated egg demonstrates the operculum, which is recessed into the shell. There is a knob or boss at the abopercular end. The egg contains a miracidium when passed and measures 29 by 16 μm. The ova of *Clonorchis sinensis* have the same configuration.

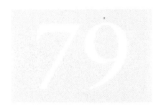

GASTROINTESTINAL MANIFESTATIONS OF SYSTEMIC DISEASES

JOEL S. LEVINE ■ GARRY A. NEIL ■ JOEL V. WEINSTOCK

Many systemic disorders have gastrointestinal manifestations caused by inflammatory infiltration. Granulomas are specialized, focal inflammations that form around poorly degradable foreign substances. The inciting factor may be either antigenic or a bland foreign body. Granulomas sequester toxic and antigenic materials released from the inciting nidus. They also wall off and destroy the nidus and eliminate the debris.

Granulomas are complex, dynamic lesions composed of a variety of inflammatory cells. As illustrated in Figs. 79-1 through 79-12, granulomas that form in response to various inciting factors may have distinctive morphologic features. The following six case reports are unusual and are good examples of how systemic illness can manifest problems in the gastrointestinal tract (Figs. 79-13 through 79-17).

CASE 1

A 23-year-old Hispanic woman with achy upper abdominal discomfort was referred because of hepatomegaly and abnormal liver tests. She did not drink alcohol, and her mother had died of complications of cirrhosis. The patient was obese (100 kg), her liver span was 21 cm at the midclavicular line, and she had no stigmata of chronic liver disease. Alanine aminotransferase (ALT) level was 110 IU (normal, <40 IU), and aspartate aminotransferase (AST) level was 140 IU (normal, <35 IU). Prothrombin time and bilirubin and alkaline phosphatase levels were normal. Viral hepatitis studies, urine copper excretion, and serum iron level were normal. The patient had mild diabetes. A liver biopsy was performed. A low-power view of the liver (see Fig. 79-13A) showed marked steatosis. At higher power (see Fig. 79-13B) the prominent macrovesicular fat with fibrosis and focal inflammatory change was evident. The patient had nonalcoholic steatonecrosis.

CASE 2

A 60-year-old woman with long-standing rheumatoid arthritis was found to have a rock hard, 20-cm liver at physical examination. Liver biochemical findings were normal. A computed tomographic scan of the liver showed focal filling defects that suggested cancer. A liver biopsy was performed. A low-power view (see Fig. 79-14*A*) showed multiple homogeneous eosinophilic densities in the liver surrounding the blood vessels. A high-power view (see Fig. 79-14*B*) showed expansion of portal area. The eosinophilic material is amyloid protein. Nodular deposition of amyloid is unusual.

CASE 3

A 22-year-old man had fever and abdominal pain. His liver was large and painful. A white blood cell count demonstrated 45,000 cells/mL with immature myelocytes. Bone marrow examination was diagnostic of acute myelogenous leukemia. Combination chemotherapy was begun, but the patient died of overwhelming sepsis within 2 days. At autopsy the liver (see Fig. 79-15) demonstrated leukemic cells throughout the sinusoids.

CASE 4

A 50-year-old man arrived in the emergency department with a 3-day history of "easy bruising," fever, and new onset of hematemesis. Physical examination revealed multiple areas of characteristic palpable purpura without necrosis (see Figs. 79-16*A*, *B*). The platelet count and bleeding time were normal. Upper gastrointestinal endoscopy revealed multiple similar lesions (see Fig. 79-16*C*) in the stomach. Skin biopsy revealed leukocytoclastic vasculitis compatible with Henoch-Schönlein purpura. A cause was not identified. Lesions resolved with time and steroid therapy. There were no recurrences.

CASE 5

A 29-year-old man arrived at the emergency department and reported passing dark red blood through the rectum. He said that this had been happening episodically over the past 4 years. He explained that multiple needlesticks on his arms were related to a recent hospital admission. He had undergone multiple tests in a variety of different hospitals in the area and in four surrounding states without receiving a diagnosis. He passed a large amount of dark clotted blood in the emergency room, was found to have a hematocrit of 24%, and was admitted to the intensive care unit.

While the patient was being admitted, the attending gastroenterologist obtained the names of several hospitals the patient had visited and called the medical record departments. During 2 hours on the phone the physician found 19 admissions for rectal bleeding that led to transfusion of 42 units of blood, 20 colonoscopic examinations, 7 angiographic studies, 19 upper gastrointestinal endoscopic examinations, 15 tagged red blood cell scans, 10 Meckel scans, and an exploratory laparotomy. The colonoscopic examinations always demonstrated blood in the colon, but no cause was ever identified.

After conducting the phone research, the attending gastroenterologist sent the patient to the radiology suite. In the presence of the hospital attorney, the patient's room was searched, and the objects shown in Fig. 79-17 were found among the patient's possessions. Included were multiple syringes and needles containing clotted blood, lancets, and a plastic bag containing clotted blood. When confronted with the findings, the patient refused further treatment and left the hospital against medical advice. The blood in the plastic bag was later found to be from nonhuman sources. It was hypothesized that this patient had a case of factitious hematochezia caused by rectal insertion of both self-derived and animal blood compatible with the diagnosis of Munchausen syndrome.

CASE 6

A 42-year-old woman was referred for endoscopy by her general internist because of chronic recurrent food impactions. She described episodic solid food dysphagia felt in the upper chest for 10 years. At times she needed to induce vomiting to get the food out. By chewing her food well and taking her time eating, she had reduced the number of these episodes to 1 to 2 per year. She denied any heartburn, indigestion, gastrointestinal bleeding, or weight loss. She had mild chronic fatigue that was attributed to her active lifestyle of work and caring for her three children. She had no other health problems. Her physical examination was normal. An upper endoscopy was performed. Multiple esophageal webs (Fig. 79-18) were identified, and were the only findings. The webs were dilated. The dysphagia resolved. A blood count revealed a microcytic anemia and iron studies confirmed her iron deficiency. With oral iron therapy her anemia resolved and she has had no further dysphagia. This was a case of Plummer-Vinson syndrome.

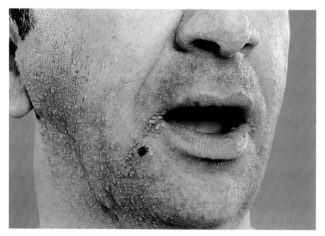

FIGURE 79-1. Verrucous and papillomatous papules on the face of a patient with Cowden syndrome.

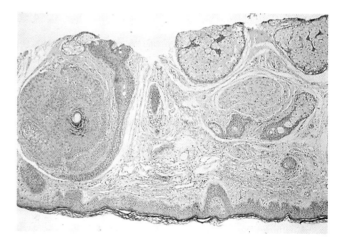

FIGURE 79-2. Skin biopsy specimen from a patient with Cowden syndrome demonstrates cutaneous trichilemmoma.

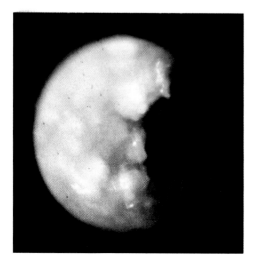

FIGURE 79-3. Endoscopic view of the stomach of a patient with Cowden syndrome reveals multiple hamartomatous polyps.

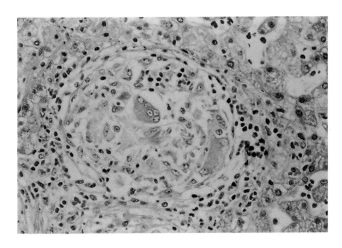

FIGURE 79-4. Sarcoidosis. One well-formed epithelioid granuloma with a thin lymphocytic halo is present in an otherwise normal-appearing liver (H&E stain; original magnification × 100).

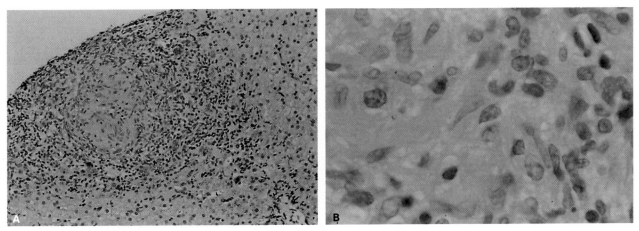

FIGURE 79-5. **A:** Liver granuloma of tuberculosis. **B:** Acid-fast stain of granuloma in **A** demonstrates *Mycobacterium tuberculosis* (H&E stain; **A** original magnification × 50, **B** original magnification × 330).

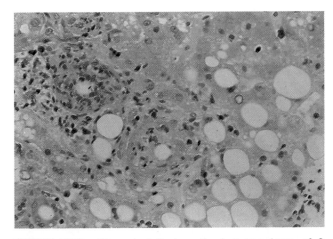

FIGURE 79-6. Characteristic hepatic ring granuloma of Q fever. The fibrin ring encircles a central vacuole (H&E stain; original magnification × 100).

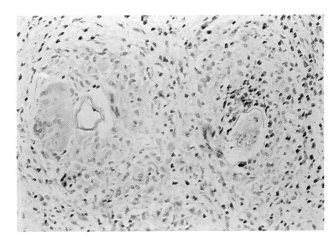

FIGURE 79-7. Eosinophilic hepatic granulomas induced by ova of *Schistosoma mansoni* (H&E stain; original magnification × 100).

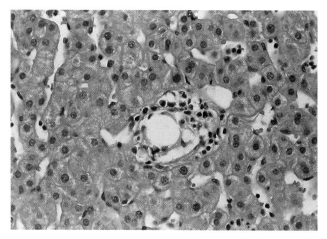

FIGURE 79-8. Lipogranuloma located in hepatic parenchyma near a central vein. The granuloma contains distinctive fat vacuoles (H&E stain; original magnification × 100).

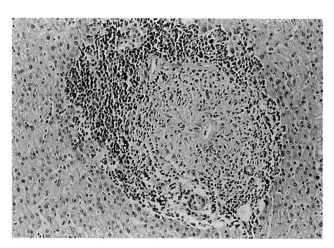

FIGURE 79-9. Portal granuloma from a patient with primary biliary cirrhosis. The relationship of the granuloma to a damaged bile duct is depicted (H&E stain; original magnification × 100).

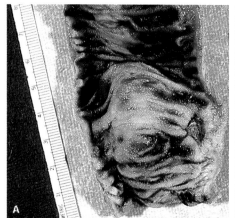

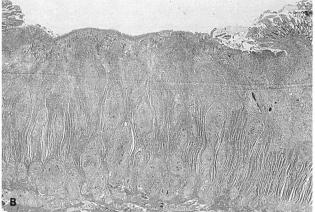

FIGURE 79-10. Enteric tuberculosis. **A:** Photograph of specimen from colonic resection reveals a tuberculous ulcer. **B:** Tuberculous ulcer underlying focal granulomas (H&E stain; original magnification × 10).

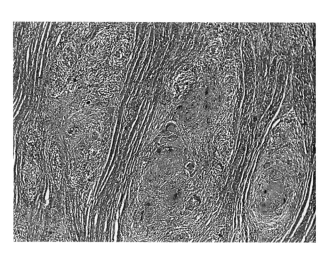

FIGURE 79-11. Enteric tuberculosis. Lesion depicted in Fig. 59-10*B* reveals granulomas with central necrosis and large giant cells (H&E stain; original magnification × 40).

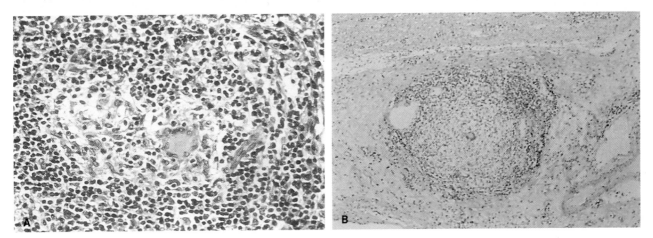

FIGURE 79-12. Crohn's disease. **A:** Loosely aggregated ileal granuloma. **B:** Mature ileal granuloma.

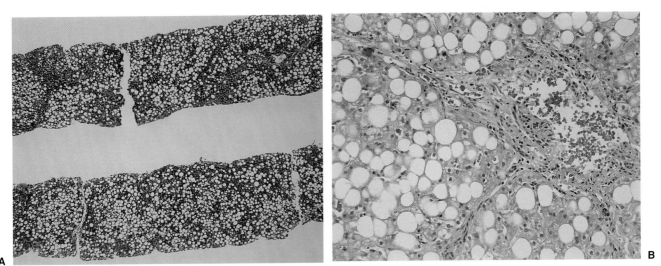

FIGURE 79-13. Nonalcoholic steatonecrosis in a patient with diabetes. **A:** Low-power view of liver biopsy specimen shows marked fatty infiltration. **B:** High-power view of biopsy specimen depicted in **A**. Mild fibrosis and inflammatory changes are visible.

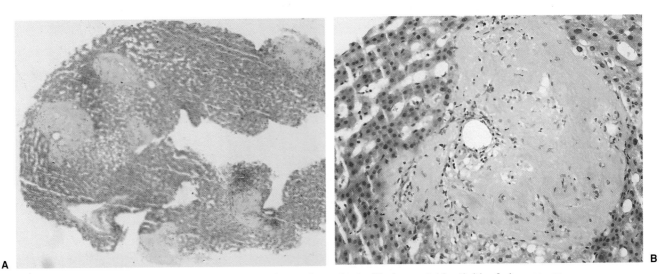

FIGURE 79-14. Liver biopsy specimen of a patient with rheumatoid arthritis. **A:** Low-power view of liver biopsy specimen shows nodular eosinophilic infiltration. **B:** High-power view of biopsy specimen depicted in **A**. The pale eosinophilic extracellular deposits surrounding blood vessels are consistent with the presence of amyloid.

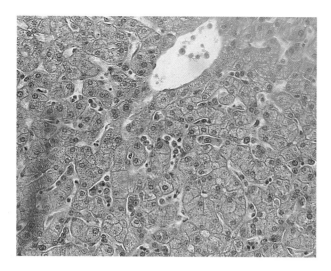

FIGURE 79-15. Liver biopsy specimen from patient with acute myelogenous leukemia. Formed blood elements are present within the sinusoids.

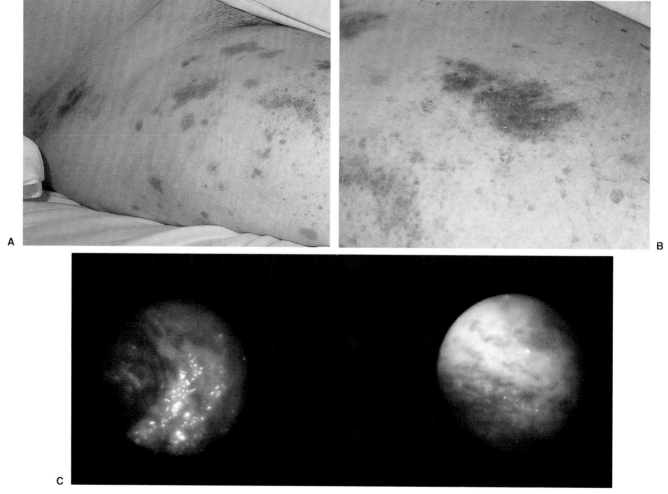

FIGURE 79-16. Vascular lesions of a patient with Henoch-Schönlein purpura. **A, B:** Veins of macular and papular purpuric lesions on the thigh. **C:** Endoscopic view of gastric mucosa demonstrates purpura.

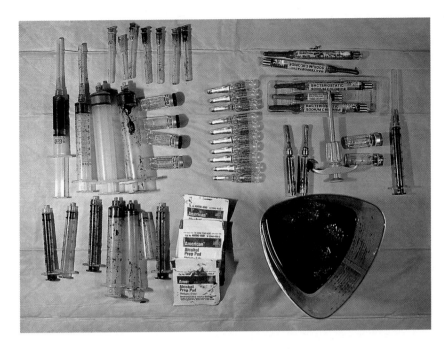

FIGURE 79-17. View of needle and syringes used by a patient with Munchausen syndrome to produce the factitious presentation of colonic bleeding.

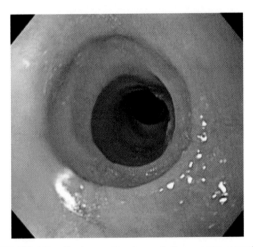

FIGURE 79-18. Endoscopic view of the upper esophagus demonstrating multiple webs in a patient with Plummer-Vinson syndrome.

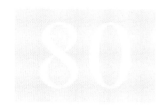

GASTROINTESTINAL MANIFESTATIONS OF IMMUNOLOGIC DISORDERS

FERGUS SHANAHAN ■ **STEPHAN R. TARGAN**

IMMUNODEFICIENCY

Immunodeficiency disorders are a heterogeneous group of conditions that may be classified broadly into primary and secondary syndromes. Selective immunoglobulin A (IgA) deficiency and common variable hypogammaglobulinemia (Figs. 80-1 and 80-2) are the most common primary immunodeficiency syndromes among adults. Secondary immunodeficiencies are much more common than primary disorders. Causes include malnutrition, protein-losing enteropathy (Fig. 80-3), cancer, and iatrogenic immunosuppression. The most important secondary immunodeficiency disorder is acquired immunodeficiency syndrome (AIDS) caused by human immunodeficiency virus (HIV) (see Chapter 76).

The gastrointestinal tract is a primary target organ in both primary and secondary immunodeficiency disorders because of its large surface area and constant exposure to environmental pathogens. The principal gastrointestinal consequence of immunodeficiency is increased susceptibility to infection. This includes infection with unusual agents, atypical manifestations of infection with commonly encountered pathogens, and bacterial overgrowth with organisms normally present in the gastrointestinal tract. There also is an increased prevalence of autoimmune disorders or chronic inflammatory conditions such as atrophic gastritis and celiac disease. In some immunodeficiency states, there is an increased incidence of malignant tumors, particularly lymphoma. Benign diffuse nodular lymphoid hyperplasia may occur among some patients, whereas lymphoid atrophy may be a feature among others. Patients with severe immunodeficiency may have graft-versus-host disease caused by transplacentally acquired maternal lymphocytes or unintentional transfusion of nonirradiated blood products. It is important for the clinician to know, however, that patients with mild or selective forms of immunodeficiency, such as selective IgA deficiency, frequently are free of infections or other manifestations.

776

NODULAR LYMPHOID HYPERPLASIA

Diffuse nodular lymphoid hyperplasia occurs among approximately 20% of patients with common variable hypogammaglobulinemia. The lymphoid nodules are in the lamina propria and submucosa and produce a nodularity that is visible on barium radiographic studies (Fig. 80-4) and at endoscopy. They are most prevalent in the small bowel, in some cases extend into the colon, and rarely extend into the stomach. At microscopic examination, the nodules consist of large lymphoid follicles with germinal centers (Fig. 80-5). Plasma cells usually are absent. Lymphoid hyperplasia is believed to be caused by proliferation of B cells that are unable to undergo full differentiation to immunoglobulin secretion and therefore are unresponsive to feedback regulation of proliferation. Unlike the situation with common variable hypogammaglobulinemia, nodular lymphoid hyperplasia does not occur in X-linked hypogammaglobulinemia, probably because there is defective pre–B-cell to B-cell differentiation with hypoplasia of peripheral lymphoid tissue and a paucity of mature B cells. It is important to recognize that localized forms of nodular lymphoid hyperplasia, particularly in the large bowel, may occur among apparently healthy immunocompetent persons. Small nodules of lymphoid tissue on a background of normal folds of small bowel are normal and are a common finding among children and young adults.

EOSINOPHILIC GASTROENTERITIS

The term eosinophilic gastroenteritis is used to describe a group of poorly defined disorders characterized by diffuse eosinophilic infiltration of a portion of the gastrointestinal tract in the absence of other disorders, such as intestinal parasitism, vasculitis, neoplasia, and other causes of eosinophilia and eosinophilic tissue infiltration (Figs. 80-6 and 80-7). Thus, disorders known to be associated with eosinophilia and eosinophilic tissue infiltration must be excluded before the diagnosis of eosinophilic gastroenteritis is made. The cause of this disorder is unclear. Although an allergic basis has been considered, the evidence for this hypothesis is limited. Clinical manifestations depend on the site primarily affected and the layer of bowel wall predominantly involved. Mucosal involvement presents itself like other forms of inflammatory bowel disease, submucosal infiltration tends to lead to intestinal obstruction, and serosal involvement may be associated with eosinophilic ascites.

GRAFT-VERSUS-HOST DISEASE

Gastrointestinal complications occur among virtually all patients at some stage during recovery from bone marrow transplantation. In addition to graft-versus-host disease, causes of gastrointestinal symptoms after bone marrow transplantation include the effects of chemotherapy and chemoradiation therapy given before bone marrow grafting and opportunistic infections that may be caused by the immunosuppressive protocol or the immunodeficiency associated with graft-versus-host disease. The gastrointestinal and liver damage associated with chemoradiation therapy usually resolves within 20 to 30 days after transplantation. Opportunistic infections may occur at any stage after bone marrow transplantation; bacterial and fungal infections tend to be more common during the first month, and viral infections more common thereafter.

The clinical severity and extent of gastrointestinal involvement with acute and chronic graft-versus-host disease are highly variable. Acute graft-versus-host disease usually occurs 20 to 60 days after transplantation and primarily affects the skin, liver, and gastrointestinal tract. Chronic graft-versus-host disease is a multisystem disorder with clinical features resembling those of sicca syndrome and systemic sclerosis. Gastrointestinal involvement occurs particularly in the oral mucosa (mucositis), esophagus, and small bowel. Chronic graft-versus-host disease usually occurs 80 to 400 days after transplantation.

The earliest morphologic feature of acute intestinal graft-versus-host disease at light microscopic examination is apoptosis of individual cells in the intestinal crypts (Fig. 80-8). This characteristic finding is diagnostic, if obtained from normal-appearing mucosa, at least 20 days after transplantation (when the effects of chemoradiation therapy have resolved). Inflammatory cells or microorganisms are not present in adjacent mucosa. Later, the histopathology can progress to total denudation of the mucosa; the apoptotic lesion is no longer evident, and changes are not specific.

The radiographic appearance of graft-versus-host disease also varies with the severity and with the stage of the disease. During the acute phase there is mucosal and submucosal edema, particularly in the distal small bowel. The barium is often diluted because of excess lumenal fluid loss, and transit is rapid. In addition to thickening of the bowel wall, there may be mucosal ulceration, sloughing, and pneumatosis cystoides intestinalis. The changes are not specific and may be mimicked by coexisting cytomegalovirus (CMV) infection. The radiologic changes of intestinal graft-versus-host disease may resolve completely or occasionally may progress to a striking ribbon-like pattern of diffuse or segmental involvement of the jejunum and ileum. This finding appears to be unique to intestinal graft-versus-host disease (Fig. 80-9).

The endoscopic appearance of acute graft-versus-host disease may be normal, show patchy erythema, or show extensive mucosal sloughing, particularly in the ileum, cecum, and ascending colon, with relative sparing of the rectal and gastric mucosa. In contrast, esophageal involvement is particularly common in chronic graft-versus-host disease. Lesions include desquamation of the upper esophagus and upper esophageal webs; the distal esophagus usually is spared.

CYTOMEGALOVIRUS INFECTION

Gastrointestinal infection with CMV occurs in several clinical settings. It may be associated with primary or secondary immunodeficiency states, particularly when there is defective cell-mediated immunity. CMV infection is seen increasingly among patients with iatrogenic immunosuppression associated with cancer therapy, transplantation, or chronic inflammatory disorders such as lupus or inflammatory bowel disease. Infection with CMV occurs in as many as one third of patients undergoing transplantation. After oroesophageal candidiasis, it is probably the most common gastrointestinal infection among patients with AIDS. CMV infection also has been described among apparently immunocompetent persons with a variety of disorders including hypertrophic gastropathy, self-limited colitis, and ulcerative colitis, particularly when complicated by development of toxic megacolon. Although the manifestations of gastrointestinal CMV infection are highly variable, severity tends to correlate with the degree of immunosuppression. Inflammation with ulceration may be focal or diffuse (Fig. 80-10A), superficial or deep (Fig. 80-10B), and may lead to bleeding and perforation. Any part of the esophagus and small or large intestine may be involved. Multifocal involvement with CMV is usual among patients with AIDS, whereas CMV often is limited to the cecum (typhlitis) and ascending colon after transplantation.

Endothelial cells are the most frequent cell types infected (Figs. 80-10C, D). Smooth muscle cells and the myenteric plexus occasionally are involved. Infected macrophages also may be seen in the lamina propria, whereas epithelial cells are seldom involved. CMV-infected cells are large with a granular cytoplasm and nuclei that are filled with intranuclear (Cowdry type A) inclusions, often with a periinclusion halo. Unlike infections with herpes simplex virus, which tend to be superficial, characteristic CMV-infected cells usually are found in the deeper layers of resected or biopsy specimens (Fig. 80-10E). Identification of CMV infection may be facilitated by in situ hybridization or immunocytochemical analysis with virus-specific antibodies (see Figs. 80-10D, E).

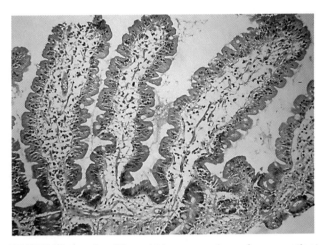

FIGURE 80-1. Small-bowel biopsy specimen from a patient with hypogammaglobulinemia shows a paucity of plasma cells in the lamina propria. Among patients with selective immunoglobulin A (IgA) deficiency, the absence or paucity of IgA-producing cells is compensated for by an increase in IgM-producing cells. (Courtesy of Dr. Klaus Lewin.)

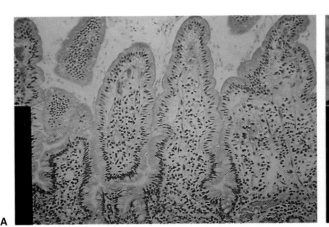
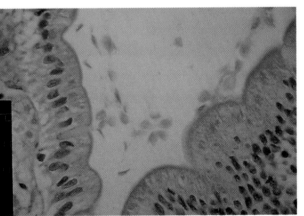

A   B

FIGURE 80-2. A, B: Giardiasis (*Giardia lamblia*) is the most common gastrointestinal parasitic infection in primary immunodeficiency syndromes. It occurs most frequently among patients with common variable hypogammaglobulinemia. Giardiasis usually does not distort villous structure but may do so among patients with immunodeficiencies. Although the diagnosis of giardiasis can be made from inspection of histological sections of small bowel, finding the organism by means of this method is difficult and tedious when the infection is scanty. The diagnosis is made more conveniently by examination of the stools for cysts, or identification of the trophozoite form in intestinal fluid or smears of mucus adherent to the biopsy specimen.

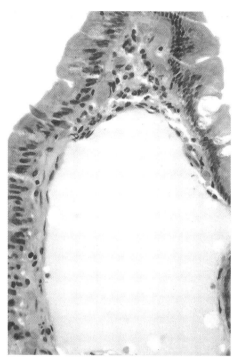

FIGURE 80-3. Secondary immunodeficiency–intestinal lymphangiectasia. Immunodeficiency caused by enteric protein loss may be a component of any severe inflammatory disorder of the gastrointestinal tract. The most severe cases of gastrointestinal protein loss occur with lymphangiectasia, which may be primary or secondary to lymphatic obstruction. Protein loss from the gastrointestinal tract is nonselective, and hypogammaglobulinemia is always accompanied by hypoalbuminemia. Among patients with lymphangiectasia, there is also loss of lymphocytes, particularly T cells, and immunoglobulins.

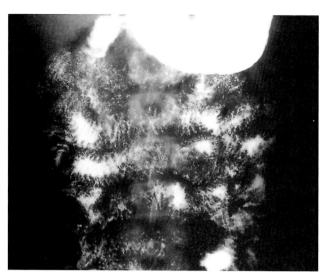

FIGURE 80-4. Upper gastrointestinal barium study of a patient with common variable hypogammaglobulinemia shows multiple diffuse filling defects caused by nodular lymphoid hyperplasia.

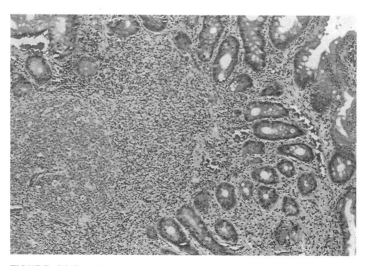

FIGURE 80-5. Histological features of diffuse nodular lymphoid hyperplasia in a patient with immunodeficiency. This jejunal biopsy specimen contains lymphoid tissue with germinal centers. Plasma cells were not identified. Radiographic evidence of nodular lymphoid hyperplasia was present. A cluster of *Giardia* organisms are present (**top right**).

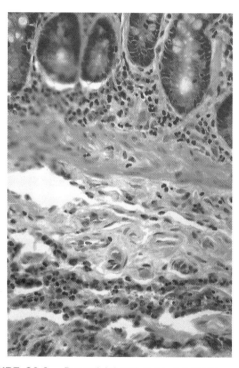

FIGURE 80-6. Peroral jejunal mucosal biopsy specimen from a patient with typical clinical findings of eosinophilic gastroenteritis. The biopsy specimen includes an involved area of submucosa that contains a characteristic band-like infiltrate of eosinophils.

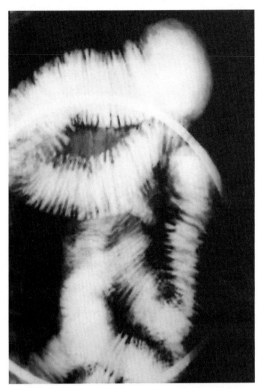

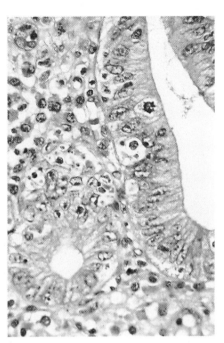

FIGURE 80-7. Upper gastrointestinal barium study of a patient with diffuse eosinophilic gastroenteritis. The thickening of jejunal folds with a "stack of coins" pattern is characteristic of submucosal infiltration but is not specific. It may occur with any cause of submucosal fluid (edema or blood) accumulation such as ischemia, hemorrhage, or inflammation. Depending on the depth of bowel wall involved, the folds may be irregular and nodular. There may be separation of bowel loops. The radiographic appearance of eosinophilic gastroenteritis may be difficult to differentiate from that of other infiltrative or inflammatory disorders, such as Crohn's disease.

FIGURE 80-8. Rectal biopsy specimen from a patient with acute graft-versus-host disease after bone marrow transplantation. The individual crypt cell apoptosis (karyolytic debris in vacuoles near crypt base) is characteristic if found after day 20, when damage from chemoradiation therapy has resolved. (Courtesy of Dr. Klaus Lewin.)

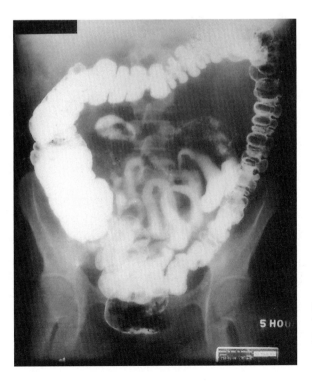

FIGURE 80-9. Upper gastrointestinal barium study shows characteristic ribbon-like pattern of small bowel that may occur among some patients with graft-versus-host disease if the early intestinal lesions do not resolve completely. This change is diagnostic and represents submucosal fibrosis and edema.

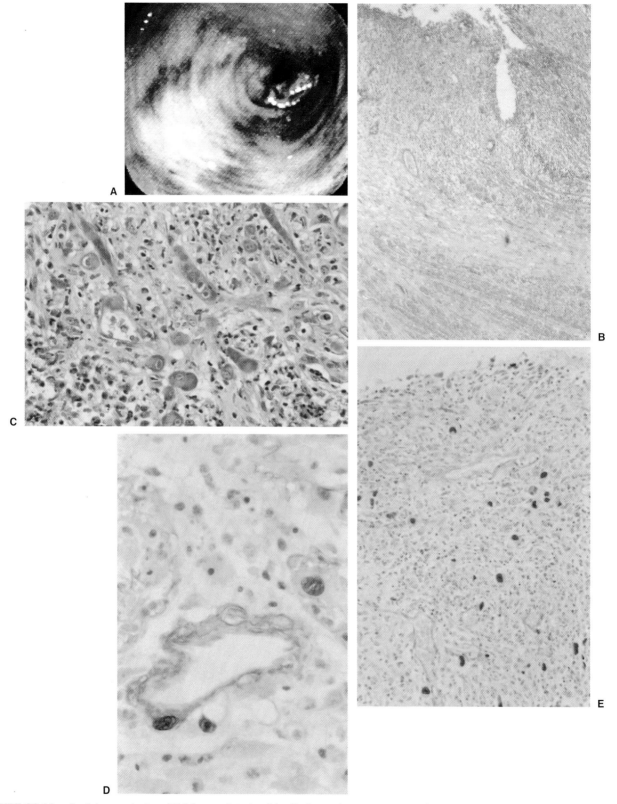

FIGURE 80-10. A: Cytomegalovirus (CMV)-associated colitis. Endoscopic appearances of patchy erythematous mucosa with linear streaks. **B:** CMV-associated colitis. Histopathological section of surgically resected colonic tissue shows penetrating ulceration with transmural inflammation in an immunodeficient patient with bloody diarrhea, abdominal pain, and peritoneal signs. **C:** High-power light microscopic image of resected colonic tissue shown in **B** shows CMV-infected cells with characteristic nuclear inclusions within the lamina propria and submucosa. CMV has a propensity to infect endothelial cells, although smooth muscle cells, macrophages, and the myenteric plexus may be involved. **D:** CMV-associated colitis. Immunocytochemical analysis with CMV-specific monoclonal antibody showed CMV within endothelial cells. **E:** Full-thickness resected tissue stained immunocytochemically with viral-specific antibody shows that CMV-infected cells usually are found in the deeper layers of gastrointestinal specimens.

81

GASTROINTESTINAL VASCULAR MALFORMATIONS OR NEOPLASMS:
Arterial, Venous, Arteriovenous, and Capillary

MITCHELL S. CAPPELL

Intrinsic vascular gastrointestinal lesions are divided, according to pathophysiology, into structural, neoplastic, and inflammatory; they are subdivided, according to most affected vessel, into arterial, arteriovenous, venous, and capillary. The structural vascular lesions are clinically important because of their propensity to bleed, whereas the neoplastic lesions are clinically important because of their tendency to bleed and/or metastasize. Inflammatory vascular lesions tend to cause mesenteric ischemia. Most vascular lesions are rare, except for angiodysplasia, which is common, and the Dieulafoy lesion, gastric antral vascular ectasia (GAVE), and Kaposi sarcoma, which are uncommon. Familiarity with the endoscopic, radiologic, and pathologic appearance of vascular gastrointestinal lesions is important for diagnosis and management.

STRUCTURAL VASCULAR LESIONS

Dieulafoy Lesion

Dieulafoy lesions cause about 1.5% of upper gastrointestinal bleeding and about 0.3% of lower gastrointestinal bleeding. Microscopic examination of the lesion reveals a thrombus attached to a large superficial artery at the base of a small mucosal erosion (Fig. 81-1). At endoscopy, the lesion appears as a pigmented protuberance, representing the vessel stump, with minimal surrounding erosion and no ulceration (Fig. 81-2). The Dieulafoy lesion most commonly occurs in the proximal stomach.

Pseudoxanthoma Elasticum

Gastrointestinal bleeding frequently occurs in pseudoxanthoma elasticum, a rare genetic disorder of elastin synthesis in which patients have yellowish xanthomatoid papules (pseudoxanthomas) on the skin. This bleeding most commonly arises from a characteristic lesion: endoscopy reveals numerous petechiae or erosions predominantly in the gastric fundus, as well as yellowish xanthomatoid gastric nodular lesions that resemble the cutaneous lesions. The gastric bleeding is attributed to elastin degeneration in small gastric arteries.

Angiodysplasia

Angiodysplasia account for about 3% to 6% of lower gastrointestinal bleeding and about 2% to 5% of upper gastrointestinal bleeding. Angiodysplasia most commonly cause chronic occult gastrointestinal bleeding, particularly in the elderly. They are usually diagnosed by endoscopy. At endoscopy angiodysplasia appear as dense, macular, and reticular networks of angiodysplastic vessels (vascular tufts), each of which is typically arranged in a fern tree, star burst, or stellate pattern (Figs. 81-3 and 81-4). Angiodysplasia are intensely red because of the high oxygen content in erythrocytes within vessels supplied by arteries without intervening capillaries. The vascular tuft is well demonstrated by microscopic analysis of a cleared preparation of gastrointestinal mucosa after silicone injection (Fig. 81-5). Sometimes, a prominent feeding artery or draining vein is observed (Fig. 81-6). Sometimes, a pale (anemic) mucosal halo is observed around angiodysplasia, attributed to shunting of blood (vascular steal) from surrounding mucosa by the low-resistance arteriovenous shunt (Fig. 81-7). Histologically, angiodysplasia consist of dilated, distorted, tortuous, and thin-walled vessels lined by endothelium with little or no fibrosis. Congenital arteriovenous malformations in young adults, unlike angiodysplasia in the elderly, typically have thick-walled arteries (Fig. 81-8). Angiodysplasia are often multiple. When multiple, they tend to be clustered (Fig. 81-9). Despite local clustering, about 15% to 20% of patients with colonic angiodysplasia have upper gastrointestinal angiodysplasia, and vice versa.

The angiographic hallmarks of angiodysplasia are a vascular tuft or tangle resulting from the local mass of irregular vessels best visualized in the arterial phase; an early and intensely filling vein resulting from a direct arteriovenous connection without intervening capillaries; and persistent opacification beyond the normal venous phase (slowly emptying vein), possibly resulting from venous tortuosity (Fig. 81-10). About 60% to 90% of patients have each of these signs. Angiodysplasia occasionally bleed acutely (Fig. 81-11A). Sometimes, bleeding angiodysplasia are first injected with alcohol or epinephrine to slow the bleeding, as was done in the illustrated case (see Fig. 81-11A). At esophagogastroduodenoscopy or colonoscopy, isolated actively bleeding angiodysplasia are treated by endoscopic thermocoagulation, electrocoagulation, or photocoagulation (Fig. 81-11B).

Hereditary Hemorrhagic Telangiectasia

The endoscopic appearance of gastrointestinal telangiectasia in patients with hereditary hemorrhagic telangiectasia (HHT) may be identical to that of angiodysplasia, except that the lesions of HHT tend to be greater in number, occur in all bowel wall layers, and occur in all bowel segments (Fig. 81-12). Patients with these telangiectasia are also distinguished from patients with angiodysplasia by the presence of a positive family history, epistaxis, and orocutaneous telangiectasia which frequently occur on the lips, tongue, and oral mucosa (Fig. 81-13).

Gastrointestinal Telangiectasia Associated With Scleroderma and Calcinosis, Raynaud Phenomenon, Esophageal Dysmotility, Sclerodactyly, and Telangiectasia of the Mucous Membranes Syndrome

Patients with calcinosis, Raynaud phenomenon, esophageal dysmotility, sclerodactyly, and telangiectasia of the mucous membranes (CREST) syndrome sometimes have gastrointestinal telangiectasia, which tend to be punctate (1 to 5 mm wide), circular, and numerous (Fig. 81-14).

Gastric Antral Vascular Ectasia

Gastric antral vascular ectasia is uncommon, and occurs in only 3 cases among 10,000 consecutive endoscopies. Patients typically present with iron deficiency anemia from chronic occult gastrointestinal bleeding. Endoscopy reveals multiple parallel prominent longitudinal folds that traverse the antrum and converge to the pyloric sphincter, and that contain intensely erythematous linear streaks at their apices (Fig. 81-15). The alternative name of watermelon stomach derives from the resemblance of these erythematous linear streaks to the stripes on a watermelon rind. Histological analysis of endoscopic biopsy samples taken from the apices of the longitudinal folds reveals hypertrophied mucosa, dilated and tortuous mucosal capillaries, often occluded by bland fibrin thrombi, and dilated and tortuous submucosal veins (Fig. 81-16).

Colonic Varices

Patients with portal hypertension rarely develop varices in the alimentary tract outside the esophagus or stomach. The varices can occur anywhere in the intestines, but most commonly occur in the rectum or sigmoid colon. At endoscopy, intestinal varices, like esophageal varices, appear as purple, serpiginous superficial vessels that are covered by normal appearing mucosa and that project into the lumen (Fig. 81-17). Intestinal varices can also be diagnosed by selective mesenteric angiography as dilated, tortuous portosystemic collaterals connecting mesenteric veins to retroperitoneal veins during the venous phase (Fig. 81-18).

NEOPLASTIC VASCULAR LESIONS

Hemangioma Syndromes

Blue Rubber Bleb Nevus Syndrome

About one half of intestinal hemangiomas are associated with cutaneous hemangiomas; the condition is called the blue rubber bleb nevus syndrome. Intestinal hemangiomas are either capillary or cavernous. Histologically, cavernous hemangiomas are clinically more significant because of their propensity to bleed. Histologically, cavernous hemangiomas consist of large, dilated, blood-filled, thin-walled, vessels lined by a thin layer of well-differentiated cuboidal endothelium and surrounded by scant fibrous stroma with occasional smooth muscle cells.

The blue rubber bleb nevus syndrome is suspected when characteristic dermatologic lesions occur in conjunction with gastrointestinal bleeding. Patients present with multiple violet-blue, slightly raised, and elastic cutaneous hemangiomas ranging in size from 0.5 to 5 cm in diameter (Fig. 81-19), together with multiple gastrointestinal hemangiomas (Fig. 81-20). The syndromic name is derived from the tactile and visual similarity of the hemangiomas to a rubber nipple. The cutaneous lesions have a wrinkled surface (see Fig. 81-19), and can be emptied of blood by manual pressure, leaving a wrinkled blue or white sac that slowly refills with blood after the pressure is released.

Abdominal radiographs or computerized tomography demonstrate phleboliths from thrombosis and calcification in about half of intestinal hemangiomas (Fig. 81-21). Typically, the phleboliths are arrayed as a cluster that outlines part of the bowel wall, and they maintain a constant distance between each other when the entire cluster shifts position within the abdomen when the patient is turned. At endoscopy, intestinal hemangiomas appear as bluish, compressible submucosal polyps that resemble the cutaneous lesions (Fig. 81-22). Cutaneous and intestinal hemangiomas in association with occluded deep veins and varicose superficial veins in one lower extremity is denoted the Klippel-Trenaunay syndrome.

Disseminated Hemangiomatosis

Rarely patients present with intestinal hemangiomas as part of disseminated hemangiomatosis involving three or more organ systems. Patients typically present at birth with numerous cutaneous hemangiomas (Fig. 81-23). Untreated patients have about 60% mortality during infancy from massive gastrointestinal bleeding or other complications.

Nonsyndromic Hemangiomas

Intestinal Hemangiomas Without Cutaneous Hemangiomas

Intestinal hemangiomas without cutaneous lesions present similarly to intestinal hemangiomas that are part of blue rubber bleb nevus syndrome, as described above. The main difference is that the diagnosis may not be suspected before endoscopy in the absence of cutaneous hemangiomas.

Phlebectasia

Intestinal phlebectasia are venous varicosities consisting of a markedly dilated and tortuous vein, with a normal vascular wall, and scant connective tissue stroma. They are sometimes classified as multiple, small hemangioma. Phlebectasia may also occur in the oral cavity, mostly at the base of the tongue, where they are called caviar spots (varices) or sublingual phlebectasia (Fig. 81-24); and in the genitalia, where they are called Fordyce lesions or scrotal phlebectasia. Intestinal phlebectasia are dark bluish-black and range from several to 10 mm in size (Fig. 81-25). They are characteristically multiple, submucosal, soft, and compressible. They blanch with pressure. Although usually asymptomatic and an incidental finding, they occasionally produce chronic occult or acute gross intestinal bleeding.

Nonhemangiomatous Vascular Neoplasms

Hemangiopericytomas

Hemangiopericytomas are uncommon, richly vascular neoplasms composed of pericytes, which are mesenchymal cells that are normally closely apposed to endothelial cells. The stomach is the most commonly involved gastrointestinal organ, but the small intestine, colon, and rectum can be involved. Endoscopy or laparotomy may reveal a solitary, fairly well-circumscribed submucosal mass or polyp covered by normal or ulcerated mucosa. Pathological examination of endoscopic biopsies may be diagnostic. Light microscopy typically reveals tightly packed spindle-shaped cells (neoplastic pericytes), surrounding intercommunicating vascular channels of variable caliber and shape. The channels are lined by a thin wall composed of flattened endothelial cells, which stain for factor VIII–related antigen by immunohistochemistry.

Kaposi Sarcoma

Although rare in the general population, Kaposi sarcoma is relatively common in homosexual patients with the acquired immunodeficiency syndrome. Patients with cutaneous lesions frequently develop gastrointestinal lesions that may cause gastrointestinal bleeding. At endoscopy, gastrointestinal lesions frequently appear as purple or red nodules, sometimes with central ulceration, and occasionally appear as sessile masses or as hemorrhagic maculae (Fig. 81-26). Histological examination reveals spindle cells and irregular, jagged, slitlike spaces lined by atypical endothelial cells.

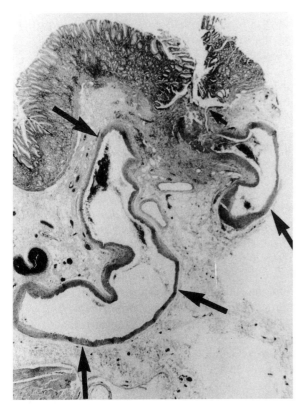

FIGURE 81-1. Histology of Dieulafoy lesion. Low-power photomicrograph shows the sinuous path of an enlarged caliber, but otherwise normal, artery (Dieulafoy lesion) in the submucosa (*large arrows*) of the gastric fundus. A recent thrombus is attached to the artery at the base of a deep mucosal erosion (*small arrow*). No enlarged vein accompanies the enlarged artery, as would occur in an arteriovenous malformation.

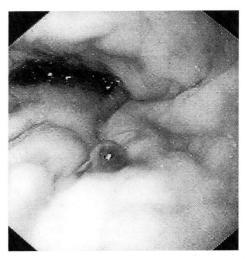

FIGURE 81-2. Endoscopic appearance of an esophageal Dieulafoy lesion. The lesion appears as a small, pigmented protuberance that represents the vessel stump, with no surrounding ulceration or erosion.

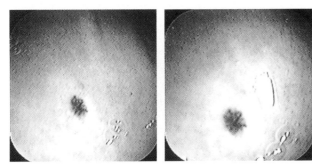

FIGURE 81-3. Vascular tuft of angiodysplasia. Endoscopic videophotograph of the gastric antrum demonstrates the intense erythema and the complex internal reticular structure (in a star burst or stellate pattern) characteristic of an angiodysplasia in a far-away (**left**) and close-up (**right**) view. Note the irregular lesion margin (also in a stellate pattern).

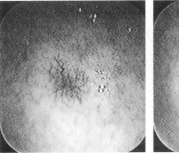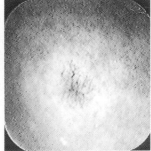

FIGURE 81-4. Arachnoid network of angiodysplasia. Endoscopic videophotograph showing an intensely red and complex reticular (arachnoid) network characteristic of an angiodysplasia in the antrum of a middle-aged female presenting with epigastric pain.

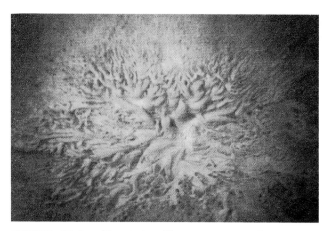

FIGURE 81-5. "Coral head" appearance of advanced angiodysplasia. Stereophotomicrograph shows the typical coral head appearance of a vascular tuft in an advanced right colonic mucosal angiodysplasia after arterial injection with silicone.

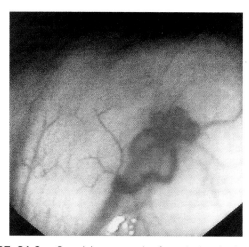

FIGURE 81-6. Supplying vessel of angiodysplasia. Endoscopic photograph showing a large vessel supplying an angiodysplasia in the ascending colon, and the well-defined internal structure (vascular tuft) of the angiodysplasia.

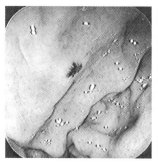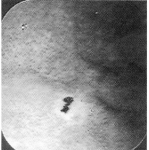

FIGURE 81-7. Anemic halo of angiodysplasia. **Left:** Endoscopic videophotograph showing an intensely red and complex finely reticular network characteristic of an angiodysplasia in the gastric antrum of an elderly male presenting with iron deficiency anemia. **Right:** Mucosa immediately around the angiodysplasia is pale. This anemic halo is attributed to shunting of blood from the surrounding tissue by the low-resistance arteriovenous shunt. Note that the anemic halo is also apparent, although less conspicuous in Fig. 81-3, particularly in the **bottom** figure.

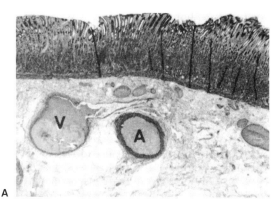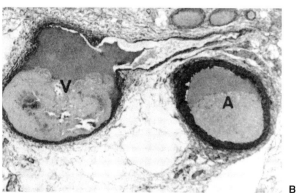

FIGURE 81-8. Histology of arteriovenous malformation. Low- (**A**) and medium- (**B**) power photomicrographs of a gastric fundal arteriovenous malformation. Note the dilated submucosal artery (*A*) and vein (*V*), the close proximity of the vein and artery, and the digitiform projection from the vein toward the artery. The arteries have a thick muscular wall and a continuous, prominent internal elastic membrane (stained black in the tunica media). (van Gieson-Verhoeff stain; original magnification ×20 and ×40, respectively.)

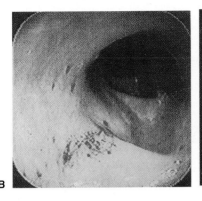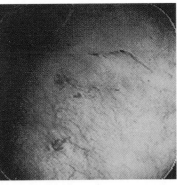

A, B

FIGURE 81-9. Clustering of angiodysplasia. **A:** Videophotograph demonstrates that the multiple angiodysplasia were all clustered in the descending colon on colonoscopy in an elderly female with iron deficiency anemia. **B:** Close-up views demonstrate the characteristic endoscopic appearance of angiodysplasia: an intensely red color, an intricate reticulonodular structure, and communication with prominent feeding arteries.

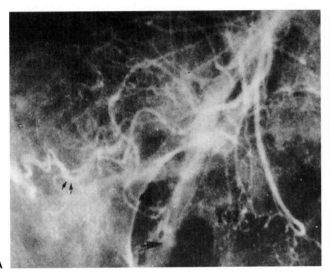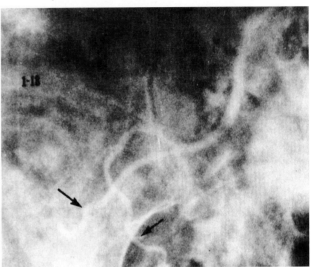

A   B

FIGURE 81-10. Angiographic findings in angiodysplasia. **A:** Arterial phase, 6 seconds after contrast injection into the superior mesenteric artery, in a patient with vascular ectasia shows a vascular tuft (*large arrow*) and two early-filling veins (*small arrows*) that have filled with contrast before other veins. **B:** Late phase, 14 seconds after contrast injection, from the same angiogram reveals two densely opacified, dilated, and tortuous late-draining cecal veins (*arrows*) that still retain contrast after other veins have cleared.

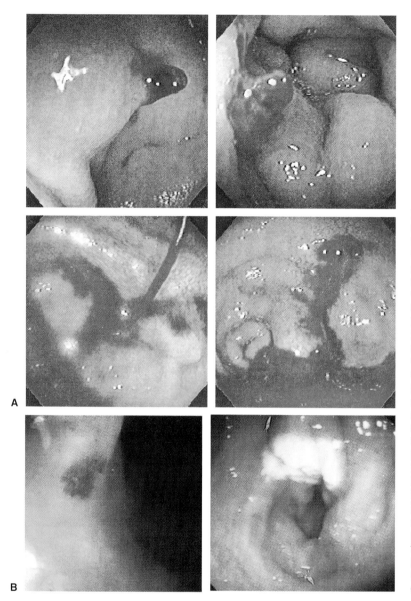

A

B

FIGURE 81-11. A: Active bleeding from angiodysplasia. At colonoscopy, blood is oozing from a nonulcerated pigmented protuberance that appears to be a visible vessel in the cecum (**upper left** profile view; **upper right** close-up profile view). Lesion irrigation prior to electrocautery washes away an overlying clot, and reveals blood spurting from a small-elevated mound that resembles a Dieulafoy lesion (**bottom left** en face view). The bleeding slows after sclerotherapy (**bottom right** en face view). Note in this videophotograph the appendiceal orifice at the 8 o'clock position, about 2 cm away from the lesion at the 1 o'clock position. Pathological examination of the resected specimen after subsequent segmental colonic resection reveals an angiodysplasia and not a Dieulafoy lesion. (Courtesy of Dr. Roger Mendes, Director of Gastroenterology Fellowship Training Program, Long Island College Hospital & Woodhull Hospital, Brooklyn, New York; and Dr. Vanada Vedula, Long Island College Hospital & Woodhull Hospital, Brooklyn, New York.) **B:** Endoscopic electrocoagulation of angiodysplasia. Endoscopic videophotographs show (**left**) an angiodysplasia in the duodenal bulb. **Right:** A white coagulum is present after Gold Probe (Microvasive, Boston Scientific Corporation, Watertown, MA) electrocoagulation.

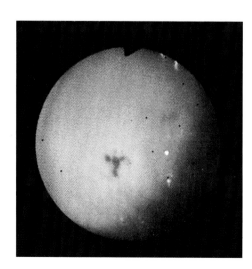

FIGURE 81-12. Endoscopic appearance of gastric antral telangiectasia in hereditary hemorrhagic telangiectasia. Videophotograph shows the characteristic findings: intense erythema, well-demarcated maculae, fine internal reticular (fernlike) structure, and irregular stellate (fernlike) margin. The endoscopic appearance is virtually identical to that of nonsyndromic angiodysplasia. (Courtesy of Dr. Burton Shatz.)

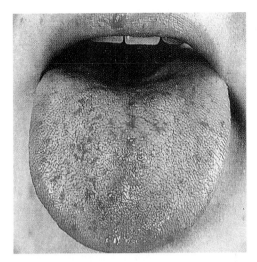

FIGURE 81-13. Mucocutaneous lesions in hereditary hemorrhagic telangiectasia. Photograph shows the typical appearance of telangiectasias on the lips and tongue in a patient with hereditary hemorrhagic telangiectasia as intensely red maculae with an abrupt but irregular (stellate) border.

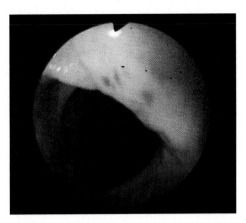

FIGURE 81-14. Endoscopic appearance of gastric antral telangiectasia in calcinosis, Raynaud phenomenon, esophageal dysmotility, sclerodactyly, and telangiectasia (CREST) syndrome. Videophotograph shows the characteristic endoscopic findings: intense erythema, well-demarcated maculae, fine internal reticular (fernlike) structure, and irregular stellate (fernlike) margin. The endoscopic appearance closely resembles that of nonsyndromic angiodysplasia.

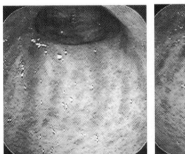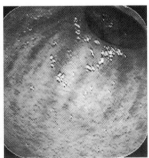

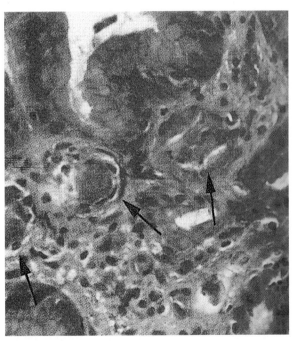

FIGURE 81-15. Endoscopic appearance of gastric antral vascular ectasia (GAVE). Videophotograph shows the characteristic endoscopic finding in GAVE of linear, intensely erythematous lesions at the apices of longitudinal antral folds radiating to the pylorus. The alternative lesion name of watermelon stomach derives from the resemblance of these erythematous linear streaks to the stripes on a watermelon rind.

FIGURE 81-16. Histology of gastric antral vascular ectasia. Findings include multiple dilated capillaries, many of which contain bland fibrin thrombi (*arrows*), and normal capillary endothelium (H&E stain; original magnification ×200).

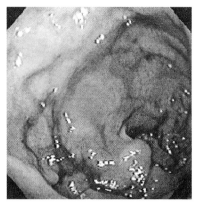
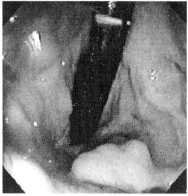

FIGURE 81-17. Endoscopic appearance of rectal varices. **Left:** Rectal varices at colonoscopy appear as superficial serpiginous bluish lesions covered by normal mucosa that project from the mucosa into the lumen, as shown on direct colonoscopic view. **Right:** Same varices shown on colonoscopic rectal retroflexion in an elderly female with cirrhosis from chronic hepatitis C infection. (Courtesy of Dr. Roger Mendes, Director of Gastroenterology Fellowship Training Program, Long Island College Hospital & Woodhull Hospital, Brooklyn, New York; and Dr. Vanada Vedula, Long Island College Hospital & Woodhull Hospital, Brooklyn, New York.)

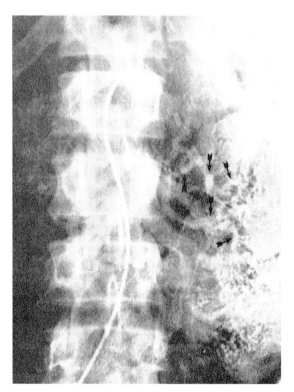

FIGURE 81-18. Angiographic findings in intestinal varices. Contrast injection via a catheter in the superior mesenteric artery shows in the venous phase dilated, tortuous portosystemic collaterals (*arrows*) communicating between the superior mesenteric vein and a massive network of retroperitoneal veins in a patient with jejunal varices proven at laparotomy.

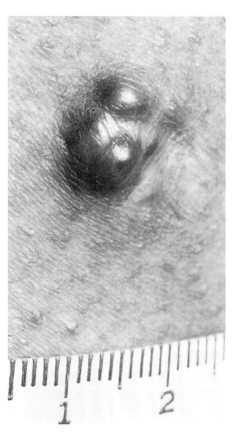

FIGURE 81-19. Appearance of a cutaneous hemangioma in the blue rubber bleb nevus syndrome. Close-up view of a dark blue, nodular, and rubbery skin lesion on the left thigh in a patient with the blue rubber bleb nevus syndrome.

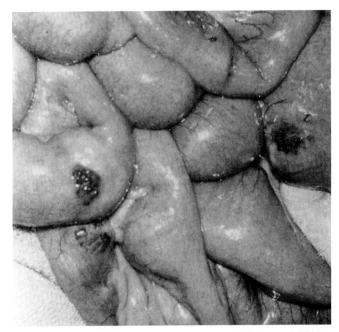

FIGURE 81-20. Intraoperative appearance of intestinal hemangiomas. At laparotomy, multiple hemangiomas appear as bluish, round, smooth, and well-demarcated sessile polypoid lesions on the serosal surface of the small intestine.

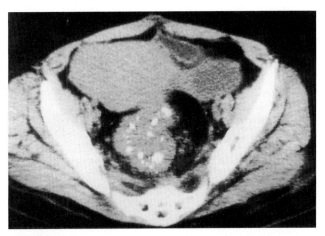

FIGURE 81-21. Radiographic findings of phleboliths. Dense calcifications on computerized tomographic scan represent phleboliths in a colonic hemangioma. The calcifications characteristically are clustered, arranged in a pattern partly outlining the bowel wall, and maintain a constant distance from each other when the entire cluster shifts in position when the patient is turned.

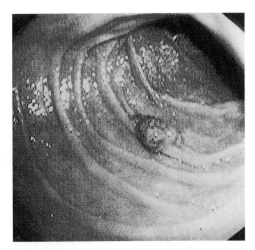

FIGURE 81-22. Endoscopic appearance of a colonic hemangioma in the blue rubber bleb nevus syndrome. Lesion appears as a bluish, round, smooth, and well-demarcated sessile polypoid lesion.

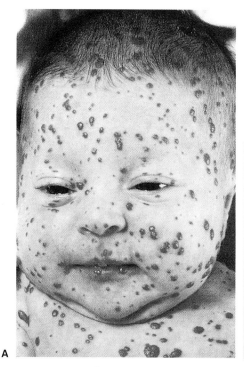

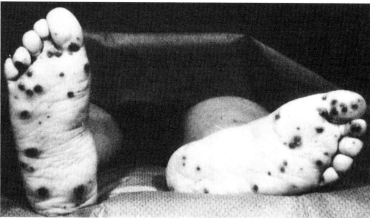

A   B

FIGURE 81-23. **A:** Disseminated cutaneous hemangiomas. Numerous bluish, nodular, and rubbery cutaneous lesions occur on the face of a child with disseminated hemangiomatosis. Patients characteristically have multiple intestinal hemangiomas. **B:** Photograph of numerous bluish-black, nodular, and rubbery skin lesions on the plantar surface of both feet in a child with diffuse hemangiomatosis.

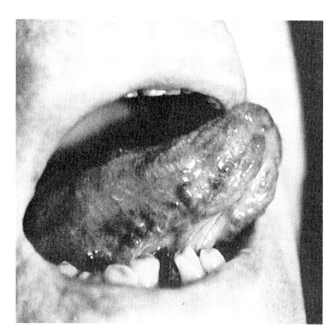

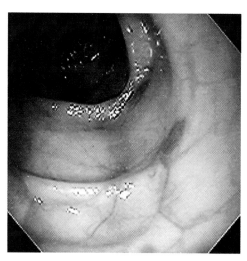

FIGURE 81-24. Sublingual phlebectasia (caviar spots). Curling and extension of the tongue demonstrates multiple purplish or bluish-gray nodular to oblong venous varicosities on the undersurface of the tongue.

FIGURE 81-25. Endoscopic appearance of phlebectasia. Phlebectasia appear at endoscopy as bluish oblong venous varicosities. In this case, a cluster of these lesions was localized to the transverse colon.

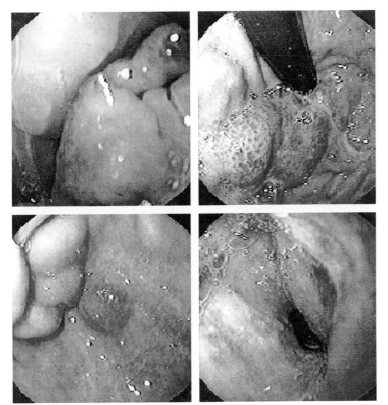

FIGURE 81-26. Spectrum of endoscopic appearance of upper gastrointestinal Kaposi sarcoma. Esophagogastroduodenoscopy revealed a reddish purple oral mass near several teeth (**upper left**), a multinodular cardial mass with superficial punctate erythema noted on gastric retroflexion (**upper right**), a small reddish nodular mass at the pylorus (**lower left**), and a violaceous circumferential mass with an overlying whitish exudate producing irregular constriction of the descending duodenum (**lower right**). (Courtesy of Dr. Roger Mendes, Director of Gastroenterology Fellowship Training Program, Long Island College Hospital & Woodhull Hospital, Brooklyn, New York; and Dr. Vanada Vedula, Long Island College Hospital & Woodhull Hospital, Brooklyn, New York.)

INTESTINAL ISCHEMIA

JULIÁN PANÉS ■ JOSEP M. PIQUÉ

Intestinal ischemia represents a broad spectrum of diseases with various clinical, radiological, and pathological manifestations. These range from localized transient ischemia to extensive necrosis of the gastrointestinal tract. Despite better insights into the pathophysiology of intestinal ischemia, some ischemic syndromes continue to have high morbidity; for example, a greater than 60% rate of mortality exists from acute ischemia of the small intestine. Diagnosis before the occurrence of intestinal infarction is the most important factor in improving survival for patients with intestinal ischemia.

ANATOMY OF THE INTESTINAL CIRCULATION

Arterial Anatomy

The celiac artery arises from the abdominal aorta at about the level of the T12 or L1 vertebral body. It branches into the left gastric, common hepatic and splenic arteries (Fig. 82-1). The left gastric artery supplies the stomach. The common hepatic artery divides into the hepatic artery, which supplies the liver; the right gastric artery, which supplies the stomach along the lesser curvature; and the gastroduodenal artery, which supplies the antrum, duodenum, and pancreas. The splenic artery supplies the spleen and body and tail of the pancreas.

The superior mesenteric artery (SMA) arises from the aorta approximately 1 cm below the celiac artery, usually at the level of L1. It courses inferiorly and toward the right to terminate at the level of the cecum as the ileocolic artery (see Fig. 82-1). The inferior pancreaticoduodenal artery supplies the pancreatic head, and anastomoses with the corresponding superior branches from the celiac axis. Generally, there are more SMA branches to the distal small bowel than to the more proximal portions, thus providing greater potential for distal anastomotic communication. The middle colic artery arises from the proximal SMA to supply the transverse colon and communicates with branches of the IMA. The right colic artery supplies the distal ascending colon and right colonic (hepatic) flexure. The ileocolic artery is the terminal branch of the SMA and supplies the distal ileum, cecum, and ascending colon.

The inferior mesenteric artery (IMA) is the smallest of the mesenteric vessels and arises from the ventral aorta approximately 6 to 7 cm below the SMA at the level of L3 (see Fig. 82-1). The artery branches into the left colic, which supplies the left transverse colon and splenic flexure; several arteries that supply the sigmoid and descending colon; and the superior rectal artery, which supplies a large part of the rectum.

Extensive anastomotic and collateral circulation exists within each and between the three major intestinal vessels, as well as between the mesenteric vessels and the nonmesenteric systemic circulation. Despite the presence of collateral channels, the vasculature has several points susceptible to poor perfusion (watershed areas). The middle part of the small intestine, in the middle of the area perfused by the SMA, is far away from collaterals from the celiac axis to the proximal SMA and from collaterals from the IMA to the distal SMA. This area is the most vulnerable to develop ischemia from SMA occlusion. Narrow terminal branches of the SMA supply the splenic flexure, and the rectosigmoid junction is supplied by terminal branches of the IMA. These two watershed areas are most vulnerable to develop ischemia during systemic hypotension if the collateral anastomoses are small or tenuous.

Venous Anatomy

The venous system generally parallels the arterial distribution. The inferior mesenteric vein (IMV) drains the rectum through the superior rectal vein, the sigmoid through the sigmoid veins, and the descending colon through the left colic vein. The superior mesenteric vein (SMV) drains the small intestine, cecum, ascending colon, and transverse colon via the jejunal, ileal, ileocolic, right colic, and middle colic veins. The SMV also drains the greater omentum and distal stomach with the right gastroepiploic vein, and drains part of the pancreas and duodenum via the inferior pancreaticoduodenal vein. The IMV drains into the splenic vein, which then joins the SMV to form the portal vein.

MECHANISMS OF ISCHEMIC INJURY

The mechanisms that are believed to participate in ischemic and reperfusion injury include the infiltration of postischemic tissues by inflammatory cells, an increased production of reactive oxygen species, alterations in vascular permeability, and inhibition of local cytoprotective mechanisms (Fig. 82-2).

CLINICAL SYNDROMES

The spectrum of intestinal ischemia comprises a number of syndromes which include acute mesenteric ischemia as a result of emboli, arterial or venous thrombi, vasoconstriction secondary to low-flow states, or small bowel loop strangulation; chronic mesenteric ischemia (also named intestinal angina) caused by transient, recurrent episodes of inadequate intestinal blood flow to sustain metabolic needs or to support increased metabolic demands, such as that associated with digestion; and ischemic colitis, in which a circulatory insufficiency of the colon results in varying degrees of local tissue necrosis and systemic manifestations.

Acute Mesenteric Ischemia

Acute insufficiency of the blood supply to the intestine can result from emboli, arterial and venous thrombi, or vasoconstriction secondary to low-flow states. Embolization to the SMA comprises about 5% of peripheral emboli and accounts for roughly 50% of all cases of acute mesenteric ischemia (AMI) (Fig. 82-3). The SMA is anatomically susceptible to embolism because it has a large caliber and arises from the aorta at a narrow angle. The most common precipitant of thrombus dislodgment and embolization is a cardiac arrhythmia, especially atrial fibrillation.

Emboli tend to obstruct mesenteric flow acutely and completely, not allowing sufficient time to develop protective mesenteric collaterals.

Thrombosis accounts for about 15% of cases of acute intestinal ischemia. Thrombosis of the SMA or celiac artery is generally associated with a preexisting stenosis, usually at the origin of the arteries (Fig. 82-4). About 30% of patients have histories consistent with chronic mesenteric ischemia, including postprandial pain, malabsorption, and weight loss before the acute episode.

Nonocclusive mesenteric ischemia (NOMI) causes 20% to 30% of episodes of acute mesenteric ischemia. Mesenteric ischemia without anatomic arterial or venous obstruction is due to mesenteric vasospasm that can occur during periods of relatively low mesenteric flow, especially if there is underlying arterial atherosclerotic disease (Fig. 82-5). Vasoconstrictive drugs, particularly α-adrenergic agents, vasopressin, ergotamine, diuretics, and digitalis glycosides, can contribute to NOMI.

Thrombosis of the SMV causes 5% to 10% of the causes of AMI. Symptomatic SMV thrombosis is about 20-fold more common than symptomatic IMV thrombosis because of the larger caliber and flow of the SMV. Risk factors for mesenteric venous thrombosis include hypercoagulable syndromes, portal hypertension, abdominal infections, perforated viscus, pancreatitis, and trauma.

Chronic Mesenteric Ischemia

Chronic mesenteric ischemia (intestinal angina) is a clinical syndrome characterized by recurrent abdominal pain and weight loss as a result of repeated transient episodes of insufficient intestinal blood flow. Clinical manifestations are related to limitations of the ability of the celiac artery or SMA to supply increased blood flow in response to metabolic demands after a meal, mainly because of atherosclerotic vascular lesions. Intestinal angina is an uncommon process that only occurs when severe atherosclerotic narrowing of a major splanchnic vessel exists in association with occlusion of one or two of the remaining vessels. This is because the very efficient collateral circulatory network in the small bowel and colon can successfully overcome the single occlusion of a major vessel.

Ischemic Colitis

Ischemic colitis is the most common form of ischemic injury to the gut and occurs more frequently in elderly people. It can result from either occlusive or nonocclusive events, mainly in the territory of the IMA, in colonic branches of the SMA, and in the superior and IMVs. Thus, ischemic colitis is predominantly seen in the left colon. The splenic flexure and rectosigmoid junction, where low perfusion exists (watershed areas), are commonly affected, whereas the rectum is not usually compromised because of excellent collateral perfusion. Right colon ischemic colitis is rare, is mainly due to low-flow states, and it is associated with poor prognosis.

A wide spectrum of disorders can be seen as a consequence of colonic ischemia. These include acute, transient, self-limited ischemia (reversible colopathy characterized by mucosal and submucosal hemorrhage), acute fulminant ischemia (which is transmural and progresses to necrosis), and chronic ischemic colitis (partially reversible vascular disease usually manifested by late colonic stenosis).

DIAGNOSIS

Plain X-ray Films of the Abdomen

Plain abdominal radiography is most useful to exclude other potential causes of abdominal pain rather than confirming the diagnosis of acute mesenteric ischemia.

Completely normal plain radiographs have been reported in more than 25% of patients with mesenteric ischemia. Subtle signs of AMI on plain abdominal radiographs include adynamic ileus and distended, air-filled loops of bowel (Fig. 82-6), but these abnormalities most commonly are due to other causes such as pancreatitis, mechanical obstruction, or colonic pseudoobstruction. More specific radiographic findings occur in 25% of cases, usually with advanced disease. These findings include mural thumbprinting resulting from edema or hemorrhage (Fig. 82-7). In advanced stages of ischemia, pneumatosis of the bowel wall can be detected (Fig. 82-8). Specifically, portal vein gas on abdominal radiography portends an extremely poor prognosis (Figs. 82-9 and 82-10).

Intralumenal barium contrast evaluations are contraindicated because residual contrast can limit visualization of the mesenteric vasculature during diagnostic angiography. On the rare occasion when barium studies are performed in a patient with abdominal pain not initially thought to have AMI, thumbprinting, stricture, or ulcerations can be found. After an ischemic episode, contrast radiology may be helpful in identifying residual stenotic lesions (Fig. 82-11).

Duplex Sonography (Doppler Ultrasonography)

Duplex ultrasonography may be of some benefit in visualizing flow in the SMA and celiac axis. With expert technical assistance, these tests can document proximal stenoses in the SMA (Fig. 82-12) or celiac axis or complete occlusion of these vessels (Fig. 82-13). In significant vascular stenosis, duplex ultrasonography shows high flow velocity and poststenotic turbulence reflected by modifications on spectral waveform and mixture of colors in the duplex image. In stenosis of the SMA greater than 50% to 70%, the sensitivity of the technique is greater than 90%, with marginal improvement with postprandial study. Sensitivity for lesions in celiac axis is slightly lower (85%–87%). When performed by skilled operators, duplex ultrasonography may be a useful screening tool. Unfortunately, duplex sonography is of no value in detecting emboli beyond the proximal main vessel or in diagnosing NOMI. Moreover, identification of significant arterial stenosis does not establish the diagnosis of intestinal ischemia because total occlusion of two or even all three splanchnic vessels can be present in asymptomatic patients.

Computed Tomography (CT)

Abdominal CT may be useful in diagnosing intestinal ischemia caused by arterial occlusion or NOMI, but is very effective for in excluding mesenteric venous thrombosis and other abdominal disorders in the differential diagnosis. As on plain radiography of the abdomen, most abnormalities on CT associated with AMI are nonspecific and occur late in the course of the disease. Nonspecific findings in a contrast-enhanced CT scan examination may include the presence of bowel wall thickening and diffuse mesenteric haziness caused by edema (Fig. 82-14). Highly suggestive findings for AMI, including portal venous gas and pneumatosis intestinalis, are seen only after infarction has developed (Figs. 82-15 and 82-16). In patients with chronic mesenteric ischemia, CT scan may demonstrate the presence of calcified atheromatous lesions (Fig. 82-17) and collateral circulation (Fig. 82-18).

In contrast to the limited role of CT in the diagnosis of arterial mesenteric ischemia, CT diagnosis of mesenteric venous thrombosis has proven more valuable (Fig. 82-19). All studies report sensitivities ranging from 90% to 100%. Abnormal bowel characteristics on CT (bowel wall thickening, pneumatosis) strongly suggest the diagnosis of acute mesenteric venous thrombosis.

Angiography

Angiography should be performed early when intestinal ischemia is suspected. Because the diagnosis before bowel ischemia becomes irreversible is the most important factor in improving patient survival, and only angiography or surgery enables such early diagnosis, angiography has become a cornerstone in the evaluation of patients with abdominal pain who are at high risk for intestinal ischemia. However, prompt laparotomy should be performed in patients with suspected intestinal ischemia in whom expeditious angiography is not available.

In cases of SMA embolization, most emboli are impacted 3 to 10 cm from the origin of the SMA, distal to the origin of the middle colic artery (see Fig. 82-3). The classic meniscus sign can often be visualized at the point of occlusion, which is different from the planar defect produced by a thrombus (see Fig. 82-4). Contrast is typically poorly visualized distal to emboli because the rapidity of embolic occlusion provides insufficient time to develop collateral flow. Other angiographic findings favoring embolus over thrombus include minimal atherosclerosis in mesenteric vessels, multiple lesions in mesenteric arterial branches, and simultaneous extramesenteric emboli.

Symptomatic thrombosis of the SMA is generally associated with a high-grade stenosis or occlusion of the celiac axis (Fig. 82-20). The stenosis usually slowly progresses and permits reconstitution of vascular flow because of development of collaterals (Fig. 82-21). Aortography is essential in these patients to evaluate potential inflow and outflow sites for bypass grafts as well as to clarify the extent and location of other atherosclerotic lesions in the iliac and inferior mesenteric arteries (Fig. 82-22). When the SMA distal to thrombotic occlusion fills from large collaterals, the SMA thrombus is probably chronic and not the cause of acute symptoms.

In patients suffering NOMI, angiography usually reveals multiple areas of narrowing and irregularity in major branches. The small and medium arterial branches may be decreased or absent, producing a "pruned" arterial tree, and there is also impaired intramural vascular filling (see Fig. 82-5). The diagnosis of NOMI is strongly favored over the diagnosis of arterial thrombosis by an absence of extramesenteric atherosclerosis and by an increase in SMA caliber after transcatheter vasodilator therapy.

Endoscopy

Colonoscopy or flexible sigmoidoscopy is the method of choice for the diagnosis of ischemic colitis because it allows direct visualization of the mucosa and tissue sampling. Colonoscopy is preferable to sigmoidoscopy because 50% of the ischemic lesions are proximal to the sigmoid colon, except for ischemic injury after aortic surgery, in which lesions always involve the distal colon. The endoscopy examination must be performed with caution and air insufflation must be minimized to avoid perforation. The mucosa of the affected segment usually appears edematous, hemorrhagic, friable (Fig. 82-23), and ulcerated (Figs. 82-24 and 82-25). When bowel necrosis is present, colonoscopy reveals cyanotic, gray or black mucosa.

HISTOPATHOLOGY OF INTESTINAL ISCHEMIA

When infarction occurs, the bowel becomes edematous and plum colored (Fig. 82-26). The mucosa is necrotic and has a nodular surface because of extensive submucosal hemorrhage, but the deep muscle layers may initially appear well preserved. As necrosis becomes more complete or gangrene develops, all layers of the intestinal wall are affected. The external surface has a mottled purple or greenish hue and the tissues of the bowel are thin and friable.

Microscopic examination of specimens with early mucosal lesions usually shows a patchy distribution with almost normal mucosa surrounding diseased areas in which crypts show necrosis, and with the formation of a surface membrane composed of mucus, fibrin, blood cells, and necrotic tissue (Fig. 82-27). There is vascular congestion with edema and occasional hemorrhages in the submucosal layer (Fig. 82-28). It is common to see fibrin thrombi within the blood vessels. With increasing severity of ischemia, the deeper layers of the bowel wall become affected (Fig. 82-29). Infarction is manifested by hemorrhage into the bowel wall, particularly the submucosa, and intravascular thrombosis and mucosal ulceration are present (Fig. 82-30). All features of ischemic necrosis can go through a process of resolution and repair. Granulation tissue replaces the layers of the bowel. The entire process is essentially the same for the small intestine and colon, and stricture is often the end result.

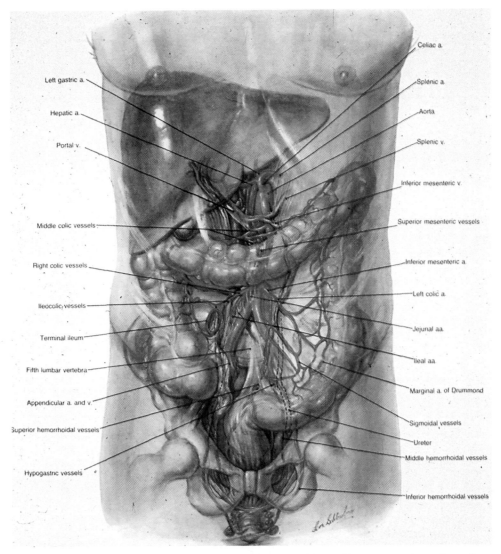

FIGURE 82-1. Anatomy of the intestinal circulation. The celiac artery arises from the abdominal aorta and branches into the left gastric, common hepatic, and splenic arteries. The superior mesenteric artery (SMA) exits the aorta 1 cm below the celiac artery. It supplies the entire small intestine except for the superior part of the duodenum, and supplies the right and transverse colon and part of the pancreas. Branches include the inferior pancreaticoduodenal artery, numerous jejunal and ileal branches, the ileocolic artery, and the middle colic artery. The inferior mesenteric artery (IMA) arises from the aorta 3 cm proximal to the aortic bifurcation. The artery branches into the left colic, several sigmoid (inferior left colic) arteries, and the superior rectal (hemorrhoidal) artery. The arcades of the SMA and IMA interconnect at the base and border of the mesentery. The connection at the base of the mesentery provides a potential collateral channel between SMA and IMA called the arc of Riolan. The connection along the mesenteric border provides another potential collateral channel called the marginal artery of Drummond.

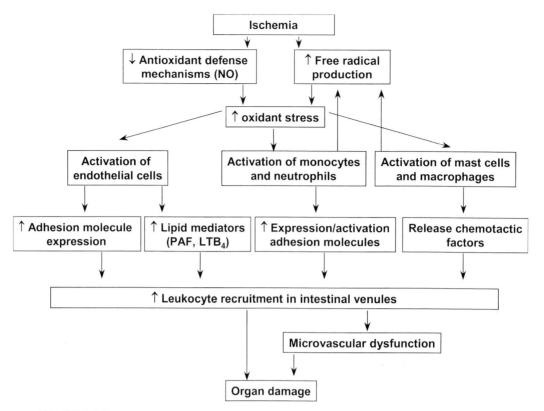

FIGURE 82-2. Mechanisms involved in ischemia-induced intestinal damage. Ischemia results in an increased production of oxidants, with a corresponding reduction in the synthesis of nitric oxide (NO) by endothelial NO synthase (eNOS). The enhanced generation of oxidants results in the activation of endothelial cells and leukocytes. Firm adhesion of leukocytes, which is mediated by β2-integrins (CD11/CD18), is induced by engagement of activated leukotriene B_4 (LTB_4) and platelet activating factor (PAF) with their receptors on rolling leukocytes. Sustained rolling and adhesion of leukocytes on endothelial cells are ensured by an oxidant-dependent synthesis of endothelial cell adhesion molecules, such as P-selectin and intercellular adhesion molecule-1 (ICAM-1). The inflammatory responses to ischemia are further amplified by oxidants derived from reduced nicotinamide adenine dinucleotide phosphate (NADPH) oxidase in leukocytes, and by mediators released from mast cells and macrophages that normally reside in close proximity to postcapillary venules.

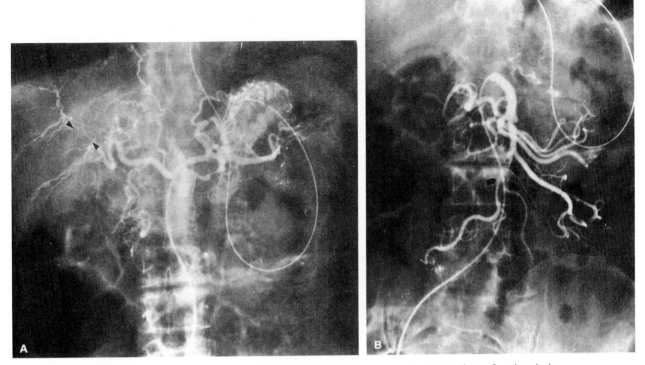

FIGURE 82-3. Visceral embolic disease. Arteriographic demonstration of splanchnic embolic disease. These two views of the same patient demonstrate emboli in two different splanchnic vessels. **A:** Hepatic artery embolus (*arrowheads*). **B:** Superior mesenteric artery embolus (*arrow*).

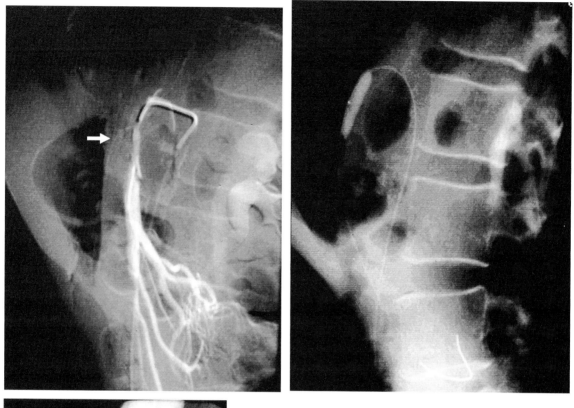

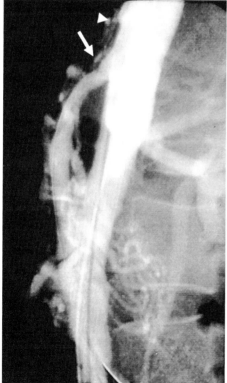

FIGURE 82-4. Abdominal angiogram of a 70-year-old patient with severe periumbilical pain of sudden onset. **A:** Selective angiogram of the superior mesenteric artery (SMA) demonstrating an 80% occlusion of the lumen (*arrow*) with poor filling of distal branches. An abdominal angiogram showed total obstruction of the celiac trunk. **B:** Transluminal angioplasty. Balloon inflated at the level of the SMA stenosis. No residual waste in the balloon is present. **C:** Abdominal angiogram after transluminal angioplasty shows a good perfusion of the SMA (*arrow*), and persistence of proximal occlusion of the celiac trunk (*arrowhead*).

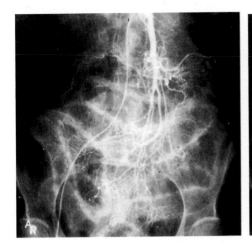

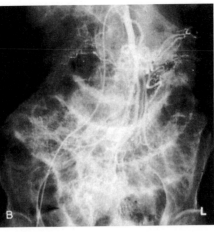

FIGURE 82-5. Nonocclusive intestinal ischemia–arteriographic findings. **A:** Initial mesenteric arteriogram of a patient with nonocclusive intestinal ischemia shows vasospasm and irregularities of the celiac and superior mesenteric arteries. The normal arterial blush of the intestinal wall is lost. **B:** After infusion of papaverine, substantial vasodilation is visible at both the macrovascular and microvascular levels. This radiograph is compatible with a normal superior mesenteric arteriogram but is diagnostic for nonocclusive mesenteric ischemia when compared with **A.**

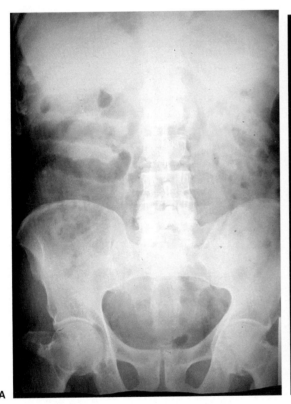

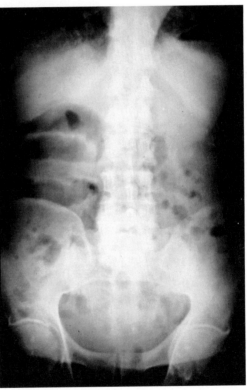

FIGURE 82-6. A 58-year-old patient with abdominal pain. **A:** Plain abdominal x-ray film showing three horizontal distended air-filled loops with mural thickening on the right upper quadrant. **B:** A second x-ray abdominal film of the same patient taken after a 3-hour interval shows persistence of the same distended loops. This finding is suggestive, although not pathognomonic, of intestinal ischemia. The patient underwent urgent surgery because peritoneal signs were present. Necrosis of 70 cm of the ileum associated with a thrombosis of the superior mesenteric artery was diagnosed.

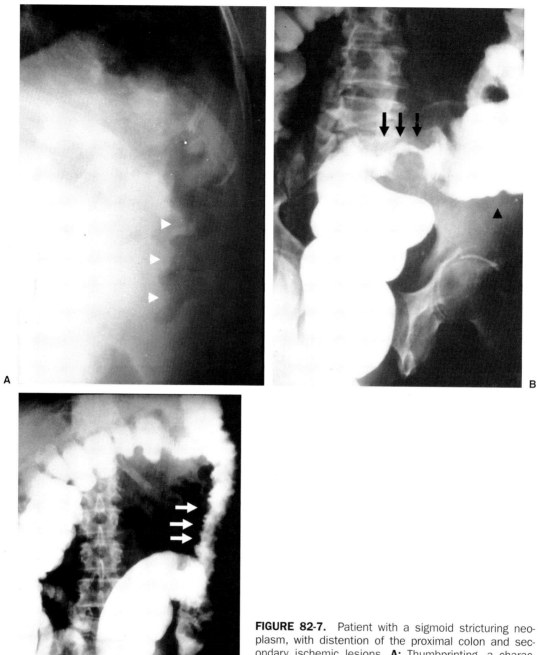

FIGURE 82-7. Patient with a sigmoid stricturing neoplasm, with distention of the proximal colon and secondary ischemic lesions. **A:** Thumbprinting, a characteristic radiologic feature of ischemia colitis, is observed in the descending colon (*arrowheads*). Projections of the intestinal wall toward the intestinal lumen result from edema or hemorrhage. **B:** Barium enema examination discloses the stricturing sigmoid neoplasm (*arrows*) and proximal distention (*arrowhead*). **C:** Thumbprinting lesions on the wall of the ascending colon are confirmed by the barium study (*arrows*).

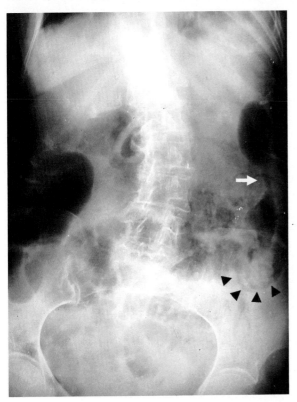

FIGURE 82-8. A 75-year-old female with ischemic colitis. Intramural air (pneumatosis) is present in the lower part of the descending colon (*arrowheads*). There is tapering of the lumen in the mid-portion of the descending colon (*arrow*).

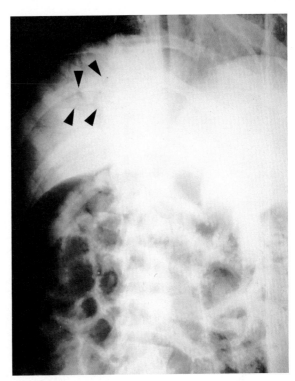

FIGURE 82-9. A 53-year-old man with atrial fibrillation that came to the emergency department because of abdominal pain. Plain x-ray film of the abdomen shows a generalized dilation of the small and large intestine and presence of gas in the portal branches (*arrowheads*). Arteriography demonstrated an embolus lodged on the superior mesenteric artery. At surgery, lesions of transmural bowel necrosis affecting the distal ileum and right colon were observed.

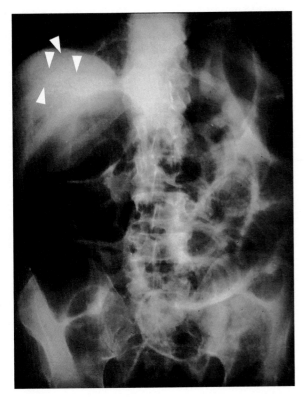

FIGURE 82-10. A 72-year-old male with superior mesenteric artery ischemia caused by thrombosis. The plain abdominal x-ray film demonstrated a marked dilation of the colon and small intestine, along with presence of gas in intrahepatic branches of the portal vein (*arrowheads*).

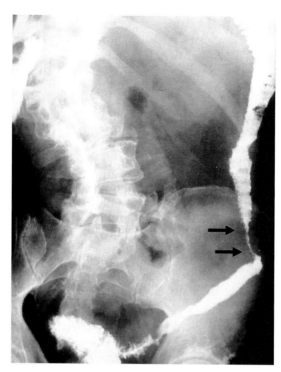

FIGURE 82-11. Barium enema of a 76-year-old female that had suffered ischemic colitis resolved with conservative measures. The patient had episodes of left-sided abdominal pain that were relieved by defecation. Barium enema was performed 2 months after the ischemic episode and revealed a stricturing lesion in the descending colon that corresponds with the location of the ischemic region (*arrows*).

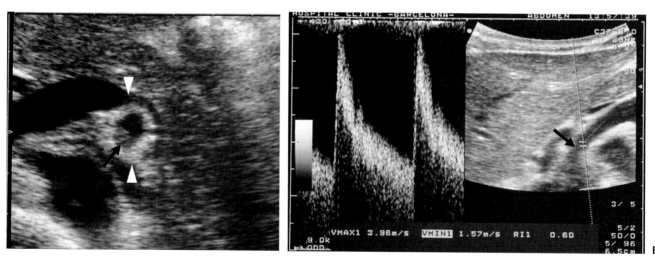

FIGURE 82-12. Ultrasound examination in a patient with celiac artery occlusion and superior mesenteric artery (SMA) stenosis. **A:** Gray-scale ultrasound showing a partial thrombus at the origin of SMA (*arrowheads*) occluding 50% of the arterial lumen (*arrow* shows thrombus). **B:** Pulsed Doppler study of the SMA origin of the same patient. **Left half** reveals a very high peak systolic velocity (3.84 m/s) resulting from the SMA stenosis (**right half,** *arrow*).

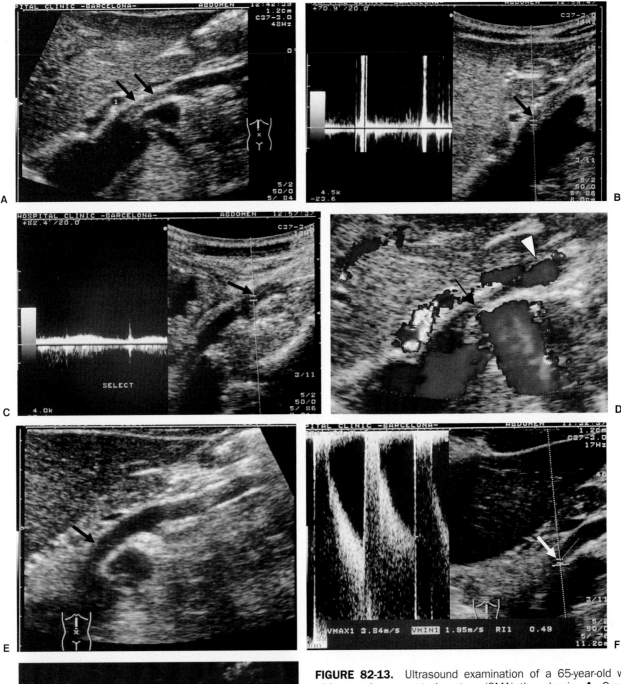

FIGURE 82-13. Ultrasound examination of a 65-year-old woman with superior mesenteric artery (SMA) thrombosis. **A:** Gray-scale ultrasound examination demonstrates an echogenic image filling the entire lumen of the superior mesenteric artery (SMA) that corresponds to an occluding thrombus (*arrows*). **B:** Assessment of SMA flow by pulsed Doppler reveals absence of flow (**left half**) in the thrombosed area (*arrow*). **C:** A low flow is detected in more distal branches (*arrow*); arteriography examinations demonstrated distal filling from the celiac axis through the pancreaticoduodenal branches. **D:** Color Doppler ultrasound confirms the absence of flow signal in the thrombosed area (*arrow*), along with presence of flow in the more distal segment (*arrowhead*). **E:** Ultrasound examination of the same patient following percutaneous angioplasty. The echogenic signal in the lumen of the SMA has disappeared (*arrow*). **F:** Doppler ultrasound demonstrates pulsatile flow (**left half**) in the region previously thrombosed (*arrow*). **G:** Color Doppler also confirms patency of the SMA (*arrows*), with normal caliber of the vessel.

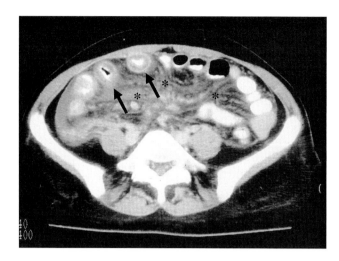

FIGURE 82-14. Ischemia of the ileum after blunt trauma in a 66-year-old woman. Contrast-enhanced computed tomography scan shows bowel wall thickening (*arrows*) in the ileum with diffuse mesenteric haziness caused by edema (*asterisks*).

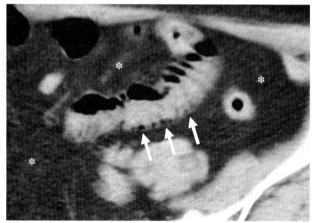

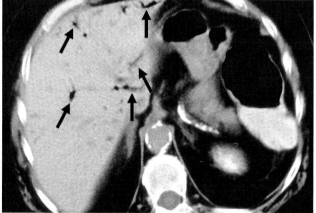

FIGURE 82-15. Contrast-enhanced computed tomography (CT) scan in a 72-year-old man with intestinal infarction caused by superior mesenteric artery embolus. **A:** Intestinal pneumatosis (*arrows*) and extensive infiltration of the mesentery (*asterisks*) are present. **B:** CT scan obtained at an upper level shows presence of gas in numerous portal branches (*arrows*).

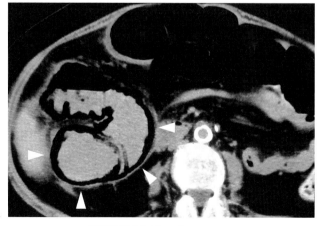

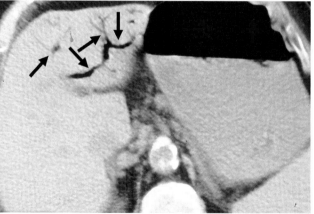

FIGURE 82-16. Severe ischemic colitis in a patient with septic shock. **A:** Transverse computed tomography scan section shows extensive pneumatosis in the colonic wall (*arrowheads*). **B:** Transverse section obtained at an upper level shows the presence of portal venous gas (*arrows*).

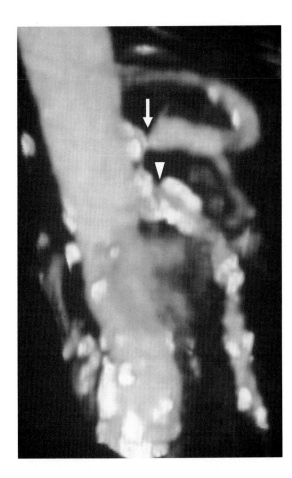

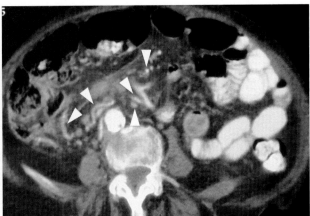

FIGURE 82-17. Lateral computed tomography scan angiogram of a 81-year-old patient with chronic intestinal ischemia. Calcified atheromatous plaques are widely distributed in the wall of the aorta, celiac axis, and superior mesenteric artery. A 95% reduction of the lumen of the origin of the celiac axis is observed (*arrow*), along with a 60% decrease in the lumen of the proximal superior mesenteric artery (*arrowhead*).

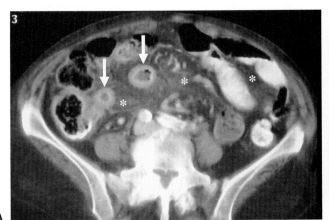

A

B

FIGURE 82-18. Contrast-enhanced computed tomography scan in a 72-year-old woman with chronic intestinal ischemia. **A:** Mural thickening of the ileal intestinal loops (*arrows*) and regional mesenteric haziness caused by edema (*asterisks*) are present. **B:** Abundant collateral circulation through aberrant vessels (*arrowheads*) is observed in this image obtained at an upper level. Angiogram (not shown) demonstrated complete occlusion of the celiac axis and an 80% occlusion of the superior mesenteric artery.

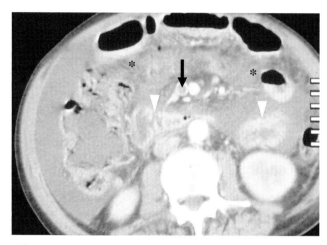

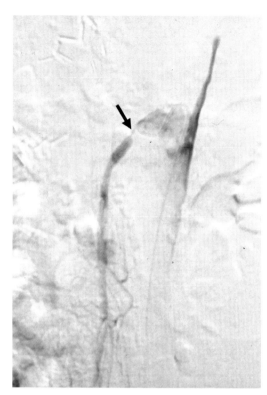

FIGURE 82-19. Contrast-enhanced computed tomography (CT) scan of the abdomen in a patient with acute pancreatitis and mesenteric venous thrombosis. CT scan shows mural thickening of small bowel loops (*arrowheads*) and a hypoattenuating thrombus of the superior mesenteric vein (*arrow*). Ascites is also present (*asterisks*).

FIGURE 82-20. Arteriography of the superior mesenteric artery in a 59-year-old male with chronic abdominal pain. Selective injection demonstrates a 90% proximal stenosis (*arrow*) with poor filling of the distal branches.

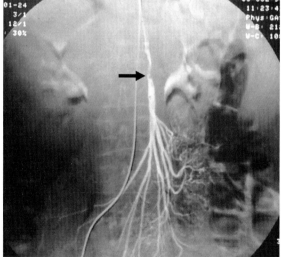
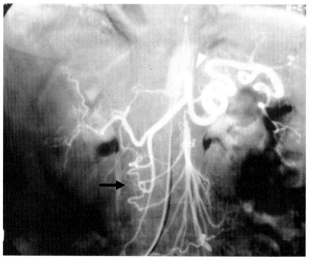

FIGURE 82-21. **A:** Selective digital subtraction angiography (DSA) of the superior mesenteric artery (SMA), showing a long and high-grade stenosis of the proximal artery (*arrow*). **B:** DSA injection of the celiac axis (*arrowhead*) of the same patient demonstrating collateral filling of the distal SMA through pancreaticoduodenal collaterals (*arrow*).

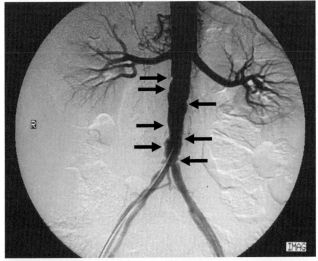

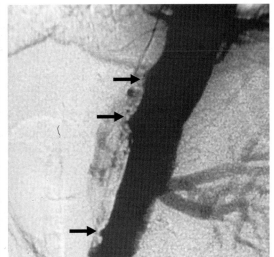

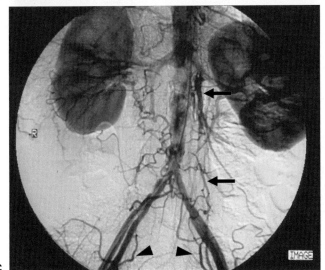

FIGURE 82-22. A 66-year-old male with long-standing postprandial abdominal pain and significant weight loss. **A:** Aortography shows diffuse atheromatous lesions in the abdominal aorta (*arrows*). **B:** The three mesenteric vessels (celiac axis, superior mesenteric artery, and inferior mesenteric artery) have a proximal thrombotic occlusion (*arrows*). **C:** Profuse collateral circulation fill the superior mesenteric artery (*thick arrow*) and inferior mesenteric artery (*thin arrow*) through the hypogastric vessels (*arrowheads*).

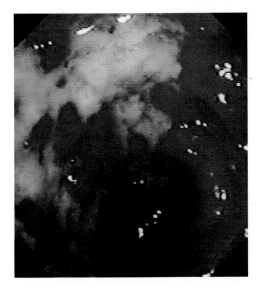

FIGURE 82-23. An 83-year-old female that presented with abdominal pain and bloody diarrhea. Colonoscopy revealed the presence of large ulcerations in the splenic flexure. Biopsies were compatible with the diagnosis of ischemic colitis. This region is commonly affected in colonic ischemia because of its relatively low perfusion (watershed area). Colonoscopy is the method of choice for the diagnosis of ischemic colitis, because it allows direct visualization of the mucosa and tissue sampling.

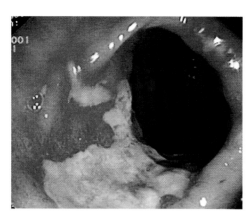

FIGURE 82-24. Large ulceration in the sigmoid region caused by ischemia. The sigmoid colon is another area that is particularly susceptible to ischemic lesions because of its relatively low perfusion. Although this lesion can be reached by a sigmoidoscopy, complete colonoscopy should be performed in patients suspected of having ischemic colitis because 50% of the ischemic lesions are proximal to the sigmoid colon.

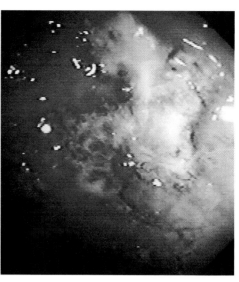

FIGURE 82-25. Endoscopic findings in a 62-year-old female with ischemic colitis associated with a low-flow state (sepsis). The mucosa of the affected segment appears edematous, hemorrhagic, friable, and ulcerated.

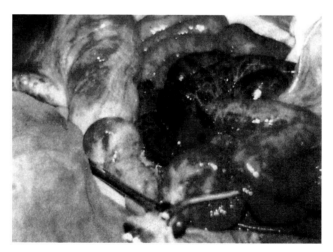

FIGURE 82-26. Gross findings at laparotomy on a patient with nonocclusive mesenteric ischemia. Although the bowel wall is mottled, it remains viable. The patient had undergone angiography and vasodilator infusion, but irreversible bowel necrosis had already occurred, necessitating laparotomy and resection.

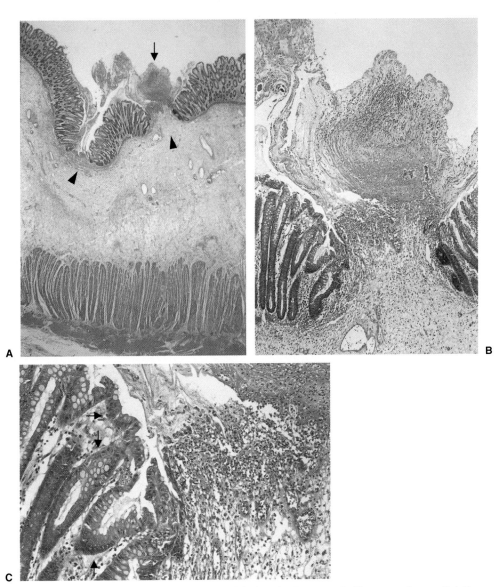

FIGURE 82-27. Early stages of intestinal ischemic damage. **A:** There are two well-delimited erosions of the mucosa (*arrowheads*), with formation of a pseudomembrane (*arrow*). The remaining mucosa is normal. The submucosa has a marked edema and discrete infiltration by inflammatory cells. **B:** Close-up view of the pseudomembrane composed of fibrin and leukocytes. **C:** Detail of inflammatory cell infiltration at the erosion site. At this magnification, reactive changes in the mucosal epithelium can be observed (*arrows*).

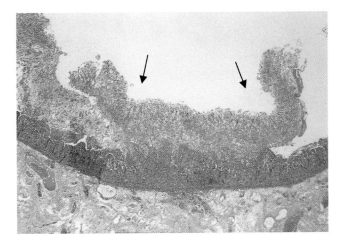

FIGURE 82-28. More extensive ischemic damage, with formation of a surface exudate (*arrows*). There is vascular congestion and presence of an inflammatory infiltrate in the lamina propria, and edema of the submucosa.

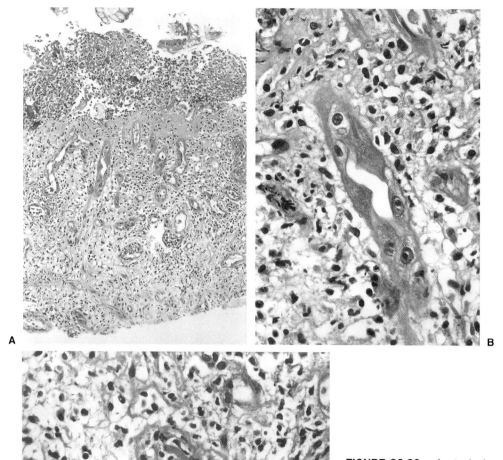

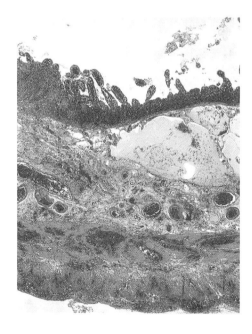

FIGURE 82-29. Acute ischemic necrosis. This illustrates a more advanced stage of ischemic damage. **A:** Villi have completely disappeared and are replaced by a membrane composed of fibrinous exudate, necrotic epithelial cells, and inflammatory cells. **B:** The crypts are severely affected and only the most basal parts have survived, at higher magnification, reactive changes can be observed in the remaining portions of the crypts. **C:** A fibrin thrombus in one of the submucosal small vessels (*arrow*).

FIGURE 82-30. Transmural hemorrhagic necrosis in a patient with superior mesenteric vein thrombosis. The mucosa, submucosa, and muscularis have congestive dilated vessels, and extravasated red cells infiltrating the tissue. There is marked edema of the submucosa and muscularis propria layers.

RADIATION INJURY IN THE GASTROINTESTINAL TRACT

STEVEN M. COHN ■ **STEPHEN J. BICKSTON**

The gastroenterologist will continue to encounter and treat patients with gastrointestinal or hepatic complications resulting from the therapeutic use of ionizing radiation. The histopathological analysis of tissue specimens can often aid in establishing the diagnosis and excluding other etiologies for a patient's symptoms. The histological appearance of lesions observed in tissue specimens is often characteristic of acute or delayed radiation injury. However, no individual histological feature is pathognomonic for radiation-induced damage. Therefore, histological findings may mimic other pathological conditions and must be interpreted carefully within the appropriate clinical context for a given patient. Patients may present with acute symptoms in days to weeks after radiation therapy is initiated or with delayed clinical syndromes that may occur years after therapy. The early effects primarily involve the mucosa, which is lined by rapidly proliferating epithelial cells that are sensitive to the acute effects of radiation injury. Clinical symptoms include odynophagia, diarrhea, nausea, vomiting, or gastrointestinal bleeding; the symptoms depend on the location of the radiation field, the dose of irradiation, and the fractionation schedule. The delayed effects of therapeutic irradiation are more likely to present with chronic diarrhea, fibrosis, ulcer formation, or bleeding, and are thought to be secondary to damage to the vasculature of the organs involved. The figures that follow illustrate selected histopathological features of acute and chronic radiation injury in the gastrointestinal tract and liver.

The histopathological features of acute radiation injury are dominated by evidence of acute injury to the mucosa. Apoptosis of lamina propria lymphocytes and epithelial cells and the cessation of epithelial cell replication occur within hours of a radiation dose. Mature, differentiated epithelial cells continue to be lost in the absence of replacement by replication of the progenitor cells within these epithelia, resulting in the subsequent loss of mucosal function. Acute diarrhea may result under these circumstances. Mucosal and submucosal edema may also be observed within the radiation field as a result of endothelial dysfunction.

Specimens from patients with acute hepatic injury secondary to therapeutic irradiation for solid neoplasms are rarely obtained. However, venoocclusive disease is not uncommon in bone marrow transplant patients following cytoreductive therapy with combined chemotherapy and irradiation (see below). Onset of venoocclusive disease in this setting usually occurs before 5 weeks posttransplant. Changes in hepatic histology include vascular congestion that is most prominent in centrilobular areas, subendothelial edema, endothelial destruction, sinusoidal dilation, and centrizonal hepatocyte necrosis with attenuation of the hepatocellular cords.

Evidence of vascular injury and regeneration is a hallmark of chronic radiation injury and is often observed in pathological specimens. Myointimal proliferation in medium-sized muscular arteries may lead to chronic ischemic injury and ulceration caused by the marked decrease in the luminal diameter of these vessels. The presence of lipophages or foamy macrophages in the intima of small arterioles is also a characteristic finding of delayed radiation injury, although these lesions may also result from other etiologies. Telangiectatic vessels in the lamina propria or submucosa are another frequent finding and account for the diffuse bleeding sometimes observed in radiation enteritis. Sclerosis or medial fibrosis indicative of healing vasculitic lesions may also be observed.

Changes in the mucosa and submucosa are also frequently observed in chronic radiation injury and are thought to be secondary to the chronic vascular changes described above. Cellular atypia may be observed in the epithelium lining any region of the alimentary tract that was within the radiation field. Mucosal atrophy resulting in impaired mucosal function is also sometimes observed. Fibrosis may be confined to the submucosa or extend through the muscularis propria and accounts for luminal strictures seen in chronic radiation injury. These strictures may occur within any irradiated region of the alimentary tract. The appearance of these fibrotic lesions in the small intestine may resemble that of Crohn's disease both on gross inspection and on radiologic examination, although fistulae and creeping fat are rarely observed.

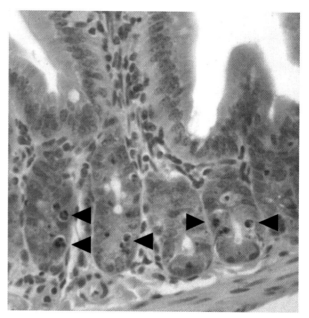

FIGURE 83-1. Acute radiation injury 6 hours after 8 Gy γ-irradiation. Apoptotic cells (programmed cell death; *arrowheads*) appear within the small intestinal crypt epithelium by 3 to 6 hours after irradiation (FVB/n mouse; H&E stain; original magnification ×200). The remaining crypt epithelial cells undergo cell cycle arrest and migrate onto the villi, depleting the crypt of cells over the next 24 hours. This experimental sample is from the laboratory mouse because tissue is rarely obtained during this time frame after irradiation in humans.

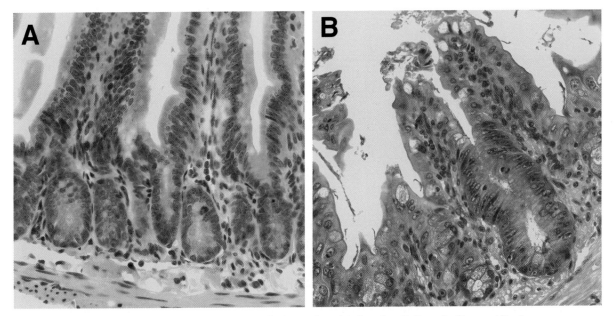

Figure 83-2. Acute radiation injury 3 days after 14 Gy γ-irradiation. **A:** The architecture of normal epithelium in the adult mouse small intestine. **B:** The histological features found in the small intestine 3 days after irradiation. Note the marked shortening of the intestinal villi, which results from cessation of crypt epithelial replication and lack of replacement of villous epithelial cells after irradiation. The loss of differentiated epithelial cells associated with villous blunting can result in impaired mucosal absorptive function. Expanded regenerative crypts first appear at this time and are composed of rapidly proliferating basophilic cells that are somewhat larger than those found in normal uninjured crypts (H&E stain; original magnification ×400). As in Fig. 83-1, this experimental sample was obtained from the laboratory mouse to illustrate the regenerative process after irradiation because tissue is rarely obtained during this time frame after irradiation in humans.

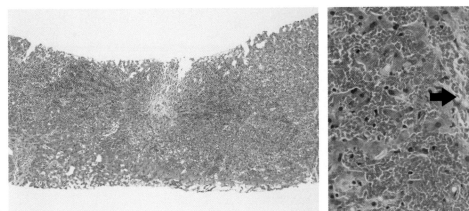
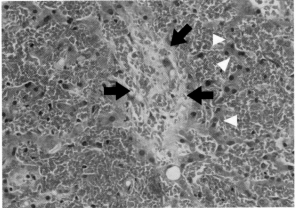

FIGURE 83-3. Hepatic venoocclusive disease occurring in a 24-year-old woman after cytoreductive therapy for bone marrow transplantation with combined chemotherapy and irradiation. **A:** A low-power view of a core biopsy that shows sinusoidal congestion with increased numbers of red blood cells in the centrolobar region (H&E stain; original magnification ×40). (Courtesy of Dr. Christopher Moskaluk.) **B:** A higher-power view of the same biopsy that demonstrates fibrinous deposits in a central vein (*arrows*), atrophy of the hepatic cords (*arrowheads*), and congestion of the sinusoids, which are packed with red blood cells (H&E stain; original magnification ×200). (Courtesy of Dr. Christopher Moskaluk.)

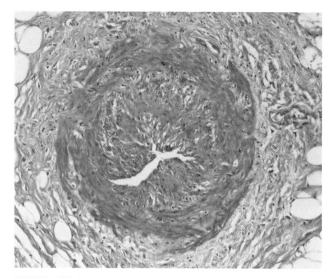

FIGURE 83-4. Myointimal proliferation nearly occludes the lumen of a moderate-sized mesenteric artery. This process usually occurs over several years after radiation injury and may lead to chronic ischemic injury caused by the marked decrease in the lumenal diameter of these vessels. Ulceration of the overlying mucosa can occur in areas of localized ischemia (H&E stain; original magnification ×100). (Courtesy of Dr. Christopher Moskaluk.)

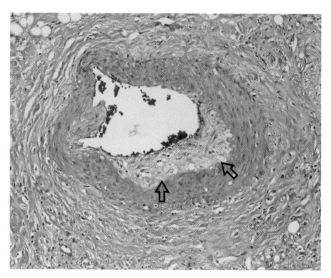

FIGURE 83-5. Intimal lipophage accumulation in intestinal arteriole following irradiation. These foam cells (*arrows*) may be seen in the intima of small arteries and arterioles of the intestine several years after irradiation, and may contribute to luminal narrowing of these vessels and subsequent ischemic injury to the mucosa (H&E stain; original magnification ×100). (Courtesy of Dr. Christopher Moskaluk.)

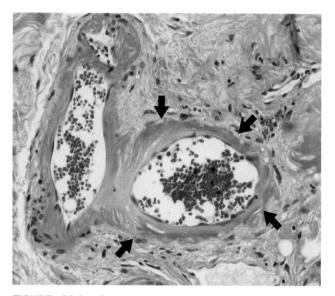

FIGURE 83-6. Radiation-induced sclerosis of small- to medium-sized blood vessels in the mesenteric vasculature. Sclerosis or medial fibrosis is a histological feature associated with healing vasculitic lesions. Note the hyalinization of the vessel walls (*arrows*) with prominent vascular ectasia (H&E stain; original magnification ×200). (Courtesy of Dr. Christopher Moskaluk.)

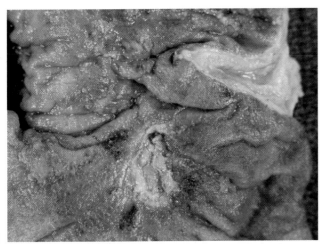

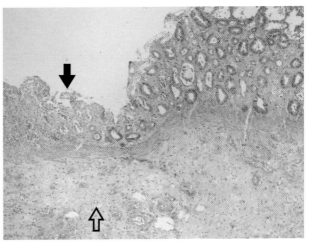

FIGURE 83-7. Radiation-induced ulceration in the colon. **A:** The gross appearance of a well-demarcated ulcer present in the rectum years after external radiation for an adjacent neoplasm. **B:** The histological appearance with chronic ulceration, mucosal necrosis similar to that seen in ischemic injury (*closed arrow*), and dense submucosal fibrosis (*open arrow*). The fibrosis may be confined to the submucosa or extend through the muscularis propria, and accounts for the thickening or strictures noted on gross examination. These strictures may occur within any irradiated region of the alimentary tract. The lesion is notable because of the absence of a prominent inflammatory infiltrate (H&E stain; original magnification ×20). (Courtesy of Dr. Christopher Moskaluk.)

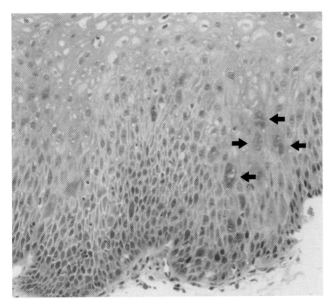

FIGURE 83-8. Epithelial atypia in the esophagus secondary to chronic radiation injury. Note the presence of enlarged atypical nuclei with irregular nuclear contours (*arrows*). Hyperchromasia of these atypical cells is rare in contrast to the cellular atypia that is characteristic of neoplastic processes and is an important histological feature distinguishing these two processes (H&E stain; original magnification ×800). (Courtesy of Dr. Christopher Moskaluk.)

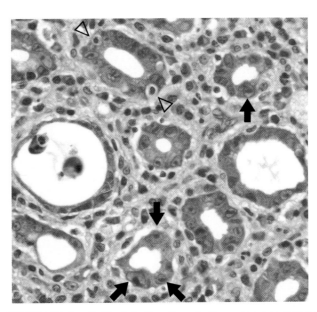

FIGURE 83-9. Epithelial alterations in the colon secondary to chronic radiation injury. Note the cells with enlarged irregular nuclei with prominent nucleoli (*arrows*). As in the esophagus in Fig. 83-8, the epithelial cellular atypia characteristic of chronic radiation injury is not associated with the nuclear hyperchromasia that is commonly observed in atypia associated with neoplastic processes. Apoptotic cells are noted in some glands (*arrowheads*). Atrophic glands with flattened and sloughing epithelial cells are also prominent (H&E stain; original magnification ×400). (Courtesy of Dr. Christopher Moskaluk.)

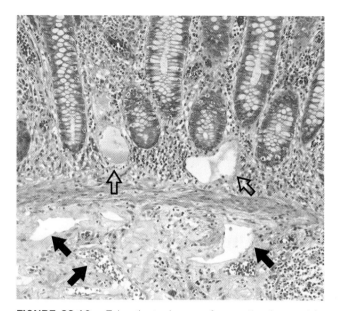

FIGURE 83-10. Telangiectasias are frequently observed in delayed radiation injury. Dilated venules and lymphatic channels may be seen in the lamina propria (*open arrows*) or in the submucosa (*solid arrows*) underlying relatively normal appearing colonic epithelium. These lesions likely account for the diffuse bleeding sometimes observed in chronic radiation enteritis (H&E stain; original magnification ×40). (Courtesy of Dr. Christopher Moskaluk.)

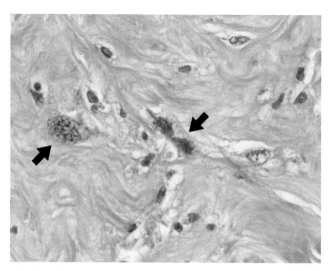

FIGURE 83-11. Atypical fibroblasts in radiation injury. Bizarre appearing fibroblasts with large pyknotic nuclei (*arrows*) are frequently seen in delayed phase of radiation injury in the alimentary tract. Although these atypical fibroblasts are frequently observed, their presence is not specific for radiation injury (H&E stain; original magnification ×400). (Courtesy of Dr. Christopher Moskaluk.)

PART THREE

DIAGNOSTIC AND THERAPEUTIC MODALITIES IN GASTROENTEROLOGY

UPPER GASTROINTESTINAL ENDOSCOPY

GUIDO N.J. TYTGAT

Endoscopy has had great impact on the management of diseases of the esophagus, stomach, and small intestine. Endoscopists must constantly strive to improve their skills in interpreting the endoscopic appearance of mucosal disease. Student endoscopists initially are concerned with their ability to introduce the endoscope into the esophagus to perform the examination. Concern with correct identification of a lesion begins gradually as experience grows. However, experienced endoscopists know that it is not always easy to be certain what is causing a lesion seen at endoscopy.

If the mucosa is red and the folds are heavy and do not flatten with distention, an experienced endoscopist knows that one of several diseases may be present. The differential diagnosis may include gastric varices. In this instance, obtaining a large snare biopsy specimen of the structure may be dangerous. Therefore, it is essential to continue to expand one's interpretative skills and to learn what further tests are indicated in a particular instance.

It is also important to appreciate the role of biopsy in differential diagnosis. The endoscopic appearance may seem pathognomonic for a particular lesion, but with experience it becomes apparent that the differential diagnosis may include several diseases. Often this is resolved with a biopsy.

As one learns endoscopic interpretation, it becomes apparent that new technology may prove helpful to improve our diagnostic capabilities. For example, having equipment (either attached to an endoscope or as a probe passable through the biopsy channel) available for ultrasound scanning during endoscopy may allow the endoscopist to acquire information about structures beneath the mucosal surface. Ultrasound scanning can help an examiner readily differentiate between gastric varices and the thickened mucosa of Ménétrier disease.

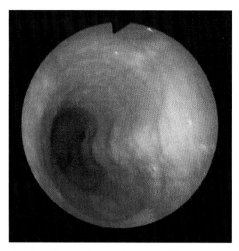

FIGURE 84-1. Normal esophagus with extrinsic impression caused by the vertebral column. The covering mucosa is normal.

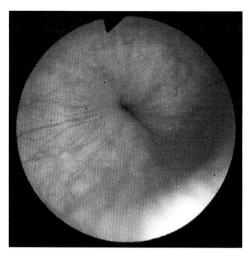

FIGURE 84-2. Normal vascular structures in the distal esophagus.

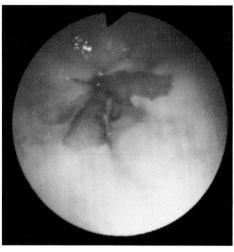

FIGURE 84-3. Squamocolumnar mucosal junction appears slightly irregular but is normal. The location is just above the diaphragmatic hiatus.

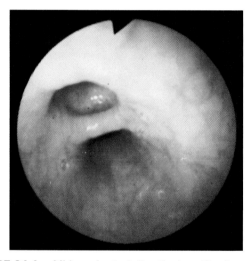

FIGURE 84-4. Midesophageal diverticulum. The lumen is in the center of the field.

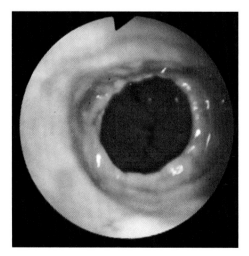

FIGURE 84-5. Schatzki B ring in the distal esophagus. The junction between the squamous mucosa of the esophagus and the columnar mucosa of the stomach is at the level of the ring.

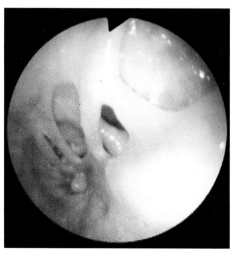

FIGURE 84-6. Congenital mucosal bands in the distal esophagus.

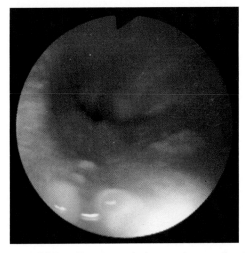

FIGURE 84-7. Esophageal glycogenic acanthosis.

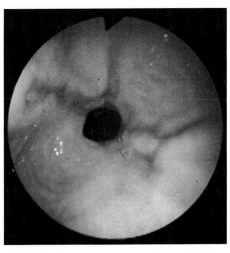

FIGURE 84-8. Esophagitis caused by gastroesophageal reflux with erosions in the distal esophagus just proximal to the squamocolumnar junction.

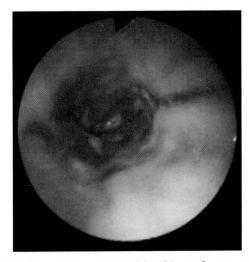

FIGURE 84-9. Reflux esophagitis with confluent erosions.

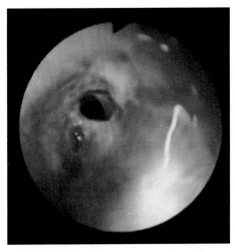

FIGURE 84-10. Stricture of the distal esophagus caused by gastroesophageal reflux. This tight stricture resulted in dysphagia.

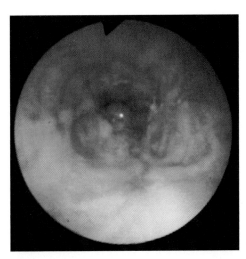

FIGURE 84-11. Reflux esophagitis evidenced by erythema erosions and scarring. A small protrusion in the distance is a sentinel polyp associated with reflux and located just distal to the squamocolumnar junction.

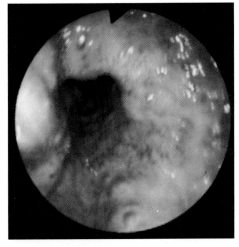

FIGURE 84-12. Esophageal varices. The varices are not large, but the bluish color is apparent, as are red spots that suggest recent bleeding from the varices.

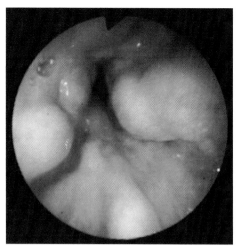

FIGURE 84-13. Esophageal varices. The venous structures are tortuous in appearance. No red signs are visible.

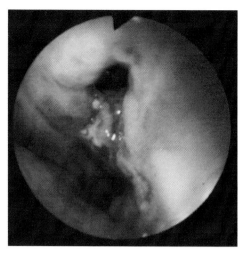

FIGURE 84-14. Perforated esophagus after sclerotherapy. The site of the perforation is above the lumen.

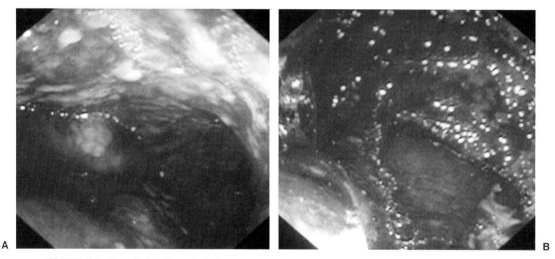

FIGURE 84-15. **A, B:** Caustic injury to the esophagus caused by ingestion of ammonia.

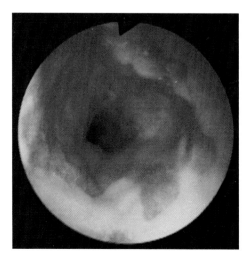

FIGURE 84-16. Barrett metaplasia of the esophagus. The ora serrata or squamocolumnar junction is located abnormally proximally in the esophagus with a segment of tubular esophagus below the junction containing Barrett metaplastic mucosa.

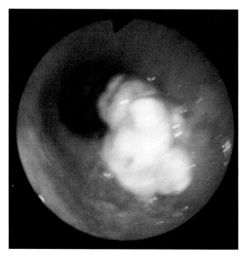

FIGURE 84-17. Barrett metaplasia of the esophagus with adenocarcinoma appearing as a protuberant white mass surrounded by Barrett metaplastic mucosa.

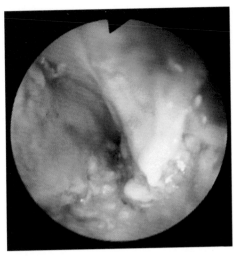

FIGURE 84-18. Obstructing esophageal carcinoma. The mucosa is irregular and nodular with stenosis of the lumen.

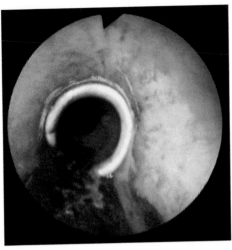

FIGURE 84-19. Same patient case as in Fig. 84-18. The obstructing esophageal carcinoma has been palliated with a prosthesis. The proximal end of the prosthesis is visible as a ring.

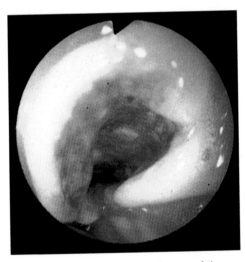

FIGURE 84-20. Squamous cell carcinoma of the esophagus presenting as an esophageal ulcer with heaped-up margins. The base of the ulcer is irregular, discolored, and covered with an exudate.

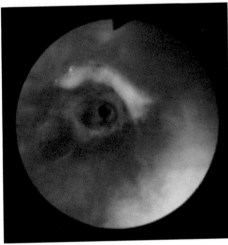

FIGURE 84-21. Postirradiation tight esophageal stricture. The mucosa proximal to the stricture is erythematous.

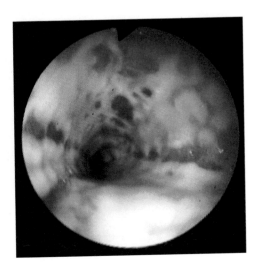

FIGURE 84-22. Esophageal ulceration following endolumenal radiation therapy. The ulceration and inflammation are extensive.

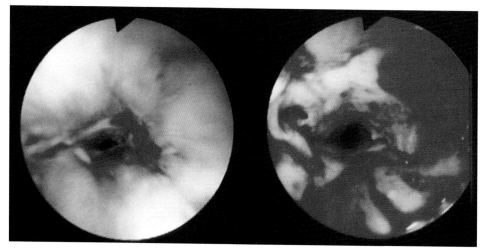

FIGURE 84-23. Caustic stricture of the esophagus (**left**). The stricture was dilated and then reexamined endoscopically. The area was friable and bled from the disruption of the stricture (**right**).

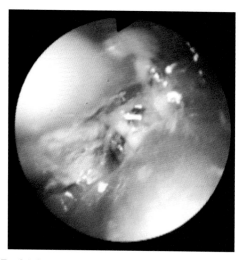

FIGURE 84-24. Anastomosis after total gastrectomy. Suture material is visible at the level of the anastomosis.

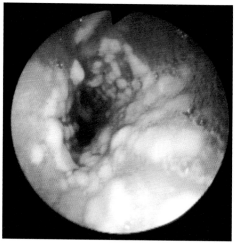

FIGURE 84-25. *Candida* esophagitis with raised, white exudative plaques.

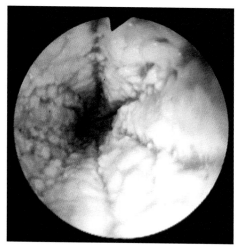

FIGURE 84-26. Severe candidiasis of the esophagus in a patient with acquired immunodeficiency syndrome. The exudate is nearly confluent.

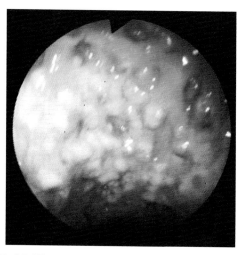

FIGURE 84-27. Esophageal intramural diverticulosis in association with candidiasis.

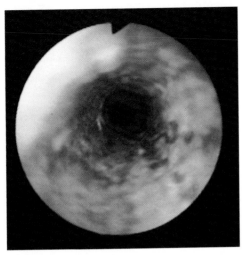

FIGURE 84-28. Herpes infection of the esophagus with severe, confluent superficial ulceration.

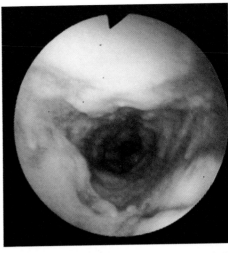

FIGURE 84-29. Cytomegalovirus esophagitis of the distal esophagus in a patient with acquired immunodeficiency syndrome. The borders of the ulcers are minimally raised.

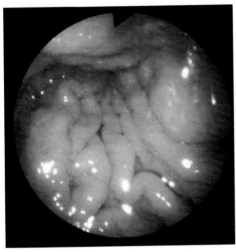

FIGURE 84-30. Normal gastric folds along the greater curvature of the stomach.

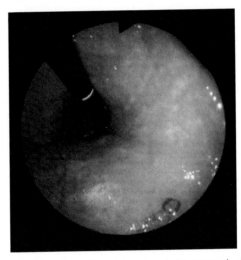

FIGURE 84-31. Retroflexed image of the normal stomach in examination of the gastric fundus. This maneuver is essential to see the cardia and fundus of the stomach.

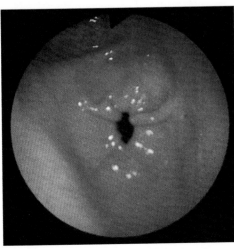

FIGURE 84-32. Endoscopic appearance of normal antrum and pylorus.

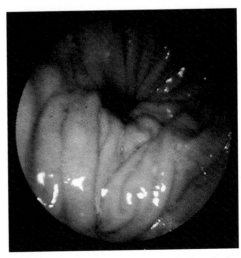

FIGURE 84-33. Axial hiatal hernia. This hernia is an outpouching above the diaphragmatic hiatus and covered with normal-appearing gastric mucosa.

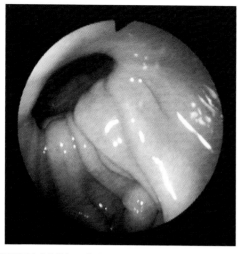

FIGURE 84-34. Subcardial gastric diverticulum.

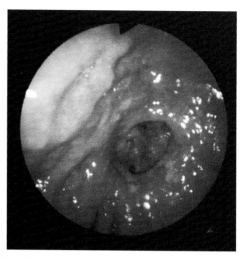

FIGURE 84-35. Billroth II stomach. The anastomosis is in the distance. The mucosa of the stomach is erythematous, probably because of alkaline reflux gastritis after this type of operation.

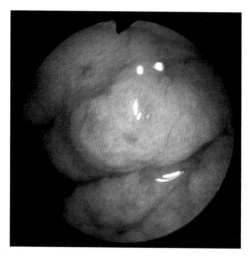

FIGURE 84-36. Giant gastric folds of hypertrophic gastropathy. Histological examination is necessary for the differential diagnosis, which includes Ménétrier disease.

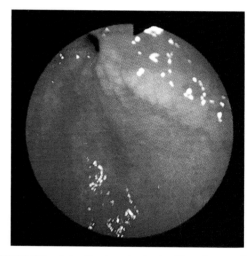

FIGURE 84-37. Intestinal metaplasia. The abnormal gastric mucosa appears pale on a background of erythematous mucosa in a patient with gastric mucosal atrophy.

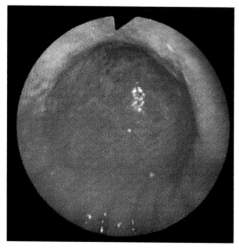

FIGURE 84-38. Advanced atrophic gastritis with extensive intestinal metaplasia in the distal stomach visible as white patches.

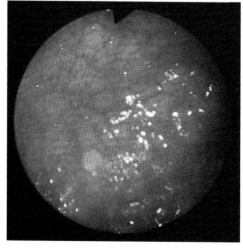

FIGURE 84-39. Atrophic gastritis of the fundus of the stomach. The mucosa is thin, and the submucosal vessels are visible. A small xanthelasma is surrounded by atrophic mucosa.

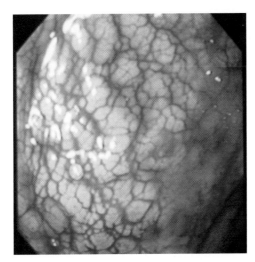

FIGURE 84-40. Abnormal prominent areae gastricae pattern accentuated with methylene blue staining.

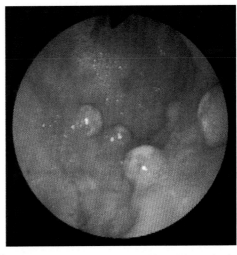

FIGURE 84-41. Varioliform gastritis with typical lesions showing a depression in the center with a white exudate.

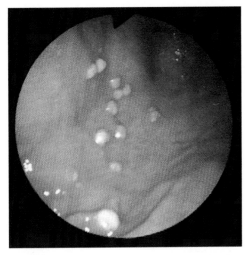

FIGURE 84-42. Gastric xanthoma involving the lower body and antrum.

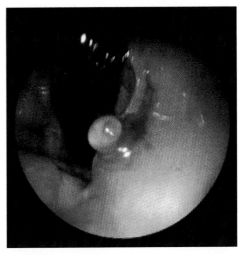

FIGURE 84-43. Mallory-Weiss tear of the stomach just distal to the esophagogastric junction. The area was best seen with the endoscope retroflexed. An organizing clot is visible adherent to the tear.

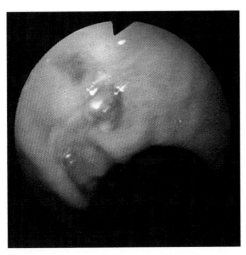

FIGURE 84-44. Dieulafoy lesion of the stomach. Arterial spurting is visible in the base of the lesion.

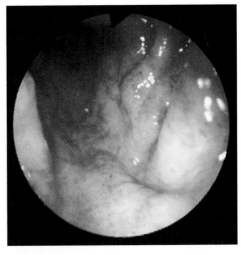

FIGURE 84-45. Gastric antral angiomatosis, or watermelon stomach.

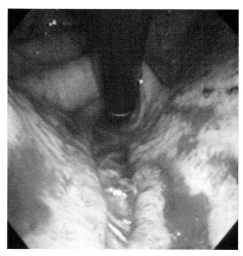

FIGURE 84-46. Gastric trauma that occurred at endoscopic examination as the result of violent retching (multiple hemorrhagic streaks are present).

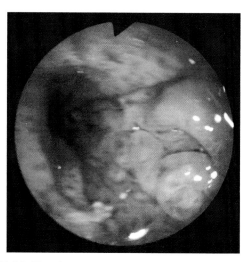

FIGURE 84-47. Congestive gastropathy often seen in association with portal hypertension.

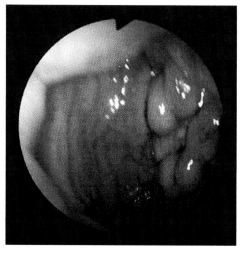

FIGURE 84-48. Gastric fundic varices. These varices appear as heavy folds in the stomach. The color may be similar to that of the surrounding gastric mucosa. Caution is indicated before acquisition of a large biopsy specimen of gastric folds if varices are suspected. Endoscopic ultrasound scanning can be used to resolve this issue.

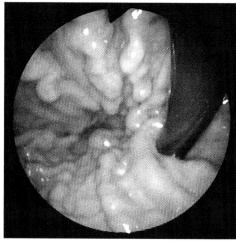

FIGURE 84-49. Gastric varices. The endoscope is retroflexed, and the varices are adjacent to the endoscope in the fundus.

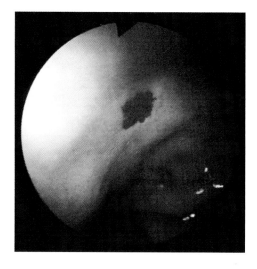

FIGURE 84-50. Gastric angiodysplastic lesion with a typical bright red appearance and a slightly irregular margin caused by underlying blood vessels.

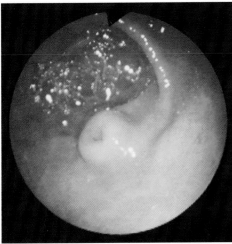

FIGURE 84-51. Ectopic pancreas in the gastric antrum with the typical apical dimple characteristic of this lesion. A rudimentary ductal system may empty into this depression.

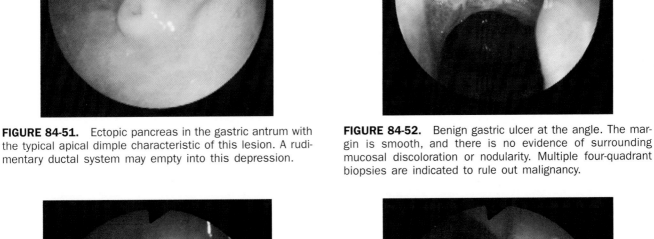

FIGURE 84-52. Benign gastric ulcer at the angle. The margin is smooth, and there is no evidence of surrounding mucosal discoloration or nodularity. Multiple four-quadrant biopsies are indicated to rule out malignancy.

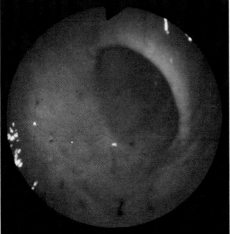

FIGURE 84-53. Mucosal hemorrhage typical of acute lesions induced by nonsteroidal antiinflammatory drug injury.

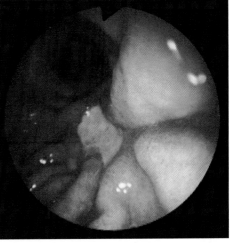

FIGURE 84-54. Nonsteroidal antiinflammatory drug–induced gastric ulcer on the greater curvature of the stomach. This ulcer has a typical benign appearance with radiating folds and no evidence of nodularity or mucosal irregularity.

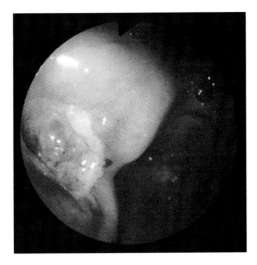

FIGURE 84-55. Gastric ulcer induced by nonsteroidal antiinflammatory drugs (NSAIDs). It is not possible to differentiate an NSAID ulcer from that not associated with NSAID use on the basis of endoscopic appearance. Biopsy is indicated to rule out malignancy.

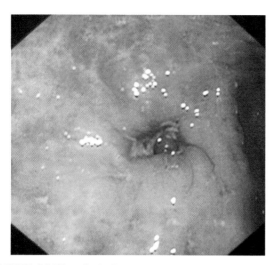

FIGURE 84-56. Crohn's disease of the gastric antrum.

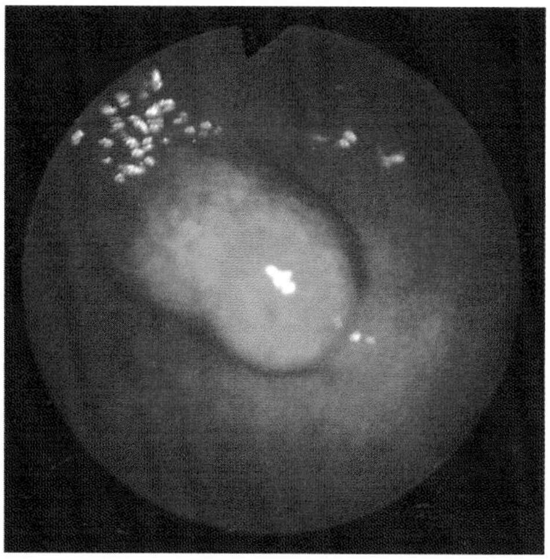

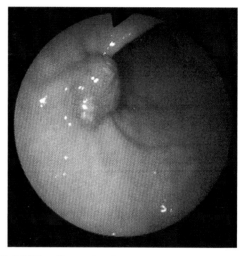

FIGURE 84-57. Gastric leiomyoma. This is a typical intramural mass. The mucosa over the surface is normal. There are often bridging folds adjacent to the mass.

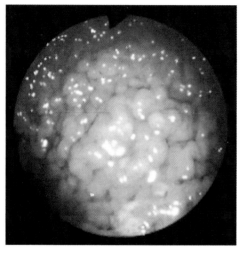

FIGURE 84-58. Gastric polyposis in a patient with Turcot disease. This syndrome is characterized by adenomatous polyposis coli in association with a cerebral tumor.

FIGURE 84-59. Hyperplastic gastric polyp. It is not possible to differentiate a hyperplastic gastric polyp from an adenomatous polyp at endoscopic examination. Removal for histologic sampling is necessary to differentiate a hyperplastic from an adenomatous polyp.

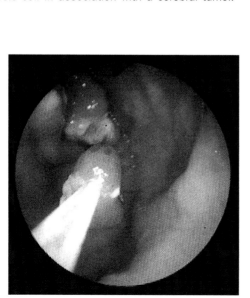

FIGURE 84-60. Gastric polyp being removed after snare resection by means of radiofrequency electrical current.

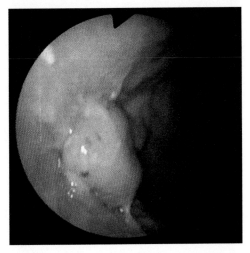

FIGURE 84-61. Gastric villous adenoma. This lesion is sessile and covers several centimeters of the gastric mucosa. Biopsy is essential to diagnose adenoma.

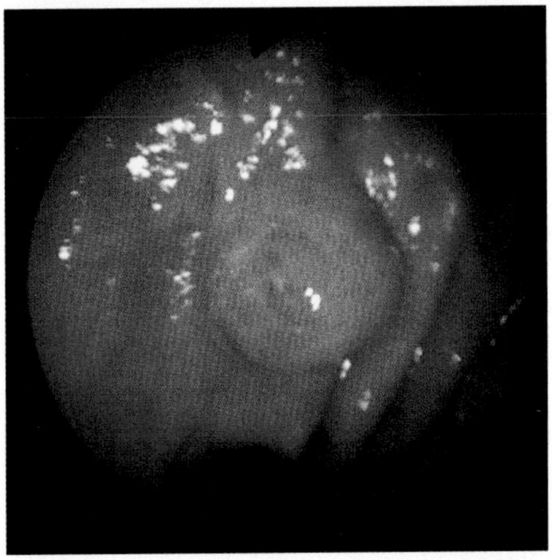

FIGURE 84-62. Gastric carcinoid. The tip of the small, sessile lesion suggests early ulceration that is typical of this tumor.

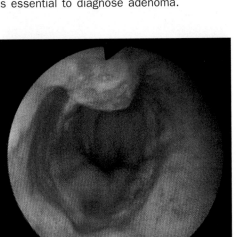

FIGURE 84-63. Early cancer of the cardia. In the distal esophagus at the top of the image, just distal to the squamocolumnar junction, a nodule is present that is early cancer of the cardia.

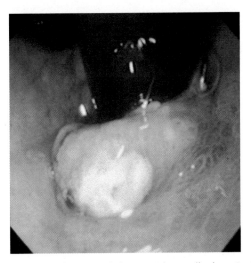

FIGURE 84-64. Cancer of the gastric cardia in retroflexed view.

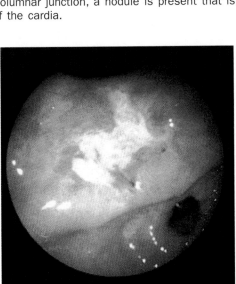

FIGURE 84-65. Malignant gastric ulcer. This ulcer contains an adenocarcinoma. There are endoscopic clues to the presence of a tumor. The margins of the ulcer are irregular, discolored, and nodular. The gastric folds do not merge with the ulcer margin adjacent to the ulcer base but are separated by the nodularity. Multiple biopsies of all quadrants are indicated to establish the histological diagnosis.

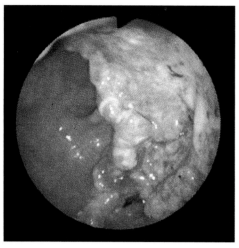

FIGURE 84-66. Advanced gastric cancer. A large discolored mass is visible. The adjacent mucosa is somewhat irregular. The surface of the lesion appears irregular and consists of tumor nodules.

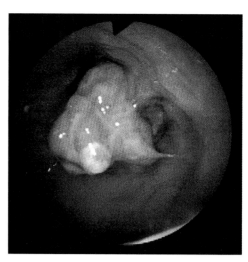

FIGURE 84-67. Pedunculated gastric cancer.

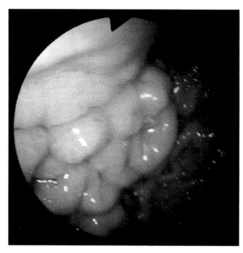

FIGURE 84-68. Linitis plastica. This type of gastric adenocarcinoma often is very difficult to diagnose at endoscopic examination. The mucosa covering the tumor is nodular in this instance and has made the wall less pliable and distensible. Biopsy is most productive if areas of tumor breakthrough are sampled.

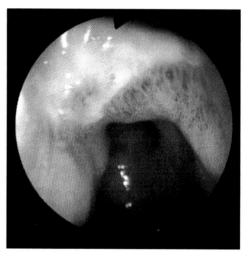

FIGURE 84-69. Gastric lymphoma presenting itself as gastric ulcer with atypical, erythematous surrounding mucosa.

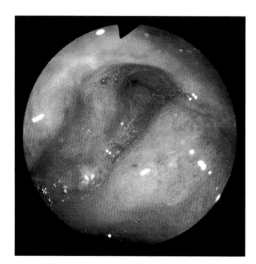

FIGURE 84-70. Non-Hodgkin lymphoma of the stomach. This tumor is covered by nodular, red, irregular mucosa. Ultrasound scanning is an excellent way to study the gastric wall beneath the mucosa to determine the extent of the lymphoma.

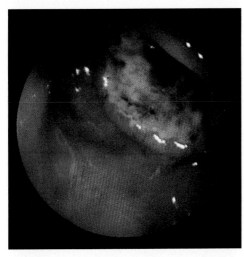

FIGURE 84-71. Non-Hodgkin lymphoma of the stomach presenting as an irregular large ulcer. There are stigmata of hemorrhage in the base of the ulcer.

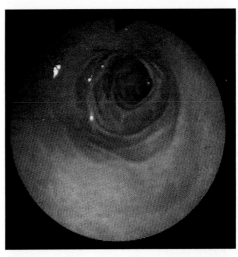

FIGURE 84-72. The duodenal bulb is slightly white because of the presence of lipid in the lamina propria. This is a normal variation. The apex of the duodenal bulb is visible in the distance.

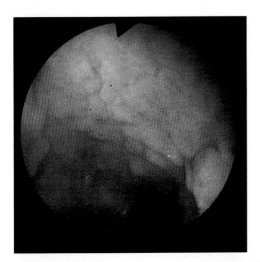

FIGURE 84-73. Heterotopic gastric mucosa in the duodenal bulb.

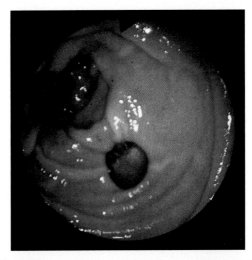

FIGURE 84-74. Duodenal diverticulum. If the diverticulum is in the area of the papilla of Vater, it is often immediately adjacent to the papilla. In other instances the papilla may be inside the diverticulum.

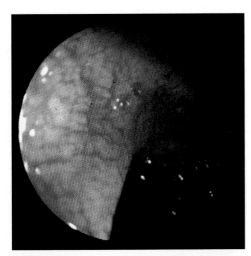

FIGURE 84-75. Celiac sprue. The mucosa appears atrophic and flat; villous atrophy is present. Biopsy is necessary to confirm the histological appearance of the mucosa.

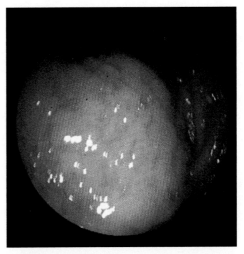

FIGURE 84-76. Celiac disease showing villous atrophy before the area is stained with methylene blue.

837

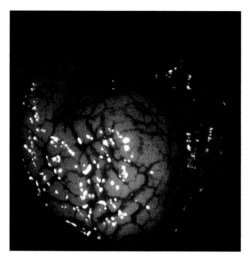

FIGURE 84-77. Celiac disease. Same case as in Fig. 84-76. After the area is stained with methylene blue, a characteristic mosaic pattern is visible.

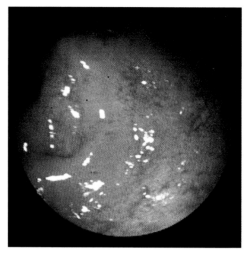

FIGURE 84-78. Pseudo-Whipple disease of the duodenum caused by *Mycobacterium avium* complex in a patient with acquired immunodeficiency syndrome. The mucosa appears coarsened and slightly white compared with normal.

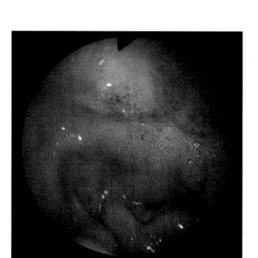

FIGURE 84-79. Duodenal bulb with a linear scar caused by previous ulceration. The scar is surrounded by endoscopic evidence of mild inflammation.

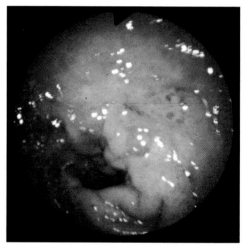

FIGURE 84-80. Duodenitis with erythema and petechiae.

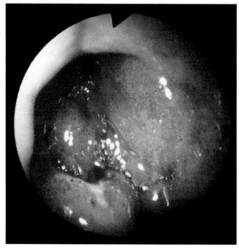

FIGURE 84-81. Duodenitis with small duodenal ulcer.

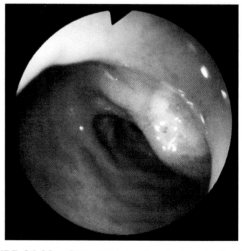

FIGURE 84-82. Recurrent duodenal ulcer in the bulb.

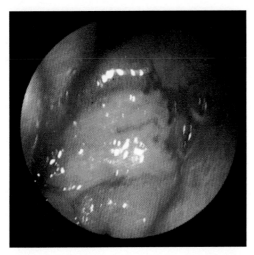

FIGURE 84-83. Large duodenal ulcer with bile staining of the exudate in the base.

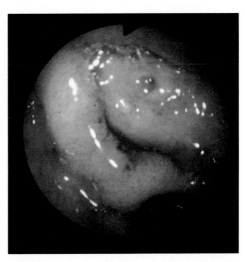

FIGURE 84-84. Large duodenal ulcer with protrusion in the upper aspect. This protrusion was a visible vessel.

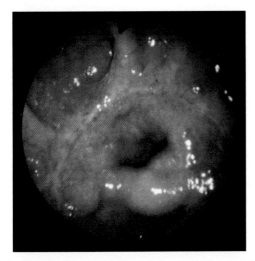

FIGURE 84-85. Duodenal bulb with scarring and deformity caused by previous ulcer disease.

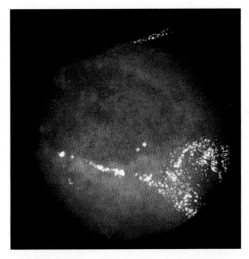

FIGURE 84-86. Flat duodenal hemangioma.

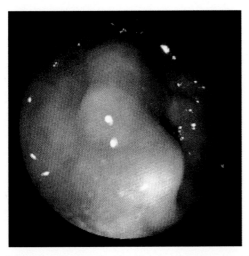

FIGURE 84-87. Varices in the duodenal bulb appearing as submucosal serpiginous structures covered with normal mucosa in a patient with portal hypertension.

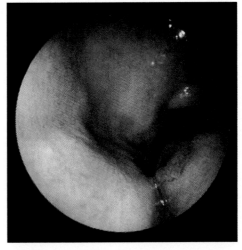

FIGURE 84-88. Kaposi sarcoma involving the duodenum. The elevation in the right lower aspect is a sarcomatous lesion.

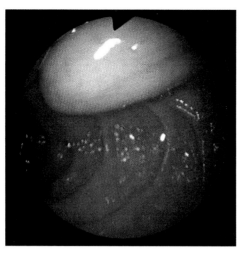

FIGURE 84-89. Duodenal leiomyoma appears as a smooth intramural mass covered with normal-appearing mucosa. There is a suggestion of adjacent bridging folds.

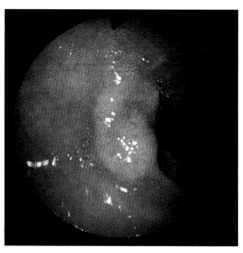

FIGURE 84-90. Brunner adenoma of the duodenum. The adenoma appears as a sessile lesion with a smooth surface.

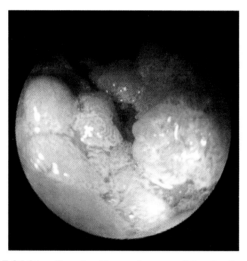

FIGURE 84-91. Sessile villous adenoma of the duodenal bulb appears as a multilobular mass with erythematous mucosa.

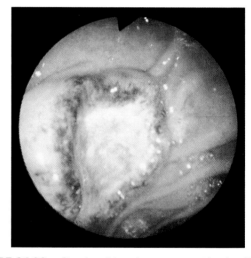

FIGURE 84-92. Duodenal lymphoma presenting itself as an ulcer with red, slightly irregular surrounding mucosa.

85

COLONOSCOPY AND FLEXIBLE SIGMOIDOSCOPY

JEROME D. WAYE ■ CHRISTOPHER B. WILLIAMS

Inflammation of the colon is commonly encountered during colonoscopy. The cause of inflammatory changes ranges from infection to idiopathic inflammatory bowel disease. The process may be acute or chronic and may be localized or diffuse. No matter what the cause, the colon does not respond differently to each inflammatory insult. The result is that most inflammatory reactions can be categorized into two main types of surface changes caused by either ulcerative colitis or Crohn's disease.

Whenever mild inflammatory disease affects the mucosa, edema causes the superficial layer to become opaque, hiding the normal branching vascular pattern of the submucosa from view. As vascular congestion proceeds, the surface lining may become hyperemic, erythematous, or may bleed whenever the endoscope contacts the mucosa. This pattern of response is most often seen with ulcerative colitis, which may progress to both small and large ulcerations. In contrast to the diffuse type of mucosal response in ulcerative colitis, the inflammatory component of Crohn's disease typically originates in the submucosa, and as the inflammation burrows onto the mucosal surface, individual aphthous ulcerations form, which are the hallmark of granulomatous colitis. This type of discrete ulceration with intervening normal mucosa is never seen with ulcerative colitis but may be present with amebiasis, tuberculosis, and other inflammatory processes in the large bowel.

With prolonged inflammation, ulcerations can become deeper and may interlink; with healing, the intervening islands of inflamed but not ulcerated mucosa exhibit a different growth pattern than the thin, reepithelialized mucosa that regenerates over ulcerated segments. This difference in growth pattern may cause polyps to appear. These are postinflammatory polyps that have no malignant potential. A cap of white slough suggests that a polyp is inflammatory, although some juvenile (hamartomatous) polyps may have similar features. Inflammatory polyps that are small, shiny, and worm-like may be diagnosed as inflammatory on visual grounds alone, although biopsies may be necessary when there is any question about the nature of polyps observed at colonoscopy.

The terminal ileum can be intubated in most patients, and entry into the small bowel may be especially important in the differential diagnosis of inflammation of the large bowel. For the most part, patients with ulcerative colitis have completely normal-appearing small bowel. Among patients with Crohn's disease of the ileum, however, the small bowel has an appearance similar to that of the large bowel, ulcers being the most prominent feature. Inflammatory polyps may occur with either ulcerative colitis or Crohn's disease but are rarely seen in the terminal ileum.

In contrast to the ulcerations of inflammatory bowel disease, pseudomembranous colitis caused by *Clostridium difficile* infection may cause patchy clumps of creamy plaques on the mucosal surface. When the history is consistent with previous exposure to antibiotics, the endoscopic appearance is virtually diagnostic and mandates bacteriologic or toxin studies in addition to routine histological examination.

Diverticulosis is common among patients older than 50 years. Diverticular orifices may range from small to a size that admits the tip of an endoscope. Muscular hypertrophy may be pronounced in some instances, causing the lumen to become narrow with spasm and marked tortuosity. Intubation may be difficult and tedious. Severe muscular hypercontractility often may result in a superficial subepithelial hematoma, which can become a small nidus of intra- or submucosal blood that can lead to further blood accumulation as a result of muscular hypercontractility. This may result in a cycle of further bleeding, hematoma, and with peristaltic activity, even appearance of a polypoid mass. When a diverticular red fold is seen, the surface mucosa is red or magenta. As red blood corpuscles break down in the tissue, hemosiderin is formed. A biopsy allows differentiation from adenoma. A request for the pathologist to stain for hemosiderin in the tissue often assists in the differential diagnosis.

Ischemic colitis presents a wide array of mucosal appearances depending on the elapsed time from the ischemic episode to endoscopic examination. The ischemic segment may be quite friable and purplish-black in its initial phase, in which the mucosa has lost its blood supply. In less severe cases, erythema alone may be encountered in the area of the descending colon or splenic flexure. Subsequent sloughing of the edematous mucosa may be associated with local or widespread ulceration. The involved segments tend to heal rapidly, leaving superficial ulcerations that may appear similar to the lesions of Crohn's disease. Biopsies often provide the correct histopathological diagnosis when ischemia of the bowel is suspected.

Vascular abnormalities of the mucosa tend to be present at opposite ends of the large bowel, with radiation changes in the rectum and vascular ectasia in the right colon. Telangiectasia caused by radiation is more frequently encountered in the rectum, because the diagnosis of prostate cancer is being made earlier, and patients are undergoing radiation therapy for tumor ablation. Radiation changes are confined to the area of radiation therapy. They consist of multiple, small, interlacing blood vessels. Biopsies are not necessary for confirmation of this diagnosis. For patients whose radiation is delivered by means of radon seed implantation, an extremely localized segment of telangiectasia may occur over the area of the prostate. External beam radiation usually is associated with diffuse damage to the rectal mucosa. Radiation telangiectasia most often occurs after a latent period following radiation therapy treatment. Persistent surface bleeding may ensue, which can be quite resistant to therapeutic endeavors. Angiodysplasia or focal vascular ectasia, probably of degenerative origin, may develop in the proximal colon of elderly patients. These may be a cause of bleeding or anemia and may be single or multiple. They vary from small, flat blebs to large, elevated collections of blood vessels with a span of 15 mm. A draining vein often is visible at endoscopic examination and represents the hallmark angiographic descriptor of this vascular malformation.

Polypoid protuberances above the normally flat surface mucosa are a common finding at colonoscopy. Such elevations may be on or underneath the surface mucosa. A biopsy specimen usually has to be submitted to a pathologist for correct designation of structure and significance. The most common submucosal tumor of the colon is lipoma, which usually has a broad base and is covered by normal mucosa, often with a recognizable surface vascular pattern with a slightly yellowish hue caused by the underlying fatty tissue. The surface indents easily with a biopsy forceps (pillow sign), and fat may be extruded from the surface during the course of obtaining multiple, progressively deeper biopsy specimens. Small, discrete submucosal nodules in the rectum may be carcinoid tumors. These firm tumors often are adherent to the deeper layers of the superficial mucosa, so a biopsy of the surface often leads to the proper diagnosis. Diffuse submucosal nodules are uncommon but may be present in lymphoma or in pneumatosis coli. Deep biopsies may cause air cysts to collapse, as may aspiration with a needle.

Hyperplastic polyps are elevated above the flat surface lining, but they arise from the mucosa and are most commonly pale and translucent. Large hyperplastic polyps may occur in the right colon. In this location the polyps frequently look like an ear with a small, narrow footprint. Hyperplastic polyps have no stroma. In the rectum, they may disappear with air insufflation, which causes mucosal stretching, but they can be revisualized as air is aspirated from the rectum.

Adenomas may occur singly or in any distribution throughout the colon. When more than 100 adenomas are present, the diagnosis of familial adenomatous polyposis (FAP) can be made, even if there is no family history of polyposis. Other than sheer number of polyps, there is nothing about the configuration of polyps that would set aside patients with FAP from those with sporadic adenomas. There is no need to remove any of these polyps except to confirm that they are adenomatous. Among patients without FAP, removal of small and pedunculated polyps can be accomplished with the snare and cautery technique, but larger sessile polyps may be more easily and safely removed after submucosal injection of saline solution at the base of the polyp. This technique is especially useful in the right colon, where the wall is thin. Placing a saline load into the submucosa provides an additional safety factor for polypectomy by means of increasing the distance between snare application (and thermal tissue injury) and the serosal surface of the bowel. A sufficient volume of saline solution should be given to elevate the polyp away from the wall, after which the polyp is removed with electrocautery current.

Dye spray may be used to add definition to the extent of a polyp. This technique, called chromoendoscopy, generally involves squirting dye (indigo carmine 0.1% or methylene blue 1%) onto the surface of a polypoid lesion. Because hyperplastic polyps and adenomas have different surface configurations, dye spraying may enhance the surgeon's visual ability to differentiate these two types of polyps. It may also aid delineation of the edges of polyps to ensure total endoscopic ablation. A magnifying colonoscope helps in assessment of surface structure.

The location of lesions in the colon may be marked with a permanent marker, such as dilute sterilized India ink, to ensure the location for a subsequent operation or for the endoscopist to reidentify the site at subsequent endoscopic examinations. Submucosal injection of India ink results in a stain that lasts for the life of the patient.

Bleeding during polypectomy may be controlled with various techniques, including injection with dilute epinephrine. A loop ligature can be placed on a bleeding pedicle or can be used to ensure hemostasis for patients with a bleeding diathesis. Hemostasis also may be achieved with application of clips to the surface through the channel of the colonoscope. Endoscopic clips are relatively easy to apply and have been found to be efficacious in the control of postpolypectomy bleeding.

Malignant tumors of the colon grow in a haphazard manner. Ulceration is a frequent finding, as is sloughing of a portion of the surface. The endoscopic appearance may vary from an apparent indentation on the top of a polyp to an obvious, fungating tumor. The cancer may be bulky or may ulcerate and become relatively flat in configuration. After colonic resection, colonoscopy may reveal that the anastomosis is healed completely, but most anastomoses are identifiable as a ridge. Sometimes staples or sutures may be identified at the margin of the anastomosis.

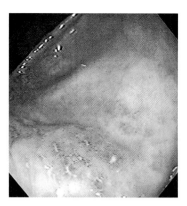

FIGURE 85-1. Crohn's disease. Multiple aphthous ulcerations in an area of otherwise unremarkable mucosa.

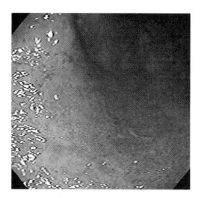

FIGURE 85-2. Early ulcerative colitis. Erythema, granularity, loss of the normal vascular pattern, and slight friability.

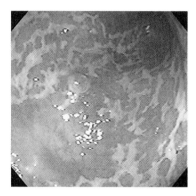

FIGURE 85-3. Severe ulcerative colitis. Linear ulcerations, erythema, and multiple interlacing ulcers.

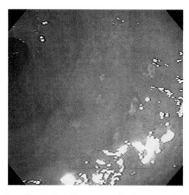

FIGURE 85-4. Crohn's disease of the terminal ileum with aphthous ulcers.

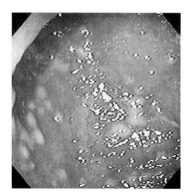

FIGURE 85-5. Antibiotic colitis pseudomembranes.

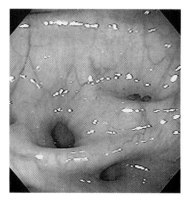

FIGURE 85-6. Diverticulosis. Multiple diverticular orifices. *Highlights* indicate that the lumen is at the 12 o'clock position.

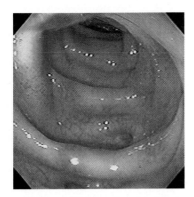

FIGURE 85-7. Reddened folds related to intramucosal bleeding from muscular activity in diverticular disease. Redness on several folds is associated with muscular hypertrophy.

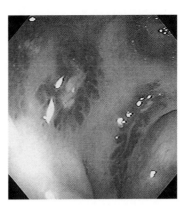

FIGURE 85-8. Ischemic bowel disease. Marked edema and erythema.

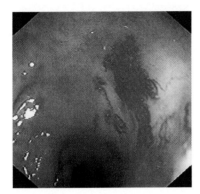

FIGURE 85-9. Radiation "colitis." Radiation therapy effect in the rectum caused by an implant for cervical carcinoma.

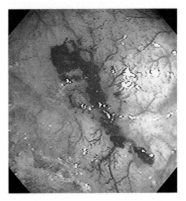

FIGURE 85-10. Vascular malformation.

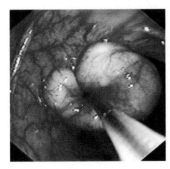

FIGURE 85-11. Lipoma. Fatty tumors can be indented with a biopsy forceps, resulting in a cushion or pillow sign.

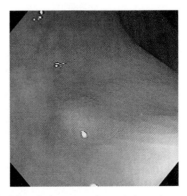

FIGURE 85-12. Submucosal rectal polyp: a carcinoid tumor.

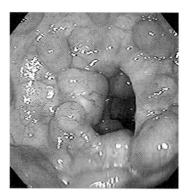

FIGURE 85-13. Pneumatosis cystoides intestinalis: multiple gas cysts.

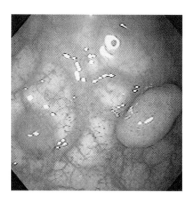

FIGURE 85-14. Hyperplastic polyps in the rectum.

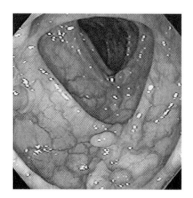

FIGURE 85-15. Familial polyposis. Multiple polyps of varying sizes throughout the colon.

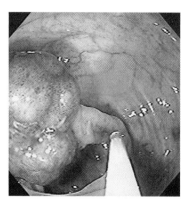

FIGURE 85-16. Pedunculated polyp on a slender pedicle (with snare).

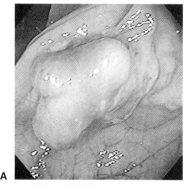

A

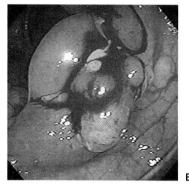

B

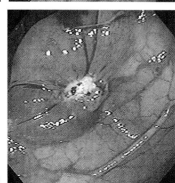

C

FIGURE 85-17. Submucosal injection polypectomy. **A:** Sessile polyp. **B:** After large-volume saline submucosal injection. **C:** Polypectomy site. A small amount of residual tissue is present at the edge of the polypectomy site, which was removed with another snare application.

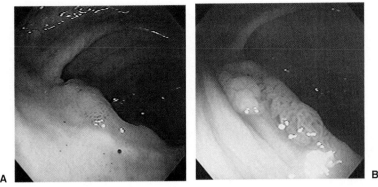

FIGURE 85-18.   Dye spray. **A:** Polyp in the right colon. **B:** Same polyp after dye spray with methylene blue. The extent of polyp is easier to see after dye spray.

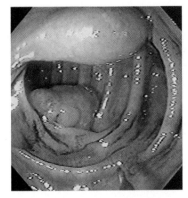

FIGURE 85-19.   India ink stain. Blebs from India ink immediately after injection of mucosa near colon cancer.

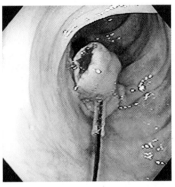

FIGURE 85-20.   Endoscopic loop on pedicle that began to bleed after snare polypectomy.

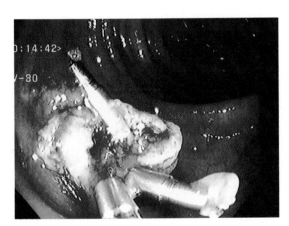

FIGURE 85-21.   Three endoscopic clips applied to a pedicle that bled immediately after transection.

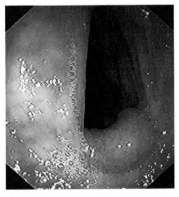

FIGURE 85-22.   Cancer—small bean-shaped carcinoma in the transverse colon.

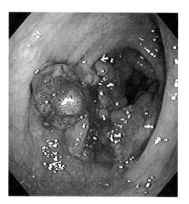

FIGURE 85-23. Cancer. Fungating carcinoma.

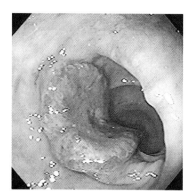

FIGURE 85-24. Cancer. Flat, saucer-shaped carcinoma.

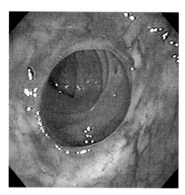

FIGURE 85-25. Colonic anastomosis. Normal stapled anastomosis.

86

ENDOSCOPIC RETROGRADE CHOLANGIOPANCREATOGRAPHY, ENDOSCOPIC SPHINCTEROTOMY AND STONE REMOVAL, AND ENDOSCOPIC BILIARY AND PANCREATIC DRAINAGE

STUART SHERMAN ■ GLEN A. LEHMAN

Since its inception and initial application in the early 1970s, endoscopic therapy has revolutionized the approach to a variety of biliary tract disorders. Before that time, interventional management of hepatobiliary and pancreatic diseases was primarily surgical. The capability of rendering definitive therapy at endoscopic retrograde cholangiopancreatography (ERCP) was the first development in the current movement of minimally invasive treatment. Innovations in instrumentation and refinements in technique rapidly ensued once the enormous potential of ERCP was appreciated. Paralleling these advances was a critical assessment of the application of ERCP. The cornerstone of therapeutic ERCP, endoscopic sphincterotomy, emerged relatively rapidly as the preferred management of common duct stones among patients who had undergone cholecystectomy. Techniques learned in the management of stones were rapidly and effectively used to treat patients with benign and malignant biliary strictures, gallstone pancreatitis, acute cholangitis, biliary fistulas, sphincter of Oddi dysfunction, and rarer problems, such as sump syndrome and biliary infestation with parasites.

Although the first pancreatic sphincterotomy was performed in 1976, ERCP was used primarily as a diagnostic modality in the setting of pancreatic disease because of concerns about prohibitive morbidity rates. Once the relative safety of ERCP and endoscopic sphincterotomy in the setting of gallstone pancreatitis was recognized, the indications for endoscopic therapy for pancreatic disorders were expanded. Endoscopic therapy is being applied in the setting of acute pancreatitis, chronic pancreatitis, complications of acute and chronic pancreatitis, pancreas divisum, and pancreatic and ampullary tumors. The role of therapeutic ERCP in the treatment of patients with pancreatic disease is still evolving. Further experience is needed to determine the place of this modality in the care of these patients. Figures 86-1 through 86-63 illustrate the range of diagnostic and therapeutic uses of ERCP.

849

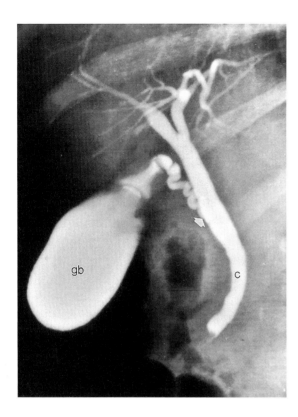

FIGURE 86-1. A normal common bile duct (*c*) becomes the common hepatic duct proximal to the insertion of the cystic duct (*arrow*). The common hepatic duct bifurcates into the right and left hepatic ducts. The cystic duct has a spiral shape owing to the valves of Heister and connects the gallbladder (*gb*) to the bile duct.

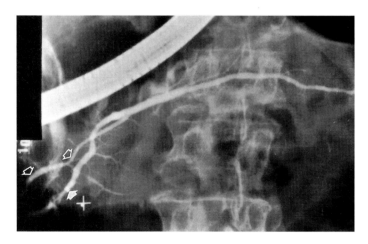

FIGURE 86-2. A normal pancreatogram obtained by means of placing a metal-tipped cannula (*solid arrow*) in the duct of Wirsung. Gradual tapering of the main pancreatic duct and the delicate side branches is visible. The duct of Santorini (*open arrows*) is filled by its connection with the main duct.

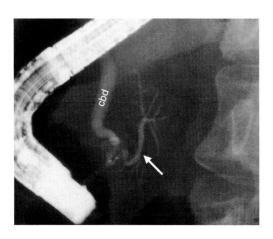

FIGURE 86-3. Normal ventral pancreatogram of pancreas divisum (*arrow*). The common bile duct (*cbd*) has been filled simultaneously with injection through the major papilla.

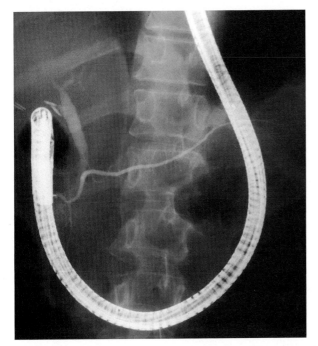

FIGURE 86-4. Cannulation of the minor papilla achieved from the long-scope position. Approximately 100 cm of endoscope has been advanced through the patient's mouth, and the endoscope lies along the greater curve of the stomach. The dorsal pancreatogram is normal.

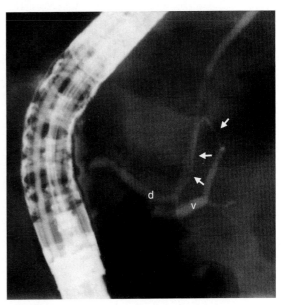

FIGURE 86-5. Incomplete pancreas divisum with a filamentous branch (*arrows*) connecting the dorsal (*d*) and ventral (*v*) ducts during ventral injection.

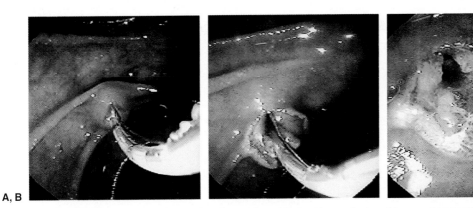

A, B

C

FIGURE 86-6. Sequence of endoscopic sphincterotomy. **A:** A pull-type sphincterotome has been introduced into the bile duct through a normal major papilla. **B:** The roof of the papilla is cut open by means of first bowing and then passing electrosurgical current through the sphincterotome wire. **C:** The completed sphincterotomy is shown.

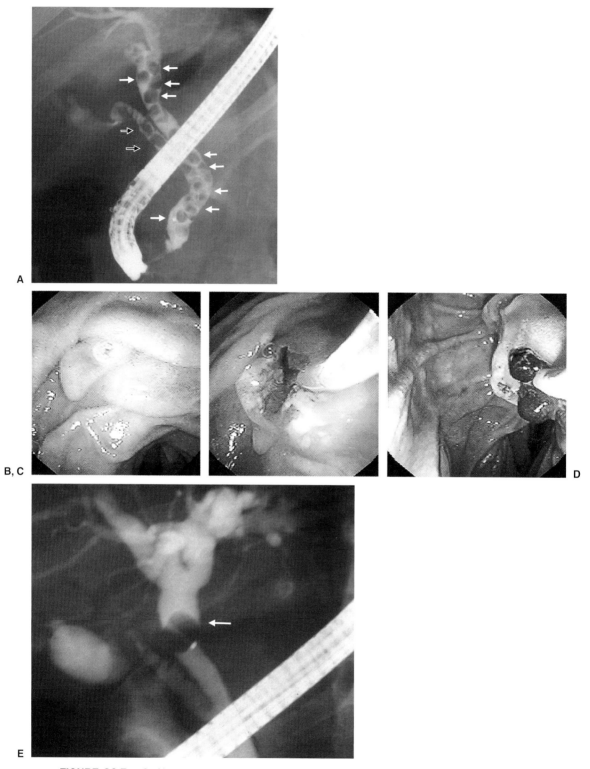

FIGURE 86-7. **A:** Numerous small stones (3 to 6 mm in diameter) in the common duct (*solid arrows*), left and right hepatic ducts, and cystic duct (*open arrows*). **B:** Endoscopic view of normal major papilla. **C:** A biliary sphincterotomy has been performed with a standard pull-type sphincterotome. **D:** A balloon catheter is inflated, and the stones are removed from the bile duct through the sphincterotomy. **E:** Repeat cholangiogram with a balloon catheter (*arrow*) shows no residual stones in the biliary tract.

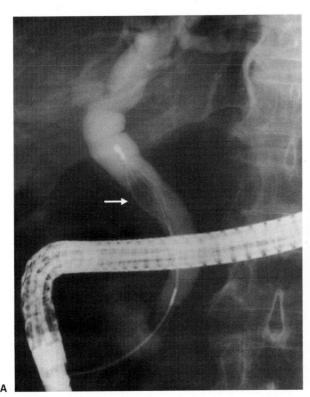
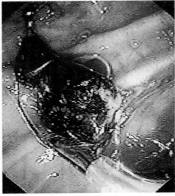

FIGURE 86-8. **A:** A Dormia basket is used to capture a bile duct stone (*arrow*). The wires have been partially tightened around the stone. **B:** Endoscopic view. After sphincterotomy is performed, a Dormia basket has been used to capture the stone and remove it through the sphincterotomy.

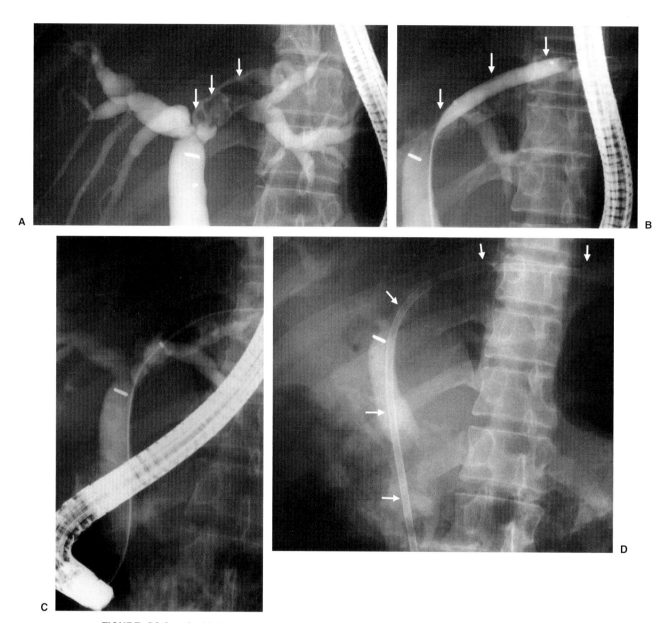

FIGURE 86-9. **A:** Multiple stones are impacted in the left hepatic duct (*arrows*) in a patient with cholangitis. **B:** A stone retrieval basket could not be advanced around the stones. Therefore, the duct adjacent to the stones was dilated with a 6-mm hydrostatic balloon (*arrows*). **C:** With a stone retrieval basket (with mechanical lithotripsy) and balloon, the stones were successfully removed. **D:** A 10F stent was placed into a branch of the left hepatic duct (*arrows*).

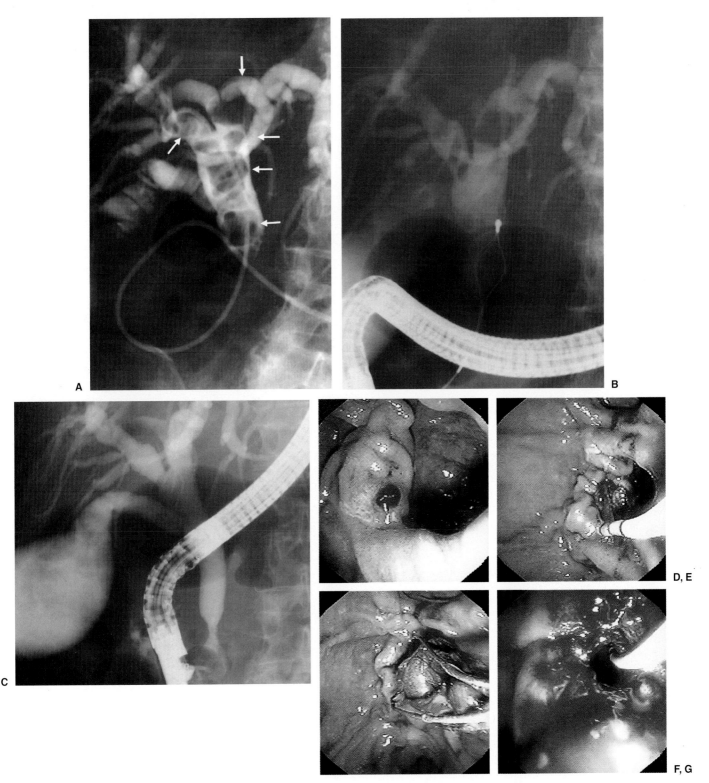

FIGURE 86-10. **A:** Numerous large stones (*arrows*) are present in the common duct and left and right hepatic ducts of a patient with cholangitis. A nasobiliary tube was placed for duct decompression. **B, C:** After the cholangitis resolved, the nasobiliary tube was removed. The stones were removed with a stone retrieval basket (**B**) and balloon (**C**) after sphincterotomy was performed. Endoscopic views. **D:** After removal of the nasobiliary tube, a small clot is present at the papillary orifice. The major papilla is on the rim of a duodenal diverticulum. **E:** Sphincterotomy is performed with a pull-type sphincterotome. **F:** Most of the stones were removed with a stone retrieval basket. **G:** The biliary orifice is gaping after sphincterotomy and stone removal.

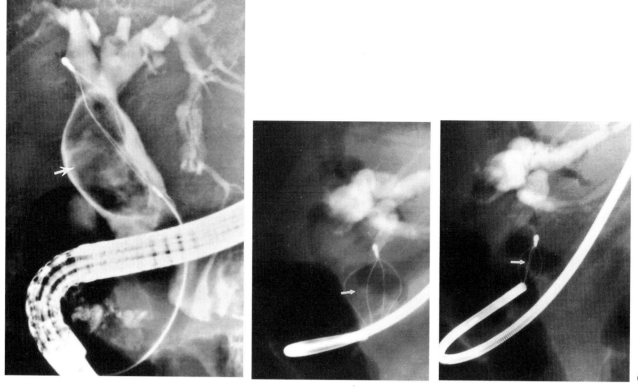

A, B   C

FIGURE 86-11.   A: This common bile duct stone (*arrow*) is too large for a conventional Dormia basket. A larger basket is used to capture the stone. A Soehendra mechanical lithotriptor (Wilson-Cook Medical Inc., Winston-Salem, NC) has replaced the endoscope to allow greater force to be applied to this common bile duct stone (*arrow*), shown before (**B**) and after (**C**) breakage.

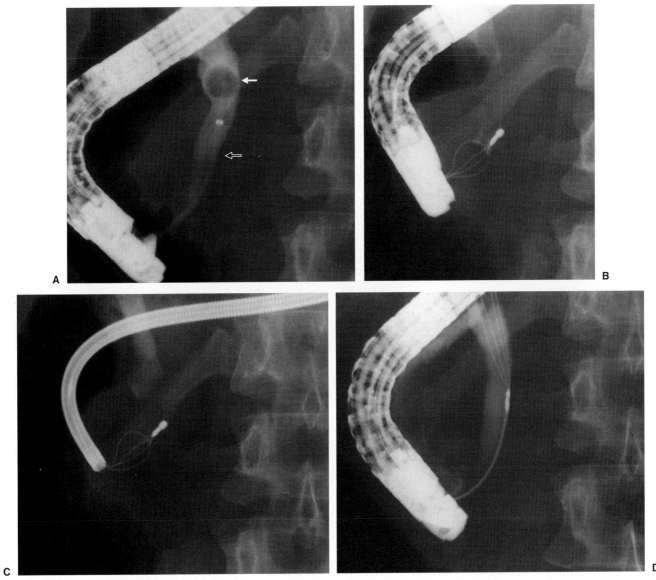

FIGURE 86-12. **A:** A 10-mm common bile duct stone (*closed arrow*) is proximal to a relatively narrow distal common bile duct segment (*open arrow*). **B:** The stone was captured with a stone retrieval basket but could not be removed through the distal common bile duct segment. **C:** A Soehendra mechanical lithotriptor (Wilson-Cook Medical Inc., Winston-Salem, NC) has replaced the endoscope to allow fragmentation of the stone. **D:** The fragments have been removed with a conventional Dormia basket. The common bile duct is clear of stone fragments.

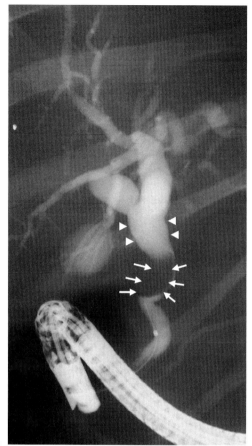

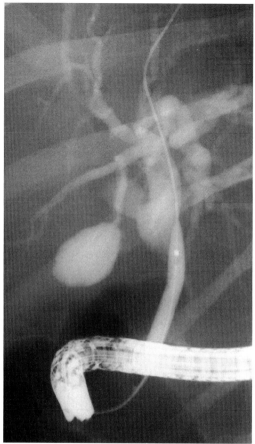

A   **B**

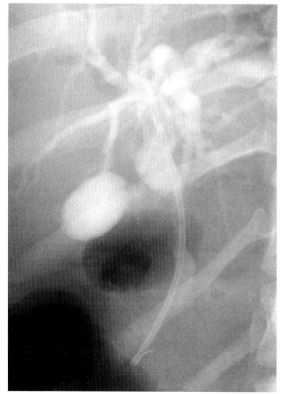

FIGURE 86-13. Mirizzi syndrome. Patient had right upper quadrant pain and jaundice. **A:** Cholangiogram demonstrates a stone in the cystic duct (probably partially in the common duct) (*arrows*) compressing the common duct and causing proximal dilation (*arrowheads*). **B:** A 6-mm hydrostatic balloon is used to dilate the bile duct adjacent to the stone. **C:** A 7F stent was placed for biliary decompression. The patient was treated surgically.

C

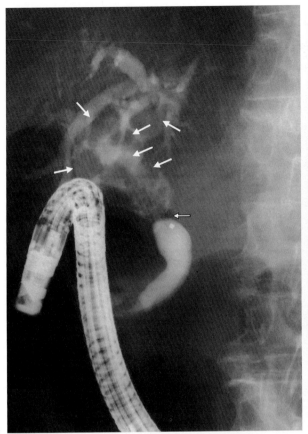

A

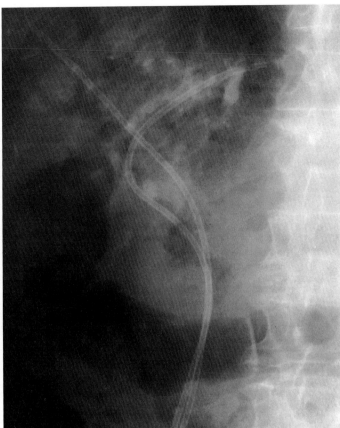

C

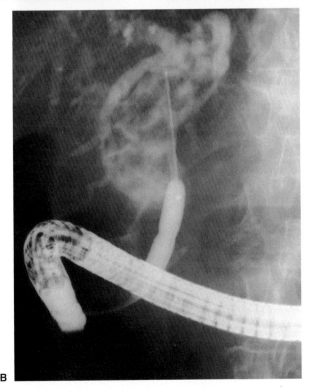

B

FIGURE 86-14. This patient, who underwent cholecystectomy 25 years earlier, presented with biliary colic and jaundice. **A:** Cholangiogram demonstrates a common duct stricture (*bottom arrow*). Proximal to the stricture are numerous stones (*top white arrows*) in a dilated biliary tract. **B:** Because of the stricture, the stones were not removable with a stone retrieval basket or balloon. The stricture was dilated with an 8-mm hydrostatic balloon opacified with contrast medium. **C:** Two 7F stents were placed through the stricture into the intrahepatic ducts.

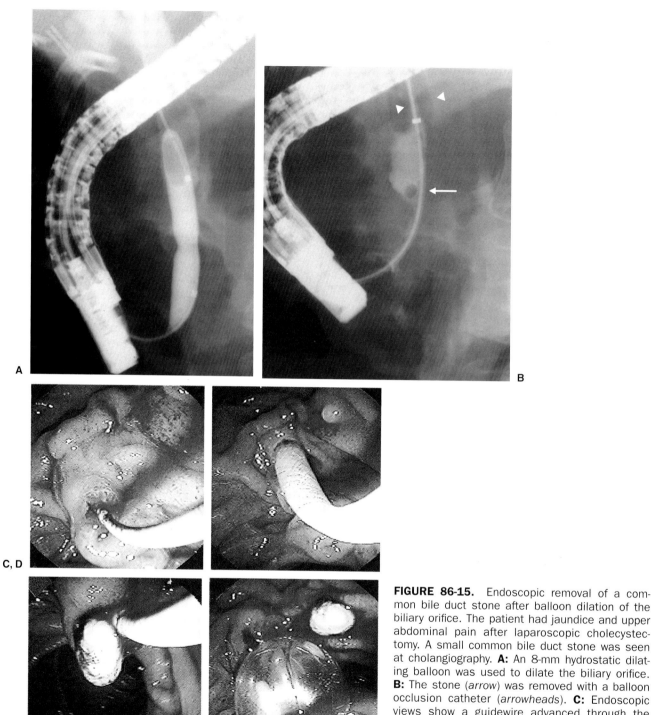

FIGURE 86-15. Endoscopic removal of a common bile duct stone after balloon dilation of the biliary orifice. The patient had jaundice and upper abdominal pain after laparoscopic cholecystectomy. A small common bile duct stone was seen at cholangiography. **A:** An 8-mm hydrostatic dilating balloon was used to dilate the biliary orifice. **B:** The stone (*arrow*) was removed with a balloon occlusion catheter (*arrowheads*). **C:** Endoscopic views show a guidewire advanced through the major papillary orifice into the bile duct. **D:** The biliary orifice was dilated with an 8-mm hydrostatic balloon. **E, F:** The stone is removed with a balloon occlusion catheter.

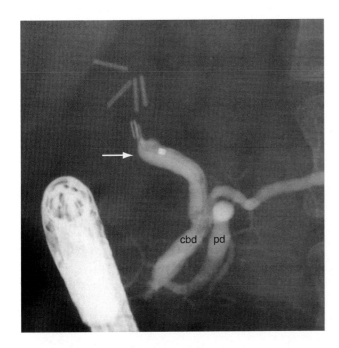

cbd   pd

FIGURE 86-16. Cholangiogram of a patient with obstructive jaundice and abdominal pain 4 days after laparoscopic cholecystectomy shows total cutoff (*arrow*) of the common bile duct (*cbd*). Clips are visible at the cephalic margin of the visualized segment of common bile duct. The pancreatic duct also is visible (*pd*). The patient was treated by means of choledochojejunostomy.

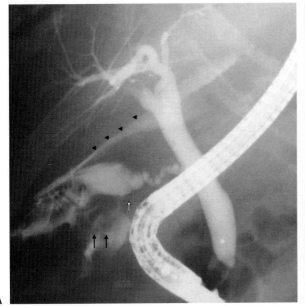

A

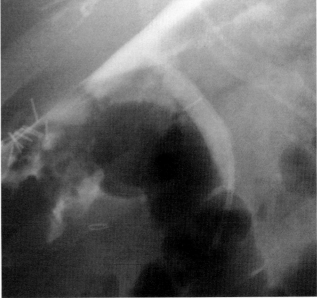

B

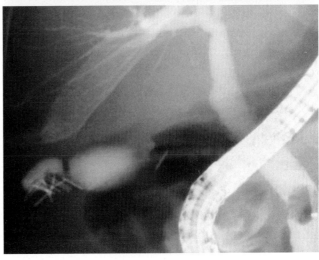

C

FIGURE 86-17. A patient who had undergone laparoscopic cholecystectomy for acute cholecystitis sought treatment 10 days later with fever, chills, and abdominal pain. **A:** Cholangiogram shows extravasation of contrast medium (*black arrows*) from a residual gallbladder remnant (*white arrow*). Subhepatic collection of contrast medium is depicted (*arrowheads*). **B:** Endoscopic sphincterotomy was performed, and a 7F stent was placed with the tip of the stent proximal to the cystic duct takeoff. **C:** The patient's symptoms rapidly resolved after stent placement. Endoscopic retrograde cholangiopancreatogram at stent removal 5 weeks later showed the fistula was closed.

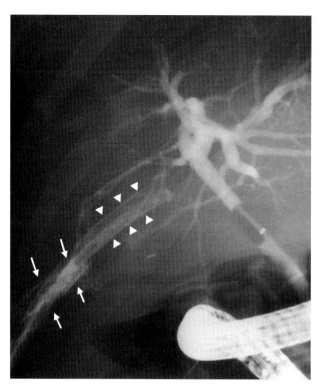

FIGURE 86-18. Cholangiogram of a patient with persistent bile drainage from a Jackson-Pratt drain (*arrowheads*) after laparoscopic cholecystectomy shows a leak of the duct of Luschka (*arrows*). This resolved after endoscopic sphincterotomy and biliary stent placement.

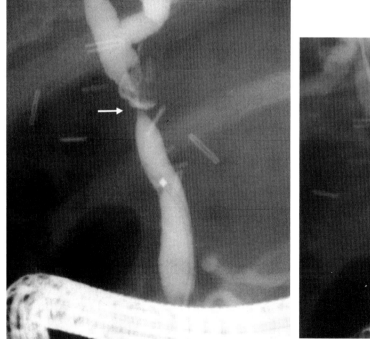

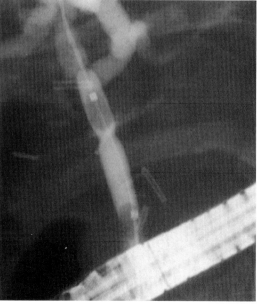

FIGURE 86-19. Obstructive jaundice 2 months after laparoscopic cholecystectomy. **A:** Cholangiogram shows a common duct stricture (*arrow*). Clips are present in the region of the common duct. **B:** The stricture was dilated with an 8-mm hydrostatic balloon. *(Continued)*

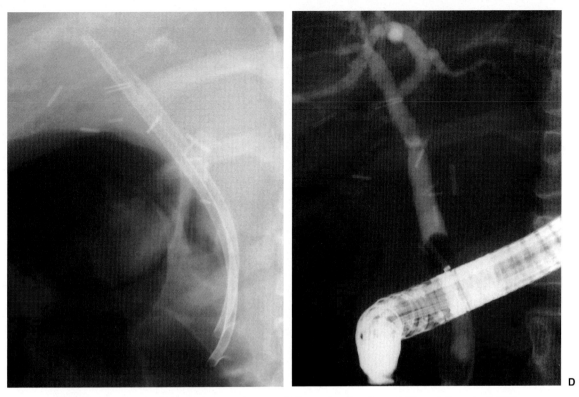

C

D

FIGURE 86-19. **C:** The patient underwent biliary stenting (one 10F and then two 10F stents) for 1 year (two 10F stents are shown). **D:** At stent removal, the stricture has resolved.

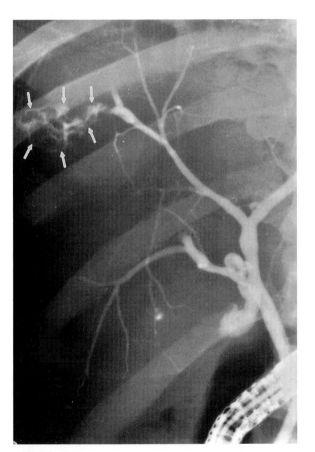

FIGURE 86-20. A collection of extravasated intrahepatic contrast material (*arrows*) identifies a bile duct leak caused by surgical trauma.

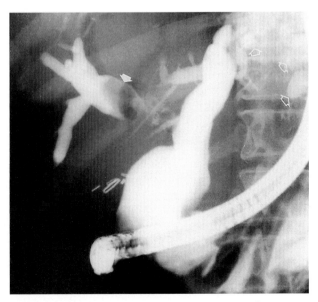

FIGURE 86-21. Patient with recurrent pyogenic cholangitis and recurrent stone formation has a stone in the right hepatic duct (*solid arrow*) and a branch of the left hepatic duct (*open arrows*).

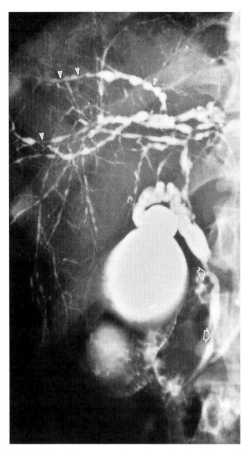

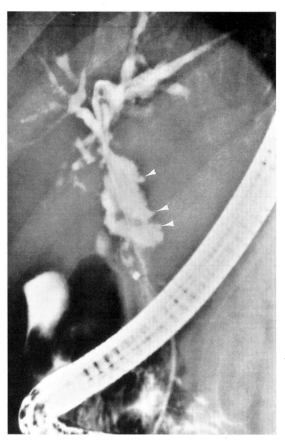

FIGURE 86-22. Primary sclerosing cholangitis with both extrahepatic and intrahepatic involvement with multiple strictures of the common bile duct (*open arrows*) and the intrahepatic ducts (*arrowheads*).

FIGURE 86-23. Cholangiogram of a patient with primary sclerosing cholangitis had pseudodiverticula (*arrowheads*) as a prominent feature.

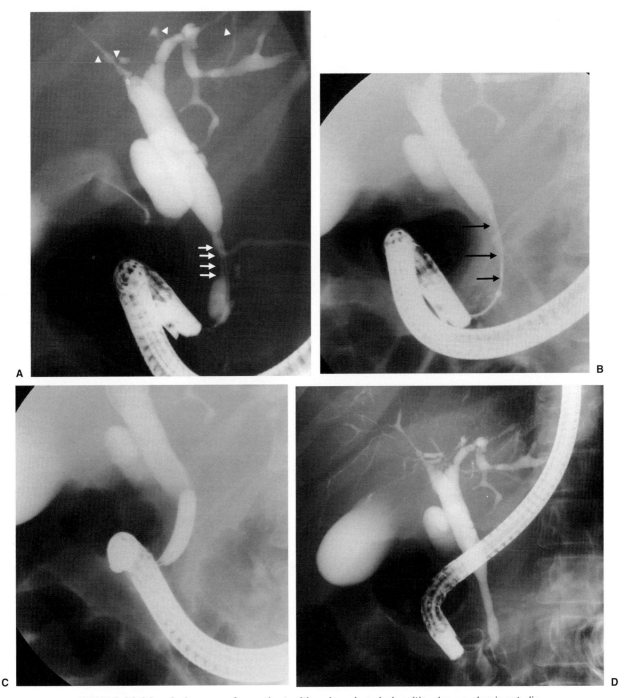

FIGURE 86-24. **A:** Images of a patient with sclerosing cholangitis show a dominant distal common bile duct stricture (*arrows*) with proximal dilation. The intrahepatic biliary tract is underfilled, but multiple strictures (*arrowheads*) are visible. **B:** A cytologic brush (*arrows*) was used to sample the distal common bile duct stricture. **C:** The stricture was then dilated with an 8-mm hydrostatic balloon. **D:** After stricture dilation, the caliber of the stricture is markedly improved. Radiograph shows diffuse intrahepatic strictures.

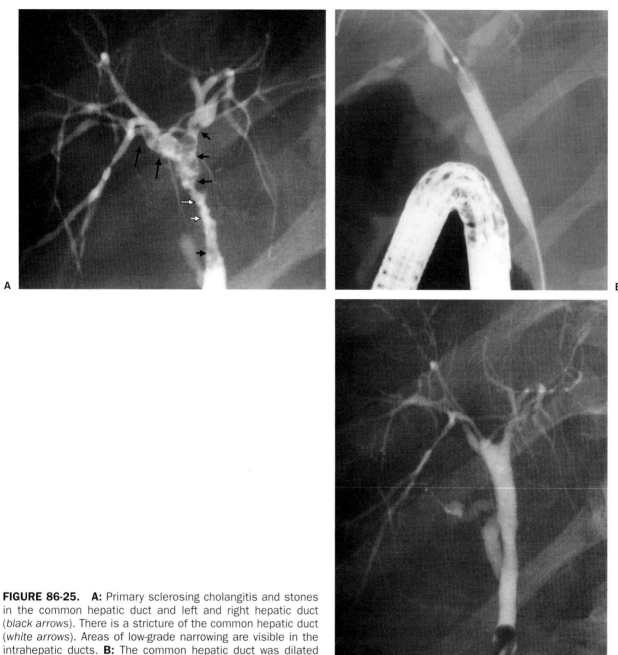

FIGURE 86-25. **A:** Primary sclerosing cholangitis and stones in the common hepatic duct and left and right hepatic duct (*black arrows*). There is a stricture of the common hepatic duct (*white arrows*). Areas of low-grade narrowing are visible in the intrahepatic ducts. **B:** The common hepatic duct was dilated with a 6-mm hydrostatic balloon. **C:** After dilation and stone removal, the common duct is of normal caliber.

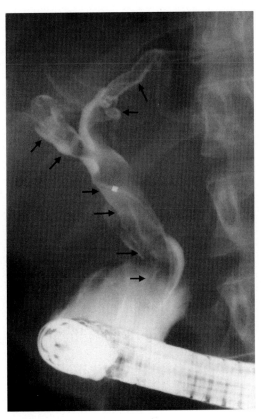

FIGURE 86-26. Cast-like filling defect (*arrows*) in the entire visualized biliary tract of a patient with jaundice and a decreasing hemoglobin level after liver biopsy. The filling defect represents a blood clot.

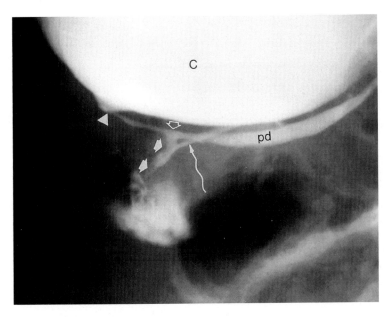

FIGURE 86-27. The distal portion of a choledochal cyst (*C*) highlights the associated anomalous connection of the pancreatic and bile ducts. The origin of the cyst from the distal common bile duct is marked with an *arrowhead*. The common bile duct and pancreatic duct (*pd*) emerge at right angles (*open arrow*) from a common connection with the duodenum (*solid arrows*). An anomalous accessory pancreatic duct (*wavy arrow*) also inserts into this common channel.

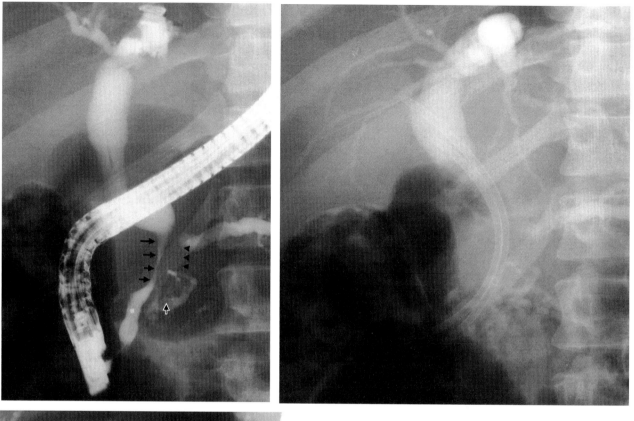

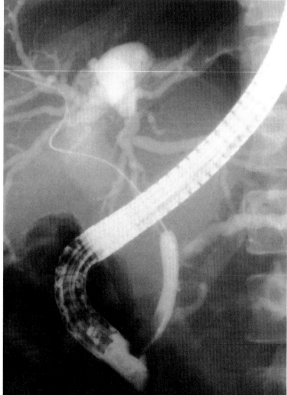

FIGURE 86-28. Common bile duct stricture induced by chronic pancreatitis. **A:** Cholangiogram shows a 2-cm common bile duct stricture (*closed arrows*) with proximal dilation. A pancreatic duct stone (*open arrow*) and stricture (*arrowheads*) are visible. **B:** Stricture being dilated with a 6-mm hydrostatic balloon. **C:** Two 10F stents have been deployed to bridge the stricture.

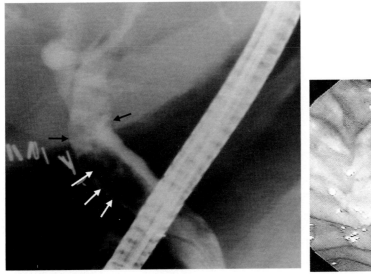

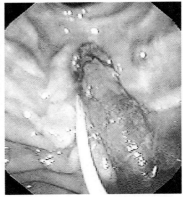

FIGURE 86-29. Sump syndrome. The patient underwent choledochoduodenostomy with removal of a large common duct stone 4 years before seeking treatment because of recurrent episodes of cholangitis. **A:** Cholangiogram shows numerous large filling defects (*arrows*). **B:** Endoscopic view. Biliary sphincterotomy was performed. Using a balloon occlusion catheter, bile-colored vegetable matter was removed from the biliary tract.

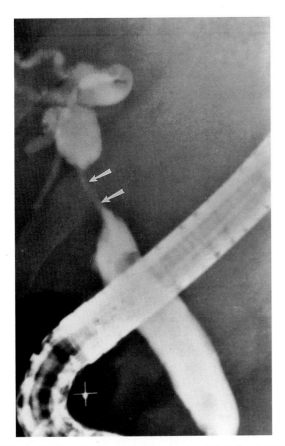

FIGURE 86-30. Cholangiocarcinoma involving the common hepatic duct below the bifurcation (type I) is of the sclerosing type because it produces concentric ductal narrowing (*arrows*).

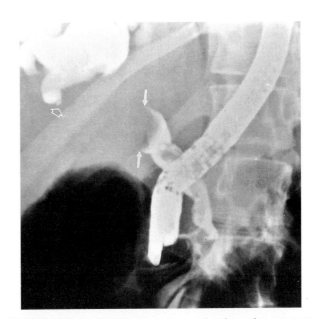

FIGURE 86-31. Cholangiocarcinoma involves the common hepatic duct but has a polypoid growth pattern with splaying of the common bile duct at the distal tumor margin (*between arrows*). The proximal extent of the tumor (*open arrow*) is just below the bifurcation.

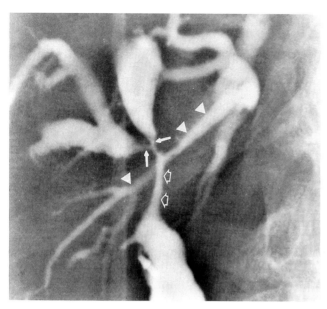

FIGURE 86-32. Bifurcation cholangiocarcinoma classified as a type II because it involves both the common hepatic duct (*open arrows*) and the origins of the left and right hepatic ducts (*solid arrows*). The left hepatic duct branch (*arrowheads*) that courses behind the common hepatic duct is not involved in the stricture.

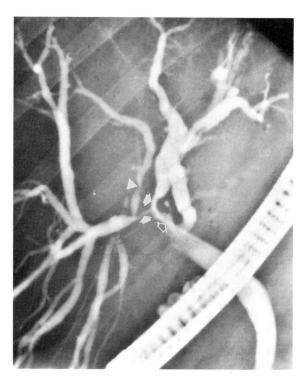

FIGURE 86-33. Type III cholangiocarcinoma of the bifurcation involves the common hepatic duct (*open arrow*), left and right hepatic duct (*solid arrows*), and a branch of the right hepatic duct (*arrowhead*).

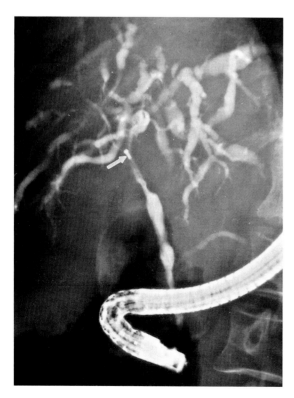

FIGURE 86-34. Injection of contrast medium through a metal-tipped cannula (*arrow*) wedged into a common hepatic duct stricture reveals diffuse involvement of the intrahepatic ducts by infiltrating cholangiocarcinoma.

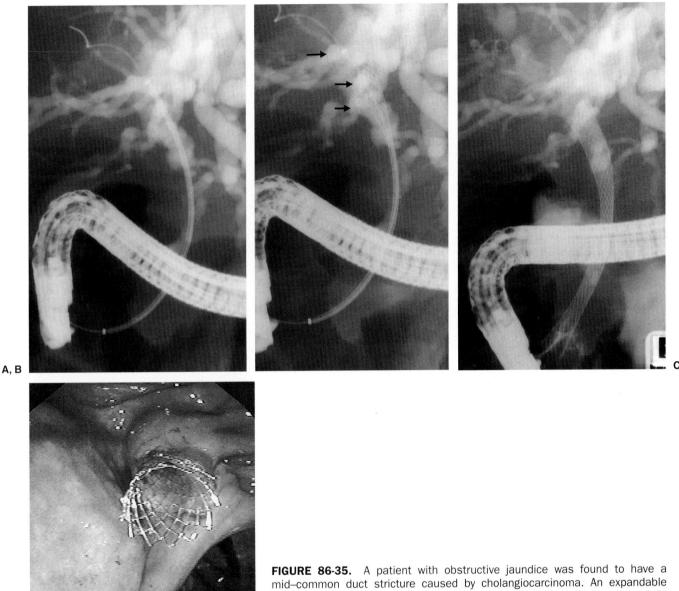

FIGURE 86-35. A patient with obstructive jaundice was found to have a mid–common duct stricture caused by cholangiocarcinoma. An expandable metal stent was placed. **A:** Stent in constrained form. **B:** Stent partially deployed (*arrows*). **C:** Stent fully deployed. **D:** Endoscopic view shows metal expandable stent protruding into the duodenum through the major papilla.

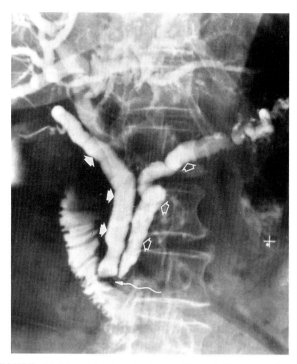

FIGURE 86-36. Malignant obstruction at the ampulla of Vater (*wavy arrow*) causing dilation of the bile duct, cystic duct stump (*solid arrows*), and pancreatic duct (*open arrows*).

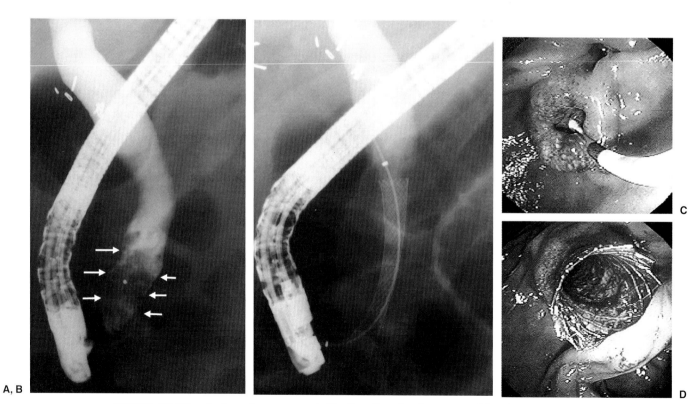

FIGURE 86-37. A: Ampullary cancer infiltrating the distal common bile duct (*arrows*). **B:** Metal expandable stent was used. **C:** Endoscopic view of ampullary cancer enlarging the papillary orifice. **D:** Deployed metal expandable stent.

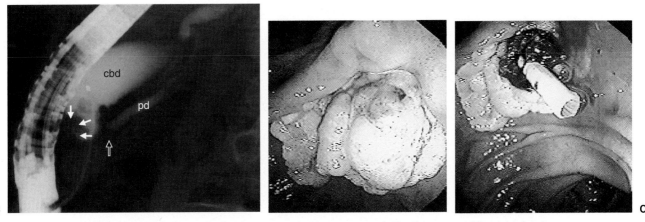

FIGURE 86-38. **A:** Ampullary cancer with involvement of distal common bile duct (*cbd*) (*closed arrows*) and pancreatic duct (*pd*) (*open arrow*). **B:** The ampullary cancer has spread along the adjacent duodenal wall. **C:** A 10F biliary stent was placed.

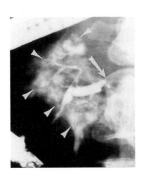

FIGURE 86-39. Contrast medium injected into the pancreatic duct caused acinarization of the head of the pancreas (*arrowheads*) because ductal obstruction (*arrow*) by a carcinoma prevented filling of the rest of the pancreatic duct.

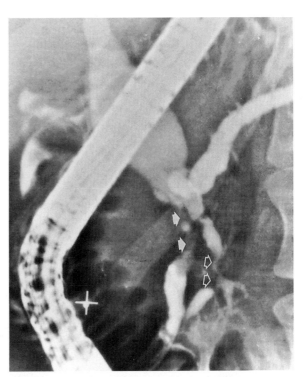

FIGURE 86-40. Pancreatic duct (*open arrows*) and bile duct (*closed arrows*) strictures caused by pancreatic carcinoma constitute the double-duct sign.

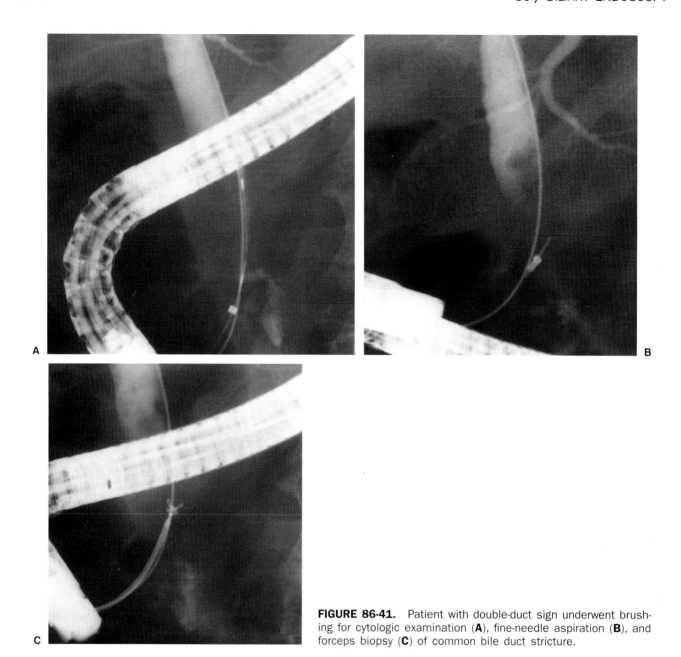

A

B

C

FIGURE 86-41. Patient with double-duct sign underwent brushing for cytologic examination (**A**), fine-needle aspiration (**B**), and forceps biopsy (**C**) of common bile duct stricture.

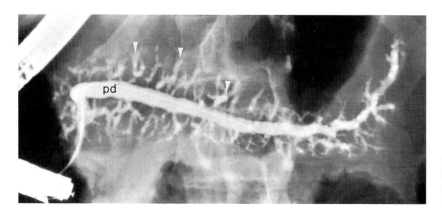

pd

FIGURE 86-42. Main pancreatic duct (*pd*) is of normal caliber, but the side branches (*arrowheads*) are dilated in a patient with mild chronic pancreatitis.

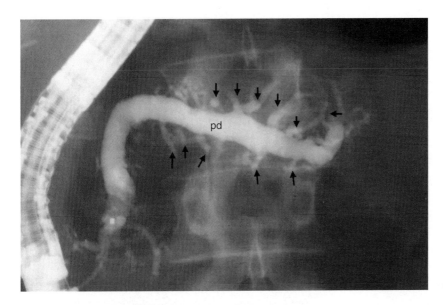

FIGURE 86-43. Pancreatogram demonstrates dilation of the main pancreatic duct (*pd*) and side branches (*arrows*), consistent with moderate chronic pancreatitis.

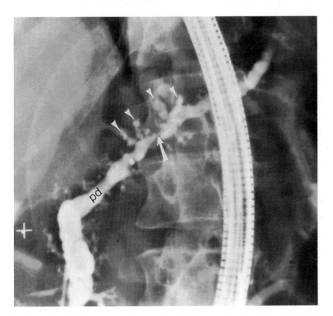

FIGURE 86-44. In addition to dilation of the main pancreatic duct (*pd*) and side branch (*arrowheads*), focal stenosis (*arrow*) of the main pancreatic duct is visible in a patient with severe chronic pancreatitis.

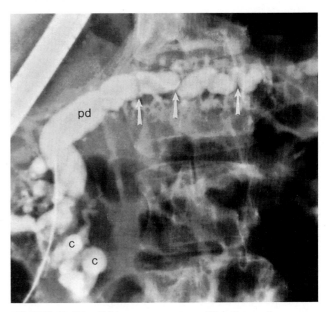

FIGURE 86-45. With severe pancreatitis, the main pancreatic duct (*pd*) has strictures (*arrows*) and is dilated, and some of the side branches are (*c*) cystically dilated.

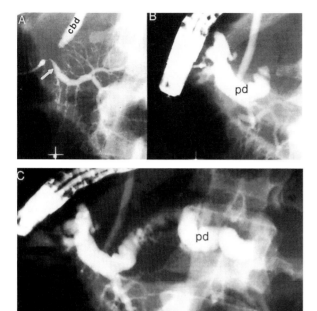

FIGURE 86-46.   A: Ventral duct (*arrow*) of a patient with pancreas divisum. The duct is dilated, as are the side branches, consistent with chronic pancreatitis. A limited portion of the common bile duct (*cbd*) also is visible. **B, C:** Injection of the minor papilla demonstrates dilation of the dorsal pancreatic duct (*pd*) caused by chronic pancreatitis.

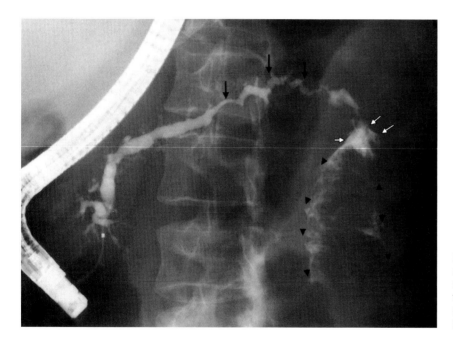

FIGURE 86-47. Pancreatogram demonstrates severe chronic pancreatitis with strictures (*black arrows*) in the region of the body and tail and a pancreatic fistula (*white arrows*) communicating with the bowel (*arrowheads*).

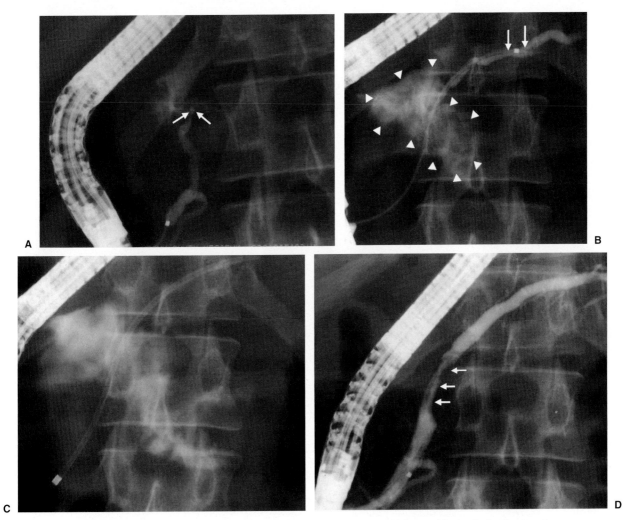

FIGURE 86-48. Pancreatic duct disruption after motor vehicle accident. **A:** Leakage of contrast material from the pancreatic duct at the level of the genu (*arrows*). **B:** Catheter (*arrows*) advanced proximally to the area of disruption. The proximal duct is normal. Contrast medium has collected in the region of the genu (*arrowheads*). **C:** A 6F, 10-cm pancreatic stent with tip proximal to the area of disruption. **D:** Pancreatogram 8 weeks after stent placement shows resolution of the disruption. However, there is narrowing of the main pancreatic duct at the site of disruption (*arrows*).

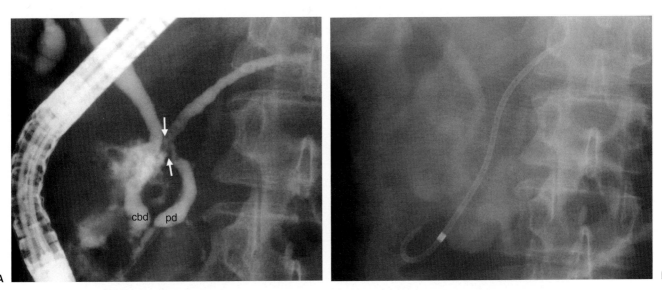

FIGURE 86-49. Severe pancreatitis and pancreatic ascites. **A:** Pancreatogram demonstrates disruption of the pancreatic duct (*pd*) from the head of the pancreas (*arrows*). The upstream duct is normal. The common bile duct (*cbd*) also is visible. **B:** A 7F stent was placed through the area of disruption.

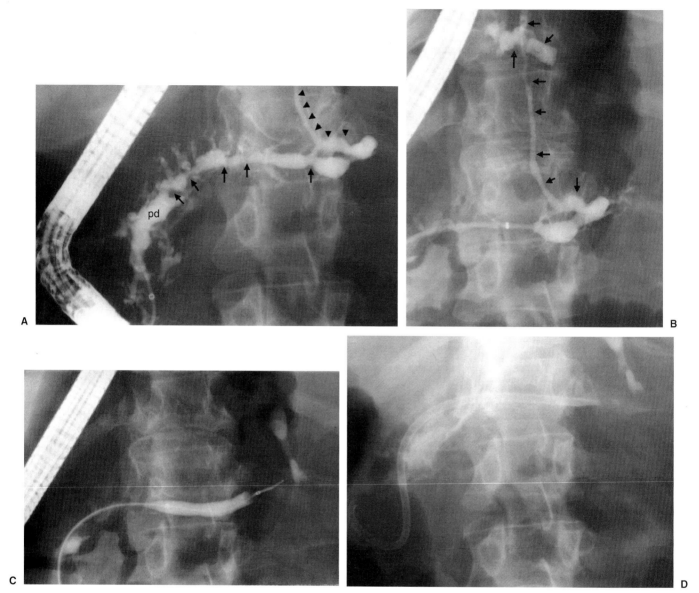

FIGURE 86-50. Severe chronic pancreatitis with pancreatic fistula. **A:** Pancreatogram demonstrates areas of main pancreatic duct (*pd*) dilation and narrowing (*arrows*). A fistula from the region of the tail (*arrowheads*) is depicted. **B:** Radiograph shows pancreatic fistula (*arrows*) arising from the tail of the pancreas. **C:** The strictures were dilated with a 6-mm hydrostatic balloon. **D:** A 10F pancreatic stent was placed through the strictures into the tail of the pancreas.

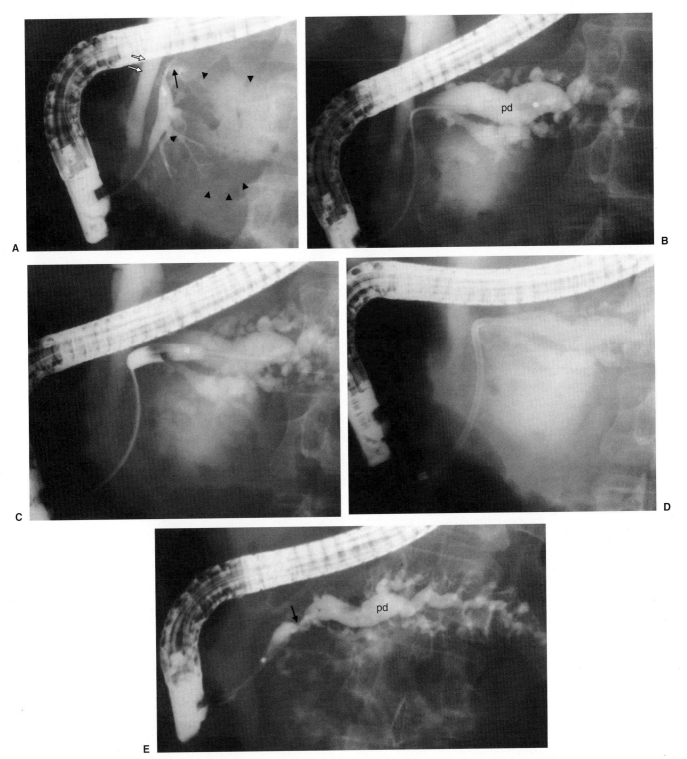

FIGURE 86-51. Recurrent pancreatitis with a 5-cm pseudocyst on a computed tomographic (CT) scan. **A:** Pancreatogram demonstrates severe chronic pancreatitis with a 5-cm communicating pseudocyst (*arrowheads*) arising from the region of the genu (*black arrow*). A narrowed segment is visible immediately downstream from the site of the pancreatic duct leak (*white arrows*). **B:** The upstream duct is markedly dilated (*pd*) and demonstrates advanced changes of chronic pancreatitis. **C:** Stricture dilated with a 6-mm hydrostatic balloon. **D:** A 12-cm, 7F, multiple sidehole, pancreatic stent was placed. **E:** Three months later pancreatogram shows resolution of the pseudocyst. There is residual narrowing (*arrow*) in the region of the genu. The pancreatic duct (*pd*) is decompressed compared with the prior study.

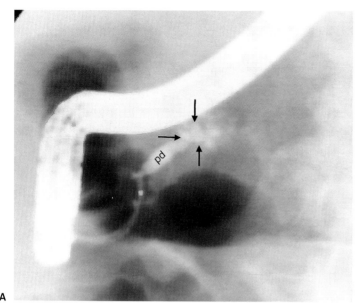

A

FIGURE 86-52. Severe gallstone pancreatitis with a large pseudocyst that increased in size was seen on serial computed tomographic scans. **A:** Pancreatogram demonstrates 1.5 cm segment of normal pancreatic duct (*pd*). The duct is disrupted above this location (*arrows*). **B:** Guidewire advanced through the papilla and looped within the pseudocyst cavity. The biliary tree is visible and is normal after cholecystectomy. **C:** 10F and 7F double-pigtail endoprostheses were placed through the papilla into the pseudocyst cavity. **D:** Endoscopic views show distortion of the major papilla, probably by the adjacent pseudocyst. **E:** Pancreatic sphincterotomy has been performed with a standard pull-type sphincterotome. **F:** The 10F and 7F double-pigtail stents are deployed.

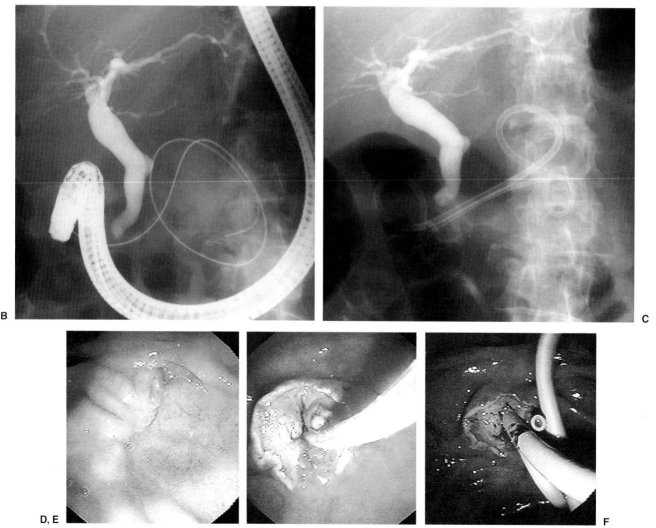

B

C

D, E

F

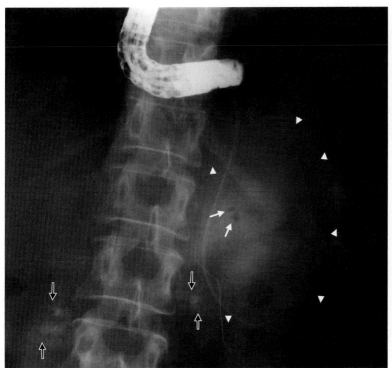

A

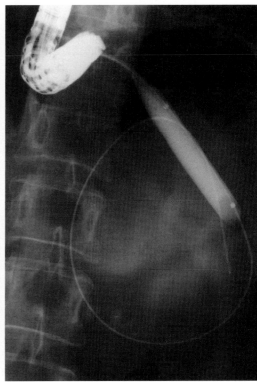

B

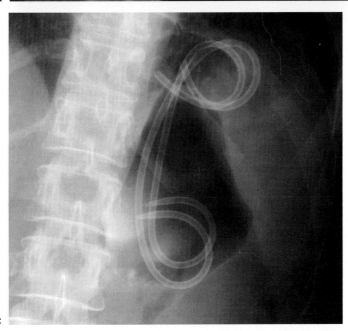

C

FIGURE 86-53. Chronic pancreatitis with a 7-cm nonre-solving pseudocyst. **A:** Puncture of the pseudocyst through the transgastric approach. Contrast injection reveals filling of a 7-cm pseudocyst (*arrowheads*) containing filling defects (*arrows*). Pancreatic calcifications (*open arrows*) are present in the region of the pancreas. **B:** Track between stomach and pseudocyst is dilated with a 10-mm hydrostatic dilating balloon. **C:** Two 10F, double-pigtail stents bridge the stomach and pseudocyst. Endoscopic views show the technique. *(Continued)*

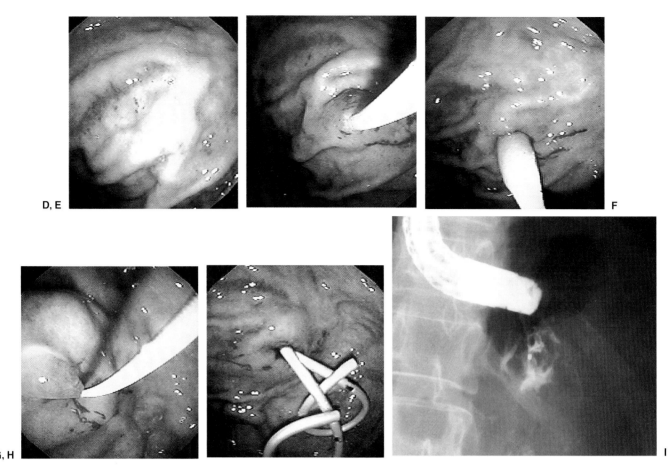

FIGURE 86-53. **(Continued)** **D:** Visible bulge on the posterior wall in the body of the stomach. **E:** Pseudocyst punctured with a double-lumen needle-knife cystoenterotome. **F:** Tract dilated with a 10-mm balloon. **G:** Close-up view demonstrates clear fluid draining from pseudocyst. **H:** Two 10F, double-pigtail stents bridge the stomach and pseudocyst. **I:** Follow-up computed tomographic scan 5 weeks later showed resolution of the pseudocyst. The stents were removed. Image demonstrates injection of the transgastric tract. No pseudocyst filling is seen.

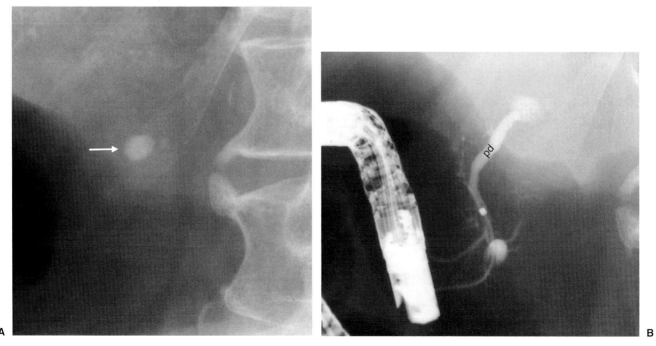

FIGURE 86-54. Recurrent pancreatitis. **A:** Plain radiograph shows 6-mm calcification in the region of the pancreatic head (*arrow*). **B:** Pancreatogram demonstrates that the stone totally obstructs the pancreatic duct (*pd*). *(Continued)*

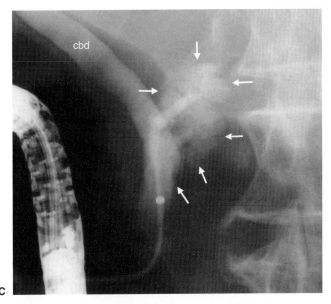

FIGURE 86-54.   C: Attempts to fill the duct proximal to the stone resulted in acinarization (*arrows*). The common bile duct (*cbd*) is visible.

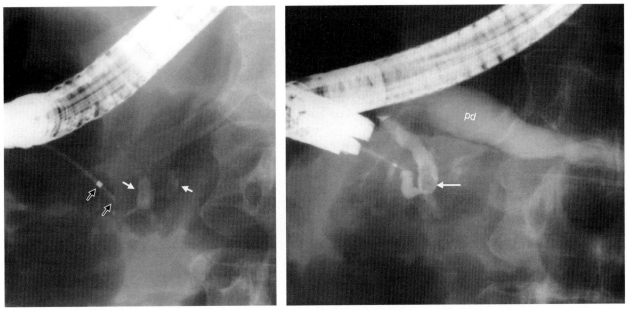

FIGURE 86-55. Chronic calcific pancreatitis with clinical episodes of acute pancreatitis. **A:** Calcifications in the region of the pancreatic head (*closed arrows*). Proximity of the stones to the papilla, which is marked by a catheter (*open arrows*). **B:** The stone is impacted (*arrow*) in the main pancreatic duct in the head of the pancreas. There is marked proximal dilation of the duct (*pd*).

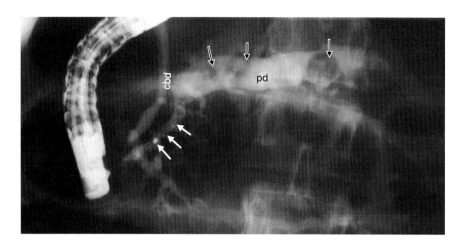

FIGURE 86-56. Pancreatogram demonstrates narrowing of the main pancreatic duct in the head of the pancreas (*closed arrows*) with marked proximal dilation (*pd*). There were at least three filling defects (pancreatic stones) in the body of the pancreas (*open arrows*), the largest measuring 10 mm. The common bile duct (*cbd*), which is narrow, is visible.

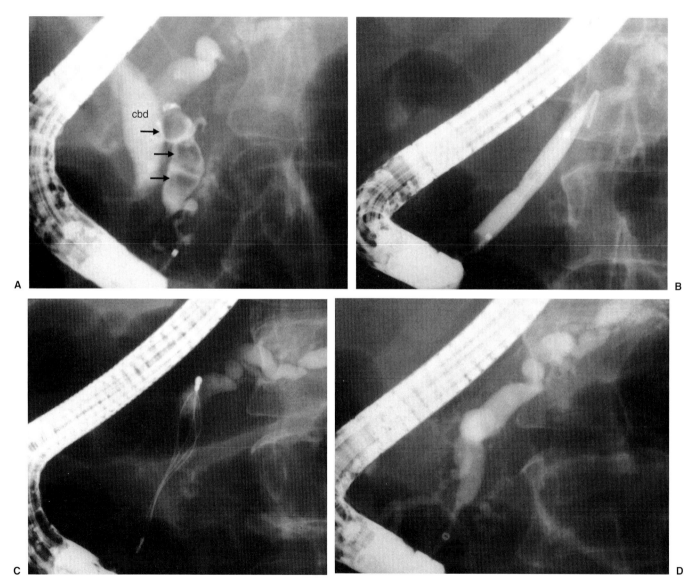

FIGURE 86-57. **A:** Pancreatogram demonstrates three stones in the main pancreatic duct in the pancreatic head (*arrows*). The common bile duct (*cbd*) is normal. **B:** Duct is dilated adjacent to the stones with a 6-mm hydrostatic balloon. **C, D:** Stones were removed with a basket (**C**) and stone retrieval balloon (**D**). The main pancreatic duct is totally cleared. *(Continued)*

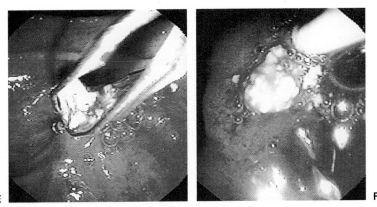

FIGURE 86-57. **E:** Endoscopic views. Pancreatic sphincterotomy has been performed and a stone captured in the basket. **F:** Stone being removed with a balloon occlusion catheter.

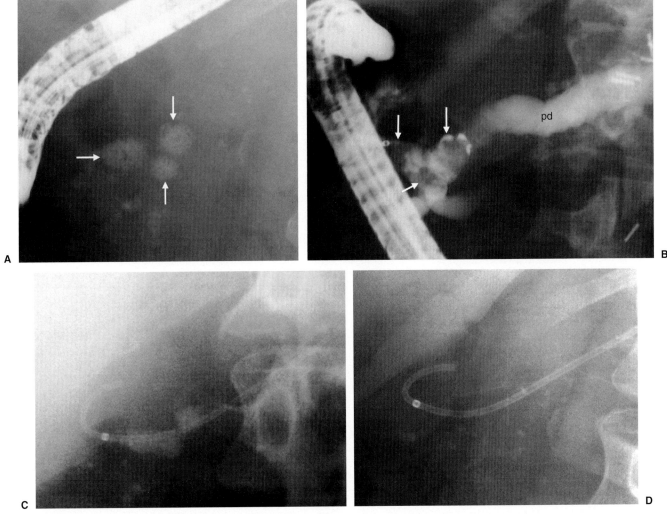

FIGURE 86-58. **A:** Alcohol-induced chronic pancreatitis complicated by episodes of clinical pancreatitis and chronic abdominal pain. Spot radiographs show three 5- to 8-mm pancreatic duct stones in the region of the pancreatic head (*arrows*). Several small adjacent stones are visible. **B:** The patient was found to have pancreas divisum. On injection of the minor papilla, the stones were found to be impacted (*arrows*) with upstream dilation of the pancreatic duct (*pd*). **C:** Minor papilla pancreatic sphincterotomy was performed. The stones could not be removed with stone retrieval balloons or baskets. A 6F pancreatic stent was used to decompress the dorsal duct. The tip of the stent is in the body of the pancreas. **D:** Extracorporeal shockwave lithotripsy was performed with fluoroscopic targeting. The stones were fragmented. Spot radiograph shows only a few residual fragments (most have passed spontaneously). *(Continued)*

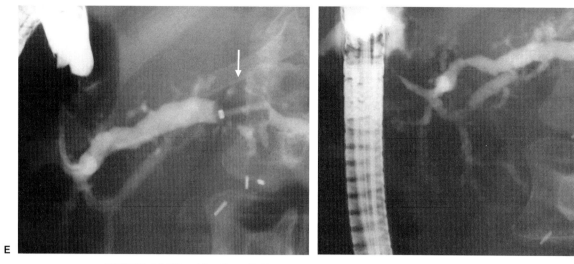

E   F

FIGURE 86-58. **(Continued)** **E:** Fragments being removed with a stone retrieval balloon (*arrow*). **F:** Repeat pancreatogram shows no residual stones and marked decompression of the dorsal pancreatic duct.

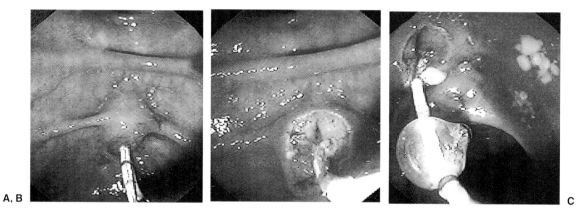

A, B   C

FIGURE 86-59. Endoscopic views demonstrate removal of pancreatic duct stones after pancreatic sphincterotomy. **A:** Pull-type sphincterotome in the pancreatic duct. **B:** Pancreatic sphincterotomy was performed with electrocautery. **C:** Stone removal with a balloon occlusion catheter.

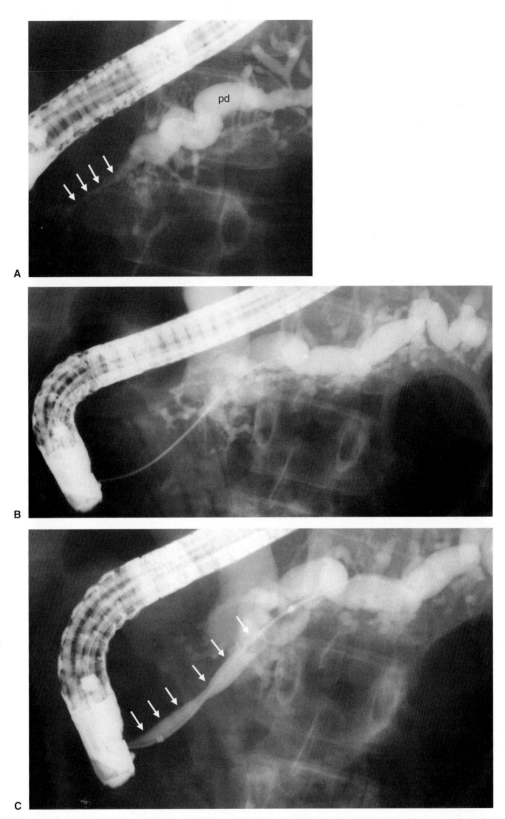

FIGURE 86-60. A 35-year-old man with alcohol-induced chronic pancreatitis and clinical episodes of acute pancreatitis sought treatment because of a clinical episode of pancreatitis and jaundice. **A:** Pancreatogram shows severe chronic pancreatitis with a distal pancreatic duct stricture (*arrows*) in the head and upstream dilation of the pancreatic duct (*pd*). **B:** Hydrophilic guidewire is advanced proximal to the stricture. **C:** After pancreatic sphincterotomy, the stricture was dilated with a 6-mm hydrostatic balloon (*arrows*). *(Continued)*

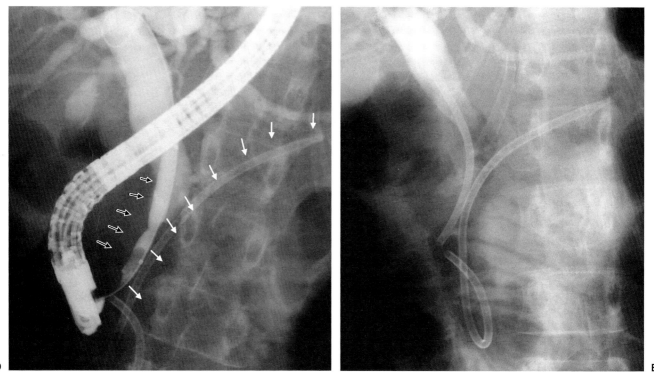

D   E

FIGURE 86-60. **(Continued) D:** A 10F, single-pigtail, multiple sidehole, pancreatic stent (*closed arrows*) was placed. The patient also had a distal common bile duct stricture. After biliary sphincterotomy, the common bile duct stricture was dilated with a 6-mm hydrostatic balloon (*open arrows*). **E:** A 10F, Amsterdam-type biliary stent was placed to bridge the common bile duct stricture.

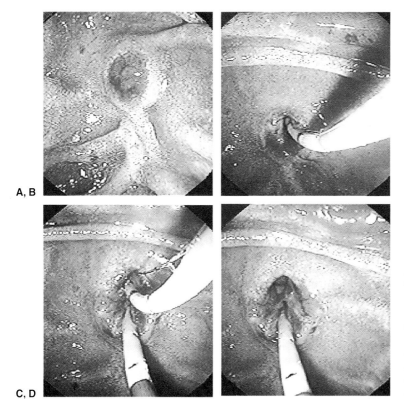

A, B

C, D

FIGURE 86-61. Technique of combined pancreaticobiliary sphincterotomy with a standard pull-type sphincterotome. **A:** Normal major papilla. **B:** Completed pancreatic sphincterotomy with standard pull-type sphincterotome. **C:** After pancreatic sphincterotomy, a 6F, multiple sidehole, pancreatic stent was placed. Biliary sphincterotomy is being performed with a standard pull-type sphincterotome. **D:** Completed biliary and pancreatic sphincterotomy with placement of a pancreatic stent.

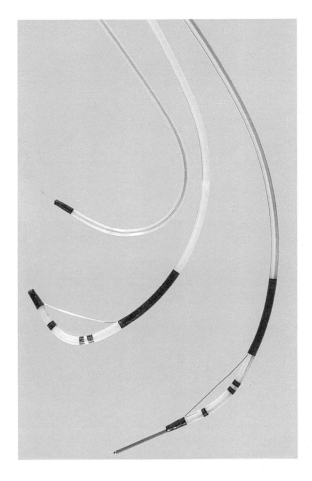

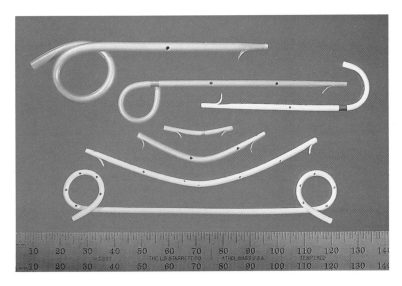

FIGURE 86-62. Three types of sphincterotomes. **Top:** Needle-knife sphincterotome. **Center:** Standard pull-type sphincterotome. **Bottom:** Standard pull-type sphincterotome with guidewire in place.

FIGURE 86-63. Commercially available straight, half-pigtail, three-quarter pigtail, full-pigtail, and double-pigtail pancreatic stents (5F to 10F). Stents longer than 2.5 cm usually have multiple sideholes to drain side branches.

ENDOSCOPIC MUCOSAL BIOPSY

CYRUS E. RUBIN ■ **RODGER C. HAGGITT***

Endoscopic mucosal biopsy of the esophagus, stomach, small bowel, and colon has greatly expanded the diagnostic capabilities of gastroenterologists and gastrointestinal pathologists. Many of the lesions that can be diagnosed with endoscopy are illustrated herein, and a summary is provided of the histological and clinical features of mucosal diseases in the several organs accessible to endoscopy. The accuracy of the diagnostic information provided by biopsy is directly related to the precision of targeting the lesion and the adequacy of the size and number of biopsy specimens obtained. The additional effort of orientation, proper fixation, separate labeling, step-serial sectioning, and informative staining greatly enhances diagnostic sensitivity and specificity.

(figures begin on page 895)

---

*Deceased

TABLE 87-1
Premalignant Lesions

TYPE OF DYSPLASIA	HISTOLOGICAL FEATURES	CLINICAL FEATURES
Esophageal squamous dysplasia	Noninvasive neoplastic basal cells that do not mature as they move superficially	Early diagnosis of squamous cancer requires biopsy of grossly invisible dysplasia in predisposed patients
Barrett esophageal dysplasia	Loss of mucous secretion, neoplastic nuclear changes, nuclear stratification, distorted architecture, no invasion of the lamina propria	Esophageal adenocarcinoma is rapidly increasing in frequency among Caucasian men in the United States; early diagnosis requires extensive biopsy of all Barrett specialized metaplasia
Cardia dysplasia	Same as Barrett esophageal dysplasia	Cardia carcinoma among Caucasian U.S. men is rapidly increasing in frequency and is often associated with a short segment of Barrett specialized metaplasia and dysplasia
Gastric dysplasia	Same as Barrett esophageal dysplasia; associated with progressive intestinalized pangastritis	Intestinalized carcinoma of the distal stomach is disappearing in the West but is still common in nonindustrialized nations; early gastric cancer can be diagnosed endoscopically
Colonic adenoma	Enlarged, pallisading, cigar-shaped nuclei; tubular, villous, or tubullovillous patterns of dysplasia within an adenoma	Precursor to sporadic colon cancer and familial polyposis coli; patients with distal colonic adenoma revealed with flexible sigmoidoscopy may have carcinoma or premalignant polyps proximally
Chronic ulcerative colitis	Dysplasia in a flat nonpolypoid area, similar to that seen in an adenoma, occasionally produces a gross lesion	Dysplasia appears after 8–10 y of extensive ulcerative colitis; it is an indication for colectomy when confirmed by an experienced gastrointestinal pathologist

TABLE 87-2
Diffuse Benign Gastric Mucosal Abnormalities

DIAGNOSIS	HISTOLOGICAL FEATURES	CLINICAL FEATURES
Diffuse antral-predominant gastritis	Antral: 100% *Helicobacter pylori*–positive diffuse interfoveolar inflammation, deeper pyloric glands intact, mild and focal intestinal metaplasia in 10–20%. Fundic: mild or no interfoveolar inflammation, no intestinal metaplasia	Caused by HP infection; asymptomatic or associated with duodenal prepyloric ulcer; associated with decreased risk for distal gastric cancer; gastritis reversible and ulcer curable with eradication of HP
Multifocal intestinalized pangastritis	Starts in multiple foci at antrofundic junction, with extensive lesser curvature intestinal metaplasia spreading to antral and fundic mucosa, more extensive than NUP, inflammation reverses with management of HP but extensive intestinal metaplasia is irreversible	Caused by HP; associated with non-NSAID gastric ulcer and increased risk for intestinal type gastric cancer; eradication of HP cures gastric ulcer, reverses inflammatory gastritis; unknown whether it can prevent cancer
Nonulcer pangastritis	Slowly progressive multifocal pangastritis with less intestinal metaplasia than PIP The type of HP gastritis present in >90% of patients with HP	Caused by HP; no ulcer, usually asymptomatic Not known whether this gastritis ever progresses to MIP

(continued)

TABLE 87-2.   *(Continued)*

DIAGNOSIS	HISTOLOGICAL FEATURES	CLINICAL FEATURES
Diffuse corporal atrophic gastritis	Lymphocytic inflammation and destruction of the oxyntic glands progressing to partial or complete loss of parietal and chief cells and possible replacement by diffuse intestinal or pyloric gland metaplasia Pyloric glands of the antrum are unaffected	Probably autoimmune and genetic with parietal cell destruction leading to loss of secretion of HCl and intrinsic factor with resultant pernicious anemia and achlorhydria
Hemorrhagic-erosive gastropathy	Erosions, superficial hemorrhage; edema and little or no inflammation There may be superficial necrosis and pseudomembranes suggestive of ischemia Regenerative epithelial changes may be seen	Multiple causes: NSAIDs, alcohol, stress, gastric hypoperfusion, iatrogenic injury
Reactive gastropathy	No interfoveolar inflammation or HP foveolar hyperplasia adjacent to an NSAID gastric ulcer or erosion	Aspirin and other NSAIDs are most common cause in United States
	Postgastrectomy stoma may show active regenerative changes in the foveolar epithelium and cystic glands extending into the submucosa	Reactive stomatitis after gastrectomy must not be confused with dysplasia or carcinoma
Vascular ectasia	Red spots or stripes containing dilated mucosal capillaries Arteriovenous anastomoses in submucosa	Can be idiopathic but is seen more often in cirrhosis and renal failure; can bleed substantially
Infection (opportunistic)	CMV, HSV, *Candida* infection, TB, syphilis, etc.	Most common in AIDS and other immunosuppressed states
Hypertrophy	Ménétrier disease: few or no parietal and chief cells, foveolar hyperplasia	Protein-losing enteropathy, viscid mucus secretion
	Gastrinoma: many parietal and chief cells	Elevated blood gastrin and excess watery gastric acid secretion
	Severe duodenal ulcer diathesis: "hypertrophic hypersecretory gastropathy"; many parietal and chief cells	Normal blood gastrin, excess acid secretion
Postgastrectomy	Stomach: normal oxyntic glands or HP-NUP–type fundal gastritis, little or no intestinal metaplasia	Not a carcinoma precursor in United States
	Stoma: foveolar hyperplasia with epithelial regenerative and cystic changes	May have HP gastritis
Granulomatous gastritis	Crohn's disease: gastric and duodenal epithelioid granulomas, isolated giant cells suggest diagnosis; rare, cause of duodenal flat lesion, more actively inflamed than celiac sprue, may be focally normal	Most common granulomatous gastritis; isolated gastric disease rare, usually proven ultimately to be generalized disease with the passage of time and repeated biopsy
	Sarcoidosis	Pulmonary or other systems involved
	Tuberculosis	Multiple large granulomas with necrotic centers and acid-fast bacilli
	Isolated granulomatous gastritis	Most rare, isolated to stomach, age older than 40 years

AIDS, acquired immunodeficiency syndrome; CMV, cytomegalovirus infection; HP, *Helicobacter pylori* infection; HSV, herpes simplex virus infection; MIP, multifocal intestinalized pangastritis; NSAIDs, nonsteroidal antiinflammatory drugs; NUP, nonulcer pangastritis; TB, tuberculosis.

TABLE 87-3
Discrete Gastric Lesions

TYPE OF POLYP	HISTOLOGICAL FEATURES	CLINICAL FEATURES
Hyperplastic	Few, if any, parietal and chief cells, foveolar hyperplasia, irregular cystic glands, inflamed edematous stroma, and frequent erosions	Endoscopically multiple mesa-like sessile lesions; superficial erosions on the crests of folds; may contain dysplastic areas or carcinoma rarely
Fundic	Sessile, small, multiple polyps in the body of the stomach, cysts often lined by mucous, parietal or chief cells	Seen in familial polyposis coli and with increasing frequency sporadically; not premalignant
Adenomatous	Usually solitary, >2 cm, antral	Rare; premalignant or already malignant; often associated with dysplasia and cancer elsewhere in stomach
Juvenile polyposis	Cystic glands, smooth surface	Cancer rare in isolated juvenile polyps, but adenomas and cancer may be seen in generalized juvenile polyposis
Peutz-Jeghers syndrome	Excess arborized smooth muscle, disorganized glands	Pigmented buccal and lip spots, small-intestinal polyps, increased frequency of cancer in the stomach, colon, and especially in nongastrointestinal sites
Cronkhite-Canada syndrome	Cystic glands, edematous lamina propria	Age >60 y, diarrhea, protein loss, skin changes; not premalignant
Inflammatory fibroid	Benign spindle cell tumor with inflammation and infiltration with eosinophils	May obstruct gastric outlet (prior misnomer was eosinophilic granuloma)
Other rare tumors		

TABLE 87-4
Diffuse Proximal Lesions of the Small Bowel

DIAGNOSTIC CLASSIFICATION	DISEASE	CLINICAL FEATURES
Nondiagnostic flat lesion	Celiac sprue	Responds to gluten-free diet
	Refractory sprue	Untreatable
Histologically diagnostic flat lesion	Collagenous sprue	Untreatable, often fatal
	Hypogammaglobulinemic sprue	Treat giardiasis; villi and absorption return, immunodeficiency irreversible
Nondiagnostic, variably abnormal villi	Stasis syndrome	Antibiotics help
	Geographic variation	Histologic improvement after prolonged residency in a developed country
	Tropical sprue	Folate and antibiotics curative
	Zollinger-Ellison syndrome	Proton pump inhibitors effective
	Graft versus host disease	May respond to cyclosporine, tacrolimus, and steroids
Histologically diagnostic, variably abnormal villi	Whipple's disease	Responds to antibiotics; macrophages are acid-fast negative
	Mycobacterium avium complex	Opportunistic infection in AIDS; macrophages have acid-fast bacilli in them
	Duodenal Crohn's disease	Can be confused with celiac or refractory sprue, but epithelioid granulomas or giant cells make the diagnosis
	Eosinophilic gastroenteritis	Focal small intestine abnormality necessitating many biopsies; clumps of eosinophils; blood eosinophils increased; intermittent nonspecific digestive symptoms
	Lymphangiectasia	Congenital or acquired
	Primary intestinal lymphoma	Confined to intestine and its lymph nodes; disease in socioeconomically depressed areas
	Common variable immunodeficiency	Treat giardiasis; villi return, malabsorption improves
	Rare conditions	

AIDS, acquired immunodeficiency syndrome.

TABLE 87-5
Types of Colitis

DIAGNOSIS	HISTOLOGICAL FEATURES	CLINICAL FEATURES
Early nonspecific colitis	Mild, nonspecific, active inflammation with preserved architecture, i.e., focal active inflammation, focal cryptitis	Differentiates obscure organic from functional diarrheas; true diagnosis emerges with the passage of time, i.e., some disappear, others become inflammatory bowel disease or collagenous colitis, etc.
Ulcerative colitis	Diffuse inflammation and crypt distortion, basal lymphoplasmacytosis, and distortion of crypt architecture Can have foreign body granulomas associated with crypt abscesses	Rectum almost always involved along with a variable length of contiguous colon
Crohn's colitis	Epithelioid granuloma or focal active inflammation	Disease usually segmental; rectal sparing frequent
ASLC	Crypt architecture intact	Mostly infectious
Opportunistic infections	CMV, MAC, *Cryptosporidium,* HSV, TB, histoplasmosis	Defects in humoral or cell-based immunity
Other infections	Amebiasis, schistosomiasis	Migrant, traveler
Antibiotic related	Pseudomembranes or only ASLC-like lesions	*Clostridium difficile* toxin–positive
Solitary rectal ulcer syndrome	Diffuse collagen, erosions, excess muscle bands, pleated hyperplastic crypts	Confused with Crohn's colitis or cancer; often caused by mucosal prolapse
Ischemic colitis	Superficial, hemorrhagic necrosis; can progress or reverse	Any cause of colonic hypoperfusion
Collagenous colitis	Subepithelial collagen band >10–15 μm thick	Idiopathic watery diarrhea
Other		
Diversion	Mild colitis	Reversed by restoring intestinal continuity
Radiation	Ischemia and vascular wall thickening	Unpredictable time of clinical onset after irradiation
Iatrogenic	Acute colitis, variable severity	Enema or laxative preparation for colonoscopy; contaminated wash fluids; chemotherapy

ASLC, acute self-limited colitis; CMV, cytomegalovirus; HSV, herpes simplex virus; MAC, *Mycobacterium avium* complex; TB, tuberculosis.

TABLE 87-6
Colonic Polyps

TYPE OF POLYP	HISTOLOGICAL FEATURES	CLINICAL FEATURES
Hyperplastic	Benign, hyperplastic epithelial layer with serrated lumens	No malignant potential
Adenoma		
Tubular	Branching neoplastic glands	Most common; least likely to contain cancer if small
Villous	Villi predominate	Uncommon; often sessile; most likely to contain cancer when large and sessile
Tubulovillous	Mixed tubular and villous	Common; if >2 cm diameter, more likely to contain cancer
Hamartoma		
Single juvenile	Pedunculated, cystic	Can self-amputate; can bleed; benign
Multiple juvenile	May have associated adenomas	Stomach and small intestine also may be involved; rare cancer in adenomas
Peutz-Jeghers	Ramified smooth muscle bundles	Labial and buccal melanotic spots; small intestine most involved; rare cancer in associated adenomas
Pseudopolyp	Residual inflamed island of mucosa	No malignant potential

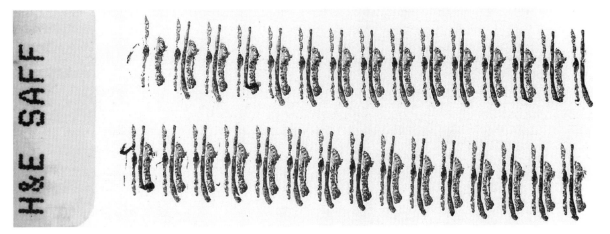

FIGURE 87-1. Single microscopic slide containing two ribbons of serial sections of three biopsy specimens with a total of 87 sections. Such serial sections make it easier to detect focal lesions, including small granulomas, cryptitis, and early carcinomatous invasion of the lamina propria.

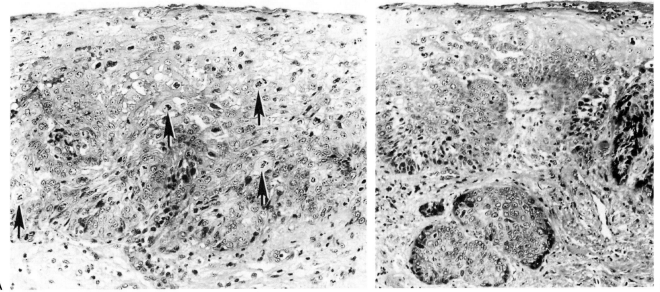

FIGURE 87-2. Esophageal squamous dysplasia and early carcinoma. **A:** Squamous dysplasia. The papillae of the lamina propria are irregular, and the mucosa has an increased number of epithelial cells per unit area. The nuclei of these epithelial cells are crowded, hyperchromatic, and overlap each other. The cells do not mature while they move toward the lumenal surface, and numerous mitotic figures are present at all levels of the mucosa (*arrows*). **B:** Esophageal biopsy specimen from another mucosal area of the same patient shows both esophageal squamous dysplasia and early invasion of the lamina propria. This section shows tongues of dysplastic squamous epithelium extending into the lamina propria, some of which have become detached to form discrete nests of early invasive carcinoma.

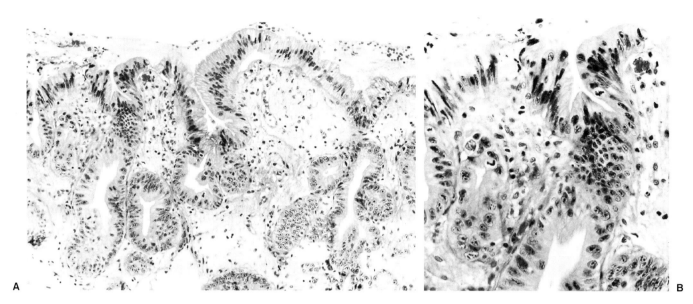

FIGURE 87-3. **A:** Barrett esophagus with high-grade dysplasia. The glandular architecture is distorted, as evidenced by the irregular contour of the glands and their lumens and by epithelial buds projecting from glands. The cells lining the glands have abnormal nuclei that are enlarged and hyperchromatic and have a focal loss of polarity. Epithelium with these nuclear abnormalities extends onto the mucosal surface. **B:** The cytologic abnormalities are seen at higher power. The image shows irregularly shaped nuclei with prominent nucleoli and crowding of abnormal cells on the mucosal surface.

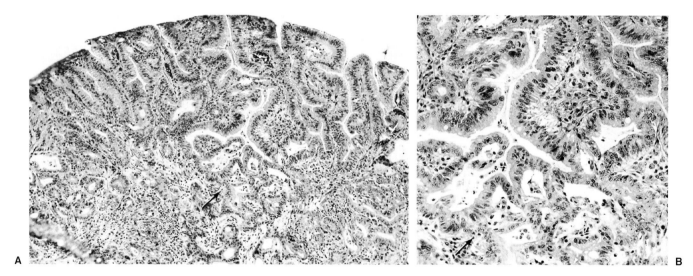

FIGURE 87-4. **A:** Gastric biopsy specimen shows high-grade dysplasia without invasion in its upper portion but with gross distortion of glandular architecture forming a complex network of gland-like spaces deeper in the biopsy specimen (*arrow*). **B:** The architectural distortion at higher magnification of the area marked with the *arrow* in **A.** The cytologic abnormalities of the nuclei lining the distorted glands are better depicted. This gross distortion of the architectural pattern suggests possible invasion of the lamina propria.

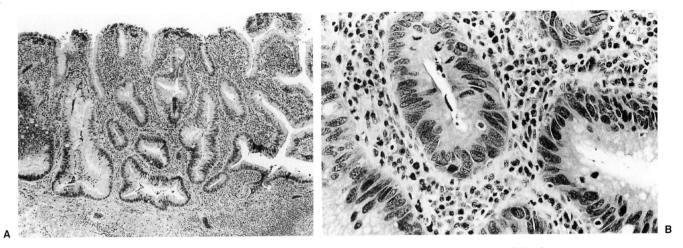

FIGURE 87-5. **A:** High-grade dysplasia complicating chronic ulcerative colitis. Image shows distorted glandular architecture, almost complete absence of goblet cell mucous, and marked crowding and stratification of nuclei. **B:** At higher power the cytologic abnormalities are readily visible. The nuclei are markedly enlarged compared with the size of the nuclei in the lamina propria, and they vary markedly in size and shape. Beginning loss of nuclear polarity also is visible.

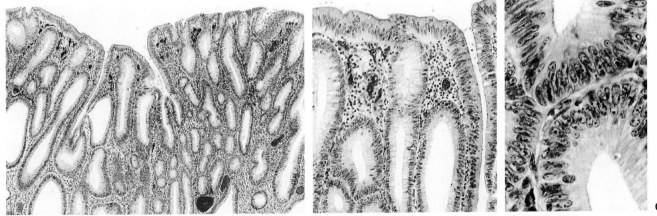

FIGURE 87-6. Colonic tubular adenoma. **A:** Characteristic tubular architecture. **B, C:** Cytologic features of the neoplastic cells lining the tubules. Nuclear enlargement, crowding, stratification, and focal diminution in mucous production are visible.

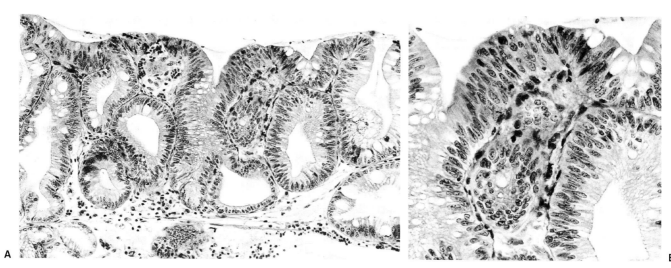

FIGURE 87-7.   Barrett esophagus with low-grade dysplasia. **A:** The dysplastic glands (**right of center**) are irregular in size and shape and have decreased mucous production. The characteristic goblet cells of the nonneoplastic, Barrett specialized metaplastic epithelial precursor to dysplasia are visible (**left** and **right**). **B:** Crowding, stratification, and enlargement of the dysplastic nuclei extend to the lumenal surface. The changes are less severe than those of high-grade dysplasia.

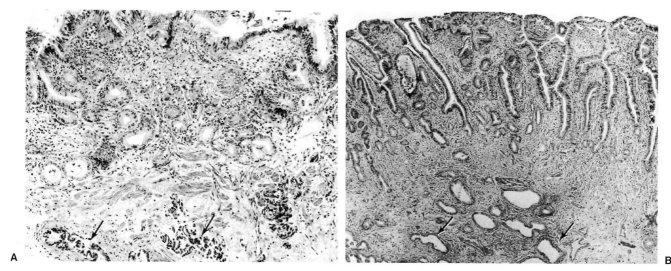

FIGURE 87-8.   Possible invasive cancer in a biopsy specimen from a patient with Barrett esophagus. The corresponding area in the surgical specimen shows definite submucosal invasion. **A:** The upper portion of the biopsy specimen above the muscularis mucosae shows only high-grade dysplasia, whereas in the lower portion of the specimen, slightly dilated, darkly stained glands (*arrows*) extend into a widened and splayed muscularis mucosae. Because of the limited depth of the specimen, invasion through the muscularis mucosae into the submucosa cannot be confirmed, but it was suspected. **B:** Surgical specimen from the same area shows dilated glands invading the submucosa (*arrows*).

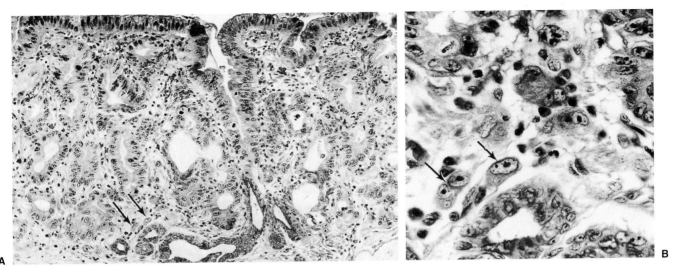

FIGURE 87-9. Low-power (**A**) and high-power (**B**) views of Barrett esophagus with high-grade dysplasia and intramucosal carcinoma. Marked distortion of the glandular architecture and prominent nuclear abnormalities are visible. Invasion of the lamina propria by individual glandular epithelial cells represents intramucosal carcinoma (*arrows*).

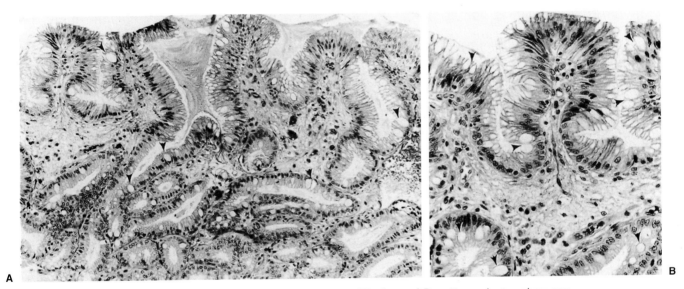

FIGURE 87-10. Low-power (**A**) and high-power (**B**) views of Barrett esophagus show specialized metaplastic epithelium with diagnostic goblet cells (*arrowheads*). The cells between the goblet cells resemble gastric surface cells at light microscopic examination. No evidence of dysplasia is visible.

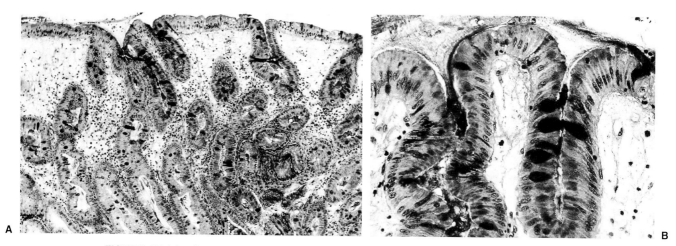

FIGURE 87-11. Low-power (**A**) and high-power (**B**) views of multifocal intestinalized pangastritis caused by *Helicobacter pylori* that has progressed to diffuse intestinal metaplasia. The biopsy specimen was obtained from the lesser curvature at the level of the angulus. No residual normal gastric glands are present; they have been replaced by glands with goblet cells containing mucin stained with Alcian blue at pH 2.5 (*black*). Between the goblet cells are cells that resemble gastric surface cells, some of which contain Alcian blue–positive acid mucous.

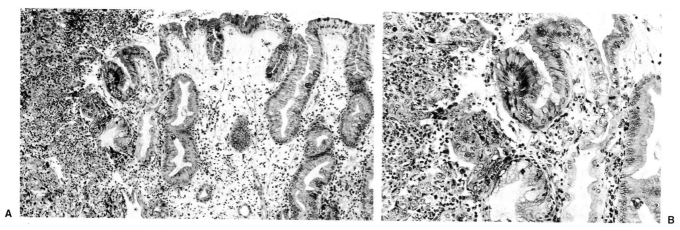

FIGURE 87-12. Low-power (**A**) and high-power (**B**) views of advanced *Helicobacter pylori*–caused multifocal intestinalized pangastritis with decreased glands, intestinal metaplasia, and associated adenocarcinoma. The normal gastric glands have been replaced with intestinal metaplasia, as evidenced by the goblet cells (**right**). Sheets of malignant-appearing cells infiltrate the lamina propria (**left**).

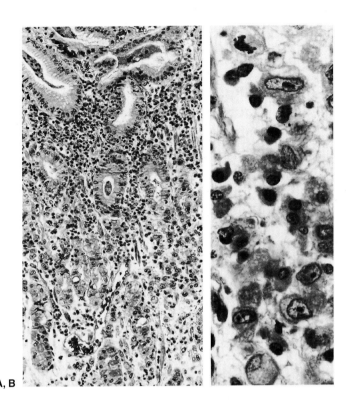

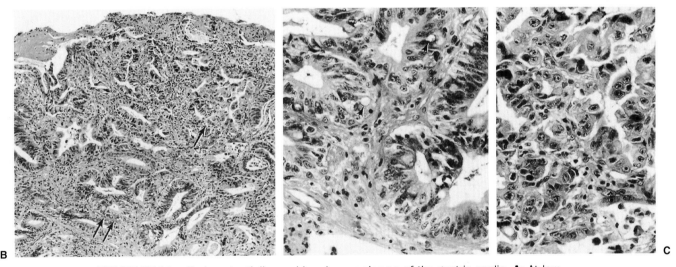

FIGURE 87-13. Gastric biopsy specimen of a minute lesion that was barely visible at endoscopy. **A:** Low-power magnification illustrates how subtle adenocarcinoma of the stomach can be. The inflamed lamina propria contains infiltrating malignant cells that are difficult to recognize because they are interspersed with inflammatory cells. **B:** The high-power view makes these infiltrating, malignant cells more apparent.

FIGURE 87-14. Early, potentially curable adenocarcinoma of the gastric cardia. **A:** At low-power magnification both high-grade dysplasia and a focus of intramucosal carcinoma (*single arrow*) are present. Residual goblet cells suggest the presence of Barrett specialized metaplastic epithelium (*double arrows*). **B:** The area previously marked with double arrows shows the enlarged goblet cells that define this dysplastic epithelium as originating from Barrett specialized metaplasia (*arrowheads*). **C:** In the area marked in **A** with a *single arrow*, malignant cells infiltrating the lamina propria are evident. This patient was alive and well 5 years after local surgical resection of this lesion. Lymph nodes were free of tumor, and the carcinoma did not extend beyond the mucosa.

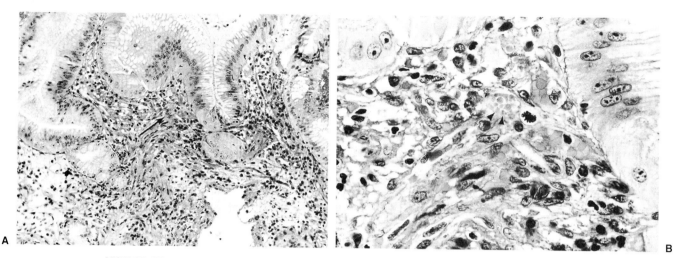

FIGURE 87-15. Gastric biopsy specimen from a patient with Kaposi sarcoma. **A:** The lamina propria contains infiltrating spindle cells of the sarcoma and a dilated vessel at the bottom. *Arrow* marks the area shown at higher power in **B.** Spindle cells comprise the lesion, and red blood cells are present in the slitlike spaces between individual spindle cells. Intracytoplasmic hyaline inclusions (*arrowheads*) are highly characteristic of Kaposi sarcoma. A mitotic figure is also depicted (**right** of *arrowheads*).

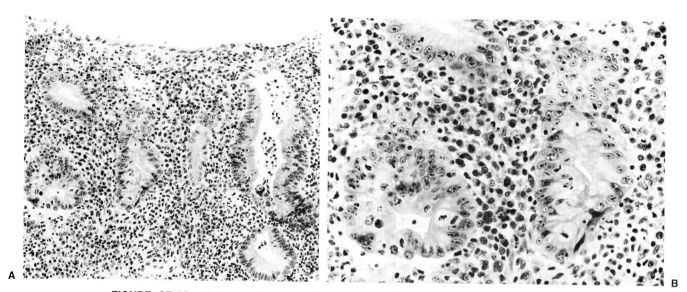

FIGURE 87-16. Colonic biopsy specimen from patient with active ulcerative colitis. **A:** Image shows polymorphonuclear leukocytes within the crypt epithelium, the crypt abscess, distortion of the crypt architecture, basal lymphoplasmacytosis, and marked chronic inflammatory infiltrate within the lamina propria. **B:** Reactive epithelial changes that can be confused with dysplasia. There are occasional polymorphonuclear leukocytes within the crypt epithelium with enlarged, crowded, stratified nuclei containing numerous mitotic figures.

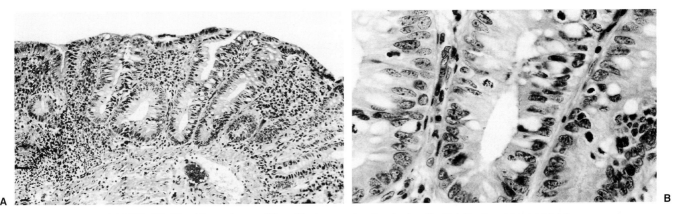

FIGURE 87-17. Ulcerative colitis with low-grade dysplasia. **A:** Relatively well-preserved crypt architecture and mild chronic inflammatory infiltrate within the lamina propria. There is no evidence of active inflammation. There are a decreased number of goblet cells, and nuclear crowding and stratification involve the crypts and extend to the surface epithelium. **B:** At high-power magnification of the crypts, the nuclear enlargement, hyperchromatism, crowding, and stratification are readily visible. Some dystrophic goblet cells do not communicate with the lumenal surface. Such goblet cells are characteristic but not diagnostic of dysplasia.

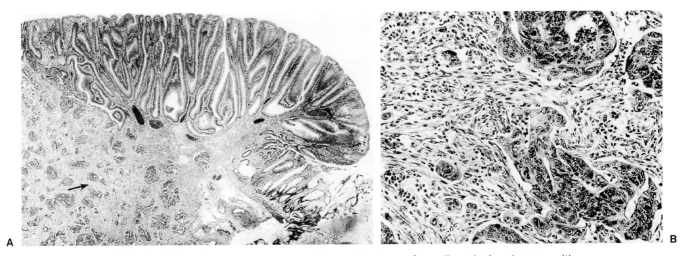

FIGURE 87-18. Electrocautery snare biopsy specimen of sessile colonic adenoma with invasive carcinoma. **A:** Normal mucosa distorted by electrocautery artifact (**lower right**). The upper portion of the tissue is composed of villous adenoma, and an invasive adenocarcinoma (**lower left**) infiltrates below the muscularis mucosae into the submucosa. **B:** High-power view (*arrow* in **A**) shows the prominent desmoplastic stromal reaction elicited by the invading carcinoma.

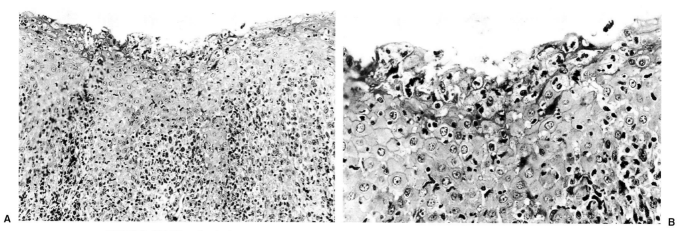

FIGURE 87-19. **A:** Active esophagitis in gastroesophageal reflux disease in which poly-morphonuclear neutrophils and lymphocytes infiltrate the surface of the squamous mucosa and the lamina propria to obscure the interface between the mucosa and the underlying lamina propria. **B:** View at higher magnification. Prominent epithelial hyperplasia is evi-denced by the enlarged, hyperchromatic, and more numerous nuclei.

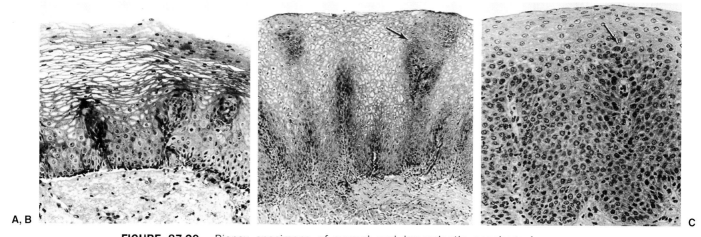

FIGURE 87-20. Biopsy specimens of normal and hyperplastic esophageal mucosa. **A:** Normal squamous mucosa of the esophagus. The papillae of the lamina propria extend through approximately 50% of the thickness of the mucosa, and the basal zone occupies a small portion of the mucosa. **B:** Hyperplasia of the mucosa is indicated by lengthening of the papillae of the lamina propria, some of which extend close to the lumenal surface (*arrow*). In addition, the basal zone is markedly hyperplastic and occupies more than 25% of the thickness of the mucosa. **C:** Profound degree of hyperplasia. The basal zone occu-pies two thirds of the thickness of the mucosa, and papillae of the lamina propria extend a similar distance through the mucosa (*arrow*).

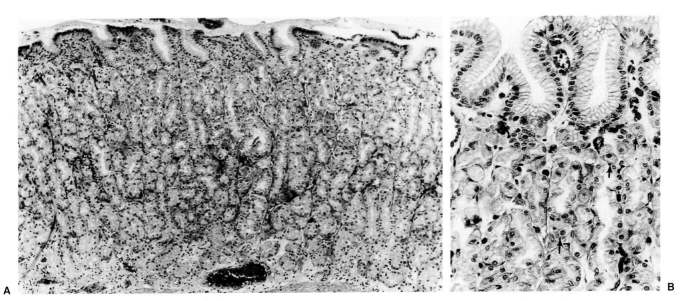

FIGURE 87-21. Biopsy specimen of a typical hiatal hernial pouch. **A:** The gastric oxyntic (fundic) glands are normal. The surface is covered by normal gastric surface mucous cells that dip into normal shallow foveolae. **B:** The lamina propria contains no recognizable inflammatory infiltrate, and numerous parietal cells are present in the normal oxyntic glands (*arrows*).

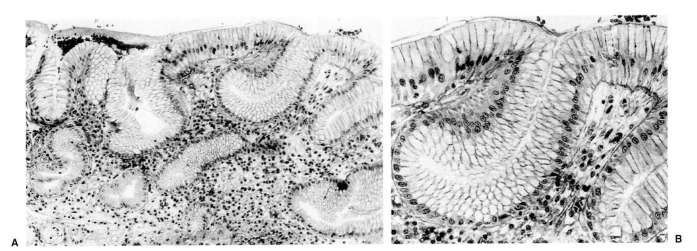

FIGURE 87-22. Normal gastric cardiac gland mucosa. **A:** The surface epithelium, foveolae, and glands are lined by cells that produce mucous. The lamina propria contains a mild increase in lymphocytes and plasma cells, a feature found in most normal biopsy specimens from this portion of the stomach. **B:** Epithelial mucous cells covering the surface and lining the foveolae at higher magnification. The lengthened columnar cells are characteristic but not diagnostic of cardiac glands.

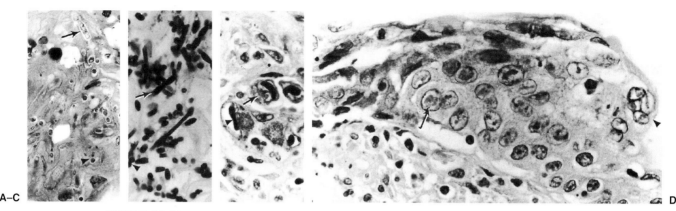

FIGURE 87-23. Esophageal biopsy specimens from various opportunistic infections. **A:** High-power image illustrates esophageal squamous mucosa in which there are budding yeast (*arrowhead*) and infiltrating pseudohyphae of *Candida* organisms (*arrow*) (H&E stain). **B:** Periodic acid-Schiff stain for carbohydrates highlights the budding yeast (*arrowhead*) and pseudohyphae of *Candida* organisms (*arrow*) more clearly than H&E stain. **C:** High-power photomicrograph of esophageal mucosa in which cytomegalovirus is present. A diagnostic inclusion body with a surrounding halo within the nucleus of an enlarged mesenchymal cell is shown (*arrowhead*). This cell and the one marked by the *arrow* also contain granular cytoplasmic inclusions. **D:** Characteristic findings of herpes simplex virus infection: ground glass nuclei, Cowdry type A inclusion body (*arrow*), and multinucleated giant cells (*arrowhead*).

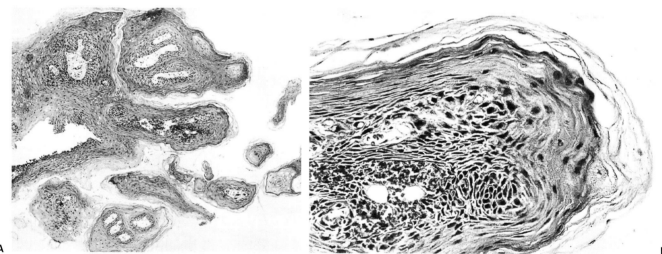

FIGURE 87-24. Esophageal biopsy specimen of squamous papilloma. **A:** Papillary (finger-like) projections are characteristic. **B:** Central fibrovascular cores of the papillae are covered by lamellated, benign, squamous epithelium.

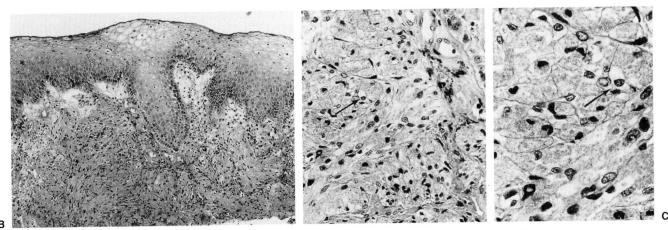

FIGURE 87-25. Biopsy specimen of a granular cell tumor of the esophagus. **A:** Lamina propria contains sheets of polygonal cells with granular cytoplasm, as evident in progressive magnifications (**B** and **C**).

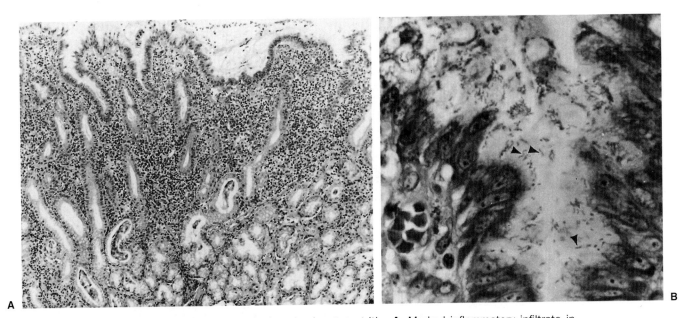

FIGURE 87-26. Diffuse antral-predominant gastritis. **A:** Marked inflammatory infiltrate in the lamina propria between the foveolae in the upper portion of the mucosa is associated with an apparent, but not real, reduction in the number of pyloric glands. Ample numbers of pyloric glands are present in the uninflamed basal portion of the mucosa. Although they cannot be recognized at this magnification, neutrophils infiltrate the glandular epithelium. **B:** At higher power, mucous in the lumen adjacent to the surface and foveolar epithelium discloses numerous *Helicobacter pylori* bacilli (*arrowheads*). Bacteria are present only in the mucous layer adjacent to gastric surface mucous cells.

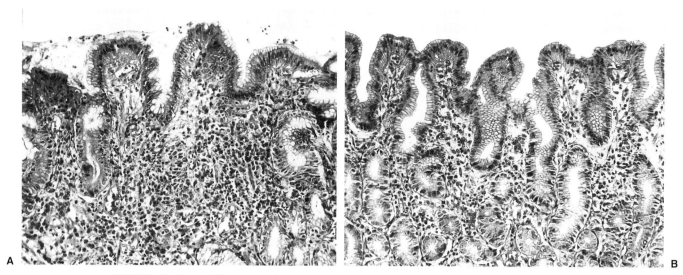

FIGURE 87-27. Diffuse antral-predominant gastritis associated with duodenal ulcer before (**A**) and 8 months after (**B**) successful eradication of *Helicobacter pylori*. **A:** Prominent interfoveolar inflammation with the pyloric glands pushed basally. **B:** Marked reduction in the number of mononuclear cells in the interfoveolar lamina propria. The pyloric glands of the antrum have resumed their normal position, and the antral mucosa has returned to a normal appearance.

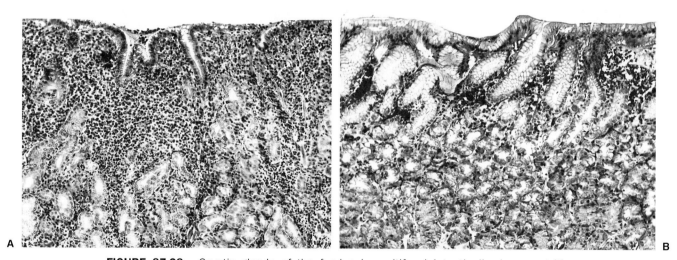

FIGURE 87-28. Oxyntic glands of the fundus in multifocal intestinalized pangastritis before (**A**) and after (**B**) eradication of *Helicobacter pylori*. **A:** Inflammatory infiltrate in the upper half of the mucosa pushes the parietal and chief cells of the oxyntic glands basally. **B:** Complete restitution of normal oxyntic glands after eradication of *H pylori*. Other focal areas of intestinal metaplasia lost the inflammation but did not reverse the metaplasia after eradication of *H pylori*.

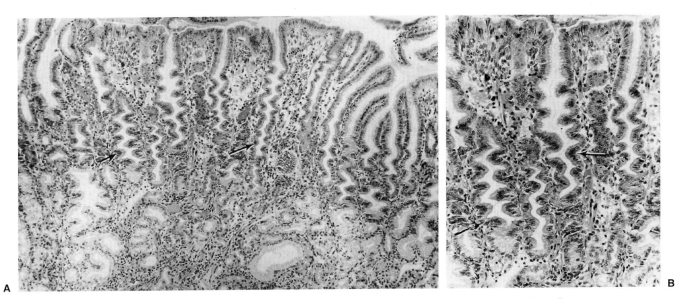

FIGURE 87-29. Reactive gastropathy associated with ingestion of nonsteroidal antiinflammatory drugs. **A:** Foveolar hyperplasia evidenced by the corkscrew or pleated configuration of the elongated gastric foveolae (*arrows*). The lack of gastritis is indicated by the paucity of inflammatory cells within the interfoveolar lamina propria. **B:** Foveolar hyperplasia with lengthened corkscrew configuration at higher magnification (*arrow*). Image shows nuclear crowding and decreased quantity of mucous in the foveolar epithelium. *Helicobacter pylori* was not present.

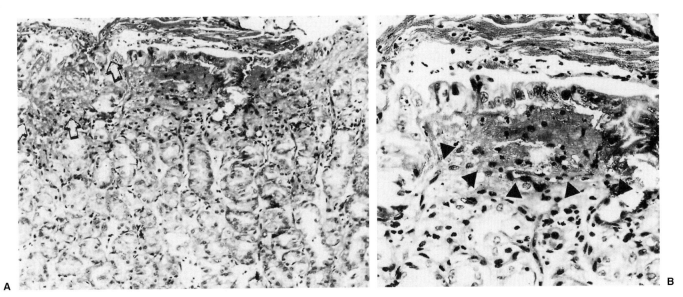

FIGURE 87-30. Gastric fundic mucosa in hemorrhagic (erosive) gastropathy. **A:** Focus of erosion (*open arrows*) of the surface epithelium with fibrinopurulent exudate adherent to the mucosal surface. There is no inflammation within the gastric mucosa proper. **B:** Adjacent to the erosion is a focus of subepithelial hemorrhage (*arrowheads*) at higher magnification.

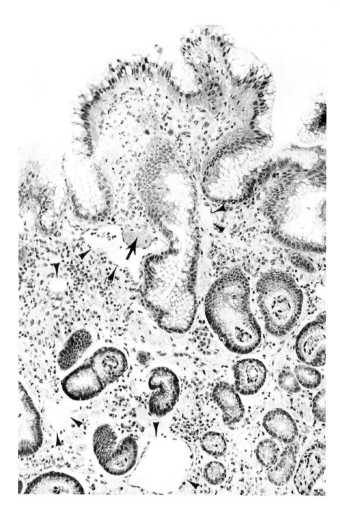

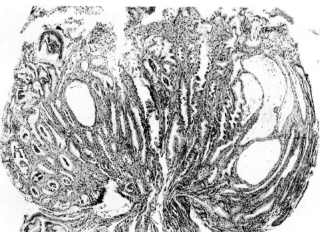

FIGURE 87-31.   Gastric antral vascular ectasia. Dilated capillaries are present in the lamina propria (*arrowheads*). In one of these is a small fibrin thrombus attached to the capillary wall (*arrow*).

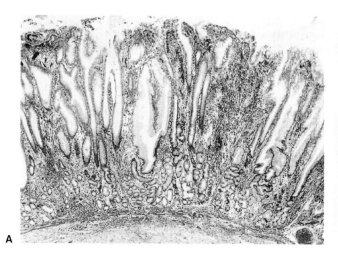

A

B

FIGURE 87-32.   Ménétrier disease. **A:** Section of the gastric body obtained from a resected stomach. The gastric pits or foveolae are strikingly elongated and irregular in configuration. This appearance is produced by profound hyperplasia of the foveolar cells that extend into the glands and replace the parietal and chief cells so that the body mucosa is now composed exclusively of mucous-producing foveolar cells. **B:** Endoscopic biopsy specimen from a patient with Ménétrier disease. In addition to the marked foveolar hyperplasia that produces a corkscrew appearance of the pits, there are dilated glands, another feature common in Ménétrier disease.

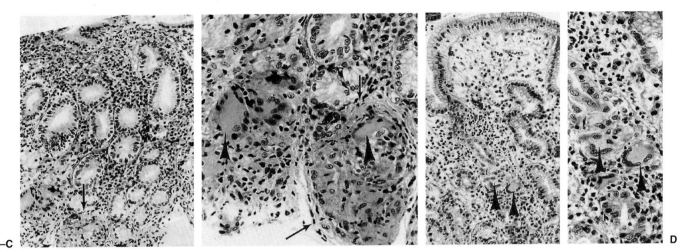

FIGURE 87-33. Granulomatous gastritis in a patient with Crohn's disease. **A:** Discrete epithelioid granuloma (*arrow*). **B:** Granuloma (*arrows*) at higher magnification. This granuloma is composed of a compact aggregate of epithelioid histiocytes with a multinucleated giant cell (*arrowhead*). In the stomach, such granulomas usually prove to be associated with Crohn's disease. Isolated multinucleated giant cells are present just to the left of the discrete granuloma (*arrowhead*). **C, D:** Multinucleated giant cells (*arrowheads*) associated with a few epithelioid histiocytes but no discrete granuloma. Giant cells like these in the stomach and duodenum are strongly suggestive of Crohn's disease, unlike giant cells in the colon.

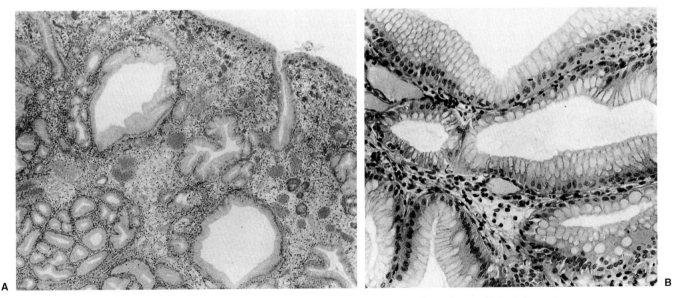

FIGURE 87-34. Hyperplastic gastric polyp. **A:** Low-power view shows dilated, irregular-shaped gastric glands lined with hyperplastic foveolar cells. Image shows inflamed, edematous stroma in which there are numerous dilated capillaries. **B:** Higher magnification shows the hyperplastic foveolar cells lining the glands that comprise the polyp.

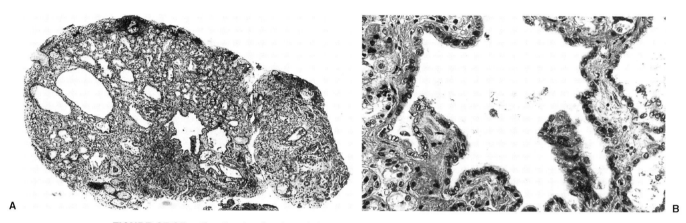

FIGURE 87-35. Fundic gland polyp of the stomach. **A:** Endoscopic biopsy specimen from a small polyp shows dilated, irregular fundic glands. **B:** The nature of the cells lining the cystic glands can be recognized. The cells include parietal cells and chief cells. Although not visible in this particular field, foveolar cells also may be present.

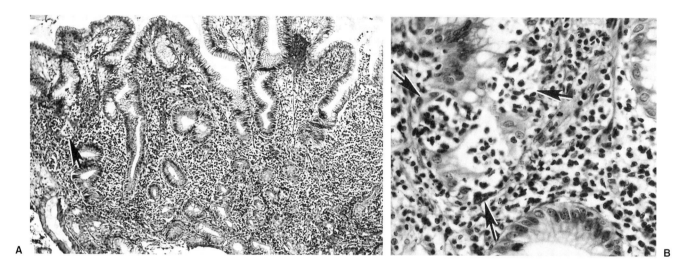

FIGURE 87-36. Gastric mucosa-associated lymphoid tissue (MALT) lymphoma. **A:** Low-power appearance can be confused with that of *Helicobacter pylori* diffuse antral-predominant gastritis, but there is a lymphoid infiltrate, a reduction in the number of glands, and lymphoepithelial lesions (*arrow*). **B:** High-power view of lymphoepithelial lesion shows small, cleaved lymphocytes infiltrating and destroying the epithelium (*arrows*).

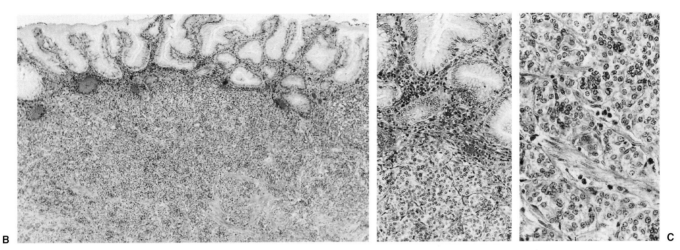

FIGURE 87-37. Gastric carcinoid. **A:** Small nests, glands, and sheets of neoplastic cells have replaced most of the mucosa and invade into the muscularis mucosae and submucosa. **B:** Higher magnification reveals nests of carcinoid cells in the lamina propria beneath the gastric pits. **C:** Highest magnification shows small, round, uniform nuclei with a finely stippled chromatin pattern characteristic of carcinoid.

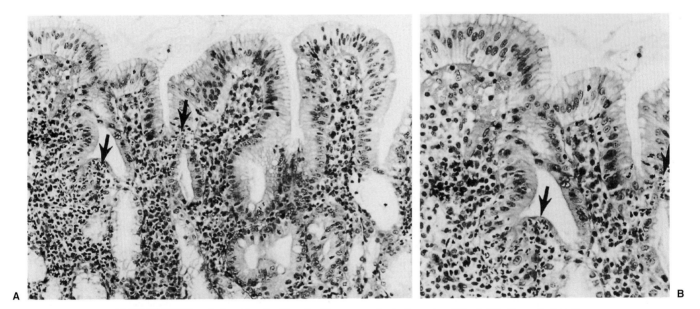

FIGURE 87-38. Active duodenitis. **A:** There are foci of neutrophilic infiltration of glands (*arrows*). Gastric surface cell metaplasia involves most of the surface cells of this biopsy specimen. Two glands (**right of center**) contain goblet cells and are normal intestinal glands, whereas the remainder of the glands are lined completely with cells that contain clear mucous and represent gastric surface cells. Brunner glands that have extended into the lamina propria are visible below; such findings also are seen in normal biopsy specimens of the duodenal bulb. **B:** Higher magnification shows gastric surface cells more clearly and glands infiltrated by neutrophils, indicating active inflammation (*arrows*).

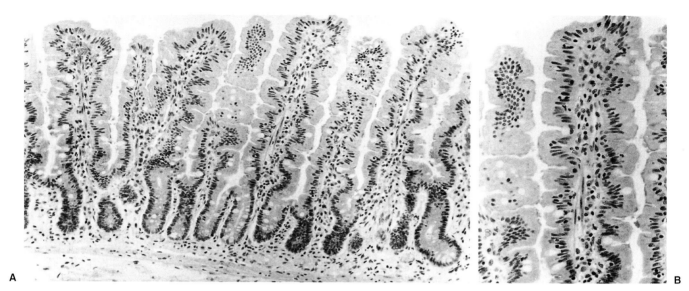

FIGURE 87-39. Biopsy specimen of normal distal duodenum. **A:** The tall, slender villi are about three times as tall as the crypts are deep. Epithelial cells covering the villi consist predominantly of absorptive cells with scattered goblet cells. The nuclei of the surface epithelial cells are lined up in a uniform, picket fence–like arrangement. The lamina propria contains small numbers of lymphocytes, and plasma cells are normally seen. **B:** Normal surface epithelium and lamina propria at higher magnification. The slender, fusiform cells in the lamina propria represent smooth muscle cells normally found in the cores of small bowel villi.

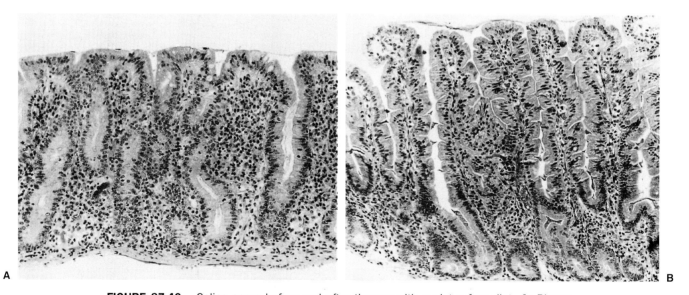

FIGURE 87-40. Celiac sprue before and after therapy with a gluten-free diet. **A:** Biopsy specimen shows flat mucosal surface. The villi are effaced, and the crypts have become elongated. The lamina propria contains a prominent infiltrate of chronic inflammatory cells, and lymphocytes infiltrate the surface epithelium. **B:** Appearance of the mucosa of patient depicted in **A** after an absolutely gluten-free period of 3 weeks, during which total parenteral nutrition was administered. The villi have returned to a normal appearance, and the inflammatory infiltrate within the lamina propria and surface epithelium has receded.

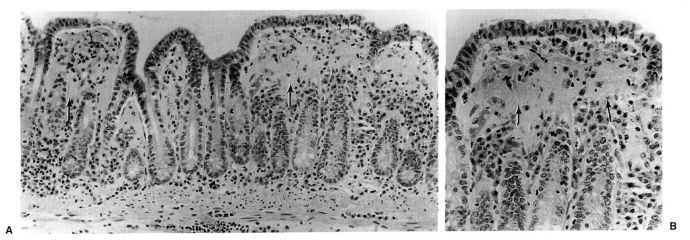

FIGURE 87-41. Collagenous sprue. **A:** The mucosal surface is flat, the villi are absent, and the crypts are elongated. An abnormally thick layer of collagen lies beneath the surface epithelium (*arrows*). Lymphocytes and plasma cells infiltrate the lamina propria, collagen, and surface epithelium. **B:** Markedly thickened subepithelial collagen table (*arrows*) is visible at higher power. Surface epithelium is abnormal.

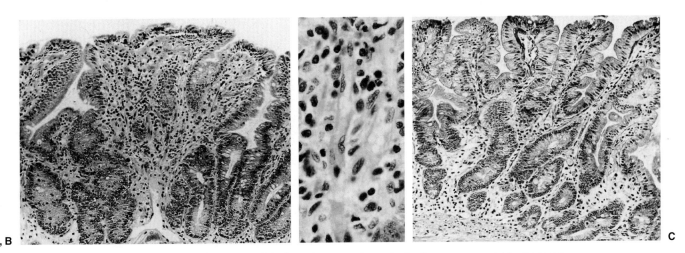

FIGURE 87-42. Hypogammaglobulinemic sprue (a variant of common variable immunodeficiency) before and after eradication of *Giardia lamblia*. **A:** Biopsy sample of the small intestine has a flat mucosal surface with marked elongation of the crypts and an inflammatory infiltrate within the lamina propria. At this magnification, it is indistinguishable from the flat biopsy specimens shown in Fig. 87-40A from a patient with celiac sprue. **B:** At higher magnification, inspection of the inflammatory infiltrate in the lamina propria reveals mostly lymphocytes with no plasma cells, a finding indicative of hypogammaglobulinemic sprue. *Giardia* organisms were identified in a Giemsa-stained smear made from the mucous adherent to the biopsy specimen. **C:** After therapy for giardiasis, the mucosal villi began to return, and malabsorption disappeared. Virtual absence of plasma cells from the lamina propria was not reversed by means of eradication of *G lamblia*.

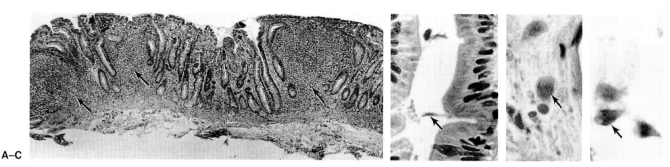

A–C   D

FIGURE 87-43. Typical appearance of a mixed lesion in a biopsy specimen of the small intestine in common variable immunodeficiency. **A:** The biopsy specimen shows mild lymphoid hyperplasia (*arrows*) and an abnormality of the villous architecture. **B:** Longitudinal sections of *Giardia lamblia* are visible (*arrow*). **C:** Pear-shaped organisms that have been sectioned en face in the paraffin-embedded biopsy specimen (*arrow*). Intracytoplasmic detail is unclear. **D:** Giardiasis is detected most easily in Giemsa-stained smears of mucus adherent to the biopsy. A characteristic pear-shaped organism in which two nuclei are barely visible is shown (*arrow*).

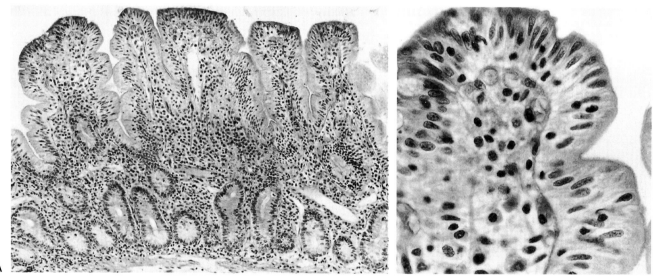

A   B

FIGURE 87-44. Geographic variation in morphologic features of the small bowel. **A:** Biopsy specimen from a symptom-free inhabitant of a developing country shows villi with mild, nonspecific abnormality in architecture. **B:** Higher magnification shows slightly blunted, shortened villi and prominent infiltrate of lymphocytes and plasma cells in the lamina propria and the surface epithelium.

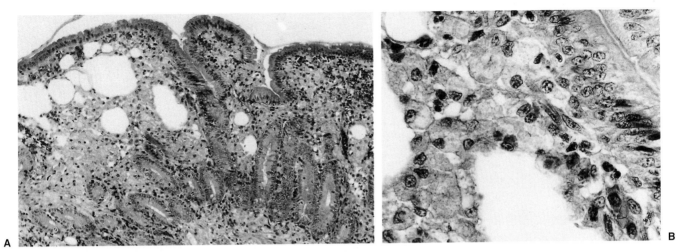

FIGURE 87-45. Whipple disease. **A:** Loss of villi and heavy infiltration of the lamina propria by macrophages with abundant cytoplasm. The clear spaces represent dilated blocked lacteal vessels filled with lipid. The surface epithelium remains essentially normal. **B:** Higher magnification shows foamy macrophages. Electron microscopy shows the abundant pale cytoplasm of these macrophages, which contains bacilli and breakdown products of bacterial cell membranes within lysosomes. Surface epithelium is completely normal (**upper right**).

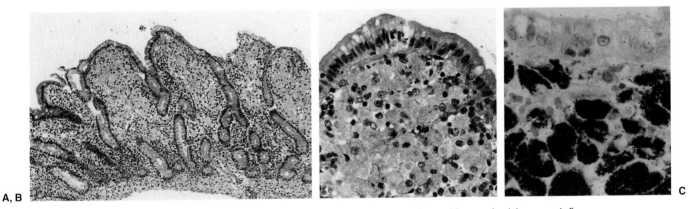

FIGURE 87-46. Small bowel biopsy specimen from a patient with acquired immunodeficiency syndrome and *Mycobacterium avium* complex infection. **A:** Shortened, broad villi and the lamina propria packed full of macrophages. **B:** Higher magnification shows macrophages within the lamina propria. With H&E stain, this appearance is almost indistinguishable from that of Whipple disease except for absence of lacteals. **C:** Ziehl-Neelsen stain shows the acid-fast nature of the bacilli within the macrophages and in the lamina propria.

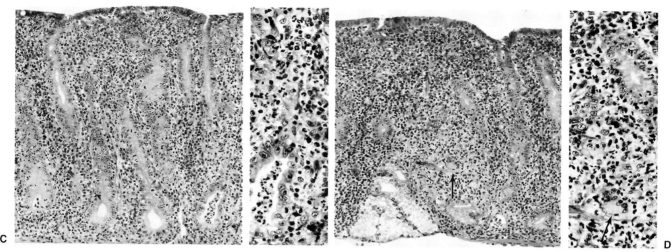

A–C

D

FIGURE 87-47. Duodenal biopsy specimen from a patient with Crohn's disease. **A:** Flat mucosal surface and markedly elongated crypts. **B:** The intense inflammatory infiltrate includes numerous neutrophils that have produced a crypt abscess, shown here at higher magnification. **C:** Another biopsy specimen from the same patient shows a focus of granulomatous inflammation. A multinucleated giant cell is surrounded by macrophages and neutrophils (*arrow*). **D:** Higher-power magnification of the giant cell shown in **C** (*arrow*).

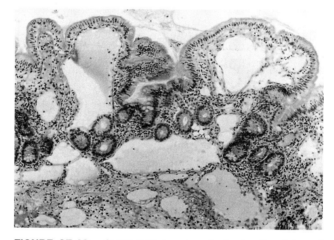

FIGURE 87-48. Congenital lymphangiectasia. Small bowel biopsy specimen shows villous architecture distorted by dilated lymphatic channels that extend through the muscularis mucosae into the submucosa (**bottom of photograph**). Apart from the dilated lymphatic vessels and distorted architecture, the mucosa is normal.

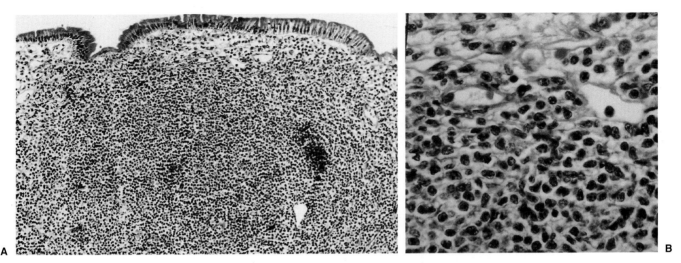

FIGURE 87-49. Primary small intestine lymphoma (immunoproliferative small intestine disease). **A:** The absence of crypts is noteworthy and probably reflects destruction of the glandular architecture by the diffuse infiltrate of small lymphocytes. **B:** Higher magnification shows the monotonous, atypical appearance of the lymphoid infiltrate.

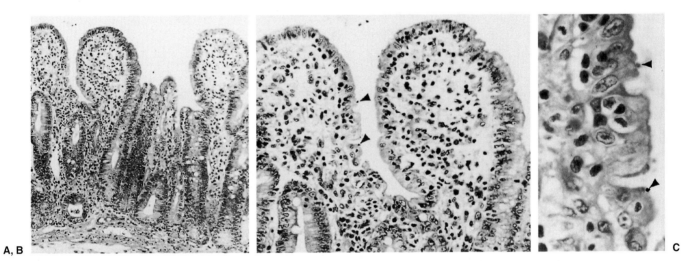

FIGURE 87-50. Cryptosporidiosis in an immunosuppressed person. **A:** Low-power view illustrates shortened, blunted villi, elongated crypts, and an inflammatory process in the mucosa. **B:** Infiltration of the lamina propria and surface epithelium by lymphocytes. *Cryptosporidium* organisms are barely visible at this magnification (*arrowheads*). **C:** The organisms are best visible at high-power magnification. They appear as small, round, gray dots adherent to the apical surface of the absorptive cells. *Cryptosporidium* organisms also may produce disease among persons with normal immune systems, but the process is acute and self-limited rather than chronic, as it may be in acquired immunodeficiency syndrome.

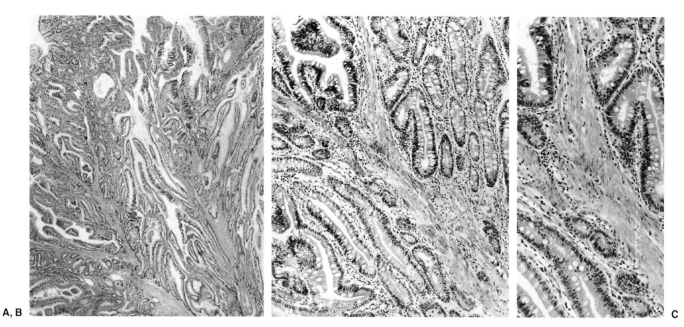

FIGURE 87-51. Small-bowel hamartomatous polyp from a patient with Peutz-Jeghers syndrome. **A:** Low-power view shows the complex, branched configuration of the hamartoma. **B, C:** Abnormal arrangement of normal tissue elements. Normal-appearing epithelium lines tubules and covers villi. A thick band of smooth muscle divides the field diagonally. **C:** Smooth muscle band and normal-appearing epithelium at higher magnification.

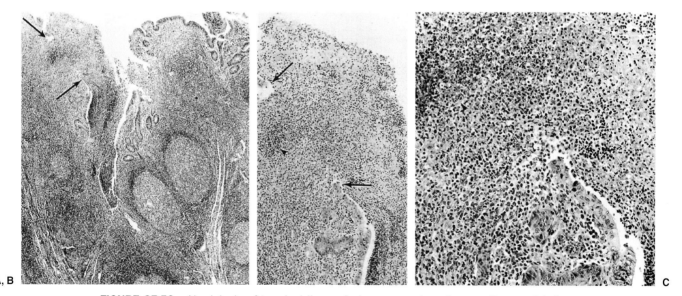

FIGURE 87-52. Yersiniosis of terminal ileum. **A:** Low-power view shows a Peyer patch in which there is erosion of the surface epithelium with adherent exudate (*arrows*). **B:** Erosion at higher power. Margins of the eroded surface epithelium are shown (*arrows*). Inflammatory exudate extends into the underlying lymphoid tissue, in which there is a focus of necrosis (*arrowhead*). **C:** Higher-power view of focal necrosis.

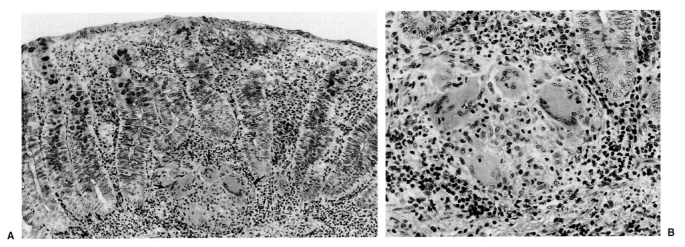

FIGURE 87-53. Crohn's disease of the colon. **A:** Biopsy specimen contains a discrete epithelioid granuloma (*arrows*) composed of multinucleated giant cells and epithelioid histiocytes. **B:** View at higher power. Although inflammation surrounds the granuloma and involves some of the lamina propria, the mucosa at the left side of **A** is essentially normal, showing that Crohn's colitis is commonly focal in distribution.

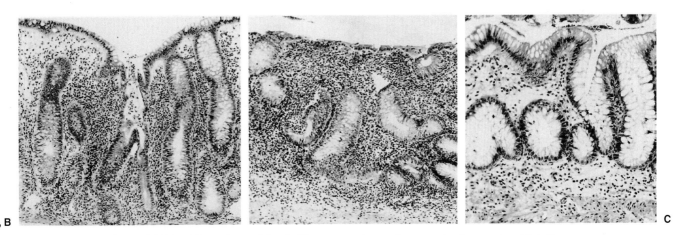

FIGURE 87-54. Ulcerative colitis. **A:** Biopsy specimen shows early disease in which the inflammatory infiltrate varies in intensity and distortion of the crypt architecture has not yet become diffuse. Crypt in the center of the biopsy sample is branched and contains neutrophils infiltrating the epithelium and lumen. **B:** Biopsy specimen from a patient with fully developed disease with diffuse inflammation, distortion of the crypt architecture, and basal lymphoplasmacytosis. **C:** Atrophic mucosa from a patient with inactive ulcerative colitis; there is distortion of the crypt architecture but no inflammation.

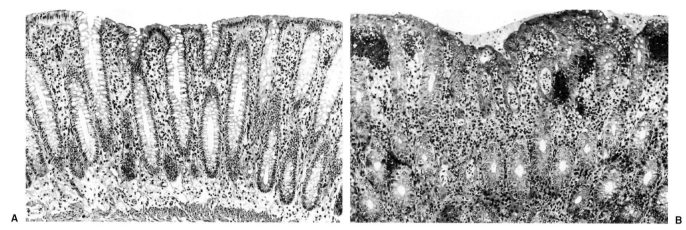

FIGURE 87-55. Acute self-limited colitis in a patient with salmonellosis. **A:** Normal mucosa. **B:** Histological appearance of the mucosa in acute self-limited colitis. In acute self-limited colitis, there is no distortion of crypt architecture, and this differentiates it from idiopathic inflammatory bowel disease. The crypts remain straight, evenly spaced tubules, but there is a mixed inflammatory infiltrate in the lamina propria in which neutrophils predominate over round cells. Accumulation of neutrophils within the crypt lumen to form crypt abscesses is evident, but this is a nonspecific finding seen in all kinds of colitis, as is the absence of mucous secretion in the actively inflamed mucosa.

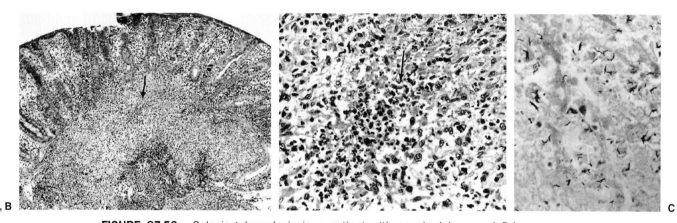

FIGURE 87-56. Colonic tuberculosis in a patient with acquired immunodeficiency syndrome. **A:** Biopsy specimen shows inflammation of the colonic mucosa with multiple, large, confluent granulomas. A focus of necrosis within a granuloma is indicated (*arrow*). **B:** View at higher power. Necrosis within granulomas (*arrow*) always suggests an infectious agent. **C:** Ziehl-Neelsen stain in which acid-fast bacilli of *Mycobacterium tuberculosis* are evident. The tissue response to *Mycobacterium avium* complex differs in that granuloma and diffuse granulomatous inflammation with discrete aggregates of epithelioid histiocytes are not visible; rather, there is diffuse infiltration of macrophages with foamy cytoplasm filled with acid-fast bacilli (see Fig. 87-46).

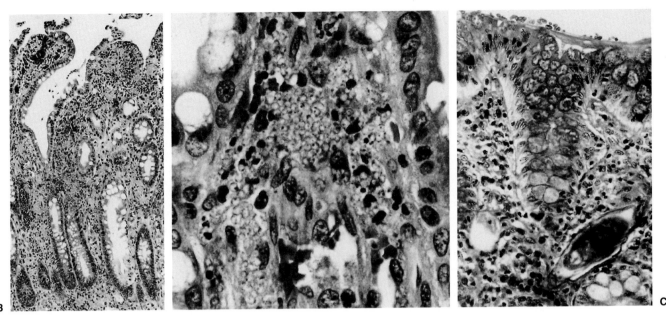

FIGURE 87-57. **A, B:** Colonic histoplasmosis in a patient with disseminated histoplasmosis and acquired immunodeficiency syndrome. **A:** Distorted glandular architecture and an inflammatory infiltrate in the lamina propria. **B:** View at higher power of inflamed lamina propria shows a foamy or bubbly appearance caused by numerous *Histoplasma* organisms within the cytoplasm of macrophages. The organisms are visible as clear vacuoles, many of which contain a dark central dot representing the nucleus. **C:** Biopsy specimen from a patient with schistosomiasis. The ovum is clearly visible in the lamina propria and can be confirmed to be a schistosome, but identification of species is not possible except in the rare circumstance in which the plane of the section passes through a lateral spine of *Schistosoma mansoni.*

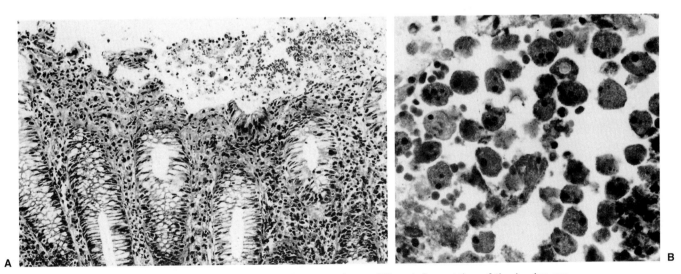

FIGURE 87-58. Amebic colitis. **A:** Mucosa shows diffuse inflammation of the lamina propria and an eroded surface. The material adherent to the surface includes erythrocytes and numerous amebic organisms. **B:** High-power view. The organisms are large cells, measuring approximately 30 μm in diameter. They have a relatively small nucleus compared with the cytoplasmic volume. Phagocytized red blood cells are visible as black, round structures within several of the amebae.

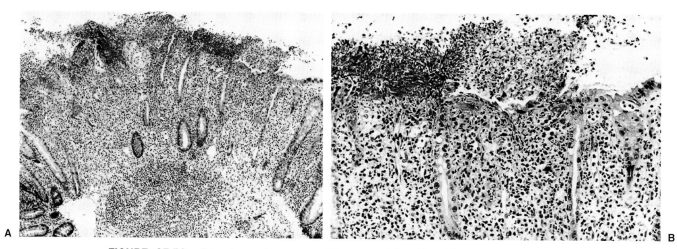

FIGURE 87-59. Pseudomembranous colitis caused by *Clostridium difficile* infection. **A:** Biopsy specimen shows features of acute self-limited colitis with active inflammation of the lamina propria, erosion of the surface epithelium, and adherent fibrinopurulent exudate (pseudomembrane) but preservation of the crypt architecture. Most of the inflammatory cells are neutrophils. **B:** High-power magnification shows erosion of the surface epithelium, the pseudomembrane, and the predominantly neutrophilic infiltration. The features also are seen with ischemic colitis.

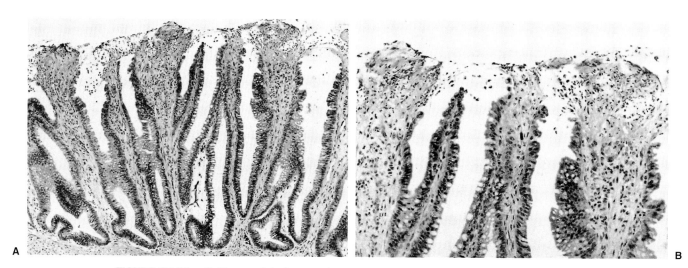

FIGURE 87-60. Solitary rectal ulcer syndrome. **A:** Biopsy specimen shows erosion of the surface epithelium, obliteration of the lamina propria by fibrosis, granulation tissue, and smooth muscle, and gross distortion of the glandular architecture. Hyperplasia of the glandular epithelium is visible. **B:** View at higher power shows eroded surface epithelium and obliteration of the lamina propria by collagenous granulation tissue and fibroblasts. Epithelial hyperplasia is present that occasionally results in misinterpretation of these lesions as adenoma or even cancer.

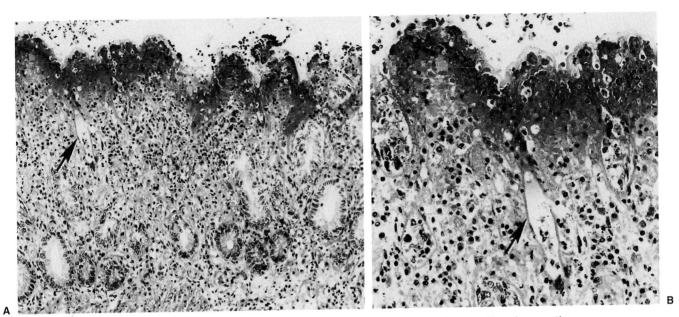

FIGURE 87-61. Ischemic colitis. **A:** Upper part of the mucosa is necrotic, whereas the deeper portion is viable. The dark band along the surface of the mucosa represents hemorrhage. Crypt basement membrane (*arrow*) is devoid of epithelial cells because they have become necrotic and have sloughed (crypt ghost). The inflammatory infiltrate is relatively mild. **B:** View at higher power shows eroded surface epithelium, superficial hemorrhage, and crypt ghosts (*arrow*).

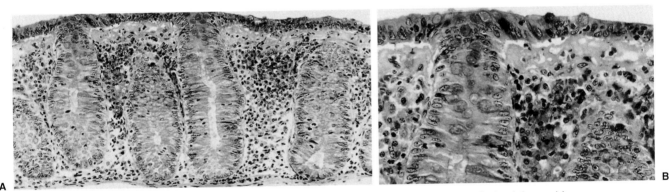

FIGURE 87-62. Collagenous colitis. **A:** Biopsy specimen shows normal glandular architecture, a possible increase in the number of plasma cells in the upper portion of the lamina propria, and a markedly thickened subepithelial collagen plate. The surface epithelium is abnormal and infiltrated by lymphocytes. **B:** View at higher power shows lacy or reticulated appearance of the thickened subepithelial collagen table.

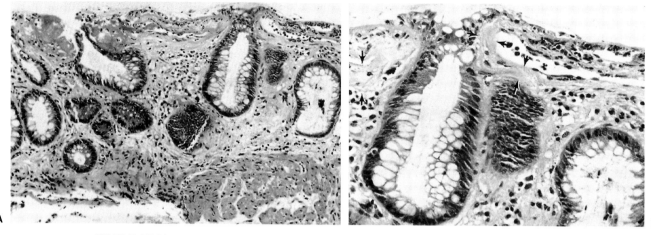

FIGURE 87-63. Colitis after therapeutic radiation. **A:** After radiation the chronic changes in the mucosa are atrophic and may resemble those of inactive ulcerative colitis. **B:** Fibrosis of the lamina propria and hyalinization of vascular walls (*arrows*) are shown. These ectatic vessels with hyalinized walls help differentiate radiation colitis from inactive ulcerative colitis. The surface epithelium in this biopsy sample is eroded; this may be an artifact because it is not a consistent finding in radiation colitis. Acute radiation changes, not shown, may be indistinguishable from ischemia.

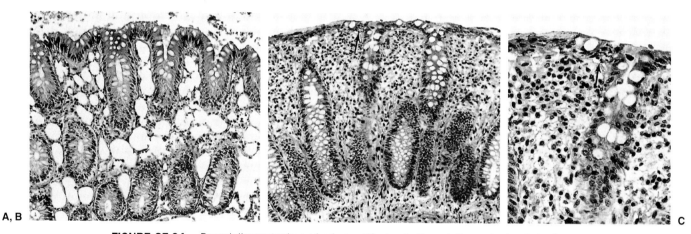

FIGURE 87-64. Pseudolipomatosis and other artifacts. **A:** Pseudolipomatosis of the lamina propria after unintentional exposure to hydrogen peroxide left after cleaning of the wash channel of a colonoscope. The bubbles in the lamina propria represent gas bubbles caused by the release of nascent oxygen when hydrogen peroxide contacted the mucosa. These bubbles can be differentiated from fat cells because they lack a cell membrane and vary markedly in size. **B:** Mucosa of a patient who received a bisacodyl enema. The surface epithelium is flattened and contains focal infiltrates of neutrophils (*arrow*). **C:** Focal neutrophilic infiltration of the abnormal surface epithelium at higher power (*arrow*).

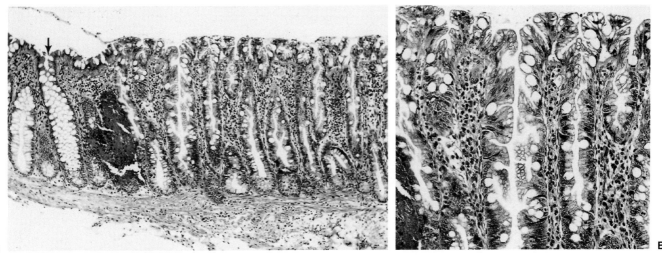

FIGURE 87-65. Hyperplastic colonic polyp. **A:** Section through the junction of normal mucosa and the hyperplastic polyp (*arrow*). The lumens of the normal crypts are straight, whereas crypt lumens within a hyperplastic polyp have a serrated or stellate profile. **B:** View at higher power shows that this serrated appearance is caused by crowding of excess numbers of normal, nonneoplastic epithelial cells, causing them to form tufts that project into the lumen.

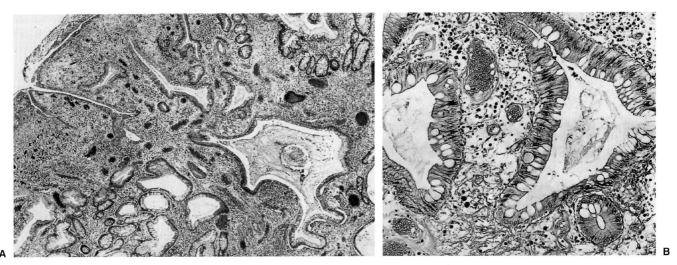

FIGURE 87-66. Juvenile polyp. **A:** Lesion composed of dilated, irregular-shaped glands (**B**) lined by epithelium of an essentially normal appearance. The lamina propria is inflamed and edematous and contains numerous congested vessels.

Acknowledgment

We appreciate the artistic printing of our photomicrographic illustrations by our senior histology technician, Rosmarie Mayes.

LIVER BIOPSY AND HISTOPATHOLOGICAL DIAGNOSIS

SUGANTHA GOVINDARAJAN

Evaluation of liver biopsy requires that the pathologist recognize the architecture and identify the pathological changes, and correlate the changes with clinical and laboratory data. Although some histological diagnosis can be made without the help of the clinical or laboratory data, most meaningful information is obtained with a proper clinical-pathological correlation.

Special stains such as Masson trichrome demonstrate fibrosis or cirrhosis of the liver, an indication of a chronic process. Other routine stains include stains for iron, reticulin, and diastase-resistant periodic acid-Schiff–positive material. Granulomas of the liver require special stains for the etiologic agent such as acid-fast organisms and fungi. Shikata or orcein stain identify hepatitis B surface antigen as well as copper-binding protein, metallothionein. Immunoperoxidase stains detect viral and nonviral protein in the biopsy material using specific antibodies directed against the proteins.

Routine hematoxylin and eosin stain sections are the most valuable tools in the diagnosis. Well-embedded (3 μm) sections with good hematoxylin and eosin stain will provide great cellular details of hepatocytes such as inclusions in the cytoplasm or the nuclei as well as features such as fat, cholestasis, or dysplasia.

Initial assessment of the architecture is followed by a closer review of the portal tract or the fibrous septa if cirrhosis is present. Elements to be examined are the bile ducts, epithelial abnormalities or their absence or proliferation, cellular types of the inflammatory infiltrates, and the infiltrates' involvement of the bile ducts, the parenchymal limiting plate, or the vessels (vasculitis). The portal tracts or the fibrous septa should also be examined under polarized light for foreign material in the macrophages, which is usually seen in patients with a history of intravenous drug addiction.

The parenchyma is examined for cord sinusoidal pattern; normal one cell thickness is altered in hepatocellular carcinoma to three to four or more cells that thicken the trabeculae. Parenchymal cytoplasmic inclusions such as Mallory bodies, mega-mitochondria, α_1-antitrypsin, or ground-glass cytoplasmic appearance are identified under higher magnifications in the review process. Irregular or regular bulging of the parenchymal lobule indicates regeneration that appears as a precursor to regenerative nodules. Areas of hepatocytolysis often appear as focal punched-out or spotty necrosis with an accumulation of Kupffer cells and lymphocytes or as large areas of collapsed reticulin with loss of hepatocytes.

Hepatocytolysis is often localized in the perivenular zones. Individual cell necrosis is seen as acidophil bodies or apoptotic cells.

Attention should also be paid to the sinusoidal lining cells, Ito cells, and the space of Disse. In alcoholic liver disease, there is collagen deposition of the sinusoidal space, which stands out on Masson trichrome stain. Amyloid is also seen in this space, either as reticular or globular type, and is demonstrated by Congo red stain.

In addition to the histological diagnosis to confirm the clinical diagnosis, the liver biopsy has become a very important prognostic tool to assess the responses to treatment of chronic viral hepatitis B and C. The histological activity index (HAI) is measured using several standardized methods on pretreatment and 1- to 2-year follow-up biopsies. This quantitative measurement of necroinflammation and fibrosis either by Knodell or Ishak score (Table 88-1) has been applied to many long-term therapeutic protocols. Standardization of the scoring has been helpful in studies that compare different treatment modalities. Its application for individual cases also helps the clinician with patient follow-up and monitoring of other serologic viral markers.

Liver biopsies are also extremely valuable in post–liver transplant settings. Standard protocols of liver biopsies help confirm the clinical diagnoses from rejection to opportunistic infections. Post–liver transplantation management of patients is largely dependent on the liver biopsy interpretations in conjunction with the other laboratory studies.

With proper indications and carefully chosen technique, a needle biopsy of the liver is an invaluable tool. Most often, the biopsy provides the final diagnosis when the pathology interpretation is made using the combined expertise of the pathologist and the hepatologist.

TABLE 88-1
Histology Activity Index (HAI): Ishak Score

MODIFIED HAI GRADING NECROINFLAMMATORY SCORES	SCORE
A. Periportal piecemeal necrosis	
Absent	0
Mild (focal, few portal areas)	1
Mild/moderate (focal, most portal areas)	2
Moderate (continuous around <50% of tracts or septa)	3
Severe (continuous around >50% of tracts or septa)	4
B. Confluent necrosis	
Absent	0
Focal confluent necrosis	1
Zone 3 necrosis in some areas	2
Zone 3 necrosis in most areas	3
Zone 3 necrosis + occasional portal-central (P-C) bridging	4
Zone 3 necrosis + multiple P-C bridging	5
Panacinar or multiacinar necrosis	6
C. Focal necrosis and focal inflammation	
Absent	0
One focus or less per 10× objective	1
Two to four foci per 10× objective	2
Five to ten foci per 10× objective	3
More than ten foci per 10× objective	4
D. Portal inflammation	
None	0
Mild, some or all portal areas	1
Moderate, some or all portal areas	2
Moderate/marked, all portal areas	3
Marked, all portal areas	4

MODIFIED STAGING: FIBROSIS AND CIRRHOSIS

CHANGE	SCORE
No fibrosis	0
Fibrous expansion of some portal areas	1
Fibrous expansion of most portal areas	2
Fibrous expansion with occasional portal to portal (P-P) bridging	3
Fibrous expansion with marked bridging	4
Marked bridging with occasional nodules, incomplete cirrhosis	5
Cirrhosis, probable or definite	6

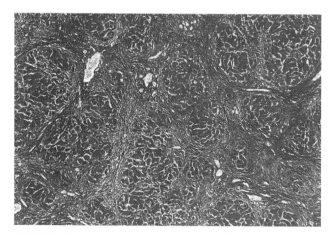

FIGURE 88-1. Cirrhosis of liver with fibrous septa and regenerative nodules (Masson stain, ×40).

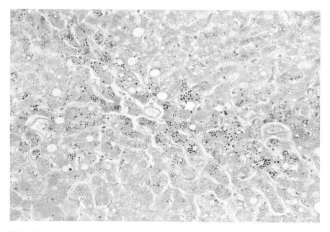

FIGURE 88-2. α_1-Antitrypsin globules in the periportal hepatocytes: diastase-resistant periodic acid-Schiff (PAS) positive (Diastase-PAS stain; original magnification ×200).

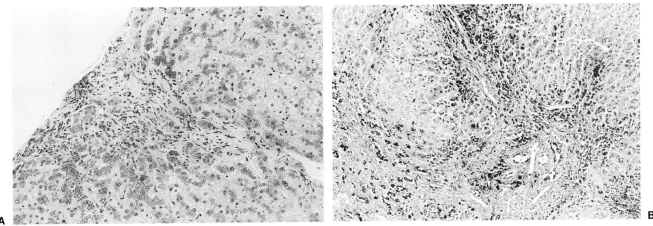

FIGURE 88-3. **A, B:** Perls iron stain demonstrating bright blue granules in hepatocytes and duct epithelial cells in hemochromatosis (original magnification ×100).

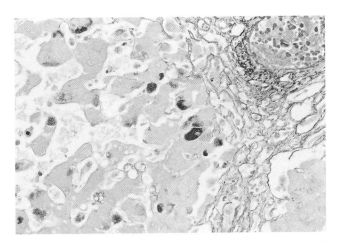

FIGURE 88-4. Shikata stain demonstrating the presence of hepatitis B surface antigen in the hepatocytes in chronic hepatitis B virus (Shikata stain; original magnification ×400).

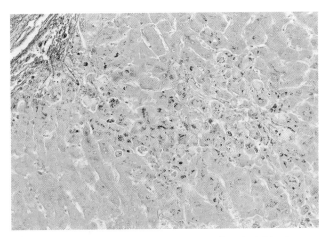

FIGURE 88-5. Shikata stain demonstrating dark black granules of copper binding protein in periseptal hepatocytes in Wilson disease (original magnification ×200).

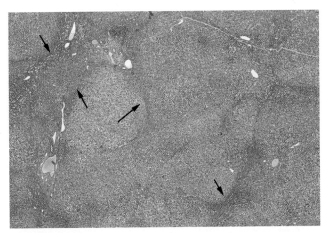

FIGURE 88-6. Nodular regenerative hyperplasia demonstrating regeneration of parenchyma (*arrows*) compressing the surrounding parenchyma without fibrous septa formation (H&E stain; original magnification ×40).

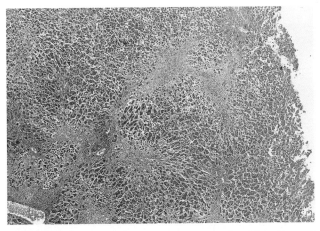

FIGURE 88-7. Submassive hepatic necrosis with collapsed perivenular reticulum network (H&E stain; original magnification ×40).

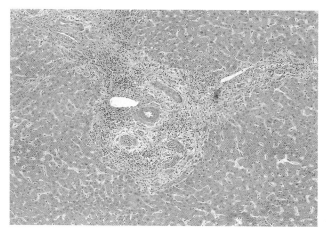

FIGURE 88-8. Portal area with prominent neutrophils in close proximity to the dilated interlobular bile duct in acute cholangitis (H&E stain; original magnification ×100).

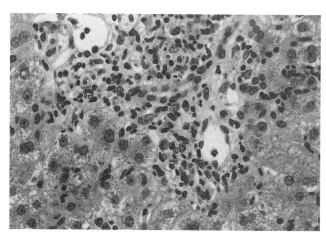

FIGURE 88-9. Portal area with prominent eosinophils among the inflammatory infiltrates in a case of phenytoin (Dilantin)-induced hepatotoxicity (H&E stain; original magnification ×200).

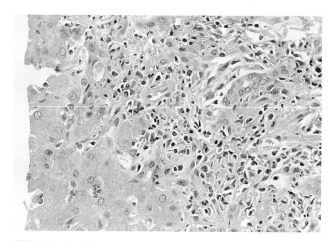

FIGURE 88-10. Portal area with increased number of eosinophils in a case of early rejection of orthotopic liver transplantation (H&E stain; original magnification ×200).

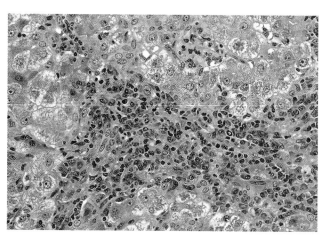

FIGURE 88-11. Prominent plasma cells among the infiltrates in portal tract of autoimmune chronic hepatitis (H&E stain; original magnification ×400).

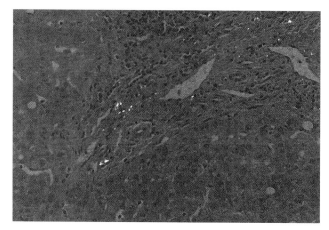

FIGURE 88-12. A portal area under polarizing light to demonstrate polarizable crystals in an intravenous drug abuser (H&E stain; original magnification ×200).

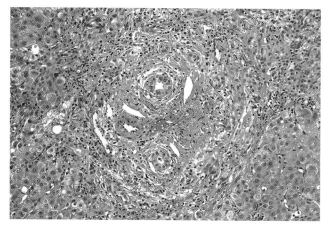

FIGURE 88-13. Lamellar periductal fibrosis in chronic bile duct obstruction (H&E stain; original magnification ×100).

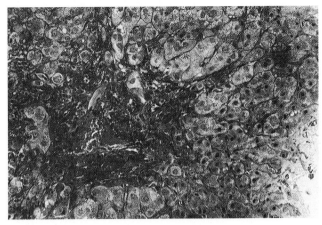

FIGURE 88-14. Arachnoid portal fibrosis with periportal extension of collagen in chronic alcoholic liver disease (H&E stain; original magnification ×100).

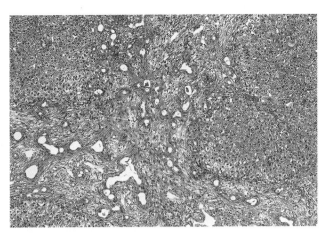

FIGURE 88-15. Portal area with marked cholangiolar proliferation in mechanical duct obstruction (H&E stain; original magnification ×100).

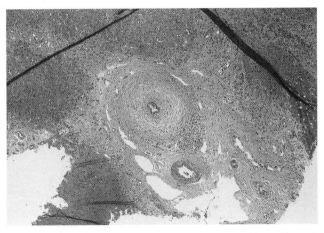

FIGURE 88-16. Primary sclerosing cholangitis with evidence of periductal fibrosis and chronic inflammatory infiltrate (H&E stain; original magnification ×100).

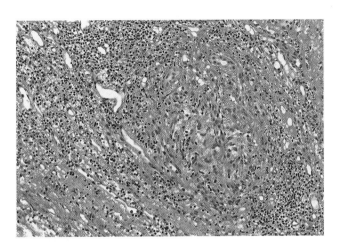

FIGURE 88-17. Primary biliary cirrhosis with granuloma (×200).

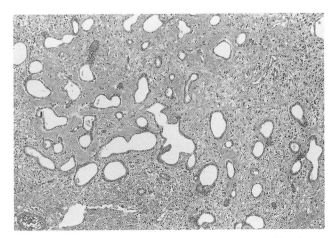

FIGURE 88-18. A few dilated duct structures with abnormal epithelium surrounded by loose collagen representing Meyenburg complex (H&E stain; original magnification ×100).

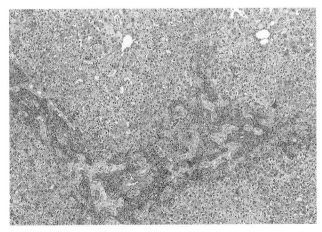

FIGURE 88-19. Biliary fibrosis and ductular proliferation in a 3-month-old child with extrahepatic biliary atresia (H&E stain; original magnification ×100).

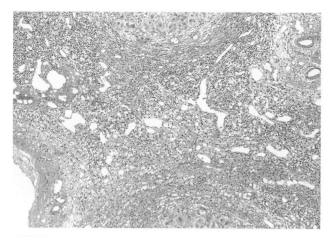

FIGURE 88-20. Increased number of thin-walled vascular structures representing portal venous radicles reflective of portal hypertension (H&E stain; original magnification ×100).

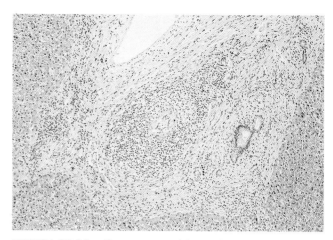

FIGURE 88-21. Severe necrotizing inflammatory reaction around hepatic arteriole in polyarteritis nodosa (H&E stain; original magnification ×100).

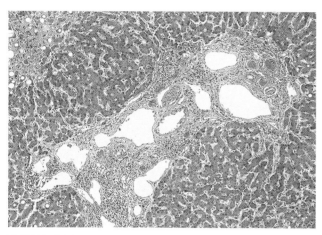

FIGURE 88-22. Increased number of abnormal vascular structures in a portal tract in Osler-Weber-Rendu syndrome (H&E stain; original magnification ×100).

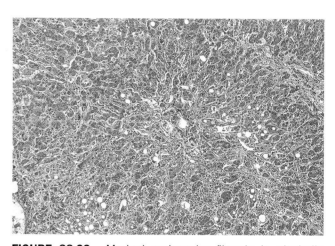

FIGURE 88-23. Marked perivenular fibrosis in alcoholic liver disease (H&E stain; original magnification ×100).

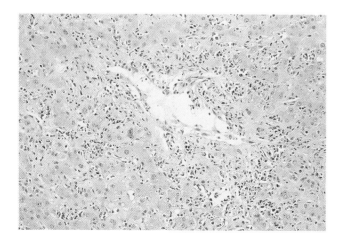

FIGURE 88-24. Endothelialitis showing inflammatory changes of a terminal hepatic venule in acute rejection of orthotopic liver transplantation (H&E stain; original magnification ×200).

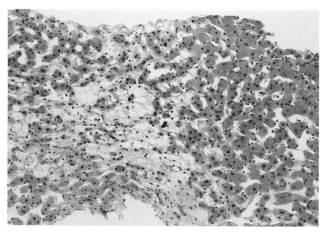

FIGURE 88-25. Budd-Chiari syndrome with perivenular sinusoidal dilation and atrophic hepatic cords (H&E stain; original magnification ×200).

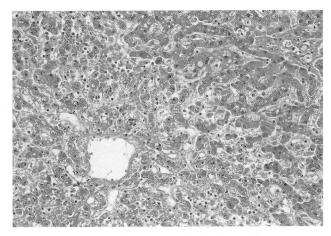

FIGURE 88-26. Confluent necrosis in the perivenular zone caused by anoxia (H&E stain; original magnification ×200).

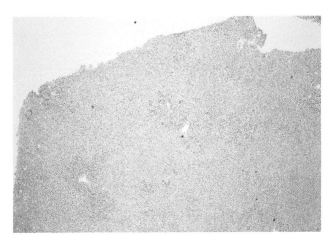

FIGURE 88-27. Massive hepatic necrosis involving the entire parenchyma with islands of portal tracts remaining (H&E stain; original magnification ×40).

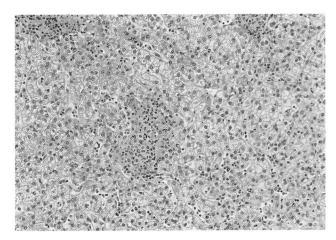

FIGURE 88-28. Punched-out granulomatous necrosis of the parenchyma in mononucleosis caused by Epstein-Barr virus (H&E stain; original magnification ×200).

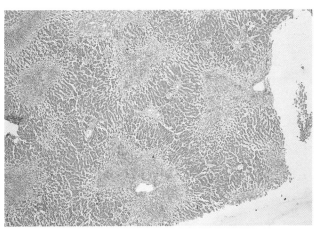

FIGURE 88-29. Acetaminophen toxicity resulting in perivenular coagulative necrosis without hepatocyte swelling (H&E stain; original magnification ×100).

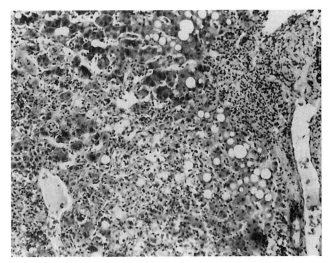

FIGURE 88-30. Halothane-induced perivenular and midzonal coagulative necrosis (H&E stain; original magnification ×100).

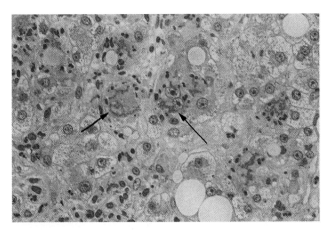

FIGURE 88-31. Perivenular hepatocytes containing Mallory hyaline (*arrows*) with neutrophilic reaction around them (H&E stain; original magnification ×200).

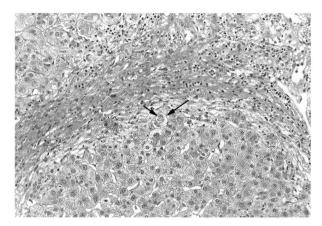

FIGURE 88-32. A periportal hepatocyte containing Mallory hyaline (*arrows*) in primary biliary cirrhosis (H&E stain; original magnification ×200).

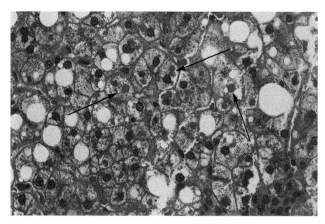

FIGURE 88-33. Hepatocytes containing spherical megamitochondria (*arrows*) in alcoholic liver disease (H&E stain; original magnification ×200).

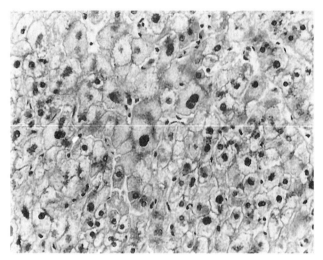

FIGURE 88-34. Focal dysplastic change consisting of enlarged cells and large nuclei in chronic hepatitis B (H&E stain; original magnification ×200).

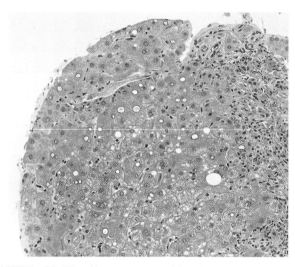

FIGURE 88-35. Hepatocytes with glycogen vacuolated nuclei (H&E stain; original magnification ×200).

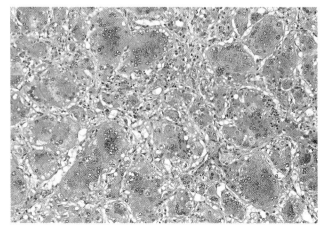

FIGURE 88-36. Syncytial hepatocytes in neonatal hepatitis (H&E stain; original magnification ×200).

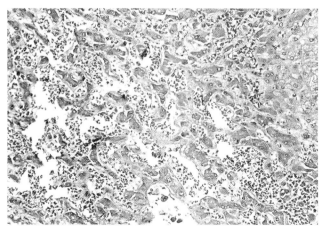

FIGURE 88-37. Chronic passive congestion causing perivenular sinusoidal dilation and atrophic hepatic cords (Masson trichrome; original magnification ×400).

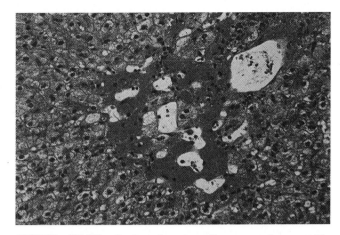

FIGURE 88-38. Perivenular hepatic parenchyma with dilated sinusoids and the presence of red blood cells within the hepatic cords in left-sided heart failure (H&E stain; original magnification ×100).

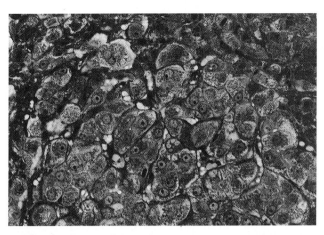

FIGURE 88-39. Collagen fibers along the sinusoids in the space of Disse in alcoholic liver disease (Masson trichrome stain; original magnification ×200).

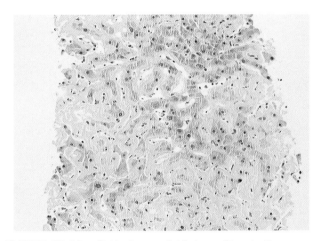

FIGURE 88-40. Reticular amyloid deposition in the space of Disse (H&E stain; original magnification ×200).

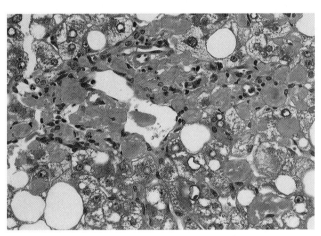

FIGURE 88-41. Globular amyloid deposition (H&E stain; original magnification ×400).

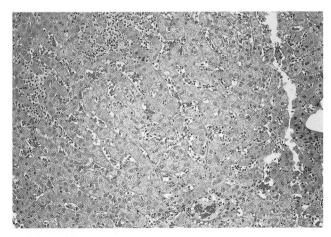

FIGURE 88-42. Hypertrophic Kupffer cells in salmonellosis (H&E stain; original magnification ×200).

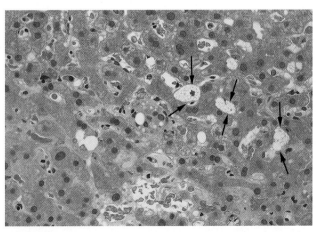

FIGURE 88-43. Ito cells with foamy fatty cytoplasm (*arrows*) along the sinusoidal surface in hypervitaminosis A (H&E stain; original magnification ×400).

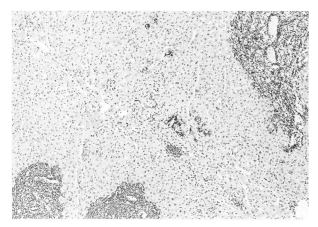

FIGURE 88-44. Leukemic cells in the sinusoidal blood space in a case of lymphocytic leukemia (H&E stain; original magnification ×200).

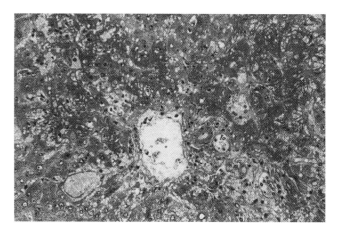

FIGURE 88-45. Periportal sinusoidal space filled with fibrin thrombi in toxemia of pregnancy (H&E stain; original magnification ×100).

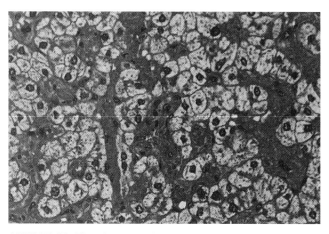

FIGURE 88-46. Clumps of sickled red blood cells packed in the sinusoidal spaces (H&E stain; original magnification ×200).

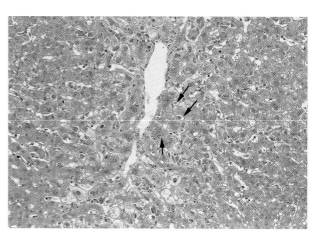

FIGURE 88-47. Cholestasis (*arrows*) in dilated canaliculi in zone 3 in chlorpromazine-induced liver disease (H&E stain; original magnification ×200).

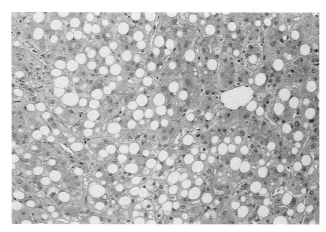

FIGURE 88-48. Macrovesicular fatty change of hepatocytes in alcoholic liver disease (H&E stain; original magnification ×200).

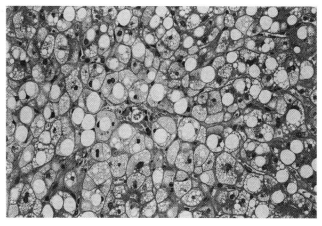

FIGURE 88-49. Diffusely enlarged hepatocytes with foamy fatty change in acute alcoholic liver disease (H&E stain; original magnification ×100).

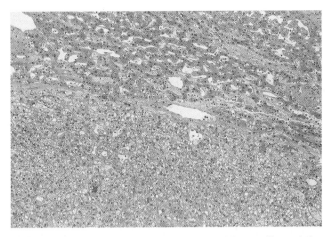

FIGURE 88-50. Liver cell adenoma with clear cells and the adjacent normal parenchyma (H&E stain; original magnification ×100).

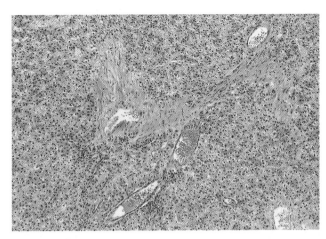

FIGURE 88-51. Liver cell adenoma with thick-walled vessels and lack of portal tracts (H&E stain; original magnification ×100).

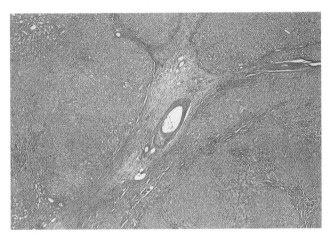

FIGURE 88-52. Focal nodular hyperplasia with central stellate scar (H&E stain; original magnification ×40).

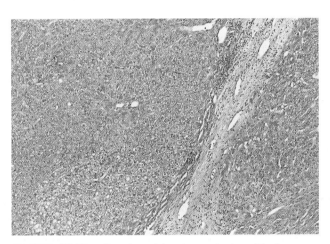

FIGURE 88-53. Focal nodular hyperplasia with the scar exhibiting lack of bile ducts and presence of vascular structures. Liver cells are uniform and regenerative in appearance (H&E stain; original magnification ×100).

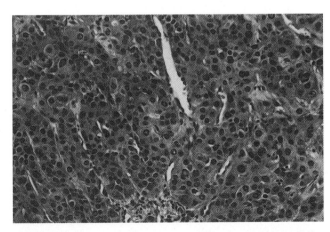

FIGURE 88-54. Well-differentiated trabecular hepatocellular carcinoma with endothelial lining (H&E stain; original magnification ×100).

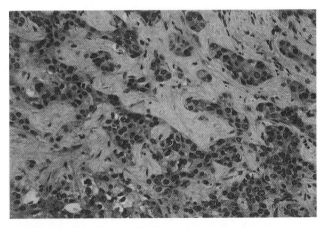

FIGURE 88-55. Sclerosing hepatic carcinoma with dense fibrous stroma (H&E stain; original magnification ×100).

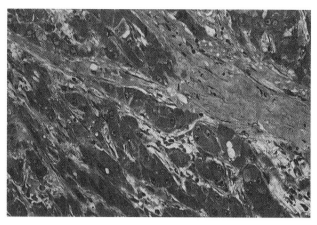

FIGURE 88-56. Eosinophilic neoplastic hepatocytes with lamellar fibrous stroma in fibrolamellar hepatocellular carcinoma (H&E stain; original magnification ×100).

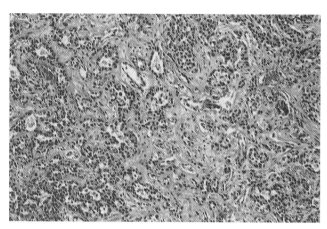

FIGURE 88-57. Neoplastic ductal structures with fibrous stroma in cholangiocarcinoma (H&E stain; original magnification ×100).

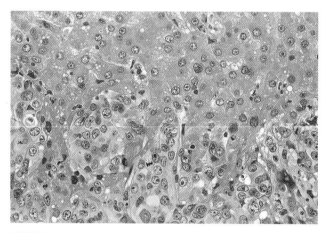

FIGURE 88-58. Metastatic, poorly differentiated adenocarcinoma infiltrating into the sinusoids (H&E stain; original magnification ×400).

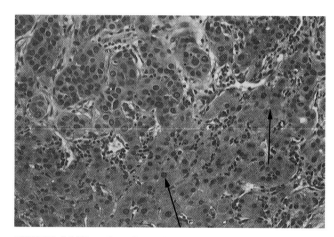

FIGURE 88-59. Junction of tumor and nontumor liver in hepatocellular carcinoma. The tumor cells grow into the hepatic cords (*arrows*) (H&E stain; original magnification ×100).

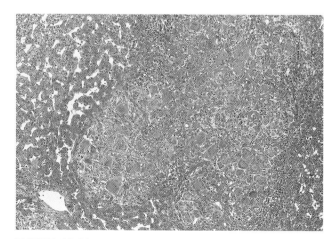

FIGURE 88-60. Partially segmented, exuberant epithelioid granuloma of sarcoidosis (H&E stain; original magnification ×100).

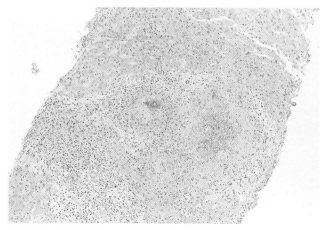

FIGURE 88-61. Epithelioid granuloma of Langhans giant cells and one cell showing central necrosis (**left**) in *Mycobacterium tuberculosis* of liver (H&E stain; original magnification ×100).

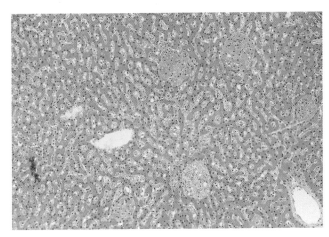

FIGURE 88-62. Well-circumscribed clusters of large foamy histiocytes in *Mycobacterium avium-intracellulare* infection of the liver. These cells contain abundant acid-fast organisms on special stain (not shown) (H&E stain; original magnification ×100).

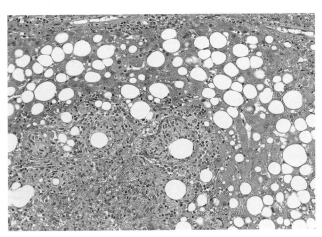

FIGURE 88-63. Granulomatous lesion with central vacuolization surrounded by a fibrin ring in Q fever (H&E stain; original magnification ×200).

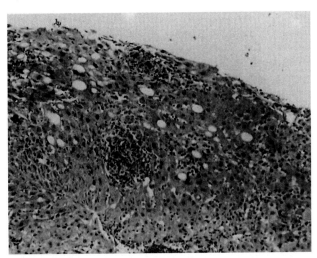

FIGURE 88-64. Small well-circumscribed granuloma in sulfonamide-induced hepatic necrosis (H&E stain; original magnification ×100).

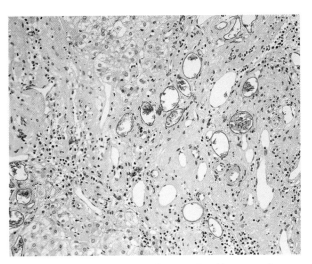

FIGURE 88-65. Remnants of ova of schistosomal organisms in a fibrous portal area (H&E stain; original magnification ×200).

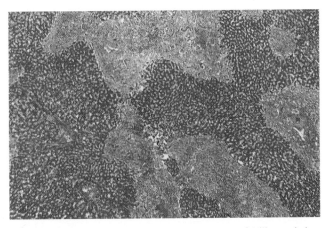

FIGURE 88-66. Jigsaw-puzzle appearance of biliary cirrhosis (Masson trichrome stain; original magnification ×40).

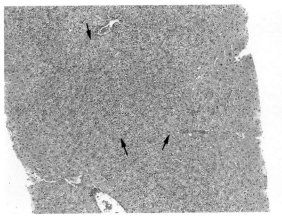

FIGURE 88-67. Scattered ground-glass cells (*arrows*) in chronic hepatitis B (H&E stain; original magnification ×100).

FIGURE 88-68. Perivenular zone in acute viral hepatitis demonstrating hydropic hepatocytes, hepatocytolysis, inflammatory exudate, and rare acidophilic bodies (H&E stain; original magnification ×200).

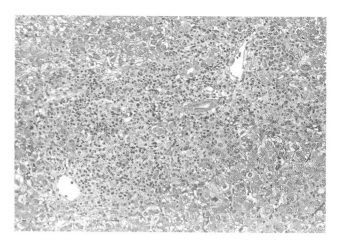

FIGURE 88-69. Portal area in acute viral hepatitis with mononuclear infiltration extending to the periportal regions (H&E stain; original magnification ×200).

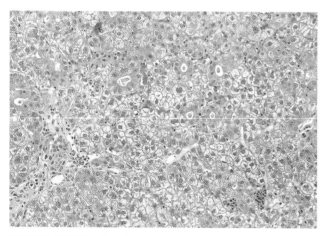

FIGURE 88-70. Prominent acinar transformation of hepatocytes in enterically transmitted acute hepatitis E (H&E stain; original magnification ×200).

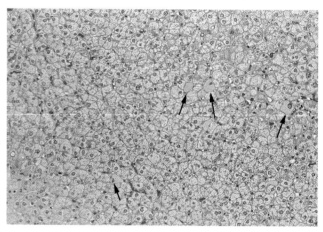

FIGURE 88-71. Uniform cobblestone appearance of parenchyma in chronic hepatitis B. A few ground-glass cells are seen (*arrows*) (H&E stain; original magnification ×200).

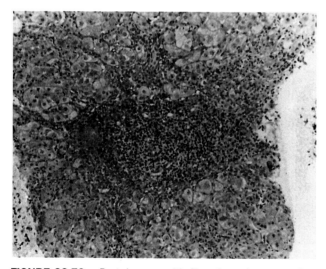

FIGURE 88-72. Portal areas with fibrosis and mononuclear inflammation extending to the parenchyma, exhibiting piecemeal necrosis in chronic hepatitis (H&E stain; original magnification ×100).

FIGURE 88-73. Chronic hepatitis C showing portal fibrosis with lymphoid nodule and inflammation in the adjacent parenchyma (H&E stain; original magnification ×100).

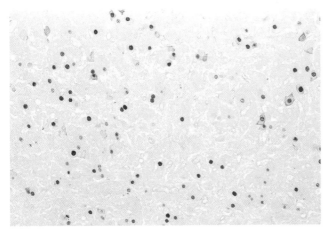

FIGURE 88-74. Immunoperoxidase stain demonstrating hepatitis delta antigen in the nuclei of hepatocytes in chronic hepatitis D (×100).

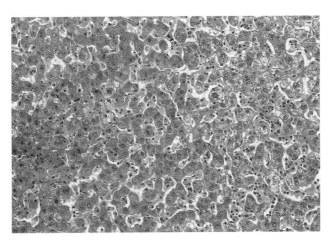

FIGURE 88-75. Striking sinusoidal lymphocytosis of atypical type in Epstein-Barr virus–induced mononucleosis (H&E stain; original magnification ×200).

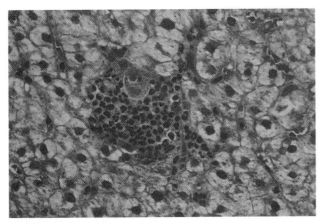

FIGURE 88-76. Intranuclear and cytoplasmic inclusions of cytomegalovirus (CMV) in a hepatocyte surrounded by polymorphonuclear leukocytes in an orthotopic liver transplant infected with CMV (H&E stain; original magnification ×200).

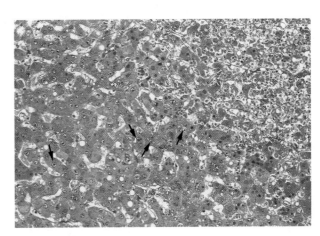

FIGURE 88-77. Intranuclear inclusions (*arrows*) of Cowdry type A of herpes simplex seen in hepatocytes (H&E stain; original magnification ×200).

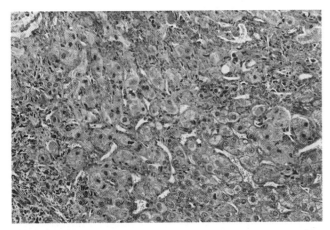

FIGURE 88-78. Diffuse interstitial fibrosis in chronic alcoholic liver disease (Masson trichrome stain; original magnification ×100).

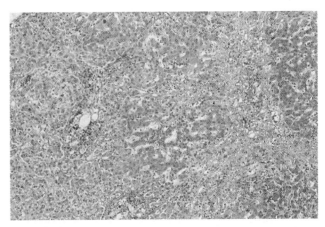

FIGURE 88-79. Marked perivenular fibrous scarring with mild portal fibrosis and lack of regenerative nodules in progressive perivenular fibrosis of alcoholic etiology (Masson trichrome stain; original magnification ×100).

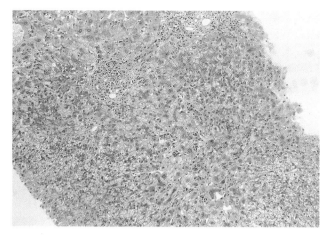

FIGURE 88-80. Hepatitis-like activity resembling acute viral hepatitis in methyldopa (Aldomet)-induced hepatotoxicity (H&E stain; original magnification ×200).

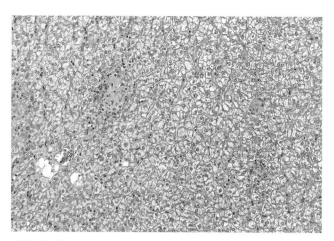

FIGURE 88-81. Phenytoin (Dilantin)-induced hepatic changes resembling mononucleosis (H&E stain; original magnification ×100).

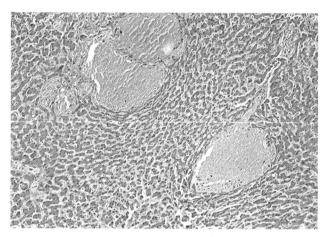

FIGURE 88-82. Peliosis hepatis with blood-filled spaces without endothelial lining (H&E stain; original magnification ×100).

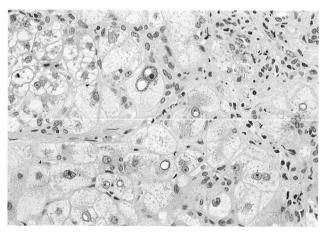

FIGURE 88-83. Sinusoidal fibrosis and nuclear dysplastic changes in methotrexate toxicity (H&E stain; original magnification ×400).

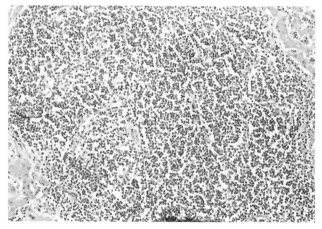

FIGURE 88-84. Portal infiltrate in non-Hodgkin lymphoma. (H&E stain; original magnification ×100).

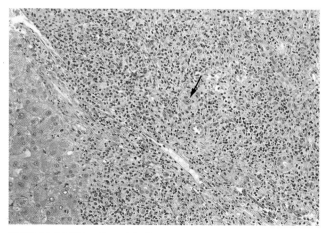

FIGURE 88-85. Portal infiltrate in Hodgkin lymphoma with an atypical Reed-Sternberg cell (*arrow*) (H&E stain; original magnification ×200).

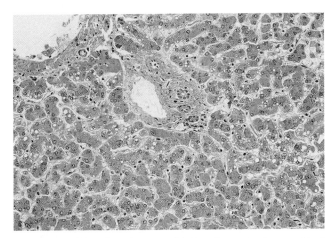

FIGURE 88-86. Portal area with lymphopenia in a patient with acquired immunodeficiency syndrome. (H&E stain; original magnification ×200).

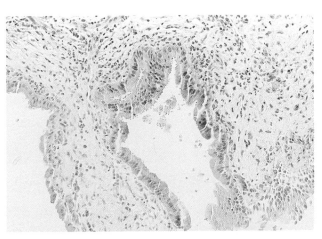

FIGURE 88-87. Bile duct epithelium, along the lumenal surface, demonstrates the presence of cryptosporidiosis of 3- to 4-μm size (H&E stain; original magnification ×400).

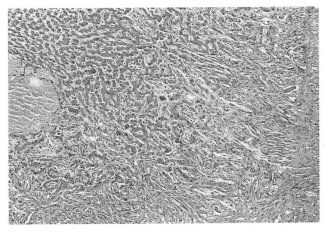

FIGURE 88-88. Kaposi sarcoma involving the liver (H&E stain; original magnification ×100).

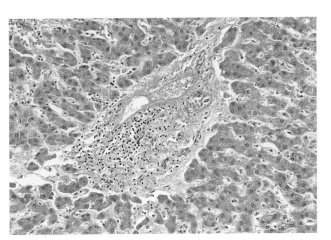

FIGURE 88-89. Portal inflammatory infiltrate with loss of bile ducts in chronic transplant rejection (H&E stain; original magnification ×200).

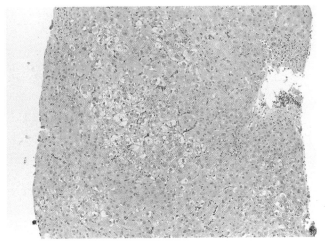

FIGURE 88-90. Marked ballooning of the hepatocytes in acinar zone 3 representing harvest injury (H&E stain; original magnification ×100).

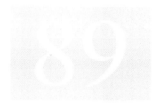

GASTROINTESTINAL DILATION AND STENT PLACEMENT

RICHARD A. KOZAREK

Although dilation of gastrointestinal strictures has been limited historically to the esophagus and anorectum, the development of polyethylene balloons has expanded the endoscopist's therapeutic horizons. Passed over a guidewire or directly through an endoscope, such balloons allow access to stenotic lesions of the stomach, small intestine, colon, and pancreaticobiliary tract. Paralleling our ability to dilate previously inaccessible stenoses has been the development of newer dilating systems for use in the esophagus. Polyvinyl dilators have virtually supplanted the Eder-Puestow metal olives (Pauldrach Medical, Garben, Germany), and lesions previously considered "undilatable" have been recategorized.

These expanded capabilities have led endoscopists into widespread dilation therapy for a variety of stenoses, despite absence of data or contradictory studies regarding risks and benefits of dilation compared with more conventional therapy such as surgical intervention. For example, lesions such as ulcerated pyloric channel strictures or stenoses with deep ulcerations caused by Crohn's disease increasingly are being dilated by endoscopists.

Expandable stent therapy has virtually supplanted conventional prosthesis placement in the esophagus, given the relative ease of placement and improved safety profile during insertion. Nevertheless, critical evaluation of this technology suggests that the need for intervention actually may increase after placement of expandable esophageal stents. This reintervention is a direct consequence of stent design: uncovered stents elicit granulation tissue and allow tumor ingrowth. Completely covered prostheses have a penchant for migration. All prostheses have the capability of causing erosion with fistulization, gastrointestinal bleeding, or occlusion by food bolus.

Even though expandable stent technology allows at least the potential to open obstructed lumenal orifices for patients at high risk and patients with widespread metastases and to open nonesophageal locations, the exact role of the technology remains ill-defined. Part of this uncertainty is the paucity of data regarding placement of these stents into locations other than the esophagus or biliary tract. Another part of the uncertainty includes the ongoing evolution of the various stents themselves and their respective delivery systems. Finally, additional uncertainty revolves around the cost of this technology—$1000 to $2000 per device depending on stent design and length. It is hoped that in the future, the various stent types can be better placed into perspective with each other and other potential therapies.

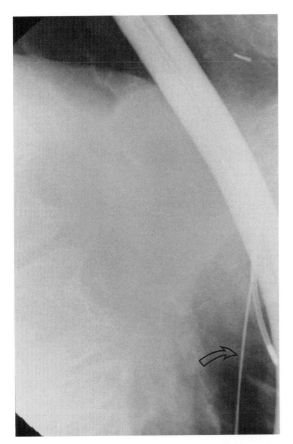

FIGURE 89-1. Barium-impregnated Savary-type dilator (American Dilator; Bard, Mentor, OH) passed over a guidewire (*arrow* shows distal portion of free guidewire in stomach) and through an obstructing distal esophageal cancer. Wire-guided polyvinyl dilators are the preferred treatment modality for acutely angulated, complex stenoses of the esophagus.

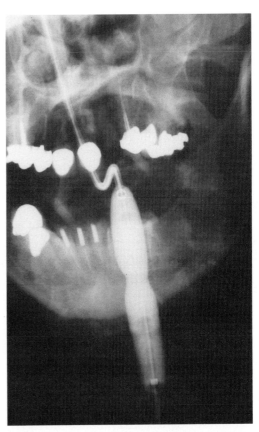

FIGURE 89-2. Balloon dilation of radiation stricture at cervical inlet. Location of stenosis precludes use of through-the-scope technology. The waist is present near midportion of balloon.

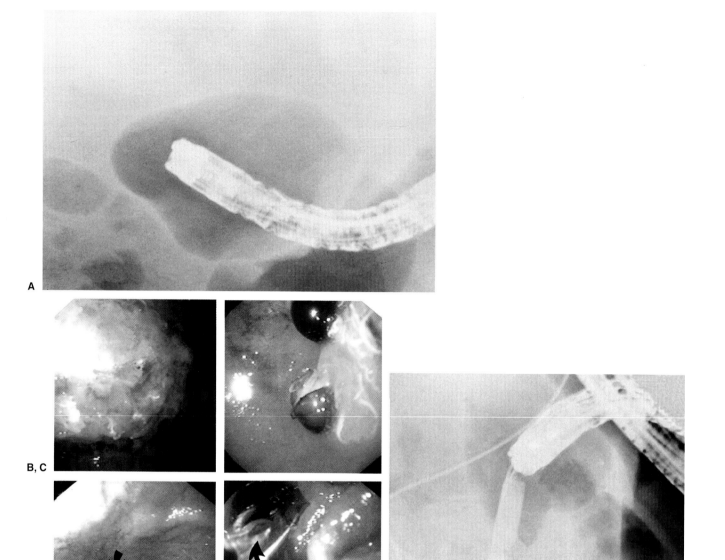

FIGURE 89-3. Dilated duodenal bulb of a patient with high-grade stricture of apex (**A**). Retained food is present in stomach (**B**) and bulb (**C**). A guidewire (*small arrow*) is inserted through the stricture (**D**) to allow proper positioning of balloon (Microvasive, Natick, MA) (*large arrow*) (**E**). Radiograph shows balloon dilation (**F, G**). *(Continued)*

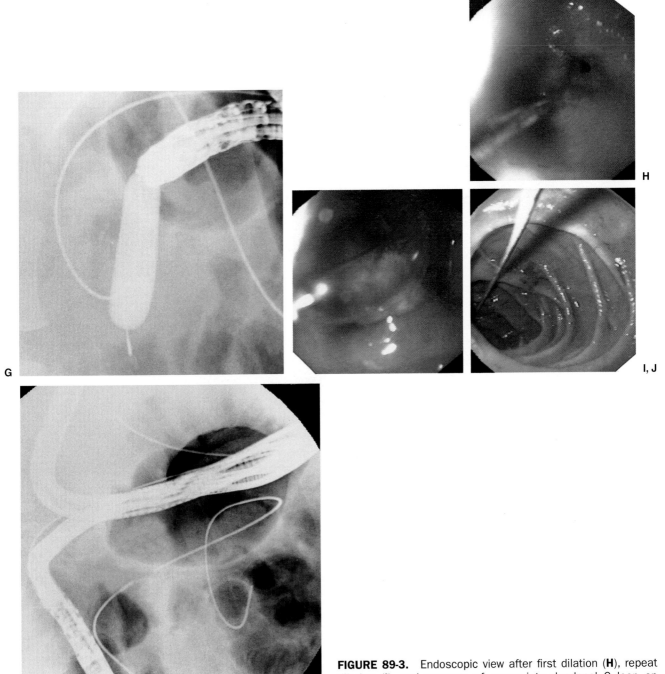

FIGURE 89-3. Endoscopic view after first dilation (**H**), repeat dilation (**I**), and passage of scope into duodenal C loop on endoscopic image (**J**) and radiograph (**K**).

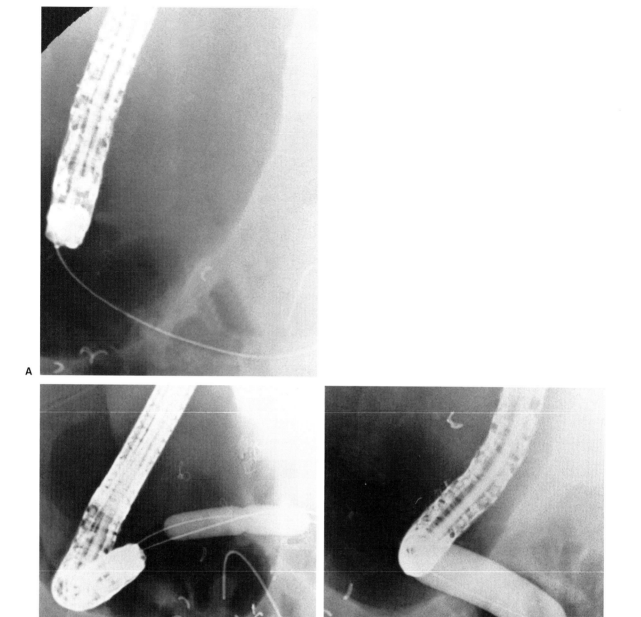

FIGURE 89-4. High-grade gastric outlet obstruction in patient with previous gastrectomy. Billroth I anastomosis for chronic abuse of aspirin (**A**). A guidewire was passed to ascertain direction of bowel beyond the level of stenosis. Anastomosis dilated with 10-mm (**B**) and 12-mm balloons (Microvasive, Natick, MA) (**C**) in initial setting.

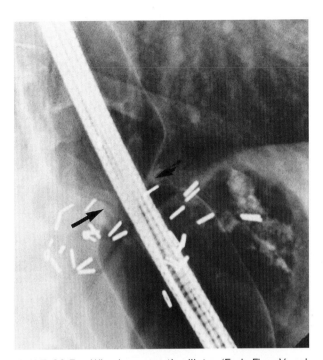

FIGURE 89-5. Witzel pneumatic dilator (Endo-Flex, Voerde, Germany) placed across the esophagogastric junction for patient with intractable dysphagia after laparoscopic antire-flux operation. The dilator is a balloon hybrid with a central channel in balloon accepting a pediatric endoscope to ensure proper position. The balloon waist is also shown (*arrows*).

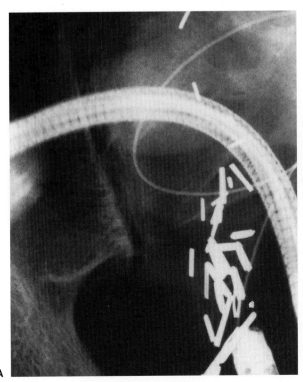

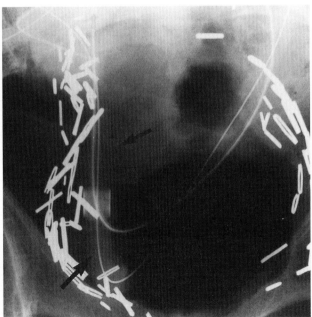

A

B

FIGURE 89-6. **A:** Endoscope inserted percutaneously into ileal conduit in a patient with total cystectomy for bladder carcinoma. Patient has ureteral ileostomies and conduit obstruction from recurrent neoplasm necessitating the use of bilateral nephrostomy tubes. Note guidewire and cystectomy clips. **B:** Savary-type dilators (Bard, Inc., Mentor, OH) (*arrows*) are passed through extrinsic neoplasm. *(Continued)*

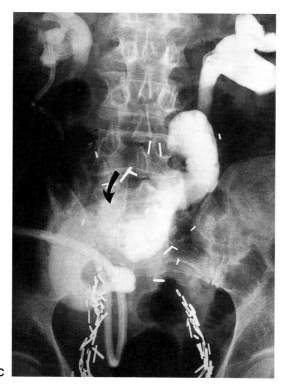

C

FIGURE 89-6. **(Continued) C:** The Savary-type dilators allow passage of decompression tube into the ileal conduit (*arrow*). This allowed nephrostomy tube retrieval, and the decompression tube functioned until patient died 2 years later.

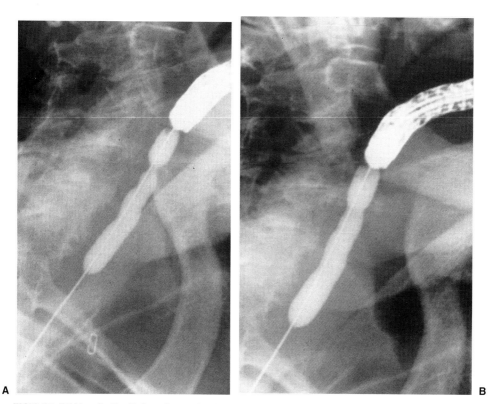

A   B

FIGURE 89-7. **A–C:** Eight-, 9-, and 10-mm controlled radial expansion (CRE) balloons (Microvasive, Natick, MA) used to treat tight irradiation stricture of the esophageal inlet. *(Continued)*

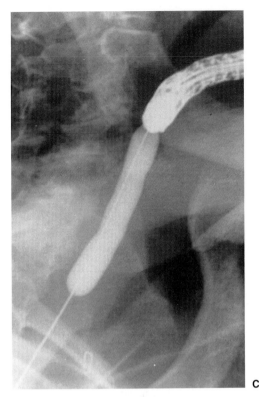

FIGURE 89-7. (Continued)

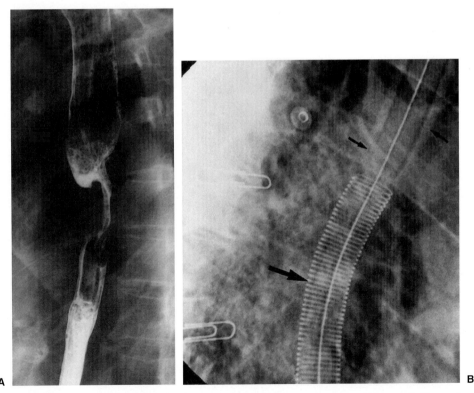

FIGURE 89-8. Stricture caused by midesophageal squamous cell carcinoma (**A**). The stricture was managed with conventional prosthesis (Wilson-Cook Inc., Winston-Salem, NC) (*large arrow*) pushed into position with Drummond introducer (*small arrows*) (**B**). (Continued)

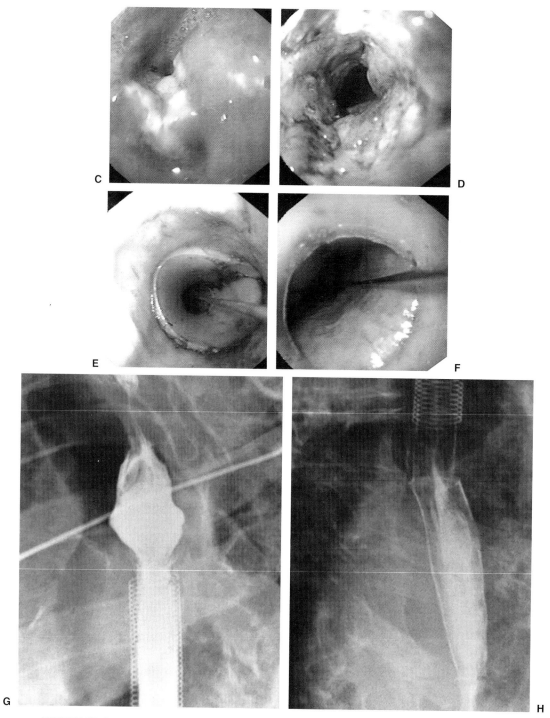

FIGURE 89-8.   (Continued) Endoscopic photographs show original neoplasm (**C**), appearance after dilation (**D**), and proximal (**E**) and distal (**F**) stent margin. Proper proximal (**G**) and distal (**H**) stent position and function at barium swallow.

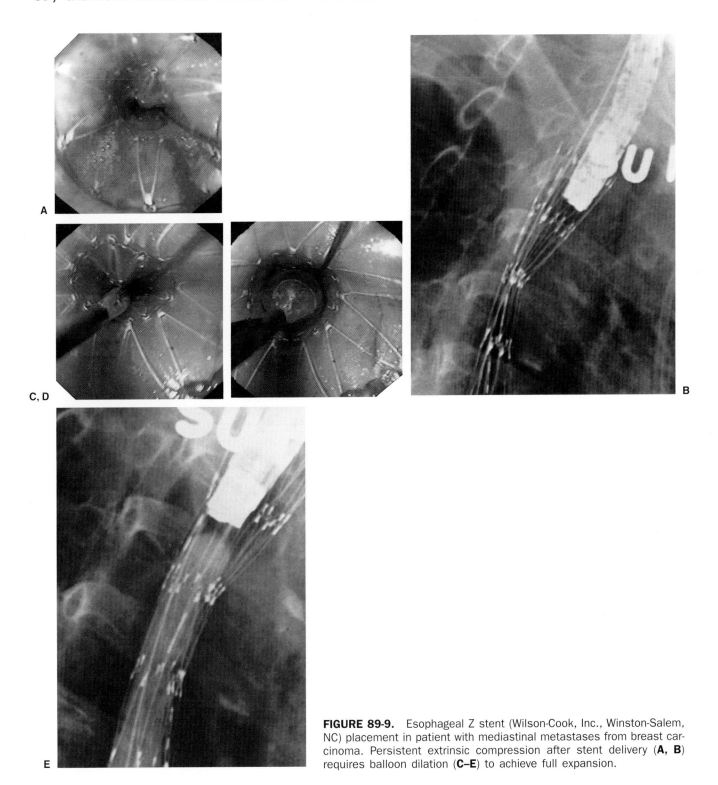

FIGURE 89-9. Esophageal Z stent (Wilson-Cook, Inc., Winston-Salem, NC) placement in patient with mediastinal metastases from breast carcinoma. Persistent extrinsic compression after stent delivery (**A, B**) requires balloon dilation (**C–E**) to achieve full expansion.

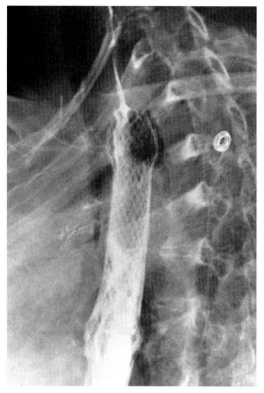

FIGURE 89-10. Barium swallow radiograph of a patient with malignant tracheoesophageal fistula from previously resected and recurrent lung carcinoma. Wallstent endoprosthesis (Microvasive, Natick, MA) is in place. There is good flow of barium distally and no demonstrable leak.

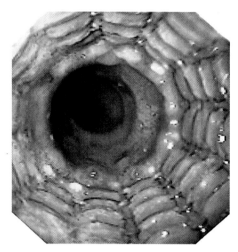

FIGURE 89-11. Endoscopic image of Ultraflex (Microvasive, Natick, MA) esophageal stent 1 month after insertion. Granulation tissue is present at the distal end, and Schatzki ring is visible in the distance.

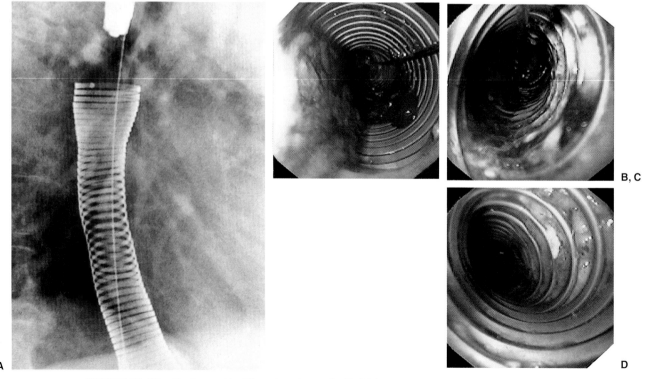

A   B, C

                                                                       D

FIGURE 89-12. Radiographic (**A**) and endoscopic (**B–D**) images of Esophacoil (Medtronics, Eden-Prairie, MN) stent inserted for midesophageal malignant tumor. Spacing between wires makes this stent less than ideal to manage esophagus-airway fistulae.

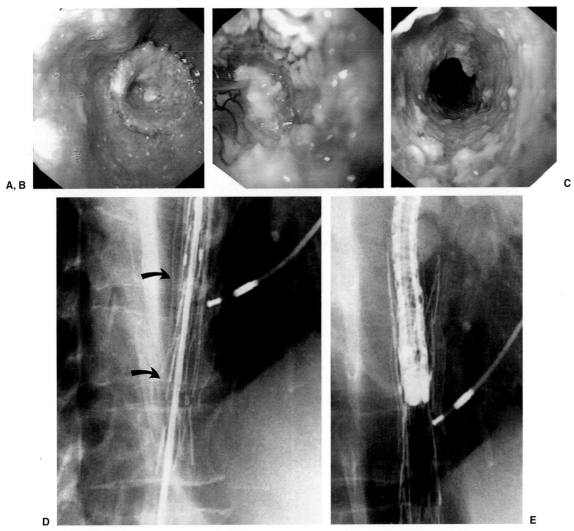

FIGURE 89-13. Problems encountered with expandable prostheses. Endoscopic photographs of a patient with esophageal cancer treated with an Ultraflex stent (Microinvasive Inc., Natick, MA) depict foodstuff (**A**), tumor ingrowth (**B**), and reactive inflammatory changes (**C**). Tumor ingrowth was managed by means of insertion of a Gianturco-Rösch (European) Z stent (Wilson Cook, Inc., Winston-Salem, NC) (**D**). An Ultraflex stent through which the Z stent has been inserted is shown (*arrows*). The pacemaker wire is visible. Deployment was followed by endoscopic visualization (**E**).

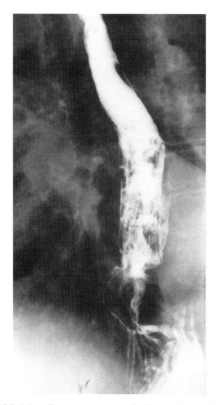

FIGURE 89-14. Tumor overgrowth through both ends of completely covered Z stent (Wilson-Cook Inc., Winston-Salem, NC) in a patient with Barrett esophagus and distal adenocarcinoma of the esophagus.

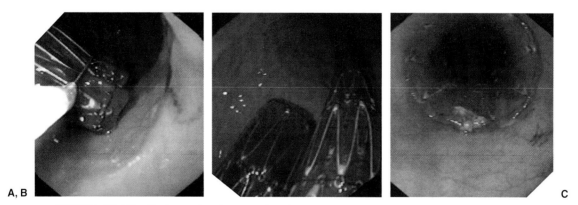

A, B   C

FIGURE 89-15. Endoscopic photographs demonstrate spontaneous migration of two 22-mm flanged Z stents (Wilson-Cook Inc., Winston-Salem, NC) into the stomach (**A**) of a patient with adenocarcinoma of the esophagogastric junction. Stents were retrieved (**B**) and replaced with a 25-mm flanged prosthesis (**C**).

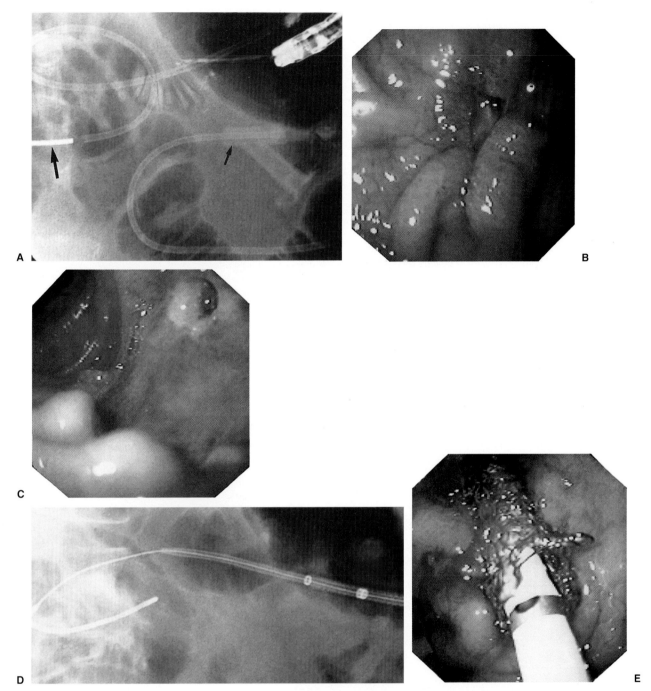

FIGURE 89-16. A: Decompressive gastrostomy (*small arrow*) and feeding nasojejunal tube (*large arrow*) in a patient with ongoing gastric outlet obstruction after gastrojejunostomy for lymphoma. Endoscopy demonstrated efferent limb obstruction and malignant gastric ulcers (**B**) and duodenal ulcers (**C**). Ultraflex prosthesis (Microinvasive Inc., Natick, MA) was placed across efferent limb stenosis over an endoscopically placed guidewire (**D**), followed by deployment (**E**) and full expansion (**F, G**). *(Continued)*

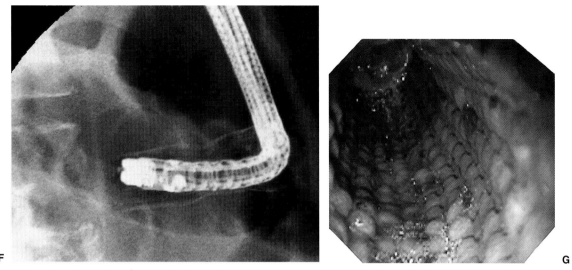

F   G

FIGURE 89-16.   **(Continued)**

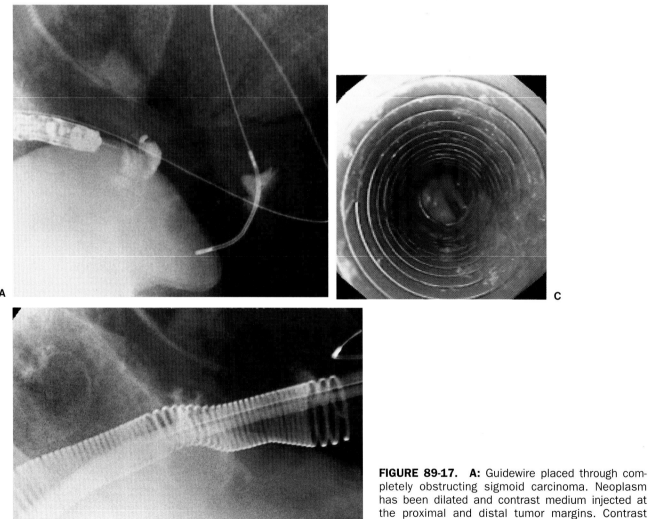

A

B

C

FIGURE 89-17.   **A:** Guidewire placed through completely obstructing sigmoid carcinoma. Neoplasm has been dilated and contrast medium injected at the proximal and distal tumor margins. Contrast material is present in the bladder. **B, C:** The neoplasm was stented with Esophacoil prosthesis (Medtronics Inc., Eden-Prairie, MN) to allow bowel preparation and one-stage colon resection.

ENDOSCOPIC THERAPY FOR UPPER GASTROINTESTINAL VARICEAL HEMORRHAGE

JAMES Y.W. LAU ■ JOSEPH J.Y. SUNG

Bleeding from esophageal and gastric varices is associated with high morbidity and mortality (Figs. 90-1 and 90-2*A, B*). Endoscopic therapy is the mainstay of treatment of patients with bleeding from esophageal varices. Endoscopic appearances of varices are prognostic and provide means of selecting patients for treatment. Endoscopic treatment in the form of sclerotherapy or band ligation is effective in the acute control of bleeding and the long-term treatment to eradicate varices and prevent recurrent bleeding.

Endoscopic findings in varices are prognostic. Several indices are in common use. The Japanese Research Society for Portal Hypertension proposed a detailed descriptive classification on the basis of variceal size, form, and the presence of red color signs (Fig. 90-3). In addition to the morphologic appearance of varices, the North Italian Endoscopic Club (NIEC) index incorporated patients' Child-Pugh class to derive a prognostic score.* These predictive indices are subject to observer variations. They may, however, be useful, especially for selection of high-risk patients for prophylactic therapy for varices.

Injection sclerotherapy was once the most widely used endoscopic therapy worldwide. There are wide variations in its technique and the choice of sclerosants. Sclerosants can be injected intravariceally using a free-hand technique, into mucosa around the varix (paravariceal), or a combination of both locations. Injection sclerotherapy leads to ulceration, tissue fibrosis, and obliteration of variceal channels. Stiegmann and Goff introduced the use of band ligation in the endoscopic treatment of esophageal varices (Fig. 90-4). Variceal band ligation is an extension of the band ligation technique in hemorrhoids. The variceal column is sucked into the ligating chamber before a plastic ring is released to strangulate the vascular channel (Fig. 90-5). From randomized studies and their metaanalysis, band ligation is safer than sclerotherapy and results in fewer associated systemic and local complications,

---

*Prediction of the first variceal hemorrhage in patients with cirrhosis of the liver and esophageal varices. A prospective multicenter study. The North Italian Endoscopic Club for the Study and Treatment of Esophageal Varices. N Engl J Med 1988;319:983.

most notably esophageal strictures. Band ligation also appears to eradicate varices more quickly. For these reasons, band ligation is becoming the preferred endoscopic treatment. Multiple banding devices are available to simplify the procedure and obviate the need of multiple intubations of the endoscope (Fig. 90-6).

As a result of the relatively high rate of complications, sclerotherapy is not used for primary prophylaxis because treatment morbidities outweigh the potential benefit. On the other hand, variceal band ligation is being evaluated as the primary prophylaxis against first bleed in high-risk patients. Evidence is growing to support its use in this clinical context. Long-term recurrence of varices, however, is more frequent after band ligation alone. It is postulated that band ligation induces less tissue fibrosis and does not lead to obliteration of perforating veins between submucosal varices and the larger paraesophageal collaterals. This has led to the combined use of band ligation and low-volume sclerotherapy, which offers the advantages of both techniques and reduces treatment-related morbidities. There are two approaches: the synchronous and metachronous approach. The synchronous approach involves the injection of a small volume of sclerosant proximally into a ligated varix. The metachronous approach uses ligation initially to reduce varices into a small size for later injection sclerotherapy. The synchronous approach has not been shown to further reduce variceal recurrence. In some studies, this synchronous approach led to an increased rate of complications when compared to variceal ligation alone. A metachronous approach, however, may be worthwhile. With repeated ligations resulting in fibrosis, small residual varices are often difficult to aspirate into the suction chamber of the banding device. In such instances, a low-volume sclerotherapy may reduce future variceal recurrences.

Gastric varices can be seen contiguous to esophageal varices or in isolation (Fig. 90-7). Isolated fundal varices carry a substantial rate of bleeding and mortality. Cyanoacrylate injection is the most effective endoscopic therapy for the condition. The adhesive admixed with lipiodol, a radiologic contrast, is injected intravariceally under fluoroscopic control (Fig. 90-8).

In the management algorithm of bleeding esophagogastric varices, endoscopic therapy maintains a central role. Prior administration with vasoactive drugs stops or slows bleeding and allows easier endoscopic therapy. Vasoactive drugs should then be continued to prevent early rebleeding. In the elective treatment of varices, weekly band ligation should be performed until eradication of varices. When endoscopic and pharmacological therapies fail, surgical or radiologic shunting is used as a salvage therapy. The use of a transjugular intrahepatic portosystemic shunt (TIPS) is an effective therapy to stop variceal hemorrhage (Fig. 90-9). However, its use is limited by subsequent hepatic encephalopathy. TIPS should be reserved for patients with recurrent bleeding not controlled by endoscopic therapies. TIPS is also an ideal stop-gap therapy for patients who require liver transplantation. In patients with good hepatic reserve who are unlikely to require liver transplantation in the near future, surgery in the form of a selected shunt (for example, a distal splenorenal shunt) can be offered.

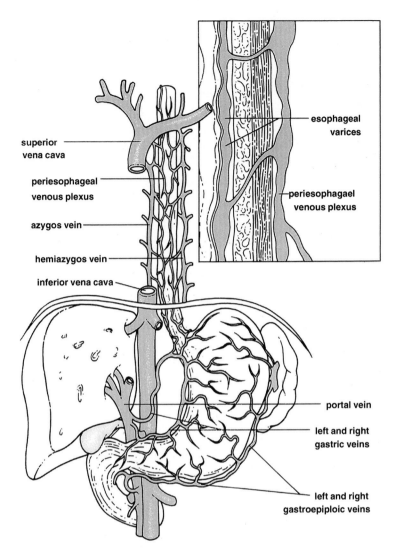

superior
vena cava

periesophageal
venous plexus

azygos vein

hemiazygos vein

inferior vena cava

esophageal
varices

periesophagael
venous plexus

portal vein

left and right
gastric veins

left and right
gastroepiploic veins

FIGURE 90-1. Schematic of the vessels of the portal venous system that are important in the formation of esophageal varices. In patients with portal hypertension and cirrhosis, esophageal collaterals dilate as a result of increased blood flow from the short gastric and coronary veins, and retrograde flow from engorged periesophageal veins; the blood enters the venous trunks of the distal esophagus. A cross section of this region of the esophagus (**inset**) shows the location of these varices in the submucosa.

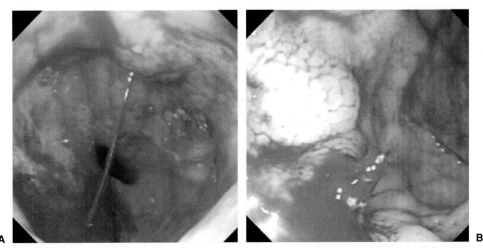

FIGURE 90-2. Bleeding gastric and esophageal varices. **A:** Active spurting from a column of esophageal varix. **B:** Fresh blood clot on gastric varix after spontaneous cessation of bleeding.

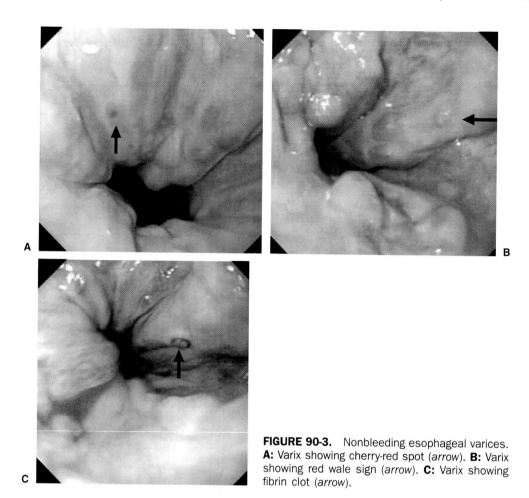

FIGURE 90-3. Nonbleeding esophageal varices. **A:** Varix showing cherry-red spot (*arrow*). **B:** Varix showing red wale sign (*arrow*). **C:** Varix showing fibrin clot (*arrow*).

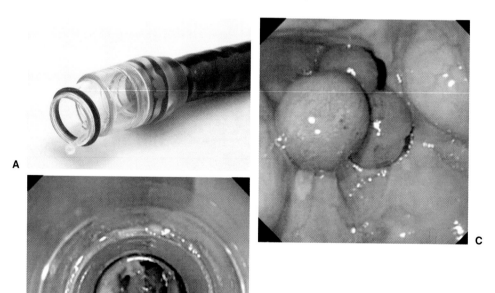

FIGURE 90-4. Esophageal ligator modified from Stiegmann and Goff. **A:** Ligation chamber, trip wire, and elastic ring. **B:** Esophageal varices seen through the endoscope with ligation device. **C:** Endoscopic view after banding ligation is completed.

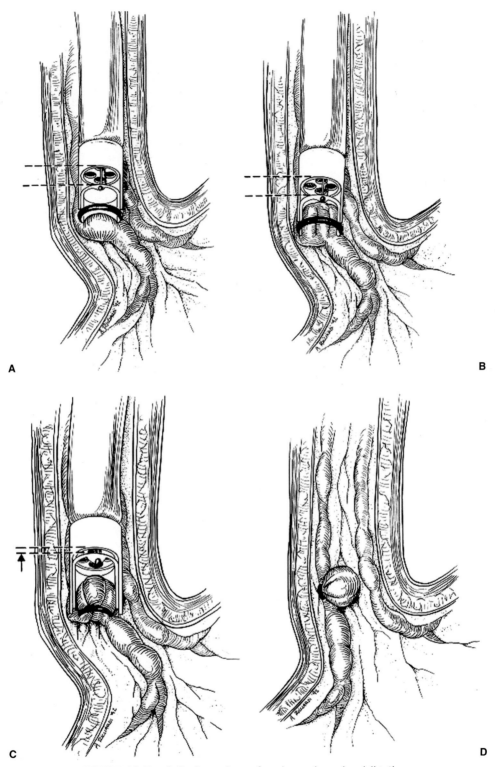

A

B

C

D

FIGURE 90-5. **A–D:** Procedure of endoscopic variceal ligation.

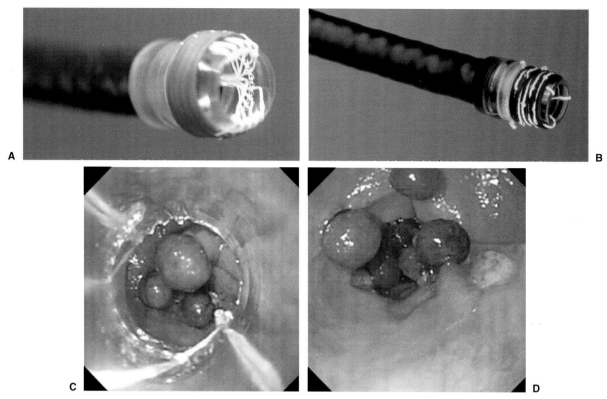

FIGURE 90-6. Multiple banding devices. **A:** Speedband (Boston Scientific, Natick, MA). **B:** Six-shooter (Wilson-Cook, Winston-Salem, NC). **C:** Endoscopic view after ligation is completed using the Speedband device. **D:** Endoscopic view after ligation is completed using the Six-shooter device.

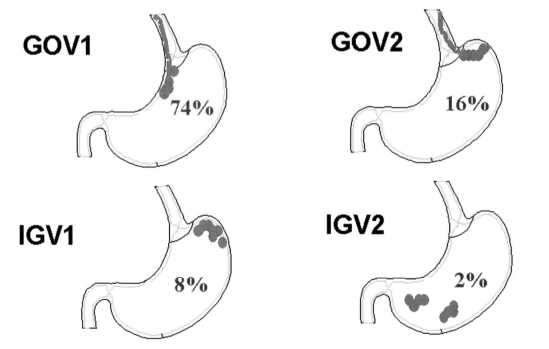

FIGURE 90-7. Classification of gastric varices according to Sarin.

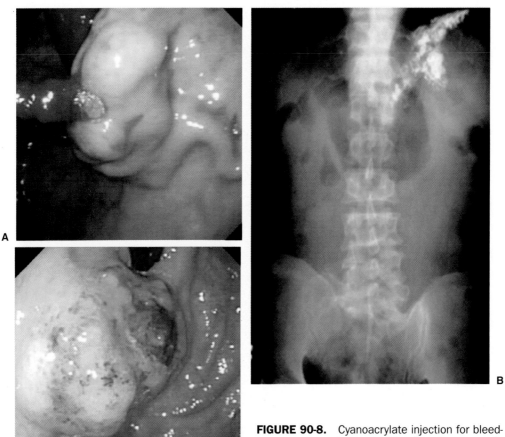

FIGURE 90-8. Cyanoacrylate injection for bleeding gastric varices. **A:** Bleeding from gastric varices. **B:** Cyanoacrylate injected under fluoroscopic control. **C:** One week after endoscopic injection of cyanoacrylate injection.

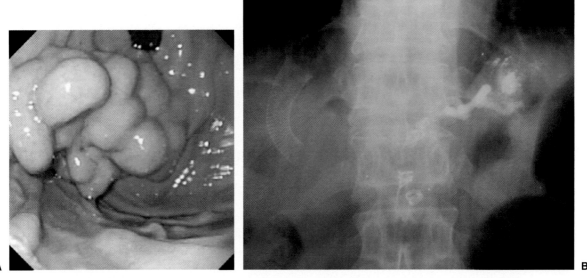

FIGURE 90-9. Transjugular intrahepatic portosystemic shunt. **A:** Gastric varices. **B:** Self-expanding metallic stent inserted across one of the hepatic veins to a branch of the portal vein to create a shunt between portal and systemic circulation. Coil embolization of splenic vein and collateral branches of the portal vein performed after failed cyanoacrylate injection.

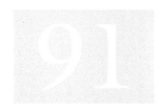

ENDOSCOPIC THERAPY FOR NONVARICEAL UPPER GASTROINTESTINAL HEMORRHAGE

DAVID J. BJORKMAN

Upper gastrointestinal (UGI) bleeding from peptic ulcer disease and other nonvariceal causes is a frequent cause for hospitalization (250,000–300,000 hospital admissions/year in the United States). Advances in endoscopic diagnosis and therapy have not substantially affected the overall mortality of this disorder, which remains in the range of 5% to 15%, depending on age and comorbid medical conditions.

Endoscopic diagnosis and therapy after vigorous volume resuscitation is the optimal approach to upper gastrointestinal bleeding. It is clear that the best predictor of persistent or recurrent bleeding, the need for surgical intervention, and mortality is the endoscopic appearance of the bleeding lesion, particularly in peptic ulcer disease, which is the most common cause of nonvariceal UGI bleeding. Lesions with active bleeding or a visible vessel have a high likelihood of rebleeding (40%–55%) and a mortality that exceeds 10%. On the other hand, lesions with a clean base have a very low risk of rebleeding (<5%) and a mortality that approaches 0%. Early endoscopic evaluation can, therefore, determine the optimal treatment approach for each patient.

Endoscopic therapy is indicated for all lesions that are considered to have a high risk of rebleeding. These include those with active bleeding, visible vessel, and potentially those with adherent clots that obscure the bleeding site. There are a variety of therapeutic modalities available to treat these lesions, all of which have a high rate (90%) of success in stopping active bleeding and significantly reduce the risk of rebleeding. Endoscopic therapy also reduces morbidity, mortality, transfusion requirements, and the costs of care.

Endoscopic therapies can be thermal (electrocoagulation, direct heat application, or laser therapy), involve injection using various agents, or employ mechanical compression of the bleeding site (hemostatic clips or bands). The technique of choice for a specific patient depends on the clinical situation, the location of the lesion, and the skill of the endoscopist.

This chapter demonstrates some of the endoscopic findings predictive of the outcome of a bleeding lesion, some of the devices used to treat the lesions, and the results of therapy.

968

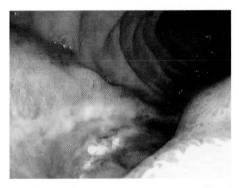

FIGURE 91-1. Deep duodenal ulcer with flat pigmented spots in the base. This lesion, despite its depth, has a low (<10%) risk of rebleeding and a mortality of less than 5%. Endoscopic therapy is not indicated in this lesion.

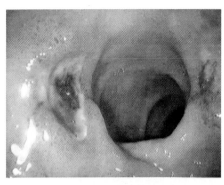

FIGURE 91-2. A duodenal ulcer with a central smooth-surfaced protuberance indicating a visible vessel. Despite the absence of active bleeding, the risk of rebleeding in this lesion is greater than 40% and the mortality is greater than 10%. Both of these figures can be considerably reduced by appropriate endoscopic therapy.

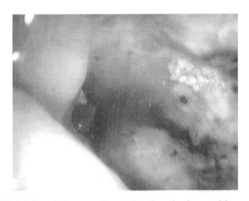

FIGURE 91-3. A large, deep duodenal ulcer with a visible vessel with bleeding is seen in the center of the base of the ulcer. The position of this lesion is ideal for direct application of thermal therapy to coagulate the vessel. The ulcer also has a flat red spot in the base, which in the absence of the visible vessel, would not indicate a high risk of rebleeding.

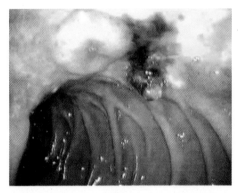

FIGURE 91-4. This large ulcer at the apex of the duodenal bulb shows a visible vessel extending into the lumen. The risk of rebleeding from this lesion is very high without endoscopic therapy.

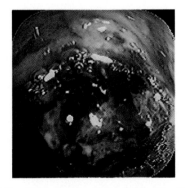

FIGURE 91-5. This large ulcer has an adherent clot (remains after vigorous washing) that obscures the ulcer base. The risk of rebleeding in this setting depends on the underlying lesion. Removal of the clot may precipitate active bleeding. Optimal treatment of this lesion remains controversial. If the clot is removed to evaluate the underlying lesion, injection therapy with epinephrine should be performed prior to clot manipulation to limit or prevent active bleeding. (Courtesy of Dr. D. Jensen.)

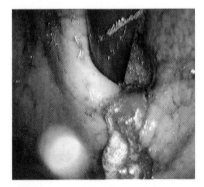

FIGURE 91-6. This clot extending from the gastroesophageal junction into the cardia of the stomach overlies and obscures a Mallory-Weiss tear. There is oozing at the superior aspect of the clot from the Mallory-Weiss tear. The endoscope is retroflexed with the proximal part of the scope seen entering the stomach from the esophagus. Although Mallory-Weiss tears usually stop bleeding spontaneously, endoscopic therapy is indicated for actively bleeding lesions, such as this.

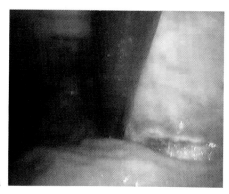
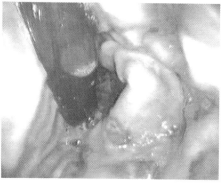

A

B

FIGURE 91-7. **A, B:** Two Mallory-Weiss tears at the gastroesophageal junction are demonstrated in these images. The flat pigmented spots in the base of the tears does not increase the risk for rebleeding; thus no endoscopic therapy is indicated for either lesion.

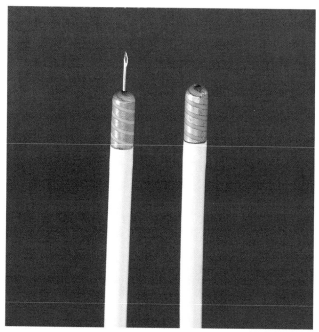

FIGURE 91-8. Bipolar electrocoagulation catheters with electrodes that circle the end of the catheter and a central channel for vigorous water irrigation. This catheter also has a retractable central injection needle to allow combined electrocoagulation and injection therapy. The probe is inserted through the working channel of the endoscope and applied directly to the bleeding lesion while electrical energy is repeatedly passed between the electrodes through the tissue. The resistance of the tissue results in heat that cauterizes the lesion and seals the walls of the bleeding vessel together in what is called coaptive coagulation. Control of the energy delivery and water irrigation is achieved by foot pedals attached to the electrical generator and the probe. (Courtesy of Dr. D. Jensen.)

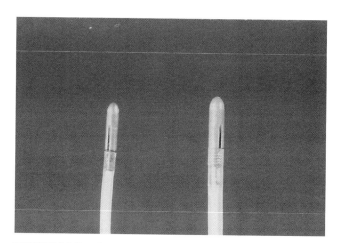

FIGURE 91-9. Two heater probes of different diameters are pictured. Each is a flexible catheter that is tipped with a heating element that is placed directly on the tissue for coaptive coagulation. No electrical current passes through the patient. Vigorous water irrigation is possible through the central channel of the catheter. As with the bipolar catheter, the probe is applied directly to the bleeding lesion, and the repeated delivery of heat is controlled by foot pedals accessible to the operator. (Courtesy of Dr. D. Jensen.)

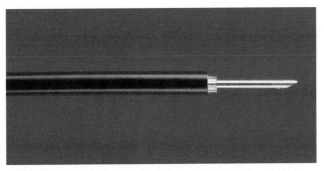

FIGURE 91-10. Endoscopic injection needle. This needle is attached to a syringe with the desired solution for injection. The needle is retracted into the catheter and then passed through the working channel of the endoscope. The needle is then advanced out of the catheter and repeated injections are made around the bleeding lesion. When saline or dilute epinephrine is used, large volumes of injected fluid (10 mL or more) can be used to tamponade the bleeding lesion. Smaller volumes (0.1- to 0.2-mL aliquots) should be injected when absolute alcohol is used. Injection of saline or epinephrine is very helpful in slowing active bleeding in preparation for more definitive thermal or injection therapy. Recent data suggest that saline injection alone is not as effective as contact thermal methods in preventing rebleeding.

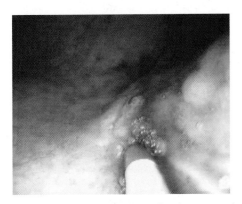

FIGURE 91-11. Direct application of a heater probe to an actively bleeding ulcer in the duodenum. Blood can be seen oozing from beneath the tip of the probe. Heat is then repeatedly applied to the tissue while pressure of the probe is maintained on the lesion.

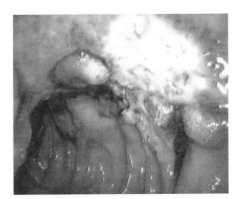

FIGURE 91-12. Appearance of a duodenal ulcer after successful thermal therapy. The bleeding site and the surrounding area have been successfully heated, leaving the white coagulated tissue behind with no evidence of a persistent visible vessel or bleeding. The surrounding edema is the result of thermal therapy and may also help reduce blood flow to the area.

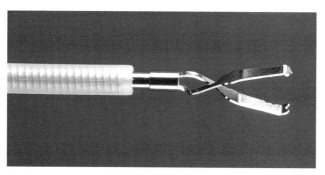

FIGURE 91-13. A hemostatic clip attached to the delivery catheter. The clip is similar to that used in surgery and is applied to a bleeding vessel to close it. After several days, the clip sloughs into the lumen and is passed. The clip can be rotated to provide better position for application. The clip is then closed via the handle on the delivery catheter and released from the delivery device. Because the bleeding vessel is not always visible or accessible, multiple clips are often required to achieve the appropriate hemostatic effect.

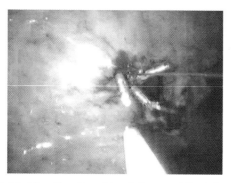

FIGURE 91-14. Spurting blood from a Dieulafoy lesion. These lesions are dilated aberrant vessels that can erode through the mucosal surface to cause recurrent vigorous bleeding. The absence of an overlying ulcer makes these lesions difficult to identify. In this case, three hemostatic clips have been applied in an attempt to stop the bleeding. The clip delivery device can be seen in the foreground. (Image courtesy of Dr. James DiSario.)

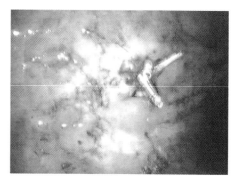

FIGURE 91-15. Successful treatment of the Dieulafoy lesion seen in Fig. 91-14. The removal of one clip (furthest to the **left** in Fig. 91-14) to allow more optimal positioning of a substitute has sealed the vessel. Note the absence of ulceration at the site of the lesion. (Image courtesy of Dr. James DiSario.)

92

ENDOSCOPIC THERAPY FOR POLYPS AND TUMORS

DOUGLAS K. REX ■ EMAD Y. RAHMANI

Endoscopic techniques can be used to resect polyps and tumors in the gastrointestinal tract or to ablate them. Successful endoscopic therapy depends on sufficient experience to recognize lesions correctly and choose the most appropriate form of therapy, and on sufficient training to execute the appropriate endoscopic technique. Examples of the use of endoscopic and ablative methods for management of polyps and tumors of the gastrointestinal tract are provided in this chapter. The chapter also includes examples of lesions that should not be managed with endoscopic resection or ablation.

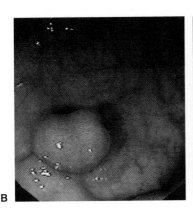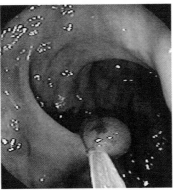

A, B

FIGURE 92-1. Removal of pedunculated polyps. **A:** Small pedunculated polyp on a short stalk. **B:** The polyp generally is grasped close to the polyp head. This allows complete resection of the neoplastic tissue and leaves a residual stalk to be grasped if immediate hemorrhage begins. In addition, it reduces the chance that the burn will spread far enough into the wall to result in post-polypectomy syndrome or perforation. If the polyp is highly likely to be malignant, grasping farther down the stalk may be preferable, because it increases the chance for having a margin that is histologically free of cancer.

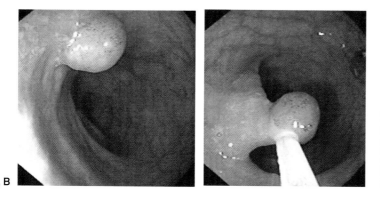

FIGURE 92-2. Creation of "pseudostalk." **A:** The small polyp is apparently sessile. **B:** After the polyp is grasped and lifted into the lumen, there is a pseudostalk. Creation of the pseudostalk by means of tenting should reduce the risk for a deep burn.

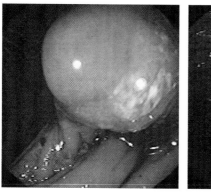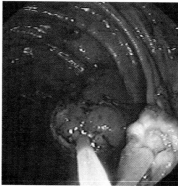

FIGURE 92-3. Retrieval of pedunculated polyps. **A:** Large pedunculated polyp. **B:** Polyp head after removal being grasped with a polypectomy snare. The lesion is removed from the colon several centimeters in front of the scope while the examination continues. An advantage of using a polypectomy snare rather than a retrieval basket is that if another small lesion is encountered, the large, previously transected polyp can be dropped in the lumen. The small lesion can be removed and suctioned into a trap. The large lesion can be regrasped, and the examination can continue.

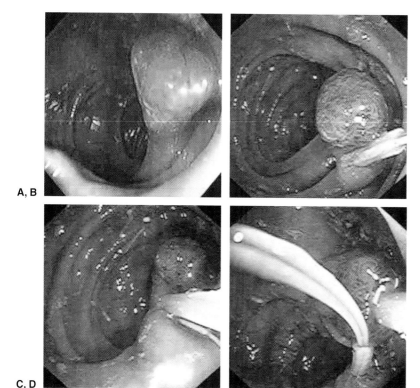

FIGURE 92-4. Prevention of bleeding by detachable snares. Some experts recommend adjunctive methods to prevent bleeding in pedunculated polyps with stalks greater than or equal to 1 cm thick or patients requiring re-anticoagulation. Detachable snares are the only method proven in a randomized trial. **A:** Pedunculated sigmoid polyp in a patient with a prosthetic valve. He was to be heparinized 6 hours after colonoscopy. **B:** Detachable snare (Endoloop; Olympus Corp., Lake Success, NY) on the polyp stalk. **C:** Monopolar cautery snare positioned between the polyp head and the detachable snare. **D:** Detachable snare on the stalk after resection. Cautery snare has picked up the resected polyp head for retrieval.

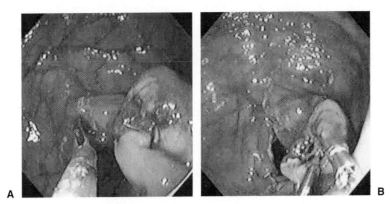

FIGURE 92-5. Prevention of bleeding by hemostatic metal clips. This alternative is anecdotally effective in preventing bleeding from pedunculated or sessile polyps. **A:** Polyp base immediately after snare resection of pedunculated polyp in a patient to be re-anticoagulated. **B:** Same base after placement of two metal clips.

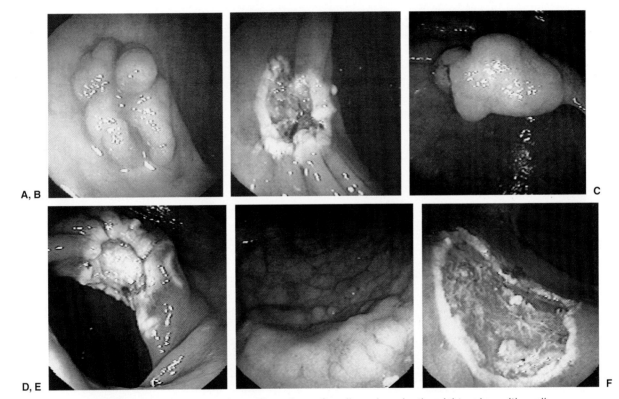

FIGURE 92-6. Removal of sessile polyps. Sessile polyps in the right colon with well-demarcated and raised edges (**A, C**). Such lesions can be readily removed in a single piece or by means of piecemeal polypectomy without submucosal saline injection (**B, D**). The decision to use submucosal saline injection is based, first, on whether injection would facilitate polypectomy by means of moving a portion of the polyp on the proximal side of a fold to a more en face position and, second, on whether, because the polyp is sufficiently large, there is risk for perforation if the entire lesion is removed in one session. Removal without saline injection leaves a mucosal defect and exposure of the submucosa. Without saline injection, this defect often tends to be deeper and more irregular (**B, D**) than when submucosal saline injection is performed. **E:** The lesion has edges that are less raised and more indistinct. **F:** Complete resection of such a lesion often is facilitated by submucosal saline injection. *(Continued)*

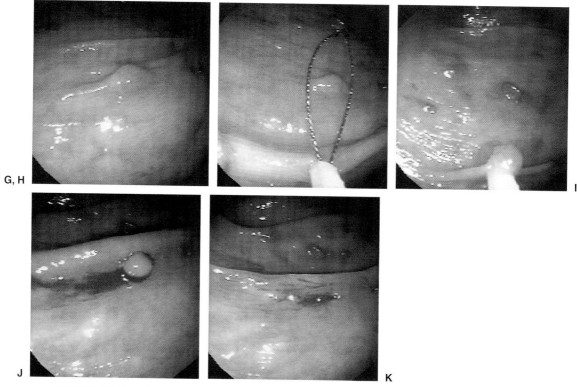

FIGURE 92-6. **(Continued)** **G–K:** Cold snare polypectomy is an appropriate method for resection of polyps smaller than 5 mm. **J:** Transection of the polyp base usually is accompanied by a few drops of bleeding, which rarely requires therapy. **K:** Site after suctioning of the polyp.

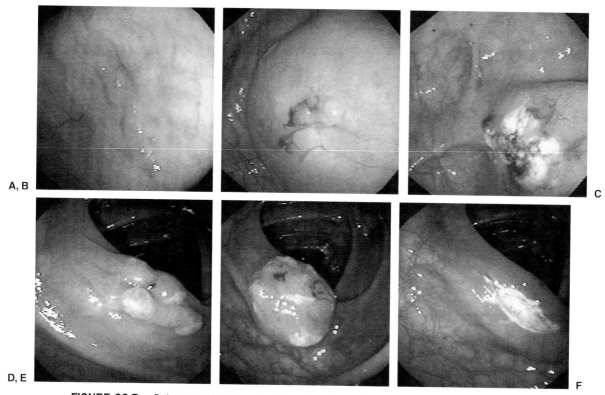

FIGURE 92-7. Submucosal saline injection. Sessile polyps from three separate patients are shown before injection (**A, D, G**), after submucosal injection of saline solution to make a large mound (**B, E, H**), and after snare resection in a single piece (**C, F, I**). The injection should produce a large submucosal mound. Once the submucosal mound has been made, it is quite acceptable for normal tissue to be included in the specimen if it facilitates complete resection. However, this step should not be taken unnecessarily. *(Continued)*

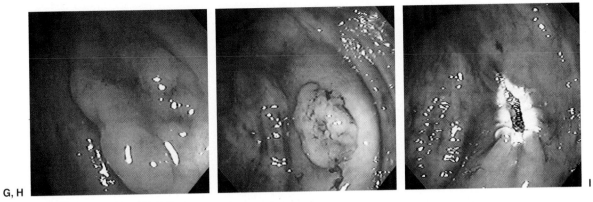

G, H

FIGURE 92-7. (Continued)

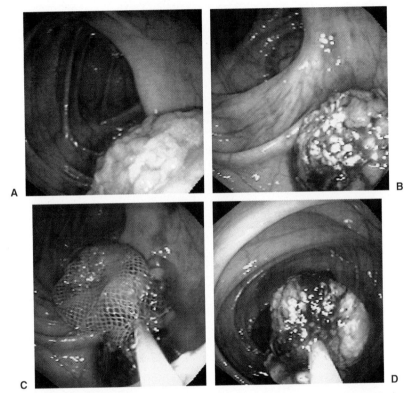

A

B

C

D

FIGURE 92-8. Retrieval of sessile lesions. When a sessile polyp is removed piecemeal, the approach to retrieval depends on the size of the fragments. If multiple small fragments are present, they all can be removed by suction into a trap. If there is one large fragment, the small fragments can be retrieved first by suction and the large fragment then can be retrieved with a polypectomy snare. When multiple large fragments are present, use of a Roth basket facilitates retrieval. **A:** Large sessile polyp in the right colon. **B:** Multiple fragments. **C:** Opening of Roth retrieval basket successfully over these fragments. **D:** Enclosed fragments all are removed at one time while the examination continues. This obviates multiple intubations to retrieve fragments.

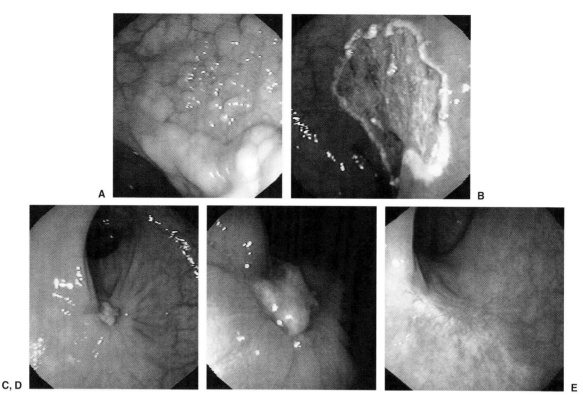

FIGURE 92-9. Natural history of polypectomy scars. **A:** Large, multilobulated sessile polyp in the rectum. **B:** Polypectomy site immediately after removal by means of submucosal saline injection and piecemeal polypectomy. **C, D:** Site 1 month later with contraction of the scar and granulation tissue in the base. It is essential to recognize granulation tissue because of its inflamed and abnormal surface, which is not epithelialized. There is no clear-cut evidence of residual polyp. **E:** Polyp site 5 months after polypectomy with complete healing of the site. Biopsies of the site demonstrated no residual adenomatous tissue. All patients with sessile polyps should be observed for recurrence, which may develop even when the polypectomy appears to be complete. The timing of follow-up examinations should allow enough time for healing but not be long enough to allow any recurrence time to grow to substantial size. The best interval is 2 to 6 months. Even after complete polypectomy has been apparently verified, it may be wise to repeat an examination in 1 year, because some recurrences are late. In our experience, biopsy findings at a polypectomy site after apparently complete resection, as in **E,** which shows dysplastic tissue, often are predictive of subsequent overt recurrence.

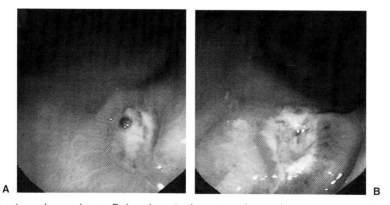

FIGURE 92-10. Postpolypectomy hemorrhage. Delayed postpolypectomy hemorrhage may occur from a few hours to as long as 3 weeks after polypectomy. About two thirds of hemorrhages stop spontaneously, but about one third of patients return for treatment because of active bloody bowel movements. In our experience, colonoscopy can be successfully performed without repeating intestinal preparation. Inspection of the polypectomy site may demonstrate active arterial hemorrhage, adherent clots, or an ulcer with a visible vessel (**A**). We manage these lesions essentially as we would upper gastrointestinal tract bleeding, by means of injection of epinephrine diluted 1:10,000 in normal saline solution typically followed by bipolar cauterization. The amount of cauterization that should be applied is not well established (as it is for procedures on the upper gastrointestinal tract). In the right colon, it is probably preferable subjectively to eradicate an apparent vessel or other bleeding point (**B**), but the thin wall of the right colon should be kept in mind, and aggressive tamponade and cauterization may be inappropriate. If there are concerns about wall integrity, simple injection followed by careful clinical observation is appropriate.

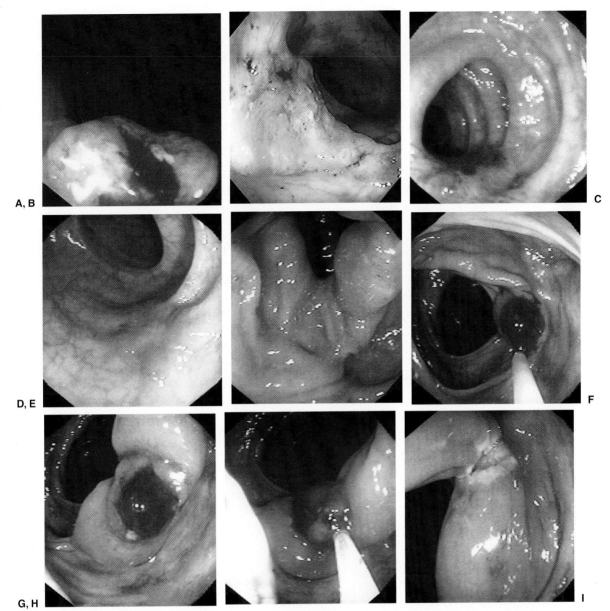

FIGURE 92-11. Malignant polyps. Sessile lesions that have surface ulceration are almost invariably malignant. **A, B:** Polyps with central areas of depression; both patients had Dukes stage A cancer. Our approach is to perform biopsy on such lesions in anticipation of surgical resection. **C, D:** Typical sessile polyp without surface ulceration may also prove to be malignant. One endoscopic feature that can be used to identify a malignant polyp is the nonlifting sign. **E:** A 1.5-cm sessile polyp in the right colon. **F:** The lesion after biopsy, which produced a blood clot on the surface of the polyp. Submucosal injection was performed. **G:** In the left-hand aspect of the polyp, a small portion remained tethered in the submucosa and would not lift, forming a notch in the submucosal saline cushion. **H:** The lesion was removed by means of snare cauterization in a single piece. **I:** Inspection revealed complete polypectomy. Pathological examination showed that the entire lesion was carcinoma extending to the resection margin along one edge. The patient underwent right hemicolectomy.

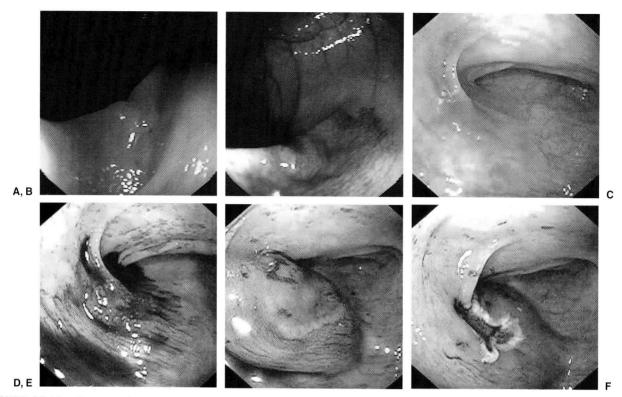

A, B

C

D, E

F

FIGURE 92-12. Dye spraying. In Japan, chromoendoscopy often is used to assist in identification of polyps. The most common practice in Japan is not to systematically spray the entire colon but to spray dye onto small erythematous spots and other surface irregularities as they are encountered during routine endoscopy. **A:** Subtle, poorly defined lesion from a person in a western population. **B:** Image after dye spraying with indigo carmine shows central pit and surrounding raised mucosa. This lesion meets the morphologic criteria for flat adenoma. It was removed by means of submucosal injection and strip biopsy and found to be tubular adenoma without severe dysplasia. **C:** Different flat adenoma barely visible with standard endoscopy. **D:** The same lesion—more apparent but still subtle after spraying with 0.8% indigo carmine. **E:** The same lesion again after washing off indigo carmine and injecting submucosal saline with a few drops of methylene blue. The methylene blue defines the polyp edges, removing the need for chromoscopy. **F:** Resection site after snare removal in a single piece.

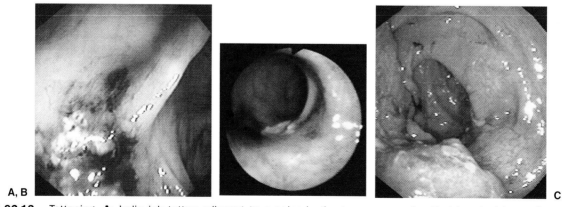

A, B

C

FIGURE 92-13. Tattooing. **A:** India ink tattoo adjacent to a polyp in the transverse colon that has just been destroyed with a Neodymium:yttrium-aluminum-garnet laser. The tattoo assists in identification of the cauterization site for subsequent follow-up examinations. **B:** Tattoos on either side of a polypectomy site. If the purpose of staining is to mark a lesion for subsequent endoscopic follow-up examinations, tattoos are placed only on either side of the polyp. However, if there is concern that the lesion is malignant and the marking is being done to facilitate subsequent surgical treatment, tattoos are placed in all four quadrants at the level of the lesion. **C:** India ink tattoos in all four quadrants immediately proximal to ulcerated tumor in the sigmoid colon. Tattooing is preferred for any lesion in which the ileocecal valve is not still in the endoscopic view or is proximal to the distal sigmoid colon.

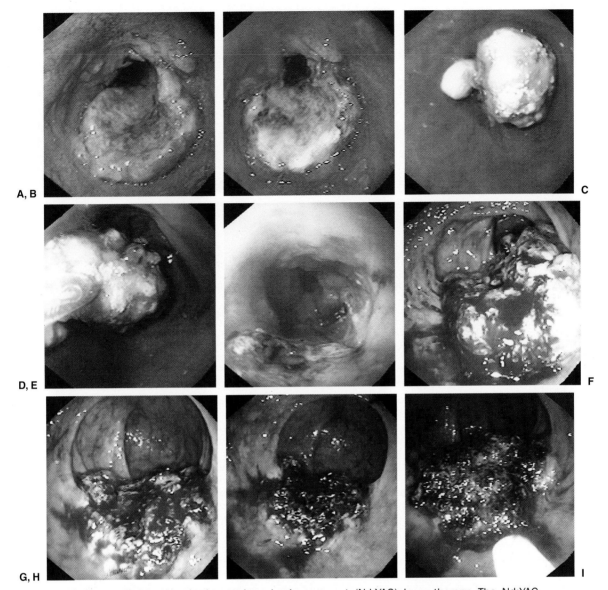

FIGURE 92-14. Neodymium:yttrium-aluminum-garnet (Nd:YAG) laser therapy. The Nd:YAG laser produces deep tissue necrosis relative to other probe-delivered endoscopic ablative modalities. **A, B:** Esophageal cancer before and after laser treatment. The therapy usually is repeated at about 4-week intervals. **C:** Relatively avascular esophageal cancer that is occluding the lumen and has the appearance of a meat impaction. **D:** Such a bulky lesion often is first managed by means of debulking with a polypectomy snare. **E:** After debulking, the laser is applied. Final result shows excellent recanalization of the lumen. In both the colon and the rectum, Nd:YAG laser therapy for obstruction is being supplanted with placement of self-expanding metal stents. However, Nd:YAG laser therapy is still an excellent option for control of hemorrhage from inoperable tumors. **F:** Rectal cancer. **G:** Same tumor as in **F** after debulking with a polypectomy snare. **H:** Tumor after treatment of the remaining surface with the Nd:YAG laser. This treatment provided excellent palliation of bleeding for 6 weeks. **I:** Final result after management of a similar rectal cancer with debulking and surface electrocauterization with an argon plasma coagulator. In our experience, the argon plasma coagulator has the advantages of being very easy to apply in a tangential manner relative to an Nd:YAG laser, produces a very dry (nonbloody) field during therapy, and is a much less expensive piece of equipment. The Nd:YAG laser can be used effectively to manage large benign sessile polyps. *(Continued)*

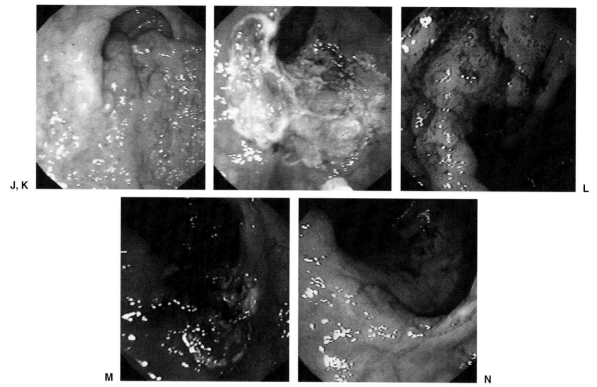

FIGURE 92-14. (Continued) J: Large villous adenoma of the rectum occupies about two thirds of the circumference. We prefer to debulk such lesions by means of submucosal saline injection and snare cauterization. This method preserves the specimen for pathological examination. An Nd:YAG laser is used to destroy tissue at the margins or elsewhere that cannot be removed. **K:** Dark eschar at the edges of the lesion represents tissue treated with a YAG laser. Anecdotal reports indicate the argon plasma coagulator can be effectively used to treat residual flat tissue. Multiple sessions may be needed to manage a lesion. **L, M:** Sessile polyp near the ileocecal valve before and after therapy with strip saline polypectomy and Nd:YAG laser (areas of black eschar). **N:** Inspection 6 weeks later revealed residual polypectomy scar and residual, flat adenoma. Follow-up treatment necessitated application of Nd:YAG laser.

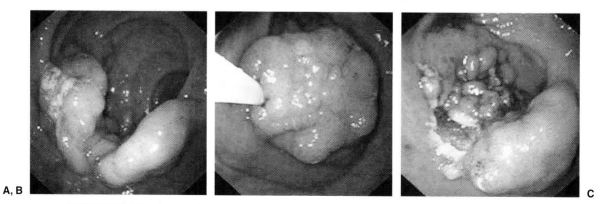

FIGURE 92-15. Argon plasma coagulation (APC) ablation of residual flat adenoma. Our approach, as in Fig. 92-14, is to resect as much polyp as possible by snare cautery, and destroy the residual very flat tissue by APC. **A:** Large sessile rectal adenoma. **B:** Saline with a few drops of methylene blue has been injected and the snare is in place to remove the first fragment. **C:** Immediately after resection of the first fragment. *(Continued)*

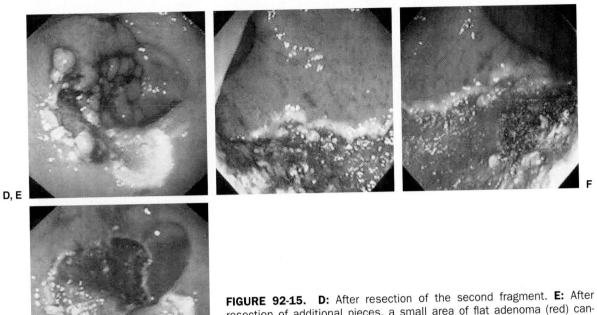

FIGURE 92-15. **D:** After resection of the second fragment. **E:** After resection of additional pieces, a small area of flat adenoma (red) cannot be snare resected. **F:** After ablation of this tissue with APC at power of 65—lower power settings of 40 to 45 are more appropriate in the right colon. **G:** Final appearance of the polypectomy site. The small portion that required ablation is not visible—it is in a poorly accessible area proximal to the rectal valve.

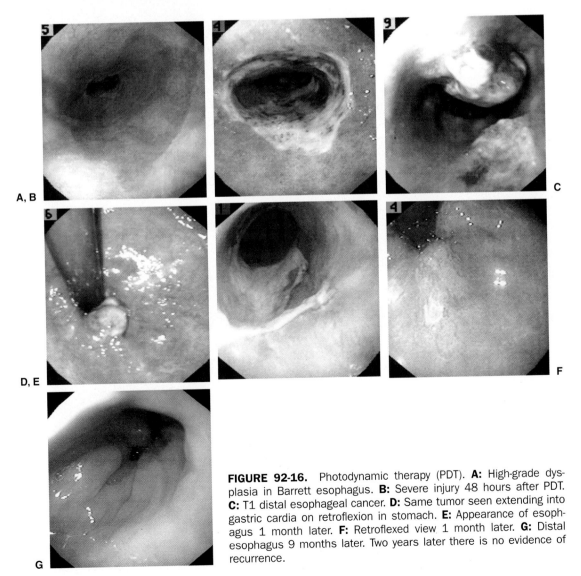

FIGURE 92-16. Photodynamic therapy (PDT). **A:** High-grade dysplasia in Barrett esophagus. **B:** Severe injury 48 hours after PDT. **C:** T1 distal esophageal cancer. **D:** Same tumor seen extending into gastric cardia on retroflexion in stomach. **E:** Appearance of esophagus 1 month later. **F:** Retroflexed view 1 month later. **G:** Distal esophagus 9 months later. Two years later there is no evidence of recurrence.

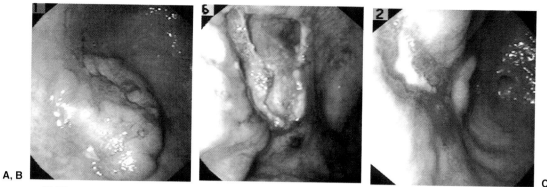

FIGURE 92-17. Endoscopic mucosal resection of early gastric cancer followed by photodynamic therapy (PDT). **A:** T1 cancer in antrum. **B:** Site after endoscopic mucosal resection. **C:** One month later the site was treated by PDT. Photo shows the site 2 months after initial resection. At 18 months there is no evidence of recurrence.

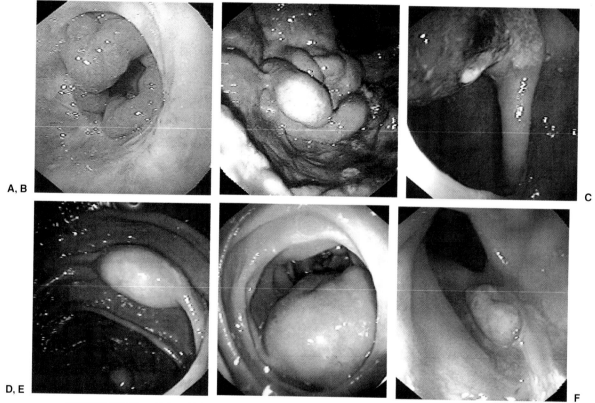

FIGURE 92-18. Polypoid lesions for which polypectomy is not indicated. Many polypoid or tumor-like lesions may appear to be endoscopically removable, but polypectomy might result in serious complications. These examples of lesions considered by trainees to be candidates for endoscopic removal are only a sampling of lesions that must be recognized as being inappropriate for endoscopic treatment. **A:** Redundant mucosa at the esophagogastric anastomosis of a patient who had undergone esophagectomy for esophageal cancer. **B:** Cluster of gastric varices. **C:** Proximal patch of ulcerative colitis. **D:** Colonic lipoma. **E:** Small bowel leiomyoma. **F:** Granulation tissue in a polypectomy site near the dentate line. *(Continued)*

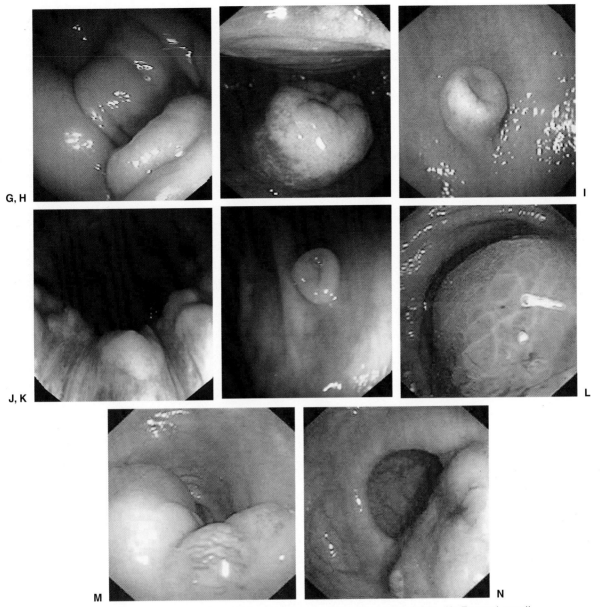

FIGURE 92-18. **G:** Everted small bowel mucosa at the ileocecal valve. **H:** Everted small bowel mucosa at the ileocecal valve; patient has melanosis coli. **I:** Pancreatic rest in the gastric antrum. **J:** Rectal adenoma overgrowing the dentate line. **K:** Everted colonic diverticulum. **L:** Bladder cancer eroding into rectum. **M:** Renal cell cancer eroding into the sigmoid. **N:** Endometrioma in rectovaginal septum.

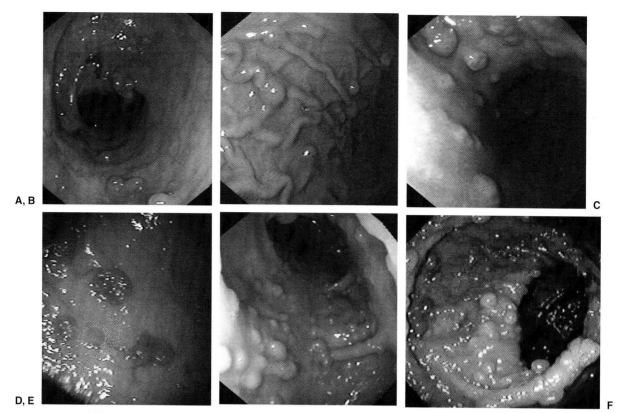

A, B

C

D, E

F

FIGURE 92-19. In some instances polypoid lesions are so numerous that they cannot be removed. The appropriate treatment is surgical. In some instances, removal is unnecessary because the lesions are not neoplastic. Examples include pseudopolyps in a patient with quiescent inflammatory bowel disease (**A**), fundic gland polyps in the stomach of a patient undergoing long-term therapy with proton-pump inhibitors (**B**), inflammatory polyps in the stomach (**C**), multiple lesions of Kaposi sarcoma in the stomach (**D**), and innumerable adenomas in the colon of a patient with familial polyposis (**E**), and multiple hamartomas in the colon of a patient with Cowden syndrome (**F**).

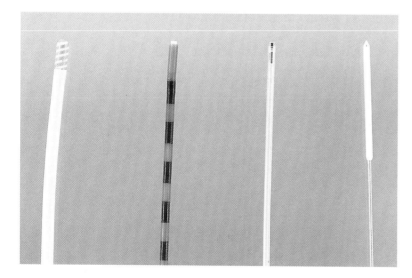

FIGURE 92-20. Probes used in ablative therapy in the gastrointestinal tract. Multipolar electrocoagulation probe, argon plasma coagulation probe, neodymium:yttrium-aluminum-garnet laser probe, and 2.5-cm photodynamic therapy probe are depicted (**left to right**).

93

EVALUATION OF GASTROINTESTINAL MOTILITY

JOHN W. WILEY ■ TIMOTHY T. NOSTRANT ■ CHUNG OWYANG

The goal of gastrointestinal motility testing is to generate information that improves understanding of the normal and abnormal motor patterns in different regions of the gastrointestinal tract. This knowledge may be helpful in making a diagnosis or evaluating responses to therapeutic intervention. The manometric and electrogastrographic procedures discussed in this chapter are generally performed in conjunction with conventional radiologic or endoscopic procedures and nuclear scintigraphic studies.

We begin with examples of esophageal manometry and 24-hour pH monitoring that illustrate our approach to performing these important studies. We chose this "how to do it" focus for these procedures because of their widespread interest to gastroenterologists and the relative paucity of literature with this emphasis. This is followed by sections on ambulatory manometry of the small intestine and electrogastrography, in which are presented examples of how these techniques elucidate the pathophysiological mechanisms that underlie gastrointestinal motility disorders. The final section is devoted to sensorimotor evaluation of anorectal function. The section includes examples of how these techniques can be used to reveal abnormalities associated with incontinence and constipation.

ESOPHAGEAL MANOMETRY AND 24-HOUR pH MONITORING

Esophageal manometry is indicated in the care of patients who have persistent symptoms associated with difficulty in swallowing. The technique can be particularly helpful in identifying achalasia, diffuse esophageal spasm, hypertensive or so-called nutcracker esophagus, and disorders associated with a hypoperistaltic lower esophagus such as scleroderma. At present, 24-hour pH monitoring is the standard for identifying abnormal gastroesophageal reflux. It is also a useful technique for evaluating responses to medical and surgical intervention.

STANDARD ESOPHAGEAL MANOMETRICS AND pH TESTING

Standard testing involves eight distinct examinations. These include measurement of the following:

1. Lower esophageal sphincter pressure (LESP)
2. Lower esophageal sphincter relaxation
3. Esophageal body amplitude, duration, and percentage abnormal contractions
4. Upper esophageal sphincter pressure (UESP)
5. Upper esophageal sphincter relaxation
6. Acid clearance
7. Standard acid reflux testing (basal and acid loaded)
8. Provocative testing

Performance of esophageal manometrics requires close attention to detail. Pressure values differ from laboratory to laboratory and are developed by each esophageal motility unit by means of examining healthy subjects, including persons younger than 40 years and older than 60 years. After normal values have been determined and personnel trained to perform the procedure, preparation of the patient for testing is crucial in obtaining consistent results. Describing the procedure step by step to the patient before testing frequently allows a complete examination, even if the patient is mildly uncomfortable.

Nasal anesthesia with lidocaine or topical cocaine is important because most of the patient's discomfort is centered on catheter movement through the nasal passage. Pharyngeal anesthesia should be avoided because it affects normal swallowing, but it can be used to improve patient comfort if upper sphincter measurements are not needed. After esophageal intubation is accomplished, all three recording transducers are placed in the stomach, as seen with a marker at 65 cm (Fig. 93-1). The position of the catheters can be checked by observing positive deflection of all transducers during abdominal breathing.

The recording catheter is pulled back at a rate of 1 cm/s. The proximal transducer records the proximal edge of the lower esophageal sphincter (LES) at 55 cm. The middle and distal transducers measure LESP at 50 and 45 cm, respectively. The catheter assembly is then returned to the stomach and the process repeated three times. LESP measurements are recorded as the mean of the nine recordings. All measurements are obtained during end expiration, as seen with a flat pneumograph. The pH probe is in the esophagus and records typical esophageal pH as more than 5. Paper speed is 2.5 mm/s and pressure range is 0 to 80 mm Hg.

After LESP measurements are completed, the proximal transducer is placed 5 cm above the LESP (as determined by means of the LESP pull-through) (see Fig. 93-1). The patient is asked to swallow (seen on the pneumograph as darkened squiggles). The middle transducer records immediate relaxation to gastric baseline followed by esophageal body contraction. After esophageal body contraction, LESP returns to baseline. Paper speed is 2.5 mm/s and pressure range is 0 to 200 mm Hg (Fig. 93-2).

All transducers are pulled back into the esophageal body. The distal transducer is placed 2 cm above the LES. The middle and proximal transducers are 7 and 12 cm above the LES, respectively. The patient is asked to swallow. The transducers record sequential movement from proximal to distal transducers (peristalsis) (Fig. 93-3). Some portions of esophageal body contraction may be simultaneous, but the primary wave should be peristaltic (90% or more).

The next manometric values to be measured are UESP, upper esophageal sphincter relaxation, and coordination of the swallowing mechanism. The technique is similar to that of LES measurement. All transducers are first placed in the esophageal body as seen with a marker at 40 cm (Fig. 93-4). The transducers are pulled back at a rate of 1 cm/s. The proximal transducer records UESP at 35 cm. The middle transducer records UESP at 30 cm. Because removal of the distal transducer requires reintubation of the esophagus, only two recordings are made. The process is performed three times, and UESP is recorded as the mean of six measurements. Paper speed is 2.5 mm/s and pressure range is 0 to 200 mm Hg.

After UESP measurements are completed, the proximal transducer is placed in the hypopharynx 5 cm above the recorded upper esophageal sphincter (UES). The middle transducer is in the UES, and the distal transducer is in the proximal esophageal body (Fig. 93-5). Each swallow should be followed by complete UES relaxation and then by hypopharyngeal contraction. After hypopharyngeal contraction ends, UESP returns to baseline, followed by proximal esophageal body contraction. Paper speed is 10 mm/s and pressure range is 0 to 200 mm Hg to record this rapid event adequately.

Conventional esophageal manometric and pH studies are next. The first study is acid clearance. A bolus of 15 mL of 0.1 N hydrochloric acid is placed 10 cm above the pH probe, which is located 5 cm above the LES. Esophageal pH drops to 1, as indicated by the pH probe (Fig. 93-6). The patient is asked to dry swallow every 20 to 30 seconds, as shown by the swallow indicator. Normal values are 15 or fewer dry swallows to return pH to greater than 4. Paper speed is 0.5 to 1.0 mm/s to decrease paper use.

To ascertain the presence of gastroesophageal reflux, standard acid reflux testing is performed after acid clearance studies are completed. The patient is placed in the supine, right decubitus, left decubitus, and prone positions. In each of these positions, the abdomen is compressed, and the patient is asked to perform the Valsalva maneuver. Most healthy persons have no reflux (denoted by pH ≥4 throughout basal studies). This study is performed after loading the stomach with 300 mL 0.1 N hydrochloric acid. After acid loading, healthy persons demonstrate acid reflux in one position at most (Fig. 93-7). To help define an esophageal source for patients with noncardiac chest pain, provocative testing with either edrophonium (80 g/kg) or bethanechol (50 g/kg × 2 separated by 15 minutes) can be performed.

MANOMETRIC EXAMPLES

Achalasia

Achalasia of the esophagus is defined by complete aperistalsis of the esophageal body and impaired LES relaxation. Figure 93-8 demonstrates incomplete relaxation of the LES in example 1, and example 2 shows absent relaxation. Figure 93-9 demonstrates complete absence of esophageal peristalsis. LESP may be increased, but this is not required for the diagnosis.

Diffuse Esophageal Spasm

Simultaneous contractions of the esophagus are the hallmark of diffuse esophageal spasm. Multipeaked waves and contractions of the esophagus not associated with swallowing (spontaneous contractions) also are important findings. At least 30% of contractions with wet swallows should be abnormal (simultaneous, spontaneous, or multipeaked). Peristalsis, however, should be present to some degree. Figures 93-10 through 93-12 show a pattern of progressively worsening diffuse esophageal spasm.

Nutcracker Esophagus

High amplitude of contraction with normal esophageal peristalsis defines nutcracker esophagus (Fig. 93-13). LESP and relaxation are normal. This manometric finding is seen among as many as 50% of patients with noncardiac chest pain.

Hypertensive Lower Esophageal Sphincter

LESP greater than 45 mm Hg and an otherwise normal esophageal manometric examination are the criteria for hypertensive LES (Fig. 93-14). High LESP occurs among 40% of patients with dysphagia.

Progressive Systemic Sclerosis

Multiorgan muscular fibrosis characterizes progressive systemic sclerosis, and the esophagus is the most commonly affected viscus. Esophageal body abnormalities, including simultaneous contractions, spontaneous waves, multipeaked contractions, and even aperistalsis, can be seen early in the disease and produce no symptoms. Involvement of the LES (decreased pressure) usually heralds symptoms of gastroesophageal reflux and dysphagia. Figure 93-15 shows typical manometric findings of this disorder.

Cervical Dysphagia

Cervical dysphagia is seen in a constellation of different diseases that patients relate to "difficulty with swallowing." These include difficulty with initiating swallowing, as with glossopharyngeal dysfunction with cerebrovascular disease, true obstruction caused by UES fibrosis, upper esophageal web formation, or esophageal stricture. Every area from the central nervous system (cerebrovascular disease) to the upper motor neurons (poliomyelitis) to the nerve end plate (myasthenia gravis) and the muscle (dermatomyositis) can be involved and produce similar symptoms. Cerebrovascular disease and UES fibrosis (nemellitine rods) are the most common causes. Manometry is useful only to the small number of patients with definable poor muscle movement, poor UES relaxation, or discoordination of movement between the hypopharynx, UES, and upper esophageal body. Figures 93-16 through 93-18 give classic manometric findings in these conditions.

Gastroduodenal and Small Intestine Manometry

In its present state of refinement, gastroduodenal manometry has been useful in revealing motor patterns in the antroduodenal region during the interdigestive and fed states. In the fasting state, periodic peristaltic activity that migrates caudad from the stomach to the ileocolonic junction occurs approximately every 90 minutes. This has been named the interdigestive migratory motor complex (IMMC), or phase III activity, which is preceded by periods of motor quiescence designated phase I and the irregular, nonperistaltic contractions characteristic of phase II (Fig. 93-19). Ingestion of food results in replacement of the IMMC with an irregular motor pattern (see Fig. 93-19). The pathophysiological significance of putative abnormalities in the normal contractile patterns present in the antrum, pylorus, and duodenum is an area of intensive research.

Gastroduodenal and small intestine manometry has been touted as a potentially useful technique to differentiate primary dysfunction of the intrinsic (enteric) or extrinsic nerves from myopathic disorder. In general, patients with enteric neuropathies have abnormalities in the configuration and propagation of IMMC complexes, poorly propagating bursts or sustained uncoordinated phase activity, and problems in converting from a fasting to a fed postprandial pattern. Diseases that primarily affect gastrointestinal smooth muscle, such as dystrophia myotonica, often result in low-amplitude contractions in the fasting and fed states and an abnormal increase in tonic contractions in the small intestine. For example, patients with diabetic autonomic neuropathy may have abnormalities in generating phase III of the IMMC and postprandial reduction in the frequency and amplitude of antral contractions. Representative tracings of abnormal postcibal antral motility are shown in Fig. 93-20.

An interesting finding among some patients with diabetes and gastroparesis is the presence of pylorospasm (Fig. 93-21). Some patients with diabetes, gastroparesis, and quiescent fasting motor activity respond well to prokinetic agents. Figure 93-22 shows a normal phase III activity front in such a patient after intravenous administration of 10 mg of metoclopramide.

Patients who have undergone upper gastrointestinal operations may demonstrate abnormal postprandial gastrointestinal motility. Abnormal motor patterns have been reported after partial gastrectomy with Roux-en-Y anastomosis. An example of the motor disturbances reported among this group of patients is shown in Fig. 93-23. Gastrointestinal manometry also can be useful in identifying myogenic-type motor abnormalities. An example is shown in Fig. 93-24 from a patient with hereditary hollow visceral myopathy and symptoms of intestinal pseudoobstruction.

Refinements in recording technology allow long-term ambulatory recordings of small intestine motor activity. With the use of this approach, differences in IMMC patterns during sleep versus the awake state have been observed. When a patient is awake, the IMMC cycle typically shows a brief phase I and a prolonged phase II, which are reversed during sleep (Fig. 93-25). Compared with normal healthy subjects, patients with irritable bowel syndrome have a shorter duration of postprandial motor activity. The intervals between IMMCs occurring while awake are shorter among patients with diarrhea predominance than among patients with constipation predominance (Fig. 93-26). Episodes of clustered contractions often are associated with transient abdominal pain in both groups (Fig. 93-27).

Electrogastrography

Smooth muscle cells in the distal two thirds of the stomach demonstrate cyclical electrical activity that is always present and referred to as basal electrical rhythm (BER), or electrical control activity. When basal electrical rhythm is associated with contractions, the amplitude of the electrogastrographic signal is increased and called electrical response activity. In the healthy human stomach, the basal electrical rhythm occurs at a frequency of contractions. Electrogastrography is used to measure the electrical signal emanating from the distal two thirds of the stomach during fasting and stimulated conditions. Patients with persistent unexplained nausea, vomiting, and gastroparesis (chronic idiopathic gastroparesis) demonstrate a variety of electrical abnormalities when examined with electrogastrography and manometry. For example, compared with myoelectric and manometric recordings obtained from the antrums of healthy subjects (Fig. 93-28), patients with chronic idiopathic gastroparesis can demonstrate tachyarrhythmia (Fig. 93-29), bradyarrhythmia (Fig. 93-30), or complex tachyarrhythmia and bradyarrhythmia (Fig. 93-31). In the presence of these electrical abnormalities, no pressure waves are observed. Therefore, the electrical abnormalities may underlie the antral motor dysfunction associated with chronic idiopathic gastroparesis. The sensitivity, specificity, and predictive value of electrogastrographic abnormalities in various clinical settings are the subject of ongoing research. An important feature of the BER is that it represents cyclic depolarization of the smooth muscle cells in the absence of associated peristaltic contractions (Fig. 93-32). Rapid depolarization of the smooth muscle membrane is necessary for a contraction to occur. This event is referred to as an action potential or electrical response activity (see Figure 93-32). Tachygastria and other dysrhythmias have been reported in patients with unexplained nausea, bloating, and vomiting (Fig. 93-33); patients with symptomatic ulcer; children with nonulcer dyspepsia and delayed gastric emptying; pregnant women experiencing nausea (Fig. 93-34); diabetics with chronic nausea, vomiting, and delayed gastric emptying in the fasting state; patients with chronic renal failure; patients with chronic intestinal pseudoobstruction; patients with Parkinson disease; patients with gastric involvement in systemic sclerosis; patients with end-stage liver disease; and normal subjects in whom motion sickness is induced experimentally.

Electronic Barostat

Conventional recording techniques with water-perfused catheters or pressure-sensitive transducers can be used for accurate measurement of changes in intralumenal pressure that reflect phasic contractile activity. However, these recording techniques are less reliable in capacious regions of the gastrointestinal tract, such as the gastric fundus, cecum, and rectum. In addition, conventional intralumenal recording methods provide less reliable measurements of relaxation. The electronic barostat was developed specifically to address these issues (Fig. 93-35). In barostat studies, the objective is to isolate a segment of the gastrointestinal tract without interfering with its function and to follow the movements of the wall. The barostat maintains constant pressure within an air-filled bag positioned in the lumen of the organ being studied. The barostat aspirates air to maintain constant intrabag pressure during contraction and injects air during relaxation. The volume of air entering or leaving the bag is an indirect measurement of changes in the tone of the organ.

A barostat has been used to measure changes in visceral tone in several regions of the gastrointestinal tract. The technique has proved useful in several areas, including assessment of sensory thresholds in the gastrointestinal tract; establishing the role of altered visceral perception in functional bowel disorders; and evaluation of new therapeutic modalities.

A barostat has been used to study gastrointestinal reflex behavior, such as the gastrocolonic reflex and peristaltic reflex. The ability of a barostat to record reliably both increases and decreases in visceral tone makes the instrument suitable for examination of the peristaltic reflex; that is, ascending contraction and descending relaxation. One approach involves placement of a three-balloon catheter in the region of interest (Fig. 93-36). To monitor the peristaltic reflex, the proximal and distal balloons are inflated to the minimal distending pressure. Inflation of the middle stimulus balloon elicits an ascending contraction that is recorded with the proximal recording balloon. To measure the descending response, tone in the distal recording balloon is measured during inflation of the middle stimulus balloon. This method has been used to examine the effect of hyperglycemia on peristaltic reflex in the colons of healthy subjects (Figs. 93-37 and 93-38).

Anorectal Manometry

Disorders of defecation and continence are relatively common, which contributes to the potential usefulness of tests used to evaluate anorectal function. A combination of anorectal manometry, sensory testing (often performed with balloon distention), and electrophysiological recordings can be quite helpful in identifying the cause of problems involving defecation and continence. This approach allows the physician to assess the various components of the neuromuscular circuitry that control defecation and continence under resting and stimulated conditions. Figure 93-39 depicts the anorectal pressure and electrical activity of the external anal sphincter and internal anal sphincter (IAS) of a healthy female subject before, during, and after rectal balloon distention. Balloon distention of the rectum results in decreased sphincter pressure associated with a loss of electrical slow wave oscillation. These findings can be contrasted to those shown in (Fig. 93-40), which shows the recordings obtained from a woman with fecal incontinence. Resting anal pressures are abnormally low and increase during rectal distention, and there is no electrical oscillation of the IAS.

Patients with nonprolapsing hemorrhoids often say they have "constipation" because of difficulties with defecation. Figure 93-41 shows the anorectal manometric and sphincter electrical activities of a patient with nonprolapsing hemorrhoids. The recordings from the outermost channels (outer aspect of the anal canal) indicate no anal relaxation during rectal distention, and the electrical activity of the sphincters is normal. This elevated residual pressure may be caused by high pressure within the vascular spaces.

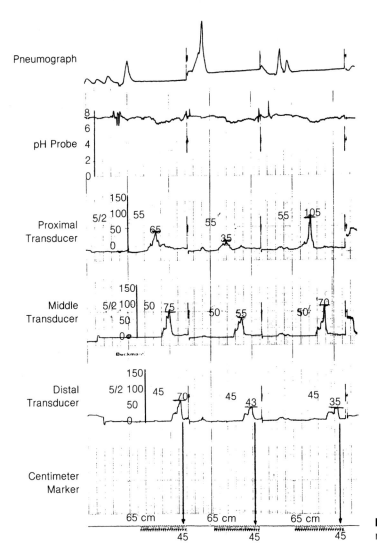

FIGURE 93-1. Lower esophageal sphincter pressure measurements.

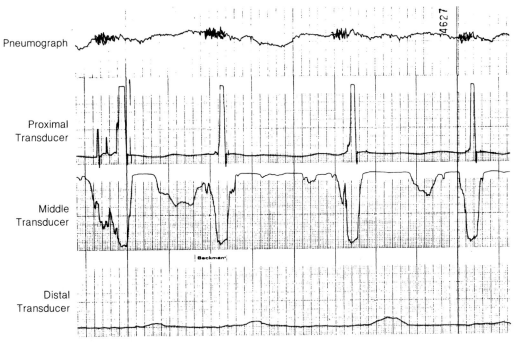

FIGURE 93-2. Lower esophageal sphincter relaxation, normal values. More than 90% of wet swallows are associated with complete relaxation.

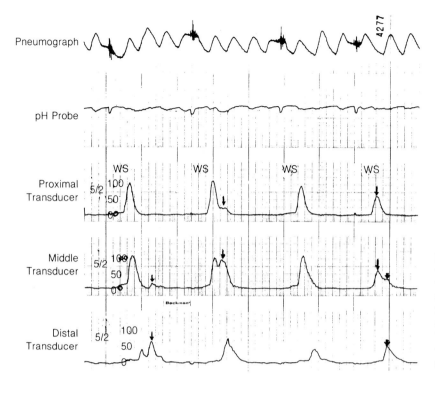

FIGURE 93-3. Esophageal body contractions and peristalsis. Normal values are as follows: amplitude of contraction 30 to 130 mm Hg (persons 40 years of age or older), 30 to 180 mm Hg (persons older than 60 years); duration of contraction less than 7 seconds; percentage abnormal contractions less than 10%; paper speed 2.5 mm/s and pressure range 0 to 200 mm Hg.

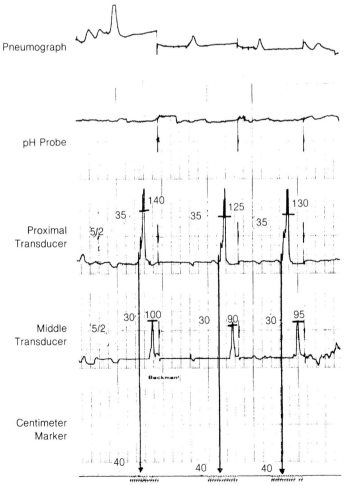

FIGURE 93-4. Upper esophageal sphincter pressure measurement. Normal values are difficult to define. Mean values less than 30 mm Hg or more than 200 mm Hg probably are abnormal.

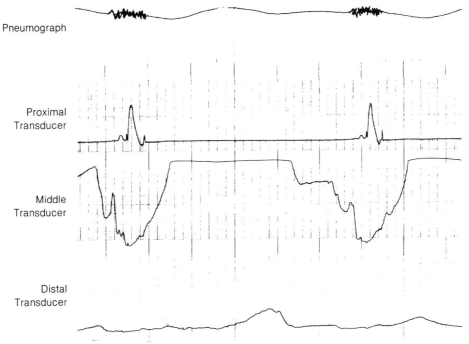

Pneumograph

Proximal
Transducer

Middle
Transducer

Distal
Transducer

FIGURE 93-5. Upper esophageal sphincter relaxation, normal values. More than 90% of wet swallows have complete upper esophageal sphincter relaxation.

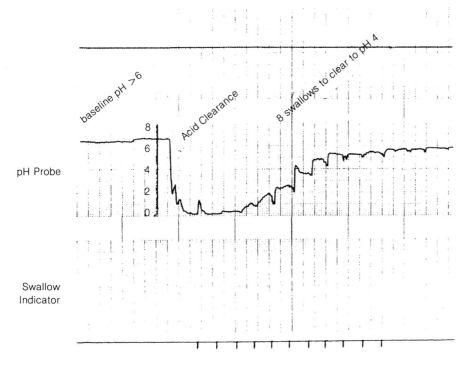

pH Probe

Swallow
Indicator

FIGURE 93-6. Acid clearance. pH is restored to 4 or more in a stepwise manner with each dry swallow. This stepwise pH increase represents salivary neutralization of adherent mucosal acid.

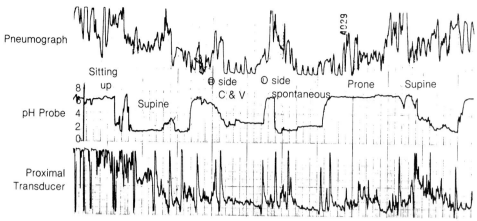

FIGURE 93-7. Standard acid reflux testing. Acid-loaded state. This test starts with placement of 300 mL 0.1 N hydrochloric acid into the stomach and placement of a pH probe 5 cm above the lower esophageal sphincter. The patient is examined in the supine, right decubitus, left decubitus, and prone positions. In each of these positions, the abdomen is compressed, and the patient is asked to perform the Valsalva maneuver (C + V). Most healthy persons have no reflux. In this figure, acid reflux (denoted by drops in pH to 2) occurs in all positions. Paper speed was 2.5 mm/s. This test can be performed without acid loading of the stomach (basal study). Healthy subjects should have no acid reflux during the basal study and acid reflux in no more than one position after acid loading.

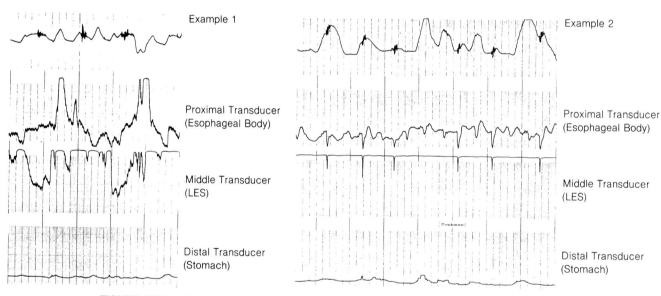

FIGURE 93-8. Achalasia. Incomplete relaxation of the lower esophageal sphincter is shown in example 1, and absent relaxation is shown in example 2.

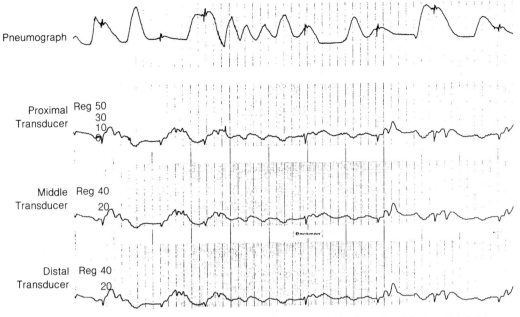

FIGURE 93-9. Achalasia. Complete absence of esophageal body peristalsis (aperistalsis).

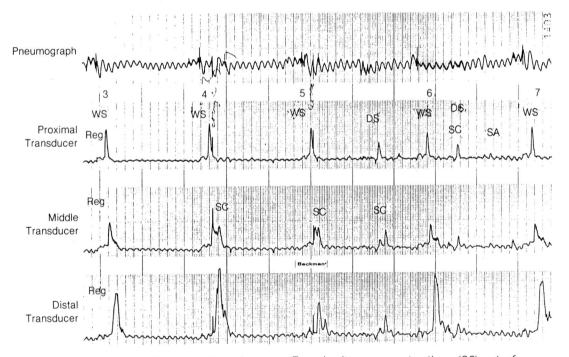

FIGURE 93-10. Diffuse esophageal spasm. Two simultaneous contractions (SC) out of five wet swallows (WS). Peristalsis is still present in three swallows. Triphasic (three-peaked waves) are present in second and third swallows (**left to right**). Spontaneous activity (SA) is present.

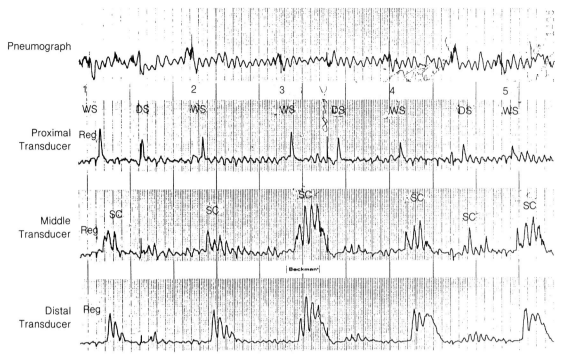

FIGURE 93-11. Diffuse esophageal spasm. Progressively more simultaneous contractions (SC), more multipeaked waves, more spontaneous activity, and longer duration (>15 seconds, paper speed 1 mm/s) contractions are present.

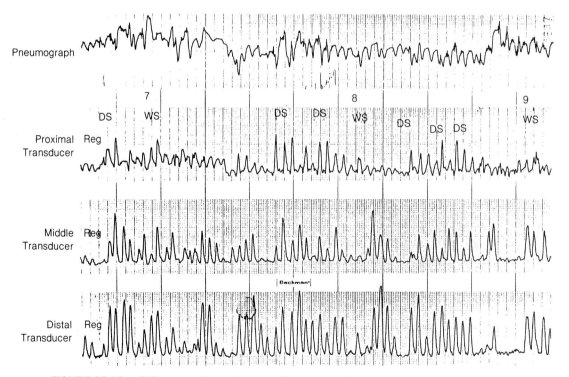

FIGURE 93-12. Diffuse esophageal spasm. Almost complete esophageal body spasm (no return to baseline absence of pressure).

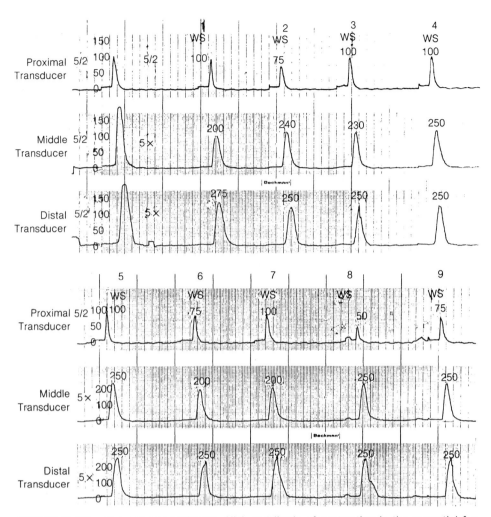

FIGURE 93-13. Nutcracker esophagus. High amplitude of contraction is the essential feature. Peristalsis and lower esophageal sphincter pressure and relaxation are normal. Recordings are taken in the smooth muscle portion of the esophagus. Paper speed is 2.5 mm/s and pressure range is 0 to 400 mm Hg.

Hypertensive LES

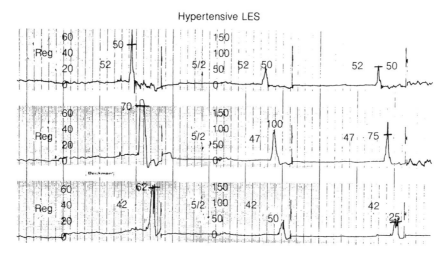

Normal Relaxation   Normal Peristalsis

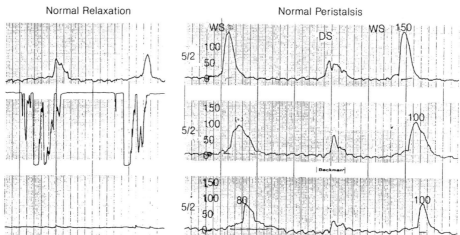

FIGURE 93-14. Hypertensive lower esophageal sphincter. Increased lower esophageal sphincter pressure (>45 mm Hg) is the criterion for diagnosis. Lower esophageal sphincter relaxation and esophageal body peristalsis are normal. If the initial pressure range (**left side**) is 0 to 80 mm Hg, lower esophageal sphincter pressure is not accurately measured. Pressure range is changed to 0 to 200 mm Hg (increased physiographic sensitivity) (**right side of graph**).

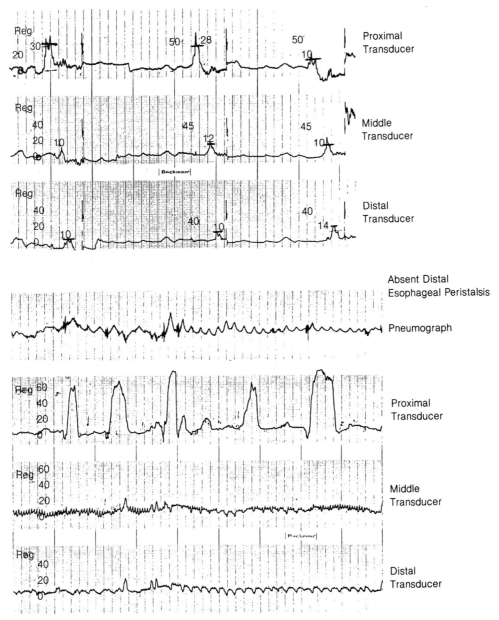

FIGURE 93-15. Progressive systemic sclerosis. Image shows involvement of the lower esophageal sphincter and esophageal body. Lower esophageal sphincter pressure is decreased, and esophageal body contraction is absent in the smooth muscle portion of the esophagus (middle and distal transducers) but normal in the proximal skeletal portion (proximal transducer). Paper speed is 2.5 mm/s and pressure range is 0 to 80 mm Hg.

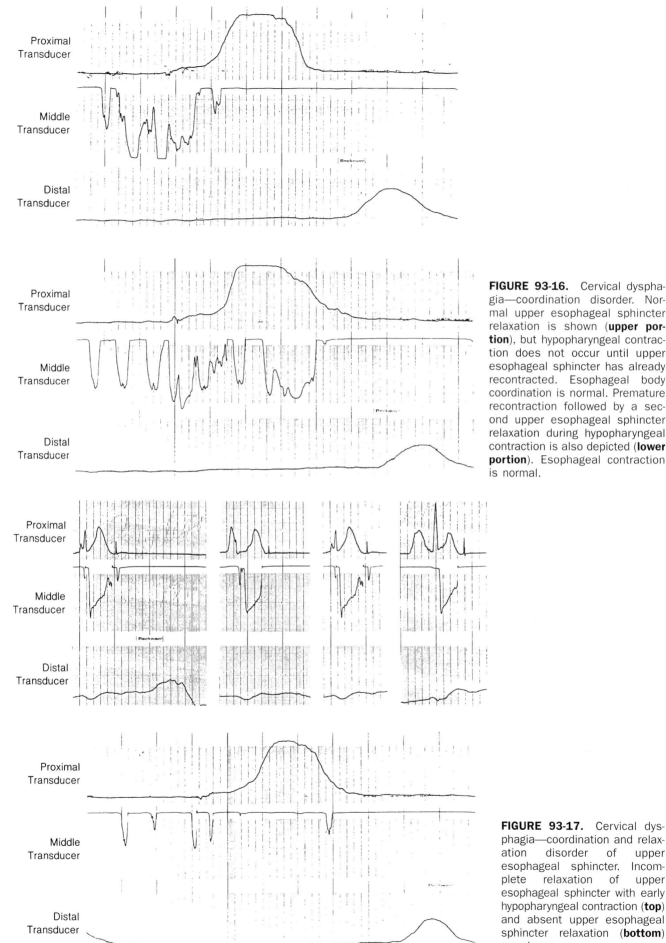

Proximal
Transducer

Middle
Transducer

Distal
Transducer

FIGURE 93-16. Cervical dysphagia—coordination disorder. Normal upper esophageal sphincter relaxation is shown (**upper portion**), but hypopharyngeal contraction does not occur until upper esophageal sphincter has already recontracted. Esophageal body coordination is normal. Premature recontraction followed by a second upper esophageal sphincter relaxation during hypopharyngeal contraction is also depicted (**lower portion**). Esophageal contraction is normal.

FIGURE 93-17. Cervical dysphagia—coordination and relaxation disorder of upper esophageal sphincter. Incomplete relaxation of upper esophageal sphincter with early hypopharyngeal contraction (**top**) and absent upper esophageal sphincter relaxation (**bottom**) are shown.

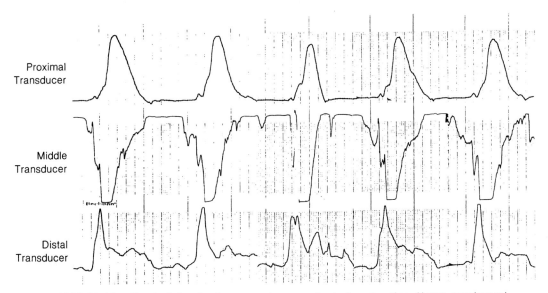

FIGURE 93-18. Cervical dysphagia—premature esophageal contraction. Upper esophageal sphincter relaxation and coordination with hypopharyngeal contraction is normal. Esophageal body contraction occurs with upper esophageal sphincter relaxation, which prevents bolus movement.

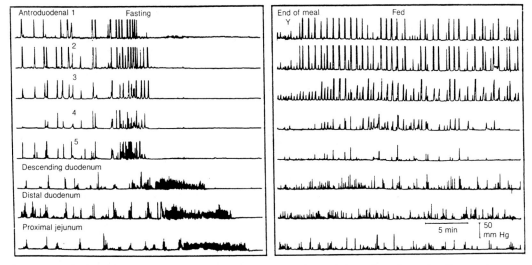

FIGURE 93-19. Normal gastrointestinal motility. Normal interdigestive migrating motor complex (fasting) is shown (**left**). Tracing shows phase III activity in the antrum, pressure activity gradually moving into the duodenum, and gradual change in configuration of the waves as they move through the antroduodenal junction. Normal fed activity is also shown (**right**). Irregular but persistent phasic pressure activity is present in the distal antrum and proximal small bowel.

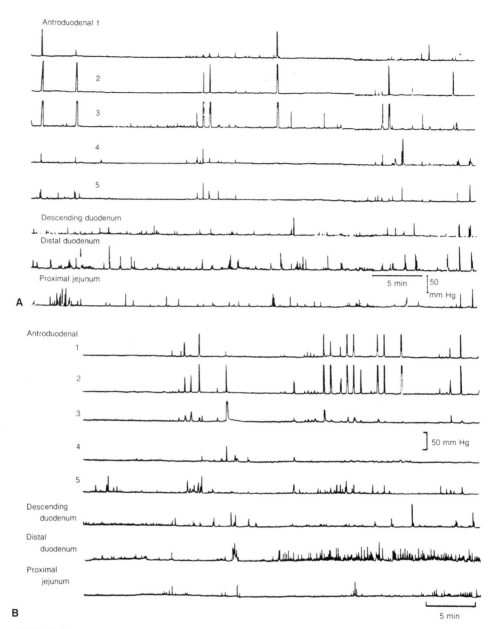

FIGURE 93-20. **A:** Diabetic gastroparesis with decreased frequency of postcibal antral contractions. A 19-year-old woman had a history of insulin-independent diabetes and associated peripheral neuropathy for 10 years, and anorexia and nausea for 6 months. Antral waves that are visible are of normal amplitude and duration but are separated by prolonged gaps. An esophageal motility study (not shown) indicated imperfect propagation of deglutition waves; swallows sometimes were followed by a propagated wave and sometimes were not. **B:** Diabetic gastroparesis with antral hypomotility. A 27-year-old woman had juvenile-onset diabetes (at age 12 years) and retinopathy. Severe episodes of nausea and vomiting associated with constipation had occurred during the previous year. Tracing shows postcibal hypomotility characterized mainly by absence of phasic pressure activity alternating with periods of normal-amplitude phasic pressure activity. Intestinal fed pattern is normal.

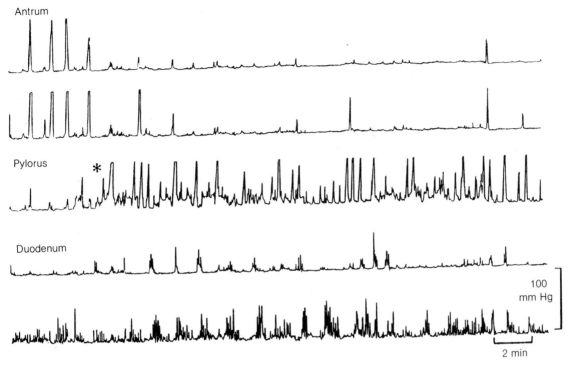

FIGURE 93-21. Episode of pylorospasm in 28-year-old woman with diabetes and gastroparesis syndrome. A marked increase in baseline pressure with associated phasic activity consists of mixed antral-type and duodenal-type waves (*asterisk*).

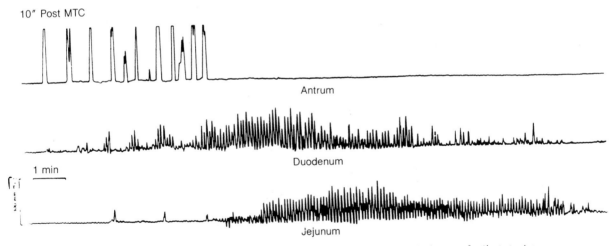

FIGURE 93-22. Effect of 10 mg metoclopramide in intravenous bolus on fasting gastroduodenal motor pattern in a patient with diabetic gastroparesis. The patient did not generate an interdigestive migratory motor complex during the hours of recording before administration of the drug. Phase III shows normal antral and intestinal contractions and propagation.

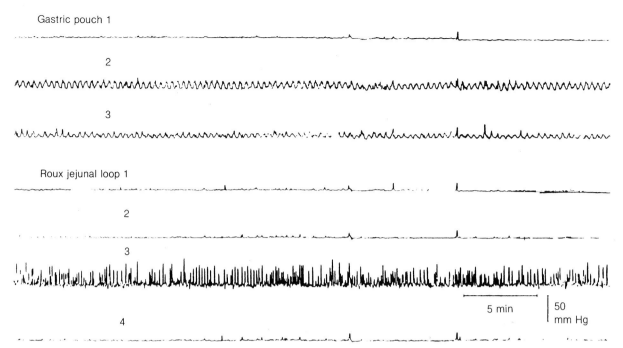

FIGURE 93-23. Postsurgical intestinal dysmotility in a 59-year-old woman. The history, covering 25 years, began with symptoms consistent with gastric outlet obstruction caused by peptic ulcer disease. A succession of gastric operations, ending in partial gastrectomy with Roux-en-Y anastomosis, did not relieve the nausea and vomiting. Tracing shows low-amplitude broad-based waves at slightly less than three per minute in the gastric pouch. In the intestine is a band of continuous activity in the jejunum alternating with others of quiescence.

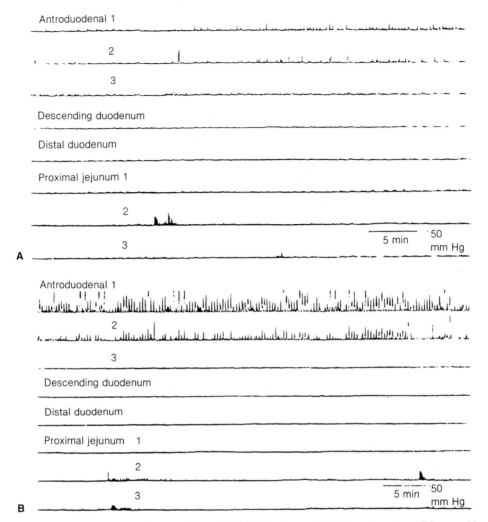

FIGURE 93-24. Myogenic-type idiopathic intestinal pseudoobstruction in a 73-year-old woman with hereditary hollow visceral myopathy. Over a 20-year period, she had multiple operations for recurrent episodes of small bowel obstruction (lysis of adhesions) and constipation. One year previously, a total colectomy was performed. Several relatives had the same condition. **A:** Fast tracing shows marked paucity of phasic pressure activity in the intestine except for small groups of contractions. Distal antrum and duodenal cap show more intense activity. **B:** Postprandially, normal-appearing antropyloric activity is visible. In contrast, the intestine shows a marked paucity of activity with a few groups of contractions and resembles the fasting pattern.

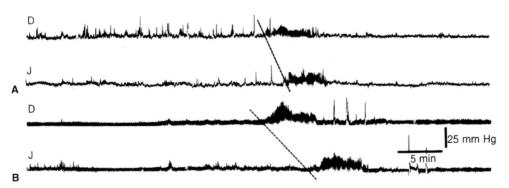

FIGURE 93-25. Typical interdigestive migratory motor complex in an awake subject (**A**) and a subject during nocturnal sleep (**B**). The *diagonal lines* connect the time of onset of phase III at the duodenal (*D*) and jejunal (*J*) sensors. There is diminished propagation velocity of phase III and a virtual absence of phase II activity during sleep.

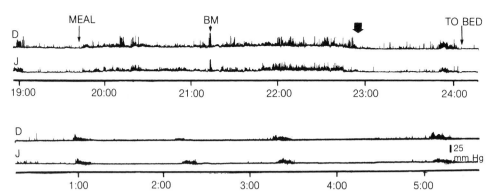

FIGURE 93-26. Continuous recording of duodenal (*D*) and jejunal (*J*) motor activity for a walking healthy subject. After a phase III activity front, the subject ate the evening meal at 7:45 PM, and postprandial duodenojejunal motor activity was established. Termination of the postprandial motor pattern (*large arrow*) was identified with the onset of motor quiescence, which marked reestablishment of fasting motor activity. After the patient went to bed, interdigestive migratory motor complexes occurred regularly. There is a virtual absence of phase II motor activity during the nocturnal period. A bowel movement (*BM*) occurred 90 minutes after the meal.

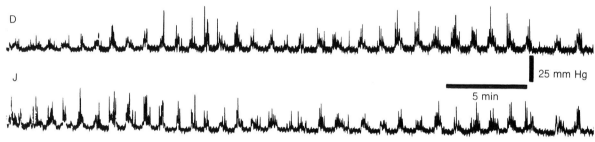

FIGURE 93-27. Clustered contractions during phase II fasting activity recorded in both the duodenum (*D*) and jejunum (*J*) of a patient with irritable bowel syndrome.

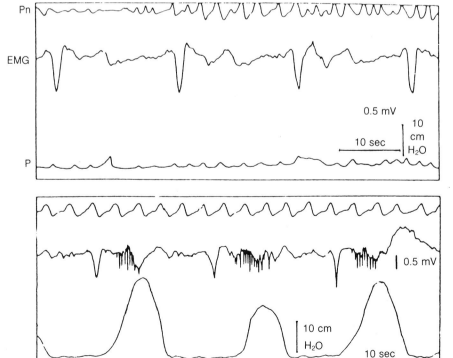

FIGURE 93-28. Myoelectric (*EMG*) and manometric (*P*) recordings obtained from the gastric antrum of a healthy subject during a period of absence of pressure waves (**top**) and a period of contractile activity (**bottom**). The electrical control activity has a frequency of about 3 cycles/min, and the action potentials appear after the control potential in correspondence with the appearance of pressure waves (time constant = 1 second; monopolar). *Pn,* pneumogram.

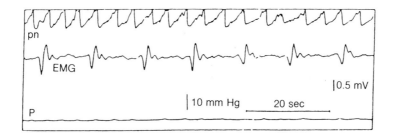

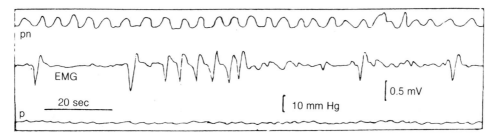

FIGURE 93-29. Tachygastria recorded from the gastric antrum of a patient with chronic idiopathic gastroparesis (**top**) is shown. Short run of tachyarrhythmia at a frequency greater than 10 cycles/min was recorded for the same subject (**bottom**). Pressure waves are absent in both instances (time constant = 1 second; monopolar). *p,* manometry; *pn,* pneumogram.

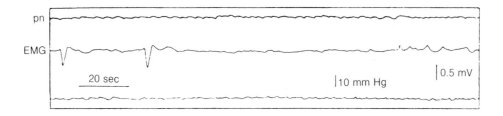

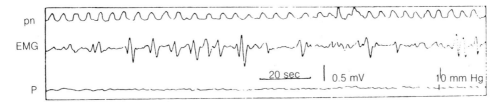

FIGURE 93-30. Examples of severe myoelectric arrhythmia recorded for a patient with chronic idiopathic gastroparesis. Electrical "asystole" after a period of bradygastria (**top**) and complete disorganization of myoelectric activity (**bottom**) are shown (time constant = 1 second; monopolar). *P,* manometry; *pn,* pneumogram.

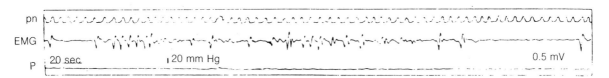

FIGURE 93-31. Complex arrhythmia formed by periods of tachyarrhythmia and bradyarrhythmia, disorganized electrical activity, and electrical "asystole" recorded for a patient with chronic idiopathic gastroparesis. No pressure wave was recorded during this period (time constant = 0.3 second; monopolar). *P,* manometry; *pn,* pneumogram.

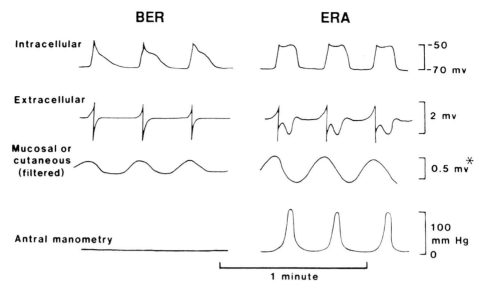

FIGURE 93-32. Stylized representation of intracellular, extracellular, and mucosal or cutaneous (filtered) electrogastrographic signals, with accompanying manometric activity. Basal electrical activity (BER) and electrical response activity (ERA) are represented. Basal electrical activity may cause some contractile activity but does not result in gastric peristalsis and usually is not detected by manometry. (*Voltage shown is for cutaneous recording; mucosal recordings approach 2 mV.)

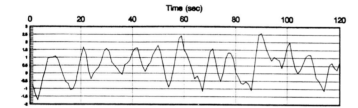

A

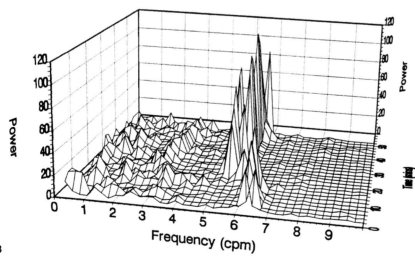

B

FIGURE 93-33. Electrogastrography (EGG) was used to evaluate a 28-year-old woman with persistent nausea, bloating, and fullness who had previously undergone a solid-phase gastric emptying scan, which yielded normal results. **A:** A low-amplitude raw EGG signal after ingestion of a 250-kcal liquid meal with a period of approximately 10 seconds. The raw EGG signal was evaluated with power spectral analysis. **B:** The pseudo–three-dimensional plot demonstrates the presence of a dominant slow-wave frequency that is higher (5–6 cpm) than in the healthy volunteer. This patient showed evidence of tachygastria, which was associated with antral hypomotility on a simultaneously performed manometric study. (Courtesy of William L. Hasler, M.D., Ann Arbor, MI.)

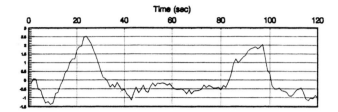

A

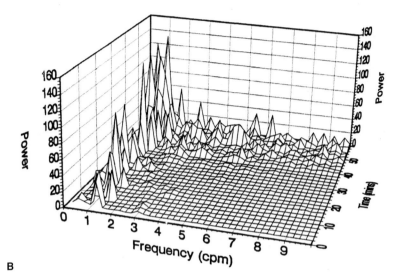

B

FIGURE 93-34. Women with nausea in the first trimester of pregnancy can exhibit marked slow wave disturbances. Electrogastrography was performed on a 22-year-old woman in the 11th week of pregnancy. **A:** Large but infrequent slow waves are seen on the raw tracing. **B:** Pseudo–three-dimensional plotting of the power spectral analysis demonstrates that the bulk of the slow-wave signal is in the frequency range from 0.75 to 2 cpm. This pregnant patient exhibited bradygastria in association with her first trimester nausea. (Courtesy of William L. Hasler, M.D., Ann Arbor, MI.)

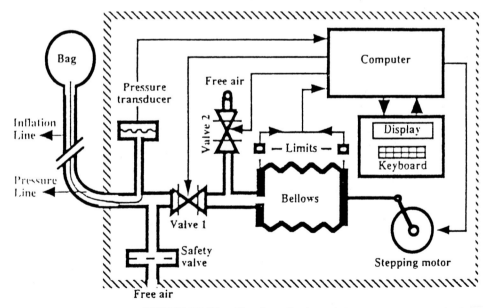

FIGURE 93-35. Circuitry of a barostat.

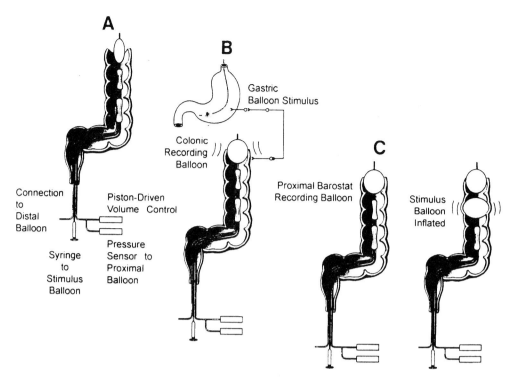

FIGURE 93-36.   Apparatus used for induction and measurement of the gastrocolonic response and the peristaltic reflex. **A:** Three-balloon catheter connected to a barostat and inflation devices is in the descending colon. **B:** Through activation of an extrinsic neural pathway, mechanical distention of the gastric antrum (100–300 mL) results in a volume-dependent increase in tonic motor activity in a recording balloon in the descending colon that is inflated to the minimal distending pressure. **C:** For the peristaltic reflex, the proximal balloon is inflated to the minimal distending pressure. Inflation of the middle stimulus balloon elicits an ascending contraction that is recorded with the proximal recording balloon. To measure the descending response, tone in the distal recording balloon is measured during inflation of the middle stimulus balloon.

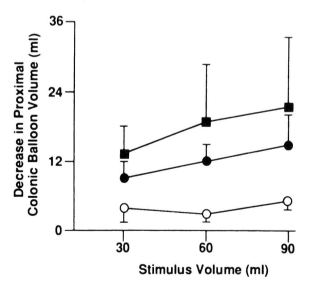

FIGURE 93-37.   The ascending contractile limb of the peristaltic reflex is quantified as a decrease in proximal balloon volume after stimulation. Inflation of the stimulus balloon results in volume-dependent decreases in proximal balloon volume under control conditions (v), which are blunted during hyperglycemic clamping (j; $P < 0.05$). In contrast, euglycemic, hyperinsulinemic clamping (m) has no effect on the ascending contraction compared with control value. All results are mean $\pm$SEM; $n = 4$.

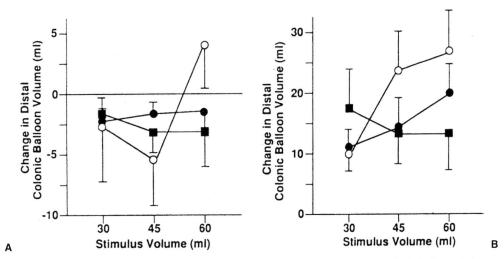

FIGURE 93-38. The descending components of the peristaltic reflex. **A:** Inflation of the stimulus balloon produces initial relaxation quantified as an increase in distal balloon volume, which is followed by **B,** an intense contraction quantified as a decrease in distal balloon volume. In contrast to the situation with the ascending contraction, hyperglycemic clamping (*j*) does not blunt descending relaxation or contraction compared with control conditions (*v*). Similarly, euglycemic, hyperinsulinemic clamping (*m*) does not modify either descending response. All results are mean ±SEM; *n* = 4.

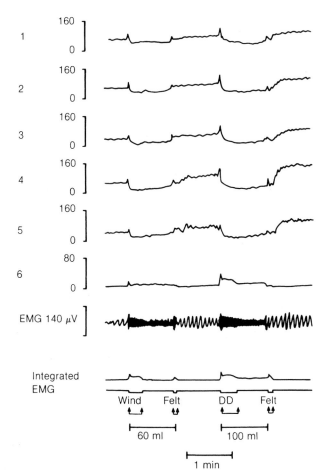

FIGURE 93-39. Recordings of anorectal pressure and the electrical activity of the external anal sphincter (EAS) and internal anal sphincter (IAS) of a typical healthy female subject before, during, and after inflation of a rectal balloon with 60 and 100 mL of air. Channels 1 to 6 represent ports situated 0.5, 1.0, 1.5, 2.0, 2.5, and 4.5 cm from the anal margin. Rectal distention (60, 100 mL) induces relaxation in sphincter pressure associated with abolition of the electrical oscillations, produced by IAS activity, and an increase in electrical activity of the EAS. Deflation produces a rebound increase in pressure associated with a marked increase in slow-wave oscillation. The point when the subject experienced rectal sensation is indicated (*bars*). *DD,* desire to defecate.

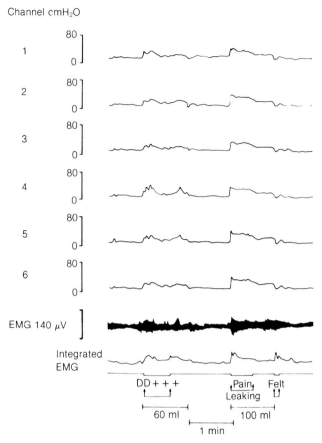

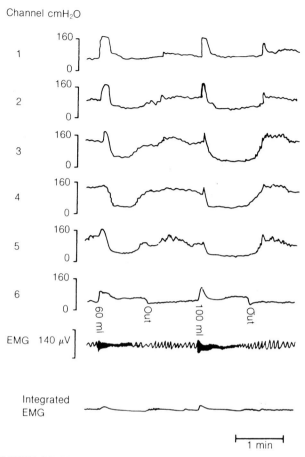

FIGURE 93-40. Recordings of anorectal pressure and electrical activity of the sphincter of a female patient with fecal incontinence. Recordings were made before, during, and after inflation of a rectal balloon with 60 and 100 mL of air. Channels 1 to 6 represent ports situated 0.5, 1.0, 1.5, 2.0, 2.5, and 4.5 cm from the anal margin. There is no internal anal sphincter electrical activity. Anal pressure is abnormally low and increases during rectal distension. This increase is associated with an increase in the electrical activity of the external anal sphincter. No rebound pressures occur with deflation of the rectal balloon. The point when the subject experienced rectal sensation and the severity of the sensation are indicated (*bars*). *DD,* desire to defecate.

FIGURE 93-41. Recordings of anorectal pressure and electrical activity of the external and internal anal sphincters during rectal balloon distention with 60 and 100 mL of air. Patient has nonprolapsing hemorrhoids. Channels 1 and 6 are situated at 0.5, 1.0, 1.5, 2.0, 2.5, and 4.5 cm from the anal margin. There was no anal relaxation in the outermost channels, and the electrical activity of the external and internal anal sphincters was similar to that of healthy subjects.

94

PLAIN AND CONTRAST RADIOLOGY

MARC S. LEVINE ■ STEPHEN E. RUBESIN ■ HANS HERLINGER ■ IGOR LAUFER

Plain radiographs of the abdomen are useful for evaluating abdominal pain or distention, obstructive symptoms, or clinical signs of an acute abdomen. The combination of supine and upright or decubitus horizontal beam radiographs allows the diagnosis of ileus as opposed to obstruction of the small bowel or colon, free intraperitoneal air (pneumoperitoneum) (Fig. 94-1), ischemic or necrotic bowel with air in the bowel wall (pneumatosis) (Fig. 94-2), air in the bile ducts (pneumobilia), and portal venous gas (Fig. 94-3). Nevertheless, computed tomographic (CT) scanning has been recognized as a more sensitive modality for evaluating acute abdominal symptoms (see Chapter 97).

Double-contrast radiography is a valuable technique for diagnosing a wide spectrum of pathological processes in the gastrointestinal tract. Because this technique can delineate normal mucosal surface patterns in the pharynx, upper gastrointestinal tract, small bowel, and colon, it is particularly helpful in detecting a variety of inflammatory or neoplastic diseases involving the mucosa. In some cases, barium studies may demonstrate abnormalities that are missed or misinterpreted at endoscopic examination. The double-contrast study is a less expensive and less invasive procedure than endoscopy. We therefore believe that double-contrast radiography and endoscopy should be considered complementary procedures for evaluating suspected gastrointestinal disease.

Double-contrast radiography can delineate in detail the normal anatomic features of the pharynx (Fig. 94-4). As a result, inflammatory (Fig. 94-5) or neoplastic (Figs. 94-6 and 94-7) lesions that disrupt or obliterate the normal anatomic landmarks can be demonstrated readily. In the upper gastrointestinal tract, double-contrast techniques allow detection of esophagitis caused by plaques or ulcers (Fig. 94-8), esophageal cancer (Fig. 94-9), benign gastric ulcer (Fig. 94-10), early gastric cancer (Fig. 94-11), duodenal ulcer (Fig. 94-12), erosive gastritis or duodenitis, and other inflammatory or neoplastic lesions. Radiographic enema examination of the small bowel has proved to be a much more sensitive technique than conventional small bowel follow-through examination for determining the site and cause of small bowel obstruction (Fig. 94-13) and a variety of other abnormalities in the small bowel (Figs. 94-14 through 94-16). Double-contrast barium enema examination is a valuable technique for detecting colonic polyps or carcinoma (Fig. 94-17) and for diagnosing inflammatory bowel disease (granulomatous and ulcerative colitis) or its complications (Fig. 94-18). Double-contrast studies may be performed to evaluate the colon after a surgical procedure (Fig. 94-19). Although rare, complications of these studies may be encountered (Fig. 94-20).

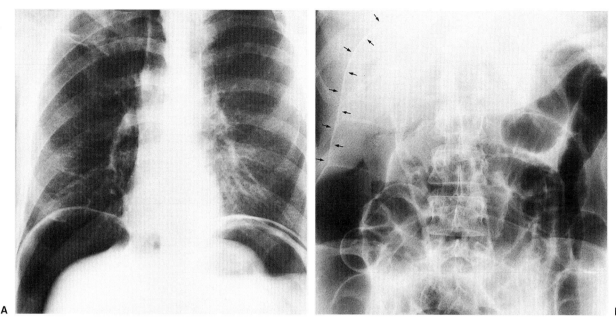

FIGURE 94-1. Pneumoperitoneum. **A:** Upright chest radiograph shows large amounts of free intraperitoneal air beneath both sides of the diaphragm of this patient with perforated duodenal ulcer. **B:** Supine plain radiograph of the abdomen of another patient shows an indirect sign of pneumoperitoneum, air on both sides of the bowel wall (Rigler sign; *arrows*), after perforation at colonoscopy.

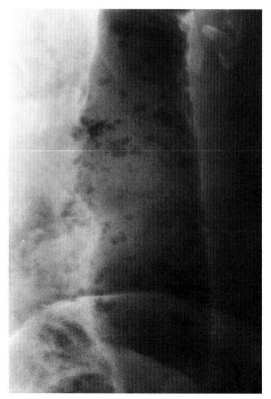

FIGURE 94-2. Pneumatosis caused by infarction of the left colon after a surgical procedure. Close-up view of supine plain radiograph of the abdomen shows tiny, mottled and linear collections of gas in the wall of the descending colon.

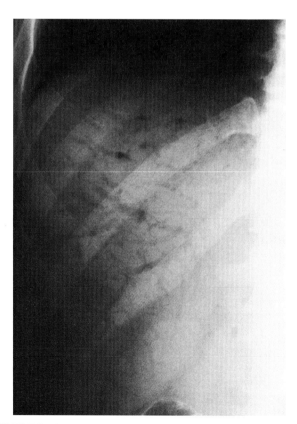

FIGURE 94-3. Close-up view of the right upper quadrant on supine plain radiograph of the abdomen shows linear, branching collections of gas in the portal venous system caused by intestinal infarction. Gas shadows extend to the periphery of the liver. This appearance is characteristic of portal venous gas.

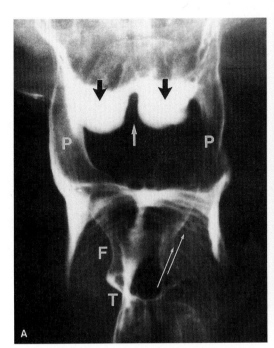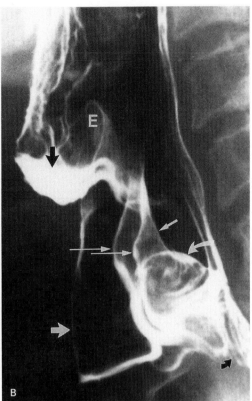

FIGURE 94-4. Normal pharyngeal anatomy. **A:** Frontal view of pharynx shows cup-shaped valleculae (*black arrows*) separated by median glossoepiglottic fold (*short white arrow*). More inferiorly, pyriform sinuses (*P*) form the anterior portion of lateral food channels. The arcuate line (*long white arrows*) is caused by normal laryngeal impression on the collapsed hypopharynx. In this case, both true (*T*) and false (*F*) vocal cords are outlined with aspirated barium in the larynx. **B:** Lateral view during phonation shows epiglottic tip (*E*), valleculae (*short black arrow*), aryepiglottic folds (*medium-length white arrow*), and anterior walls of pyriform sinuses (*long white arrows*). Redundant mucosal folds overlie the muscular process of the arytenoid cartilages (*curved white arrow*) and cricoid cartilage (*curved black arrow*). Aspirated barium outlines laryngeal vestibule (*short white arrow*) and ventricle.

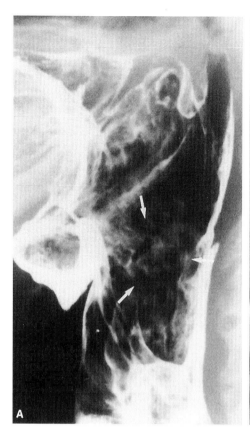
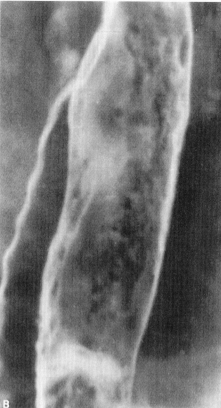

FIGURE 94-5. *Candida* pharyngitis and esophagitis in an immunosuppressed patient undergoing chemotherapy for metastatic breast cancer. **A:** Lateral view of pharynx shows small, sharply circumscribed plaques (*arrows*) in hypopharynx. **B:** Double-contrast esophagogram also shows multiple plaque-like lesions in the esophagus caused by concomitant *Candida* esophagitis.

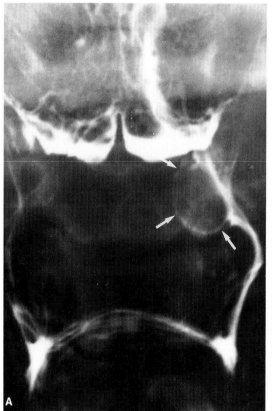
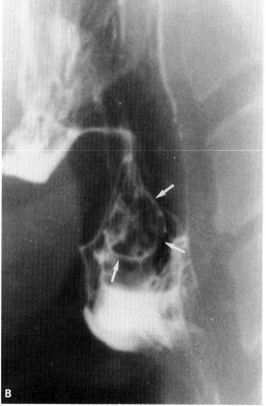

FIGURE 94-6. Aryepiglottic fold cyst. **A:** Frontal view of pharynx shows cyst as a smooth submucosal mass (*arrows*) with approximately 90° angle between the border of the mass and adjacent pharyngeal wall. **B:** Lateral view shows lesion as a round, sharply circumscribed mass (*arrows*).

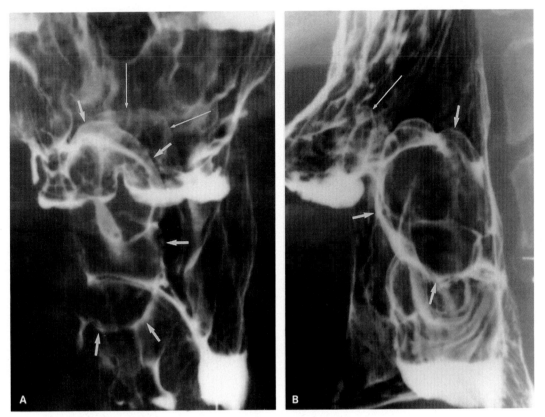

FIGURE 94-7. Squamous cell carcinoma of hypopharynx. **A:** Frontal view of pharynx shows large polypoid mass (*short arrows*) obliterating right lateral wall of hypopharynx. Tumor extends across midline. Valleculae and tip of epiglottis (*long arrows*) are preserved. **B:** Lateral view demonstrates lobulated mass (*short arrows*) in hypopharynx. Epiglottic tip (*long arrow*) is preserved.

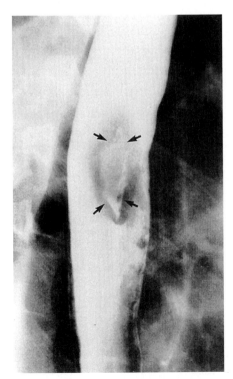

FIGURE 94-8. Single-contrast esophagram shows a giant, diamond-shaped ulcer (*arrows*) with a surrounding radiolucent rim of edema in the midesophagus. Patient has human immunodeficiency virus (HIV) infection and odynophagia. Endoscopic biopsy specimens, brushings, and cultures revealed no evidence of cytomegalovirus infection, so the ulcer probably was caused directly by HIV infection (idiopathic or HIV-related ulcer).

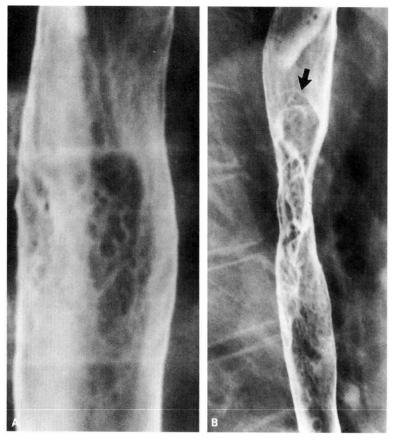

FIGURE 94-9. Esophageal carcinoma. **A:** Superficial spreading carcinoma with focal nodularity of midesophagus caused by tiny, coalescent nodules and plaques. **B:** Advanced esophageal carcinoma with irregular narrowing of lumen. Mucosal destruction and abrupt, shelf-like upper border of tumor are indicated (*arrow*).

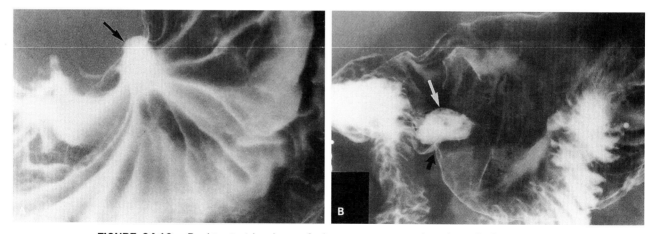

FIGURE 94-10. Benign gastric ulcers. **A:** Lesser curvature ulcer (*arrow*). Smooth folds radiate to edge of crater. This lesion fulfills the radiologic criteria for benign gastric ulcer. **B:** Greater curvature ulcer (*white arrow*) caused by aspirin ingestion. Deformity of greater curvature (*black arrow*) is depicted adjacent to ulcer.

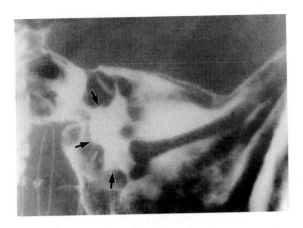

FIGURE 94-11. Early gastric cancer manifested by irregular ulcer (*arrows*) on posterior wall of antrum with scalloped borders and nodular, clubbed folds surrounding ulcer.

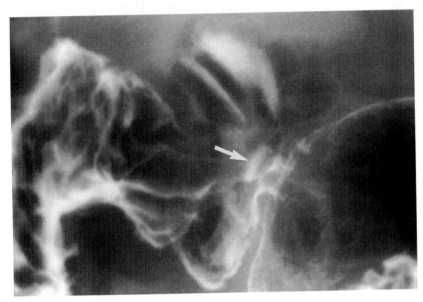

FIGURE 94-12. Linear duodenal ulcer (*arrow*) at base of bulb. Thickened folds are present above ulcer.

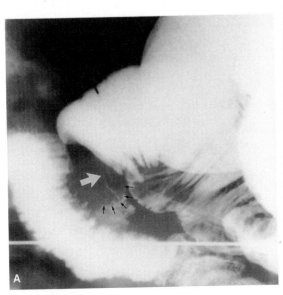

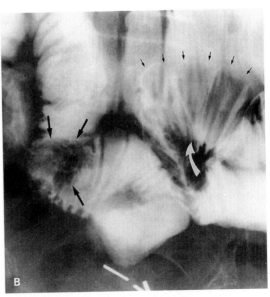

FIGURE 94-13. Small bowel metastases causing obstruction. **A:** High-grade small bowel obstruction caused by annular metastasis from gastric carcinoma. Tight, constricted segment (*white arrow*) and distal mass effect (*black arrows*) are visible. **B:** Partially obstructing metastases from sigmoid carcinoma. One metastasis causes spiculation and fixation of small bowel wall (*white arrow*) with normal distensibility of opposite wall (*small black arrows*). Another metastasis appears en face as a filling defect (*large black arrows*) causing distortion of folds.

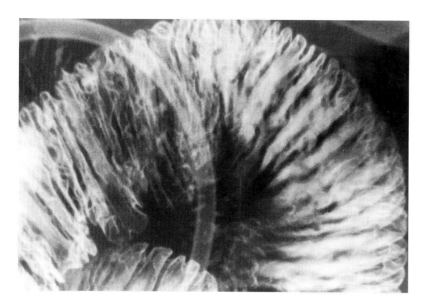

FIGURE 94-14. Intestinal lymphangiectasia manifested by thickened, mildly irregular folds and tiny nodules representing engorged villi.

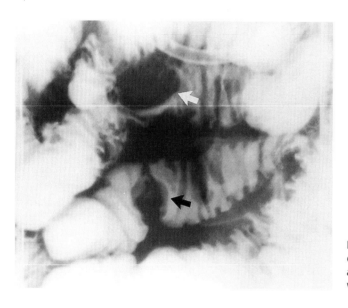

FIGURE 94-15. Carcinoid tumors in ileum. The smaller, more distal lesion appears as smooth submucosal mass (*black arrow*). However, a larger lesion (*white arrow*) is associated with outward extension into the mesentery.

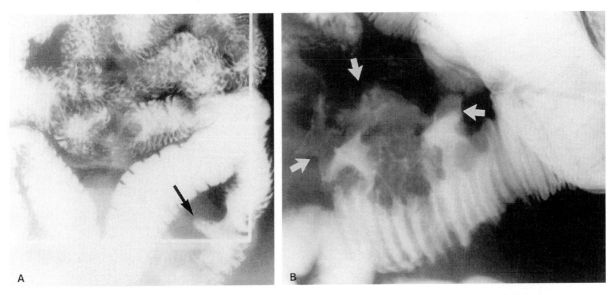

FIGURE 94-16. Non-Hodgkin lymphoma of small bowel. **A:** Radiograph from small-bowel meal follow-through study shows focal obliteration of folds of small bowel with associated ulcer (*arrow*) on mesenteric border of bowel. Because of a history of systemic lupus erythematosus, these findings were attributed to lupus-related vasculitis. **B:** Spot radiograph from enema examination of the small bowel performed during later hospital admission shows exoenteric excavation (*arrows*) from previously ulcerated area. This finding is characteristic of non-Hodgkin lymphoma involving the small bowel.

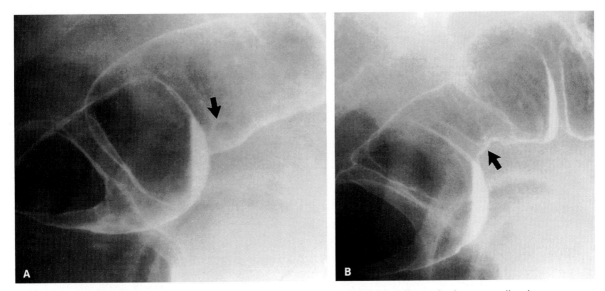

FIGURE 94-17. Development of colonic carcinoma. **A:** Initial radiograph shows small polypoid lesion (*arrow*) on anterior wall of distal sigmoid colon. **B:** Repeat radiograph from double-contrast barium enema several years later shows how polyp has developed into infiltrating carcinoma (*arrow*).

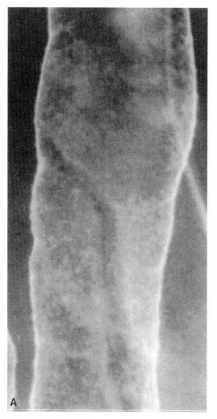

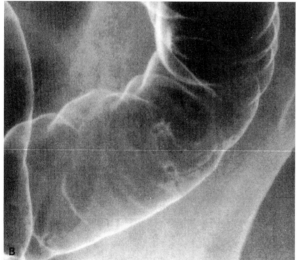

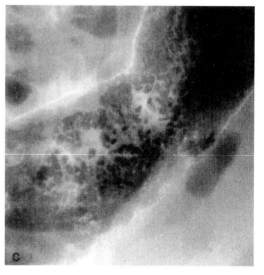

FIGURE 94-18.   Ulcerative colitis. **A:** Stippling of colonic mucosa caused by superficial erosion in acute ulcerative colitis. **B:** Postinflammatory (filiform) polyposis in a patient with quiescent colitis. **C:** Epithelial dysplasia (precancerous) in a patient with chronic ulcerative colitis. Faceted, angular filling defects are characteristic of dysplasia. (Courtesy of Dr. F.M. Kelvin.)

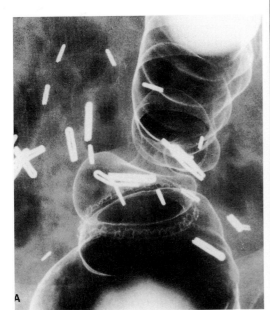
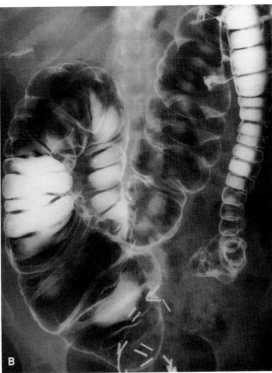

FIGURE 94-19. Postoperative colons of two patients. **A:** Normal double-contrast appearance of colorectal anastomosis. The site of anastomosis is indicated by the staple line. **B:** Radiograph from double-contrast colostomy enema examination shows normal postoperative colon. This examination is important for detecting recurrent or metachronous carcinoma.

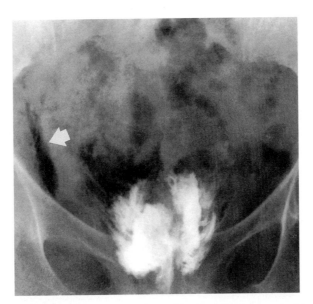

FIGURE 94-20. Complication of barium enema caused by laceration of rectum by inflated rectal balloon. Radiograph shows extravasation of barium into perirectal tissue. Retroperitoneal air (*arrow*) is visible along the right lateral wall of the pelvis.

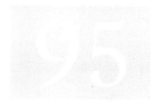

ULTRASONOGRAPHY

PHILIP W. RALLS ■ R. BROOKE JEFFREY JR. ■ ROBERT A. KANE
MICHELLE L. ROBBIN

Diagnostic sonography is experiencing the most vigorous and revolutionary period of technological advancement of any imaging modality. Current systems make use of sophisticated technology to produce high-resolution pictures that incorporate anatomic and pathologic features and color-coded blood flow into a single moving real-time image.

DOPPLER SONOGRAPHY

Doppler sonography is a virtually routine component of many modern sonographic examinations. It adds dynamic, real-time flow information to the morphologic images provided by gray-scale imaging. Color flow sonography (CFS) passively and automatically superimposes color-coded flow information on all or a selected portion of gray-scale images. CFS facilitates comparison of flow in different anatomic locations and minimizes the chance of missing flow in an unexpected area. Spectral Doppler sonography is used to acquire detailed flow information from a small area when quantitative information about flow velocity or fluctuation in flow is important.

ROLE OF SONOGRAPHY IN GASTROENTEROLOGY

Sonography is an important, often primary imaging modality for the biliary tract, liver, and pancreas. High-resolution transabdominal visualization of the gastrointestinal tract is vital in appendicitis and increasingly useful for the remaining gastrointestinal tract from esophagus to anus. Its abilities ensure an increasing role in evaluating gastrointestinal problems.

STRENGTHS AND WEAKNESSES OF SONOGRAPHY COMPARED WITH OTHER MODALITIES

When sonography can depict the area of clinical interest, it is nearly an ideal modality. The ability of diagnostic sonography to display flow and soft tissue in real time is unique among imaging techniques. Its spatial resolution is superior to that of computed tomographic (CT) scanning and magnetic resonance imaging (MRI). Because diagnostic sonography is safe and tolerated well by patients, it can be performed serially when necessary to follow the progress of treatment. When needed, ultrasound examinations can be performed quickly and at the bedside.

Unfortunately, there are many circumstances in which optimal or even adequate images cannot be obtained. The single most important problem is the inability of sonography to show what is beyond gas–soft tissue or bone–soft tissue interfaces. This makes comprehensive survey scanning essentially impossible. CT scanning, in particular, and MRI are better survey modalities. The other main limitation of sonography is its relatively poor contrast resolution, which provides a limited ability to display differences between normal and abnormal tissue. CT scanning and MRI have inherently better contrast resolution, which is further improved with use of oral and intravenous contrast agents. Contrast agents for ultrasound imaging are still in an early stage of development and currently have no clinical importance. Many abnormalities displayed automatically on whole-body CT scans or magnetic resonance images are either impossible or very difficult to visualize with sonography.

Sonography often is superior to CT scanning and MRI in examinations of patients who are uncooperative, unable to hold their breath, or unable to remain relatively still. It is often superior in examinations of patients with little body fat. This makes sonography very useful in pediatric imaging, for example. Patient factors that impede optimal sonography include extreme obesity and factors that limit cutaneous acoustic access, such as burns, incisions, dressings that cannot be removed, and cutaneous gastrointestinal enterostomies.

THE LIVER

Liver sonography has many uses as a primary and secondary imaging examination. Primary indications include suspected or known cirrhosis (Fig. 95-1), suspected abscess (Fig. 95-2), suspected tumor (Figs. 95-3 through 95-5), suspected vascular abnormalities (Figs. 95-6 and 95-7), trauma, and transplantation. Sonography can be used to characterize abnormalities found at other imaging examinations, such as CT scanning or MRI. Its safety and relatively modest cost make it an ideal means of assessment of the therapeutic response of known lesions or sequential follow-up evaluation of liver lesions of questionable importance.

Sonography is often a simple and effective way to guide percutaneous aspiration, drainage, biopsy, or tumor ablation. Unsuspected liver lesions often are incidental findings during sonography performed for nonhepatic indications. Sonography can guide further evaluation or management of these lesions. The main strengths of hepatic sonography are the ability to help characterize common benign lesions (cysts, hemangiomas) and guide percutaneous procedures, safety, excellent patient tolerance, and low cost. Weaknesses include inability to image the entire liver in some patients and inferiority to CT scanning in detecting extrahepatic disease.

Sonography, like CT scanning, can be used effectively to guide percutaneous procedures. MRI and nuclear medicine studies lack this ability. When performed by an expert, sonographically guided liver biopsy often is quicker and easier than biopsy with CT guidance. Sonography can directly depict the needle tip as it is placed in the lesion, facilitating biopsy of small lesions and lesions in uncooperative patients. Ultrasound-guided biopsy is more efficient and cost effective, even when lesions are initially detected with another modality. Despite the advantages of sonography, CT biopsy is more popular with radiologists because it almost always shows the needle location. Sonographic needle visualization may be difficult or impossible when the liver is echogenic or when acoustic access is imperfect. Newer sonographic techniques that enhance needle-tip visualization and improved biopsy guides promise to make sonographically guided biopsy easier.

Sonography may be used to evaluate resectability of primary or metastatic liver tumors (see Fig. 95-3). The ability of sonography to provide images in any oblique plane often makes it superior to CT scanning and MRI in localizing lesions to an anatomic hepatic segment. Sonography can be used to guide biopsy of newly detected lesions that might preclude curative hepatic resection. Intraoperative sonography is the most sensitive means of detecting focal liver lesions. At many centers where hepatic resections are performed, intraoperative sonography is routine before resection. When a questionable lesion is found at intraoperative ultrasound scanning, sonographically guided biopsy can be performed.

Although less sensitive than CT scanning or MRI, hepatic sonography can be used to seek focal lesions. When a liver abscess (see Fig. 95-2) is suspected clinically, sonography is the preferred screening modality. Hepatic sonography can be used to screen for metastases, if extrahepatic staging is not needed. When an optimal sonographic examination cannot be performed on an individual patient, CT scanning or MRI should be performed. CT scanning is preferred when extrahepatic staging is needed.

THE GALLBLADDER AND BILIARY TRACT

Sonography is the imaging method of choice for the initial evaluation of all clinically suspected diseases of the gallbladder. It is particularly valuable to patients with acute right upper quadrant pain and possible acute cholecystitis. Sonography is highly reliable in the detection of tiny gallstones (Fig. 95-8) and is useful for evaluating focal or diffuse abnormalities of the gallbladder wall (Figs. 95-9 and 95-10). Biliary sonography has several distinct advantages compared with scintigraphy and CT scanning. It is less expensive than both modalities and can be performed rapidly without patient preparation or use of contrast agents. Unlike biliary scintigraphy, sonography is not organ specific and may provide important diagnostic information regarding the liver, pancreas, and peritoneal cavity. Sonography can be performed readily on patients with abnormal liver tests, which often preclude scintigraphy. Finally, sonography may be used to guide percutaneous cholecystostomy in the care of critically ill patients at the bedside. When the gallbladder is normal, sonography can be used for a rapid survey of the remainder of the abdomen to search for an alternative cause of right upper quadrant pain.

One of the most important technical improvements in the last decade has been the increasing sensitivity of color Doppler imaging and the development of power Doppler sonography. Although some initial studies have suggested that mural hyperemia may accompany some cases of more advanced forms of acute cholecystitis, it remains to be seen whether color Doppler imaging will have a role in differentiating normal from abnormal gallbladder perfusion (see Fig. 95-9). The development of ultrasound contrast agents affords an opportunity to evaluate gallbladder perfusion much more easily. The most problematic area in gallbladder imaging is that of acalculous cholecystitis. It is unclear whether future developments will enhance diagnostic efficacy.

The ability of sonography to depict dilated bile ducts and the level of biliary obstruction makes it the technique of choice for examining patients with jaundice. Sonography can depict the cause of obstruction (Fig. 95-11), albeit with limited accuracy. Infectious cholangitis and conditions such as cholangiopathy caused by human immunodeficiency virus infection are indications for sonography. Sonography can be used to detect and assess, with the help of color Doppler imaging, the resectability of cholangiocarcinoma and other tumors of the bile ducts.

Sonography routinely displays the normal intra- and extrahepatic ducts. The internal diameter of the normal extrahepatic bile duct is 5 mm or less, although elderly patients and patients with gallstones may have ducts 6 to 9 mm in internal diameter. Ten or more millimeters is abnormal dilation. The distal common duct is usually seen within the pancreatic head and has a somewhat smaller caliber.

The intrahepatic bile ducts may be ventral to the left and right portal veins. The normal internal diameter of the main left and right intrahepatic bile ducts is about 1 mm.

THE PANCREAS

Sonography is indicated in the care of all patients with acute pancreatitis, not to evaluate the pancreas itself but to detect gallstones and biliary dilation. Complications of pancreatitis are best sought with CT scanning, but sonography may be used to detect and follow complications of acute pancreatitis (Fig. 95-12). Sonography can be used to guide biopsy, drainage, or aspiration of selected pancreatic lesions. Sonography is the primary imaging method to screen patients with jaundice or abdominal pain. Sonography may be used to detect acute or chronic pancreatitis or reveal pancreatic masses. Sonography may be more effective than CT scanning in determining whether a lesion is pancreatic or contiguous with the pancreas. Sonography occasionally is useful to characterize abnormalities found at CT scanning, to determine, for example, whether a lesion is cystic or solid.

Although CT scanning remains the most sensitive means of evaluating pancreatic disease, modern ultrasound technology and new scanning techniques (oral contrast administration, compression scanning) are reestablishing sonography as a useful and clinically relevant pancreatic imaging technique. Although sonography cannot be used to diagnose pancreatic necrosis, it can be used to follow known pancreatitis-associated fluid collections and guide interventional techniques to treat patients with pancreatitis. Color Doppler sonography shows great promise as a tool to assess the resectability of pancreatic tumors (Fig. 95-13), potentially lessening the role of both CT and endoscopic ultrasound scanning.

THE GASTROINTESTINAL TRACT

The most common indication for gastrointestinal sonography is evaluation of right lower quadrant pain and possible appendicitis (Fig. 95-14). Sonography may be useful in the diagnosis of diverticulitis (Figs. 95-15 and 95-16), obstruction of the small bowel (Fig. 95-17), and bulky mesenteric (Fig. 95-18) or gastrointestinal neoplasms. Not infrequently, a gastrointestinal tract abnormality is discovered incidentally during a screening examination of the upper abdomen or pelvis. High-resolution intralumenal probes routinely depict five discrete layers of bowel wall. With conventional abdominal transducers, however, it is not possible to resolve all five layers. The echogenic submucosal layer, however, is clearly visible and serves as a constant anatomic feature that is an extremely useful landmark to identify an intraabdominal structure as a bowel loop.

Pathological processes that cause ulceration and necrosis of the bowel lead to focal or global loss of visualization of the echogenic submucosa. Primary neoplasms involving the bowel wall may result in focal thickening of the bowel wall referred to as the target sign or pseudokidney sign (Fig. 95-19). Tumor infiltrating the bowel wall appears as a hypoechoic mass (mimicking the cortex of the kidney). The echogenic mucosal surface lumen is preserved and mimics the fat-containing hilum of the kidney. Gas trapped within ulcerating lesions involving the bowel wall may result in high-amplitude echoes with acoustic reverberation artifacts within the submucosal layers of the bowel wall.

Color Doppler sonography may be a useful adjunct to gray-scale imaging in the evaluation of focal thickening of the bowel wall. Increased arterial flow within the involved segment suggests inflammation or infection; diminished flow or absence of flow suggests intramural hemorrhage (Fig. 95-20), ischemia, or infarction (Fig. 95-21).

The vascularity of gastrointestinal tumors is variable, but adenocarcinoma typically is hypovascular.

THE PERITONEAL CAVITY

The most common indication for evaluation of the peritoneal cavity with sonography is to search for intraperitoneal fluid collections such as ascites, abscesses, or hemorrhage. Sonography is useful not only to identify intraperitoneal fluid collections but also to guide percutaneous needle aspiration for definitive diagnosis. Solid peritoneal masses representing either primary or metastatic tumors may be detected on occasion. For patients with a clinical likelihood of peritoneal metastases, however, CT scanning is the preferred imaging modality.

INTRAOPERATIVE ULTRASOUND

Intraoperative ultrasonography (IOUS) provides indispensable information that influences clinical management and choice of surgical procedure. Several technical advances have made IOUS even more effective. These advances include miniaturization of transducers, use of spectral and color flow Doppler ultrasound, and the development of laparoscopic ultrasonography.

Optimal IOUS requires considerable technical expertise and, more important, experience in interpreting subtle real-time sonographic abnormalities. If surgeons perform intraoperative scanning, it is imperative that they be appropriately trained and sufficiently experienced to use IOUS effectively. In gastroenterology, IOUS is most often used in examining patients who are candidates for surgical resection of primary or metastatic malignant tumors of the liver. IOUS is essential for optimal detection of all liver lesions. It is far superior to all preoperative imaging modalities, including MRI and CT portography. It is even better than surgical inspection and palpation (Fig. 95-22).

IOUS also is important in intraoperative pancreatic imaging to search for small occult tumors (Fig. 95-23), assess tumor extension, and detect metastatic disease in draining lymph nodes and the liver. Laparoscopic ultrasonography is important in gallbladder surgery; it has replaced intraoperative cholangiography at some centers. Laparoscopic ultrasonography also has been used to stage malignant bowel tumors, particularly gastric tumors.

IOUS facilitates accurate and safe biopsy of deep-seated, nonpalpable lesions and small lesions adjacent to critical vascular structures; is an effective guide to drainage of cysts, pseudocysts, and other fluid collections encountered intraoperatively; and is useful for tumor ablation with cryosurgery, alcohol injection, or hyperthermic ablation with radio frequency, laser, or microwave energy sources. Increased awareness of the abilities of IOUS has resulted in the development of new applications.

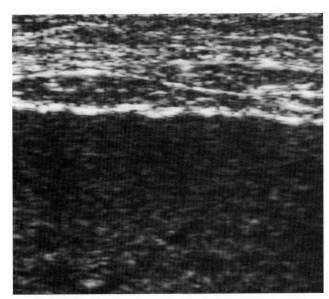

FIGURE 95-1. Cirrhosis with nodular liver surface. Image obtained with a high-resolution linear array transducer shows liver nodules several millimeters in size. The normal liver surface is smooth. This nodularity usually indicates cirrhosis. Micronodular cirrhosis may have a smooth-appearing surface on ultrasound scans. On occasion, subcapsular tumor nodules cause surface nodularity.

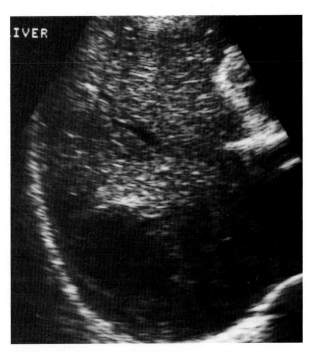

FIGURE 95-2. Pyogenic liver abscess. Transverse sonogram of the right lobe of the liver shows a mixed-echogenicity, predominantly hypoechoic liver abscess at the hepatic dome. The lesion is not well defined medially, which is a sonographic feature of pyogenic liver abscess.

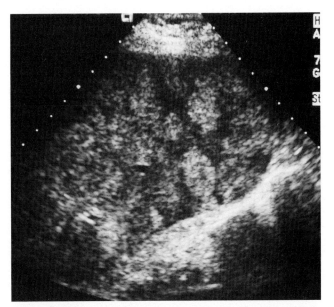

FIGURE 95-3. Echogenic liver metastases. Hepatic metastases can have any sonographic pattern. In this patient, the metastases are primarily hyperechoic compared with the normal liver parenchyma. Some hypoechoic lesions are present.

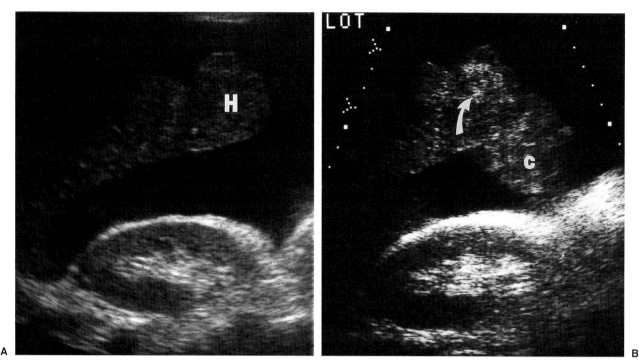

A

B

FIGURE 95-4. Hepatocellular carcinoma with acute intraperitoneal hemorrhage. **A:** Longitudinal sonogram shows an exophytic hepatocellular carcinoma (*H*) extending out of the tip of the right lobe of the liver. **B:** Sonogram performed 1 week later shows increased echogenicity within the lesion (*curved arrow*) and an acute clot (*c*). This represents acute hemorrhage of a hepatocellular cancer, a fairly common occurrence.

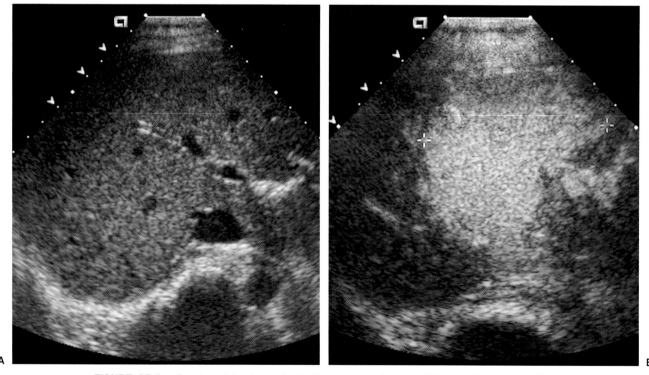

A

B

FIGURE 95-5. Focal nodular hyperplasia: transverse ultrasound image through the right lobe. **A:** Precontrast gray-scale image does not demonstrate a definite mass. **B:** Postcontrast gray-scale interval delay image shows the now easily visualized hypervascular mass (*cursors*).

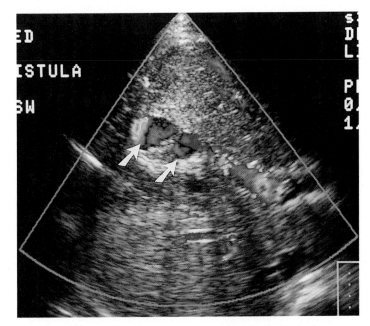

FIGURE 95-6. Hepatic pseudoaneurysm after gunshot wound. This patient had fever and pain 3 weeks after being released from the hospital after treatment of a liver injury associated with a gunshot wound. Color Doppler sonogram demonstrates two hepatic artery pseudo-aneurysms (*arrows*). Color Doppler sonography is useful in the diagnosis of vascular abnormalities such as this. The patient later underwent therapeutic angiographic embolization.

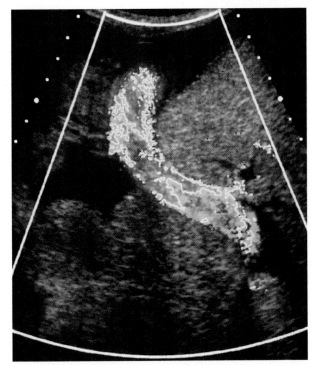

FIGURE 95-7. Recanalized paraumbilical vein. Transverse sonogram of a patient with cirrhosis, ascites, and portal hypertension shows an enlarged paraumbilical vein that serves as a hepatofugal collateral vessel. Paraumbilical veins are the easiest portosystemic collaterals to image because of their superficial location as they arise from the left portal vein to communicate with superficial abdominal collateral vessels. The most common type of collateral vessel, the left gastric-coronary vein, is extremely difficult to identify at sonography.

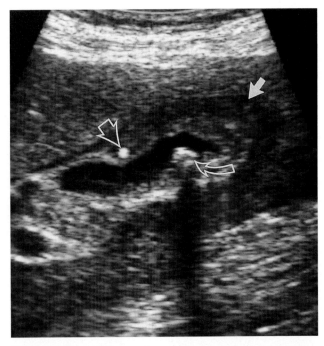

FIGURE 95-8. Gallstone in a patient with adenomyomatosis. An intralumenal gallstone (*curved open arrow*) is visible, and an intramural gallstone (*straight open arrow*) is present within a diffusely thickened gallbladder wall (*arrow*). Surgical findings confirmed gallstone disease and adenomyomatosis.

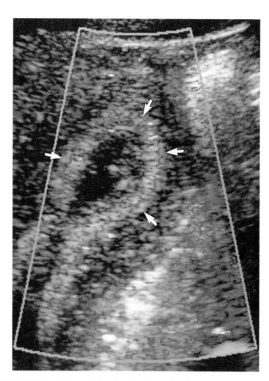

FIGURE 95-9. Hepatitis A with fundic flow. Not all patients with fundic color Doppler flow have acute cholecystitis. This image shows a patient with hepatitis A who has thickening of the gallbladder wall related to inflammation caused by the hepatitis. Mural color flow (*small arrows*) is displayed on the color Doppler image.

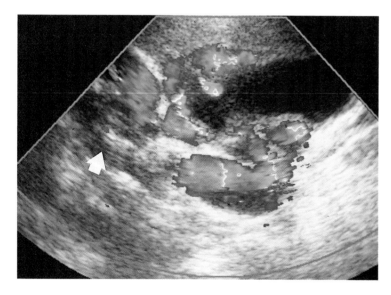

FIGURE 95-10. Prominent color-coded gallbladder wall varices in a patient with main portal thrombosis. The occluded portal vein is visible adjacent to the gallbladder (*arrow*). Hepatopetal collateral vessels after portal vein thrombosis may involve the gallbladder wall and produce gallbladder varices, as in this patient.

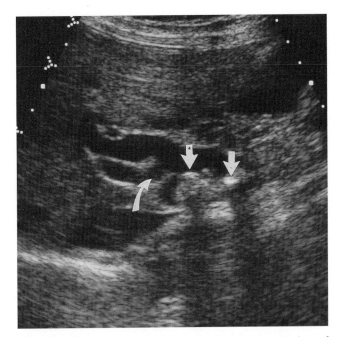

FIGURE 95-11. Common bile duct stone. Long-axis view of the intra- and extrahepatic bile ducts reveals two echogenic common duct stones (*arrows*). The cystic duct (*curved arrow*) enters the common duct dorsally.

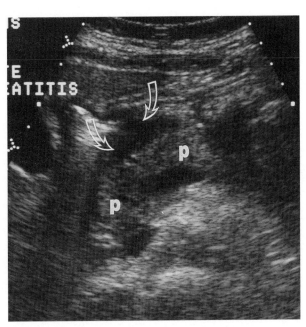

FIGURE 95-12. Acute pancreatitis with peripancreatic abnormality. Transverse sonogram reveals hypoechoic inflammation (*curved open arrows*) ventral to the pancreas (*p*). The pancreas itself appears normal. Peripancreatic abnormality may be the only sonographic evidence of acute pancreatitis.

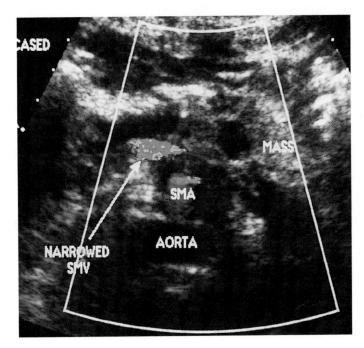

FIGURE 95-13. Pancreatic carcinoma encases the celiac artery. The hypoechoic pancreatic mass (*MASS*) encases the superior mesenteric artery (*SMA*) and narrows the superior mesenteric vein (*long-tailed arrow*). This renders the tumor unresectable. Sonography, especially with color Doppler imaging, is an effective tool in assessing resectability of periampullary neoplasms.

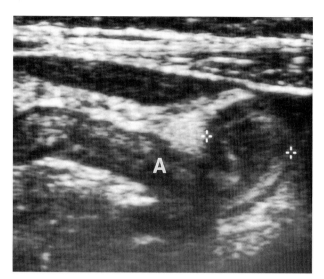

FIGURE 95-14. Acute appendicitis. Distended appendix (*A*) has a dilated tip (*cursors*).

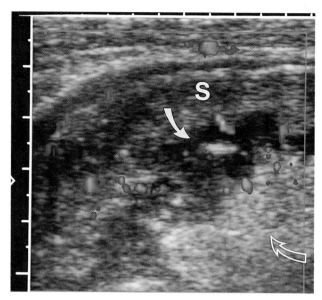

FIGURE 95-15. Sigmoid diverticulitis. Graded compression color Doppler scan of left lower quadrant reveals thickened sigmoid colon (S). Image shows echogenic sigmoid meso-colon (*open curved arrow*) and intramural abscess (*closed curved arrow*).

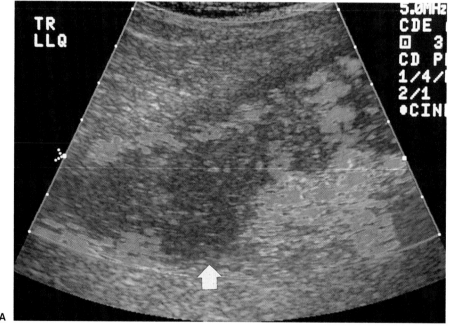

FIGURE 95-16. Diverticulitis with focal ischemia. **A:** A transverse power Doppler sono-gram obtained of the left lower quadrant reveals focal areas of hyperemia with a necrotic area where there is no flow (*arrow*). *(Continued)*

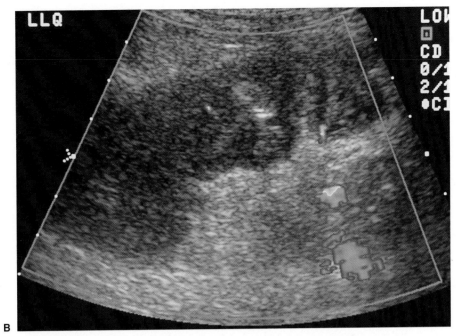

FIGURE 95-16. **B:** Conventional-velocity color Doppler image is much less useful in showing flow and is essentially nondiagnostic for this patient.

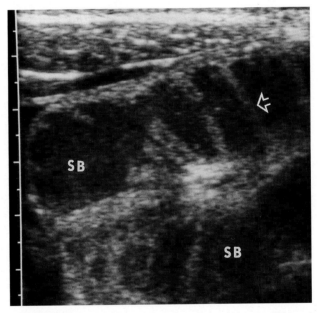

FIGURE 95-17. Closed-loop obstruction of the small bowel. Dilated U-shaped loop of small bowel (*SB*) represents closed-loop obstruction.

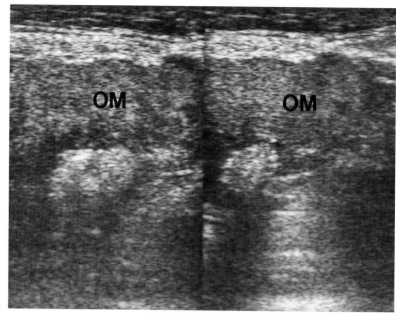

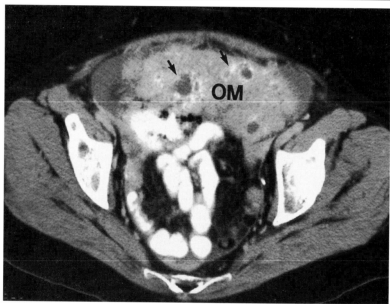

FIGURE 95-18. Omental metastases. **A:** Sonogram demonstrates an echogenic omental "cake" (*OM*) from metastatic ovarian carcinoma. **B:** Computed tomographic scan of the same patient as in **A**. Areas of calcification (*arrows*) within the omental cake (*OM*) are not apparent on sonogram.

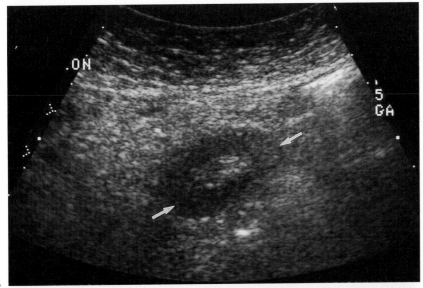

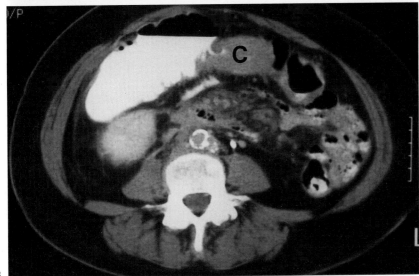

FIGURE 95-19. Pseudokidney sign of gastrointestinal tumor. **A:** Sagittal sonogram of the midabdomen demonstrates a mass (*arrows*) that resembles a kidney. **B:** Computed tomographic scan demonstrates circumferential carcinoma (*C*) obstructing hepatic flexure.

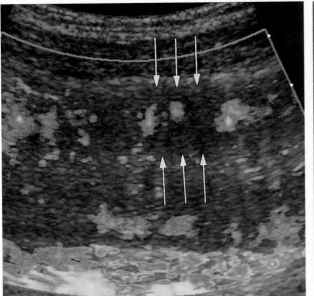

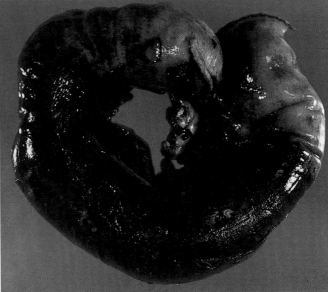

FIGURE 95-20. Intramural hemorrhage caused by warfarin therapy. **A:** A longitudinal left lower quadrant image of the small intestine reveals diffuse thickening of the bowel wall (a portion of which is outlined between the *arrows*) but intact blood flow as manifest with power Doppler imaging. **B:** Surgical specimen shows intramural hemorrhage in the same location.

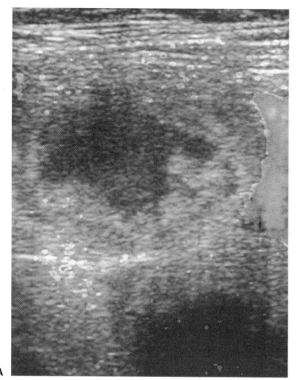

A

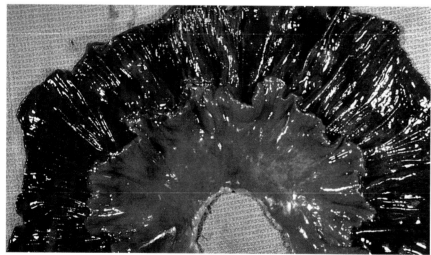

B

FIGURE 95-21. Infarction of the small bowel. **A:** Power Doppler sonogram of the left upper quadrant shows little or no flow in the edematous loop of small intestine. **B:** The pathological specimen confirms the sonographic diagnosis.

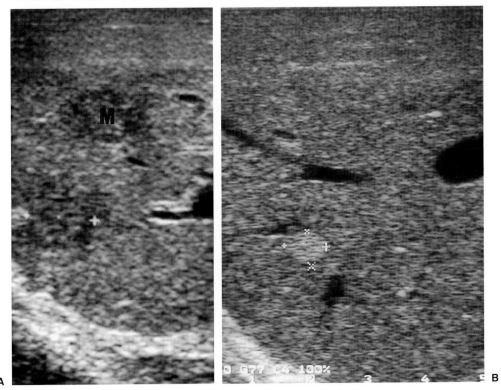

FIGURE 95-22. Intraoperative ultrasound scans show metastasis and hemangioma. **A:** Sonogram shows hepatic metastasis (*M*). **B:** Homogeneous hyperechoic hemangioma (outlined by cursors) in the same patient. A total of three hemangiomas were visualized in addition to the metastases.

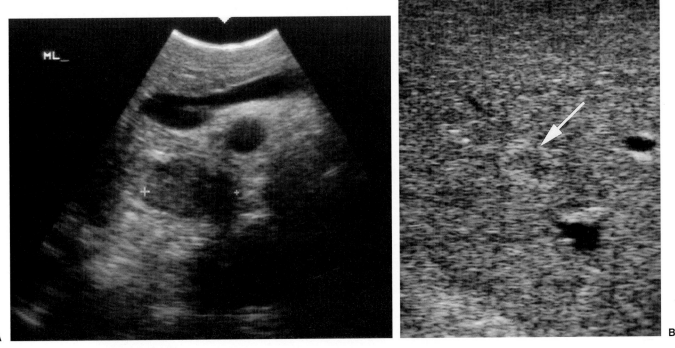

FIGURE 95-23. Intraoperative ultrasound scans show nonpalpable pancreatic insulinoma. **A:** Intraoperative ultrasound scan of the pancreas demonstrates hypoechoic insulinoma (outlined by *cursors*) in the low head and uncinate process of the pancreas. **B:** Intraoperative ultrasound scan of the liver shows a less than 1-cm liver nodule (*arrow*) in the same patient that suggests metastasis. Intraoperative ultrasound-guided biopsy is required to confirm metastasis, because other lesions, such as fibrosed hemangioma or focal nodular hyperplasia, can have a similar appearance.

ENDOSCOPIC ULTRASONOGRAPHY

MICHAEL B. KIMMEY ■ PETER VILMANN

Endoscopic ultrasound (EUS) scanning combines two commonly used diagnostic procedures: endoscopy and ultrasonography. Better ultrasound resolution of the gastrointestinal tract and its adjacent organs is made possible by endoscopic delivery of ultrasound transducers close to the target organs. The interfering effects of bone and gas are eliminated, and higher-frequency ultrasound can be used because less penetration of the ultrasound beam is required.

This field has changed rapidly as newer and better ultrasound endoscopes have been developed and more gastroenterologists have been trained to perform the procedure. Most experience was gained with radial scanning endoscopes. This instrument is still used widely but has been complemented by the development of electronic curvilinear array instruments. The curvilinear-array ultrasound endoscope has Doppler capability and allows biopsy of lesions under EUS guidance. Transendoscopic ultrasound probes continue to be developed and are clinically applicable in selected circumstances.

The indications for EUS scanning also have expanded. Definition of subepithelial gastrointestinal masses and staging of gastrointestinal cancer are still important. However, EUS scanning also is frequently used to evaluate the pancreas, retroperitoneum, and common bile duct. The added capability of EUS-guided biopsy has extended the clinical utility of this imaging modality.

The images presented in Figs. 96-1 through 96-30 represent the range of gastrointestinal abnormalities that can be approached with EUS scanning. In general, EUS is useful when more anatomic information is considered to be helpful in clinical management, including characterization of impressions on the gastrointestinal lumen that are covered by normal mucosa; accurate local and regional staging of mucosal neoplasms; and tissue diagnosis and staging of malignant tumors involving organs adjacent to the gastrointestinal tract.

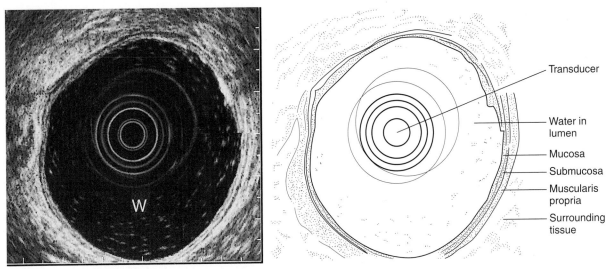

FIGURE 96-1. Normal stomach imaged with a 7.5-MHz radial scanning endoscope. Water (*W*) in the gastric lumen facilitates imaging of the wall layers that correspond to mucosa, submucosa, muscularis propria, and surrounding tissue.

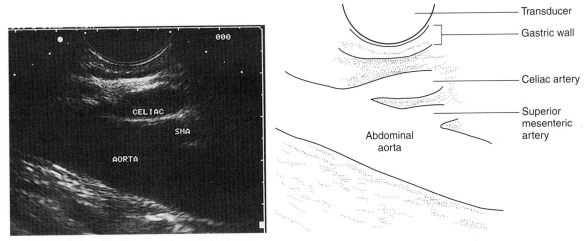

FIGURE 96-2. The abdominal aorta and the origins of the celiac and superior mesenteric arteries (*SMA*) imaged through the gastric wall with an electronic curvilinear-array ultrasound endoscope. This instrument also has Doppler capability for demonstration of blood flow in these vessels.

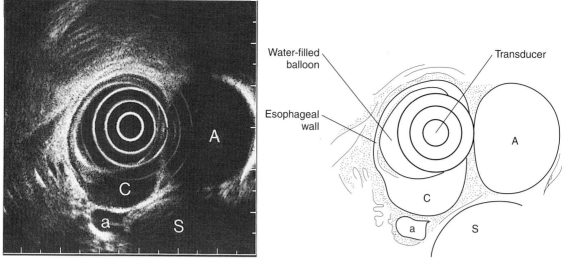

FIGURE 96-3. Image shows an intramural esophageal cyst (*C*), the descending aorta (*A*), azygous vein (*a*), and spine (*S*).

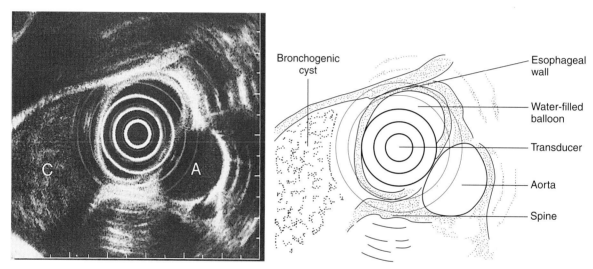

FIGURE 96-4. Image shows a bronchogenic cyst (*C*) outside the esophageal wall. Close examination reveals all wall layers. The echoes from within the cyst are caused by mucus and debris. The descending aorta (*A*) is visible on the left side of the esophagus.

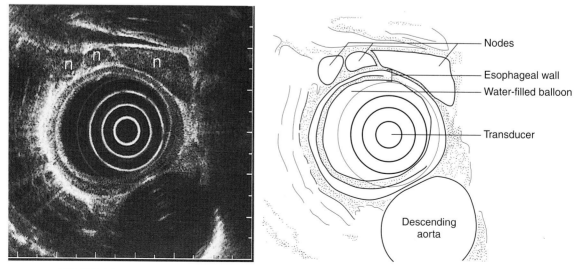

FIGURE 96-5. A cluster of benign lymph nodes (*n*). These subcarinal nodes have a heterogeneous echo pattern and seem to drape across the anterior surface of the esophagus.

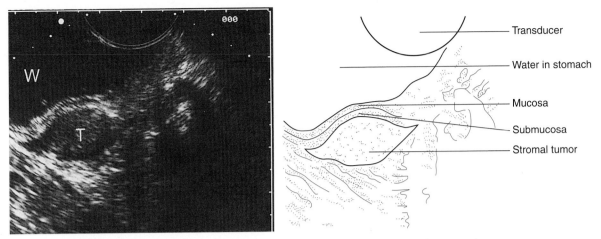

FIGURE 96-6. Image obtained with a curvilinear-array ultrasound endoscope shows a gastric stromal tumor. Water (*W*) in the gastric lumen allows good definition of gastric wall layers that correspond to mucosa and submucosa that overlie the tumor (*T*). This stromal tumor has benign characteristics: it is small (1.5 cm), has a homogeneous echo pattern, and has a smooth outer border.

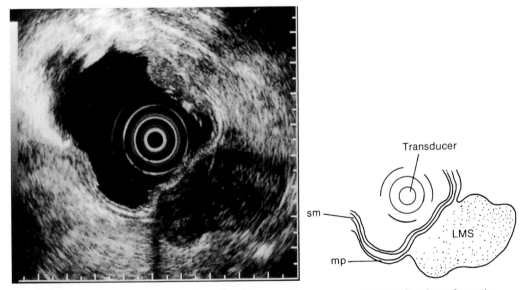

FIGURE 96-7. Malignant gastric stromal tumor (leiomyosarcoma [*LMS*]) arises from the muscularis propria (*mp*) and compresses the submucosa (*sm*). The tumor has a lobulated outer margin and an irregular and heterogeneous echo pattern.

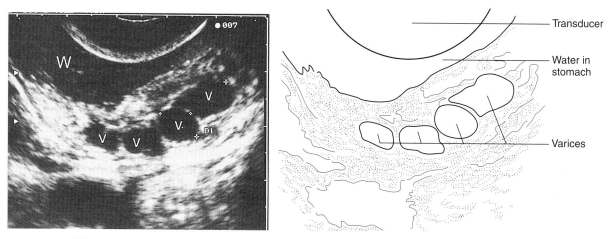

FIGURE 96-8. Image from within the stomach obtained with a curvilinear-array ultrasound endoscope shows multiple large gastric varices (*v*). Water (*W*) has been placed in the gastric lumen so that the surface layers can be easily seen.

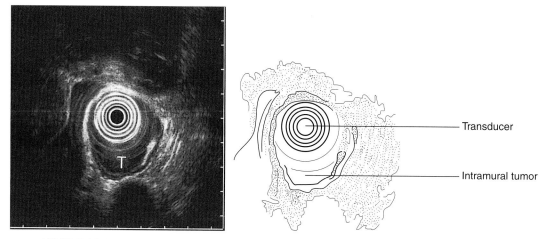

FIGURE 96-9. Elderly patient with dysphagia and radiographic and manometric evidence of achalasia. The radial scanning ultrasound endoscope could not be passed through the narrowed gastroesophageal junction. Imaging at the farthest point of insertion revealed a hypoechoic tumor (*T*) in the esophageal wall. The surgical finding was stromal tumor.

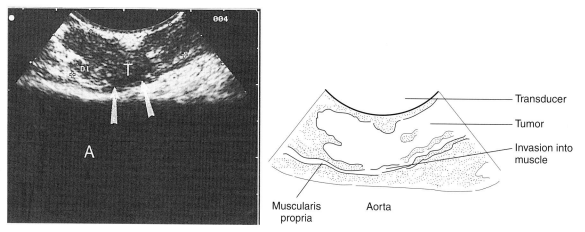

FIGURE 96-10. A carcinoma (*T*) in the midesophagus caused this hypoechoic mass, which penetrates into but not out of the muscularis propria (*arrows*). This T2 stage tumor is adjacent to the descending aorta (*A*).

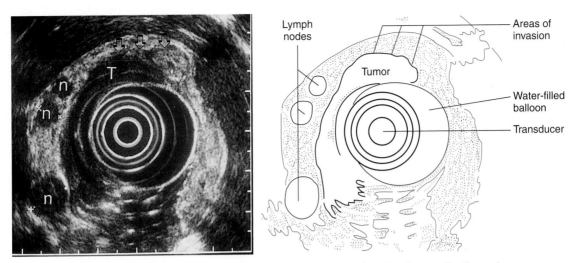

FIGURE 96-11. Hypoechoic tumor (*T*) in the esophagus invades the mediastinum (*open arrows*). The adjacent lymph nodes (*n*) probably have malignant involvement because they are round and are similar in echogenicity to the primary tumor. This would be staged as a T3N1 esophageal carcinoma.

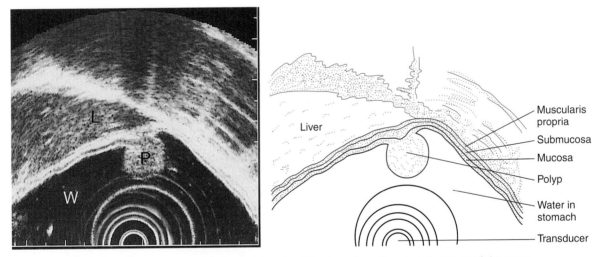

FIGURE 96-12. A hyperplastic gastric polyp (*P*) arises from the mucosal layer of the stomach. Underlying layers of the gastric wall are normal. Water (*W*) has been placed in the gastric lumen. Part of the left hepatic lobe (*L*) is visible next to the stomach wall.

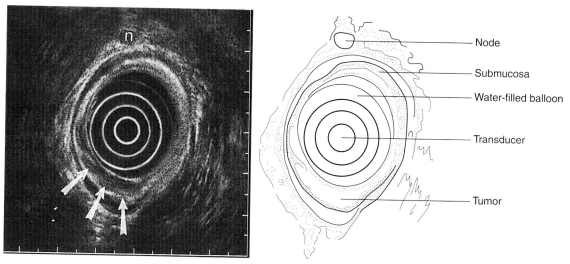

FIGURE 96-13. Mucosal thickening with penetration (*arrows*) into the submucosal layer is visible in this early carcinoma of the gastric cardia. The adjacent small round lymph node (*n*) contained malignant cells when examined with the resected stomach.

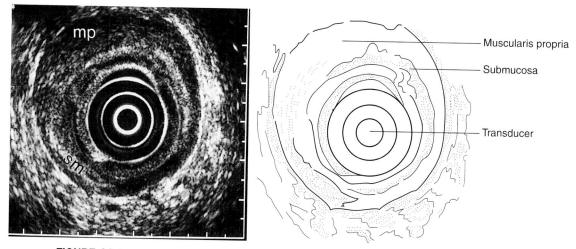

FIGURE 96-14. Radial ultrasound image shows thickening of the stomach wall (1.5 cm) caused by metastatic breast cancer. The normal layers, including submucosa (*sm*) and muscularis propria (*mp*) are thickened and distorted by the infiltrating cancer.

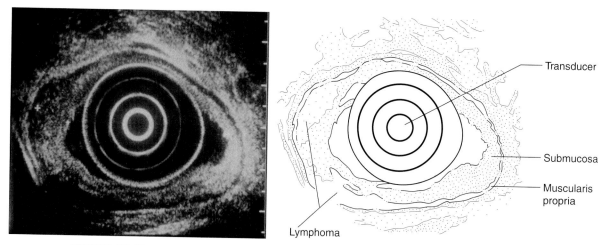

FIGURE 96-15. The radial ultrasound image obtained at 12 MHz shows an advanced gastric lymphoma producing diffuse gastric wall thickening and involving all layers of the stomach.

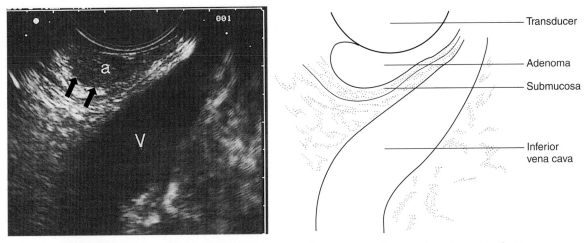

FIGURE 96-16. Image obtained with a curvilinear-array ultrasound endoscope shows ampullary adenoma (*a*). The adenoma does not invade the echogenic submucosal layer (*arrows*). The downstream duodenum is to the right in the image, which also shows part of the inferior vena cava (*V*).

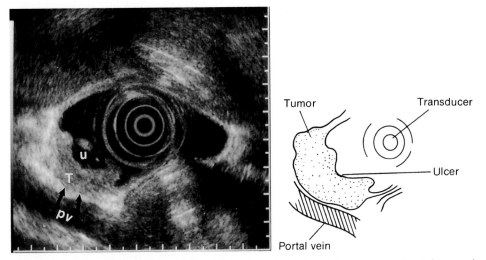

FIGURE 96-17. Ampullary carcinoma (*T*) is ulcerated (*u*) and has invaded the subserosal fat layer (*arrows*) near the portal vein (*pv*).

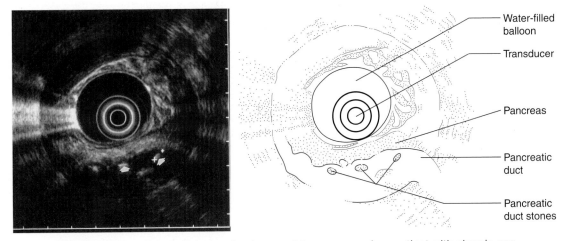

FIGURE 96-18. This radial scanning image of the pancreas in a patient with chronic pancreatitis reveals echogenic filling defects (*arrows*) caused by stones within a dilated pancreatic duct.

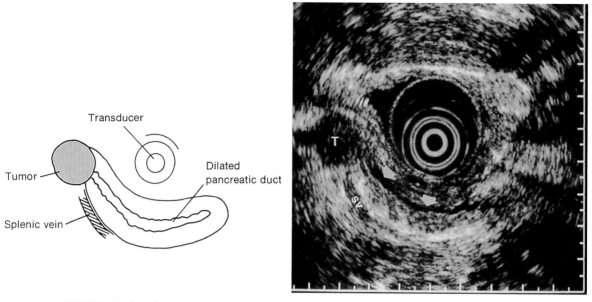

FIGURE 96-19. Carcinoma (*T*) of the head of the pancreas near the splenic vein (*sv*) has caused pancreatic ductal obstruction and dilation (*arrows*).

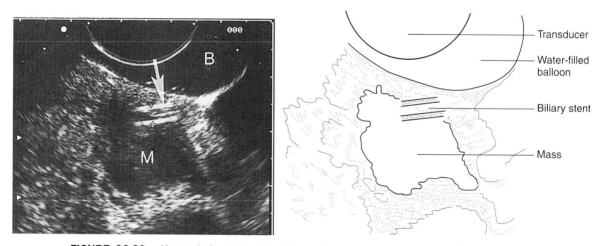

FIGURE 96-20. Hypoechoic mass (*M*) caused by pancreatic carcinoma. The walls of a previously placed biliary stent are visible (*arrow*). The image was made from the duodenum with a curvilinear-array ultrasound endoscope with a water-filled balloon (*B*) around the transducer.

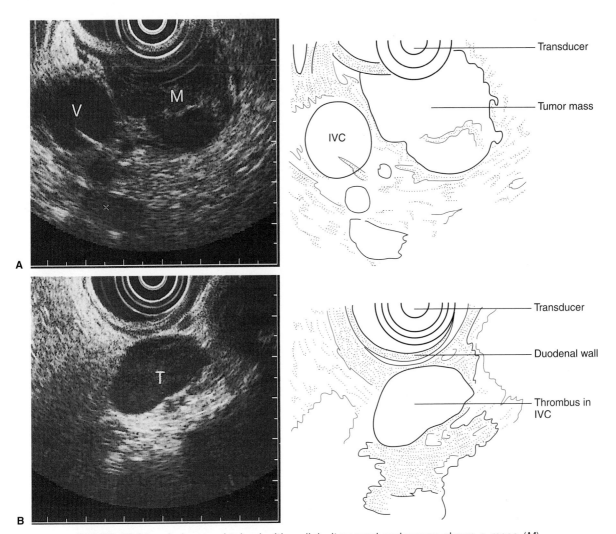

FIGURE 96-21. **A:** Image obtained with radial ultrasound endoscope shows a mass (*M*) caused by pancreatic carcinoma. The inferior vena cava (*V*) is adjacent to the mass. **B:** In the same patient depicted in **A**, the inferior vena cava (*IVC*) is shown to contain thrombus (*T*) when imaged from farther down the duodenum. The thrombus is highly suggestive of tumor invasion into the inferior vena cava.

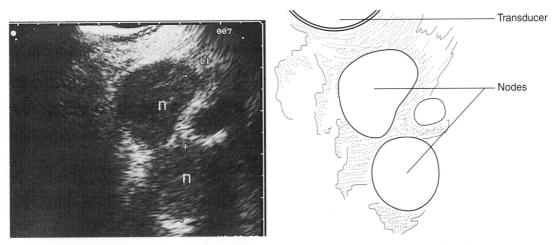

FIGURE 96-22. Image shows two large (2 cm), hypoechoic lymph nodes (*n*) adjacent to the pancreatic head in a patient with large cell lymphoma.

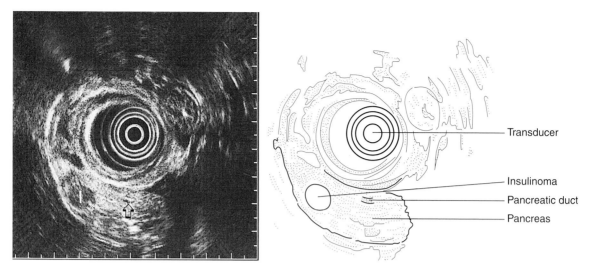

FIGURE 96-23. A 1-cm-diameter hypoechoic mass within the pancreas is caused by insuli-noma (*I*). A portion of the normal pancreatic duct is visible (*arrow*).

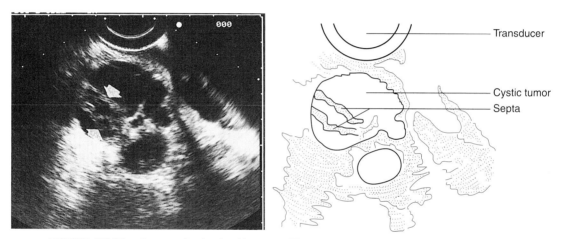

FIGURE 96-24. Image obtained with a curvilinear-array endoscope shows a complex cystic mass within the pancreatic tail. Septa (*arrows*) are present within some cystic neo-plasms, such as this one. Fluid aspirated from the cyst under endoscopic ultrasound guid-ance had the characteristics of a serous cystadenoma.

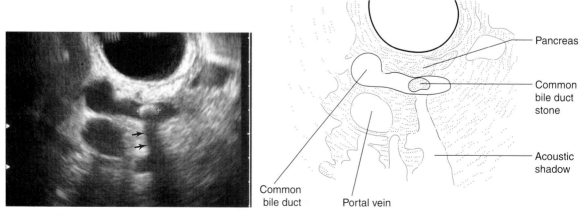

FIGURE 96-25. A 1-cm-diameter common bile duct stone (between + *signs*) with posterior acoustic shadowing (*arrows*) is imaged within a nondilated bile duct. This image was made with the electronic radial-array ultrasound endoscope using 5 MHz ultrasound frequency.

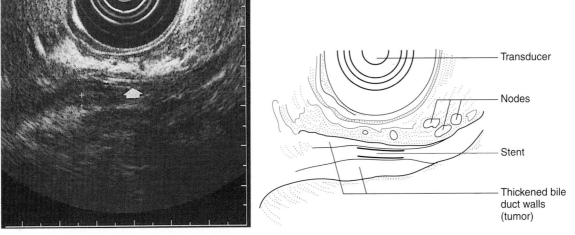

FIGURE 96-26. Image obtained from the duodenum with a radial scanning ultrasound endoscope shows cholangiocarcinoma. The bile duct wall is circumferentially thickened to 3 mm (between ×× and ++). A biliary stent is visible within the bile duct lumen (*arrow*).

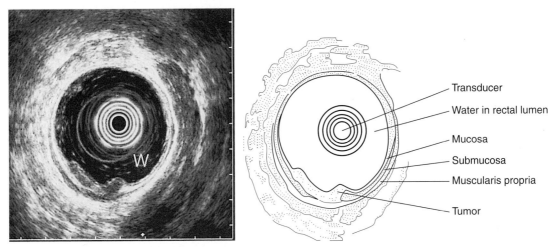

FIGURE 96-27. Image obtained with a radial scanning ultrasound endoscope shows early (stage T1) rectal cancer as a small, hypoechoic mass that penetrates into the submucosa but not the muscularis propria. Water (*W*) in the lumen allows better image resolution and delineation of surface details.

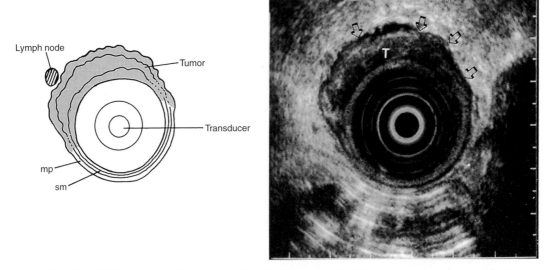

FIGURE 96-28. Advanced rectal carcinoma (*T*) has invaded the perirectal fat (*arrows*) and disrupted the normal layers that correspond to submucosa (*sm*) and muscularis propria (*mp*). It cannot be determined from this image whether a small lymph node, approximately 5 mm in diameter, contains malignant cells.

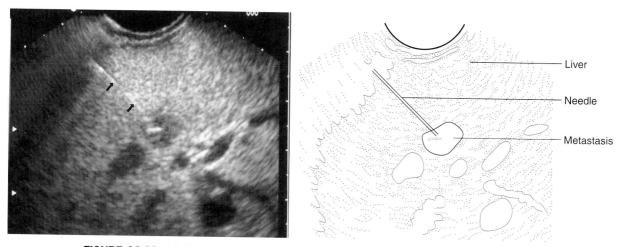

FIGURE 96-29. A 7-mm-diameter liver metastasis (*m*) in a patient with gastric cancer is sampled for cytologic examination with an endoscopic ultrasound–guided fine needle aspiration needle (*arrows*).

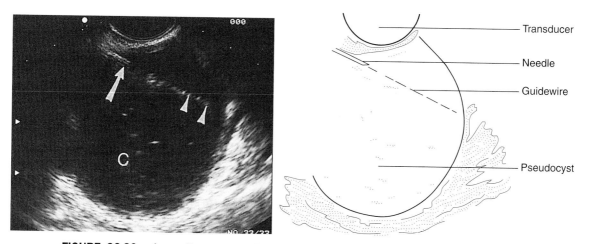

FIGURE 96-30. A curvilinear-array ultrasound endoscope was used to direct a needle (*arrow*) through the gastric wall into a pancreatic pseudocyst (*C*). An 0.018-in. guide wire (*arrowheads*) was threaded through the needle to mark the location for subsequent endoscopic cystogastrostomy in this patient who did not have an endoscopically visible bulge into the gastric lumen.

APPLICATIONS OF COMPUTED TOMOGRAPHY TO THE GASTROINTESTINAL TRACT

ALEC J. MEGIBOW

This chapter illustrates common examples of pathological conditions of the alimentary tract and solid abdominal viscera that display the wide utility of computed tomographic (CT) imaging. All of the following examples were obtained with helical or spiral acquisitions. Although these helical axial images look no different from conventional CT images, rapid acquisition allows the radiologist to use the data in a wider variety of ways. Several examples of these angiographic, cholangiographic, and virtual applications are illustrated. Above all, patients undergoing the examination can benefit from considerably shorter examination times than with older technology. A further benefit of helical CT technology may be that it will become a standard method of imaging abdominal disease, eliminating the redundant use of other modalities. We hope this benefit will be realized in definitive, accurate patient examinations and speedier access to appropriate therapy.

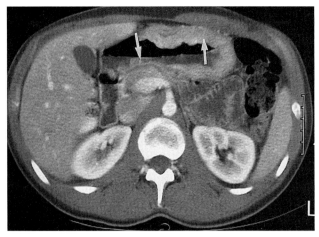

FIGURE 97-1. Scirrhous gastric carcinoma. There is focal thickening throughout the wall of the proximal stomach (*arrows*). The attenuation of the thickened tissue is greater than that of the adjacent enhanced liver parenchyma.

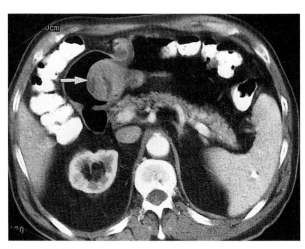

FIGURE 97-2. Gastric stromal neoplasm. A heterogenous mass arises from the lesser curvature aspect of the antrum (*arrow*). Variable attenuation and large size correlate with increasingly aggressive outcomes.

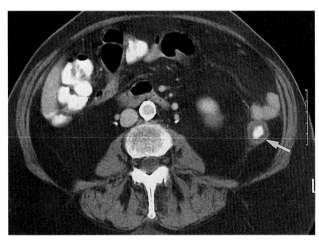

FIGURE 97-3. Crohn's disease, fat hypertrophy. A thickened edematous descending colon is depicted (*arrow*). Increase in the perienteric fat is represented by low-attenuation (dark) density.

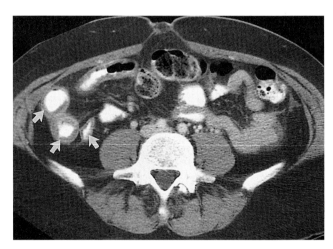

FIGURE 97-4. Cytomegalovirus ileitis. Thickened, edematous loops of small bowel (*arrows*) in the right lower quadrant of a patient with acquired immunodeficiency syndrome have an identical appearance to abnormal loops in Crohn's disease.

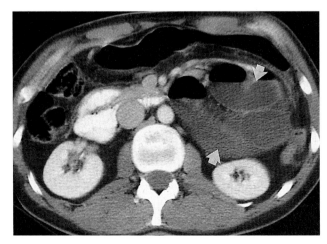

FIGURE 97-5. Obstruction of the small bowel secondary to internal hernia. Dilated, clustered jejunal loops are present posterior to the root of the mesentery of the small bowel (*arrows*). Distal air-filled loops are evident. The bowel was found in a peritoneal lined sac herniating through a rent in the posterior peritoneum (paraduodenal hernia).

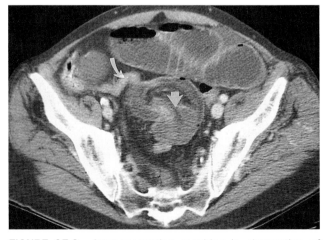

FIGURE 97-6. Intussusception resulting in obstruction of the small bowel. Dilated jejunum and collapsed ileum (*curved arrow*) are evident. An intussusception (*thick arrow*) is recognized as the cause of the obstruction. A benign stromal mass was the lead point.

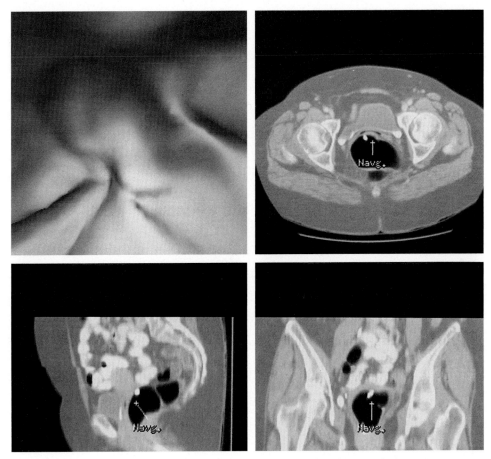

FIGURE 97-7. Rectal carcinoma. Virtual colonoscopic view of sessile, polypoid rectal carcinoma (**upper left**). Reformatted conventional computed tomographic images in axial, coronal, and sagittal planes are included in the data display to facilitate three-dimensional localization of the lesion.

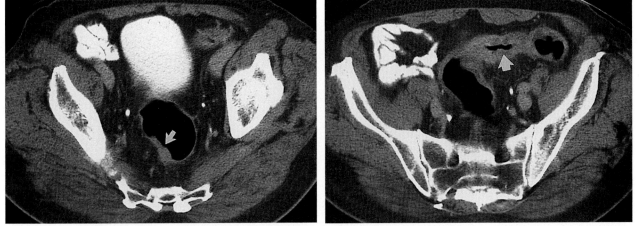

FIGURE 97-8. Synchronous carcinomas. **A:** Rectal lesion (*arrow*). **B:** Sigmoid lesion presenting itself as segmental thickening (*arrow*).

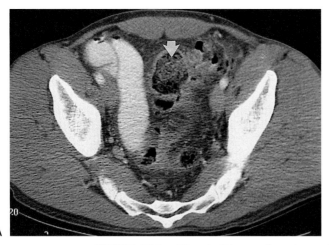
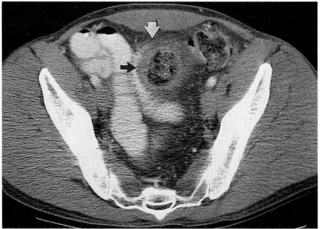

FIGURE 97-9. Diverticulitis causing obstruction of the small bowel. **A:** Large stool-filled diverticulum is apparent (*arrow*) in association with increased density within the peridiverticular fat. **B:** Extent of the process. The abscess (*white arrow*) has buried itself in the wall of adjacent jejunum (*dark arrow*). Dilated contrast medium–filled proximal loops are visible.

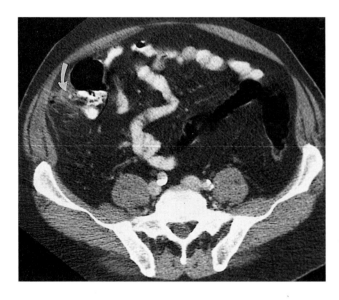

FIGURE 97-10. Cecal diverticulitis. Pericecal perforation results in a localized inflammatory response. Extralumenal air is present (*curved arrow*). At operation a normal appendix was found; the inflammation was caused by a ruptured cecal diverticulum.

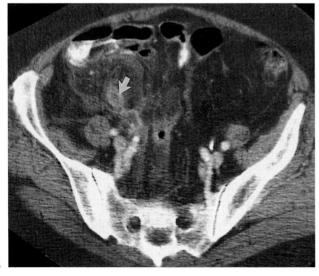
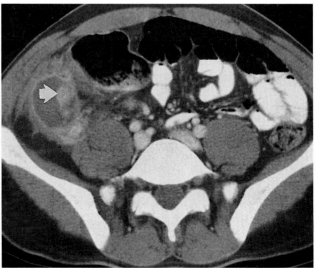

FIGURE 97-11. Acute appendicitis. **A:** Abnormal appendix (*arrow*). Bright wall is accentuated by intravenously administered contrast agent. Periappendiceal fat changes are evident. **B:** A pericecal abscess is evident. The etiology was established with identification of the abnormal appendix (*arrow*) within the cavity.

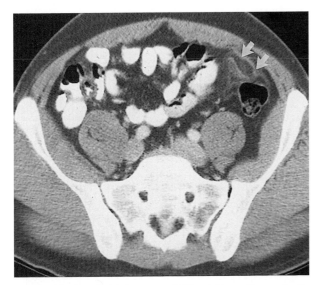

FIGURE 97-12. Epiploic appendicitis. A finger-like projection of fat is surrounded by an inflammatory rind (*arrows*). This appearance is diagnostic of torsion of epiploic appendage. When this abnormality is on the left, the differential diagnosis is diverticulitis; on the right, the diagnosis is appendicitis. This condition, if recognized, does not require surgical intervention in the absence of clinical signs of infection.

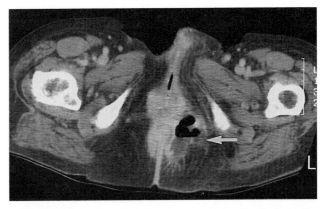

FIGURE 97-13. Perianal abscess secondary to Crohn's disease. The presence and extent of a perianal abscess are readily apparent (*arrow*). Computed tomographic scanning is an ideal technique for predrainage planning.

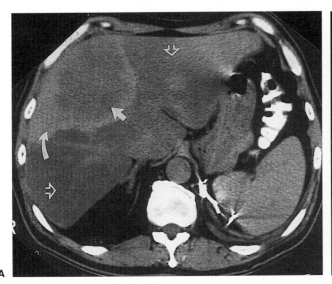

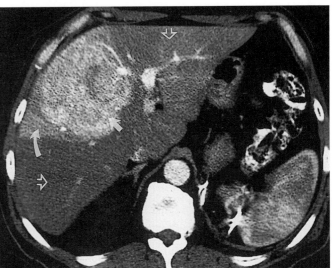

A

B

FIGURE 97-14. Three-phase liver examination. Scans show several basic principles of liver imaging with helical computed tomographic technique. **A:** Lesion seen on the non–contrast-enhanced image (*straight arrow*) is hypodense to surrounding hepatic parenchyma (*curved arrow*). This segment of parenchyma is more dense than most of the fatty infiltrated liver (*open arrows*). **B:** Arterial phase image results in bright enhancement of the lesion with less enhancement of the background liver parenchyma. *(Continued)*

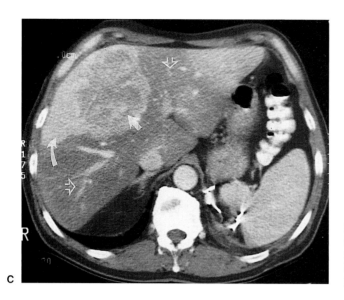

C

FIGURE 97-14. **(Continued) C:** Portal phase reveals the lesion to be almost equal in density to the surrounding normal liver parenchyma. This perilesional parenchyma is brighter than the maximally enhanced fatty liver because of perilesional circulatory effects.

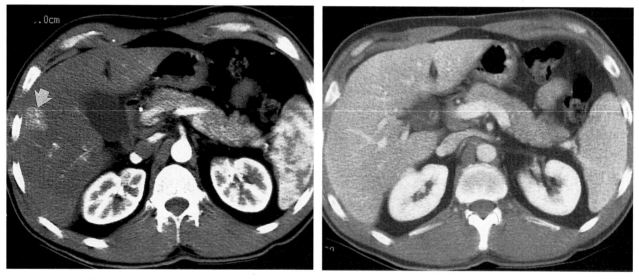

A

B

FIGURE 97-15. Hepatocellular carcinoma. **A:** Arterial phase image shows hyperdense lesion (*arrow*) in the lateral aspect of the right lobe of the liver. The appearance of the spleen is important. **B:** During the portal phase, the lesion is not visible because the normal parenchyma (predominantly supplied by the portal vein) is enhanced, rendering the lesion isodense and invisible.

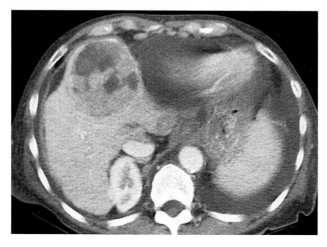

FIGURE 97-16. Hepatocellular carcinoma. A solitary lesion with a dense capsule and mosaic appearance is present.

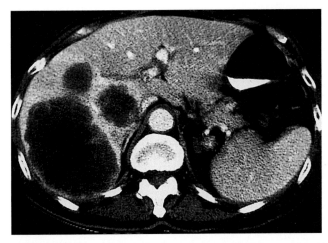

FIGURE 97-17. Metastatic lung cancer. Multiple, predominantly water-dense lesions are visible in the liver. A thickened peripheral rind of soft tissue identifies them as neoplasms as opposed to cysts. Even though the "enhanced" tissue is peripheral and variably globular, these lesions should not be confused with hemangiomas because the degree of enhancement is considerably less than that of the aorta.

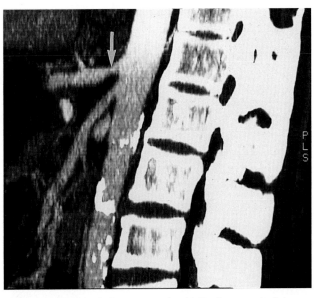

FIGURE 97-18. Celiac stenosis. Helical computed tomographic data can be used to produce diagnostic images beyond the traditional axial display. In this case, high-grade celiac stenosis (*arrow*) is depicted in a patient with suspected pancreatic disease.

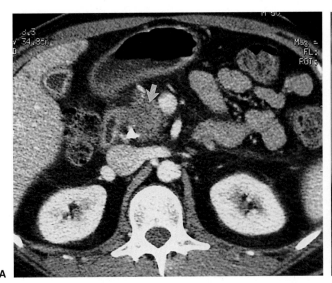

A

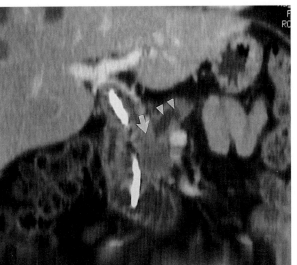

B

FIGURE 97-19. Pancreatic adenocarcinoma. **A:** Axial image reveals low-attenuation mass in head of pancreas (*arrow*). The bright density in the distal common bile duct represents a stent (*arrowhead*). **B:** Three-dimensional rendering of the data set shows the mass (*arrow*) surrounding the stent. A dilated pancreatic duct (*arrowheads*) is present proximal to the mass. Multiple liver metastases are evident.

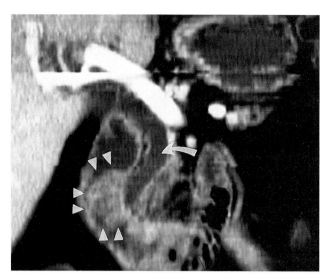

FIGURE 97-20. Ampullary carcinoma. Computed tomographic cholangiogram reveals a dilated common bile duct (*curved arrow*). This can be followed into the ampulla. The margins of a polypoid intralumenal periampullary mass are outlined (*arrowheads*).

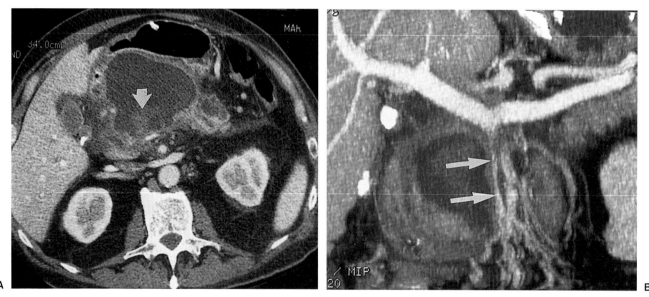

FIGURE 97-21. Hemorrhage into pseudocyst. **A:** Large fluid collection is present in the neck of the pancreas. The dependent density (*arrow*) represents blood. **B:** Angiographic rendering shows a narrowed superior mesenteric vein (*arrows*). Blood within the cyst is evident.

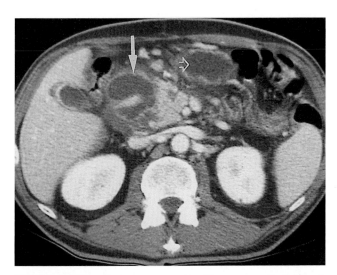

FIGURE 97-22. Groove pancreatis. The pancreatic fluid collection has accumulated between the duodenal wall and the pancreatic parenchyma (*solid arrow*). This form of acute pancreatitis can result in gastric outlet obstruction. A portion of the water-filled stomach also is identified (*open arrow*).

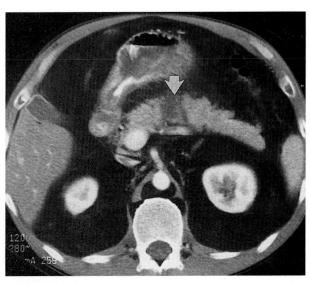

FIGURE 97-23. Central cavity necrosis. This form of acute pancreatitis results in focal necrosis within the central portion of the gland (*arrow*). Even when larger areas are affected, the outcome is usually less severe than with traditional necrotizing pancreatitis.

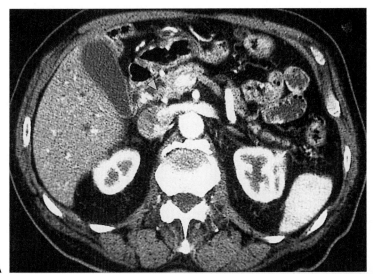

A

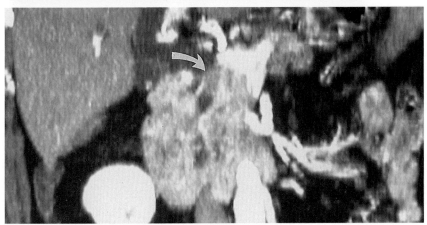

B

FIGURE 97-24. Cholangiocarcinoma of proximal common duct. **A:** Sessile polypoid mass is visible along the medial wall of the common bile duct (*arrowhead*). **B:** Cholangiographic rendering shows asymmetric density (*curved arrow*) along the medial wall of the proximal common bile duct.

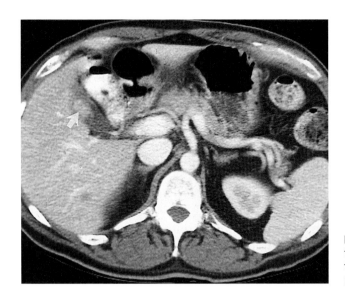

FIGURE 97-25. Melanoma metastatic to the gallbladder. Soft-tissue density (*arrow*) is present in the gallbladder secondary to a melanoma metastasis. Liver metastasis is visible in the posterior portion of the right liver lobe.

98

MAGNETIC RESONANCE IMAGING

ERIC K. OUTWATER

Magnetic resonance imaging (MRI) has been used clinically to investigate intra-abdominal diseases since 1984. The perception that MRI has serious limitations in intra-abdominal applications, when compared to computed tomography (CT) for example, is rapidly changing. The development of MRI sequences performed with suspended respiration eliminates the motion artifacts that plagued earlier MR images. Many technical advances led to the dramatic suppression of motion artifacts in non–breath-hold images. More recent technical innovations include surface coils, which improve MR imaging of the abdomen, and an array of contrast agents that selectively enhance specific organs. One result of these technical innovations is that the indications for MRI of the abdomen have expanded. MRI is now suitable for many pancreatic, biliary, and bowel disorders previously considered the domain of CT or conventional contrast radiography such as angiography or endoscopic retrograde cholangiopancreatography (ERCP).

The generation of MR images involves the spatial localization of radiofrequency signals elicited from water- or fat-containing tissue in the body. The variation in gray scale on the image from white to black represents the strength of these signals and is called the signal intensity. Tissues and structures that are bright on the MR image are described as being of high signal intensity, and tissues and structures that are black on the image are of low signal intensity. When the specific technical parameters are changed on the MR magnet system, images can be generated that probe different tissue properties. Two tissue properties, T1 and T2, are examined on T1- and T2-weighted sequences, respectively. The presence of lipid within tissue is identified using chemical shift images. Other properties, such as vascularity, capillary permeability, biliary secretion, or macrophage activity, are imaged using a wide array of different contrast agents (Fig. 98-1). Blood flow in vessels also is selectively visualized with gradient echo sequences, called magnetic resonance angiography. Last, although it is not widely used clinically, MR spectroscopy holds the potential for even more precise tissue characterization. The varied ways in which the tissue signal can be manipulated to probe the specific tissue characteristics have made MRI an exciting field for the investigation of intra-abdominal diseases.

Most research on intra-abdominal MRI has focused on the liver. Tissue contrast in the liver on MRI is particularly advantageous because normal liver shows low signal intensity, and tumors of all types show considerably higher signal intensity on T2-weighted images. Lesions showing very high signal intensity on T2-weighted images are hemangiomas or cysts (Fig. 98-2). Lesions with moderately high signal intensity on T2-weighted images are typically malignant tumors such as hepatocellular carcinomas, metastases, and other primary liver malignancies (Fig. 98-3). On the basis of this different behavior on T2-weighted images, hemangiomas and cysts can be differentiated from metastases and other malignant lesions. The pattern of enhancement after administration of intravenous contrast agents also differentiates hemangiomas from metastasis and hepatocellular carcinomas. Intravenous contrast perfuses through hemangiomas at a slow rate compared to hepatocellular carcinomas and metastases, which demonstrate rapid and heterogeneous contrast enhancement (Fig. 98-4). Many studies have examined the sensitivity of MRI for the detection of metastases, and most have found that MRI is equivalent or superior to contrast-enhanced CT scanning. It is inferior to CT portography in terms of sensitivity, but superior in specificity, because of this ability to differentiate hemangiomas and cysts from metastases.

MRI can also characterize diffuse liver diseases such as cirrhosis, fatty infiltration, and hemochromatosis. Cirrhosis is accurately diagnosed on MRI by visualization of the regenerating nodules directly separated from each other by the fibrovascular septae. Larger regenerating nodules can be differentiated from small hepatocellular carcinomas on the basis of their arterial phase enhancement during dynamic scanning. Macroregenerative nodules or adenomatous hyperplasia show low signal intensity on T2-weighted images, homogeneity, and enhancement during the portal phase. Hepatocellular carcinomas show higher, frequently inhomogeneous signal intensity on T2-weighted images (Fig. 98-5) and become enhanced during the arterial phase. The images frequently show tumor capsules (see Fig. 98-5), metastases, or vascular invasion (Fig. 98-6). Fatty infiltration of the liver is diagnosed on specific MR sequences called chemical shift imaging. Hemochromatosis causes marked low signal intensity on T2-weighted and gradient echo sequences. This finding is specific for abnormal iron deposition in the liver.

MR imaging of the pancreas and biliary tract has been greatly aided in recent years by the introduction of techniques to image the pancreatic duct and the biliary tree. These sequences are called MR cholangiography (Fig. 98-7). They selectively image fluid in the abdomen, including bile and secretions in the biliary tract and pancreatic duct. Using these sequences and displaying them in a format similar to conventional ERCP or cholangiography, one can identify obstruction of the biliary duct and pancreatic duct (Fig. 98-8). Filling defects such as calculi appear as low-signal abnormalities within the duct. Characterization of obstructing lesions is aided by dynamic gadolinium-enhanced images. Pancreatic adenocarcinomas for example, show delayed enhancement relative to normal pancreatic parenchyma (see Fig. 98-8). Furthermore, there is usually intrinsic tissue contrast on T1-weighted images between normal pancreatic parenchyma and tumors or focal chronic pancreatitis. Unlike ERCP or conventional cholangiography, no special contrast agent is needed to display the biliary tract and pancreatic ducts at MR cholangiography.

The potential of MR imaging of disorders that are primarily peritoneal or bowel in origin has only recently begun to be explored. Although peristalsis of bowel causes motion artifacts on MR images, as does respiratory motion, many peritoneal and bowel lesions are imaged well (Fig. 98-9). Bowel motion can be reduced by the intravenous injection of antiperistaltic agents such as glucagon. These techniques can differentiate bowel from pathological processes (Fig. 98-10). Intrinsic intestinal wall abnormalities such as inflammatory bowel disease can be characterized (Fig. 98-11). Several bowel contrast agents are on the market and approved by the U.S. Food and Drug Administration for delineation of the bowel lumen.

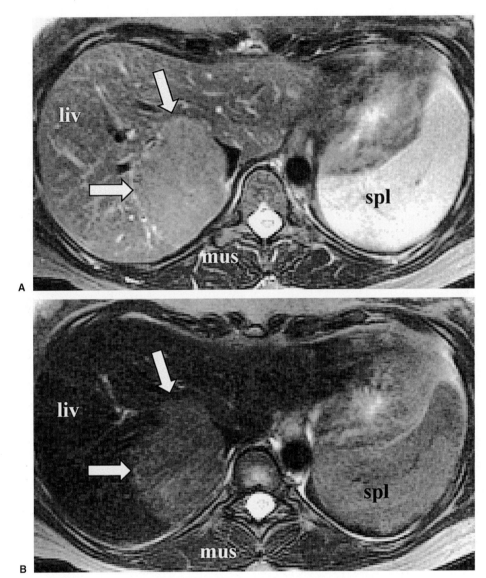

FIGURE 98-1. Characterization of a liver mass as focal nodular hyperplasia with a targeted magnetic resonance (MR) contrast agent. **A:** T2-weighted image in this 28-year-old woman with a liver mass (*arrows*) shows that the mass is hyperintense (bright) compared to muscle (*mus*). **B:** Identical T2-weighted MR image after injection of the patient with intravenous superparamagnetic iron oxide (SPIO) contrast agent shows that the liver (*liv*), spleen (*spl*), and mass (*arrows*) are darker, indicating uptake of the agent. SPIO is taken up by macrophages of the reticuloendothelial system, which occur predominantly in liver, spleen, focal nodular hyperplasia, and rarely, hepatic adenoma.

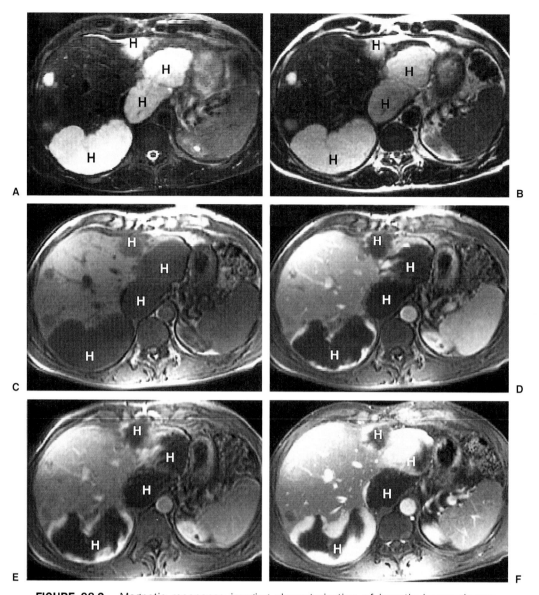

FIGURE 98-2. Magnetic resonance imaging characterization of hepatic hemangiomas. **A:** T2-weighted image shows well-defined hyperintense (bright) masses (*H*) in both lobes of the liver. **B:** Heavily T2-weighted image with a longer echo time than in **A** shows the lesions remaining hyperintense, which is typical for lesions with a high fluid content such as hemangioma and cysts. Note that the liver and spleen show a lower signal intensity (darker) on the heavily T2-weighted image in **B** compared to the standard T2-weighted image in **A**. Malignant liver lesions such as hepatocellular carcinomas and metastases have lower signal intensity than the hemangiomas on a heavily weighted T2-weighted sequence. T1-weighted breath-hold images before (**C**) and after (**D–F**) injection of a gadolinium contrast agent, gadopentetate dimeglumine. Dynamic contrast enhancement during the arterial (**D**) and portal phase (**E**) shows the peripheral nodular enhancement of the hemangiomas (*H*), which proceeds to fill in most of the lesion on the delayed image in **F**. This pattern of enhancement is diagnostic of hepatic hemangiomas.

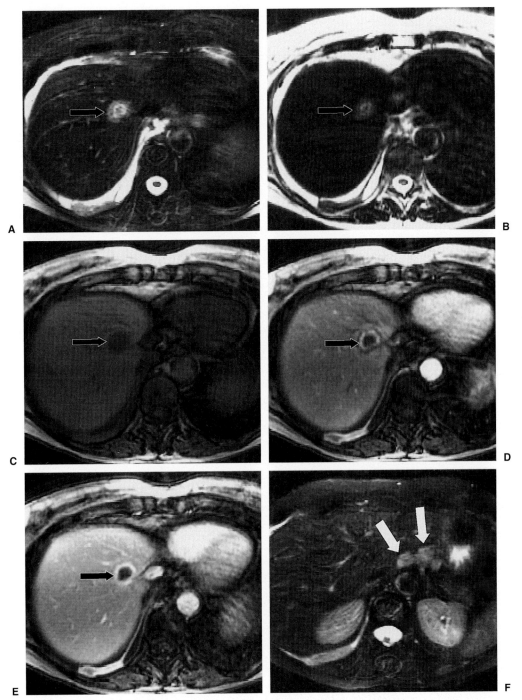

FIGURE 98-3. Magnetic resonance imaging characterization of hepatic metastases in a patient with lung carcinoma. **A:** T2-weighted image shows a metastasis from lung carcinoma in the right lobe of the liver (*black arrow*). **B:** Heavily T2-weighted image with a longer echo time than in **A** shows the lesion is heterogeneous (central hyperintensity) with a ring-like structure, features which are not seen in hemangiomas. The mass is of lower signal intensity than hemangiomas or cysts (compare the degree of signal intensity with the hemangiomas in Fig. 98-2). T1-weighted gradient echo images performed before (**C**) and after (**D, E**) intravenous injection of gadopentetate dimeglumine show ring-like peripheral enhancement of the tumor during the arterial phase (**D**) and in the delayed image (**E**), a pattern distinctly different from that of the hemangioma in Fig. 98–2. This pattern of enhancement is typical of hypervascular tumors. The darker ring surrounding the tumor in (**D**) results from compression of hepatic parenchyma, which enhances in a delayed manner (**E**). The center of the tumor does not become enhanced because of necrosis. **F:** T2-weighted image shows enlarged hyperintense lymph nodes (*white arrows*) along the celiac axis that represent nodal metastases.

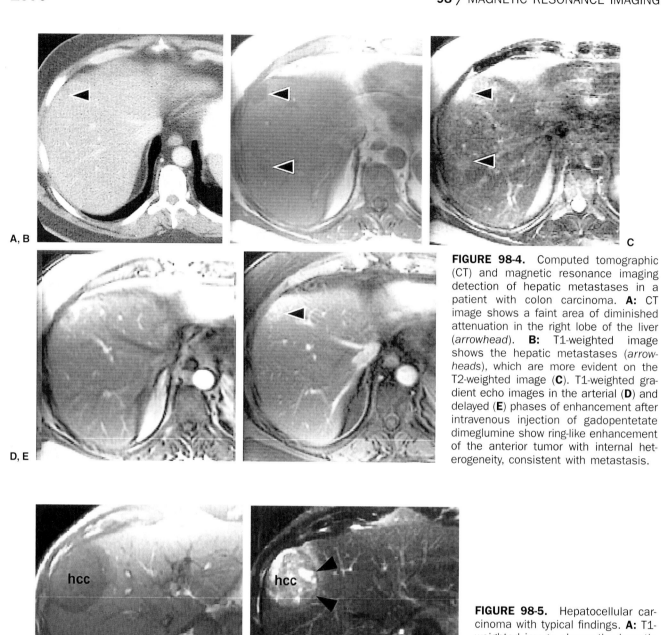

FIGURE 98-4. Computed tomographic (CT) and magnetic resonance imaging detection of hepatic metastases in a patient with colon carcinoma. **A:** CT image shows a faint area of diminished attenuation in the right lobe of the liver (*arrowhead*). **B:** T1-weighted image shows the hepatic metastases (*arrowheads*), which are more evident on the T2-weighted image (**C**). T1-weighted gradient echo images in the arterial (**D**) and delayed (**E**) phases of enhancement after intravenous injection of gadopentetate dimeglumine show ring-like enhancement of the anterior tumor with internal heterogeneity, consistent with metastasis.

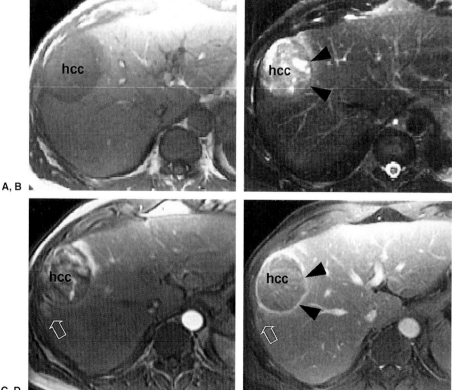

FIGURE 98-5. Hepatocellular carcinoma with typical findings. **A:** T1-weighted image shows the hepatic mass (*hcc*) in the right lobe of the liver. **B:** Internal necrosis and a thin tumor capsule (*arrowheads*) are evident on the T2-weighted image. **C:** T1-weighted image performed during the arterial phase of liver enhancement after injection with gadopentetate dimeglumine shows rapid enhancement of the hepatocellular carcinoma, as well as a satellite nodule (*open arrow*). **D:** T1-weighted image of delayed enhancement 3 minutes after injection shows the tumor capsule (*arrowheads*) to better advantage. The findings of a tumor capsule and arterial phase hypervascularity are commonly seen in hepatocellular carcinoma, which was proven at biopsy.

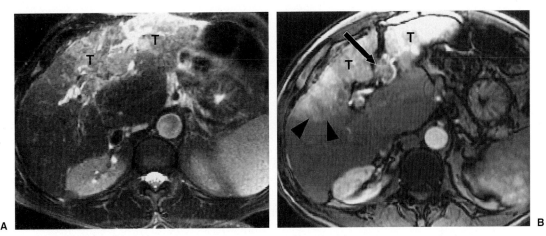

FIGURE 98-6. Hepatocellular carcinoma with portal vein invasion. **A:** T2-weighted image shows extensive tumor (*T*) in the left lobe of the liver with higher signal intensity than the normal liver in the right lobe. **B:** T1-weighted image performed immediately after gadopentetate dimeglumine injection during the arterial phase of liver enhancement shows rapid enhancement of the hepatocellular carcinoma (*T*). There is enhancement of the tumor thrombus in the left portal vein (*arrow*). Arterial enhancement of the medial segment of the left lobe (*arrowheads*) is due to obstruction of portal flow with compensatory increased arterial perfusion.

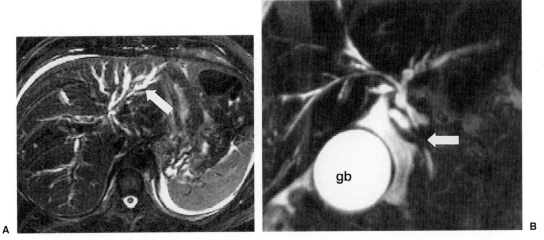

FIGURE 98-7. Magnetic resonance (MR) cholangiography in a patient with sclerosing cholangitis. **A:** T2-weighted image shows intrahepatic dilated ducts in the left lobe of the liver (*arrow*). **B:** MR cholangiogram selectively images the common bile duct, common hepatic duct, and some of the intrahepatic ducts. Multifocal intrahepatic biliary strictures and dilations are evident, as well as a dominant stricture in the common bile duct (*arrow*). *gb,* gallbladder.

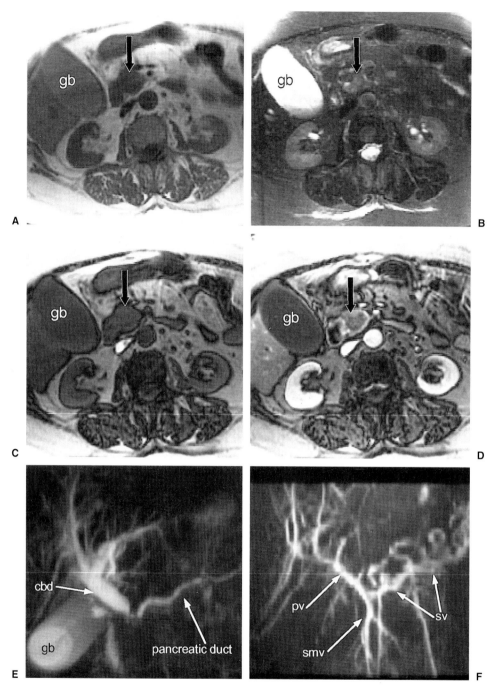

FIGURE 98-8. Evaluation of pancreatic carcinoma in an 81-year-old woman. **A:** T1-weighted spin echo image shows the focal low signal abnormality within the uncinate process (*arrow*). Normal pancreas is brighter than liver on T1-weighted images. **B:** T2-weighted image shows that the carcinoma (*arrow*) is of low signal intensity, similar to normal pancreatic parenchyma, and therefore is not well seen. T1-weighted gradient echo images performed in suspended respiration before (**C**) and after (**D**) injection of gadopentetate dimeglumine show abnormal arterial enhancement (*arrow*) of the pancreatic head caused by the tumor. Normal pancreatic parenchyma enhances intensely during the arterial phase, similar to the kidney, whereas adenocarcinoma is less enhanced, as shown here. **E:** Three-dimensional magnetic resonance (MR) cholangiogram shows obstruction of the common bile duct (*cbd*) and pancreatic duct in the pancreatic head, producing the double duct sign. **F:** Anterior projection of MR angiogram shows patent superior mesenteric vein (*smv*), portal vein (*pv*), and splenic vein (*sv*), indicating lack of encasement. *gb,* gallbladder.

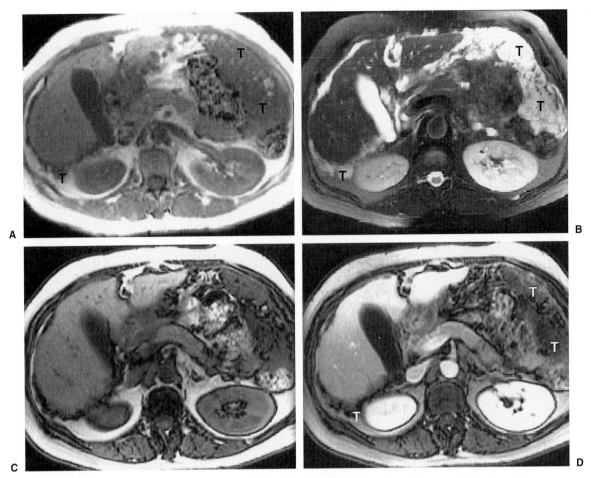

FIGURE 98-9. Peritoneal carcinomatosis (pseudomyxoma peritonei) from metastatic mucinous rectal carcinoma. T1-weighted (**A**) and T2-weighted image (**B**) shows extensive tumor
(*T*) in the left upper quadrant and perihepatic regions. The tumor shows high signal intensity, similar to that of fluid. T1-weighted images obtained before (**C**) and after (**D**) injection of gadopentetate dimeglumine show enhancement of the tumor deposits (*T*), indicating presence of a vascularized tumor and not ascites.

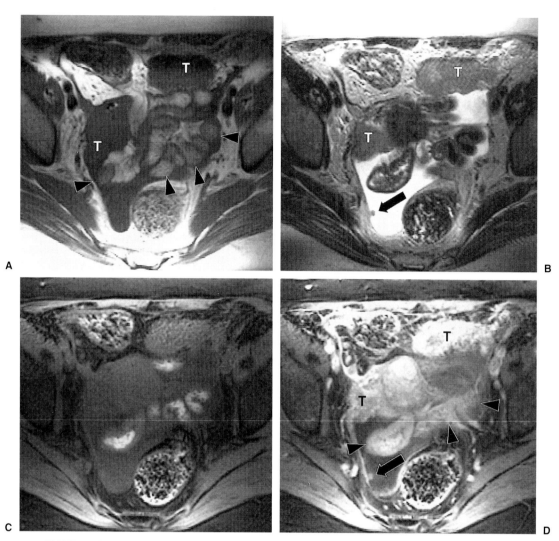

FIGURE 98-10. Peritoneal enhancement in a patient with ovarian carcinoma metastatic to the peritoneum. **A:** Axial T1-weighted spin echo image shows fluid in the cul-de-sac appearing as intermediate signal intensity surrounding the higher-signal-intensity loops of the small bowel (*arrowheads*). Tumor nodules (*T*) have different signal intensity than that of small bowel, but cannot be distinguished from the fluid. **B:** Axial T2-weighted fast spin echo image shows fluid in the cul-de-sac as bright signal. A small nodule (*arrow*) lies along the peritoneum in the cul-de-sac. Axial fat-saturated T1-weighted images before (**C**) and after (**D**) gadopentetate dimeglumine injection show peritoneal enhancement (brighter lining in **D**) surrounding the fluid, enhancement of the peritoneal implant of tumor (*straight arrow*), and the larger tumor masses (*T*). The contents of the small bowel luminal are bright in **C** and there is enhancement of the bowel wall (*arrowheads* in **D**) caused by tumor infiltration. Surgical findings confirmed peritoneal spread of tumor and tumor masses.

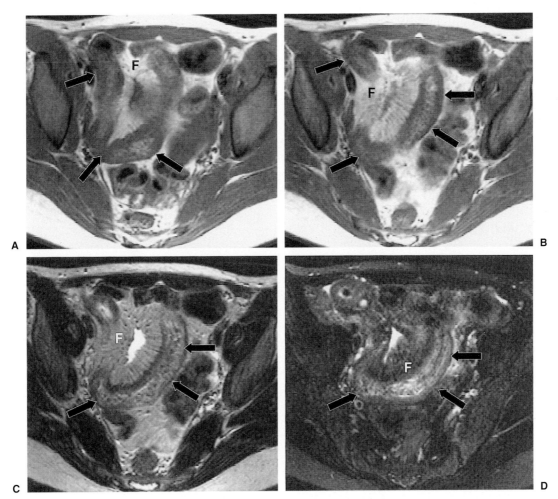

FIGURE 98-11. Crohn's disease in 26-year-old pregnant patient. Bowel wall thickening with infiltration of mesenteric fat (*F*). **A, B:** Axial T1-weighted images at different locations show bowel wall thickening in a loop of terminal ileum (*arrows*). Stranding in mesenteric fat (*F*) is evident. Axial T2-weighted fast spin echo images without (**C**) and with (**D**) fat saturation demonstrate the transmural wall thickening with higher than normal signal intensity of the wall (*arrows*) and in the mesenteric fat (*F*).

APPLICATIONS OF RADIONUCLIDE IMAGING IN GASTROENTEROLOGY

ARNOLD F. JACOBSON

Selecting the most appropriate imaging technique for a given clinical situation remains one of the more daunting tasks for both the clinician and the imaging specialist. Although the role of nuclear medicine, the imaging specialty that uses radioactive isotopes (radionuclides) in diagnostic evaluations of anatomy and particularly physiology, is often less well appreciated than that of other modalities such as ultrasound, computed tomography (CT), and magnetic resonance imaging (MRI), radionuclide imaging remains an important contributor to the provision of high-quality health care. Both agents introduced in the past decade and others that have been in use for 30 years or longer continue to expand the number of clinical applications served by this diagnostic modality.

Most radionuclide imaging agents are labeled with technetium 99m (^{99m}Tc), primarily because of its favorable physical characteristics, including a relatively short half-life (6 hours) which limits patient radiation dose, and a principal photon energy (140 keV) that is well suited to the gamma camera, the standard instrument for nuclear medicine imaging. Radiopharmaceutical chemists have proved particularly adept at incorporating technetium into a wide variety of compounds and complexes of biologic interest. Other radionuclides that are used less frequently but still play a role in routine clinical nuclear medicine imaging include indium 111 (^{111}In), gallium 67 (^{67}Ga), thallium 201, and iodine 123 and 131. In recent years, the increased availability of positron-emission tomography (PET) scanners and gamma cameras capable of performing coincidence imaging has placed the positron emitter fluorine 18 (in the form of fluorodeoxyglucose [FDG]) in the list of radionuclides routinely used in many nuclear medicine clinics.

Although the radionuclide liver-spleen scan using technetium-labeled colloid (sulfur or albumin) was one of the earliest introduced and most widely used gastrointestinal system nuclear medicine studies for many years, it is now more of historical interest than of practical clinical importance. There are multiple other radionuclide techniques in routine clinical use for imaging the liver. One such technique is hepatobiliary imaging using one of the several technetium-labeled iminodiacetic acid (IDA) compounds extracted by the liver hepatocytes and excreted in the bile. These agents have established utility for diagnosis of acute and chronic cholecystitis on the basis of the absence of or delay in bile flow through the cystic duct. They are also useful for defining the patency of the intra- and extrahepatic bile ducts and identifying the presence of posttraumatic or postsurgical bile leaks.

For identifying the presence of hepatic cavernous hemangiomas, imaging with technetium-labeled red blood cells (RBCs) has sensitivity comparable to that of contrast CT, ultrasound, and MRI for detection of lesions greater than 1.5 cm. These various radiologic modalities all depend on identification of the signal characteristics associated with the increased vascularity and blood pool in hemangiomas, which are reflected by increased accumulation of labeled RBCs during the nuclear medicine exam. Imaging of the liver for the possible presence of primary tumor or metastases may be done using a variety of agents, including gallium-, technetium-, and indium-labeled monoclonal antibodies and peptides, and FDG.

Several other notable radionuclide imaging techniques have been in routine clinical use for several decades. For patients with gastrointestinal bleeding of obscure origin, usually after at least one negative or equivocal endoscopy (upper or lower), technetium-labeled RBC imaging can be used to detect both acute and intermittent GI hemorrhage. This technique is particularly flexible because once the technetium-labeled RBCs have been injected intravenously, imaging can be performed intermittently for as long as 24 to 30 hours. This allows the detection of bleeding that occurs not only immediately after injection of the tracer, as in visualization of contrast extravasation on x-ray angiography, but also several hours later. Another source of GI bleeding, the Meckel diverticulum, can usually be identified using the tracer technetium pertechnetate, which is actively extracted by cells of the gastric mucosa, thereby allowing demonstration of Meckel diverticula and other congenital anomalies that contain ectopic gastric mucosa.

One of the strengths of nuclear medicine imaging is its quantitative capability. In the gastrointestinal tract, this is best demonstrated in the various studies used to examine gastrointestinal motility. The most common of these is the gastric emptying study, in which a radiolabeled liquid or solid meal is ingested and the clearance of the activity from the stomach is monitored over time. From the time-activity curve for the stomach, both emptying rates and half-times can be determined and compared with reference control data. Whole gut motility studies, which monitor passage of labeled substances from the stomach through the colon, may require several days of imaging and usually employ a ^{111}In rather than a ^{99m}Tc tracer because ^{111}In has a longer half-life. Other applications of quantitative radionuclide imaging in the tubular gastrointestinal tract include measurements of gastroesophageal reflux, sometimes including quantitation of pulmonary aspiration, and esophageal motility during a series of liquid swallows. Elsewhere in the abdomen, quantitation of gallbladder contraction can be readily performed using hepatobiliary scintigraphy and a cholecystagogue (cholecystokinin or a synthetic analog).

Single photon emission CT (SPECT), the nuclear medicine equivalent of tomographic radiologic techniques such as CT and MRI, is widely used to provide improved contrast resolution and anatomic detail via cross-sectional images displayed in transverse, sagittal, coronal, and other user-specified planes. SPECT is routinely performed as part of ^{99m}Tc-labeled RBC studies to identify hepatic hemangiomas, as well as in most of the applications in the abdomen involving imaging agents for infection and tumor.

Numerous radiopharmaceuticals are available for evaluating patients for the presence of infection and tumor. The prototypical agent in this category, ^{67}Ga-citrate, although still used for infection, particularly in immune-compromised patients, has been largely supplanted by FDG-PET for imaging of tumors such as hepatomas and lymphomas. Another useful agent for infection imaging is white blood cells (WBCs) labeled with either ^{111}In or ^{99m}Tc. Labeled leukocyte imaging can aid in identification of abscesses in the abdominal cavity, the tubular viscera, and the solid organs. Labeled WBC imaging can also be used to identify the presence of inflammatory bowel disease and infectious colitis, and to monitor response to therapy as a supplement to serial endoscopic evaluations.

Two categories of agents for tumor imaging that have become commonplace during the last decade are radiolabeled peptides and monoclonal antibodies. In the former category, the best characterized is indium-labeled octreotide, a somatostatin receptor agent that can be used to identify neuroendocrine malignancies such as enteropancreatic tumors and carcinoids. Octreotide scanning is particularly useful for clarifying equivocal CT results or to restage suspected occult recurrence. Monoclonal antibody agents have achieved only limited success since their introduction in the mid-1990s, and like gallium, are now primarily used in centers where PET is not readily available. These agents include indium-labeled OncoScint CR/OV (Cytogen, Princeton, NJ), a whole antibody used for colorectal cancer imaging, and technetium-labeled CEA-Scan (Immunomedics, Morris Plains, NJ), an anti–carcinoembryonic Fab′ antibody fragment that can also be used for identifying both primary and recurrent colorectal cancer.

Clinical radionuclide imaging includes a wide breadth of techniques and applications. There are many specific situations in which the nuclear medicine method can complement, supplement, or even replace other conventional radiologic modalities. Most often, however, nuclear medicine imaging serves best when used in conjunction with other imaging methods. Such imaging adds elements of physiology and function to the anatomic details delineated by other means. Scintigraphic results can be particularly helpful as an aid to characterizing the etiology of often incidental findings seen on ultrasound, CT, or MRI. With the increased use of PET and the continued development of new radiopharmaceuticals for conventional nuclear medicine imaging, particularly the peptides, radionuclide imaging techniques are well-positioned to remain an important contributor to patient assessment in clinical gastroenterology for many years to come.

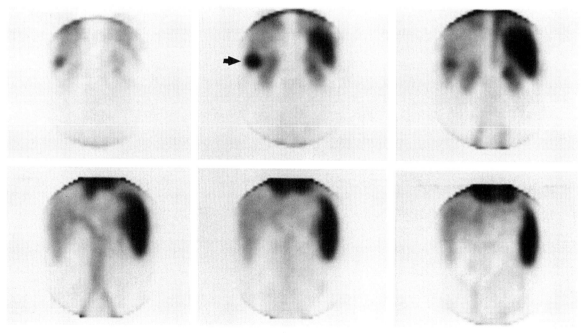

FIGURE 99-1. Cavernous hemangioma. Sequential coronal single photon emission computed tomography images (posterior to anterior, **upper left** to **lower right**) from a labeled red blood cell scan of the liver show a focal region of increased activity (*arrow*) in the right lobe representing a 3-cm cavernous hemangioma initially identified on sonography.

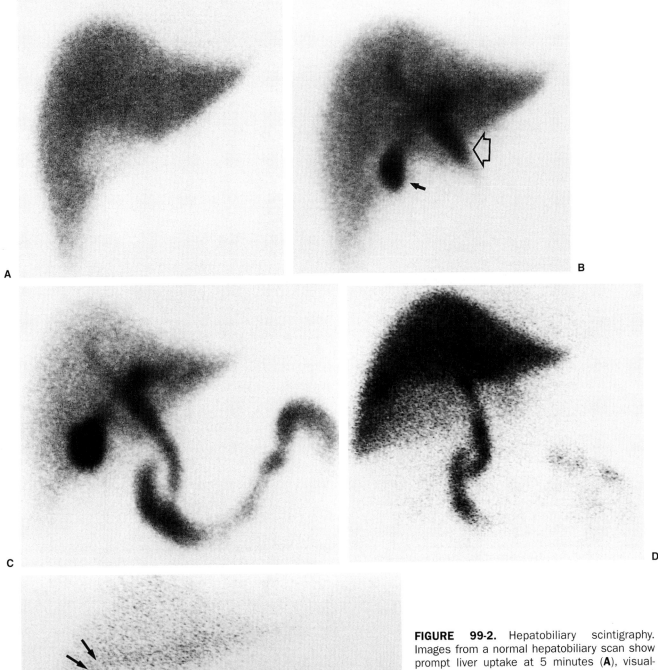

FIGURE 99-2. Hepatobiliary scintigraphy. Images from a normal hepatobiliary scan show prompt liver uptake at 5 minutes (**A**), visualization of the common bile duct (*open arrow*) and gallbladder (*arrow*) at 30 minutes (**B**), and activity in the small bowel at 50 minutes (**C**). An abnormal hepatobiliary scan shows prompt liver uptake, and bile duct and small bowel activity at 10 minutes (**D**), but the gallbladder was not visualized at 60 minutes and a rim sign (*arrows*) was observed (**E**). The surgical finding was acute cholecystitis with gallbladder necrosis.

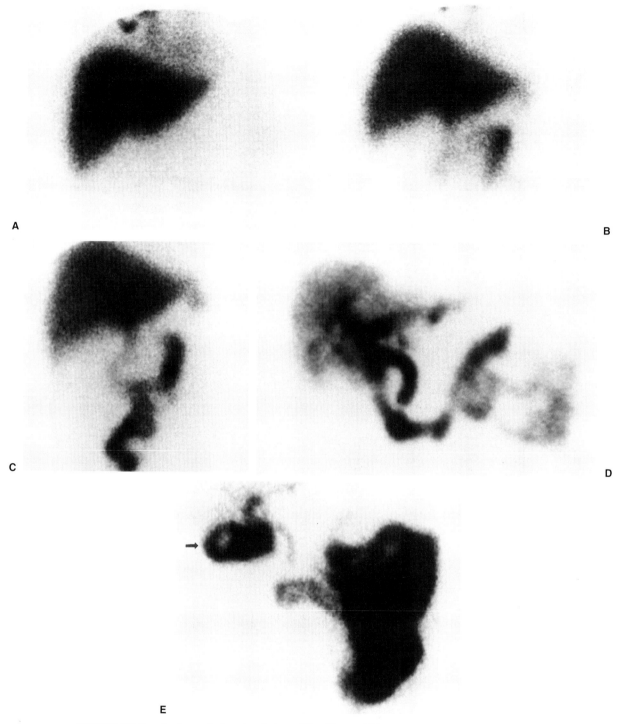

A

B

C

D

E

FIGURE 99-3. Acute and chronic cholecystitis. Hepatobiliary study on a 41-year-old man with abnormal liver function tests and equivocal gallbladder ultrasound shows a small amount of activity in the cardiac blood pool and spleen at 15 minutes after injection (**A**). At 60 minutes after injection (**B**), there is a moderate amount of activity in the proximal small bowel, with no visualization of the gallbladder. The patient was then given 3.4 mg morphine sulfate intravenously (IV), but the gallbladder still was not visualized 30 minutes later (**C**). Surgery performed several days later demonstrated acute acalculous cholecystitis. The curvilinear structure seen superior to the midportion of the liver, particularly on the 15-minute image, represents the central venous catheter through which the radiopharmaceutical was initially injected. Images **D** and **E** are from a second study in which the gallbladder was not visualized at 60 minutes, the first prior to and the second following IV administration of 4 mg morphine sulfate. The later image shows activity in the gallbladder (*arrow*), with a central photopenic region corresponding to either one large or multiple small gallstones. The visualization of tracer activity in the gallbladder following administration of morphine generally reflects chronic rather than acute cholecystitis.

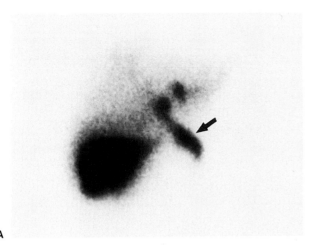
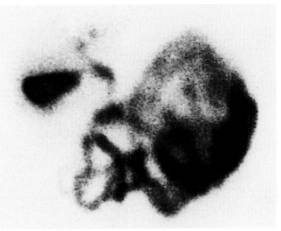

A

B

FIGURE 99-4. High resting sphincter of Oddi tone. Hepatobiliary study was performed on a 62-year-old diabetic man with right upper quadrant pain and tenderness, and poorly visualized gallbladder on ultrasound scans. Images shown are from 60 (**A**) and 90 minutes after injection (**B**). The 60-minute image shows substantial activity in the gallbladder (tracer was first seen in the gallbladder at 15 minutes [image not shown]), with only a small amount of activity remaining in the liver. The common bile duct is apparent (*arrow*), but no distinct activity is noted in the small bowel. Because there was no clinical suspicion of common duct obstruction, the patient was given a small amount of whole milk to drink. On the image 30 minutes later (**B**), a substantial amount of activity is present throughout the entire small bowel. Activity in the gallbladder is also reduced, consistent with contraction in response to the fatty stimulus. These findings are consistent with a high resting sphincter of Oddi tone in the fasting state, a normal variant seen in up to 20% of normal subjects on hepatobiliary imaging.

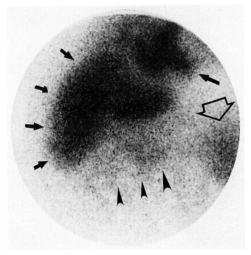
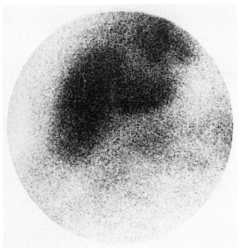

A

B

FIGURE 99-5. Liver failure. A hepatobiliary scan was performed on a 44-year-old man 2 years after orthotopic liver transplantation because of recent progressive worsening of cholestasis and liver failure. Recent endoscopic retrograde cholangiopancreatography demonstrated an anastomotic stricture of the extrahepatic bile duct, which was then stented, but the patient continued to have extremely elevated alkaline phosphatase (2628 U/L) and bilirubin (25.7 mg/dL) levels. Hepatobiliary study with 11 mCi of ^{99m}Tc-mebrofenin showed very minimal specific liver uptake. Images at 30 minutes (**A**) and 5 hours after injection (**B**) show virtually the same pattern of activity in the heart (*single arrow*), liver (*multiple arrows*), spleen (*open arrow*), and upper abdomen (*arrowheads*). This is a pattern of blood-pool activity with no significant uptake by the liver hepatocytes, consistent with overwhelming liver failure. This can be differentiated from the pattern of intrahepatic cholestasis, in which the cardiac and other vascular activity disappears over time, while activity remains in the liver because of specific uptake by hepatocytes, but without subsequent excretion into the bowel.

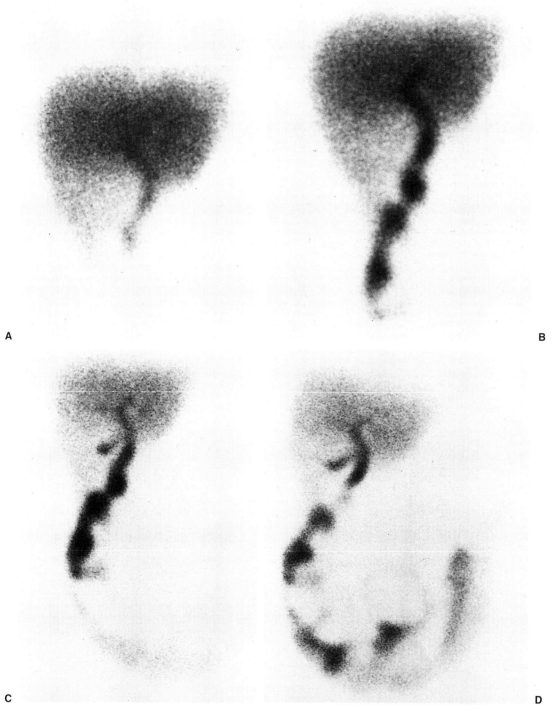

A

B

C

D

FIGURE 99-6. Bile leak. A hepatobiliary scan was performed on a 79-year-old man who had nonspecific abdominal complaints and a bilirubin level of 1.2 mg/dL. An early image at 15 minutes (**A**) shows relatively good uptake of ^{99m}Tc-mebrofenin by the liver, with depiction of the common bile duct and a small amount of activity in the proximal small bowel. On subsequent images at 30 minutes (**B**), 60 minutes (**C**) and 75 minutes after injection (**D**), however, activity is seen tracking down the right lateral abdomen, then moving medially across the pelvis to the left side. This pattern of activity is consistent with movement of radiotracer in the peritoneal cavity. There is no definite visualization of activity within the bowel beyond the duodenum near the point of entrance of the common duct into the small bowel. Activity is seen in the cystic duct on the later views, but activity is not definitely identified in the gallbladder. The patient died after completion of this study. The autopsy finding was a perforated duodenal ulcer.

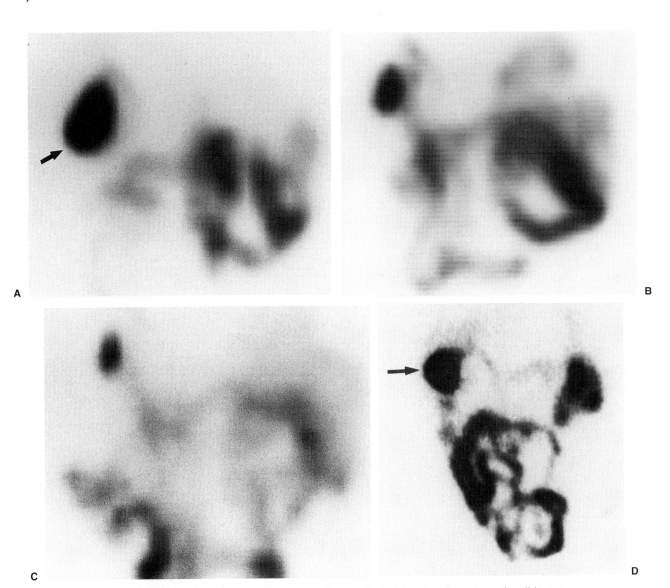

A

B

C

D

FIGURE 99-7. Gall bladder ejection fraction. Selected images from two sincalide-augmented hepatobiliary scans are shown. A 65-year-old man with nausea and anorexia and a negative gastrointestinal tract evaluation underwent a ^{99m}Tc-mebrofenin study with normal uptake by the liver and visualization of the gallbladder. After approximately 1 hour, a 0.02 μg/kg infusion of sincalide was administered intravenously (IV) over 30 minutes. Images shown are at 6 (**A**), 18 (**B**), and 30 minutes (**C**) into the infusion. On the initial image, only gallbladder (*arrow*) and small bowel activity are seen. There was prompt contraction of the gallbladder after the infusion was begun, as can be appreciated from the decreased size and intensity of activity in the gallbladder on the subsequent images. Calculated maximum gallbladder ejection fraction was 83%. The second study was performed on a 39-year-old woman with a 2-week history of abdominal pain and right upper quadrant tenderness and suspected cholecystitis. Initial images (not shown) showed rapid uptake of the pharmaceutical by the liver and gallbladder and spontaneous excretion into the gut. A sincalide infusion of 0.02 μg/kg administered IV over 30 minutes was performed to assess gallbladder contractility. Images are shown from the 2nd minute (**D**), the 19th minute (**E**), and the 31st minute (**F**) of the study. Gallbladder (*arrow*) contraction is minimal during the course of the infusion, with a calculated ejection fraction of 11%, possibly reflecting underlying hepatobiliary disease. However, comparison of the bowel pattern from the first to the last image, shows evidence of substantial progression of activity from the multiple loops of small bowel initially to a large concentration of activity in the right colon by 19 minutes and persisting to 31 minutes. This reflects an increase in bowel motility produced by the sincalide. *(Continued)*

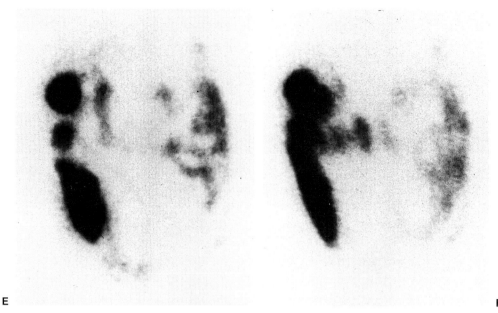

E   F

FIGURE 99-7.   (Continued)

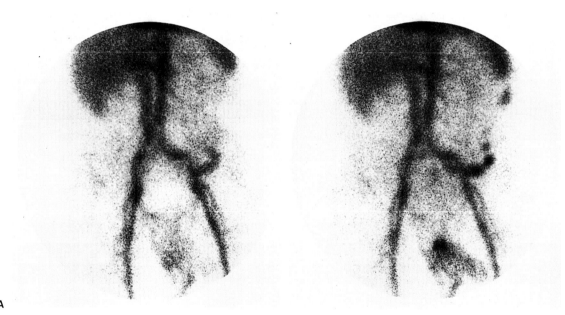

A   B

FIGURE 99-8.   Active gastrointestinal (GI) bleeding. **A–D:** Images from a ^{99m}Tc-labeled red blood cell (RBC) study on a 70-year-old man who was passing bright red blood per rectum and had a progressively decreasing hematocrit. Labeled RBC activity is seen in the left lower quadrant on the first image at 5 minutes after injection (**A**), in a pattern suggestive of distal left or proximal sigmoid colon. On the images at 30 minutes (**B**), 45 minutes (**C**), and 60 minutes (**D**), activity moves retrograde into the left colon and later appears in the midline behind the bladder (*arrows*) in a location (seen on a lateral image [not shown]) indicative of sigmoid colon and rectum. Angiographic findings subsequent to the RBC scan were negative, but colonoscopy demonstrated diverticular disease in the descending and sigmoid colon presumed to be the source of bleeding. Bleeding resolved spontaneously without surgical intervention. *(Continued)*

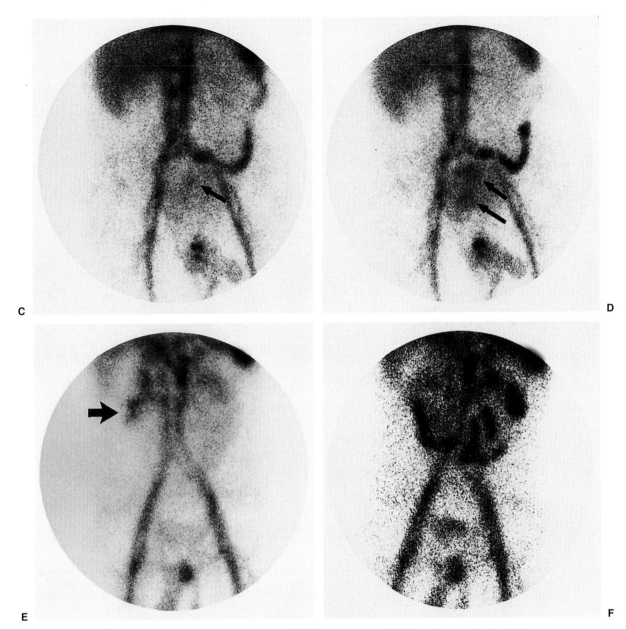

C

D

E

F

FIGURE 99-8. E–G: Images are from a ^{99m}Tc-labeled RBC GI bleeding study of a 43-year-old man with large volume passage of bright red blood per rectum over the preceding 18 hours. Upper endoscopy performed prior to this study showed duodenal ulcers that were not actively bleeding. Images shown are from 3 minutes (**E**), 15 minutes (**F**), and 40 minutes (**G**) after injection of the tracer. The initial image shows accumulation of abnormal labeled RBCs in the right upper quadrant overlying the right kidney (*arrow*). *(Continued)*

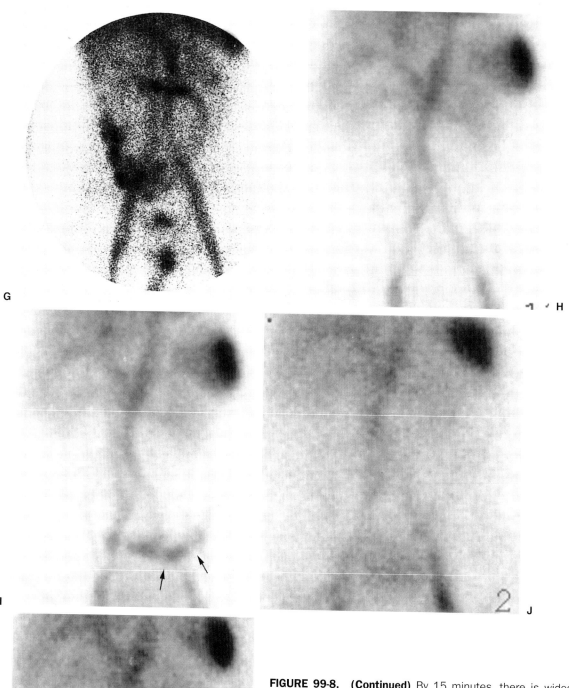

FIGURE 99-8. (Continued) By 15 minutes, there is widespread distribution of labeled RBCs throughout multiple loops of small bowel. After approximately 30 minutes, the patient passed approximately 200 mL of red blood per rectum. The image obtained shortly afterward (**G**) distinctly demonstrates activity extending from the cecum to the right, transverse, and descending colon. Endoscopic examination following a negative angiography showed evidence of gastric varices and duodenal ulcers. The presumed cause of the patient's GI hemorrhage was a combination of coagulopathy (initial international normalized ratio of 6:1), variceal bleeding, and bleeding from the duodenal ulcers. **H–K:** Images from a GI bleeding scan performed to investigate the source of bright red blood per rectum. The scan was negative (25-minute image shown in **H**) until 48 minutes, when activity began to accumulate in the lower abdomen just to the left of midline (**I,** *arrows*). Shortly thereafter, the patient passed a bloody stool. Follow-up images showed no significant intralumenal bowel activity initially (**J**), then new focal activity began to accumulate in the left lower quadrant several minutes later (**K,** *arrowhead*). Colonoscopic examination subsequently demonstrated bleeding diverticula in the sigmoid colon.

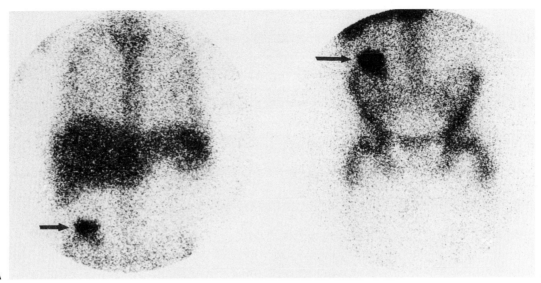

FIGURE 99-9. Abdominal abscess. Anterior chest and abdomen (**A**) and pelvis (**B**) images from ^{111}In-leukocyte scan show normal biodistribution of activity in the liver, spleen, and bone marrow, and abnormal focal increased uptake in the right lower quadrant (*arrows*). Contrast-enhanced computed tomography and subsequent surgery confirmed the presence of an abscess in this location secondary to a perforated diverticulum.

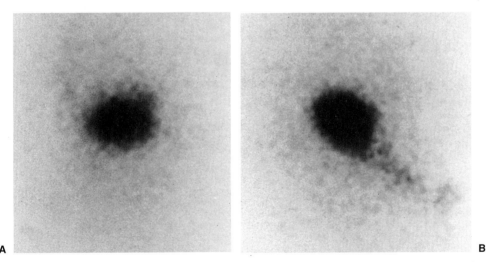

FIGURE 99-10. Normal gastric emptying study. A 52-year-old man with diabetes and history of nausea and dyspepsia underwent a gastric emptying study. Shown are anterior (**A**) and posterior (**B**) images of the abdomen obtained immediately after ingestion of 0.5 mCi ^{99m}Tc-sulfur colloid in an egg salad sandwich and images at 30 minutes (**C, D**) and 60 minutes (**E, F**). *(Continued)*

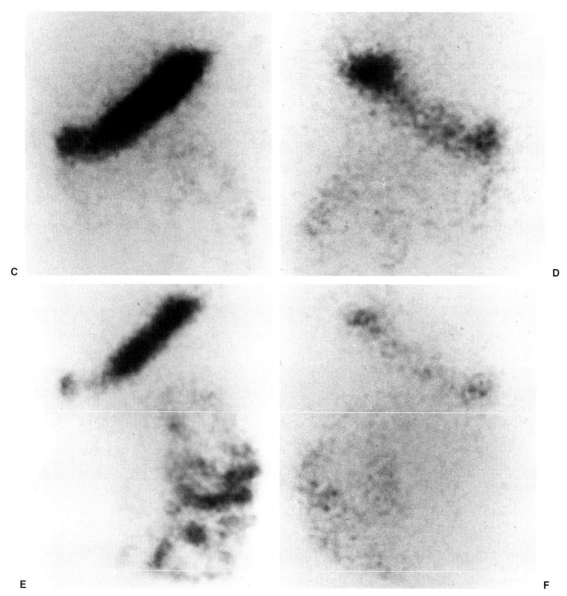

C

D

E

F

FIGURE 99-10.   (Continued) There is progressive transit of activity from the stomach into the small bowel, with a gastric emptying half-time estimated at 50 minutes, within the normal range.

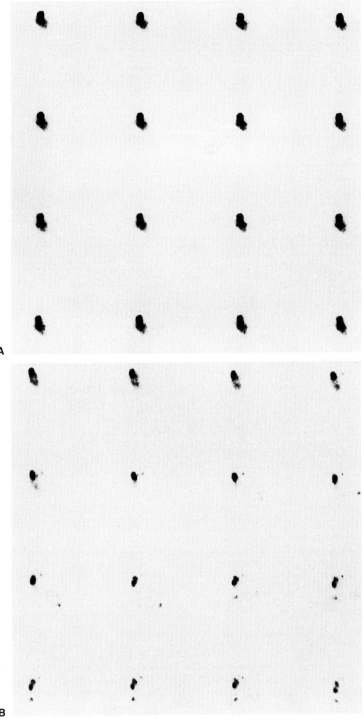

A

B

FIGURE 99-11. Gastric emptying study with prolonged lag phase. Serial posterior images (**A, B**) and time-activity curve (**C**) from a gastric emptying study using 0.5 mCi ^{99m}Tc-sulfur colloid mixed in an egg salad sandwich. Patient is a 43-year-old man presenting with nocturnal vomiting. Two series of 16 sequential images of 1 minute per frame are shown: the first shows the initial 16 minutes of the study (**A**) and the second encompasses minutes 33 to 48 (**B**). During the initial phase of the study, there is no significant emptying of the stomach, with minimal change in the time-activity curve through approximately 30 minutes. There is then a period of rapid gastric emptying, as reflected on the later images as well as the time-activity curve, which occurs over approximately 15 minutes and ends at approximately 45 minutes into the study. Bowel activity is not apparent on the second set of images (**B**) because of image scaling to the stomach contents. Calculated gastric emptying half-time is 38 minutes. However, there is no significant additional emptying of the gastric contents for the second 45 minutes of the study. This study demonstrates evidence of gastric dysmotility with a prolonged lag phase initially and persistent residual food in the stomach after a rapid emptying phase. This study illustrates why it is necessary to examine more than the emptying half-times in gastric emptying studies, because patterns of motor function may suggest dysfunction even though numeric descriptors such as emptying half-time may be normal.

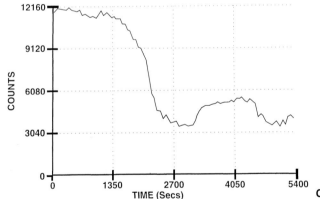

C

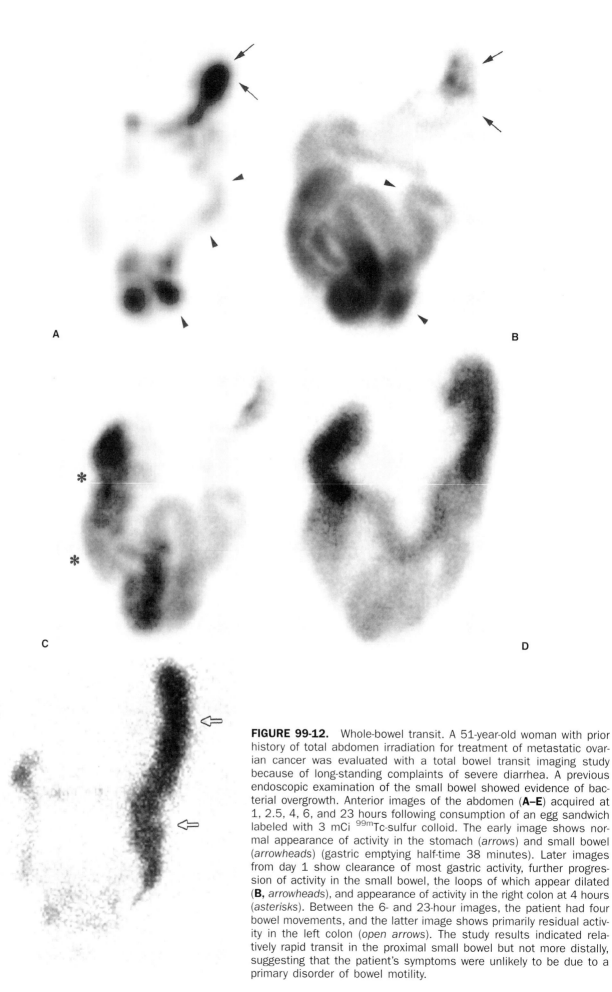

FIGURE 99-12. Whole-bowel transit. A 51-year-old woman with prior history of total abdomen irradiation for treatment of metastatic ovarian cancer was evaluated with a total bowel transit imaging study because of long-standing complaints of severe diarrhea. A previous endoscopic examination of the small bowel showed evidence of bacterial overgrowth. Anterior images of the abdomen (**A–E**) acquired at 1, 2.5, 4, 6, and 23 hours following consumption of an egg sandwich labeled with 3 mCi ^{99m}Tc-sulfur colloid. The early image shows normal appearance of activity in the stomach (*arrows*) and small bowel (*arrowheads*) (gastric emptying half-time 38 minutes). Later images from day 1 show clearance of most gastric activity, further progression of activity in the small bowel, the loops of which appear dilated (**B,** *arrowheads*), and appearance of activity in the right colon at 4 hours (*asterisks*). Between the 6- and 23-hour images, the patient had four bowel movements, and the latter image shows primarily residual activity in the left colon (*open arrows*). The study results indicated relatively rapid transit in the proximal small bowel but not more distally, suggesting that the patient's symptoms were unlikely to be due to a primary disorder of bowel motility.

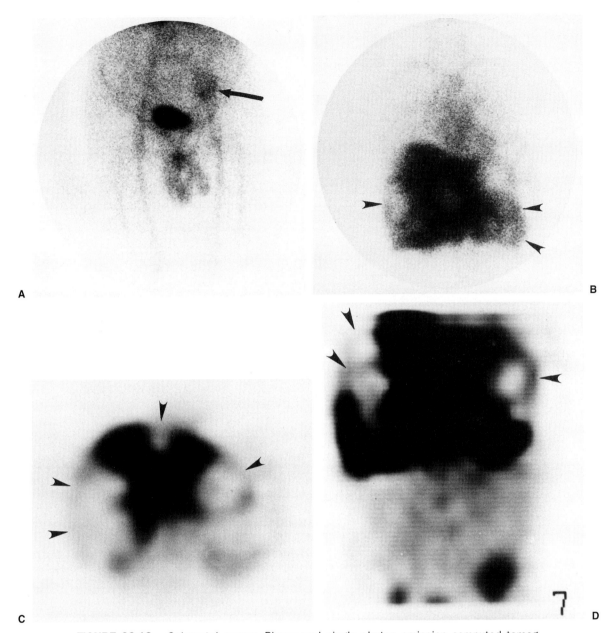

FIGURE 99-13. Colorectal cancer. Planar and single photon emission computed tomography (SPECT) images from a ⁹⁹ᵐTc-CEA-Scan study on a 61-year-old man with previously diagnosed colon cancer and hepatic metastases. Planar images of the anterior pelvis (**A**) and chest and upper abdomen (**B**) 5 hours after injection of the radiopharmaceutical demonstrate distinct increased uptake in the left lower quadrant overlying the iliac vessels, in the region of the known left colon primary (*arrow*). There are multiple large photopenic defects in both the right and left lobes of the liver (*arrowheads*), corresponding with metastatic lesions evident on computed tomographic scan. Cardiac blood pool activity is also still apparent. SPECT images of the abdomen, in both axial (**C**) and coronal planes (**D**), also show the multiple photopenic defects (*arrowheads*). It is not uncommon for larger liver metastases to appear as photopenic defects on antibody imaging. This appearance is presumed to reflect necrotic tumor and areas of metastasis with poor blood supply that limit access of the labeled antibodies.

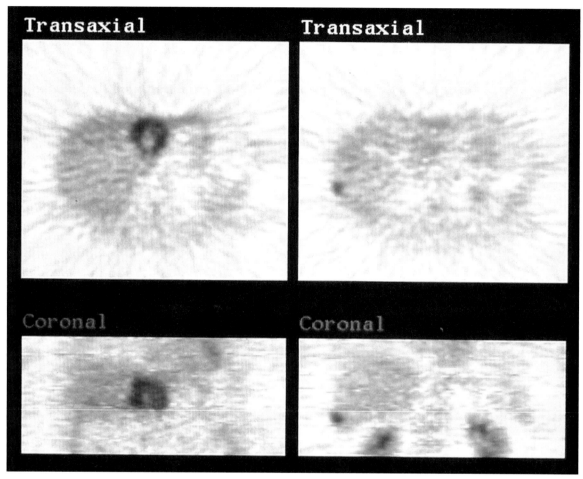

FIGURE 99-14. Positron emission tomography (PET). Selected transaxial (**top**) and coronal (**bottom**) images from a fluorodeoxyglucose (FDG) PET study on a 47-year-old man with history of colon cancer (treated with subtotal colectomy) and liver metastases (treated with laser ablation). Study was obtained because of an increasing carcinoembryonic antigen level and computed tomographic (CT) scan showing post-laser changes in the left lobe and an equivocal low attenuation area in the right lobe of the liver. There is a large area of increased uptake in the left lobe of the liver (**left**) with a central area of decreased activity likely reflecting necrotic tissue. A smaller focus of increased uptake is present more posteriorly in the inferolateral aspect of the right lobe (**right**), corresponding in location to the second CT finding. Biopsy of the left lobe abnormality confirmed presence of recurrent colon carcinoma.

100

ANGIOGRAPHY

KYUNG J. CHO

Angiography is performed to establish a specific diagnosis of neoplasm and vascular lesions, to evaluate portal hemodynamics, and to obtain specific information about vascular anatomy and variation before radiologic and surgical intervention. In this chapter the technique and use of angiography in the diagnosis and management of gastrointestinal, pancreatic, and hepatic lesions are illustrated.

PERCUTANEOUS ANGIOGRAPHY

Gastrointestinal angiography is performed by means of percutaneous retrograde femoral arterial catheterization (Seldinger technique). The common femoral artery usually is punctured with an 18-gauge (0.049-in.) double-wall puncture or 19-gauge (0.042-in.) or 21-gauge (0.032-in.) single-wall puncture needle (Fig. 100-1). The Seldinger technique for percutaneous angiography with the micropuncture set is shown in Fig. 100-2. Most visceral angiography is performed with 4F or 5F catheters with preshaped configurations. Three commonly used preshaped catheter configurations for visceral angiography are the shepherd's hook catheter, cobra, and sidewinder configurations.

Intraarterial digital subtraction angiography is commonly used for evaluation of the vascular anatomy. When vascular details are needed, conventional angiography is used (Figs. 100-3 through 100-6). Magnification angiography and photographic subtraction provide additional vascular details.

Magnetic resonance angiography (MRA) is an imaging technique that can depict the vascular system, including the heart, aorta and its branches (Fig. 100-7), peripheral arteries, and portal venous system. It requires no arterial catheterization or administration of iodinated contrast media. Magnetic resonance (MR) contrast media do not cause allergic reactions or renal toxicity. They are administered through a peripheral intravenous line.

Carbon dioxide (CO_2) has been used as an angiographic contrast agent for more than a decade. The gas is well tolerated when injected intraarterially or intravenously in small amounts. It causes no known allergic reactions, and its use reduces risk for contrast-induced renal failure. CO_2 vascular imaging is obtained with the digital subtraction technique. CO_2 angiography is used to visualize the abdominal aorta and renal, mesenteric, and peripheral arteries (Fig. 100-8) and in conjunction with therapeutic angiographic procedures. The method has been shown to be more sensitive than use of conventional contrast media in detecting minute gastrointestinal bleeding. CO_2-wedged hepatic venography is a safe and effective method of visualizing the portal vein (Fig. 100-9). It is commonly used to facilitate portal vein puncture during transjugular intrahepatic portosystemic shunt (TIPS) procedures.

The techniques used in visceral angiography are biplane aortography, selective angiography, magnification angiography (Fig. 100-10), hepatic venography (Fig. 100-11), direct portography (Fig. 100-12), splenoportography (Fig. 100-13), wedged hepatic venography (Fig. 100-14), and superselective angiography with 3F coaxial catheter systems (Fig. 100-15).

GASTROINTESTINAL ANGIOGRAPHY

Visceral angiography is used for the diagnosis of arterial occlusive disease, aneurysms (Fig. 100-16), arteriovenous fistula (Fig. 100-17), portal vein aneurysm (Fig. 100-18), and vascular impressions on the gastrointestinal tract (Fig. 100-19).

Angiography continues to play an important role in the diagnosis of upper and lower gastrointestinal bleeding (Figs. 100-20 through 100-23). Angiography is especially important for the diagnosis of chronic gastrointestinal bleeding from tumors (Fig. 100-24), vascular malformations (Fig. 100-25), and colonic vascular ectasia (Fig. 100-26). Visualization of the portal venous system is important in the evaluation of cirrhosis, portal hypertension, and pancreatic, biliary, and hepatic tumors. The portal vein can be evaluated by means of indirect portography (arterial portography) (Figs. 100-27 and 100-28) or direct portography (Fig. 100-29). Angiography is used to differentiate occlusive from nonocclusive mesenteric ischemia. It is also useful in the diagnosis of carcinoid tumor and hepatic metastases (Fig. 100-30). Percutaneous translumenal angioplasty may be used to manage intestinal angina caused by arteriosclerotic celiac and superior mesenteric artery stenosis. Transcatheter embolization is effective in arresting arterial bleeding from peptic ulceration, and vasopressin infusion is used for control of lower gastrointestinal tract bleeding.

PANCREATIC ANGIOGRAPHY

Ultrasound and computed tomographic (CT) scanning are the initial diagnostic procedures for inflammatory and neoplastic pancreatic lesions. Endoscopic retrograde cholangiopancreatography with cytologic examination is commonly performed for patients with suspected pancreatic cancer. Once pancreatic lesions have been demonstrated with the imaging methods, angiography is performed to obtain a specific diagnosis and to assess the vascular anatomy and resectability of the tumor before surgical intervention (Fig. 100-31).

Endoscopic ultrasound scanning is commonly used for localization of pancreatic islet cell tumors. When it reveals a pancreatic mass in a patient with hyperinsulinism, surgical therapy is provided without additional localization procedures. Angiography remains a useful method for localization of vascular islet cell tumors including vasoactive intestinal polypeptide-secreting tumor (VIPoma), pancreatic polypeptide-producing tumor (PPoma), somatostatinoma, and glucagonoma (Fig. 100-32). Arteriography is not sensitive in identification of gastrinoma because this tumor tends to be avascular on angiograms. Transhepatic venous sampling is indicated for localization of occult adenoma (Fig. 100-33).

Angiography is important in the diagnosis and management of gastrointestinal bleeding complicating pancreatitis and pseudocyst (Fig. 100-34). Such bleeding may originate from an aneurysm or varices associated with portal or splenic venous thrombosis.

HEPATIC ANGIOGRAPHY

Ultrasound and CT scanning, magnetic resonance imaging (MRI), and radionuclide studies are used for the diagnosis of hepatic mass lesions. CT scanning, with and without contrast enhancement, is the most frequently used modality for the diagnosis of hepatic neoplasm. Angiography is sensitive in detecting vascular tumors in the liver, including hepatoma, cavernous hemangioma (Fig. 100-35), focal nodular hyperplasia (Fig. 100-36), and bleeding associated with hepatic adenoma (Fig. 100-37).

Hepatic angiography plays an important role in the preoperative evaluation of resectability of tumors. Involvement of both lobes, regional lymph node metastases, and portal vein invasion indicate unresectability of the tumor (Fig. 100-38). The portal venous phase of high-dose superior mesenteric angiography is used to evaluate the portal venous system. Angiography is used for localization of lesions and treatment of patients with clinically significant hemobilia or bleeding after laparoscopic cholecystectomy (Fig. 100-39). Selective arterial embolization is effective in controlling bleeding from intrahepatic sources and eliminates the need for major surgical intervention (Fig. 100-40).

Panhepatic angiography is an important preoperative procedure for portosystemic shunt operations. It includes both arterial and venous examinations with manometry. Angiography is essential in the diagnosis of Budd-Chiari syndrome (Fig. 100-41). Hepatic venography with injection of contrast medium into the occluded hepatic vein or patent accessory vein usually demonstrates typical spider web collaterals. Angiographic methods used for the management of Budd-Chiari syndrome include percutaneous translumenal angioplasty, placement of metallic stents, and TIPS.

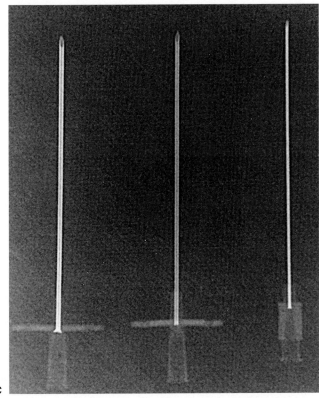

A–C

FIGURE 100-1. Digital images of the needles currently in use for arterial and venous puncture for percutaneous access. **A:** The 18-gauge Seldinger needle (shown with trocar removed) is used to puncture both walls of the artery. After the trocar is removed, the cannula is slowly withdrawn until blood spurts from the needle. A 0.035-in. guidewire is introduced through the needle, and the needle is removed. A catheter is advanced over the wire. **B:** The 19-gauge needle has no inner trocar and is slowly advanced through the anterior wall of the artery until blood spurts from the needle. A 0.035-in. guidewire is used for catheter introduction. **C:** The 21-gauge needle is advanced until the arterial blood flows, and a 0.018-in. guidewire is introduced.

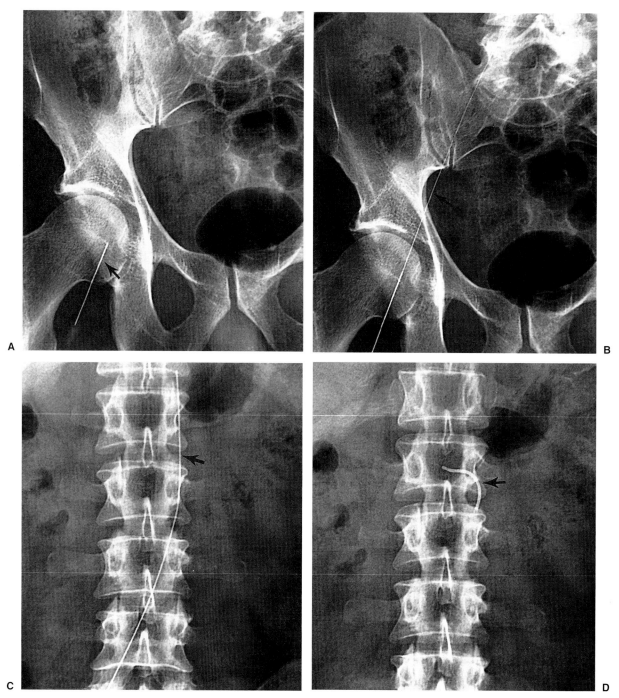

FIGURE 100-2. Seldinger technique for percutaneous angiography with micropuncture technique. **A:** The common femoral artery is accessed with a 21-gauge needle (*arrow*). **B:** The 0.018-in. (0.46-mm) stainless steel guidewire with platinum tip (*arrow*) is introduced through the iliac artery into the aorta. **C:** The 0.035-in. guidewire (*arrow*) is introduced into the aorta through a 4F coaxial dilator, which was advanced over the 0.018-in. guidewire. **D:** The 5F shepherd's hook catheter (*arrow*) has been placed in the abdominal aorta for catheterization of the branches of the aorta.

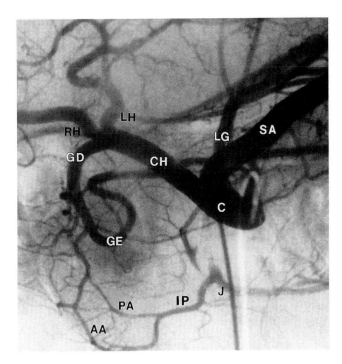

FIGURE 100-3. Celiac axis anatomy. The celiac axis (*C*) gives off the splenic (*SA*), left gastric (*LG*), and common hepatic (*CH*) arteries. The common hepatic artery divides into the gastroduodenal (*GD*) and left (*LH*) and right (*RH*) hepatic arteries. The gastroduodenal artery gives rise to the anterior arcade (*AA*) and posterior arcade (*PA*) arteries, which join to form the inferior pancreaticoduodenal artery (*IP*). The first jejunal (*J*) artery joins the latter before anastomosing with the superior mesenteric artery. The right gastroepiploic artery (*GE*) originates from the gastroduodenal artery, runs along the greater curvature of the stomach, and anastomoses with the left gastroepiploic artery from the splenic artery.

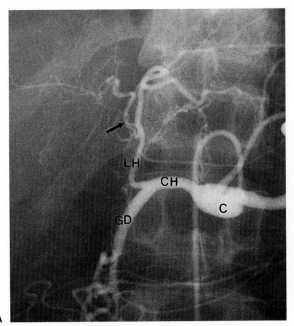

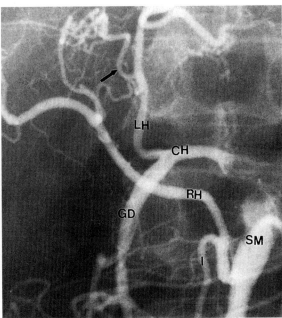

A

B

FIGURE 100-4. Aberrant right hepatic artery originating from the superior mesenteric artery. **A:** The common hepatic artery (*CH*) divides into the gastroduodenal (*GD*) and left hepatic (*LH*) arteries. The middle hepatic artery (*arrow*) originates from the left hepatic artery (*LH*). **B:** Arterial phase of superior mesenteric arteriogram of same patient. The replaced right hepatic (*RH*) originates from the superior mesenteric artery (*SM*), and the inferior pancreaticoduodenal (*I*) artery originates from the aberrant right hepatic artery. The gastroduodenal (*GD*) and left hepatic (*LH*) arteries are filled from the superior mesenteric artery because of celiac stenosis.

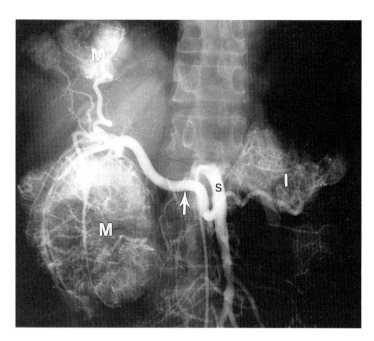

FIGURE 100-5. Hepatic artery variation. Superior mesenteric arteriogram of a patient with hepatic metastases (*M*) from nonfunctioning islet cell carcinoma of the pancreas (*I*). The right hepatic artery (*arrow*) is replaced from the superior mesenteric artery (*S*) and supplies hypervascular metastases (*M*) in the liver. The splenic, left gastric, and common hepatic arteries originate from the celiac axis (not shown).

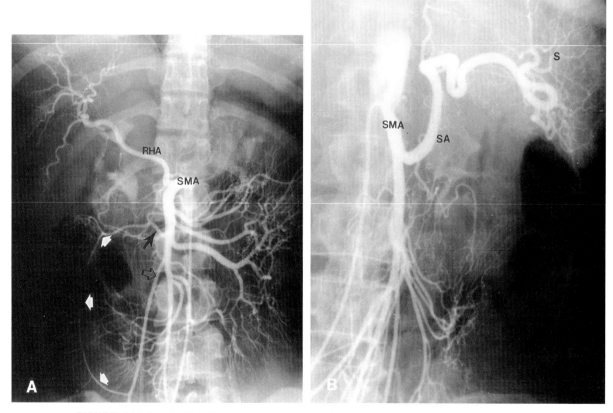

FIGURE 100-6. Celiac trunk variations. **A:** Arterial phase of a superior mesenteric angiogram. The right hepatic (*RHA*) artery has a replaced origin from the superior mesenteric artery (*SMA*). The middle colic (*black arrow*) and right colic (*black open arrow*) arteries form the paracolic arcade (*white arrows*) along the ascending colon. The common hepatic and splenic arteries arise from the celiac trunk (not shown). **B:** Arterial phase of a superior mesenteric angiogram. The splenic artery (*SA*) has a replaced origin from the superior mesenteric artery (*SMA*). In this patient, the celiac trunk gives off a left gastric artery and a common hepatic artery (not shown). *S,* spleen.

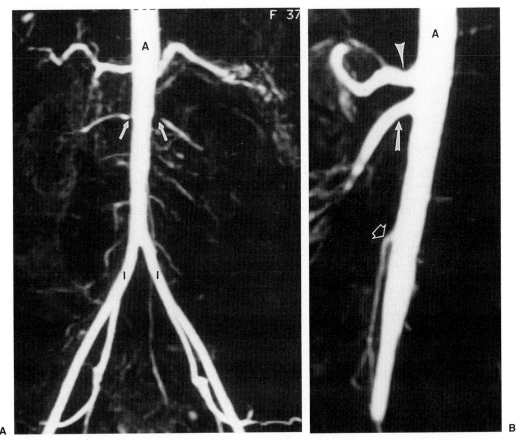

FIGURE 100-7. Three-dimensional contrast magnetic resonance angiogram. **A:** Coronal projection shows aorta (*A*) and iliac artery (*I*). There are bilateral renal artery stenoses (*arrows*). **B:** Sagittal projection shows celiac (*arrowhead*), superior mesenteric (*arrow*), and inferior mesenteric (*open arrow*) arteries.

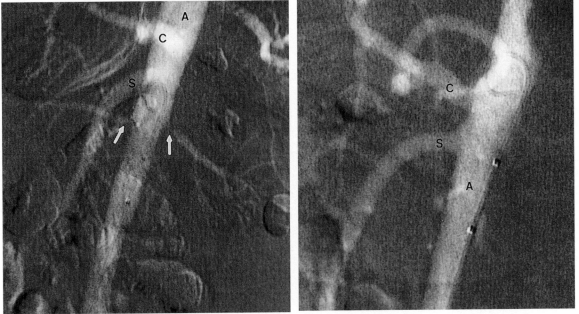

FIGURE 100-8. **A:** CO_2 digital subtraction aortogram shows aorta (*A*), bilateral renal artery stenoses (*arrows*), superior mesenteric (*S*) and celiac (*C*) arteries. **B:** Lateral image shows celiac and superior mesenteric arteries.

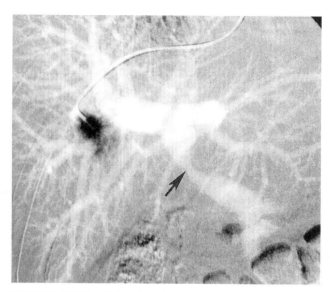

FIGURE 100-9. CO_2 digital subtraction wedge hepatic venogram in a liver transplant shows a moderate stenosis at the anastomosis (*arrow*) of the portal vein, which was successfully treated with percutaneous transhepatic balloon dilation.

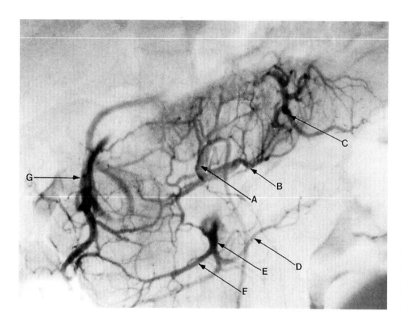

FIGURE 100-10. Normal dorsal pancreatic arteriogram (subtraction technique). Dorsal pancreatic arteriogram (arterial phase) shows all of the entire intrapancreatic arteries. Abundant intrapancreatic and peripancreatic arterial anastomoses are visible. *A*, dorsal pancreatic artery; *B*, transverse pancreatic artery; *C*, pancreatica magna artery; *D*, jejunal artery; *E*, inferior pancreaticoduodenal artery; *F*, pancreatic arcade; *G*, gastroduodenal artery.

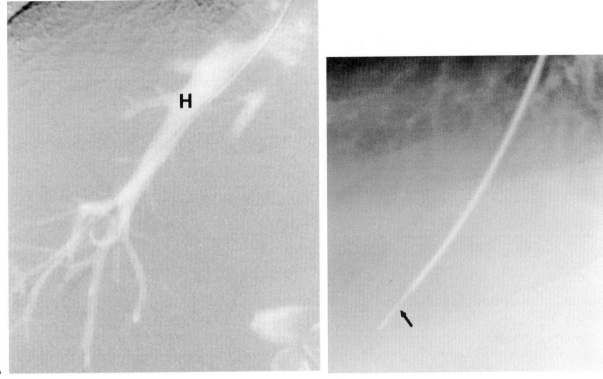

FIGURE 100-11. **A:** CO_2 digital subtraction hepatic venogram from a right jugular vein before liver biopsy shows patent right hepatic vein (*H*). **B:** Digital image taken during liver biopsy shows a Quick-Core biopsy needle (*arrow*) (Cook Inc., Bloomington, IN).

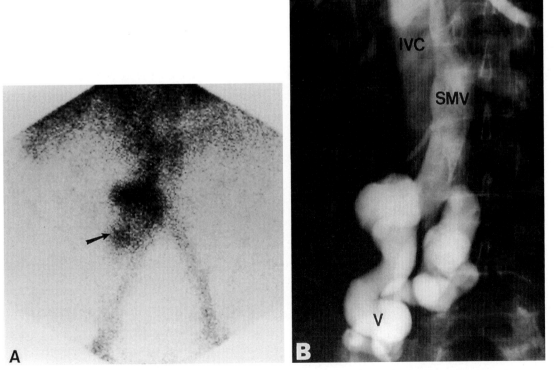

FIGURE 100-12. Intestinal varices. **A:** Radionuclide scan of a patient with cirrhosis and portal hypertension demonstrates an area of increased radionuclide uptake (*arrow*) in the lower abdomen. **B:** Percutaneous transhepatic portogram shows ileal varices (*V*) arising from the superior mesenteric vein (*SMV*) and emptying into the inferior vena cava (*IVC*).

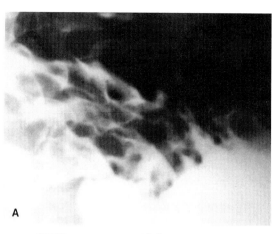
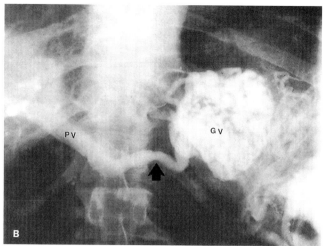
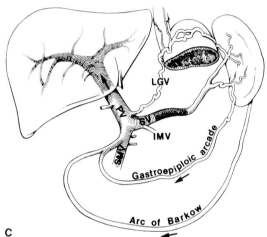

FIGURE 100-13. Isolated gastric varices secondary to splenic vein occlusion. **A:** Double-contrast view of the gastric fundus shows polypoid defects. **B:** Splenoportogram shows contrast medium injected into the spleen drains through the gastric varices (*GV*) and coronary vein (*arrow*) into the portal vein (*PV*). **C:** Diagram shows venous collateral pathways in splenic vein occlusion. Hepatopetal collateral flow develops through the left gastric (*LGV*), gastroepiploic, and omental (Arc of Barkow) veins. *PV,* portal vein; *SMV,* superior mesenteric vein; *IMV,* inferior mesenteric vein.

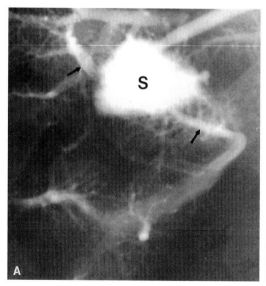
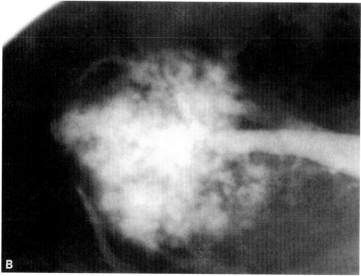

FIGURE 100-14. Wedged hepatic venograms. **A:** Normal wedged hepatic venogram. The sinusoids (S) are filled homogeneously. The intrahepatic portal vein branches (*arrows*) are filled through the sinusoids because of pressure injection. **B:** Abnormal wedged hepatic venogram of a patient with cirrhosis shows sinusoidal filling is inhomogeneous and nodular in pattern because of cirrhosis.

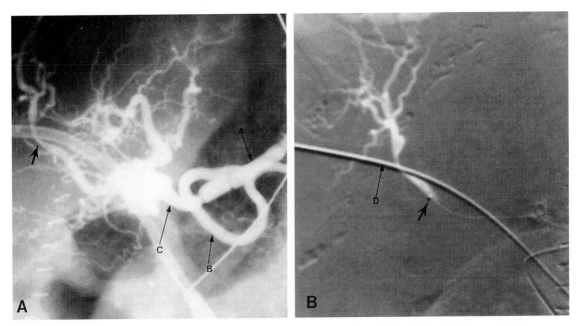

FIGURE 100-15. Superselective catheterization of a hepatic artery branch with a coaxial catheter system (Tracker-18, Boston Scientific Corporation, Natick, MA) in a patient with hemobilia subsequent to percutaneous biliary drainage. **A:** Celiac arteriogram shows biliary catheter has injured a right hepatic arterial branch (*arrow*). **B:** Digital subtraction arteriogram through a 3F catheter (*arrow*) in the bleeding artery demonstrates arterial injury. Hemobilia was controlled by means of embolization. *A,* celiac artery; *B,* splenic artery; *C,* hepatic artery; *D,* transhepatic biliary catheter.

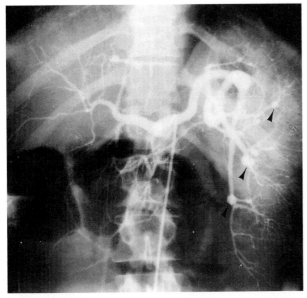

FIGURE 100-16. Splenic artery aneurysms associated with portal hypertension. Multiple aneurysms are present in the splenic artery branches (*arrowheads*). The spleen is enlarged because of portal hypertension.

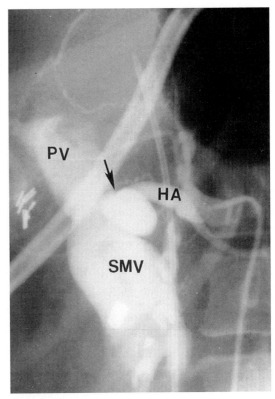

FIGURE 100-17. Arterioportal fistula that developed after a gunshot wound. Selective hepatic arteriogram (oblique view) demonstrates a large fistula (*arrow*) and aneurysm between the hepatic artery (*HA*) and portal vein (*PV*). *SMV,* superior mesenteric vein.

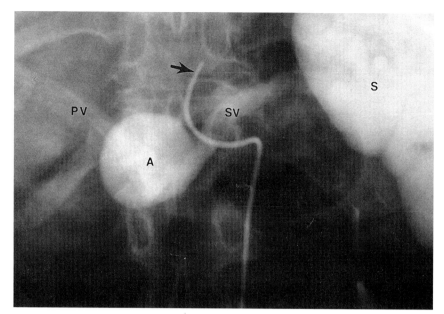

FIGURE 100-18. Portal venous aneurysm. Venous phase of a splenic angiogram shows catheter tip in the splenic artery (*arrow*). A portal vein aneurysm (*A*) arises from the junction of the splenic (*SV*) and portal (*PV*) veins. Venous aneurysms may occur in the splenic, superior mesenteric, and portal veins. Most portal vein aneurysms are found incidentally and cause no specific symptoms. The splenic parenchyma (*S*) is opacified with contrast medium.

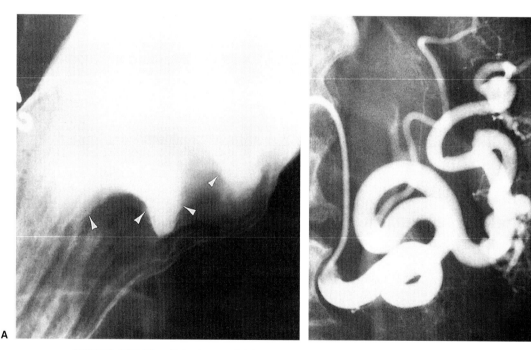

FIGURE 100-19. Splenic arterial impression on the stomach. **A:** Barium swallow image demonstrates smooth filling defects (*arrowheads*) in the body of the stomach. **B:** Splenic arteriogram (arterial phase) demonstrates markedly tortuous splenic artery causing gastric impression.

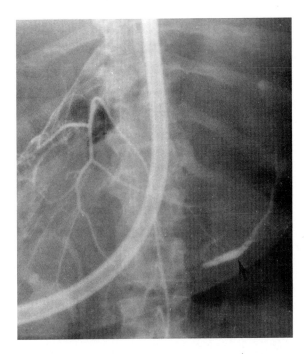

FIGURE 100-20. Arterial bleeding from peptic ulcer. The catheter has been selectively placed into the gastric artery. Angiogram shows extravasation of contrast medium in the body of the stomach near the greater curvature. The extravasated contrast medium gives the appearance of a vein ("pseudovein" sign) (*arrow*). The bleeding was successfully controlled by means of gelatin sponge (Gelfoam, Upjohn, Kalamazoo, MI) embolization.

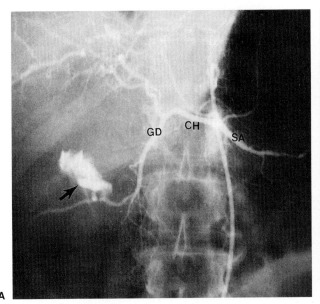

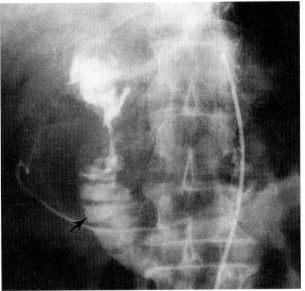

A

B

FIGURE 100-21. Massive arterial bleeding into the duodenum of a patient with peptic ulcer. **A:** Celiac arteriogram (arterial phase) shows branches of the celiac artery with severe vasoconstriction caused by hypovolemic shock. Massive contrast extravasation is demonstrated in the duodenal bulb (*arrow*) from the proximal gastroepiploic artery. *SA,* splenic artery; *CH,* common hepatic artery; *GD,* gastroduodenal artery. **B:** Venous phase of same angiogram shows extravasated contrast medium outlining the mucosal folds of the duodenum (*arrow*).

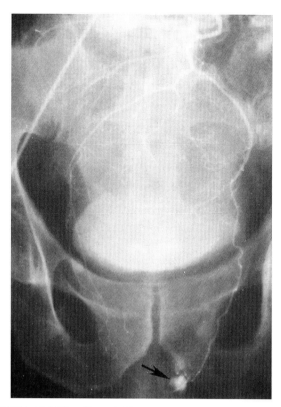

FIGURE 100-22. Rectal bleeding complicating rectal tube placement. Inferior mesenteric arteriogram shows active bleeding (*arrow*) into the distal rectum. Vasopressin infusion stopped the bleeding.

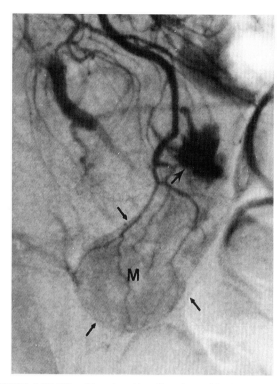

FIGURE 100-23. Massive bleeding from Meckel diverticulum. Superior mesenteric arteriogram (subtraction technique) of a 7-year-old girl with lower gastrointestinal bleeding shows Meckel diverticulum (*M, small arrows*) and extravasation of the contrast medium (*large arrow*) near its attachment to the ileum.

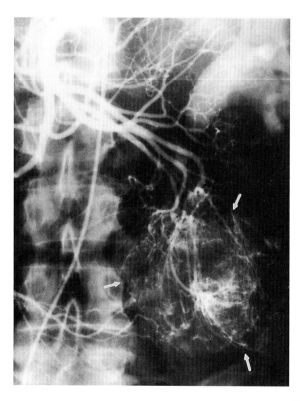

FIGURE 100-24. Intestinal leiomyosarcoma. Superior mesenteric arteriogram demonstrates a vascular tumor with dilated feeding arteries and tumor vessels (*arrows*). The inhomogeneous tumor blush and poor margin of the tumor suggest a malignant tumor.

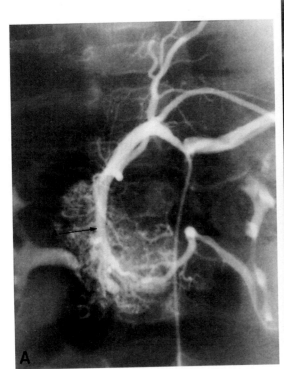

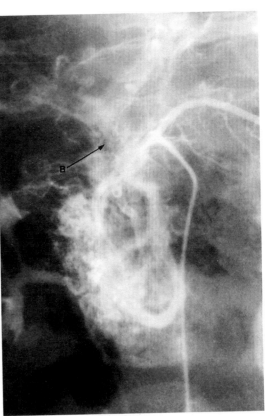

FIGURE 100-25. Pancreatic and duodenal arteriovenous malformations. **A:** Arterial phase of a gastroduodenal angiogram of a 7-month-old boy with gastrointestinal hemorrhage demonstrates tortuous abnormal vascular channels in the duodenum and pancreas. The gastroduodenal artery (*A*) and its branches supply the malformations. **B:** Parenchymal phase demonstrates mottled staining and early, dense venous opacification from the lesion. *B*, portal vein.

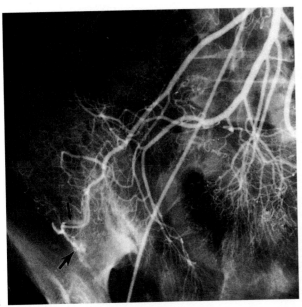

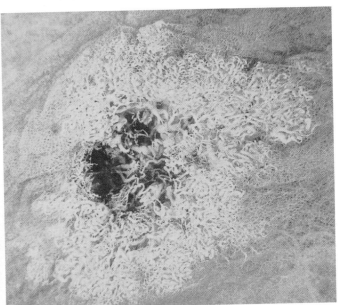

FIGURE 100-26. Vascular ectasia of the cecum. **A:** Superior mesenteric arteriogram of a 70-year-old woman with recurrent lower gastrointestinal bleeding. Dilated cecal artery feeds a small mucosal vascular ectasia (*large arrow*). An early draining vein (*small arrow*) is beginning to fill. **B:** The resected cecum has been injected with Microfil (Canton Bio-Medical Products, Inc., Boulder, CO) and has undergone the clearing process. Mucosal vascular ectasia is present.

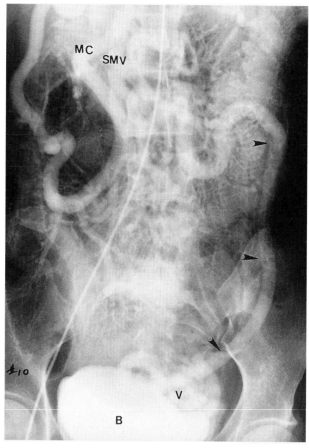

FIGURE 100-27. Varices in the wall of the urinary bladder of a patient with hematuria. Venous phase of superior mesenteric angiogram shows large varices (*V*) in the wall of the bladder (*B*) filled from the superior mesenteric vein (*SMV*) through the middle (*MC*) and left colic (*arrowheads*) veins.

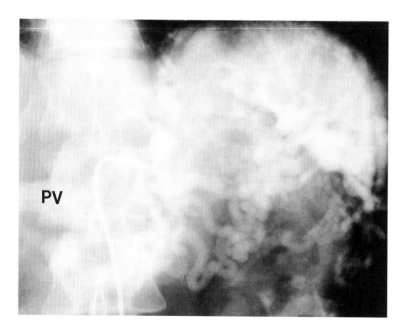

FIGURE 100-28. Gastric varices of a patient with splenic vein occlusion associated with pancreatitis. Venous phase of splenic angiogram shows varices in the wall of the stomach and upper abdomen. Varices reconstitute the portal vein (*PV*).

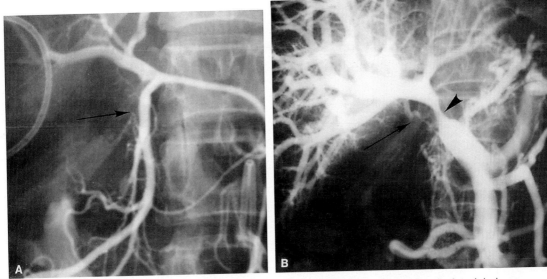

FIGURE 100-29.   Invasion of common bile duct by gallbladder carcinoma. **A:** Arterial phase of a hepatic angiogram demonstrates occlusion of the bile duct artery (*arrow*). **B:** Portal venogram through the percutaneous transhepatic approach shows that vein of the bile duct (*arrow*) and portal vein (*arrowhead*) are encased, indicating unresectability of the tumor.

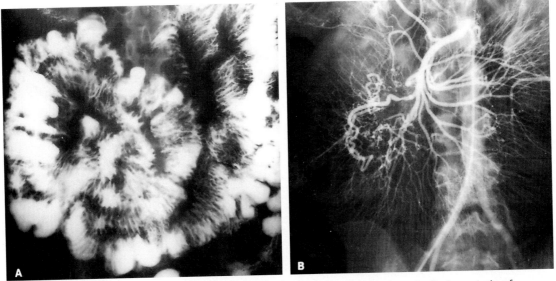

FIGURE 100-30.   Ileal carcinoid tumor with mesenteric metastases. **A:** Barium study of a 52-year-old woman with diarrhea and abdominal pain shows that loops of small bowel are retracted and their walls are thickened. **B:** Superior mesenteric arteriogram shows that right colic and ileocolic arteries are encased and the mesenteric artery branches are retracted into a stellate pattern.

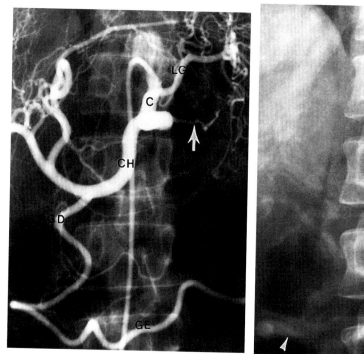
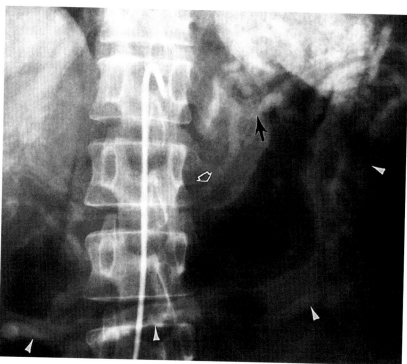

A   B

FIGURE 100-31. Splenic artery encasement and occlusion caused by pancreatic carcinoma. **A:** Celiac angiogram (arterial phase) demonstrates encasement (*arrow*) and occlusion of the splenic artery. Collateral circulation toward the spleen is visible through the left gastric (*LG*) and right gastroepiploic (*GE*) arteries. *C*, celiac axis; *CH*, common hepatic artery; *GD*, gastroduodenal artery. **B:** Venous phase of same angiogram shows splenic vein occluded (*arrow*) in the region of the body of the pancreas. Venous collateral vessels have developed through the gastroepiploic (*arrowheads*) and gastric (*open arrow*) veins.

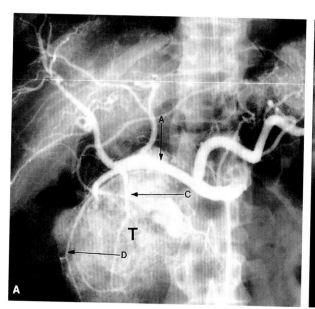
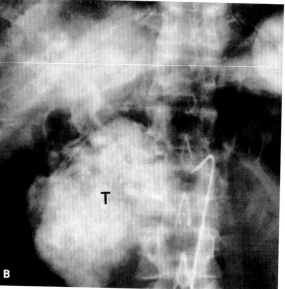

FIGURE 100-32. Glucagonoma. **A:** Arterial phase of a celiac angiogram of a 64-year-old man with dermatitis, diabetes mellitus, and anemia. Hypervascular tumor (*T*) in the head of the pancreas is supplied by the pancreatic arcade arteries. *A*, common hepatic artery; *B*, gastroduodenal artery; *C*, posterior arcade artery; *D*, anterior arcade artery. **B:** Parenchymal phase shows tumor has homogeneous dense contrast accumulation characteristic of an islet cell tumor.

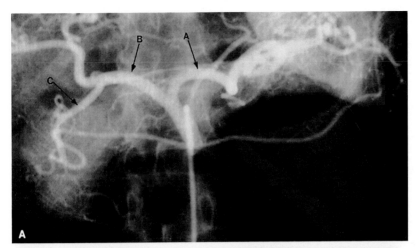

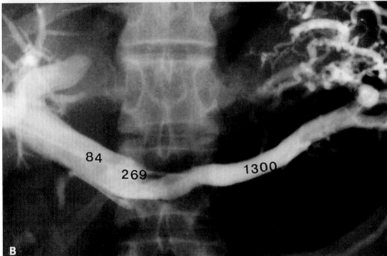

FIGURE 100-33. Transhepatic venous sampling for localization of occult islet adenoma. **A:** Arterial phase of a celiac angiogram of a 46-year-old woman with organic hyperinsulinism. The angiogram is negative for islet cell adenoma. *A,* splenic artery; *B,* common hepatic artery; *C,* gastroduodenal artery. **B:** Transhepatic splenoportogram with insulin values (μU/mL) shows abnormally high insulin level in the splenic vein, localizing the tumor to the body of the pancreas. The surgical finding was a 1-cm-diameter islet cell adenoma in the body of the pancreas.

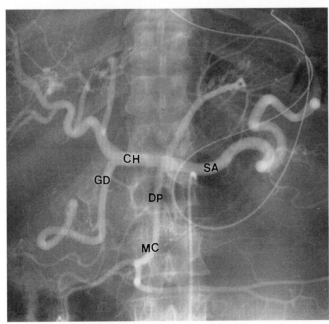

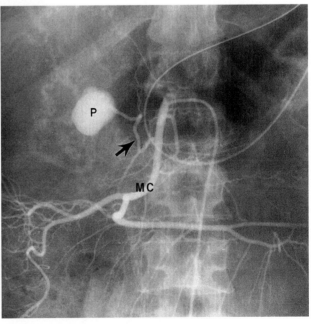

FIGURE 100-34. Bleeding into a pseudocyst. **A:** Celiac angiogram (arterial phase) shows middle colic artery (*MC*) arising from the dorsal pancreatic (*DP*) artery that originates from the celiac axis. *SA,* splenic artery; *CH,* common hepatic artery; *GD,* gastroduodenal artery. **B:** Selective injection into the dorsal pancreatic artery demonstrates a pseudoaneurysm (*P*) filled from a branch of the dorsal pancreatic artery (*arrow*).

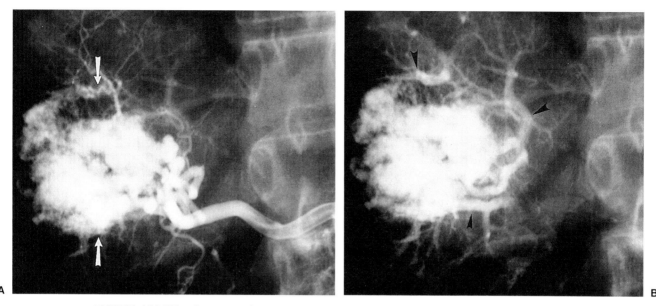

FIGURE 100-35. Cavernous hemangioma. **A:** Hepatic angiogram (arterial phase) shows dilated hepatic artery and the vascular spaces of the hemangioma filled with contrast medium (*arrows*). **B:** Vascular spaces have retained contrast medium through the venous phase, characteristic of hemangioma. Portal veins (*arrowheads*) are opacified, indicating arteriovenous shunting. Arteriovenous shunting is an unusual finding with hemangioma.

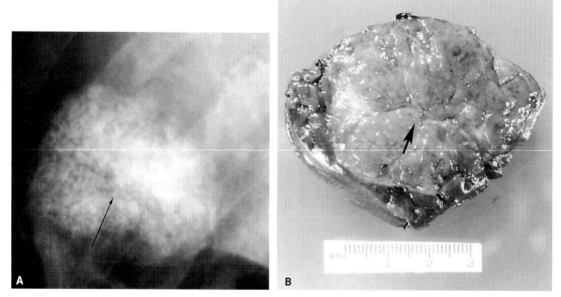

FIGURE 100-36. Focal nodular hyperplasia. **A:** Parenchymal phase of a hepatic angiogram, magnification technique, of a 26-year-old woman demonstrates nodular accumulation of contrast medium with central scar formation (*arrow*) typical of focal nodular hyperplasia. **B:** Section of the resected mass shows a nodular pattern, central scar (*arrow*), and radiating septa.

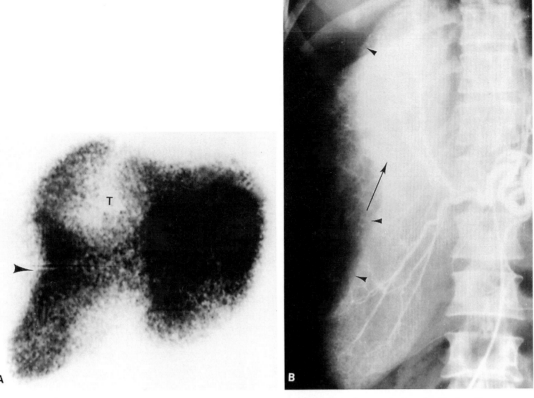

FIGURE 100-37. Ruptured hepatic adenoma with massive hemorrhage. **A:** Technetium 99m–sulfur colloid scan of a 30-year-old woman with a history of use of oral contraceptives demonstrates a photon-deficient area (*T*) and large subcapsular hematoma (*arrowhead*) in the right lobe of the liver. **B:** Arterial phase of a hepatic angiogram demonstrates an avascular mass (*arrow*) associated with a large subcapsular hematoma (*arrowheads*). Liver is displaced from the lateral abdominal wall.

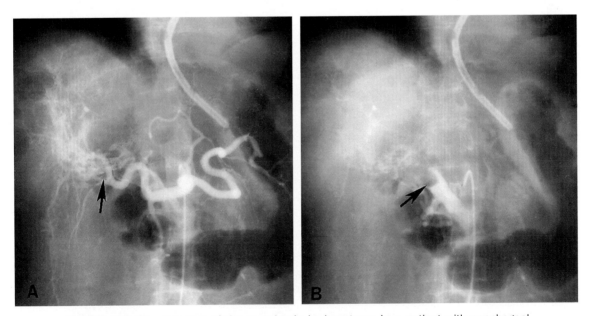

FIGURE 100-38. Invasion of the portal vein by hepatoma in a patient with esophageal variceal bleeding. **A:** Arterial phase of a celiac angiogram shows linear abnormal vessels (*arrow*) running along the portal vein. **B:** Venous phase of same angiogram demonstrates tumor thrombus (*arrow*) in the portal vein.

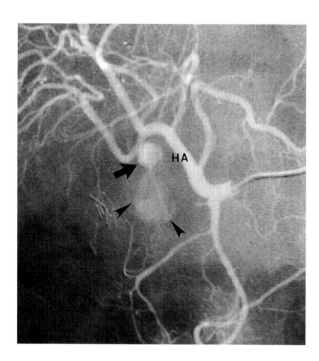

FIGURE 100-39. Massive bleeding complicating laparoscopic cholecystectomy. Hepatic angiogram (arterial phase) demonstrates bleeding (*arrowheads*) from pseudoaneurysm (*arrow*) of the right hepatic artery (*HA*).

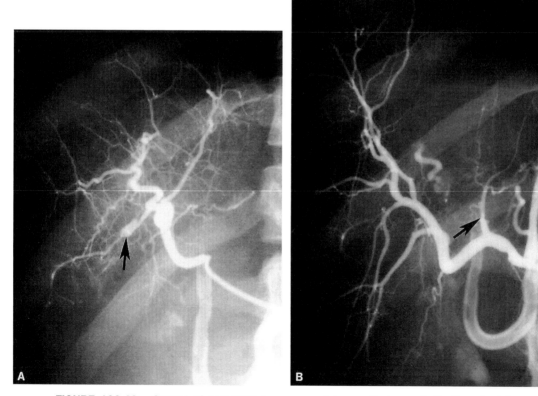

FIGURE 100-40. Control of hemobilia by means of transcatheter embolization. **A:** Arterial phase of selective hepatic angiogram demonstrates an aneurysm in the posterior segmental artery branch (*arrow*). **B:** Arteriogram after Gelfoam (Upjohn, Kalamazoo, MI) embolization demonstrates occlusion of the posterior segmental artery (*arrow*). Hemobilia was controlled by means of embolization.

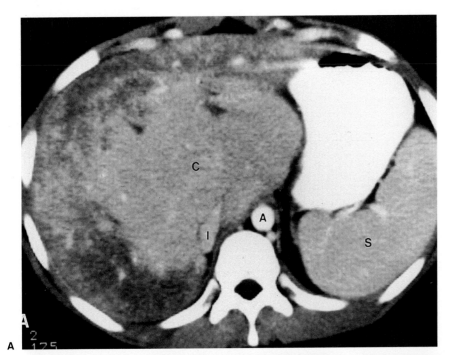

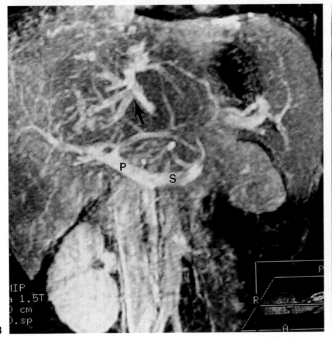

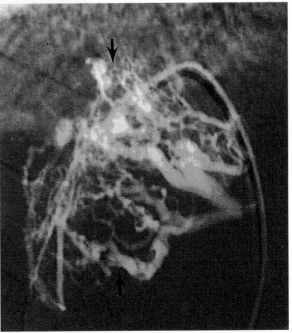

FIGURE 100-41. Budd-Chiari syndrome. **A:** Computed tomographic scan of a 23-year-old woman with ascites and pulmonary embolism demonstrates enlarged caudate lobe (C) and inhomogeneous perfusion in the periphery of the liver. A, aorta; I, inferior vena cava; S, spleen. **B:** Three-dimensional contrast magnetic resonance angiogram demonstrates obliteration of the hepatic veins. The dilated accessory hepatic veins (arrow) drain from the caudate lobe into the inferior vena cava. The splenic (S) and portal (P) veins are patent. **C:** Wedged hepatic venogram with injection of contrast medium through the occluded hepatic vein demonstrates typical spider web hepatic venous collateral vessels (arrows). The patient underwent orthotopic liver transplantation.

INTERVENTIONAL RADIOLOGY

KYUNG J. CHO ■ GRACE H. ELTA

Interventional radiologic techniques are used for the diagnosis and treatment of a variety of vascular and nonvascular disorders. They can be divided into vascular (infusion, occlusion, dilation) and nonvascular (biopsy, drainage, dilation, and ostomy formation) procedures. This chapter describes techniques and clinical applications of interventional radiology in the management of gastrointestinal disorders.

VASOPRESSIN INFUSION

Intraarterial infusion of vasopressin is effective in controlling bleeding from hemorrhagic gastritis, Mallory-Weiss tears, and lower gastrointestinal bleeding (Fig. 101-1). The method is less effective for bleeding caused by peptic ulcer disease. Once a bleeding site has been demonstrated, the catheter is placed in the bleeding artery. The infusion usually is started at the rate of 0.2 units/min, and the dosage is increased up to 0.4 units/min if necessary. The infusion should be continued for an additional 24 hours. The most hazardous complication of vasopressin infusion is myocardial infarction. For patients with coronary artery disease, concomitant administration of nitroglycerin may be beneficial. The other potential risks include arrhythmia, bowel ischemia, and oliguria. The therapeutic role of this technique in the treatment of GI bleeding has diminished as the more effective, relatively safe embolization method has become available.

SELECTIVE ARTERIAL EMBOLIZATION

Selective arterial embolization is effective treatment of patients with massive gastrointestinal hemorrhage and is the treatment of choice among patients with arterial bleeding if endoscopic treatment fails. The method is effective for both upper and lower gastrointestinal bleeding. It is essential to deliver the embolic agents as close to the bleeding site as possible to prevent embolization of normal tissue. The left gastric artery usually is embolized for gastric hemorrhage, the gastroduodenal artery for duodenal hemorrhage (Fig. 101-2), mesenteric branches for small bowel (Fig. 101-3) or colonic bleeding (Fig. 101-4), and the inferior mesenteric artery for rectosigmoid bleeding.

The other uses of selective arterial embolization are control of hemobilia and obliteration of visceral artery aneurysms. Splenic artery embolization has been used as an alternative to splenectomy to treat patients with hypersplenism, splenic vein occlusion, and traumatic splenic bleeding (Fig. 101-5). The risk of splenic artery embolization is formation of a splenic abscess. This complication can be avoided with occlusion of less than 80% of splenic arterial branches and use of antibiotic prophylaxis.

VARICEAL EMBOLIZATION

Percutaneous transhepatic variceal embolization is effective for bleeding from gastro-esophageal varices or from varices at unusual sites. Rebleeding is common because of development of new collateral veins, which historically hampered enthusiasm for this technique. Variceal embolization is rarely used because of the availability of simpler (endoscopic) or more effective techniques, such as transjugular intrahepatic portosystemic shunt (TIPS). Gelatin sponge (Gelfoam, Upjohn, Kalamazoo, MI) ethanol, and coils have been used as embolic agents. If communication between the gastro-esophageal varices and the pulmonary vein is demonstrated (Fig. 101-6), particulate embolic agents should not be used because of the risk of systemic arterial embolization. Embolic therapy may be justified if bleeding persists despite endoscopic therapy and balloon tamponade, or if stabilization is required before a TIPS procedure, shunt operation, or liver transplantation.

PERCUTANEOUS TRANSLUMENAL ANGIOPLASTY

Percutaneous translumenal angioplasty (PTA) is effective for treating patients with chronic mesenteric ischemia caused by atherosclerotic narrowing of the mesenteric vessels. PTA is justified in the treatment of patients at high surgical risk. PTA can be used to manage Budd-Chiari syndrome caused by occlusion or stenosis of the hepatic vein or hepatic segment of the inferior vena cava. PTA and stents have been used in therapy for suprahepatic caval anastomotic stenosis complicating orthotopic liver transplantation (Fig. 101-7).

TIPS insertion is a widely accepted interventional radiologic procedure for decompressing portal hypertension and for managing variceal bleeding. It has a lower mortality rate than emergency surgical shunting and is currently indicated for patients with variceal bleeding unresponsive to endoscopic therapy. The utility of TIPS as an effective bridge to treat patients with variceal bleeding while they await hepatic transplantation has been documented. A TIPS also is effective for managing intractable ascites in patients with cirrhosis and portal hypertension (Fig. 101-8). Shortening of the stent or biliary stent fistula may cause acute shunt thrombosis. Revision can be performed by means of balloon dilation, placement of metallic stents within the TIPS, or use of a mechanical thrombectomy device. The use of covered stents may be beneficial if a biliary-TIPS fistula is demonstrated. Unfortunately, development of neointimal hyperplasia leads to stenosis or occlusion of the TIPS among as many as 50% of patients within 1 year. Ultrasound surveillance is used to detect stenosis and correct the lesion to prevent occlusion. Balloon dilation or stent placement is effective management of stenosis of a TIPS (Fig. 101-9).

PERCUTANEOUS BILIARY DRAINAGE

Percutaneous transhepatic catheterization of the bile duct is an important interventional radiologic procedure. The technique is used for biliary drainage, dilation of biliary strictures, stone extraction, and intraductal biliary biopsy. A right lateral approach is used for catheterization of the right hepatic duct (Fig. 101-10), and an anterior subxiphoid approach is used for the left hepatic duct (Fig. 101-11). To minimize risk for bleeding, a peripheral bile duct is punctured in patients who need a large catheter for drainage or stone extraction.

PERCUTANEOUS ABSCESS DRAINAGE

Percutaneous techniques can be used to drain intra-abdominal abscesses and fluid collections, including hepatic cysts, hydatid cysts, pyogenic abscess, and pancreatic pseudocysts. Successful drainage of an intra-abdominal abscess (Fig. 101-12) requires accurate localization by means of computed tomographic (CT) or ultra-sound scanning. Follow-up sinograms document shrinkage of the abscess cavity and exclude an underlying fistula.

PERCUTANEOUS GASTROSTOMY AND GASTROJEJUNOSTOMY

Percutaneous gastrostomy is a safe and effective method for enteral feeding and decompression of intestinal obstruction. It is a simple technique used for nutritional support of patients unable to maintain oral intake because of neurological disorders or esophageal obstruction. Before puncture of the gastric lumen, a sufficient amount of air should be insufflated into the stomach to achieve gastric distention. This brings the anterior wall of the stomach to the abdominal wall and pushes the small bowel and colon away from the puncture site. Inserting suture anchors into the gastric lumen facilitates placement of a gastric tube (Fig. 101-13). The gastric tube is inserted between the two anchor sutures or adjacent to a single anchor, and the distal self-retaining loop is string-fixed to prevent dislodgment (Fig. 101-14). After the tube is drained for 24 hours, feeding may be started. Among patients with gastroesophageal reflux or pyloric or duodenal obstruction, a gastrojejunostomy tube is placed with the tip beyond the ligament of Treitz. When percutaneous gastrostomy is not possible because of previous gastric operations, direct percutaneous jejunostomy can be performed for enteral feeding (Fig. 101-15). Percutaneous cecostomy is effective for colonic obstruction in the care of patients who are at poor surgical risk for surgical colostomy or resection of the underlying lesion.

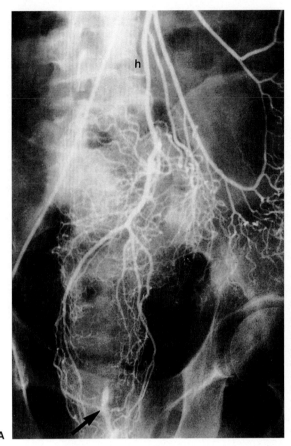
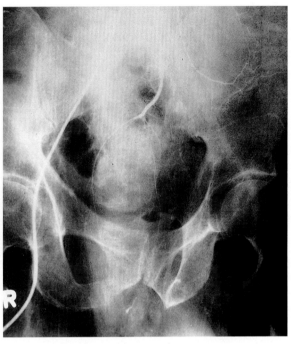

FIGURE 101-1. Vasopressin infusion into the inferior mesenteric artery in a patient with rectosigmoid bleeding. **A:** Inferior mesenteric arteriogram shows extravasation (*arrow*) of contrast medium in the rectum. The bleeding artery is a branch of the superior hemorrhoidal artery (*h*). **B:** Arteriogram 20 minutes after intraarterial infusion of vasopressin at 0.2 units/min. Most of the inferior mesenteric arterial branches reveal severe constriction. The bleeding has stopped.

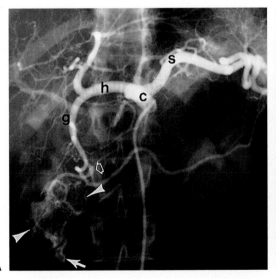
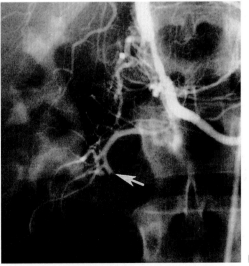

FIGURE 101-2. Control of bleeding from a duodenal leiomyoma with gelatin sponge (Gelfoam, Upjohn, Kalamazoo, MI) embolization in a 26-year-old woman. **A:** Celiac arteriogram shows a vascular mass (*arrowheads*) in the second portion of the duodenum. The tumor receives its blood supply from the anterior superior pancreaticoduodenal branch (*open arrow*) of the gastroduodenal artery (*g*). Contrast extravasation from the tumor is indicated (*arrow*). The right hepatic artery arises from the superior mesenteric artery. *c,* celiac axis; *s,* splenic artery; *h,* hepatic artery. **B:** Arteriogram after embolization with gelatin sponge pieces shows occlusion of the bleeding artery (*arrow*). The bleeding has stopped after embolization. One month later, the patient underwent surgical removal of a leiomyoma of the duodenum.

1119

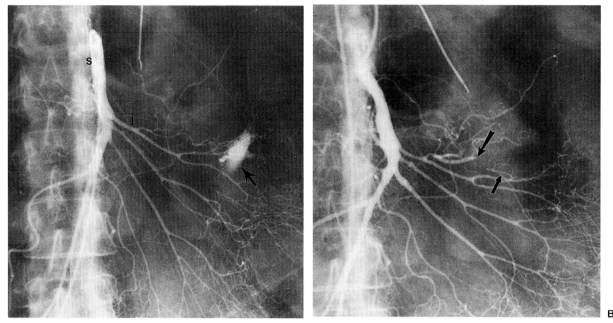

FIGURE 101-3. Jejunal bleeding controlled with Gelfoam (Upjohn, Kalamazoo, MI) embolization. **A:** Superior mesenteric (s) arteriogram shows contrast extravasation (*arrow*) in the proximal jejunum. The bleeding artery is a proximal jejunal artery (*j*). **B:** Arteriogram after embolization shows bleeding has stopped. Occlusion of the jejunal branches is indicated (*arrows*).

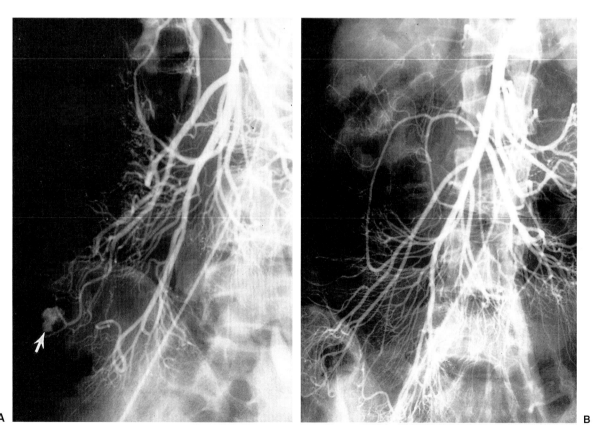

FIGURE 101-4. Embolic control of colonic bleeding in a 21-year-old woman with bright red blood per rectum. Flexible sigmoidoscopic examination showed blood in the colon. Technetium 99m–tagged red blood cell scan localized the bleeding to the right colon. After resuscitation, the patient underwent angiography and embolization. **A:** Superior mesenteric arteriogram shows a collection of contrast medium (*arrow*) in the right colon. The bleeding artery was selectively catheterized with a 3F coaxial catheter system. Polyvinyl alcohol sponge particles (250–350 μm) were injected close to the bleeding site. **B:** Arteriogram after embolization showed no contrast extravasation. The bleeding stopped. The patient underwent right hemicolectomy to prevent recurrent bleeding.

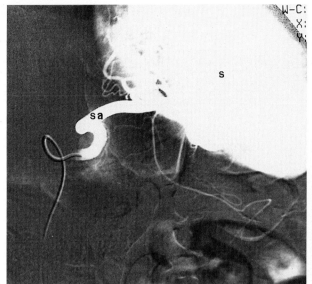

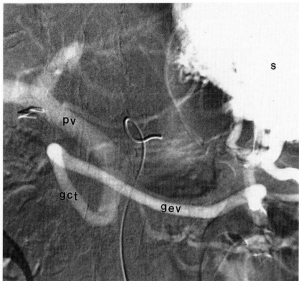

A

B

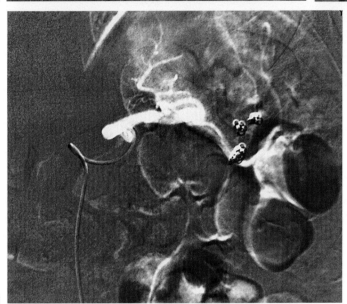

FIGURE 101-5. Splenic venous occlusion associated with pancreatitis and a pseudocyst. **A:** Digital subtraction splenic arteriogram. Contrast medium was injected into the splenic artery (*sa*). The splenic pulp (*s*) is densely filled with contrast medium. **B:** Venous phase shows evidence of splenic venous occlusion with venous collaterals through the gastroepiploic vein (*gev*) draining into the gastrocolic trunk (*gct*) and portal vein (*pv*). **C:** The splenic artery has been embolized with Gelfoam (Upjohn, Kalamazoo, MI) and coils to minimize venous bleeding during distal pancreatectomy. Most of the splenic arterial branches are occluded after embolization.

C

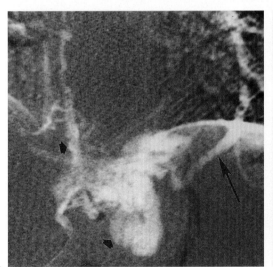

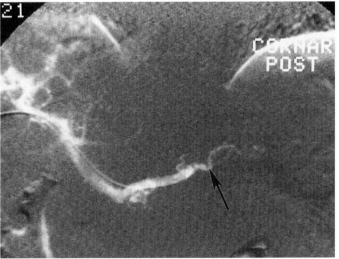

A

B

FIGURE 101-6. Embolization of bleeding esophageal varices. Percutaneous transhepatic coronary venogram of a patient with bleeding esophageal varices. **A:** Injection of coronary vein that was catheterized from the percutaneous transhepatic approach demonstrates esophageal varices (*smaller arrows*), which communicate with the left pulmonary vein (*larger arrow*). **B:** After embolization with ethyl alcohol, the varices are occluded (*arrow*) and gastrointestinal hemorrhage has ceased.

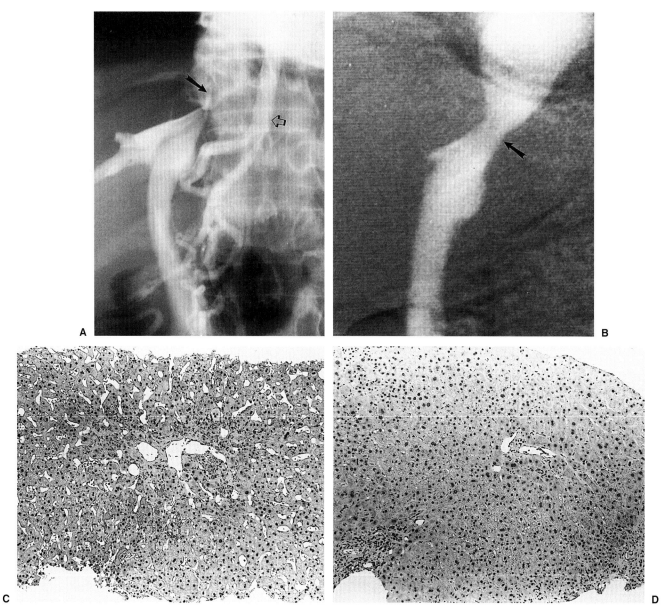

FIGURE 101-7. Suprahepatic caval anastomotic stenosis in a patient who 6 months earlier had undergone hepatic transplantation. **A:** Inferior vena cavogram shows suprahepatic caval anastomosis (*black arrow*) is nearly occluded and collateral blood flows through the azygos vein (*open arrow*). **B:** Digital subtraction venacavogram after angioplasty with 15-mm-diameter balloon catheter demonstrates substantial decrease in stenosis (*arrow*). The azygos venous collateral vessel disappeared and the abnormal cavoatrial pressure gradient was eliminated. **C:** Liver biopsy specimen before angioplasty shows chronic congestive changes and profound sinusoidal dilation consistent with high-grade venous outflow obstruction (H&E stain; original magnification ×100). **D:** Liver biopsy 2 months after angioplasty shows sinusoidal dilation has resolved (H&E stain; original magnification ×100).

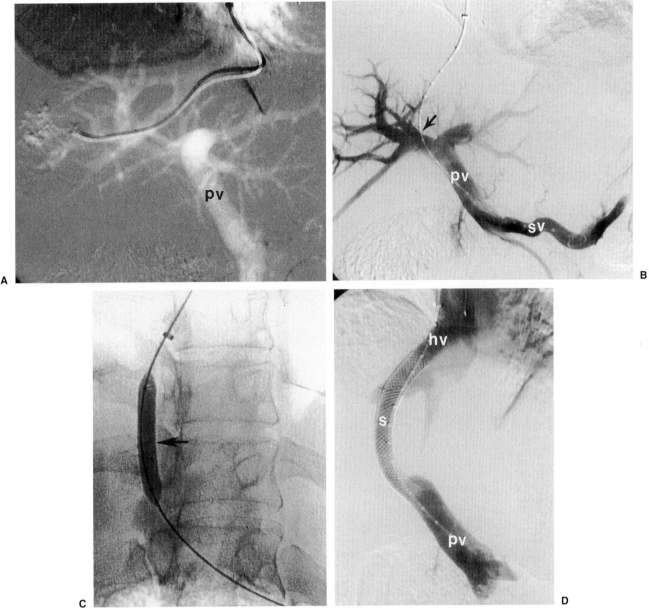

FIGURE 101-8. Transjugular intrahepatic portosystemic shunt (TIPS) placement in a patient with end-stage liver disease secondary to alcohol abuse, complicated by refractory ascites. **A:** CO_2 wedge hepatic venogram from a right jugular approach shows patent portal vein (*pv*). **B:** After successful puncture of the right main portal vein (*arrow*) using a Colapinto needle (Cook, Bloomington, Indiana), splenoportography was performed, which demonstrates patent splenic (*sv*) and portal vein (*pv*). The flow in the intrahepatic portal vein is hepatopetal. **C:** The liver parenchymal tract is dilated with an angioplasty balloon (*arrow*). **D:** After placement of a 10 mm-diameter Wallstent in the parenchymal tract, extending from the portal vein (*pv*) to the hepatic vein (*hv*), portogram demonstrates patent shunt (*s*) and reversal in the intrahepatic portal flow. Pressure gradient (portal pressure minus right atrial pressure) decreased from 20 mm Hg (pre-TIPS) to 10 mm Hg (post-TIPS). The patient's ascites has resolved but he developed mild encephalopathy.

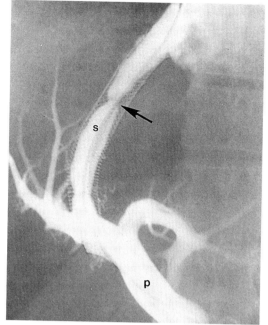

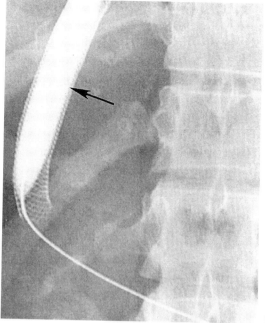

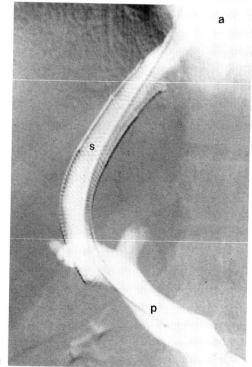

FIGURE 101-9. Stenosis of a transjugular intrahepatic portosystemic shunt (TIPS) in a 39-year-old woman who 11 months earlier had undergone a TIPS procedure for Budd-Chiari syndrome. Transjugular liver biopsy revealed chronic congestive changes and central hemorrhagic necrosis. **A:** Transjugular catheterization of the shunt. The catheter has been passed through the shunt into the portal vein. Contrast medium fills the portal vein (p) and shunt (s). Moderate stenosis (arrow) is visible in the shunt consistent with neointimal hyperplasia. **B:** The stenosis was dilated with a 10-mm-diameter balloon catheter (arrow) and stent placement. **C:** Portal venogram after revision. The shunt (s) is widely patent. Portal blood (p) flows toward the shunt into the right atrium (a). The portosystemic gradient decreased from 15 to 6 mm Hg. The patient's symptoms improved, and her liver function remained stable with patency of the shunt for 18 months.

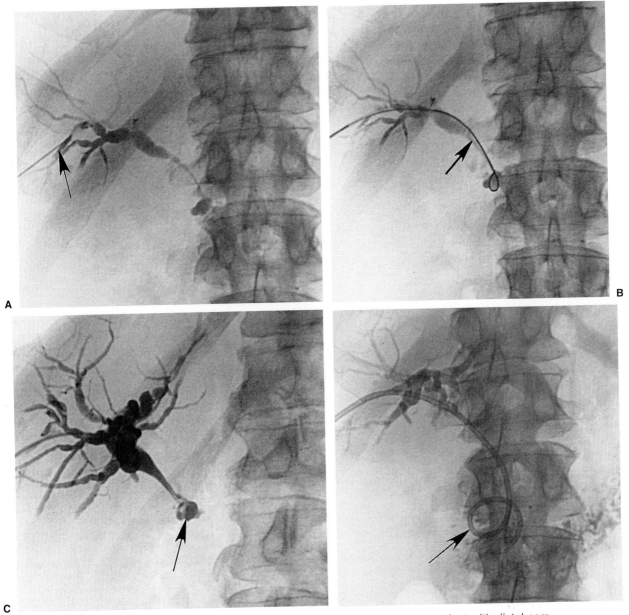

FIGURE 101-10. Percutaneous transhepatic biliary drainage in a patient with distal common bile duct obstruction caused by pancreatic cancer. **A:** Peripheral bile duct branch is punctured with a 22-gauge needle (*arrow*). **B:** The 0.018-in.-diameter guidewire (*arrow*) is introduced through the needle. **C:** After decompression of the bile duct with an introducer catheter, a 5F catheter has been introduced into the bile duct, and contrast medium shows obstruction (*arrow*). **D:** After the obstruction had been crossed, an 8.5F Cope loop catheter (*arrow*) (Cook Inc., Bloomington, IN) was introduced into the duodenum for external and internal drainage.

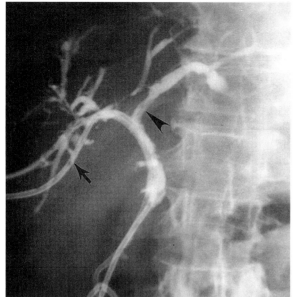

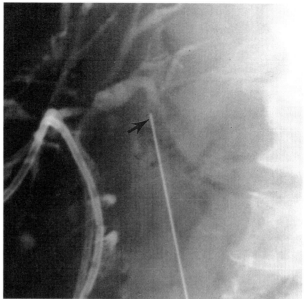

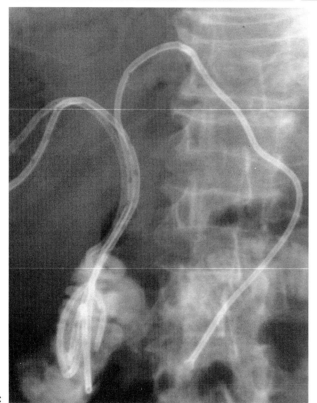

FIGURE 101-11. Percutaneous transhepatic drainage of left hepatic duct in a 53-year-old man who 5 years earlier had undergone orthotopic liver transplantation because of cryptogenic cirrhosis. The patient had recurrent cholangitis and multiple intrahepatic biliary strictures. **A:** Two percutaneous transhepatic biliary catheters (*arrow*) have been placed for right hepatic biliary strictures. Moderate stricture is present in the left hepatic duct (*arrowhead*). **B:** Opacification of the left hepatic duct with injection of contrast medium and air into the right biliary catheter in left anterior oblique view. A 22-gauge needle is placed into the left hepatic duct filled with air (*arrow*) under fluoroscopic guidance. **C:** After a guidewire was advanced through the needle, the tract was dilated. An 8.5F Cope loop catheter was placed with its distal loop in the duodenum.

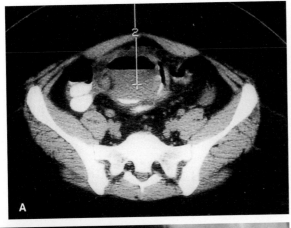

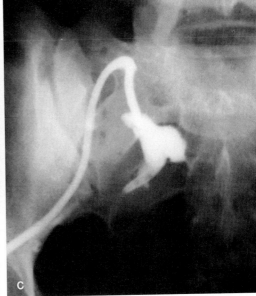

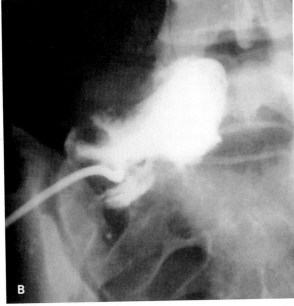

FIGURE 101-12. Successful percutaneous drainage of an intra-abdominal abscess in a 24-year-old woman. With computed tomographic guidance (**A**), a needle and then a catheter over a guidewire (**B**) were inserted into the fluid collection. **C:** Follow-up contrast sinogram shows the cavity is smaller and there is no fistula. The abscess was successfully drained, and the catheter was removed after 10 days.

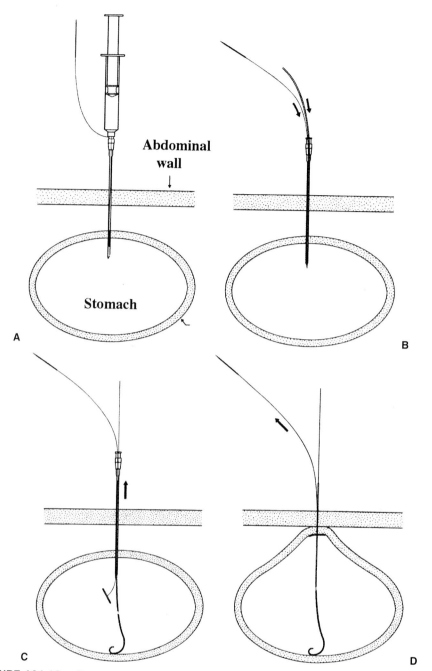

FIGURE 101-13. Suture anchor technique for percutaneous gastrostomy. **A:** The stomach (*arrow*) is insufflated with air through a nasogastric tube. The introducer needle preloaded with the gastrointestinal suture anchor is thrust into the stomach under fluoroscopic guidance. **B:** The guidewire is introduced through the needle, and the suture anchor is pushed into the gastric lumen. **C:** The needle is removed while the wire is left in the stomach. **D:** While the guidewire is in position, traction is applied to the suture to pull the anterior wall of the stomach against the abdominal wall. The guidewire is used to introduce a gastrostomy catheter. The suture may be left in place for 2 weeks, or it may be cut after placement of a gastrostomy tube.

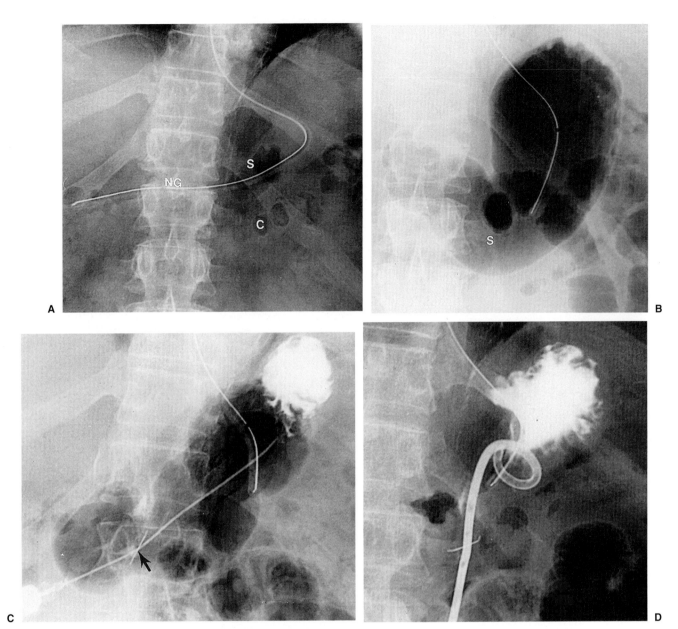

FIGURE 101-14. Percutaneous gastrostomy in a patient who is unable to swallow. **A:** Plain abdominal radiograph shows nasogastric tube (*NG*) has been placed in the stomach. The stomach (*S*) is not distended, and the transverse colon (*C*) is near the stomach. **B:** Air has been insufflated into the stomach (*S*) after intravenous administration of 1 mg of glucagon. **C:** After placement of a suture anchor (*arrow*) into the stomach, a 5F dilator was introduced into the stomach. Injection of contrast medium confirmed catheter position in the fundus of the stomach. **D:** After dilation of the tract, a 12F Cope loop gastrostomy tube (Cook Inc., Bloomington, IN) was placed.

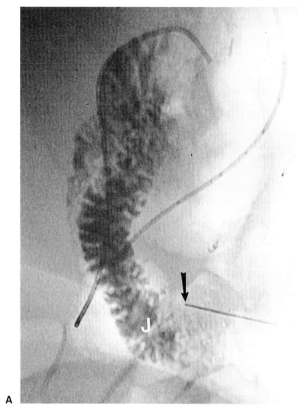

A

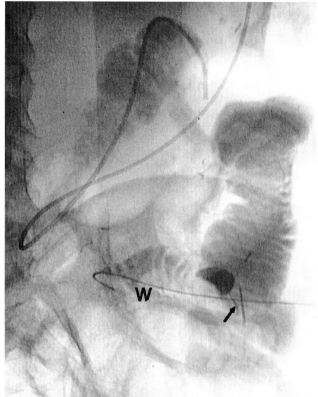

B

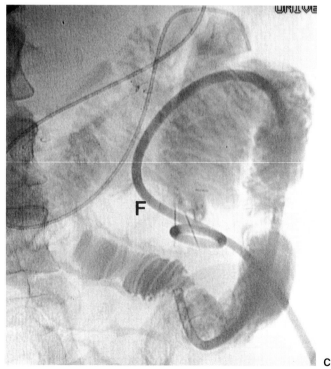

C

FIGURE 101-15. Percutaneous jejunostomy in a patient who is unable to swallow after esophagectomy and gastric pull-through for esophageal cancer. **A:** After intravenous administration of 1 mg of glucagon, proximal jejunum (J) has been visualized with contrast medium. An 18-gauge needle (arrow) was then inserted into the jejunum under fluoroscopic guidance. **B:** After placement of two suture anchors (arrow) to fix the wall of the jejunum to the abdominal wall, a wire (W) was introduced into the jejunum. **C:** After dilation of the tract, a 12F loop jejunostomy tube (F) was placed.

102

LAPAROSCOPY AND LAPAROTOMY

NATHANIEL J. SOPER ■ H. WORTH BOYCE JR. ■ H. JUERGEN NORD

Laparoscopy is a visual medium. With the advent of high-quality miniaturized television cameras, high-power light sources, and modern optics, a video laparoscope can display virtually the entire peritoneal cavity in full color at up to 15-power magnification. Laparoscopy by itself can be used only to image surface structures unless one performs operative techniques to dissect beyond the visible surface.

The application of laparoscopy as a diagnostic technique depends to a tremendous degree on visual diagnosis once access to the peritoneal cavity has been achieved. Those who perform diagnostic laparoscopy must become students of visual diagnosis by studying color prints or transparencies of laparoscopic findings. Concentrated study of such photographs considerably enhances diagnostic acumen, which otherwise would require years of practical experience to develop.

The laparoscopic photographs presented in Figs. 102-1 through 102-23 were selected to include a spectrum of diagnoses demonstrating the gross pathological features of intra-abdominal disease while providing examples of lesions that represent the main clinical appearances at laparoscopy. The laparoscopic photographs presented in Figs. 102-24 through 102-30 demonstrate surgical anatomy during the performance of therapeutic laparoscopic procedures. Although this text is not meant to be an atlas of surgical technique, these representative photographs should help physicians who are not surgeons appreciate the clarity with which therapeutic laparoscopists view a laparoscopic surgical field.

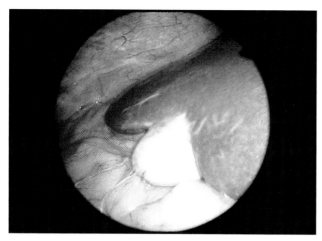

FIGURE 102-1. Normal right upper quadrant with fatty liver and chronic cholecystitis. This view of the right upper quadrant shows the inferior-lateral aspect of the right lobe. The reddish brown color, combined with the rounded edge lateral to the gallbladder, suggests a fatty liver, which was confirmed at biopsy. The niche into the inferior liver edge adjacent to the gallbladder is a normal variant. Fine adhesions from the gallbladder fundus to the omentum suggest mild chronic cholecystitis. The parietal peritoneum has a regular vascular pattern, and the omentum has a normal yellow color.

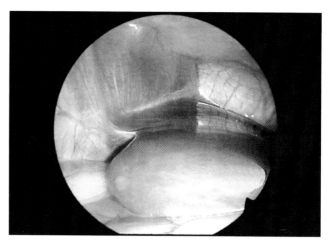

FIGURE 102-2. Normal left hepatic lobe. The left hepatic lobe has a smooth, glistening surface and rests with its sharp inferior edge on the gastric wall, which is barely visible in the foreground. The falciform ligament (*left*) has a thin sail-like transparent appearance with a fine vascular network. In portal hypertension, these vessels usually are increased and engorged. The central tendon of the diaphragm is visible in the background. Cardiac pulsations of the right ventricle are usually visible in this area.

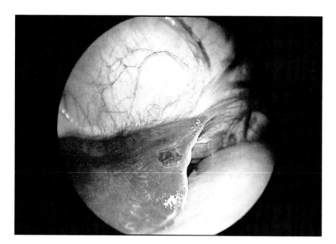

FIGURE 102-3. View of normal left lobe, anterior gastric wall, and diaphragm. A normal left hepatic lobe is suspended at the level of the diaphragm by normal peritoneal reflections (*left of center*). A slight elevation is visible in the midportion of the margin of the left lobe. This lesion was confusing on a scan. It proved to be a benign hemangioma when viewed from the anterior surface and underneath with use of a palpating probe. The anterior wall of the stomach is shown to the *right near the bottom*. At the upper end of the stomach almost in the *center* of the photograph is a patulous diaphragmatic hiatus typical of a hiatal hernia. Vascularity of the undersurface of the diaphragm is normal.

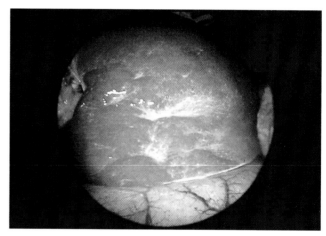

FIGURE 102-4. Dystrophic scars of the left lobe of the liver. The left lobe with its normal sharp edge shows several dystrophic scars that give the surface an irregular pattern. This picture may be seen after recovery from hepatitis and is usually of little consequence. It should not be confused with cirrhosis. Biopsy specimens should not be taken from such scars because they often contain large blood vessels. Liver function studies with this abnormality usually are normal. The gastroepiploic veins are visible in the foreground as they cross the body of the stomach.

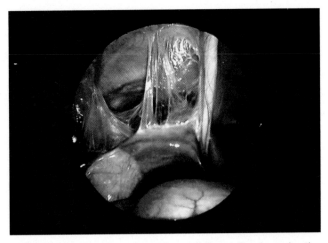

FIGURE 102-5. Multiple, thin, sail-like adhesions in the right upper quadrant. These fine, transparent avascular adhesions were found after blunt abdominal trauma. They were causing abdominal pain and had eluded detection. The round ligament, the remnant of the umbilical vein, at the free edge of the falciform ligament is visible (*right*). The adhesions hold the right hepatic lobe above the underlying structures, allowing inspection of the undersurface, which is usually hidden. The robin's egg blue structure is the infrahepatic gallbladder.

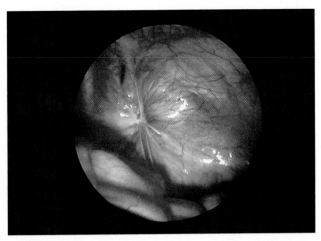

FIGURE 102-6. Right lower quadrant after herniorrhaphy. Star-like convergence of folds of the parietal peritoneum on the anterior abdominal wall in the right lower quadrant after closure of the hernial sac is visible. A black silk suture is visible (*above and to the left*). The right lateral umbilical fold is visible from the 11 o'clock position to the center of the herniorrhaphy site.

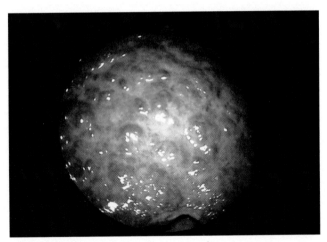

FIGURE 102-7. Micronodular cirrhosis, right hepatic lobe. This type of cirrhosis, frequently caused by alcohol abuse, is characterized by regenerating nodules, which usually do not exceed 3 mm in diameter and which are surrounded by circumferential whitish scars, in some areas in the form of broader bands. Multiple highlights from the photographic flash, each representing a regenerating nodule.

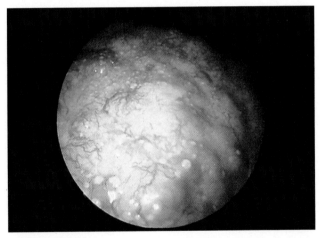

FIGURE 102-8. Micronodular cirrhosis of left lobe of the liver with lymph cysts. Tiny lymph cysts cover the nodular hepatic surface, which shows an increased vascular pattern. These cysts result from impairment of lymph flow through the surface vessels caused by cirrhotic transformation of the liver. They usually precede ascites formation.

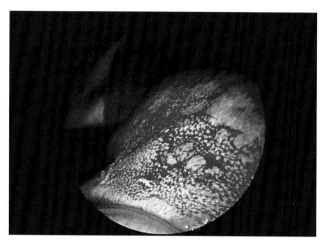

FIGURE 102-9. Right hepatic lobe with micronodular cirrhosis and ascites after guided biopsy. The micronodular pattern of the right lobe is accentuated by the blood streaking over the liver surface after guided biopsy. The liver is markedly enlarged, extending beyond the normal boundaries of the right costal margin, which is visible (*upper left*). The ascites fluid in the background covering the most dependent portion of the right lobe is stained with blood from the biopsy site.

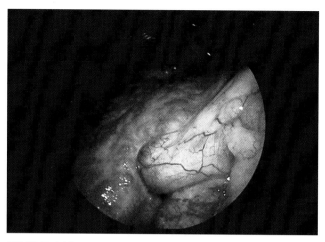

FIGURE 102-10. Micronodular cirrhosis with Cruveilhier-Baumgarten syndrome. Micronodular cirrhosis with recanalized umbilical vein at the insertion of the falciform ligament. Vasa vasorum cover the large vessels (*center*) in this view.

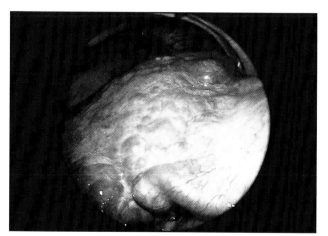

FIGURE 102-11. Micronodular cirrhosis with recanalized umbilical vein and hepatocellular carcinoma. Portions of the right lobe of the liver are visible with regenerating nodules of different size. A recanalized umbilical vein in the free edge of the falciform ligament is visible in the foreground. A bulge in the background and the redder color with larger irregular nodules indicate hepatocellular carcinoma in the medial aspect of the right lobe.

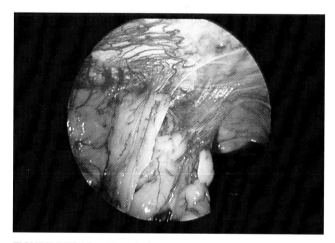

FIGURE 102-12. Postcholecystectomy adhesions and extensive collateral vessels. This view into the right upper quadrant reveals a typical fatty-fibrous adhesion that develops along the line of a cholecystectomy incision. The right upper quadrant is often completely obscured by adhesions after this type of operation. Among patients with portal hypertension, all abdominal scars are favorite sites of collateral vessel formation. This patient has extensive collateral vessels throughout the adhesion and the anterior abdominal wall. This illustration gives adequate reason to keep any puncture site well away from any abdominal scar in patients with suspected portal hypertension.

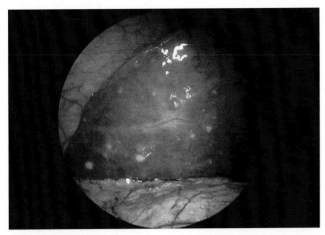

FIGURE 102-13. Tuberculous hepatitis with mild cholestasis. Elevation of the right hepatic lobe in a patient with fever of unknown cause reveals multiple whitish nodules. Biopsy specimens showed granulomas. Mild cholestasis caused by granuloma accentuating the lobular hepatic pattern is present. The patient responded to antituberculosis therapy. The gross appearance of these focal lesions is indistinguishable from that of sarcoidosis or metastatic tumor.

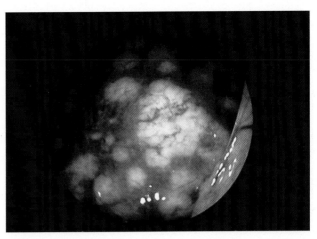

FIGURE 102-14. Metastatic adenocarcinoma. Extensive metastases of various sizes cover the surface of the right lobe. The marked neovascularity, especially of the larger lesions, is characteristic of carcinoma (in this case metastatic adenocarcinoma of the pancreas).

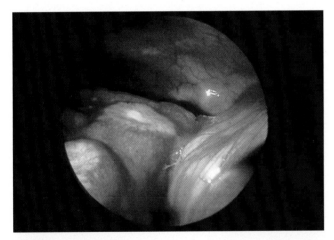

FIGURE 102-15. Metastatic adenocarcinoma. Several metastases of adenocarcinoma with central umbilication and neovascularity at their margin are visible. The central umbilication characteristic of adenocarcinoma is caused by necrosis as the enlarging tumor outgrows its vascular supply. The falciform ligament is seen (*right*).

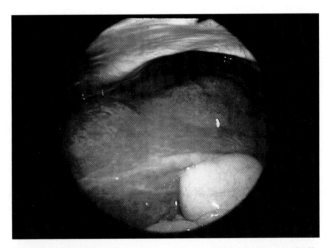

FIGURE 102-16. Focal fatty metamorphosis in alcoholic hepatitis. In this patient with chronic alcohol abuse and hepatomegaly, several filling defects were found at computed tomographic scanning. Cytologic findings of skinny-needle aspirates were designated class I. The prominent bulges of lighter, yellowish-brown color represent focal fatty infiltration and are recognized with increasing frequency. There is marked hepatomegaly as the liver extends beyond the right costal margin, which is visible (*upper right*). The under portion of the right lobe is visible, indicating infiltration, in this case caused by alcoholic hepatitis and steatosis.

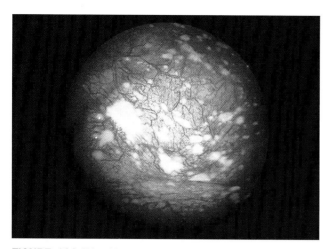

FIGURE 102-17. Metastasis from adenocarcinoma of the stomach to the parietal peritoneum. The whitish irregular plaque-like lesions represent gastric adenocarcinoma metastatic to the parietal peritoneum. There is marked neo-vascularity. These lesions are usually not visible on computed tomographic scans.

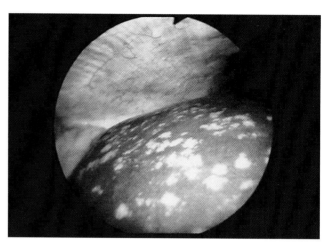

FIGURE 102-18. Diffuse sarcoidosis of the right hepatic lobe. This view of the right hepatic lobe reveals a basically normal background color of the liver. Scattered over the surface are many irregular, white lesions from 1 to 10 mm in diameter. The appearance of these lesions is nonspecific but suggestive of multiple granulomas or hepatic metastases. The absence of new vessel formation around the margins of these lesions suggests a benign cause; most large metastases show evidence of neovascularity around the periphery. Regardless of surface appearance, biopsy confirmation of such lesions is essential. The undersurface of the right diaphragm (*top*) is shown, and a small portion of greater omentum is visible at the 9 o'clock position.

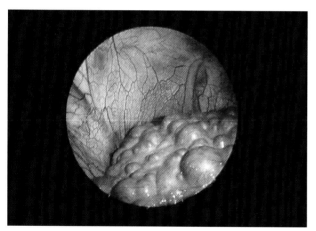

FIGURE 102-19. Macronodular hepatic cirrhosis caused by Wilson disease. This view reveals multiple, large, regenerative nodules in the left hepatic lobe. An earlier blind biopsy of the right lobe of this liver revealed only chronic active hepatitis, but laparoscopic inspection reveals classical advanced macronodular cirrhotic changes. The left side of the falciform ligament is shown with a slight increase in vascular pattern, suggesting early portal hypertension. The patient is a 15-year-old girl who had had undiagnosed progressive neurological disease for 5 years before Wilson disease was suspected.

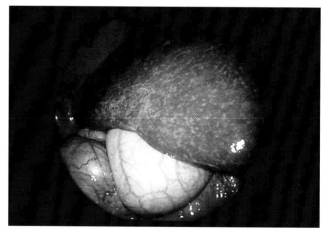

FIGURE 102-20. Intrahepatic cholestasis caused by drug-induced liver injury. View of the right lobe reveals a dark greenish-black liver color that indicates abnormality of the hepatic parenchyma. A normally distended gallbladder is visible (*lower center*) immediately under the right hepatic lobe. The appearance of the thin right-lobe margin immediately adjacent to the gallbladder suggests the absence of any increased intrahepatic pressure or infiltrative disease, such as infection, inflammation, or neoplasm.

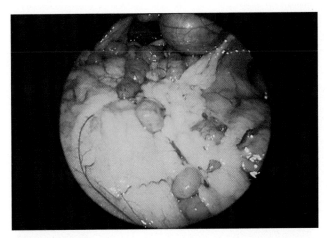

FIGURE 102-21. Multiple metastases of leiomyosarcoma. View of the right upper quadrant reveals the fundus of the normal gallbladder at the 12 o'clock position. Scattered about the greater omentum are multiple, smooth, round metastases caused by primary leiomyosarcoma of the uterus that was resected several years before this examination. These lesions were not diagnosed from a computed tomographic examination.

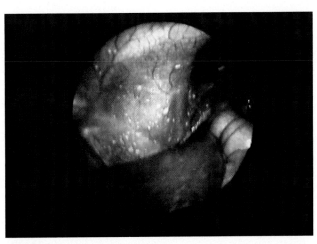

FIGURE 102-22. Diaphragmatic metastases of carcinoma of the ovary. View of the upper abdomen reveals a normal left hepatic lobe (*bottom*) and distal transverse colon (*right*). Small, multiple, white metastatic lesions of carcinoma of the ovary (*top and center*) are scattered over the peritoneal surface of the inferior aspect of the left hemidiaphragm. Diaphragmatic peritoneal metastases are a typical finding in metastatic carcinoma of the ovary.

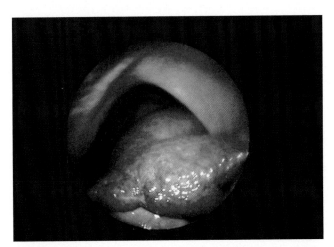

FIGURE 102-23. Indentation of Zahn. View of the right hepatic lobe reveals multiple highlights and surface changes compatible with micronodular cirrhosis and areas of dystrophic scarring. The undersurface of the diaphragm is shown (*top*). From the 12 o'clock to the 3 o'clock positions is a large band of diaphragmatic muscle that has resulted in production of a notch in the medial aspect of the right hepatic lobe. When the patient breathes, this diaphragmatic band, or fold, moves inferiorly to completely fill the notch. This view, taken in mid-inspiration, shows the notch in the right lobe only partially filled with the diaphragmatic band. This abnormality is simply a contour defect and is of no clinical significance other than that it may cause confusing findings on liver scans.

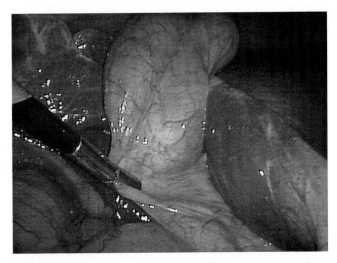

FIGURE 102-24. Appearance of gallbladder before initiation of laparoscopic cholecystectomy. The neck of the gallbladder is retracted to the patient's right.

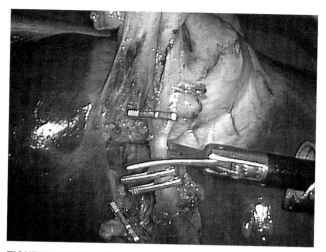

FIGURE 102-25. Clips have been placed on the cystic duct during laparoscopic cholecystectomy before division of the duct with scissors.

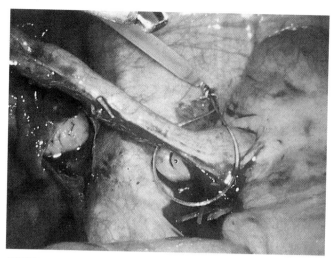

FIGURE 102-26. During laparoscopic appendectomy, a preformed loop ligature encircles the appendix and will be used to occlude its stump.

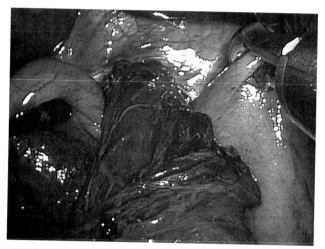

FIGURE 102-27. Intraoperative photograph during laparoscopic Nissen fundoplication. The portion of gastric fundus that has been pulled posterior to the esophagus is being elevated on the left, whereas the fundus maintaining its anatomic location is being elevated to the right of the esophagus, which is the reddish structure coursing vertically (*center*). The diaphragm (*top*) is shown, and the stomach would be the continuation of the esophagus (*bottom*).

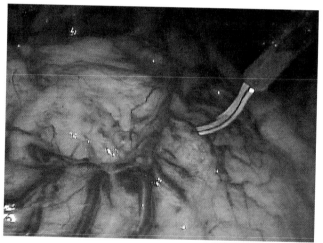

FIGURE 102-28. Laparoscopic appearance of the lesser curvature of the stomach before laparoscopic proximal gastric vagotomy. The neurovascular structures inserting into the lesser curvature of the stomach at the incisura can be clearly visualized with a scissors tip marking the "crow's foot" of the neurovascular bundles.

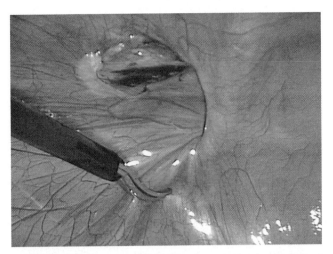

FIGURE 102-29. Intraoperative view at the beginning of laparoscopic repair of a left inguinal hernia. The scissors tip is pointing at the spermatic cord, which is visible through the peritoneum. A small transverse incision has been made at the superior border of the hernial orifice in preparation for development of a peritoneal flap. Immediately to the right of the indirect hernia the inferior epigastric blood vessels are coursing vertically behind the peritoneum.

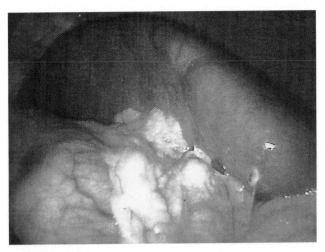

FIGURE 102-30. Appearance of the spleen just prior to laparoscopic splenectomy.

FIGURE CREDITS

CHAPTER 1

Figure 1-10A,B. Elta GH. Approach to the patient with gastrointestinal bleeding. In: Humes HD, DuPont HL, Gardner LB, et al. (eds). Kelley's textbook of internal medicine, 4th ed. Philadelphia, Lippincott Williams & Wilkins, 1997.

CHAPTER 2

Figure 2-2. Ali MA, Luxton AW, Walker WH. Serum ferritin concentration and bone marrow iron stores: a prospective study. Can Med Assoc J 1978;118:945. **Figure 2-16.** Ahlquist DA, Wieand HS, Moertel CG, et al. Accuracy of fecal occult blood screening for colorectal neoplasia: a prospective study using Hemoccult and Hemo-Quant. JAMA 1993;269:1262. **Figure 2-17A,B.** Stewart JG, Ahlquist DA, McGill DB, et al. Gastrointestinal blood loss and anemia in runners. Ann Int Med 1984;100:843. **Figure 2-20.** Young GP, St John DJB. Selecting an occult blood test for use as a screening tool for large bowel cancer. Front Gastrointest Res 1991;18:135. **Figure 2-21A.** Roche M, Perez-Gimenez ME. Gastrointestinal bleeding in hookworm infection. Am J Dig Dis 1957;2:265. **Figure 2-21B.** Roche M, Layrisse M. The nature and cause of hookworm anemia. Am Trop Med Hyg 1966;15:1029.

CHAPTER 3

Figure 3-4. Nussbaum MS. Diseases of the appendix. In: Bell RH Jr., Rikkers LE, Mulholland MW (eds). Digestive tract surgery: a text and atlas. Philadelphia, Lippincott–Raven, 1996. **Figure 3-5.** Koehler RE, Memel DS, Stanley RJ. Gastrointestinal tract. In: Lee JKT, Sagel SS, Stanley RJ, Heiken JP (eds). Computed body tomography with MRI correlation, 3rd ed. Vol. 1, Philadelphia, Lippincott–Raven, 1998.

CHAPTER 4

Figures 4-1, 4-2, 4-4A,B. Summers RW, Lu CC. Approach to the patient with ileus and obstruction. In: Yamada T, Alpers DH, Owyang C, Powell DW, Silverstein FE (eds). Textbook of gastroenterology. Philadelphia, JB Lippincott, 1991.

CHAPTER 5

Figures 5-1, 5-3. Thillainayagam AV, Hunt JB, Farthing MJ. Enhancing clinical efficacy of oral therapy: is low osmolality the key? Gastroenterology 1998;114:197. **Figure 5-2.** Kilgore PE, Holman RC, Clarke MJ, Glass RI. Trends of diarrheal disease-associated mortality in U.S. children, 1968 through 1991. JAMA 1995;274:1143. **Figure 5-5.** Crowe SE, Powell DW. Mechanisms of diarrhea: role of the neuroimmune system. Regulatory Peptide Letter 1995;6:49. **Figure 5-7.** Surawicz CM. Food poisoning: a practical approach to management. Gastrointest Dis Today 1997;6:12. **Figure 5-8.** Crane JK, Guerrant RL. Acute watery diarrhea. In: Blaser MJ, Smith PD, Ravdin JI, Greenberg HB, Guerrant RL (eds). Infections of the gastrointestinal tract. New York, Raven Press, 1995. **Figure 5-9.** DuPont HL. Persistent diarrhea in a traveling student. Gastrointest Dis Today 1993;2:1. **Figure 5-10.** DuPont HL, Marshall GD. HIV-associated diarrhoea and wasting. Lancet 1995;346:352. **Figure 5-12.** Abdulkarim AS, Murray JA. Celiac disease. Curr Treat Options Gastroenterol 2002;5:27. **Figure 5-13.** Ramzan NN. Whipple disease. Curr Treat Options Gastroenterol 1999;2:363. **Figure 5-14.** Misiewicz JJ, Forbes A, Price A, Shorvon P, Triger D, Tytgat G. Atlas of clinical gastroenterology, 2nd ed. London, Wolfe, 1994. **Figures 5-15A,B, 5-16A,B.** Dhouri MR, Huang G, Shiau YF. Sudden stain of fecal fat: new insight into an old test. Gastroenterology 1989;96:423. **Figure 5-17.** Fine KD, Fordtran JS. The effect of diarrhea on fecal fat excretion. Gastroenterology 1992;102:1936. **Figure 5-18A–D.** Jabbari M, Wild G, Goresky CA, et al. Scalloped valvulae conniventes: an endoscopic marker of celiac sprue. Gastroenterology 1988;95:1519. **Figure 5-19.** Myner TP, Moss AA. Radiologic evaluation of the malabsorption syndrome. Practical Gastroenterology 1980;4:25. **Figure 5-20.** Bayless TM. Lactose deficiency and intolerance to milk. Viewpoints on Digestive Disease 1971;3:3. **Figure 5-21.** Sellin JH. Curr Treat Options Gastroenterol 2000;3:15. **Figure 5-22.** Silverstein FE, Tytgat GNJ. Gastrointestinal endoscopy, 3rd ed. London, Mosby-Wolfe, 1997. **Figure 5-23.** O'Neill BH, Venook AP. Management of carcinoid tumors and the carcinoid syndrome. Clin Perspect Gastroenterol 2001;Sep/Oct:279. **Figure 5-24.** Wrong O, Metcalfe-Gibson A, Morrison BIR, Ng ST, Howard AV. In vivo dialysis of faeces as a method of stool analysis. Clin Sci 1965;28:357. **Figure 5-25.** Cutz E, Rhoads JM, Drumm B, et al. Microvillus inclusion disease: an inherited defect of brush-border assembly and differentation. N Engl J Med 1989;320:646.

CHAPTER 6

Figure 6-5. Original references for techniques are from Wald A. Approach to the patient with constipation. In: Yamada T, Alpers DH, Kaplowitz N, et al. Textbook of gastroenterology, 4th ed. Philadelphia, Lippincott Williams & Wilkins, 2003:901. **Figure 6-6.** Wald A. Evaluation of biofeedback in childhood encopresis. J Pediatr Gastroenterol Nutr 1987;6:554.

CHAPTER 8

Figures 8-2, 8-3. Lindsay KL, Hoofnagle JH. Serologic tests for viral hepatitis. In: Kaplowitz N, ed. Liver and biliary diseases, 2nd ed. Baltimore, Williams & Wilkins, 1996.

CHAPTER 11

Figures 11-2, 11-3, 11-4. Medical emergencies. In: Hayes PC, Mackay TW, Forrest EH, Fisken RA. Churchill's pocketbook of medicine. Edinburgh, United Kingdom, Churchill Livingstone, 2002:460.

CHAPTER 12

Figures 12-5, 12-6, 12-20, 12-26, 12-27, 12-28, 12-35, 12-53, 12-54, 12-55, 12-56. Sherertz EF, Jorizzo JL. Skin lesions associated with gastrointestinal diseases. In: Yamada T, Alpers DH, Owyang C, Powell DW, Silverstein FE (eds). Textbook of gastroenterology. Philadelphia, JB Lippincott, 1991.

CHAPTER 13

Figures 13-4, 13-5. Bresalier RS. Neoplasia of the colon and rectum. In: Feldman M (ed). Gastroenterology and hepatology: the comprehensive visual reference. Philadelphia, Current Medicine, 1997. **Figure 13-6.** Ahlquist DA. Approach to the patient with occult gastrointestinal bleeding. In: Yamada T, Alpers DH, Kaplowitz N, et al. Atlas of gastroenterology. Philadelphia, JB Lippincott, 1992. **Figures 13-7, 13-8, 13-11, 13-12, 13-13, 13-14.** Allison MC. Diagnostic picture tests in gastroenterology. London, Mosby-Wolfe, 1991. **Figure 13-9.** Habif TP. Superficial fungal infections. In: Baxter S (ed). Clinical dermatology: a color guide to diagnosis and therapy, 3rd ed. St. Louis, Mosby, 1996. **Figure 13-10.** Briggaman R. Clinical nutrition I slideset. American Gastroenterological Association, Bethesda, MD, 2000. **Figures 13-15, 13-16, 13-17, 13-18.** Weinert M, Grimes RM, Lynch DP. Oral manifestations of HIV infection. Ann Intern Med 1996;125:485.

CHAPTER 14

Figures 14-1, 14-2, 14-3. Maps adapted from Centers for Disease Control and Prevention. Health Information for International Travel, 1996-7. Washington, DC, US Government Printing Office, 1997.

CHAPTER 16

Figure 16-3. Kahrilas PJ, Lin S, Chen J, Logemann JA. Oropharyngeal accommodation to swallow volume. Gastroenterology 1996;111:297. **Figure 16-6A.** Kahrilas PJ, Ergun GA. Evaluation of the patient with dysphagia. In: Bone R (ed). Current practice of medicine. Vol. 4. Philadelphia, Current Medicine, 1996;2:2. **Figures 16-8, 16-15.** Kahrilas PJ, Dodds WJ, Hogan WJ. The effect of peristaltic dysfunction on esophageal volume clearance. Gastroenterology, 1988;94:73. **Figure 16-12.** Hirano I, Tatum RP, Shi G, Sang Q, Joehl RJ, Kahrilas PJ. Heterogeneity in the manometric criteria of idiopathic achalasia. Gastroenterology 2001;120:789. **Figure 16-22.** Stevoff C, Rao S, Parsons W,

Kahrilas PJ, Hirano I. EUS and histopathologic correlates in eosinophilic esophagitis. Gastrointest Endosc 2001;54:373.

CHAPTER 17
Figure 17-1. Locke GR 3rd, Talley NJ, Fett SL, Zinsmeister AR, Melton LJ 3rd. Prevalence and clinical spectrum of GER: a population-based study in Olmsted County, Minnesota. Gastroenterology 1997;112:1448. **Figure 17-2.** Helm JF, Dodds WJ, Pelc LR, Palmer DW, Hogan WJ, Teeter BC. Effect of esophageal emptying and saliva on clearance of acid from the esophagus. N Engl J Med 1984:310:284.

CHAPTER 18
Figure 18-14A,B. DeSilva R, Stoopack P, Raufman JP. Esophageal fistulae associated with mycobacterial infection in patients at risk for AIDS. Radiology 1990;175:449.

CHAPTER 19
Figures 19-1, 19-2, 19-3, 19-7, 19-15. Eisenberg RL. Gastrointestinal radiology: a pattern approach, 4th ed. Philadelphia, Lippincott Williams & Wilkins, 2003. **Figures 19-4, 19-11.** Silverstein FE, Tytgat GNJ. Gastrointestinal endoscopy, 3rd ed. London, Mosby-Wolfe, 1997. **Figures 19-5A–C, 19-10.** Misiewicz JJ, Bartram CI, Cotton PB, Mee AS, Price AB, Thompson RPH. Atlas of gastroenterology. London, Gower, 1988.

CHAPTER 20
Figure 20-6. Misiewicz JJ, Forbes A, Price A, Shorvon P, Triger D, Tytgat G. Atlas of gastroenterology, 2nd ed. London, Wolfe, 1994. **Figures 20-7, 20-13, 20-14, 20-17.** Eisenberg RL. Gastrointestinal radiology: a pattern approach, 4th ed. Philadelphia, Lippincott Williams & Wilkins, 2003.

CHAPTER 21
Figure 21-4. Rohen JW, Chichiro Y. Color atlas of anatomy. New York, Igaku-Shoin, 1993. **Figure 21-5.** Rosse C, Gaddum-Rosse P. Hollinshead's textbook of anatomy. Philadelphia, Lippincott–Raven, 1997. **Figure 21-6A,B.** Gartner LP, Hiatt JL. Color textbook of histology. Philadelphia, WB Saunders, 1997. **Figure 21-7.** Ross MH, Romrell LJ, Kaye GI. Histology. Baltimore, Williams & Wilkins, 1995. **Figure 21-8.** Digestive system. In: Sadler TW (ed). Langman's medical embryology, 5th ed. Baltimore, Williams & Wilkins, 1985. **Figures 21-9, 21-12.** Eisenberg RL. Gastrointestinal radiology: a pattern approach, 4th ed. Philadelphia, Lippincott Williams & Wilkins, 2003.

CHAPTER 22
Figures 22-1, 22-19. Koch KL. Diabetic gastropathy. Dig Dis Sci 1999;44:1061. **Figure 22-2.** Data from Guo J-P, Maurer AH, Urbain J-L, Fisher RS, Parkman HP. Extending gastric emptying scintigraphy from two to four hours detects more patients with gastroparesis. Dig Dis Sci 2001;46:24. **Figure 22-3.** Troncon LE, Bennett RJ, Ahluwalia NK, Thompson DG. Abnormal intragastric distribution of food during gastric emptying in functional dyspepsia patients. Gut 1994;35:327. **Figures 22-4, 22-6.** Data from Parkman HP, Urbain J-L, Knight LC, et al. Effect of gastric acid suppressants on human gastric motility. Gut 1998;42:243. **Figure 22-5.** Data from Parkman HP, Harris AD, Fisher RS. Influence of age, gender, and menstrual cycle on the normal electrogastrogram. Am J Gastroenterol 1996;91:127. **Figure 22-7.** Lin Z, Chen JD, Schirmer BD, McCallum RW. Postprandial response of gastric slow waves: correlation of serosal recordings with the electrogastrogram. Dig Dis Sci 2000;45:645. **Figure 22-8.** Hongo M, Okuno Y, Nishimura N, et al. Electrogastrography or prediction of gastric emptying state. In: Chen JZ, McCallum RW (eds). Electrogastrography: principles and applications. New York: Raven Press, 1994:257. **Figure 22-9.** Chen JD, Zou X, Lin X, Ouyang S, Liang J. Detection of gastric slow wave propagation from the cutaneous electrogastrogram. Am J Physiol 1999;277:G424. **Figure 22-10.** Lin X, Chen JZ. Abnormal gastric slow waves in patients with functional dyspepsia assessed by multichannel electrogastrography. Am J Physiol 2001;280:G1370. **Figure 22-11.** Chey WD, Shapiro B, Zawadski A, Goodman K. Gastric emptying characteristics of a novel ^{13}C-octanoate-labeled muffin meal. J Clin Gastroenterol 2001;32:394. **Figure 22-12.** Bityutskiy LP, Soykan I, McCallum RW. Viral gastroparesis: a subset of idiopathic gastroparesis—clinical characteristics and long-term treatment outcomes. Am J Gastroenterol 1997;92:1501. **Figure 22-13.** Frank JW, Saslow SB, Camilleri M, Thomforde GM, Dinneen S, Rizza RA. Mechanism of accelerated gastric emptying of liquids and hyperglycemia in patients with type II diabetes mellitus. Gastroenterology 1995;109:755. **Figure 22-14.** Hasler WL, Soudah HC, Dulai G, Owyang C. Mediation of hyperglycemia-evoked gastric slow-wave dysrhythmias by endogenous prostaglandins. Gastroenterology 1995;108:727. **Figure 22-15.** Jebbink RJ, Samsom M, Bruijs PP, et al. Hyperglycemia induces abnormalities of gastric myoelectric activity in patients with type 1 diabetes mellitus. Gastroenterology 1994; 107:1390. **Figure 22-16.** Jones KL, Kong MF, Berry MK, Rayner CK, Adamson U, Horowitz M. The effect of erythromycin on gastric emptying is modified by physiological changes in the blood glucose concentrations. Am J Gastroenterol 1999;94:2074. **Figure 22-17.** Samsom M, Salet GA, Roelofs JM, Akkermans LM, Vanberge-Henegouwen GP, Smout AJ. Compliance of the proximal stomach and dyspeptic symptoms in patients with type 1 diabetes mellitus. Dig Dis Sci 1995; 40:2037. **Figure 22-18.** Waldron B, Cullen PT, Kumar R, et al. Evidence for hypomotility in non-ulcer dyspepsia: a prospective multifactorial study. Gut 1991;32:246. **Figure 22-20.** McCallum RW, Chen JD, Lin Z, Schirmer BD, Williams RD, Ross RA. Gastric pacing improves emptying and symptoms in patients with gastroparesis. Gastroenterology 1998;114:456.

CHAPTER 23
Figure 23-3. Adapted from McGowan, Cover TL, Blaser MJ. Helicobacter pylori and gastric acid: biological and therapeutic implications. Gastroenterology 1996;110:926. **Figures 23-4, 23-5, 23-8.** Mitros FA. Atlas of gastrointestinal pathology. London, Gower, 1988. **Figure 23-7.** Scientific American: Science and Medicine. 1994; September/October: cover. **Figures 23-9, 23-10, 23-11, 23-12.** McNeil NI. Gastroenterology: an essential slide collection, slides 33, 32, 27, and 21. **Figure 23-13.** Blackstone H. Endoscopic interpretation: normal and pathologic appearances of the gastrointestinal tract. New York, Raven Press, 1984:117. **Figure 23-14.** Mifflin RC, Powell DW. Cyclooxygenases. Regulatory Peptide Letter 2001;8:49. **Figure 23-16A.** Simon LS, Weaver AL, Graham DY, et al. Anti-inflammatory and upper gastrointestinal effects of celecoxib in rheumatoid arthritis: a randomized controlled trial. JAMA 1999;282:1921. **Figure 23-16B.** Hawkey C, Laine L, Simon T, et al. Comparison of the effect of rofecoxib (a cyclooxygenase 2 inhibitor), ibuprofen, and placebo on the gastroduodenal mucosa of patients with osteoarthritis: a randomized, double-blind, placebo-controlled trial. The Rofecoxib Osteoarthritis Endoscopy Multinational Study Group. Arthritis Rheum 2000;43:370. **Figure 23-17.** Shoen RT, Vender RJ. Mechanisms of nonsteroidal anti-inflammatory drug induced gastric damage. Am J Med 1989;86:449. **Figure 23-18.** Adapted from Scheiman JM. NSAIDs, gastrointestinal injury, and cytoprotection. Gastroenterol Clin North Am 1996;25:279.

CHAPTER 25
Figure 25-1. SEER Cancer Statistics Review 1973–1998, National Cancer Institute. Bethesda, MD, 2001.

CHAPTER 26
Figures 26-1, 26-7. Debas HT, Orloff SL. Surgery for peptic ulcer disease and postgastrectomy syndromes. In: Yamada T, Alpers DH, Owyang C, et al. (eds). Textbook of gastroenterology, 2nd ed. Philadelphia, JB Lippincott, 1995. **Figure 26-5.** Macintyre IM, Millar A, Smith AN, et al. Highly selective vagotomy 5–15 years on. Br J Surg 1990;77:65. **Figure 26-6.** Adapted from Schafmayer A, Börger WH, Köhler H, et al. Recurrent ulcers after proximal gastric vagotomy: special aspects of the prepyloric ulcer. Dig Surg 1989;6:4. **Figure 26-8.** Debas HT, Orloff SL. Surgery for peptic ulcer diseases and postgastrectomy syndromes. In: Yamada T, Alpers DH, Owyang C, et al. (eds). Textbook of

gastroenterology, 2nd ed. Philadelphia, Lippincott-Raven, 1995:1523. **Figures 26-10, 26-11.** Seymour NE. Surgery of the stomach and duodenum. In: Feldman M (ed). Gastroenterology and hepatology: the comprehensive visual reference. Philadelphia, Current Medicine, 1996.

CHAPTER 27

Figures 27-1, 27-2B, 27-4, 27-7. Eisenberg RL. Diaphragmatic hernias. In: Gastrointestinal radiology, 4th ed. Philadelphia, Lippincott Williams & Wilkins, 2003. **Figure 27-5.** Castell DO, Richter JE. Hiatus hernia. In: The esophagus, 3rd ed. Philadelphia, Lippincott Williams & Wilkins, 1999. **Figures 27-8, 27-9B, 27-10B.** Eisenberg RL. Filling defects in the stomach. In: Gastrointestinal radiology, 4th ed. Philadelphia, Lippincott Williams & Wilkins, 2003. **Figure 27-9A.** Eisenberg RL. Filling defects in the gastric remnant. In: Gastrointestinal radiology, 4th ed. Philadelphia, Lippincott Williams & Wilkins, 2003.

CHAPTER 28

Figure 28-1. Larsen WJ (ed). Human embryology, 2nd ed. New York, Churchill Livingstone, 1997:241. **Figure 28-7.** Langer JC. Gastroschisis and omphalocele. Semin Pediatr Surg 1996;5:124.

CHAPTER 29

Figure 29-1. Grundy D, Camilleri M. Neurogastroenterology and motility: new millenium, new horizons. Neurogastroenterol Motil 2001;13:177. **Figure 29-2.** Mitros FA. Atlas of gastrointestinal pathology. London, Gower, 1988. **Figure 29-4.** Mueller LA, Camilleri M, Emslie-Smith AM. Mitochondrial neurogastrointestinal encephalomyopathy: manometric and diagnostic features. Gastroenterology 1999;116:959. **Figures 29-6, 29-7.** Bonsib SM, Fallon B, Mitros FA, et al. Urologic manifestations of patients with visceral myopathy. J Urol 1984;132:1112. **Figure 29-8.** Edery P, Lyonnet S, Mulligan LM, et al. Mutations of the RET proto-oncogene in Hirschsprung's disease. Nature 1994;367: 378; and Romeo G, Ronchetto P, Luo Y, et al. Point mutations affecting the tyrosine kinase domain of the RET proto-oncogene in Hirschsprung's disease. Nature 1994;367:377. **Figure 29-9.** Smith, et al. Gut 1999;45:143. **Figures 29-10, 29-11.** Lee JC, Thuneberg L, Berezin I, et al. Generation of slow waves in membrane potential is an intrinsic property of interstitial cells of Cajal. Am J Physiol 1999;277:G409. **Figures 29-12, 29-13.** He CL, Burgart L, Wang L, et al. Decreased interstitial cell of Cajal volume in patients with slow-transit constipation. Gastroenterology 2000;118:14. **Figure 29-14.** Ordog T, Takayama I, Cheung WK, et al. Remodeling of networks of interstitial cells of Cajal in a murine model of diabetic gastroparesis. Diabetes 2000;49:1731. **Figure 29-15.** Mayer EA, Schuffler MD, Rotter JI, et al. Familial visceral neuropathy with autosomal dominant transmission. Gastroenterology 1986;91:1528. **Figure 29-17.** Camilleri M. Medical treatment of chronic intestinal pseudoobstruction. Pract Gastroenterol 1991;15:10. **Figure 29-19.** Choi MG, Camilleri M, O'Brien MD, et al. A pilot study of motility and tone of the left colon in patients with diarrhea due to functional disorders and dysautonomia. Am J Gastroenterol 1997;92:297.

CHAPTER 30

Figures 30-2, 30-3C. Finlay BB, Cossart P. Exploitation of mammalian host cell functions by bacterial pathogens. Science 1997; 276:720. **Figures 30-3A,B.** Slide atlas of infectious diseases. Lambert HB, Farrar WE. Infections of the gastrointestinal tract and biliary system. Abbott Laboratory slide atlas of infectious disease, vol. 7., London, Gower. **Figure 30-3D.** Vallance BA, Finlay BB. Exploitation of host cells by enteropathogenic *Escherichia coli.* Proc Natl Acad Sci USA 2000;97:8799–8806. **Figure 30-4.** Matsumoto T, Lida M, Matsui T. Endoscopic findings in *Yersinia enterocolitica* enterocolitis. Gastrointest Endosc 1990;36:583. **Figure 30-5.** Van Trappen G, Geboes K, Ponette E. *Yersinia* enteritis. Med Clin North Am 1982;66:647. **Figure 30-8.** Agus SG, Dolin R, Wyatt RG, Tousimis AJ, Northrup RS. Acute infectious nonbacterial gastroenteritis: intestinal histopathology. Histologic and enzymatic alterations during illness produced by the Norwalk agent in man. Ann Intern Med 1973;79:18.

CHAPTER 31

Figure 31-6. Fantry GT, James SP. Whipple's disease. Dig Dis 1995;13:108. **Figures 31-11, 31-12, 31-13, 31-14, 31-15.** Fenoglio-Preiser CM, Noffsinger AE, Stemmermann GN, et al. Nonneoplastic lesions of the small intestine. In: Gastrointestinal pathology: an atlas and text, 2 ed. Philadelphia: Lippincott-Raven, 1999.

CHAPTER 32

Figure 32-5. Ferguson A. Coeliac disease (gluten hypersensitivity). J Hum Nutr 1976;30:193.

CHAPTER 35

Figures 35-16, 35-18. Silverstein FE, Tytgat GNJ. Gastrointestinal endoscopy, 3rd ed. London, Mosby-Wolfe, 1997.

CHAPTER 37

Figures 37-1, 37-2. Kodner IJ, Fry RD, Fleschman JW, Birnbaum EH. Colon, rectum, and anus. In: Schwartz SI (ed). Principles of surgery, 6th ed. New York, McGraw Hill, 1994. **Figures 37-5A,B, 37-6A,B.** Cohn SM, Birnbaum EH. Colon: anatomy and structural anomalies. In: Yamada T, Alpers DH, Owyang C, et al. (eds). Textbook of gastroenterology, 2nd ed. Philadelphia, JB Lippincott, 1995.

CHAPTER 38

Figures 38-1, 38-6, 38-12, 38-14, 38-18A,B, 38-21A,B, 38-24, 38-27A,B, 38-28. Stenson WF, MacDermott RP. Inflammatory bowel disease. In: Yamada T, Alpers DH, Owyang C, Powell DW, Silverstein FE (eds). Textbook of gastroenterology. Philadelphia, JB Lippincott, 1991. **Figures 38-2, 38-3, 38-4, 38-10.** Mitros FA. Atlas of gastrointestinal pathology. London, Gower, 1988. **Figures 38-5, 38-36, 38-37, 38-41, 38-42, 38-46, 38-48, 38-49, 38-50, 38-54.** Silverstein FE, Tytgat GNJ. Gastrointestinal endoscopy, 3rd ed. London, Mosby-Wolfe, 1997. **Figure 38-16.** Misiewicz JJ, Forbes A, Price A, Shorvon P, Triger D, Tytgat G. Atlas of clinical gastroenterology, 2nd ed. London, Wolfe, 1994.

CHAPTER 39

Figures 39-1, 39-5, 39-6, 39-8, 39-9, 39-11, 39-12. Silverstein FE, Tytgat GNJ. Gastrointestinal endoscopy, 3rd ed. London, Mosby-Wolfe, 1997. **Figures 39-2, 39-3, 39-4.** Blackstone MO. Postsurgical appearances and uncommon colonic conditions. In: Endoscopic interpretation: normal and pathologic appearances of the gastrointestinal tract. New York, Raven Press, 1984. **Figure 39-7.** Blackstone MO. Acute diarrheal illnesses and uncommon types of colitis. In: Endoscopic interpretation: normal and pathologic appearances of the gastrointestinal tract. New York, Raven Press, 1984. **Figure 39-10.** Eisenberg RL. Gastrointestinal radiology: a pattern approach, 4th ed. Philadelphia, Lippincott Williams & Wilkins, 2003. **Figure 39-13.** Misiewicz JJ, Bartram CI, Cotton PB, Mee AS, Price AB, Thompson RPH. Atlas of clinical gastroenterology. London, Gower, 1988.

CHAPTER 40

Figures 40-1, 40-12. Pemberton JH, Armstrong DN, Dietzen CD. Diverticulitis. In: Yamada T, Alpers DH, Owyang CO, et al. (eds). Textbook of gastroenterology, 2nd ed. Philadelphia, JB Lippincott, 1995:1870. **Figure 40-2.** Young-Fadok TM, Pemberton JH. Colonic diverticular disease: epidemiology and pathophysiology. In: Rose BD, ed. UpToDate in medicine [CD-ROM]. Wellesley, MA: UpToDate, 1997. **Figures 40-4, 40-6, 40-7.** Young-Fadok TM, Pemberton JH. Colonic diverticular disease: natural history, clinical features and diagnosis. In: Rose BD, ed. UpToDate in medicine [CD-ROM]. Wellesley, MA: UpToDate, 1997. **Figure 40-8.** Young-Fadok TM, Pemberton JH. Colonic diverticular disease: hemorrhage. In: Rose BD, ed. UpToDate in medicine [CD-ROM]. Wellesley, MA: UpToDate, 1997. **Figure 40-13.** Young-Fadok TM, Pemberton JH. Colonic diverticular disease: fistula. In: Rose BD, ed. UpToDate in medicine [CD-ROM]. Wellesley, MA: UpToDate, 1997.

CHAPTER 41

Figure 41-3. Modified by VK Viswanathan from Gansheroff LJ, O'Brien AD. *Escherichia coli* 0157:H7 in beef cattle presented for slaughter in the US: higher prevalence rates than previously estimated. Proc Natl Acad Sci 2000;97:2959. **Figure 41-5.** Modified from Johnson S, Gerding DN. *Clostridium difficile-associated diarrhea.* Clin Infect Dis 1998;26:1027. **Figure 41-8.** Mitros FA. Atlas of gastrointestinal pathology. London, Gower, 1988. **Figures 41-9, 41-10.** Misiewicz JJ, Forbes A, Price A, Shorvon P, Triger D, Tytgat G. Atlas of clinical gastroenterology. London, Wolfe, 1994.

CHAPTER 42

Figures 42-1, 42-2, 42-5, 42-6, 42-10, 42-13, 42-14, 42-15, 42-40, 42-41, 42-42, 42-50, 42-51, 42-52, 42-53, 42-54, 42-55, 42-57, 42-58, 42-59, 42-64, 42-65, 42-66, 42-67, 42-68, 42-69, 42-70, 42-71, 42-80, 42-81, 42-82, 42-83, 42-84, 42-85. From Luk GD, Alousi MA, Jones LA Jr, Sakr WA. Colonic polyps: benign and premalignant neoplasms of the colon. In: Yamada T, Alpers DH, Owyang C, Powell DW, Silverstein FE (eds). Atlas of gastroenterology. Philadelphia, JB Lippincott, 1992.

CHAPTER 43

Figures 43-3, 43-4. Gardener EJ, Burt RW, Freston JW. Gastrointestinal polyposis: syndromes and genetic mechanisms. West J Med 1980;132:488. **Figure 43-6.** Traboulsi EI, Krush AJ, Gardner EJ, et al. Prevalence and importance of pigmented occular fundus lesions in Gardner's syndrome. N Engl J Med 1987;316:661. **Figure 43-8.** Sogol PB, Sugawara M, Gorden HE, et al. Cowden's disease: familial goiter and skin hamartomas. West J Med 1983;139:324. **Figure 43-9.** Russell DM, Bhathal PS, St. John DJ. Complete remission in Cronkhite-Canada syndrome. Gastroenterology 1983;85:180. **Figure 43-11.** Malhotra R, Sheffield A. Cronkhite-Canada syndrome associated with colon carcinoma and adenomatous changes in C-C polyps. Am J Gastroenterol 1988;83:772.

CHAPTER 44

Figure 44-1. Miller AB. Trends in cancer mortality and epidemiology. Cancer 1983;51:2413. **Figure 44-2.** Adapted from Greenwald P. Colon cancer overview. Cancer 1992;70:1206. **Figure 44-3A.** Armstrong B, Doll R. Environmental factors and cancer incidences and mortality in different countries with special reference to dietary practices. Int J Cancer 1975;15:617. **Figure 44-3C.** Willett W. The search for the causes of breast and colon cancer. Nature 1989;338:389. **Figure 44-4.** Boland CR, Sato J, Appelman HD, et al. Microallelotyping defines the sequence and tempo of allelic losses at tumour suppressor gene loci during colorectal cancer progression. Nat Med 1995;1:902. **Figure 44-5.** Boland CR. Malignant tumors of the colon. In: Yamada T, Alpers DA, Laine L, et al. (eds). Textbook of gastroenterology, 3rd ed. Philadelphia, Lippincott Williams & Wilkins, 1999. **Figure 44-6.** Colon and rectum. In: Beahrs OH, Henson DE, Hutter RVP, Kennedy BJ (eds). Manual for staging of cancer of the American Joint Committee on Cancer, 4th ed. Philadelphia, JB Lippincott, 1992. **Figure 44-7.** Winawer SJ, Fletcher RH, Miller L, et al. Colorectal cancer screening: clinical guidelines and rationale. Gastroenterology 1997;112:594. **Figure 44-8A.** Fuchs C, Giovannucci EL, Colditz GA, et al. A prospective study of family history and the risk of colorectal cancer. N Engl J Med 1994;331:1669. **Figure 44-8B–D.** Winawer SJ, Zauber AG, Gerdes H, et al. Risk of colorectal cancer in the families of patients with adenomatous polyps. N Engl J Med 1996;334:82. **Figure 44-9.** August DA, Ottow RT, Sugarbaker PH. Clinical perspectives on human colorectal cancer metastases. Cancer Metastasis Rev 1984; 3:303. **Figures 44-16, 44-28.** Lind DS, Souba WW. Neoplasms of the colon and rectum. In: Bell RH Jr., Rikkers LF, Mulholland MW (eds). Digestive tract surgery: a text and atlas. Philadelphia, Lippincott–Raven Publishers, 1996. **Figure 44-20.** Misciewicz JJ, Forbes A, Price A, Shorvon P, Triger D, Tytgat G. Atlas of clinical gastroenterology, 4th ed. London, Wolfe, 1994. **Figures 44-21, 44-22, 44-23, 44-24, 44-25.** Blackstone MO. Colonic malignancies. In: Endoscopic interpretation: normal and pathologic appearances of the gastrointestinal tract. New York, Raven

Press, 1984. **Figures 44-26, 44-27.** Corman ML, Veidenhelmer MC, Swinton NW. Diseases of the anus, rectum, and colon. Part 1: neoplasms. New York, Medcom, 1972. **Figures 44-29, 44-30, 44-31.** Corman ML. Carcinoma of the colon. In: Colon and rectal surgery, ed 4. Philadelphia, Lippincott–Raven Publishers, 1998. **Figure 44-32.** Milsom JW, Ludwig KA. Surgical management for rectal cancer. In: Wanebo HJ (ed). Surgery for gastrointestinal cancer: a multidisciplinary approach. Philadelphia, Lippincott–Raven Publishers, 1997.

CHAPTER 45

Figures 45-6, 45-7, 45-9, 45-12. Rios Magrina E. Color atlas of anorectal diseases. Barcelona, Salvat Editores, 1980. **Figures 45-10, 45-11.** Suppurative processes. In: Rios Magrina E. Atlas of therapeutic proctology. Philadelphia, WB Saunders, 1984.

CHAPTER 46

Figures 46-1, 46-3, 46-4, 46-9. Misciewicz JJ, Forbes A, Price A, Shorvon P, Triger D, Tytgat G. Atlas of clinical gastroenterology, 4th ed. London, Wolfe, 1994. **Figures 46-5, 46-6, 46-7, 46-8.** Skandalakis JE, Gray SW, Rowe JS. Anatomical complications in general surgery. New York, McGraw-Hill, 1983.

CHAPTER 47

Figures 47-2, 47-3. Misciewicz JJ, Forbes A, Price A, Shorvon P, Triger D, Tytgat G. Atlas of clinical gastroenterology, 4th ed. London, Wolfe, 1994. **Figures 47-5, 47-6.** Banks PA, Burrell MI, Sweeting JG, Green PHR. The American Gastroenterological Association Clinical Teaching Project, Unit 5, Pancreatitis. Bethesda, MD, American Gastroenterological Association, 1990. **Figure 47-8.** Steer ML. Acute pancreatitis. In: Yamada T, Alpers DH, Owyang C, Powell DW, Silverstein FE (eds). Textbook of gastroenterology. Philadelphia, JB Lippincott, 1991.

CHAPTER 48

Figure 48-2. Misciewicz JJ, Forbes A, Price A, Shorvon P, Triger D, Tytgat G. Atlas of clinical gastroenterology, 4th ed. London, Wolfe, 1994. **Figure 48-4.** Beger HG, Buchler M, Ditschuneit H, Malfertheiner. Chronic pancreatitis. Springer-Verlag, 1990. **Figure 48-5.** Adapted from DiMagno EP, Go VL, Summerskill WH. Relations between pancreatic enzyme outputs and malabsorption in severe pancreatic insufficiency. N Engl J Med 1973; 288:813. **Figures 48-7, 48-18.** Banks PA, Burrell MI, Sweeting JG, Green PHR. The American Gastroenterological Association Clinical Teaching Project, Unit 5, Pancreatitis. Bethesda, MD, American Gastroenterological Association, 1990. **Figure 48-8.** Eisenberg RL. Gastrointestinal radiology: a pattern approach, 4th ed. Philadelphia, Lippincott Williams & Wilkins, 2003. **Figure 48-15.** Solvay Pharmaceuticals, in consultation with Banks PA, Campbell DR, Toskas PP. Chronic pancreatitis. Marietta, GA, Solvay Pharmaceuticals, 1992. **Figure 48-17.** Little AG, Moosa AR. Gastrointestinal hemorrhage from left-sided portal hypertension. An unappreciated complication of pancreatitis. Am J Surg 1981;141:153. **Figures 48-19, 48-20.** Bengtsson M, Löfström JB. Nerveblock in pancreatic pain. Acta Chir Scand 1990;156:285. **Figure 48-23.** Prinz R. Surgical drainage procedures. In: Howard JM, Idezuki Y, Ihse I, Prinz RA. Surgical diseases of the pancreas, 3rd ed. Baltimore: Williams & Wilkins, 1998:359.

CHAPTER 51

Figure 51-4. Dowsett JF, Rode J, Russell RC. Annular pancreas: a clinical, endoscopic, and immunohistochemical study. Gut 1989;30:130.

CHAPTER 52

Figures 52-1, 52-6. Pellegrini CA, Duh Q-Y. Gallbladder and biliary tree: anatomy and structural anomalies. In: Yamada T, Alpers DH, Owyang C, et al. (eds). Textbook of gastroenterology, 2nd ed. Philadelphia, JB Lippincott, 1995. **Figures 52-4, 52-11, 52-12.** Linder H. Embryology and anatomy of the biliary tree. In: Way LW, Pellegrini CA (eds). Surgery of the gallbladder and bile ducts. Philadelphia, WB Saunders, 1987. **Figure 52-13.** Soper NJ. Cystic disease of the biliary tract. In: Bell RH, Rikkers LF,

Mulholland MW (eds). Digestive tract surgery: a text and atlas. Philadelphia, Lippincott–Raven Publishers, 1996.

CHAPTER 55

Figure 55-3. Burrell MI. The American Gastroenterological Association Clinical Teaching Project, Unit 4, Hepatobiliary Disease and Jaundice. Bethesda, MD, American Gastroenterological Association, 1989. **Figure 55-4A.** Kimura K, Ohto M, Ono T, et al. Congenital cystic dilatation of the common bile duct: relationship to anomalous pancreaticobiliary ductal union. AJR Am J Roentgenol 1977;128:571. **Figure 55-5.** Hamlin JA. Anomalies of the biliary tract. In: Berk JE (ed). Bockus gastroenterology. Philadelphia, WB Saunders, 1985. **Figure 55-8.** Kaplowitz N, ed. Liver and biliary diseases. Baltimore: Williams & Wilkins, 1992.

CHAPTER 57

Figures 57-4, 57-5, 57-6, 57-7. Agur AMR. Grant's atlas of anatomy, 10th ed. Baltimore: Williams & Wilkins, 1999. **Figure 57-10.** Phillips MJ, Poucell S, Patterson J, et al. The liver. An atlas and text of ultrastructural pathology. New York: Raven Press, 1987. **Figure 57-12.** Sternberg SS. Histology for pathologists. New York, Raven Press, 1992.

CHAPTER 59

Figure 59-1. Modified by RG Gish from Scheuer PJ. Classification of chronic viral hepatitis. J Hepatology 1991;13:372. **Figure 59-8.** Centers for Disease Control.

CHAPTER 63

Figure 63-14. Adapted from Heathcote J. AASLD practice guidelines: management of primary biliary cirrhosis. Hepatology 2000; 31:1005.

CHAPTER 66

Figures 66-1, 66-2. Lumeng L, Crabb DW. Alcoholic liver disease. Curr Opin Gastroenterol 2001;17:211.

CHAPTER 68

Figure 68-1. Conn HO, Lieberthal MM. Pathogenesis of portal-systemic encephalopathy. In: The hepatic coma syndromes and lactulose. Baltimore, Williams & Wilkins, 1979:46. **Figure 68-2.** Weissenborn K, Ruckert N, Hecker H, Manns MP. The number connection tests A and B: interindividual variability and use for the assessment of early hepatic encephalopathy. J Hepatol 1998;28:646. **Figure 68-3.** Takashi M, Igarashi M, Hino S, et al. Portal hemodynamics in chronic portal-systemic encephalopathy. J Hepatol 1985;1:467. **Figures 68-4, 68-5, 68-6, 68-9.** Kaplowitz N, ed. Liver and biliary diseases, 2nd ed. Baltimore, Williams & Wilkins, 1996. **Figure 68-7.** Basile AS, Jones EA. Ammonia and GABA-ergic neurotransmission: interrelated factors in the pathogenesis of hepatic encephalopathy. Hepatology 1997;25:1303. **Figure 68-8.** Haussinger D, Kircheis G, Fischer R, Schliess F, vom Dahl S. Hepatic encephalopathy in chronic liver disease: a clinical manifestation of astrocyte swelling and low-grade cerebral edema? J Hepatol 2000;32:1035.

CHAPTER 69

Figure 69-1. UNOS data, March 2001, courtesy of John P. Roberts, M.D., Department of Surgery, University of California, San Francisco. **Figure 69-4.** Data from annual report of the U.S. Scientific Registry for Transplantation Recipients and the Organ Procurement and Transplantation Network: Transplant data: 1989–1999. Rockville, MD: Department of Health and Human Services, 2000, for the year 1998.

CHAPTER 71

Figures 71-1, 71-2, 71-3, 71-4. From Reynolds TB. Liver abscess. In: Kaplowitz N (ed). Liver and biliary diseases, 2nd ed. Baltimore: Williams & Wilkins, 1996:463.

CHAPTER 75

Figures 75-13, 75-14. Adapted from Ros PR, Olmsted WW, Moser RP Jr, et al. Mesenteric and omental cysts: histologic classification with imaging correlation. Radiology 1987;164:327.

CHAPTER 76

Figures 76-4, 76-5. Smith PD, Saini SS, Raffeld M, Manischewitz JF, Wahl SM. Cytomegalovirus induction of tumor necrosis factor-α by human monocytes and mucosal macrophages. J Clin Invest 1992;90:1642.

CHAPTER 77

Figure 77-2. Sepulveda B, Manzo N. Clinical manifestations and diagnosis of amebiasis. In: Martinez-Palomo A (ed). Amebiasis. Amsterdam, Elsevier, 1986. **Figures 77-5, 77-9.** Healy GR, Garcia LS. Intestinal and urogenital protozoa. In: Murray PR (ed). Manual of clinical microbiology. Washington, DC, ASM Press, 1995. **Figure 77-6.** Case records of the Massachusetts General Hospital. Weekly clinicopathological exercises. Case 8-1997. A 65-year-old man with recurrent abdominal pain for five years. N Engl J Med 1997;336:786. **Figures 77-10, 77-16.** Farrar WE, Wood MJ, Innes JA, Tubbs H. Infectious diseases: text and color atlas. St. Louis, Mosby-Year Book, 1992. **Figure 77-11.** Guerrant RL, Petri WA, Wanke CS. Parasitic causes of diarrhea. In: Lebenthal E, Duffey M (eds). Pathophysiology of secretory diarrhea. Boston, Raven Press, 1990. **Figure 77-12.** Soave R, Weikel CS. *Cryptosporidium* and other protozoa including *Isospora, Sarcocystis, Balantidium coli,* and *Blastocystis.* In: Mandell GL, Douglas RG Jr, Bennett JE (eds). Principles and practice of infectious diseases, 3rd ed. New York, Churchill Livingstone, 1990.

CHAPTER 78

Figures 78-1, 78-4, 78-5, 78-6, 78-8, 78-10, 78-11, 78-12, 78-13, 78-14, 78-15, 78-16, 78-17, 78-19, 78-20, 78-21, 78-22. Smith JW, Ash LR, Thompson JH Jr, et al. Intestinal helminths. In: Atlas of diagnostic medical parasitology series. Chicago, American Society of Clinical Pathologists, 1984. **Figure 78-2.** Pearson RD, Irons RP Sr, Irons RP Jr. Chronic pelvic peritonitis due to pinworm *Enterobius vermicularis.* JAMA 1981;245:1340.

CHAPTER 80

Figures 80-3, 80-5, 80-6. Mitros FA. Atlas of gastrointestinal pathology. London, Gower, 1988.

CHAPTER 81

Figure 81-1. Eidus LB, Rasuli P, Manion D, Heringer R. Caliber-persistent artery of the stomach (Dieulafoy's vascular malformation). Gastroenterology 1990;99:1507. **Figure 81-2.** Scheider DM, Barthel JS, King PD, Beale GD. Dieulafoy-like lesion of the distal esophagus. Am J Gastroenterol 1994;89:2080. **Figure 81-5.** Boley SJ, Sammartano R, Adams A, DiBiase A, Kleinhaus S, Sprayregen S. On the nature and etiology of vascular ectasias of the colon: degenerative lesions of aging. Gastroenterology 1977;72:650. **Figure 81-6.** Foutch PG. Angiodysplasia of the gastrointestinal tract. Am J Gastroenterol 1993;88:807. **Figures 81-8, 81-9.** Cappell MS. Spatial clustering of simultaneous nonhereditary gastrointestinal angiodysplasia: small but significant correlation between nonhereditary colonic and upper gastrointestinal angiodysplasia. Dig Dis Sci 1992;37:1072. **Figure 81-10.** Boley SJ, Sprayregan S, Sammartano RJ, Adams A, Kleinhaus S. The pathophysiologic basis for the angiographic signs of vascular ectasias of the colon. Radiology 1977;125:615. **Figure 81-11B.** Savides TJ, Jensen DM. Therapeutic endoscopy for nonvariceal gastrointestinal bleeding. Gastroenterol Clin North Am 2000;29:465. **Figure 81-13.** Haitjema T, Westermann CJ, Overtoom TT, et al. Hereditary hemorrhagic telangiectasia (Osler-Weber-Rendu disease): new insights in pathogenesis, complications, and treatment. Arch Intern Med 1996;156:714. **Figure 81-16.** Watson M, Hally RJ, McCue PA, Varga J, Jimenez SA. Gastric antral vascular ectasia (watermelon stomach) in patients with systemic sclerosis. Arthritis Rheum 1996;39:341. **Figure 81-18.** Cappell MS, Price JB. Characterization of the syndrome of small and large intestinal variceal bleeding. Dig Dis Sci 1987;32:422. **Figure 81-19.** Sandhu KS, Cohen H, Radin R, Buck FS. Blue rubber bleb nevus syndrome presenting with recurrences. Dig Dis Sci 1987;32:214. **Figure 81-20.** Weinstein EC, Moertel CG,

Waugh JM. Intussuscepting hemangiomas of the gastro-intestinal tract: report of a case and review of the literature. Ann Surg 1963;157:265. **Figure 81-22.** Bak YT, Oh CH, Kim JH, Lee CH. Blue rubber bleb nevus syndrome: endoscopic removal of the gastrointestinal hemangiomas. Gastrointest Endosc 1997;45:90. **Figure 81-23A.** Stratte EG, Tope WD, Johnson CL, Swanson NA. Multimodal management of diffuse neonatal hemangiomatosis. J Am Acad Derm 1996;34:337. **Figure 81-23B.** McCauley RG, Leonidas JC, Bartoshesky LE. Blue rubber bleb nevus syndrome. Radiology 1979;133:375. **Figure 81-24.** Brandt LJ. Gastrointestinal disorders of the elderly. New York, Raven Press, 1984:5.

CHAPTER 82

Figure 82-1. Schlossberg L, Zuidema GD. The Johns Hopkins atlas of human functional anatomy, 3rd ed. Baltimore, The Johns Hopkins University Press, 1986. **Figures 82-3A, 82-3B, 82-5A, 82-5B, 82-26.** Bastidas JA, Reilly PM, Bulkley GB. Mesenteric vascular insufficiency. In: Yamada T, Alpers DH, Owyang C, et al. (eds). Textbook of gastroenterology, 2nd ed. Philadelphia, JB Lippincott, 1995.

CHAPTER 87

All figures (with the exception of 87-27, 87-28, 87-36) from Rubin CE, Haggitt RC, Levine DS. Endoscopic mucosal biopsy. In: Yamada T, Alpers DH, Owyang C, Powell DW, Silverstein FE (eds). Textbook of gastroenterology. Philadelphia, JB Lippincott, 1991.

CHAPTER 88

Figures 88-1, 88-9, 88-12, 88-14, 88-30, 88-31, 88-33, 88-34, 88-38, 88-39, 88-45, 88-46, 88-49, 88-54, 88-55, 88-56, 88-57, 88-59, 88-64, 88-66, 88-72, 88-76, 88-78, 88-79. Kaplowitz N, ed. Liver and biliary diseases, 2nd ed. Baltimore, Williams & Wilkins, 1996.

CHAPTER 90

Figure 90-1. Waye JD, Geenen JE, Fleischer D, Venu RP. The slide atlas of techniques in therapeutic endoscopy. New York, Gower, 1987. **Figure 90-4.** Stiegmann GV, Goff JS, Sun JH, Davis D, Bozdech J. Endoscopic variceal ligation: an alternative to sclerotherapy. Gastrointest Endosc 1989;35:431. **Figure 90-5.** Stiegmann GV, Yamamoto M. Endoscopic management of esophageal varices. World J Surg 1992;16:1034. **Figure 90-7.** Sarin SK, Lahoti D, Saxena SP, Murthy NS, Makwana UK. Prevalance, classification and natural history of gastric varices: a long-term follow-up study in 568 portal hypertension patients. Hepatology 1992;16:1343.

CHAPTER 93

Figures 93-19, 93-20, 93-21, 93-23, 93-24. Malagelada JR, Camilleri M, Stanghellini V. Manometric diagnosis of gastrointestinal motility disorders. New York, Thieme, 1986. By permission of Mayo Foundation. **Figures 93-25, 93-26, 93-27.** Kellow JE, Gill RC, Wingate DL. Prolonged ambulant recordings of small bowel motility demonstrate abnormalities in the irritable bowel syndromes. Gastroenterology 1990;98:1208. **Figures 93-28, 93-29, 93-30, 93-31.** Bortolotti M, Santi P, Barbara L, Brunelli F. Gastric myoelectric activity in patients with chronic idiopathic gastroparesis. J Gastrointest Mot 1990;2:104. **Figure 93-32.** Abell TL, Malagelada J-R. Electrogastrography: current assessment and future perspective. Dig Dis Sci 1988;33:983. **Figures 93-36, 93-37, 93-38.** Sims MA, Hasler WL, Chey WD, et al. Hyperglycemia inhibits mechanoreceptor-mediated gastrocolonic responses and colonic peristaltic reflexes in healthy humans. Gastroenterology 1995;108:350. **Figures 93-39, 93-40, 93-41.** Read NW, Sun WM. Anorectal manometry, anal myography and rectal sensory testing. In: Read NW (ed). Gastrointestinal motility—Which test? Great Britain, Wrightson Biomedical Publishing, 1989.

CHAPTER 94

Figures 94-1, 94-3. Levine MS. Plain radiograph diagnosis of the acute abdomen. Emerg Med Clin North Am 1985;3:541. **Figures 94-4, 94-7.** Rubesin SE, Glick SN. The tailored double-contrast pharyngogram. CRC Crit Rev Diagn Imaging 1988; 28:133. **Figure 94-9A.** Levine MS, Rubesin SE, Herlinger H, Laufer I. Double contrast upper gastrointestinal examination: technique and interpretation. Radiol 1988;168:593. **Figure 94-11.** Levine MS, Creteur V, Kressel HY, Laufer I, Herlinger H. Benign gastric ulcers: diagnosis and follow-up with double contrast radiography. Radiology 1987;164:9.

CHAPTER 100

Figure 100-13. Cho KJ, Adams D. Diagnostic angiography in gastrointestinal hemorrhage. In: Fiddian-Green RG, Turcotte JG (eds). Gastrointestinal hemorrhage. New York, Grune & Stratton, 1980. **Figure 100-25.** Chuang VP, Pulmano CM, Walter JF, Cho KJ. Angiography of pancreatic arteriovenous malformation. AJR Am J Roentgenol 1977;129:1015. **Figures 100-30, 100-36, 100-37.** Inflammatory disease. In: Reuter SR, Redman HC, Cho KJ. Gastrointestinal angiography, 3rd ed. Philadelphia, WB Saunders, 1986. **Figure 100-32.** Cho KJ, Wilcox CW, Reuter SR. Glucagon-producing islet cell tumor of the pancreas. AJR Am J Roentgenol 1977;129:159.

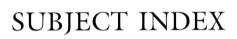

SUBJECT INDEX

Page numbers followed by *f* indicate figures; page numbers followed by *t* indicate tables.